D0121492

BLACK'S
VETERINARY
DICTIONARY

BLACK'S VETERINARY DICTIONARY

Edited by Geoffrey P. West MRCVS

Seventeenth edition
with 226 illustrations

A & C BLACK · LONDON

SEVENTEENTH EDITION 1992
A. & C. BLACK (PUBLISHERS) LIMITED
35 BEDFORD ROW, LONDON WC1R 4JH

ISBN 0-7136-3600-9

FIRST PUBLISHED 1928
SECOND EDITION 1935
THIRD EDITION, ENTIRELY RE-SET 1953
FOURTH EDITION 1956
FIFTH EDITION 1959
SIXTH EDITION 1962
SEVENTH EDITION 1964
EIGHTH EDITION 1967
NINTH EDITION 1970
TENTH EDITION 1972
ELEVENTH EDITION, ENTIRELY RE-SET 1975
TWELFTH EDITION 1976
THIRTEENTH EDITION, ENTIRELY RE-SET 1979
FOURTEENTH EDITION 1982
FIFTEENTH EDITION 1985
SIXTEENTH EDITION 1988

A CIP catalogue record for this book
is available from the British Library.

Text set in 8/9pt Compugraphic/Monotype Times by BP Integraphics, Bath
Printed and bound in Great Britain at The Bath Press, Avon, England

PREFACE TO THE SEVENTEENTH EDITION

The latest edition of this work has been thoroughly overhauled and revised. Among the many new topics included is one on the European Community, to which UK legislation has been subordinated in some instances. Numerous existing entries have been increased in length. The entry on UK law itself has been extended to cover the new Acts and Orders which concern the practising veterinary surgeon, while information on the health hazards of veterinary surgeons, stockpersons, and meat-handlers has been greatly increased to include the Spongiform Encephalopathies in people, farm animals, and cats.

Information is given on accidents of many kinds (including a few disasters), world-wide disease eradication campaigns, health promotion, the housing of animals, and pest control. In addition, technical advances in surgery have been described, e.g. gastropexy and stents.

Abstracts of the veterinary literature of many countries have been included, and the references will be found useful for further reading.

In the course of my travels in four out of the five continents, during which I visited 60 countries from Alaska in the north to New Zealand in the south, I have had glimpses of farming in eight countries in the tropics. I suggest, therefore, that the entry headed TROPICS, LIVESTOCK PRODUCTION IN THE, will prove helpful to those there already or planning to go, particularly since I have included advice from veterinary experts in the field.

During the course of revision, the opportunity has been taken to rearrange the information in many entries in order to provide a clearer layout and easier access to information.

As with the two previous editions, an appendix appears at the end of the book. Space in the Appendix is reserved for changes and developments which have taken place since the bulk of the Dictionary went to press. The user is referred to entries in the Appendix by the symbol ☞.

I should like to thank the British Veterinary Association for much helpful information, and the publishers of the Dictionary for coping with last-minute revisions and additions to the text.

1992   G. P. W.

Black's Veterinary Dictionary, first published in 1928, owes its existence to the late Professor William C. Miller, who was also responsible for the 1935 edition. When on the teaching staff of the Royal (Dick) Veterinary College, Edinburgh, he saw the need for such a book, and modelled it upon *Black's Medical Dictionary*. Professor Miller held the chair of animal husbandry at the Royal Veterinary College, London, and completed a distinguished career by becoming Director of the Animal Health Trust's equine research station at Newmarket.

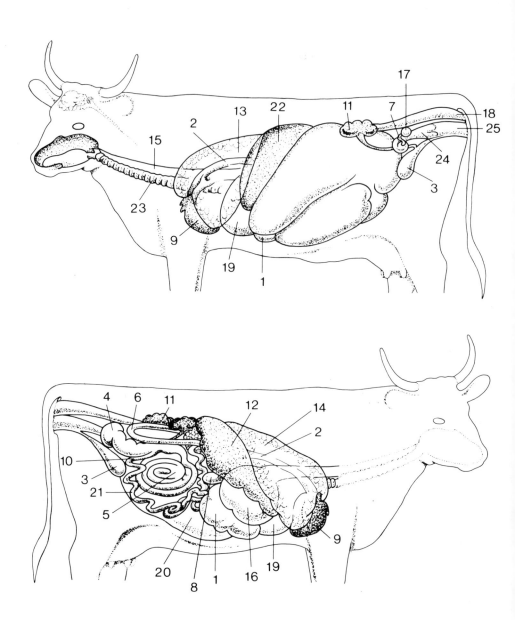

INTERNAL ORGANS OF THE COW

1 abomasum	10 ileum	18 rectum
2 aorta	11 kidney, left	19 reticulum
3 bladder	12 liver	20 rumen
4 caecum	13 lung, left	21 small intestine
5 colon	14 lung, right	22 spleen
6 duodenum	15 oesophagus (gullet)	23 trachea (windpipe)
7 Fallopian tube	16 omasum	24 uterus
8 gall bladder	17 ovary, left	25 vagina
9 heart		

A

ABDOMEN. (For a description of abdominal organs, see under appropriate headings.)

ABDOMEN, DISEASES OF (*see under* STOMACH, DISEASES OF; INTESTINE, DISEASES OF; DIARRHOEA; LIVER, DISEASE OF; PANCREAS, DISEASE OF; KIDNEYS, DISEASES OF; BLADDER, DISEASES OF; PERITONITIS; BLOAT; COLIC; ASCITES; HERNIA; etc.)

ABDOMEN, INJURIES OF. These include both injuries to the abdominal walls, and to the organs within the abdomen. Trauma may result in damage to the liver, spleen, kidneys, or urinary bladder. Apparently small external wounds of the abdominal wall may be far more serious than their appearance suggests.
DIAGNOSIS. An *exploratory laparotomy* may be necessary to establish the internal effects of such wounds, and also the cause of internal haemorrhage, free intra-peritoneal gas, peritonitis, etc.
Paracentesis is another useful diagnostic method. However, as a needle may become blocked by omentum, it is preferable to use a catheter, and peritoneal lavage. D. T. Crowe, in a study of cases involving 109 dogs and 20 cats, showed that the above method was highly accurate in detecting early intra-abdominal traumatic lesions, e.g. those mentioned above and rupture of the gall-bladder or bile-duct, prostatic abscess, uterine rupture, etc. (Crowe, D. T. (1984) *J. Amer. Anim. Hospital Association* **20** 223.)
When a stake or other pointed object has caused a large wound in the abdominal wall, the bowels may protrude through the opening, and if the incision be extensive, evisceration may take place. When only the wall of the abdomen has been damaged, there may be severe bruising, and haemorrhage into the tissues (*see* HAEMATOMA).
If exposure of the abdominal contents has taken place, or if the organs have been themselves damaged, there is risk of shock, haemorrhage, infection, and peritonitis; the latter causing great pain and usually proving fatal. For this reason the injured animal should receive promptly the expert services of a veterinary surgeon or else be humanely destroyed. Simple wounds or bruises of the abdominal walls are treated in the same way as ordinary wounds (*see* WOUNDS, SHOCK, PERITONITIS).

ABIOTROPHY. A degenerative disorder not attributable to external causes, and occurring after birth – hereditary rather than congenital. (*see* LYOSOMES – Lyosomal storage disease.)

ABNORMALITIES, INHERITED (*see under* GENETICS, DEFORMITIES).

ABOMASUM is the 4th stomach of ruminating animals. It is also called the 'true' or 'rennet stomach', and the 'reed'. It is an elongated, pear-shaped sac lying on the floor of the abdomen, on the right-hand side, and roughly between the 7th and 12th ribs.

ABOMASUM, DISPLACEMENT OF (*see* STOMACH, DISEASES OF *and* TYMPANITIC RESONANCE).

ABORTION in farm animals represents one important aspect of INFERTILITY (which see). The causes of abortion in the farm animals are shown in the tables below:

COWS
Infections
Viruses
  BVD/MD (bovine virus diarrhoea/mucosal disease); bovine herpes virus 1 (infectious bovine rhinotracheitis/infectious pustular vulvovaginitis)
Chlamydia
  C. psittaci
Rickettsiae
  Coxiella burnetti (Q fever)
  Ehrlichia phagocytophilia (tick-borne fever)
Bacteria
  Salmonella dublin, typhimurium, and other species
  Brucella abortus; also *B. melitensis* (but not in UK)
  Corynebacterium pyogenes
  Listeria monocytogenes
  Leptospira hardjo and other serovars
  Campylobacter fetus
  Besnoitia
Fungi
  Aspergillus fumigatus
  Mortierella wolfii
Protozoa
  Toxoplasma gondii
  Trichomonas fetus

Non-infectious causes
Claviceps purpurea (ergot in feed)
Stress
Recessive lethal gene
Malnutrition
Haemolytic disease

EWES
Infections
Viruses
  Border disease virus
  Thogoto
Chlamydia
  Chlamydia psittaci (*ovis*) (Enzootic abortion of ewes)
Rickettsiae
  Ehrlichia phagocytophilia (tick-borne fever)
Coxiella burnetti (Q fever)
Bacteria
  Bacillus licheniformis
  Salmonella dublin, typhimurium, and others

Listeria monocytogenes
Arizona species
Corynebacterium pyogenes
Brucella abortus and (not in the UK) *B. ovis*
Campylobacter jejuni
Fungi
  Aspergillus fumigatus
Protozoa
  Toxoplasma gondii
              Non-infectious causes
Stress (e.g. chasing/savaging by dogs; transport)
Near-starvation
Pregnancy toxaemia
Claviceps purpurea (ergot in feed)

SOWS
              Infections
Viruses*
  Swine fever virus
Bacteria
  Erysipelothrix rhusiopathiae (swine erysipelas)
  Brucella abortus suis
  Pasteurella multocida (occasionally)
  E. coli
  Leptospira species
Protozoa
  Toxoplasma gondii
              Non-infectious causes
Malnutrition, e.g. vitamin A deficiency
(*See also* CARBON MONOXIDE.)

MARES
              Infections
Viruses
  Equine herpes virus 1 (Equine rhino-
  pneumonitis)
Bacteria
  Salmonella abortus equi
  Brucella abortus (rarely)
  Leptospira species (sometimes in association
  with equine herpes virus 1)
              Non-infectious causes
Twin foals
Plant poisoning (e.g. by Locoweed)

BITCH AND CAT
  Brucellosis, toxoplasmosis, and herpes virus
  infections.

ABORTION, ENZOOTIC, OF EWES. This disease occurs in lowland flocks in S E Scotland and
N E England, as well as overseas.
CAUSE. Chlamydia, which multiplies in the
placenta where it causes necrosis of the
cotyledons. It can, however, remain latent for
long periods in non-pregnant sheep. (*See*
CHLAMYDIA PSITTACI).
SIGNS. Abortion occurs during the last 6 weeks,
usually during the last 2 or 3 weeks of the normal
period of gestation. Stillbirths and the birth of
weak full-term lambs also occur. The aborted
fetus is dropsical. The ewes often remain ill for
several weeks, but very few die. Infertility is
temporary, since usually ewes lamb normally
the following season.

* *see* SMEDI and AUJESZKY's for causes of infertility not
usually associated with abortion.

PREVENTION. Vaccines are available, including one developed in France based on a temperature-sensitive mutant of *Chl. psittaci*.

ABSCESS is a localised collection of pus. A
minute abscess is known as a pustule (*see* PUS-
TULE), and a diffused area that produces pus is
spoken of as an area of cellulitis (*see* CELLULITIS).
Abscesses in cats are usually of this type and
seldom 'point'.

An acute abscess forms rapidly and as rapidly
comes to a head and bursts, or else becomes reabsorbed and disappears – a process that is called
'abortion'. Acute abscesses generally run their
course in a week or 10 days.
CAUSES. The direct cause of an acute abscess is
either infection with bacteria, or the presence of
an irritant in the tissues, either chemical or mechanical. Bacterial invasion is the more common
cause, and even in many abscesses that are considered to be of a mechanical nature, such as the
presence of bullets or pieces of metal, thorns,
splinters, etc., in the tissues, the production of pus
is directly due to the micro-organisms that have
been introduced.
  The organisms that are most often associated
with the formation of abscesses include *staphylococci* and *streptococci*.
  An abscess may occur in virtually any organ or
tissue, e.g. liver, lung, brain, mammary gland,
bone.
  When bacteria have gained access they commence to multiply, and by the formation of
poisonous substances ('toxins'), they damage the
surrounding tissues.
  White blood-cells (leucocytes) and, in particular those called Neutrophils, gather in the area
invaded by the bacteria and engulf them. The area
of invasion becomes congested with dead or dying
bacteria, dead or dying leucocytes, dead tissue
cells which formerly occcupied the site, débris,
and a certain amount of fluid exuded from the
gorged blood-vessels in the vicinity. This constitutes the pus.
SIGNS. In an abscess there are the classic symptoms of inflammation, *rubor, calor, tumor*, and
dolor, i.e. redness, warmth, swelling, and pain;
and besides these, when the abscess is of large size
and is well developed, fever.
  'Pointing' of an abscess means that it has
reached that stage when the skin covering it is
dead, thin, generally glazed, and bulging. This is
only appreciable when the abscess is near to the
surface. If slightly deeper, the skin over the area
becomes swollen, is painful, and 'pits' on
pressure. The lymph nodes in the vicinity become
swollen and are tender. When the abscess bursts,
or when it is evacuated by lancing, the pain disappears, the swelling subsides, the temperature
falls, and the tissues around regain their normal
elasticity. If all the pus has been evacuated the
cavity rapidly heals, and only a tiny pit remains.
If, however, the abscess has burst into an internal
cavity, such as the chest or abdomen, pleurisy or
peritonitis may follow (and may prove fatal).
When an abscess is deeply seated so as to be out of
reach of diagnosis by manipulative measures, its

presence can be confirmed by blood tests. (*See* HAEMOGLOBIN REACTIVE PROTEIN.)

TREATMENT. Antibiotics may be employed as the sole means of treating multiple or deep-seated abscesses, they may be injected into a cavity following aspiration of the pus, or they may be used in addition to the lancing of an abscess. Hot fomentations, or application of a poultice, afford relief prior to lancing.

When an abscess is to be opened the following points should be kept in mind:

(1) Important arteries, veins, and nerves in the vicinity should not be damaged.

(2) The opening should be as far away from any new source of infection, such as the mouth, anus, or prepuce, as possible.

(3) The abscess cavity should always be opened by a large incision so that it will not heal over and imprison any pus which will often result in the formation of a second abscess at the same site.

(4) The opening should always be situated at the lowest part of the cavity so that its discharges will drain away by gravity. Failure to ensure this results in a collection of putrid fluid in the lower parts of the cavity, which will remain in place and form a sinus (*see* SINUS); for this reason it is sometimes necessary to make one or more 'counter-openings' by which the pus may escape.

After the abscess had been opened it is usually best to leave it uncovered.

A chronic abscess takes a long time to develop, seldom bursts, unless near to the surface of the body, and becomes surrounded by large amounts of fibrous tissue.

CAUSES. Abscesses due to tuberculosis, actinomycosis, staphylococci, and caseous abscess formation in the lymph nodes of sheep, are the most common types of cold or chronic abscesses. They may arise when an acute abscess, instead of bursting in the usual way, becomes surrounded by dense fibrous tissue.

SIGNS. Swelling may be noticeable on the surface of the body (as in actinomycosis), or it may show no signs of its presence until the animal is slaughtered (as in the case of many tuberculous abscesses and in lymphadenitis of sheep). If it is present on the surface, it is found to be hard, cold, only very slightly painful, and does not rapidly increase in size. As a rule the health of the patient remains quite good, unless the swelling is in such a position that it will interfere with some of the vital functions of the body, such as swallowing or breathing.

CHARACTERS OF THE PUS. The contained fluid varies in its appearance and its consistency. It may be thin and watery, or it may be solid or semi-solid. To this latter type the name 'inspissated pus' is given, and the process is often spoken of as 'caseation'. In certain cases, especially in tuberculous abscesses that have been in existence for a long time, the contained material may calcify.

TREATMENT. This may involve surgery, and/or the use of antibiotics, depending upon the nature of the abscess and its location.

ACACIA POISONING has been recorded in cattle and goats. Different species of acacia contain different toxic principles.

ACAPNIA means a condition of diminished carbon dioxide in the blood.

ACARICIDE. A parasiticide effective against mites.

ACARUS is a parasitic mite belonging to the natural order *Acarina*. This includes the mange mites, harvest mites, follicular mites, flour mites, etc. (*See* MITES.)

ACCIDENTAL SELF-INJECTION. This has led to human infection with BRUCELLOSIS, ORF, PLAGUE, Q FEVER, TUBERCULOSIS.

If the accident involves 'IMMOBILON' the effects can be reversed by an immediate self-injection of 'Revivon' (diprenorphine hydrochloride.) A veterinary surgeon who had no 'Revivon' with him died within 15 minutes, after accidental self-injection, when a colt made a sudden violent movement.

ACCIDENTS. Injuries include almost every possible form of wounding of the skin, of muscles, tendons, blood-vessels, nerves, and internal organs, as well as many varieties of fractures.

Dogs and cats. Road accidents and injuries resulting from falls from an upper window-ledge on to pavements, etc. The question of maliciousness sometimes arises. In some road accidents, rupture of the diaphragm occurs. (*See also* ELECTROCUTION, FRACTURES, BLEEDING, INTERNAL HAEMORRHAGE, BURNS; SHOCK; EYES, DISEASES OF.)

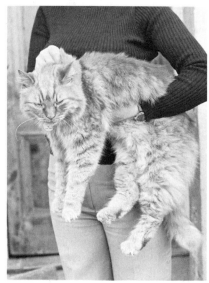

First Aid for owners: How to carry an injured cat with a suspected limb fracture. (Photo by courtesy of Marc Henrie and Pedigree Petfoods.) A dog may be carried similarly if not too large. An alternative for a bigger dog is to draw it gently on to a coat or rug, ready for lifting into the back of a car for transport to a veterinary surgeon.

ACCOMMODATION (*see* EYE).

ACEPROMAZINE is useful as a drug to give prior to anaesthesia, and enables low doses of barbiturates to be used. It is useful for tranquilising purposes; 1 to 3 mg per kg bodyweight being given by mouth a quarter of an hour or more before food, for the prevention of travel sickness in small animals.

Acepromazine lowers blood pressure, and so is contra-indicated in accident cases. Noradenaline is recommended for reversing any fall in blood pressure.

ACETABULUM is the cup-shaped depression on the pelvis with which the head of the femur forms the hip-joint. Dislocation of the hip-joint sometimes occurs as the result of 'run-over' accidents., and fractures of the pelvis involving the acetabulum frequently result from the same cause. (*See* HIP-JOINT, DISLOCATION, FRACTURE.)

ACETAMINOPHEN (*see* PARACETAMOL).

ACETIC ACID is the active principle of vinegar. Strong acetic acid is a caustic, and an irritant poison.

Acetic acid poisoning has caused the death of pigs fed a mash which had been allowed to stand. (After 24 hours in a warm place the acetic acid content of the mash reached 5 per cent.)

Acetic acid may also occur in silage and in fermenting hay, and is one of the normal breakdown products of cellulose-digesting bacteria in the rumen.

ACETONAEMIA and **KETOSIS** are names given to a metabolic disturbance in cattle and sheep. It may be defined as the accumulation in the blood plasma, in significant amounts, of ketone bodies. It may occur at any time, but is commonest in winter in dairy cows kept indoors. Many cases are shown by cows up to about 3 weeks after calving, when receiving a full ration of concentrates. With these at least 6 lb of hay should be fed daily. Heavy feeding with low-quality silage is stated to be a predisposing factor. It often follows hypomagnesaemia. It is very rare in heifers and seldom occurs before the 3rd calving.

CAUSE. Whenever the glucose level in the blood plasma is low, as in starvation or on a low carbohydrate diet, or when glucose is not utilisable, as in diabetes, the concentration of free fatty acids in the plasma rises. This rise is roughly paralleled by an increase in the concentration of ketone bodies, which provide a third source of energy. In other words the moderate ketosis which occurs under a variety of circumstances is to be looked upon as a normal physiological process supplying the tissues with a readily utilisable fuel when glucose is scarce.

By contrast, the severe forms of ketosis met with in the lactating cow and the diabetic cow, and characterised by high concentrations of ketone bodies in the blood and urine, are obviously harmful pathological conditions where the quantities of ketone bodies formed grossly exceed possible needs. (*See* KETONE BODIES.)

SIGNS. The cow ceases to feed normally, but may lick or chew the walls, chain, head-rope, or other objects. Depression is marked, but short periods of what would seem to be delirium may be shown, when the cow may become excited. Constipation and decrease in urine secretion occur, and rumination either ceases or is intermittent. Milk secretion is reduced. This may be the first symptom.

A peculiar sickly sweet odour (the odour of acetone) can be perceived from breath, urine, milk, and even from the skin in established cases. It is upon the presence of acetone in the body secretions, etc., that a diagnosis is based. To confirm the diagnosis a chemical test (Rothera's test) may be carried out.

FIRST-AID TREATMENT consists in giving half a pint of glycerine, diluted in water, or a proprietary preparation containing sodium propionate.

The feeding of cut grass, the addition of a little molasses to feed, and exercise all aid recovery. In herds prone to this condition, Molassine meal is helpful as a preventative, also a little ground maize. Resistant cases are met with which defy all treatment, the cow improves up to a point but does not feed properly and dies in 10 to 20 days.

PREVENTION. Advice from the Animal Diseases Research Institute, Compton, is as follows:

In the second half of a lactation, the diet of a dairy cow should contain a greater proportion of home-grown foods with a lower digestibility than that in the diet fed during peak lactation. In this way the animals can receive an adequate intake for their requirements and at the same time, receive an economically priced diet with a roughage content which will ensure an active rumen fermentation. Feeding in excess of requirements must be avoided at all costs during the second half of lactation.

At the beginning of the dry period, the cows should not be in a fat condition. As dry animals, they should be fed to satisfy their requirements until the beginning of the 'steaming up' period.

A prolonged period for 'steaming up' can be detrimental since the cows may no longer be on a rising plane of nutrition at the time of calving and in early lactation. 'Steaming up' should commence therefore, 4 to 5 weeks before the anticipated date of parturition.

During the 'steaming up' period the production concentrate ration should be introduced to the cow beginning with 3 to 5 lb of concentrate a day in the first week and rising to 8 to 12 lb per day in the week before calving. Throughout the whole 'steaming up' period the hay and silage to be fed during production should be included in the ration.

After calving, the quantity of production ration fed should be steadily increased as the milk production increases. For high yielding cows the production concentrate ration should contain 16 to 18 per cent crude protein. The carbohydrate in the ration should be readily digestible. The inclusion of some ground maize may be particularly helpful in ketosis-prone herds, since some of the starch escaping rumen fermentation is digested and absorbed as sugars. Production concentrates should contain a balanced vitamin and mineral supplement.

During the period when the milk yields are highest and the cows are being fed to a maximum dry matter intake, the stockman must ensure that the cows are managed in such a way that they can consume, if not all, as much of their ration as possible. They must *not* be given free access to straw; *not* given all their concentrate ration in the milking parlour where time is limited to consume the ration, but in addition fed concentrates between milkings. High yielding cows should not be penned for a long time in yards, but be given ample opportunity for exercise.

During the first 3 months of lactation, high yielders should not be subjected to sudden changes in ration. A change in the supply of a concentrate ration, i.e. from one manufacturer to another can present dietary problems. Although the crude analysis of protein, lipid, etc. may be the same, the individual cereals and oil cakes in the ration can be different so a sudden change of ration can lead to a temporary decreased efficiency of utilisation.

After the first 10 to 12 weeks of lactation, the feeding routine of the high yielders can be modified. The home grown carbohydrate cereals can be slowly increased in the ration with a corresponding decrease in the more expensive highly digestible carbohydrates. This change-over must be a gradual process.

In all stages of lactation attention must be paid to the quality of the foods fed to a dairy herd. Silage and hay quality is frequently over-rated by the farmer leading to an inadequate intake for the animal's requirements.

ACETONE. This is found in small amounts in certain samples of normal urine, and present in greater quantities during the course of diabetes, pneumonia, cancer, starvation, and diseases of disturbed metabolism.

ACETYLCHOLINE is produced in the areas of the nerve endings of the neuro-muscular system and is a link in the transmission of nerve impulse to the muscles controlled by each nerve. In cases of pain, shock, injury, etc., the normal supply may fail, so that nerve impulses cannot reach the muscle fibres and paralysis results. The administration of acetylcholine serves to correct this deficiency.

In health, acetylcholine is destroyed as soon as a nerve impulse has passed, by the enzyme cholesterinase. This, however, is itself destroyed by exposure to organic phosphorus insecticides; resulting in poisoning – convulsions and death. Excessive salivation is an important symptom in dogs so poisoned.

ACHALASIA of the oesophagus. Absence of progressive peristalsis and failure of the lower oesophageal sphincter to relax.

ACHONDROPLASIA is a form of dwarfing due to disease affecting the long bones of the limbs before birth. It is noticed in some calves of certain breeds of cattle such as the Dexter, and in some breeds of dogs, and in lambs. (*See* GENETICS, GENETIC DEFECTS.)

ACHORION (*see* RINGWORM).

ACID-FAST ORGANISMS are those which, when once stained with carbol-fuchsin dye, possess the power to retain their colour after immersion in strong acid solutions, which decolorise the non-acid-fast group. The method serves to differentiate between organisms belonging to the two classes. The more important of the acid-fast group are *Mycobacterium tuberculosis*, causing tuberculosis in man and animals; *Mycobacterium johnei*, the cause of Johne's disease; and *leprosae*, causing human leprosy. Many other non-pathogenic types are also encountered in sewage, dung, ear-wax, smegma, butter, and one, the *M. phlei*, occurs frequently on Timothy grass and may be mistaken for the *M. tuberculosis*.

ACIDOSIS. A condition of reduced alkaline reserve of the blood and tissues, with or without an actual fall in pH. Sudden death may occur in cattle from acidosis after gorging on grain, or following a sudden introduction of cereal-based concentrates. (*See also* BARLEY POISONING.) Sheep may similarly be affected.

ACIDS, POISONING BY. It occasionally happens that animals are either accidentally or maliciously poisoned.
SIGNS. Excessive salivation, great pain, and destruction of the mucous membrane lining the mouth (which causes the unfortunate animal to keep its mouth open and protrude its tongue), are seen. After a short time convulsive seizures and vomiting occur, and general collapse follows; while if a large amount of acid has been taken, death from shock rapidly supervenes.
TREATMENT. Alkaline demulcents should be given at once and in large quantities; bicarbonate of sodium given in gruels or barley-water or milk is quite useful. These neutralise the acids into harmless salts, and soothe the corroded and burnt tissues. (*See* ACETIC ACID, ARSENIOUS ACID, CARBOLIC ACID, HYDROCYANIC ACID, OXALIC ACID, etc.)

ACINUS is the name applied to each of the minute sacs of which secreting glands are composed, and which usually cluster round the branches of the gland-duct like grapes on their stems.

ACNE. An inflammation of sebaceous glands or hair follicles, with the formation of pustules. In the horse, a contagious form of acne is sometimes due to infection with *Corynebacterium ovis*. Acne often accompanies canine distemper, and is seen on the chin of the cat.

ACONITE (*Aconitum napellus*, commonly known as 'Monkshood', 'Wolfsbane', 'Blue-Rocket', etc.). Aconite is an extremely poisonous plant found in all parts of the world, but especially in

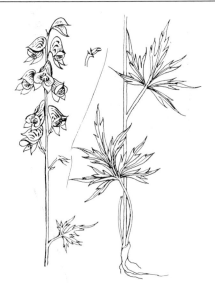

Aconite (*Aconitum napellus*). The flowers are either blue or yellow, and each has a petal which is in the shape of a helmet or hood; hence the name Monkshood which is often applied to the plant when growing in gardens. Height: 2 to 6 ft, according to variety.

the cooler mountainous parts of both hemispheres. It is frequently cultivated in gardens in Great Britain for its decorative appearance. All parts of the plant are poisonous, the parts above the ground being often eaten by stock (*see* later). Aconite owes its poisonous properties to an alkaloid (*Aconitine*), mainly found in the tuberous root, but present in smaller amounts in other parts of the plant. Aconitine is irritant in large doses, but smaller doses have a sedative and paralysing effect on the sensory nerves. It has been used as an ingredient of liniments.

ACONITE POISONING. Poisoning by aconite generally occurs when herbivorous animals gain access to gardens in which the plant is cultivated for ornamental purposes and eat its upper parts. Pigs rooting in fields where it grows (especially on the continent of Europe) sometimes eat the horse-radish-like root with toxic results.
SIGNS. The chief symptoms shown are general depression, loss of appetite, salivation, inflammation of the mucous membrane of the mouth and jaws, grinding of the teeth; pigs are nauseated and may vomit; and horses become restless and may be attacked with colic. Animals walk with an unsteady gait, and later become paralysed in their hind-limbs. The pulse becomes feeble or almost imperceptible, and unconsciousness is followed by convulsions and death.
TREATMENT. Animals which have eaten aconite should be secured at once in a convenient building. An emetic must be given to the pig, dog, and cat to induce vomiting, and the stomach-tube may be passed in the large herbivorous animals that do not vomit. Stimulants, such as strong black tea or coffee, should be given by the mouth.

ACOPROSIS. Absence or scantiness of faecal matter in the intestines.

ACORN POISONING (*see under* OAK).

ACROMEGALY. A condition caused by excess of the growth hormone STH, produced by the anterior lobe of the pituitary gland, leading to enlargement of the extremities, and to overgrowth of connective tissue, bone and viscera. (*See also* SOMATOTROPHIN.)

ACROPACHIA. A condition in which new bone is laid down, first in the limbs and later in other parts of the skeleton. It may accompany tumours and tuberculosis in the dog.

ACROSOME. A cap enclosing the head of a sperm.

ACRYLIC IMPLANTS (*see* IMPLANTS).

ACTH, ADRENOCORTICOTROPHIN. (*See* CORTICOTROPHIN.)

ACTINOBACILLOSIS is a disease of cattle similar in some respects to actinomycosis, and sometimes mistaken for it. (*See* ACTINOMYCOSIS.)
Generally only one or two animals in a herd are affected at one time.
The disease occurs also in sheep. Swellings may be seen on lips, cheeks, jaw, and at the base of the horn. Pneumonia, infection of the liver or alimentary canal may lead to death in untreated cases. ☞
CAUSE. Actinobacillosis is due to infection of the tissues with the organism *Actinobacillus lignièresi*. These are arranged at the centre of the lesions in a radiating manner. Infection occurs through injuries, abrasions, etc., of soft tissues, and when lymph nodes are affected through invasion along the lymph vessels. Occasionally subcutaneous tissue may be involved without apparent lesions in the lymph nodes. Abscesses form.
Lesions may involve the lungs, rumen, omasum, abomasum, and reticulum. A case of genital actinobacillosis in a bull was reported by the Milk Marketing Board in 1971. The semen at first appeared normal but clots formed five minutes after collection. There were no lesions which could be felt.
SIGNS. When lymph nodes in the throat are affected, the swelling and pressure caused may make swallowing and breathing difficult; if the lesion is in the skin and superficial tissues only, it may attain to a great size without causing much trouble; when the tongue is affected the animal has difficulty in mastication and swallowing and there is usually a constant dribbling of saliva from the mouth. If this is examined there may be found in it small greyish or greyish-yellow 'pus spots', in which the organism can be demonstrated by microscopic methods. Later, the saliva may become thick, purulent, and foul smelling.
In those cases where feeding or breathing are hindered, animals, especially bullocks, rapidly lose flesh, and if neglected severe emaciation may

occur, occasionally resulting in death. In cows, the yield of milk may be greatly reduced, especially where pain is severe, or feeding is difficult.

TREATMENT. The intravenous injection of sodium iodide made the treatment of this condition easier than formerly. Antibiotics may also be tried.

The treatment of actinobacillosis is not always successful, and it is sometimes advisable to slaughter a fat bullock rather than to treat it.

Pigs. The disease has been recorded both in the UK (very rarely) and also overseas, caused by *Actinobacillus equuli* (*Bacterium viscosum equi*).

Horses (*see under* FOALS, DISEASES OF).

PRECAUTIONS. The disease can be transmitted to man. Accordingly, care must be taken over washing the hands, etc., after handling an animal with actinobacillosis.

ACTINOMYCES PYOGENES. Another name for *Corynebacterium pyogenes.* A cause of fetal death and abortion in cows.

ACTINOMYCOSIS. This has been recorded in very many species of animals, including man, dogs, pigs, birds, and reptiles.

The lesions produced bear a considerable resemblance to those of actinobacillosis, and are often indistinguishable from them, but typically actinomycosis affects the cheeks, pharynx and especially the **bone** of the jaws, while actinobacillosis is more likely to attack soft tissues only. When bone and periosteum become affected by actinomycosis, the soft tissue adjacent usually become involved as the disease progresses, which may lead to a difficulty in diagnosis.

CAUSE is *Actinomyces bovis.* For many decades this was referred to as the 'ray fungus', but it is now regarded as one of the 'higher bacteria'.

This anaerobic bacterium is present in the digestive system of cattle, and it is probable that it can only become pathogenic by invading the tissues through a wound. It is common during the ages when the permanent cheek teeth are cutting the gums and pushing out the milk teeth. It may then be carried into the tooth sockets by barley awns, pieces of straw, etc. The abdominal organs, especially the liver, are sometimes affected, while actinomycosis and actinobacillosis have both been found in lungs and bronchi.

Yellow sulphur granules are found in the lesions.

SIGNS. The swelling in bone and other tissue, mainly composed of dense fibrous tissue, may reach a considerable size causing interference with mastication, swallowing, or breathing, depending on the situation of the lesion. In most cases when the mouth or throat is affected, there is a constant dribbling of saliva in varying amounts from the mouth. In the earlier stages this saliva is normal in its appearance, but later becomes offensive.

Actinomycosis of the bone of the upper and lower jaws produces an increase in the size of the part and a rarefication of its bony structure, the spaces becoming filled with the proliferation of fibrous tissue which is characteristic of the disease.

When the udder is affected, hard fibrous nodules may be felt below the skin, varying in size from that of a pea to a walnut or larger, and firmly embedded in the structure of the gland itself. These swelling enclose soft centres of suppuration which, on occasions, may either burst through the covering skin, or else into an adjacent milk sinus or duct. The milk from such a cow should not be used for human consumption because of the danger of the consumer contracting the disease.

TREATMENT. The use of penicillin or streptomycin. Sulpha drugs assist recovery. (*See also* ACTINOBACILLOSIS, PRECAUTIONS.)

ACTIVE PRINCIPLES are the substances in a drug which are responsible for its effects. For example, the alkaloid morphine is the chief active principle of the crude drug opium. (*See* ALKALOIDS, GLUCOSIDES, SAPONINS.)

ACUARIA UNCINATA. This roundworm has caused outbreaks of disease in geese, ducks, and poultry. The life-cycle of this parasite involves an intermediate host, *Daphnia pulex*, the water flea. On post-mortem examination of affected birds, worms may be found in nodules scattered over the mucous membrane of the oesophagus and proventriculus. Mortality may be high among geese and ducks.

ACUPUNCTURE. The centuries-old Chinese technique of needle insertion at certain specified points has become a part of Western veterinary medicine – for treatment, analgesia, and resuscitation.

Adaptations have been made such as the use of lasers instead of needles, obviating the need for restraint. Ultrasonics and heat have also been applied to the points.

At a symposium in London, Philip Rogers, principal research officer at the Dublin Agricultural Institute, stated that although acupuncture is mainly used to relieve painful conditions, it can also aid poor circulation, tissue damage, smooth muscle dysfunction and paralysis.

He warned that over-stimulation at the points could exaggerate the signs of disease.

Acupuncture can produce the morphine-like natural substances (*see* ENDORPHINS) which are, in effect, analgesics.

In China acupuncture has been used for surgical analgesia. In a case described by Dr White, a cow – apparently completely anaesthetised on its right flank – was conscious and standing during a laparotomy, and walked away afterwards as if nothing had happened.

Chronic back pain which did not respond to conventional treatments improved in from two to eight weeks in 13 out of 15 racehorses. An injection of sterile saline at nine acupuncture points once a week enabled training and racing to be resumed. (Martin, B. B. & others. *JAVMA* (1987) **190** 1177.)

There have been many reports of successful resuscitation, by means of acupuncture, of cats which had stopped breathing or whose hearts had stopped.

Acupuncture is not a panacea, and is not entirely free from risk.

A series of deaths in boarding kennels in America could not be accounted for at autopsy. The only common factor in each case was that an injection had been given. Dr Donald L. Pohlman suggested that perhaps the injections had been made into what acupuncturists recognise as a danger area. 'If an injection is given there, many dogs die within 48–72 hours,' he stated. (*Modern Veterinary Practice* (1976) **57** 79.)

ACUTE DISEASE. A disease is called acute in contradistinction to 'chronic' when it appears rapidly, and either causes death quickly or leads to a speedy recovery. As examples of acute diseases in the lower animals, anthrax and blackquarter (where the animal may be dead within 12 hours) acute pneumonia, and acute distemper, may be mentioned. Sometimes 'acute' is used as an indication of a very severe or painful condition. (*See also under* DEATH, SUDDEN.)

AD LIB. FEEDING is a labour-saving system under which pigs or poultry help themselves to dry meal, etc., and eat as much as they wish. The self-feeding of silage to cattle also comes under this heading. (*See also* DRY-FEEDING.)

ADDISON'S DISEASE. This has been recorded in dogs, mostly of the female sex, and is a disease of the cortex of the adrenal glands, leading to under-production of the hormone cortisol (ALDOSTERONE).

CAUSES include a congenital defect, an infection or tumour affecting the adrenal glands, prolonged steroid administration, and possibly autoimmune disease.

A case was reported (Ruben, J. M. and others (1985) *Veterinary Record* **116,** 91) in a puppy which collapsed four times when from eight to 16 weeks old, and was treated for shock. A fifth episode proved fatal. The average age of onset is stated to be four years. (*See* ADRENAL GLANDS.)

ADDITIVES. Substances added to a compound or a protein concentrate in the course of manufacture for some specific purpose other than as a direct source of nutrient.

The current list of additives is a long one, and includes such diverse products as those for treating ringworm in cattle and horses without the necessity to handle the animals; vitamin, mineral and trace element additives; those containing urea; and those for the control of worm infestations, coccidiosis, and 'scours' in pigs, respectively.

Feed antibiotics, for adding to animal feeds as growth promotants, include: Flavomycin, virginiamycin, avoparcin, zinc bacitracin, olaquindox, and tylosin.

M A F F should be consulted concerning the latest position as changes are continually being made in the regulations and policies.

The object of these regulations is to ensure as far as possible that the benefits gained from the use of antibiotics in animal feeds are not offset by hazards to human and animal health. The benefits may include a faster growth rate, a more efficient use of food, and the possibility of successfully rearing unthrifty or runt pigs. (*See also under* MEDICINES ACT, ANTIBIOTICS, OLAQUINDOX, GROWTH PROMOTERS, HORMONES IN MEAT PRODUCTION.)

ADENITIS means inflammation of a gland. (*See* LYMPHADENITIS; PAROTID GLAND, DISEASES OF.)

ADENOMA. A tumour composed of epithelial tissue, often gland-like in appearance. It may sometimes be found in positions where glandular tissue is not normally present. A malignant form is the adenocarcinoma. (*See* TUMOURS, CANCER.)

ADENOMATOSIS (*see* PORCINE INTESTINAL ADENOMATOSIS; *also* JAAGSIEKTE).

ADENOVIRUS. This is a contraction of the original term 'adenoidal-pharyngeal conjunctival agents'. (*See* VIRUSES.)

ADH (*see* ANTIDIURETIC HORMONE).

ADHESION FACTOR, bacterial. (*See* BACTERIAL ADHESIVENESS.)

ADHESIONS. Adhesions occur by the uniting or growing together of structures or organs which are normally separate and freely movable. They are generally the result of acute or chronic inflammation, and in the earlier stages the uniting material is fibrin, which later becomes resolved into fibrous tissue.

TREATMENT. Surgical division of the obstructing bands is often necessary in the abdominal cavity and in adhesions of the walls of the vagina following injuries received at a previous parturition. (*See* PLEURISY, PERITONITIS, etc.)

ADIPOSE TISSUE. Here fat is stored as an energy reserve; globules of fat forming within connective tissue cells. When additional fat is stored, each cell eventually becomes spherical, its nucleus pushed to one side.

During demanding muscular exercise, or when food is insufficient, or during a debilitating disease, the cells release the fat into the bloodstream and resume their normal shape. (*See also* next page and LIPOMA.)

ADJUVANT. A substance added to a viral vaccine, in order to localise the virus at the injection site, and to make the virus insoluble by precipitation with aluminium hydroxide or by a water-in-oil emulsion. (Russell, P. H. & Edington, N. *Veterinary Viruses.*)

ADRENAL GLANDS, also called SUPRARENAL GLANDS are two small organs situated at the anterior extremities of the kidneys, and are endocrine glands.

FUNCTION. The cortex secretes hormones which are called steroids or corticosteroids. These include Glucocorticoids, notably *cortisol,* concerned with the regulation of carbohydrate

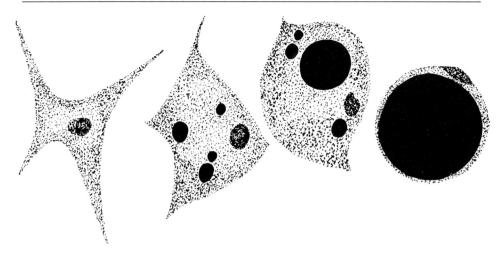

Typical fat cell formed by intake of fat globules. Reproduced with permission from R. D. Frandson: *Anatomy and Physiology of Farm Animals*, Lea & Febiger, Philadelphia, 1986. After Ham and Leeson; *Histology*, J. B. Lippincott Co.

metabolism; and Mineralocorticoids (which regulate sodium and potassium levels in body fluids), *e.g. aldosterone*. The cortex also secretes androgens; the medulla secretes *adrenalin* and *noradrenalin*.

Surgical removal of the adrenal glands (**adrenalectomy**) has been carried out in the treatment of CUSHING'S DISEASE (which see) in the dog; survival being possible through hormone implants. Otherwise removal of the adrenals usually leads to death within a matter of weeks; blood-pressure falls, temperature falls, kidney action is impaired, and the animal lacks resistance to the effects of stress or infection.

ATROPHY. 'By far the commonest cause of adrenal atrophy in the Western world is corticosteroid therapy.' (*Lancet*, 20.9.75.)

ADRENALIN is the 'fight or flight' hormone from the adrenal glands.

Its chief action is that of raising the tone of all involuntary muscle fibres, stimulating the heart, constricting the walls of the smaller arteries, and producing a rise in the blood-pressure. It is used for checking capillary haemorrhage in wounds, for warding off shock or collapse by raising the blood-pressure. (*See* ADRENAL GLANDS.)

ADRENOCORTICOTROPHIN. Commonly abbreviated to ACTH. It has been used in the treatment of acetonaemia in cattle, and is a naturally occurring hormone obtained from the anterior lobe of the pituitary gland.

AEDES (*see* MOSQUITOES *and* FLIES).

AELUROSTRONGYLUS. A lungworm of cats. (*See* ROUNDWORMS.)

AEROBE. A micro-organism which needs oxygen for its growth and multiplication.

AEROMONAS (*see* BACTERIA, Table).

AEROSOL. A liquid agent or solution dispersed in air in the form of a fine mist. If aerosols, for insecticidal and other purposes, are used over a long period, *e.g.* by a continuous evaporator, thought must be given to the effect of the chemicals used (a) on the health of the livestock; (b) on organochlorine or other residues left in the carcase to the detriment of people eating meat; (c) on the health of the stockmen.

AEROSOLS AS A MODE OF INFECTION. Viruses excreted by animals suffering from an infectious disease may be transmitted to other animals (or man) as an aerosol. ('Coughs and sneezes spread diseases.') Examples, the common cold of man, foot-and-mouth disease, rabies. ☞

AEROTROPISM. The tendency of micro-organisms to group themselves about a bubble of air in culture media.

AETIOLOGY is the cause of a disease, or the study of such causes.

AFFERENT is the name given to nerve fibres which carry impulses in towards the central nervous system to distinguish from efferent fibres which conduct impulses outwards to organs or tissues. Broadly speaking, afferent fibres have mainly sensory functions, while efferent fibres are concerned with activities of organs, such as movement, secretion, vascular changes, etc.

AFLATOXINS. Toxins produced by fungi, *e.g. Aspergillus flavus* and the cause of poisoning in animals eating contaminated GROUNDNUT MEAL (which see) or sunflower or cotton seed; or various grains stored under conditions of high humidity and temperature.

In cattle, aflatoxins may give rise to a reduced growth rate or drop in milk yield. In pigs jaundice may be a symptom, and cancer of the liver expected.

Aflatoxicosis in poultry is characterised by haemorrhages, anorexia, decreased efficiency in food utilisation, pathological changes in the liver, kidneys and bile ducts, and death. The problem can be prevented by storing grain with 13 per cent of moisture or less. The litter may also be a source of toxins and consequently it is important to keep the moisture in the litter to a minimum by ensuring that the ventilation of the house is adequate and that the waterers are operating correctly. (Cavalheiro, A. C. L. (1981) *World Poultry Science Journal* **37, 34.**)

As one of the precautions taken to maintain animal feeds free of dangerously high levels of aflatoxins, trout are used as a means of testing, since in young trout (as in pigs) aflatoxin poisoning is likely to result in cancer of the liver. (Mature cock fish become fully resistant). Equally, care has to be taken with commercial dry trout feeds, to ensure that aflatoxin level is below 0·5 parts per billion; otherwise malignant tumours are apt to develop, and later liquid-filled cysts may grow to a remarkable size (Dr H. Wunder). (*See also* MYCOTOXICOSIS *and* CIRRHOSIS.)

AFRC, the Agricultural and Food Research Council.

AFRICAN HORSE SICKNESS (*see* HORSE SICKNESS, AFRICAN).

AFRICAN SWINE FEVER (*see entry after* SWINE FEVER).

AFRICANDER. Cattle in origin about ¾ Brahman and ¼ British beef breed. (*See also under* CYTOGENETICS.)

AFRIKANER. A synonym for Brahman or Zebu cattle.

AFTERBIRTH (*see* PLACENTA).

AFTERBIRTHS, INFECTED may be a source of infection to other animals. (*See* SCRAPIE, BRUCELLOSIS, ENZOOTIC OVINE ABORTION.)

AGALACTIA. The absence of milk in the udder, following parturition. (*See* SOW'S MILK, ABSENCE OF; COW'S MILK, ABSENCE OF.)

AGALACTIA, CONTAGIOUS is a contagious disease of goats particularly, and sheep less commonly, characterised by inflammatory lesions in the udder, eyes, and joints. It is chiefly met with in France, Switzerland, the Tyrol, Italy, the Pyrenees, North Africa and India.
CAUSE. *Mycoplasma agalactiae.* The disease often occurs in the spring and the summer, and disappears with the advent of the colder weather. There appears to be some relationship between the presence of certain flies and the incidence of the disease. The infection may be carried by the hands of the milkers and by the litter in a shed becoming contaminated, while the fetus may be infected before birth.
SIGNS. Fever, mastitis, and a greatly reduced milk yield. The milk becomes yellowish-green

and contains clots. In addition to the udder, both joints and eyes may be involved; a painful arthritis, and conjunctivitis followed by keratitis (with resultant temporary blindness) worsening the animal's condition.

Emaciation and death within 10 days may occur in very acute cases; otherwise recovery usually follows within a few weeks, though the former milk yield will not have been regained.

Male animals may have orchitis as well as arthritis.

Inflammation of the lymph nodes may occur, and lesions may be found also in abdominal organs and tissues, and in the chest.
TREATMENT. Isolation of the affected animals and strict segregation of the in-contacts should be carried out.

In most instances it is more economical to slaughter all but the most valuable animals and burn their carcases.

AGAR is the gelatinous substance prepared from ceylon moss and various kinds of seaweed. It dissolves in boiling water, and, on cooling, solidifies into a gelatinous mass at a temperature slightly above that of the body. It is extensively used in preparing culture-media for use in bacteriological laboratories, and also in the treatment of chronic constipation in dog and cat, for which purpose it may be shredded and mixed with the food.

AGAR-GEL IMMUNODIFFUSION TEST (*see* COGGINS).

AGENE PROCESS. The bleaching of flour with nitrogen trichloride. The use of such flour in dog foods gave rise to nervous symptoms. (*See* HYSTERIA.)

AGES OF ANIMALS.

Horses. By the time it has reached 17 years, which generally means about 14 years of work, a horse's powers are on the wane. Many at this age are still in possession of their full vigour, but these are generally of a class that is better looked after than the average, *e.g.* hunters, carriage-horses, or favourites. On an average, the feet of the horse are worn out first, not the arteries as in man, and consequently horses with good feet and legs are likely to outlast those inferior in this respect, other things being equal. After the feet come the teeth. In very many cases a horse's teeth wear out before their time. It often happens that the upper and lower rows of teeth do not wear in the normal way; the angle of their grinding surfaces becomes more and more oblique, until the chewing of the food becomes less and less perfect, and the horse loses condition.

Instances are on record of horses attaining the age of 35, 45, 50, and one of a horse that was still working when 63 years old. These, however, are very exceptional. The average age at which a horse dies or is euthanased lies somewhere between 20 and 25 years.

Cattle. The great majority of bullocks are killed before they reach 3 years of age, and in countries where 'prime beef' is grown they are fattened and killed between 2½ and 3 years. In the majority of herds, few cows live to be more than 8 or 10 years of age. Pedigree bulls may reach 12 or 14 years of age before being discarded. Records are in existence of cows up to 39 years old, and it is claimed that one had 30 calves. Sixteen and 22 calves are claimed for other cows in Britain.

Sheep. Here again the requirements of the butcher have modified the age of the animal at death. Wether lambs are killed at ages ranging from 4 to 9 months (Christmas lambs), and older fat sheep up to 2½ years. Ewes, on the average, breed until they are from 4 to 6 or 7 years, when they too are fattened and slaughtered for mutton. Exceptionally, they reach greater ages, but unless in the case of pure breeding animals, each year over six reduces their ultimate value as carcases. Rams are killed after they have been used for two or three successive seasons at stud, that is, when they are 3 or 4 years of age, as a rule.

Pigs. In different districts the age at which pigs are killed varies to some extent, according to the requirements of local trade. Pigs for pork production are killed at about 3½ to 4 months; bacon pigs are killed between 6 and 7½ months, and only breeding sows and boars are kept longer. Ages of up to 12 years have been recorded in the case of the sow.

Dogs and cats. These are the only domesticated animals which are generally allowed to die a natural death. The average age of the dog is about 12 years, and of the cat 9 to 12, but instances are not uncommon of dogs living to 18 or 20 years of age, and of cats similarly. (*See also* BREEDING OF LIVESTOCK, DENTITION OF ANIMALS.)

Elephants. Their normal life-span is unknown, but some working elephants are employed up to the age of 65 or 70, and then retired. (Lawson, A. A. *Daily Telegraph.*)

AGGLUTINATION is the clumping together of cells in a fluid. For example, bacteria will agglutinate when a specific antiserum is added to the suspension of bacteria. Similarly, the blood serum of one animal will cause the red blood cells of another to become grouped together or agglutinated.

Agglutination is explained by the presence in the serum of an *agglutinin* which combines with an agglutinable substance, or *agglutinogen*, possessed by the organisms.

Agglutination is made use of in the Agglutination Test, which depends upon the principle that in the blood serum of an animal harbouring in its body disease-producing organisms (though it may show no symptoms) there is a far greater concentration of agglutinins than in a normal animal. Minute doses (*e.g.* dilutions of 1 part to 100 or even 1000) of such serum will cause agglutination while serum from a normal animal will not cause agglutination when diluted more than 1 part in 10. Incubation of the mixture at body heat usually hastens the results and enables a rapid diagnosis to be made.

AGGRESSIVENESS. This may be transient, as in a nursing bitch fearful for her puppies. Persistent aggressiveness can be the result of jealousy, when the birth of a baby means a decline in status for the dog. Ill-treatment, attacks by some local pugnacious dog, being kept tied up for long periods, or shut in an empty house are other causes. Heredity is an important factor, too, and it is unwise to breed from aggressive parents even if they look like Show winners. Brain disease – for example, encephalitis, or a brain tumour – may account for aggressiveness in any animal. So may pain. (*See* ENCEPHALITIS, MENINGIOMA, RABIES, BENZOIC ACID POISONING in the cat, EQUINE VERMINOUS ARTERITIS, 'VICES', CHLORINATED HYDROCARBON poisoning, acute MUSCULAR RHEUMATISM, OVARIES, DISEASES OF, FELINE HYPERAESTHESIA, BOVINE SPONGIFORM ENCEPHALOPATHY, LISTERIOSIS, ANAPLASMOSIS, ACETONAEMIA, GRASS SICKNESS, *and* HEARTWATER.)

AGONIST. A type of drug which gives a positive response (e.g. contraction or relaxation of a muscle fibre, or secretion from a gland) when its molecule combines with a **receptor**. The latter is a specific structural component of a cell, on its membrane, and usually a protein.
Antagonist. A drug which merely blocks the attachment of any other substance at the receptor, so preventing any possible active response.
Partial agonist. A drug which produces a positive response at the receptor, but only a weak one. However, since it occupies the receptor it prevents any full agonist from binding so that, in the presence of agonists, partial agonists may act as antagonists.

Many drugs are now classified according to their major action, e.g. β blockers, H_1 and H_2 receptor antagonists.

β receptors are present in the heart and smooth muscle of the bronchioles, uterus, and arterioles supplying skeletal muscle. Drugs which are selective β_1 (heart) or β_2 (elsewhere) are now available. For example, clenbuterol is a specific β_2 antagonist. (*See* CLENBUTEROL). (Marriner, S. E. *Veterinary Record* (1986) **119**, 132.)

European Commissioner Mr. Ray MacSharry has said that tighter EC controls will be sought on the use of these compounds in livestock fattening, and has warned of on-the-spot checks by EC veterinary staff.

AIR. Atmospheric air contains by volume 20·96 per cent of oxygen, 78·09 per cent of nitrogen, 0·03 per cent of carbon dioxide, 0·94 per cent of argon, and traces of a number of other elements the most important of which are helium, hydrogen, ozone, neon, zenon, and krypton, as well as variable quantities of water vapour. In addition to these normal constituents, impurities, such as soot, dust, particles of organic matter, etc., are present in larger or smaller amounts. (*See* SMOG.)

Air that has been expired from the lungs in a normal manner shows roughly a 4 per cent change in the amount of the oxygen and carbon dioxide, less of the former (16·96 per cent) and more of the latter (4·03 per cent). The nitrogen remains unaltered.

In enclosed spaces to which fresh air has not free access, it is obvious that if animals are housed for any length of time, the composition of the contained air must change; the concentration of the oxygen becomes increasingly less, while that of the carbon dioxide and water vapour gradually rises. The body reacts to such conditions, greater volumes of blood are sent to the lungs to be exposed to the respired air, the heart-beats and the rate of respiration increase, and when the reduction of the oxygen content in the air inhaled is excessive, the blood becomes imperfectly supplied with that gas. Disease-producing organisms which may be present are enabled to survive longer and their numbers increase to a much greater extent than can occur in an atmosphere which is being constantly changed by the introduction of fresh air. It is under these circumstances that respiratory diseases, such as tuberculosis, influenza, bronchitis, pneumonia, etc., gain ground. The importance of fresh air in livestock buildings is immense. (*See* VENTILATION, RESPIRATION, SMOG, OZONE, SLURRY, CARBON MONOXIDE.)

AIR FILTRATION. The effect of a recirculating air filter unit on concentrations of airborne bacteria, clinical and subclinical respiratory disease, and production performance of veal calves was studied over a period of one year, and found to be beneficial in all these respects. (D. G. Pritchard and others. *Veterinary Record* (1981), **109**, 5.)

AIRGUN INJURIES (*see* GUNSHOT WOUNDS).

AIR PASSAGES (*see* NOSE *and* NASAL PASSAGES).

AIRSAC DISEASE (*see under* SINUSITIS, INFECTIOUS of turkeys).

AKABANE VIRUS. First isolated from mosquitoes in Japan; antibodies detected in cattle, horses and sheep in Australia. A possible cause of abortion in cattle, and of birth of abnormal calves. The virus, a member of the Bunyavirus group, is teratogenic.

Some calves are born blind and walk with difficulty; some have the cerebrum virtually replaced by a water-filled cyst.

(*See also* ARTHROGRYPOSIS *under* CONGENITAL DEFECTS.)

ALBINISM is a lack of the pigment melanin in the skin – an inherited condition (Mendelian recessive).

ALBUMINS are proteins closely resembling white of egg and composing in great part all the tissue of the body. (*See* PROTEINS, CONALBUMIN, ALBUMINURIA.)

ALBUMINURIA. The presence of albumin in the urine: one of the earliest signs of inflammation of the kidneys (a common condition in the dog). It may also indicate derangement of the urinary system below the kidneys, *e.g.* cystitis. Albuminuria, however, occurs also during fevers of several types. Detected by chemical tests, it is a useful aid to diagnosis.

ALCOHOL POISONING. Acute alcoholism is usually the result of too large doses given *bona fide*, but occasionally the larger herbivora and pigs eat fermenting windfalls in apple orchards; or are given, or obtain, fresh distillers' grains, or other residue permeated with spirit, in such quantities that the animals become virtually *drunk*; or in more serious cases they may become comatose, while fatal cases are sometimes recorded. The symptoms described are great excitement, prancing and striking out with the fore-feet, an unsteady gait, and a great tendency to fall to the ground, from which the animal only recovers itself with difficulty. Intermittent or almost continuous winking with one or both eyes is often seen.

ANTIDOTES are tea or coffee for first-aid; stimulants.

ALDOSTERONE. This is a hormone secreted by the adrenal gland, probably under the control of the kidneys. Aldosterone regulates sodium retention and potassium excretion. (*See* CORTICOSTEROIDS.)

ALDRIN. An insecticide. It is a chlorinated naphthalene derivative used in agriculture against wireworms, etc. Misuse of it – as a dressing for orf affecting lambs' mouths – led to the death of 105 out of 107 lambs over a period of a week or so. Symptoms included: blindness, salivation, convulsions, rapid breathing. (*See* GAME BIRDS.)

ALEUTIAN DISEASE. First described in 1956 in the USA, this disease of mink also occurs in the UK, Denmark, Sweden, New Zealand and Canada.

Mink.
SIGNS include: failure to put on weight or even loss of weight; thirst; the presence of undigested food in the faeces – which may be tarry. Bleeding from the mouth and anaemia may also be observed. Death usually follows within a month. Mink other than the dark-grey Aleutian ones may be affected.

Ferrets. In these animals the disease is characterised by a persistent viraemia.

SIGNS include loss of weight, malaise, chronic respiratory infection, and paresis or paraplegia. (Oxenham, M. *Veterinary Record* June 9th 1990.)

Bleeding from the mouth, and anaemia may also be observed. Death usually follows within a month.

ALEXIN (*see* COMPLEMENT).

ALFALFA, fed in large quantities, has in Israel given rise to infertility in cattle – owing, it is believed, to oestrogens.

ALGAE can be a nuisance on farms when they block pipes or clog nipple drinkers. This happens especially in warm buildings, where either an antibiotic or sugar is being administered to poultry via the drinking water. Filters may also become blocked by algae.

The colourless *Prototheca* species are pathogenic for both animals (cattle, deer, dogs, pigs) and man. (*See* MASTITIS – Algal for an example of disease in cattle.)

ALGAE POISONING.

Occurs in the mid-West, USA, chiefly in the months of June to September, when a strong wind may blow a thick scum of blue-green algae from their normal habitat in the centre of a lake to the shore. In such cases an oily, paint-like layer several inches thick may accumulate. Deaths have occurred also in Canada, South Africa, and the UK (where cows died after drinking from a lake). 'Heavy summer blooms of cyanobacteria (blue-green algae) are a feature of many lakes and ponds in Britain', especially when the water has a high nitrate and phosphate content derived from farm land.

'The main toxic freshwater cyanobacteria are strains of the unicellular *Microcystis aeruginosa*, and the filamentous forms *Anabaena flos-aquae, Aphanizomenon*, and *Oscillatoria agardhii*.' These can form thick scums at lake edges.

SIGNS vary according to the dominant cyanobacterium present. *Anabaena flos-aquae*, for example, can form alkaloid neuromuscular toxins which can produce symptoms within half an hour; these being muscular tremors, stupor, ataxia, prostration, convulsions, sometimes opisthotonus, and death. Dyspnoea and salivation may also be seen.

Mycrocystis strains produce a slower-acting peptide toxin, which may cause vomiting and diarrhoea, salivation, thirst, piloerection, and lachrymation. Survivors may show LIGHT SENSITISATION, with inflamed white skin and oedema of ears and eyelids. (G. A. Codd, University of Dundee.)

Poisoning by algae has been recorded in dogs that have been in the sea off Denmark. In America a colourless alga is reported to have caused dysentery, blindness and deafness, and sometimes ataxia and head-tilting.

ALIMENTARY CANAL (*see* DIGESTION).

ALKALI

is a substance which neutralises an acid to form a salt, and turns red litmus blue. Alkalies are generally the oxides, hydroxides, carbonates, or bicarbonates of metals.

VARIETIES. Ammonium, lithium, potassium, and sodium salts are the principal alkalies, their carbonates being weak and their bicarbonates weaker. Calcium (lime), magnesium, barium, and strontium compounds are called the alkaline earths and act as alkalies, while certain substances which in the body are converted into alkalies are called indirect alkalies, the chief of these being acetates, citrates, and tartrates.

USES. In poisoning by acids, alkalies in dilute solution should be administered at once. (*See* ACIDS, POISONING BY; DYSPEPSIA; STOMACH, DISEASES OF; DISINFECTION; DETERGENTS.)

ALKALIES, POISONING BY.

Poisoning may occur as a result of the accidental administration of ammonia, caustic soda, or potash, but it is of rare occurrence. When such a case does arise it is necessary to give weak solutions of the weaker acids – for instance, vinegar and water – and follow this with substances soothing to the mucous membranes such as olive oil, beaten-up eggs and milk, etc.

ALKALOIDS

constitute a large number of the active principles of plants and all possess a powerful physiological action. Like alkalies, they combine with acids to form salts, and turn red litmus blue. Many alkaloids are used in medicine, and their names have an almost constant ending . . . *ine, e.g.* atropine, morphine, quinine, etc.

Below is a list of the most common and important alkaloids and similar substances, with the parent plant from which they are derived:

Aconitine⎫ from Monk's-hood (*Aconitum*
Aconine ⎭ *napellus*).

Arecoline, from Areca nut (*Areca catechu*).

Atropine, from Belladonna, the juice of the Deadly Nightshade (*Atropa belladonna*).

Caffeine, from the Coffee Plant (*Coffea arabica*) and from the leaves of the Tea Plant (*Thea sinensis*), also found in the Kola nut, Guarana, and species of Holly, etc.

Cocaine, from Coca leaves (*Coca erythroxylon*).

Digitoxin*⎫ from Foxglove (*Digitalis purpurea*).
Digitalin* ⎭

Ephedrine, from various species of *Ephedra.*

Ergotoxin* ⎫ (*Claviceps purpurea*).
Ergometrine⎭

Hyoscyamine, from Henbane (*Hyoscyamus niger*).

Hyoscine or ⎫ also from Henbane.
Scopolamine⎭

Morphine⎫
Codeine ⎪ from Opium, the juice of the Opium
Thebaine ⎬ Poppy (*Papaver comniferans*)
Heroin ⎭

Nicotine, from Tobacco leaves (*Nicotiana tobaccum*).

Physostigmine⎫ from Calabar Beans (*Physo-*
or *Eserine* ⎭ *stigma venenosum*)

Pilocarpine, from Jaborandi (*Pilocarpus jaborandi*).

Quinine, from Cinchona or Peruvian Bark (*Cinchona*, and *Cinchona rubra*).

Santonin*, from Wormwood (*Artemesia pauci-flora*).

Sparteine, from Lupins (*Lupulinus,* sp.) and from Broom (*Cytisus scoparius*).

Strychnine, from Nux vomica seeds (*Strychnos nux vomica*).

Veratrine, from Green hellebore (*Veratrum viridi*).

Veratrine, from Cevadilla seeds (*Cevadilla officinale*, or *Schoenocaulon officinale*).

A first-aid antidote for poisoning by an alkaloid is strong tea.

ALLANTOIS (*see* PLACENTA, PERVIOUS URACHUS, EMBRYOLOGY).

Those marked * are neutral principles.

ALLELES or ALLELOMORPHS are genes which influence a particular development process, processes, or character, in opposite ways, and can replace one another at a particular locus on a chromosome. They result from a previous mutation, and the original gene and its mutated form are called an 'allelomorphic pair'. Another definition is: one of a pair or series (multiple alleles) of genes occupying alternatively the same locus. (*See also* GENETICS and HEREDITY.)

ALLERGIC DERMATITIS is another name for eczema caused by an allergy. For example, 'Queensland Itch' is seen in horses in Australia, where it is a result of hypersensitivity to *e.g.* the bites of a sandfly; in Japan it follows bites of the stable-fly. It is a disease of the hot weather, and is intensely itchy in character. Treatment involves the use of antihistamines. In the UK 'Sweet Itch' is the name for a similar or identical condition in horses. (*See also* ECZEMA.)

ALLERGY, a specific sensitivity to *e.g.* a plant or animal product, usually of a protein nature. The tuberculin reaction is an example. In the dog and cat sensitivity occurs most commonly to agents present in bedding, carpeting, rubber products, household cleaners, plants, and some skin dressings; in pigs, soyabean protein antigens.

The three main symptoms are itching, self-inflicted damage as a result, and redness; sometimes oedema of the face, ears, vulva or extremities, or skin weals.

Many foodstuffs have caused allergy in the dog, *e.g.* cow's milk; horse, ox, pig, sheep and chicken meat; eggs. True food allergies are less common in cats. They can, however, be distressing. All constituents of the feline diet may be involved, including colouring agents and preservatives.

Tobacco smoke was reported to be the cause of an allergy in a dog.

Allergy may arise following the bites of sandflies, stable-flies, fleas and sometimes bee or wasp stings. Pollens can produce skin changes; likewise avianised vaccines, horse serum, antibiotics, and synthetic hormone preparations. (*See also* ATOPIC, ECZEMA, ANAPHYLAXIS; ANTI-HISTAMINES; LIGHT SENSITISATION; LAMINITIS.)

On the subject of human allergies in relation to IgE and parasites the *Lancet* commented (April 24, 1976): 'Parasite antigens are a potent stimulus for induction of antiparasite antibodies of the IgE class, and parasite infection can potentiate a pre-existing IgE antibody response to an unrelated antigen. IgE is also implicated in many allergic diseases, and so it is logical to seek a connection between parasites and allergies.

'There is evidence for an inverse relationship between parasites and allergy: asthma and hay-fever are rare in parts of the world where the population is highly parasitised, suggesting that some factor associated with parasite infection may block or inactivate immediate-hyper-sensitivity reactions.

'. . . Allergic diseases may be the price man has had to pay for increasing hygiene in an environment abounding in highly allergenic materials.' (*See* IMMUNOGLOBULINS, REAGINIC ANTIBODIES.)

Extrinsic allergic alveolitis (*see* 'FOG FEVER', 'FARMER'S LUNG', 'BROKEN WIND', 'BIRD-FANCIER'S LUNG').

ALLOGRAFT. A piece of tissue, or a complete organ, transplanted from one animal to another of the same species. (*See* SKIN GRAFTING.)

ALOPECIA. This has to be differentiated from loss of hair due to mange, ringworm, lice infestation, and eczema.

Alopecia may be the result of a hormone imbalance, a dietary deficiency, or selenium poisoning.

A temporary alopecia is occasionally seen in newborn animals, and also in the dams of newborn animals. A deficiency of iodine or of thyroxine may produce such hair loss. In dogs bald patches, usually symmetrical, may occur on the flanks and extend to the limbs. This type of canine alopecia usually responds to thyroid therapy. In male dogs of five years old and upwards alopecia may be accompanied by an attraction for other males, and may respond to castration but not to hormone therapy. A Sertoli-cell tumour of the testicle also causes alopecia and feminisation. Symmetrical bare patches, accompanied by other symptoms, are a feature of Cushing's disease. Senile alopecia affects some cats, and a patchy loss of fur may occur from time to time in some spayed cats. Tetracyclines may occasionally cause severe hair loss in cats.

Alopecia, with symmetrical bilateral hair loss from trunk, neck and end of tail, in dogs, may sometimes be due to a deficiency of the growth hormone SOMATROPHIN. The age group affected is 1 to 4 years. Highly pigmented skin may be a feature. Treatment with the growth hormone has proved successful. (Smith, E. K. (1985) *Veterinary Medicine* **80,** 8 48.)

ALPHACHLORALOSE is a condensation product of chloral and glucose. It is a powerful and stupefying hypnotic that retards metabolic processes, produces peripheral vasodilatation, hypothermia and death. It has been used experimentally in wood-pigeon baits and also for the destruction of mice, and has led to unintentional poisoning in dogs and cats. Treatment with methylamphetamine has been recommended.

ALPHAVIRUS. Viruses of arbovirus group A and equine encephalitis viruses bear this name.

ALTITUDE above sea level (*see* 'MOUNTAIN SICKNESS'). Fertility rates may become reduced at high altitudes. The testicles of cats, rabbits, and rats atrophy, with the reproductive tissue being replaced by connective tissue, after 6 months at 4,500 metres above sea-level; sterility resulting. Hens and geese lay infertile eggs or cease laying at high altitudes. (C. Monge, Faculty of Medicine, Lima, Peru. In E. S. E. Hafez's *Adaptation of Domestic Animals*, Lea & Febiger, Philadelphia, 1968.)

ALUMINIUM TOXICITY. In the rat, research in South Africa has shown, aluminium toxicity might be due to (experimental) porphyria. In Israel it has been shown that rats given aluminium salts and then examined under ultra-violet light, showed fluorescence of eyes, long bones, brain and peri-testicular fat. In rats at least, therefore, aluminium cannot be regarded as a harmless element.

ALVELD. A disease of lambs in Norway, associated with the eating of bog asphodel, and thought to be due to poisoning by microfungi present on the plant. (Aas, O. & others. *Vet. Record* (1989) **124**, 563.) (*See* BOG ASPHODEL.)

ALVEOLUS is a term applied to the sockets of the teeth in the jawbone. The term is also applied to the minute divisions of glands and to the air sacs of the lungs.
Alveolitis. Inflammation of an alveolus. (*See* EX-TRINSIC.)

AMAUROSIS. Impaired vision or even loss of sight, resulting from disease of the optic nerve, brain, or spinal cord.

AMOEBIC ENCEPHALITIS due to *Acanthamoeba castellani* was found after euthanasia of 4-month-old puppy examined before its final inoculation of a multiple vaccination programme. Fits and hyperkeratosis of the foot pads suggested the cause was the distemper virus, but *A. castellani* was recovered from an area of suppurative necrosis in the brain.
(In human medicine several species of this amoeba are recognised as an important cause of granulomatous encephalitis). (Pearce, J. R. & others (1985) *JAVMA* **187**, 951.)

AMBLYOPIA. Diminution of vision.

AMERICAN BOX TORTOISES. A ban on the importation into the UK of tortoises from Mediterranean countries led dealers and petshops to seek an alternative, and the choice was *Terrapene carolina*. These are terrestial, but like to take an occasional dip in water about three inches deep. Poor swimmers, they dislike water deeper than that. The recommended diet for them is 'earthworms, mushrooms, beans, beansprouts, cucumber, grapes, banana, and some leafy vegetables.' In winter a vitamin and mineral supplement is advisable. (Jackson, Oliphant F. and Lawton, Martin P. C. (1985) *Veterinary Record* **116**, 355.)

AMERICAN QUARTER HORSE. A breed derived mainly from dams of Spanish origin, for long bred by American Indians, and from Galloway sires brought by the early settlers. 'It was Barb blood spiced with a Celtic infusion and refined with a dash of Eastern blood that fashioned the present-day Quarter Horse.' – R. M. Denhardt.

AMINE. An organic compound containing NH_2.

AMINO ACIDS are the 'building blocks' into which proteins can be broken down, and with which proteins can be constructed.

Amino acids contain carbon, hydrogen, and oxygen, together with an amine group (NH_2).
The quality of a protein, in terms of its value as an animal feed, depends upon its content of *essential amino acids*. These are **lysine, methionine, tryptophane, leucine, isoleucine, phenylalanine, threonine, histidine, valine,** and **argenine.**
What are at present regarded as non-essential amino acids include glycine, cystine, alananine, serine, tyrosine, aspartic acid, glutamic acid, proline, and hydroxypyroline.
Lysine is a particularly important amino acid for growth and milk production, and is one of those prepared synthetically and added to some livestock feeds. (*See also* LYSINE.)
Some amino acids are glucogenic (glucose producing), *e.g.* leucine; some are ketogenic, forming acetic acid.
The pig and rat require, for rapid growth: lysine, tryptophane, leucine, isoleucine, methionine, threonine, phenylalanine, valine, and histidine. The chick needs glycine in addition to these. The cat needs TAURINE (*which see*).

AMINONITROTHIAZOLE. A drug used in the treatment and prevention of Blackhead in turkeys.

AMMONIA is a pungent gas formed by heating a mixture of sal-ammoniac and quicklime.
As an inhalation a few drops of ammonia on a piece of cotton-wool held a few inches from the nostrils has a good effect in reviving animals which have collapsed. (Inhalation of concentrated ammonia can prove fatal.) Ammonia fumes from litter may adversely affect poultry. (*See* DEEP LITTER.) (*See also* QUATERNARY AMMONIA COMPOUNDS.)
An excess of ammonia in the rumen has been cited as a cause of hypomagnesaemia in spring following massive applications of nitrogenous fertiliser. (*See also* UREA.)
Ammonia poisoning. Hydrolysis of urea to ammonia in the rumen may occur very rapidly in cattle receiving excessive amounts of urea. If more ammonia reaches the blood and then the liver than the latter organ can detoxify, then ammonia poisoning will result. (*See* UREA.)
Several cows died after being fed straw which had been treated with ammonia for five days only and came direct from the treatment box. (It is recommended that the treatment should be for 10 days, with a two-day interval before the product is fed to livestock.) Laryngeal oedema and emphysema of the lungs were caused.
(*See also* LITTER, OLD.)

AMNION. This is the innermost of the three fetal envelopes. It is continuous with the skin at the umbilicus (navel), and completely encloses the fetus but is separated from actual contact with it by the amniotic fluid, or the 'liquor of the amnion', which in the mare measures about 5 or 6 litres (*i.e.* 9 to 10½ pints). (*See* PLACENTA.)
This 'liquor amnii' forms a kind of hydrostatic bed in which the fetus floats, and serves to protect it from injury, shocks, extremes of temperature,

allows free though limited movements, and guards the uterus of the dam from the spasmodic fetal movements which, late in pregnancy, are often vigorous and even violent.

At birth it helps to dilate the cervical canal of the uterus and the posterior genital passages, forms part of the 'waterbag', and, on bursting, lubricates the maternal passages. (*See* PARTURITION.)

AMOXYCILLIN. This antibiotic resembles ampicillin, but is absorbed from the gut more quickly and to a greater extent, and a greater proportion is excreted in the urine.

AMPHISTOMES (*see* FLUKES).

AMPICILLIN. A semi-synthetic penicillin, active against both Gram-positive and Gram-negative bacteria. It is not resistant to penicillinase, but can be given by mouth.

AMPOULE is a small glass container having one end drawn out into a point capable of being sealed so as to preserve its contents sterile. It is used to contain solutions of drugs for hypodermic injection, while many vaccines and other biological products are also distributed in ampoules. A potential hazard of glass embolism has been recognised in human medicine, and the wisdom of allowing glass particles to settle, before filling a syringe, has been stressed.

AMPUTATIONS. If a long bone of dog or cat has been shattered into several pieces, or is the site of cancer, amputation is usually the only humane course to take (other than euthanasia).

It is certainly kinder than leaving the animal a permanent cripple, perhaps suffering some degree of pain for the rest of its life.

A three-legged dog or cat can be expected to revise its technique of balance and movement, and to become not merely nimble but fast as well; and to demonstrate a capacity for enjoying life.

A questionnaire was submitted to the owners of 55 dogs and 18 cats which had undergone amputation of a limb. In 26 animals the reason was cancer, and in the others it was severe injury.

All the owners stated that they were pleased that the operation had been performed, although many had found it a difficult decision to make.

AMYLASE (AMYLOPSIN). A starch-splitting enzyme. (*See* DIGESTION.)

ANABOLIC. Relating to anabolism, which means tissue building, and is the opposite of catabolism or tissue breakdown.

An **anabolic steroid** is one derived from testosterone in which the androgenic characteristics have been reduced and the protein-building (anabolic) properties increased in proportion. Examples are nandrolone, ethylestrenol. These are used in malnutrition, wasting diseases, virus diseases, and severe parasitism.

Synthetic anabolic steroids are used as implants in commercial beef production. It has been found that anabolic steroids can give rise to changes in the liver and its functioning in both animals and man; with, in some instances, tumour formation. (*See* STILBENES.)

ANAEMIA is a term meaning literally 'no blood', but one which refers to a deficiency of red cells or of haemoglobin.

Anaemia is a sign rather than a disease, and it is important to establish the cause (obvious only in the case of *acute* external haemorrhage due to trauma), so that a prognosis and suitable treatment can be given.

The animal may be suffering from a *chronic loss of blood* due to internal bleeding, *e.g.* from the urinary or digestive tracts; and the owner of a cat, for instance, may fail to notice the presence of blood in the urine, and so not bring the animal for treatment until other signs of illness have become obvious.

Anticoagulants, such as Warfarin, may cause internal haemorrhage and hence anaemia.

An *iron-deficient diet* (and one lacking also the trace elements cobalt and copper, which aid the assimilation of iron) is another cause of anaemia; likewise a deficiency of folic acid, vitamin B_6 and vitamin B_{12}.

Both *external and internal parasites* (lice, fleas, ticks, liver flukes, roundworms and tapeworms, can all cause anaemia.

Parasites of the bloodstream are an important cause, and include trypanosomes, piroplasms, rickettsiae. (*See also* FELINE INFECTIOUS ANAEMIA.)

For an *incompatability between the blood of sire and dam*, see haemolytic disease *(under* FOALS, DISEASES OF).

Aplastic anaemia means a defective, or a cessation of, regeneration of the red blood cells; and may be drug-induced. (*See also* RETICULOCYTES.) (In human medicine, the drugs involved have included chloramphenicol, phenylbutazone, and rarely penicillin and aspirin deaths have resulted.)

Bracken poisoning, exposure to X-rays or other forms of irradiation are other causes; also salicylates (including aspirin).

Auto-immune haemolytic anaemia, in which the animal forms antibodies against its own red cells.

Heinz-body haemolytic anaemia (see HEINZ-BODIES) may result from kale poisoning in cattle, and from paracetamol or methylene blue poisoning in cats; and sometimes from lead poisoning.

SIGNS. Pallor of the mucous membranes, loss of energy and of appetite, and pica. Dogs and cats may feel the cold more than usual, and seek warm places. In some cases fever is present, and liver enlargement. The heart rate may increase.

TREATMENT. In the smaller animals especially, vitamin B_{12} or liver extract is often a valuable method of treatment. Where cobalt or copper or iron are lacking, these must be supplied. Lice or ticks or fleas should be destroyed, and treatment against internal parasites undertaken if they are the cause. (*See* PIGLET ANAEMIA, FELINE and EQUINE INFECTIOUS ANAEMIA, CANINE BABESIOSIS, HEART WORMS, CANINE TROPICAL PANCYTOPAENIA, HOOKWORMS, ROUNDWORMS, FLUKES.)

ANAEMIA, EQUINE INFECTIOUS (*see under* EQUINE INFECTIOUS ANAEMIA).

ANAEROBE is the term applied to bacteria having the power to live without oxygen. Such organisms are found growing freely, deep in the soil, as, for example, the tetanus bacillus.

ANAESTHESIA, GENERAL. The use of general anaesthetics for operations on animals dates back to 1847, when several veterinary surgeons used ether. Chloroform was also used in 1847. Ether is still much used today in conjunction with oxygen, but chloroform has very largely been abandoned, on account of its toxicity, for the horse, dog, and cat.

'Anaesthetic drugs all act by limiting the oxygen uptake of tissues. The effect on an individual tissue is proportional to its normal oxygen requirement. Since the oxygen requirement of nervous tissues is disproportionately high, these tissues are the first to be affected by anaesthetic drugs. Unconsciousness, abolition of reflexes, muscular atony, and respiratory paralysis are due to depression of the cerebral cortices, the mid-brain, the spiral cord, and the medulla respectively.

'A constant action of any anaesthetic agent is its effect on the respiratory centre which is always depressed. This has the effect of lowering the sensitivity of the centre to its physiological stimulant – carbon dioxide.' (J. R. Campbell and D. D. Lawson.)

Endotracheal anaesthesia. This technique depends upon the introduction into the trachea of a tube which connects with the outside. The tube is passed via the mouth under a narcotic or anaesthetic, such as nembutal, given into a vein, and may then be used as the route for an inhalant anaesthetic mixture. The method ensures a clear airway throughout the period of anaesthesia, and thus obviates the danger of laryngeal obstruction (*e.g.* by the tongue falling backwards), which sometimes causes death. The method has several other advantages, *e.g.* it permits an unobstructed operation field during lengthy major operations, obviates excessive salivation, achieves better oxygenation, and even anaesthesia, and permits of positive pressure ventilation of the lungs in the event of respiratory failure.

Endotracheal anaesthesia is administered in one of two ways. *Insufflation anaesthesia* involves the use of air and a volatile anaesthetic vapour delivered into the tube by means of a pump or, more commonly, a mixture of gases supplied from cylinders (and sometimes bubbled through a volatile anaesthetic liquid in addition). *Auto-inhalation anaesthesia* involves the use of a wide bore endotracheal tube through which the animal inhales the anaesthetic mixture by its own respiratory efforts. A 'rebreathing bag' may be used.

The following general anaesthetics are described elsewhere under their respective alphabetical headings: BARBITURATES, CHLOROFORM, CYCLOPROPANE, ETHER, HALOTHANE, ISOFLURANE, NITROUS OXIDE, PROPOFOL.

As an alternative to general anaesthesia, EPIDURAL ANAESTHESIA (involving the injection of a local anaesthetic into the spinal canal) is used for some surgical procedures.

Cattle. After premedication with, for example, xylazine ('Rompun'; Bayer), chloroform or halothane are used. Cattle take chloroform well, and recovery is rapid.

ENDOTRACHEAL INTUBATION is recommended in order to preserve a free airway, and to prevent inhalation of regurgitated rumen contents.

Horses. Halothane is the preferred volatile anaesthetic. Isoflurane is also excellent. (*See also* CYCLOPROPANE.)

A combination of xylazine and ketamine hydrochloride was recommended (Hall, L. W. & Tayler, P. M. *Veterinary Record* (1981) **108,** 489).

After premedication with acepromazine or xylazine, a combination of guaicol glycerine ether with thiopentone 'gave calm, controlled inductions and smooth recoveries. Useful anaesthesia lasted for about 10 to 12 minutes. Recumbency persisted for 15 to 25 minutes.' (Brouwer, G. J. *Equine Veterinary Journal* (1985) **17,** 252).

Use of a water mattress. Anaesthetised horses when positioned in left lateral recumbency, showed least muscle or nerve injuries when lying on a water mattress. (Foam rubber was far from satisfactory.)

Sheep. Alphaxolone/alphadolone has been found useful for inducing and maintaining anaesthesia. Propofol (see below under *Dogs and cats*) has also been used.

Goats. Alphaxolone/alphadolone (Saffan; Glaxovet); etorphine (Immobilon); and halothane/oxygen have all been recommended for the disbudding of kids.

Dogs and cats. Pentobarbitone ('Nembutal') is preferred by most veterinary surgeons. Administered by intravenous injection, it is rapid in action.

Thiopentone, given intravenously, is a short-acting general anaesthetic.

Ketamine hydrochloride, given by intramuscular injection, is another choice but has the disadvantage of causing cats to become very excitable at the recovery stage, unless xylazine is included in the injection.

Saffan (CT1341) is used either for the induction of anaesthesia by other drugs, or as a short-acting anaesthetic itself.

Propofol, an alkyl phenol (Diprivan; ICI) is a useful intravenous anaesthetic for dogs. 'Recovery from it is quiet and rapid – an advantage when the patient has to be returned to the owner's care with the minimum of delay.' (Watkins, S. B. & others. *Veterinary Record* (1987) **120,** 326.)

Propofol is also an anaesthetic for cats given intravenously. Side-effects during recovery: retching, sneezing, and pawing of the face. (Brearley, J. C. & others. *Journal of Small Animal Practice* (1988) **29,** 315.)

Monkeys. Phenicyclidine, which can be given intramuscularly, has been found very suitable as a tranquillisation agent, which will prevent biting and render monkeys easy to handle. It is given by intramuscular injection. For

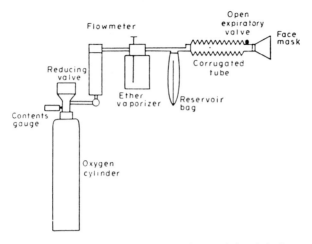

A method of administering ether oxygen in a semi-closed circuit.

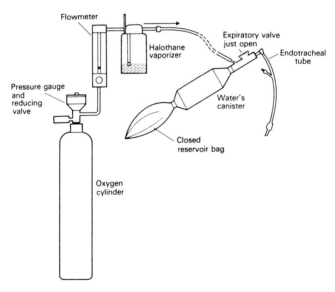

A satisfactory method of administering halothane in a closed circuit.

Both illustrations reproduced with permission from Jones's *Animal Nursing*, Pergamon.

anaesthesia, pentobarbitone sodium ('Nembutal') may then be given intravenously. Ketamine hydrochloride (*e.g.* Ketaset; C-Vet) is an alternative, given by subcutaneous, intramuscular, or intravenous injection. A mixture of ketamine and xylazine has been recommended also. Halothane is suitable.

Rabbits. The combination of fentanyl-fluanisole and diazepam 'provides good anaesthesia, is easy to administer, and is readily reversible with naloxone,' P. A. Flecknell and C. J. Green commented. 'It is certainly far safer than pentobarbitone, aphaxolone-alphadolone, or ketamine-xylazine.'

Birds. Ether may be used, or a 25 to 40 per cent mixture of cyclopropane in oxygen, or halothane. For *restraint*, the bird may be placed in a large, clear polythene bag, into which the tube for the anaesthetic gas is introduced.

For injections of ketamine hydrochloride or nembutal, the bird may be immobilised with a cylinder of paper rolled around it and secured with adhesive tape.

Reptiles. Halothane or ketamine is satisfactory.

Fish. 'Propoxate' – dl-l-(l-phenyl-ethyl)-5-(propoxy-carbomyl)-imida- zole HCl) – is a safe and powerful anaesthetic for cold-blooded vertebrates, soluble in both fresh and salt water.

In an emergency, carbon dioxide – generated by Alka Seltzer tablets in the water – has proved effective.

ANAESTHESIA, LOCAL and REGIONAL.
For minor operations, local anaesthetics are often used instead of general anaesthesia and are administered by hypodermic injection. They include cocaine, procaine, lignocaine.

Local anaesthetics are also often added to eye lotions and ear drops for pain-relieving purposes, and to prevent the animal causing further damage by scratching or rubbing the inflamed part.

For regional anaesthesia, the local anaesthetic is injected into the connective tissue around a sensory nerve trunk, *e.g.* to relieve the pain of laminitis. (For 'spinal anaesthesia', *see* EPIDURAL ANAESTHESIA, which is of help in difficult calving cases and for minor operations on uterus, vagina or rectum, etc.).

For the diagnosis of the site of lameness, local anaesthetics are sometimes used at two or more successive sites on a limb until the 'nerve block' has banished pain and indicated the approximate position of the lesion.

Local anaesthetics must not be used indiscriminately, since poisoning can result, and affect the brain and heart. Symptoms of poisoning include sudden collapse, or excitement, vomiting and convulsions.

ANAESTHETICS, LEGAL REQUIREMENTS.
The Protection of Animals (Anaesthetics) Act, 1964, amended a previous Act of 1954, especially in the matter of castration. It is now obligatory to use an anaesthetic when castrating dogs, cats, horses, asses, and mules of any age.

Castration: only a veterinary surgeon, using an anaesthetic, is permitted to castrate any farm animal more than 2 months old; with the exception of rams for which the maximum age is 3 months.

The use of rubber rings or similar devices for castrating bulls, pigs, goats, and sheep, or for docking lambs' tails, is forbidden unless applied during the first week of life. The Act of 1964 also requires that an anaesthetic be used when dehorning cattle; and also for disbudding calves unless this be done by chemical cautery applied during the first week of life.

A requirement, still in force, of the 1954 Act is the use of an anaesthetic for any operation, performed with or without the use of instruments, which involves interference with the sensitive tissues or the bone structure of an animal.

Exceptions are the rendering in emergency of first-aid to save life or relieve pain; the docking of a dog's tail or amputation of its dew claws before its eyes are open; any minor operation performed by a veterinary surgeon or veterinary practitioner, being an operation which, by reason of its quickness or painlessness, is customarily so performed without the use of an anaesthetic; any minor operation, whether performed by a veterinary surgeon or veterinary practitioner or by some other person, being an operation which is not customarily performed only by such a surgeon or practitioner.

ANAESTHETICS, RESIDUES IN CARCASES.
Dogs and cats have shown severe symptoms of poisoning after being fed on meat from animals humanely slaughtered by means of an overdose of a barbiturate anaesthetic, or chloral hydrate.

ANAL. Relating to the anus.

ANAL GLANDS (*see under* ANUS).

ANALEPTICS (*see* STIMULANTS).

ANALGESICS are drugs which cause a temporary loss of the sense of pain without a loss of consciousness, *i.e.* **analgesia**.

Analgesics include non-steroidal anti-inflammatory drugs such as aspirin, paracetamol, phenylbutazone. (They are contra-indicated if heart, kidney or liver disease is present.)

The most effective of the opiates is MORPHINE (which see.) (*See also* BUPRENORPHINE, DETOMIDINE, *and* ACUPUNCTURE.)

ANAMNESIS is the past history of a particular patient.

ANAPHRODISIA. Impairment of sexual appetite.

ANAPHYLACTIC SHOCK, ANAPHYLAXIS.
The reaction to a foreign protein which sometimes follows bee or wasp stings, injections of an antibiotic or antiserum, etc., after the patient has become hypersensitised to the substance. There is often a rapid fall in blood pressure; and anaphylactic shock can prove fatal. (*See* ANTIHISTAMINES, HYPERSENSITIVITY, WARBLES.)

ANAPLASMOSIS. This is an infectious disease of cattle, characterised by anaemia and caused by a parasite of the red blood cells, *Anaplasma marginale.*

This parasite is found in Africa, Asia, Australia, Southern Europe, South America, and the southern States of North America. *A. centrale* (in cattle) and *A. ovis* (in sheep and goats) are other species.

SIGNS. The disease resembles Texas fever and frequently anaplasmosis coexists with babesiosis, but pure infections may also occur. It is characterised by acute anaemia, fever, jaundice, and degeneration of the internal organs; haemoglobinuria does not occur as the rate of red blood-cell destruction is not fast enough to produce free haemoglobin in the circulating blood. Young animals appear to be resistant, and cases in calves under one year old are rare. In older animals the disease may be acute or chronic, and in the former case they may die within 2 to 3 days after the appearance of the first symptoms. The disease starts with a high temperature of 105° to 107°F and after a day or two anaemia and icterus appear. In the acute illness, aggressiveness and abortion are other symptoms.

TRANSMISSION artificially may be by inoculation of blood from affected animals or those in a state of premunition. Natural transmission is by ticks, and various species of the following genera act as vectors: *Boophilus, Rhipicephalus, Hyalomma, Ixodes,. Dermacentor,* and *Haemaphysalis.* Infection is passed through the egg to the next generation of ticks. In addition, several species of Tabanid flies have been shown to be mechanical carriers provided the transfer of infective material from an infected to a healthy beast is immediate and within not more than 5 minutes. Certain mosquitoes have also been incriminated.

Animals which recover from anaplasmosis are in a state of premunition, and remain carriers for long periods, probably for life.

In the South African States the less serious *A. centrale* has been found to give protection against the serious *A. marginale,* and both there and in other countries successful results follow its use as an immunising agent. In other areas where Texas fever and anaplasmosis frequently occur together, cattle are often immunised by blood of a bovine infected with *A. centrale,* which produces a mild infection, and with a mild form of *Babesia bigemina.* The inoculated cattle usually suffer from Texas fever first, as it has the shorter incubation period, and anaplasmosis later, and they then possess an increased tolerance for both diseases.

ANASARCA is a condition of oedema, particularly of the tissues below the skin.

ANASTOMOSIS is a term describing the means by which the circulation is carried on when a large vessel is severed or its stream obstructed. In anatomy the term is applied to a junction between two or more arteries or veins which communicate with each other.

ANATOXIN. A toxin rendered harmless by heat or chemical means but capable of stimulating the formation of antibodies.

ANCYLOSTOMA. A genus of hookworms. (*See* HOOKWORMS.)

ANDROGEN is the name given to those hormones which influence the growth and development of male sex organs and male characters. (*See* HORMONES.)

ANDROSTENEDIONE. While investigating the function of ovarian hormones on follicle development, it was found that ewes immunised against androstenedione (the major C19 steroid secreted by the mature Graafian follicle) surprisingly showed a high proportion of multiple ovulations. This finding led to the commercial development of 'Fecundin' by Glaxo Animal Health Ltd., to produce more lambs.

ANERGY. Failure or suppression of the cellular immune mechanism. This may occur in human brucellosis, for example, and in other chronic diseases. Anti-anergic treatment with levamisole has been found successful in some patients. (R. D. Thorne, *Vet. Rec.* (1977) **101,** 27.) (*See* IMMUNOSUPPRESSION.)

ANEUPLODY. The presence of an irregular number of chromosomes (not an exact multiple of the haploid number). It may arise through faulty cell division.

ANEURIN is the vitamin B_1, the anti-neuritic vitamin.

ANEURYSM. This is a dilatation of an artery (or sometimes of a vein) following a weakening of its walls. The result is a pulsating sac which is liable to rupture; although it may remain intact and be discovered only after death from other causes. Aneurysms occur in the abdomen, chest, and brain, and may result from a congenital weakness of the blood-vessel, from disease of its lining cells, from injury, etc.

In many cases the existence of an aneurysm is never suspected until the animal falls down dead as a result of rupture of the sac and internal haemorrhage.

If the condition is diagnosed during life, and if a surgical operation is practicable, treatment consists in ligaturing the vessel so that the blood flow is diverted through healthy, smaller vessels.

CAUSES. Sudden and violent muscular efforts are regarded as the chief factors in the production of aneurisms; and as would be expected, the horse is more subject to this trouble than any of the other domesticated animals.

'Verminous aneurysm' is a misnomer for verminous arteritis of horses caused by immature strongyle worms. (*See* EQUINE VERMINOUS ARTERITIS.)

ANGIOGENESIS: a method of treating a tumour by depriving it of its blood supply.

ANGIOGRAPHY. A technique which enables the blood flow to and from a diseased organ to be visualised with the aid of single-exposure or, preferably, serial radiography, after injection of a contrast medium.

ANGIOMA is a tumour composed of a large number of blood-vessels. They are common in the livers of cattle. (*See* TUMOURS, HAEMANGIOMA.)

ANGIOSTRONGYLUS (*see* HEART WORMS).

ANGITIS, or **ANGIITIS,** means inflammation of a vessel, such as a blood-vessel, lymph-vessel, or bile-duct.

ANGLEBERRY (*see* WARTS).

'ANGRY CAT' POSTURE. This is assumed by a cat partially crippled as a result of exostoses of neck bones due to an excess of vitamin A. The symptom may appear within one to five years of being on a virtually all-liver diet.

ANHIDROSIS. A failure of the sweat mechanism. This occurs in horses especially, but also in cattle, imported into tropical countries with humid climates.

At first, affected horses sweat excessively and their breathing is distressed after exercise. Later, sweating occurs only at the mane; the skin becomes scurfy; and breathing becomes more laboured. Heart failure may occur.

ANHYDRIDE. An oxide which can combine with water to form an acid.

ANHYDROUS. Containing no water.

ANIMAL BEHAVIOUR as a guide to animal welfare. (*See* PRODUCTIVITY, AGGRESSIVENESS, ANALGESIA, ETHOLOGY, TRANSPORT, ELECTRIC SHOCK, ANIMAL HOUSING.)

ANIMAL BOARDING ESTABLISHMENTS ACT, 1963. This requires that the owner of a boarding establishment shall obtain a licence from the Local Authority, and that this licence must be renewed annually. The applicant has to satisfy the licensing authority on certain personal points, and that the 'animals will at all times be kept in accommodation suitable as respects construction, size of quarters, number of occupants, exercising facilities, temperature, lighting, ventilation, and cleanliness'. The Act also requires that animals boarded 'will be adequately supplied with suitable food, drink, and bedding material, adequately exercised, and (so far as necessary) visited at suitable intervals'. Isolation facilities and fire precautions are covered by the Act, which empowers the Local Authority to inspect both the boarding establishment and the register which must be kept there.

ANIMAL FOOD (*see* CONCENTRATES, DIET, RATIONS, PROTEINS, POISONING, VITAMINS, ADDITIVES, TINNED FOODS; *also sections on* HORSES, CATTLE, SHEEP and DOGS, CAT FOODS, etc.).

ANIMAL HEALTH SCHEMES (*see under* HEALTH SCHEMES).

ANIMALS, HOUSING OF (*see* HOUSING OF ANIMALS and the various illustrations).

ANIMAL HUSBANDRY (*see* GRAZING, PASTURE, HOUSING, WATER, DIET, DAIRY HERD, COWS, SHEEP, PIGS, etc.).

ANIMAL NURSING (*see* VETERINARY NURSES – Lay assistants who have passed the requisite examination under the auspices of the Royal College of Veterinary Surgeons).

ANIMALS (SCIENTIFIC PROCEDURES) ACT 1986. This makes it illegal to supply animals, other than those purpose-bred in Home Office designated breeding establishments, for use in experimental procedures involving dogs, cats, and other animals. The Act requires all laboratories in the UK where animals are used in research to appoint a veterinary surgeon to be responsible for the care and welfare of their experimental animals.

On January 1, 1990 it became illegal to sell or supply pet or stray animals for use in scientific experiments.

The Act also represents the culmination of the efforts of three organisations, the British Veterinary Association (BVA), the Committee for the Reform of Animal Experimentation (CRAE) and the Fund for the Replacement of Animals in Medical Experiments (FRAME) to reform animal experimentation legislation. The new Act is firmly rooted in BVA/CRAE/FRAME proposals sent to the Home Secretary in 1983, and represents an effective compromise between the welfare needs of animals, the legitimate demands of the public for accountability, and the equally legitimate requirements of medicine, science and commerce.

The legislation gives the Home Secretary the power and the responsibility to judge the scientific merit of the work he authorises and for which he will be answerable to Parliament.

ANIMAL TRANSPORT (*see* TRANSPORT).

ANIMAL WELFARE CODES (*see under* WELFARE CODES FOR ANIMALS).

ANKYLOSIS is the condition of a joint in which the movement is restricted by union of the bones or adhesions. (*See* JOINTS, DISEASES OF.)

ANISCORIA (see EYE, DISEASES).

ANODYNES are pain-relieving drugs.

ANOESTRUS is the state in the female when no oestrus or 'season' is exhibited. It is a state of sexual inactivity. In most mares, for example, 'anoestrus occurs during the winter months, when daylight is reduced, ambient temperatures are low and, in the wild state, food is scarce. In these circumstances the pituitary gland does not release the gonadotrophins FSH and LF (*see* HORMONES) so that neither follicles nor *corpora lutea* develop in the ovaries.' (W. R. Allen, (1977), *Vet. Rec.* **100**, 68.)

Similar circumstances apply with cattle. Fear, hunger, cold, and pain may all result in anoestrus. (*See* OESTRUS.)

ANOREXIA (*see* LOSS OF APPETITE).

ANOXIA. Oxygen deficiency. Cerebral anoxia, or a failure in the oxygen supply to the brain, occurs during nitrite and prussic acid poisoning; in copper deficiency in cattle; and in the thoroughbred 'barker foal'. (*See also* ANAESTHESIA.)

ANTE-NATAL INFECTION. Examples of this may occur with the larvae of the dog hook- worm, *Ancylostoma caninum*, and with the larvae of other roundworms. (*See* TOXOCARA.) Toxoplasmosis is another example of an infection which may occur before birth.

ANTE-PARTUM PARALYSIS is a fairly common condition in the cow, has been seen in the sheep and goat, but is rare in the mare, in which the hindquarters of the pregnant animal suddenly become paralysed. It appears from 6 to 25 days before parturition, and is liable to affect animals in almost any condition – those that are well kept as well as others.
SIGNS. The condition suddenly appears without any warning. The pregnant animal is found in the lying position, and is quite unable to regain her feet.
TREATMENT. As a rule, the nearer to the day of parturition that the paralysis appears, the more favourable will be the result. Those cases that lie for two or more weeks are very unsatisfactory. The condition usually disappears after parturition has taken place, either almost at once or in 2 or 3 days. As a consequence, treatment should be mainly directed to ensuring that the animal is comfortable, provided with plenty of bedding, is turned over on to the opposite side 3 or 4 times a day, if she does not turn herself, and receives a laxative diet so that constipation may not occur. Mashes, green food, and a variety in the food-stuffs offered, are indicated. When the paralysis has occurred a considerable time before parturition is due, it is often necessary to produce artificial abortion of the foetus and so relieve the uterus of its heavy encumbrance.

ANTHELMINTICS are substances which are given to expel parasitic worms. They include levamisole, thiabendazole, methyridine, piperazine compounds, tetramisole, hygromycin B, santonin, rafoxanide, haloxon, morantel tartrate, oxyclozanide, dichlorvos, parbendazole. Niclosamide and bunamidine preparations are used against tapeworms in the dog; also praziquantel. (*See also* DRONCIT). Fenbendazole and albendazole are broad-spectrum anthelmintics usually effective against inhibited fourth-stage ostertagia larvae in cattle. (*See also* IVERMECTIN – a current anthelmintic of great efficacy.)

Certain criteria apply in anthelmintics. For example, will the drug in question kill worm eggs? Is it effective against immature worms? Is it effective against adult worms of the economically important species? Does the drug discolour or taint milk? Can it be given to pregnant, or emaciated, animals?

Methods of administration include drenching; injection (in the case of tetramisole, for example); in the feed. (*See* WORMS, FARM TREATMENT AGAINST.)

Several gastro-intestinal nematodes have developed resistance to anthelmintics.

ANTHISAN. An antihistamine.

ANTHRACOSIS. A condition of the lungs and bronchial lymph nodes due to the deposition of particles of carbon, soot, etc., from the inspired air.

ANTHRAX is commonest among the herbivora.
CAUSE: the *Bacillus anthracis.* Under certain adverse circumstances each rod-shaped bacillus is able to form itself into a spore. The spores of anthrax are hard to destroy. They resist drying for a period of at least two years. They are able to live in the soil for ten years or more and still be capable of infecting animals.

Consequently pastures that have been infected by spilled blood from a case that has died are extremely difficult to render safe for stock.

Earth-worms may carry the spores from deeper layers of the soil up to the surface. Spores have been found in bone meal, in blood fertilisers, in wool and hides and in feeds. (*See also* STREAMS.)

The bacillus itself is a comparatively delicate organism and easily killed by the ordinary disinfectants.
METHOD OF INFECTION. In cattle infection nearly always occurs by way of the mouth and alimentary system. Either the living organisms or else the spores are taken in on the food or with the drinking water. Flies can spread the disease. The disease has been caused through inoculation of vaccine contaminated by spores. Sheep should not be inoculated, therefore, in a dusty shed. Unsterilised bone-meal is an important source of infection. (*See* BONE-MEAL.)

SIGNS. Three forms of the disease are recognised: the *per-acute,* the *acute,* and the *sub-acute.*

Cattle. In most *per-acute* cases the animal is found dead without having shown any noticeable symptoms beforehand. *Acute:* a temperature of 106° or 107°F, a thin, rapid pulse, coldness of the ears, feet, and horns, and 'blood-shot' eyes and nostrils. After a few hours this picture is followed by one of prostration, unconsciousness, and death. In either of the above types there may have been diarrhoea or dysentery.

In the *sub-acute* form the affected animal may linger for as long as 48 hours, showing nothing more than a very high temperature and laboured respirations. Occasionally cattle may be infected through the skin, when a 'carbuncle' follows, similar to that seen in man. Diffuse, painless, doughy swellings are seen in other cases, especially about the neck and the lower part of the chest.

As sudden death of an animal is often wrongly attributed to lightning stroke a farmer should consult a veterinary surgeon (who will carry out a rapid blood test) to make sure that the cause of death is not anthrax – before handling the carcase, cutting into it, moving it, or letting farm dogs, hounds, cats, etc., feed upon it.

Sheep and goats. Anthrax in these animals is almost always of the per-acute type.

Horses. There are two notable forms of anthrax in the horse; one in which there is a marked swelling of the throat, neck, and chest.

In the second form of equine anthrax a fit of shivering ushers in the fever. The pulse-rate becomes increased, the horse lies and rises again with great frequency; shows signs of slowly increasing abdominal pain by kicking at his belly, by gazing at his flanks, or by rolling on the ground.

Pigs. The disease may follow the feeding of slaughter-house refuse or the flesh of an animal that has died from an unknown disease, which has really been anthrax, or raw bone-meal intended as a fertiliser. There is sometimes swelling of the throat; or the intestine may be involved. In this abdominal form the symptoms may be very vague. Otherwise the pigs are dull, lie a good deal, show a gradually increasing difficulty in respiration, present in the early stages a swelling of the throat and head which later invades the lower parts of the neck.

Recovery is not unknown.

Dogs and cats. A localised form, with oedema of the head and neck (similar to that in the pig) is characteristic.

PREVENTION AND TREATMENT. In Great Britain, as in most developed countries, anthrax is a NOTIFIABLE DISEASE. In so far as its prevention is concerned, the important points to remember are (1) disposal of the carcase by efficient and safe means (*see* DISPOSAL OF CARCASES) and (2) frequent observation of other animals which have been in contact with the dead one; and their isolation if showing a rise in body temperature.

Bleaching powder in a hot 10 per cent solution kills both bacilli and the spores almost instantaneously.

The prompt use of anti-anthrax serum in large doses has been useful in proportion of animals already showing symptoms, but it is essential that it is given at once. Penicillin may be used; also sulpathiozole.

The milk from in-contact animals must be regarded as dangerous until such time as these are considered to be out of danger. The law forbids any one who is not authorised to cut an anthrax carcase for any purpose whatsoever. Cases of death from this procedure are by no means unknown, and illness following the dressing of a carcase must always be considered suspicious of anthrax until the contrary has been established. The need for reporting illness to the medical authorities, by all persons whose work brings them into contact with carcases of animals cannot be too strongly stressed.

Anthrax in human patients. Between 1961 and 1980, 145 cases of anthrax in human patients were notified in England and Wales. There were 12 fatalities. Of the 145 cases, 122 were associated with occupational exposure. There was a decline in the numbers of people exposed to wool, hair or bristle. Most of the occupationally acquired cases (82) were in industries other than those traditionally associated with anthrax; 32 cases were in the meat trade, 15 handled bone meal and four handled sacks probably contaminated with bone meal. The remaining 36 cases included farm or horticulture workers (12), dock workers or sailors (9) and lorry drivers (7). The cases presented as pulmonary anthrax in one person and cutaneous anthrax in 121. The lesions were usually detected on the arms, hands, neck and face. Of the 23 cases of non-occupational anthrax 15 were in people who handled bone meal in their gardens. (Communicable Disease Surveillance Centre (1982), *British Medical Journal* **284**, 204.)

ANTHROPONOSES. Diseases transmissible from man to lower animals. Such diseases include: tuberculosis; mumps (to dogs); scarlet fever (giving rise to mastitis in dairy cows); tonsillitis (giving rise to calf pneumonia, etc.); infestation with the beef tapeworm; influenza in pigs and birds. (Compare ZOONOSES.)

ANTIBIOTIC. A chemical compound derived from living organisms (or synthesised) which is capable, in small concentration, of inhibiting the life process of micro-organisms. To be useful in medicine an antibiotic must (1) have powerful action in the body against one or more types of bacteria; (2) have specific action; (3) have low toxicity for tissues; (4) be active in the presence of body fluids; (5) not be destroyed by tissue enzymes such as trypsin; (6) be stable; (7) be not too rapidly excreted; (8) preferably not give rise to resistant strains of organisms.

'Antibiotics can be divided, on a basis of their mode of action, into three groups: (1) those acting on the bacterial cell wall, such as the penicillins and bacitracin; (2) those affecting the cell membrane in a manner similar to that of detergents, and including polymixin, novobiocin, and nystatin; (3) this group appears to act by interfering with protein synthesis in bacteria and includes the tetracyclines, chloramphenicol, neomycin, streptomycin and erythromycin.

'*The antibacterial activities of all antibiotics require the intervention of the cellular and humoral defence mechanisms of the body.* Evidence of this requirement is shown by the fact that in diseases such as agranulocytosisis, leukaemias, etc., the administration of even a competent antibiotic such as penicillin is useless, although the organism causing the infection is penicillin-sensitive.' – Professor F. Alexander.

Antibiotics are much used in veterinary medicine to overcome certain infections, and they have been of notable service, for instance, in the control of certain forms of mastitis in dairy cattle, in the avoidance of septicaemia following badly infected wounds, deep-seated abscesses, peritonitis, etc. Abdominal and other surgery has been rendered safer by the use of antibiotics. They must not, however, be used indiscriminately, be regarded as a panacea, or given in too low a dosage. It is unwise to use antibiotics of the tetracycline group in either pregnant or very young animals owing to the adverse effects upon bone and teeth which may result.

SELECTION OF ANTIBIOTIC. It is often necessary to begin antibiotic therapy before the results of bacteriological examinations are available, and therapy must depend on the clinical features. However, the taking of material for culture and carrying out sensitivity tests are most important procedures. Another factor in veterinary practice is the cost of the drug.

Only in a very few instances are mixtures of antibiotics superior to a single drug, and the use of fixed dose mixtures can be very misleading. In those cases in which more than one antibiotic is required, it is much better to use full doses of each of the individual antibiotics. Moreover, there is a degree of antagonism between penicillin and the tetracyclines. Combined antibiotic therapy does not improve the outlook in chronic urinary infections or, indeed, many chronic infections. Mixtures of antibiotics have been most successful when used in local applications or in infections of the alimentary canal. (*See* ADDITIVES, *and under* MILK.) Ten of the most widely used antibiotics in veterinary medicine are: BENZYLPENICILLIN, METHYCYLLIN, AMPICILLIN, AMOXYCILLIN, STREPTOMYCIN, NEOMYCIN, TETRACYCLINES, CHLORAMPHENICOL, ERYTHROMYCIN, GRISEOFULVIN. (*See under these headings.*) (*See also* CEPHALOSPORIN, TIAMULIN, SALINOMYCIN; *and below.*)

For advice on selection of these for treatment, *see* Knifton, A. (1984) *Veterinary Record* **114**, 357.

ANTIBIOTIC RESISTANCE. Bacteria can become drug-resistant in one of two ways. The first to be discovered was chromosomal resistance which develops through mutation and is probably rare. Bacteria which achieve this kind of resistance are unable to transfer it to other bacteria, but pass it on to their own future generations through the ordinary process of cell division.

The second method is transmissible drug resistance (TDR). This (discovered by Watanabe and his colleagues in 1963) is achieved by means of PLASMIDS (which see).

Many bacteria carry, in their cytoplasm, *resistance* or *R factors*. These are pieces of DNA which include genes coding for resistance to antibiotics and other genes which facilitate the transit of the R factor to other bacteria. Both groups of genes are carried on plasmids.

A Gram-negative bacterium which possesses an R factor is able to conjugate with other Gram-negative bacteria. This involves intimate contact through a protoplasmic bridge called a *sex pilus*. When this occurs a duplicate of the R factor is transmitted to the second, recipient, cell, which thereby acquires both the drug resistance and the ability to transmit it to other bacteria.

Inside the gut of an animal being dosed with an antibiotic, these resistant bacteria survive and multiply at the expense of the antibiotic-sensitive bacteria. 'Moreover, the resistant bacteria persist as that animal's dominant gut flora. Cross-infection can then bring about a similar situation in other animals – possibly in man also,' A. H. Linton has stated. (*Vet. Rec.* (1976), **99**, 370.)

The persistence of TDR in the animal gut has been related to the pattern of antibiotic usage. Again quoting Dr Linton, this includes both the route and the duration of administration. In dairy herds administration of an antibiotic via the teat, over short periods of time, or as a preventative during the dry period, had little or no effect on drug-resistance in *E. coli* in the herd. Several other research workers have shown that in calves and pigs, when antibiotics were given by the oral route, for brief periods, the high initial levels of drug resistance which arose in the gut flora soon decreased.

However, in contrast, on farms where antibiotics were fed continuously at low (subtherapeutic) levels, the incidence of resistant organisms in the gut and the frequency of multiple antibiotic-resistance was greater and persisted. Dr Linton and his colleagues demonstrated this in calves and pigs after feeding the antibiotic tetracycline. Such drug resistance did not occur in calves and pigs receiving the non-antibiotic growth-promoters nitrovin and quindoxin.

Other authorities have published figures showing the prevalence of antibiotic-resistant organisms. For example, writing in the *Veterinary Journal* (1976) W. J. Sojka (a senior research officer at MAFF's Central Veterinary Laboratory) and E. R. Hudson reported that they had examined 2166 Salmonella strains isolated from farm animals in 1972, and that 90 per cent of these strains were resistant to streptomycin.

Resistance to tetracycline, chloramphenicol, neomycin and ampicillin were found in a much smaller percentage of strains. (*See also* the entry under COLIFORM INFECTIONS.)

Dr Linton, after referring to the great benefits which antibiotics have brought to both human and veterinary medicine, pointed out that antibiotic-resistant bacterial populations arise in man and animals by the use of antibiotics for all three purposes: (1) therapy; (2) disease-prevention; and (3) growth promotion. 'The non-therapeutic uses therefore have come under heavy criticism by those concerned with the treatment of infectious disease. The immense value of anti-microbial agents for disease-prevention, particularly in intensive livestock production, and the improvement in feed conversion through the use of antibiotic growth-promoters, has to be balanced against these disadvantages. There is no simple answer to this problem, since it is in essence a political one, balancing one advantage for a community against another.'

It was the 'heavy criticism' and anxiety about TDR which led to the setting up of the Swann Committee by the British government. (*See under* ADDITIVES.)

ANTIBIOTIC SUPPLEMENTS are subject to certain Government regulations in the U K. (*See under* ADDITIVES.)

ANTIBIOTICS, ADVERSE REACTIONS TO. (*See* PENICILLIN, SENSITIVITY TO; NEOMYCIN; CHLORAMPHENICOL; TETRACYCLINES; TYLOSIN.)

ANTIBODY. A substance in the blood-serum or other body fluids formed to exert a specific restrictive or destructive action on bacteria, their toxins, viruses, or any foreign protein.

Antibodies are not produced, like hormones, by a single organ, the blood then distributing them throughout the body. Antibody production has been shown to occur in lymph-nodes close to the site of introduction of an antigen, in the skin, fat, and voluntary muscle, and locally in infected tissues.

Chemically, antibodies (belonging to a group of proteins called Immunoglobulins) are protein molecules of complex structure. In the IMMUNE RESPONSE (which see) antibody and antigen molecules combine together in what is called a complex. These complexes are removed from the body by the RETICULO-ENDOTHELIAL SYSTEM (which see). Agglutination of bacteria and precipitation of soluble protein antigens both occur following combination of antibody and antigen molecules, and are made use of in laboratory tests.

Antibodies are not always protective; some join mast cells and eosinophils – later exposure to the specific antigen resulting in the release of histamine, as happens in ALLERGY. (*See also* REAGINIC ANTIBODIES.)

ANTICOAGULANTS. Agents which inhibit clotting of the blood. They include dicoumarol and heparin. They have been used in the treatment of coronary thrombosis in humans, but not without a number of fatalities. (*See also* WARFARIN.)

ANTICOAGULINS. These are substances secreted by hookworms in order to prevent clotting of the blood, which they suck.

ANTICONVULSANTS (*see* ANTISPASMODICS *and* PHENYTOIN SODIUM).

ANTIDIURETIC HORMONE (ADH). This is secreted by the posterior lobe of the PITUITARY GLAND (which see). A deficiency of A D H leads to Diabetes Insipidus.

ANTIDOTES neutralise the effects of poisons either (*a*) by changing the poisons into relatively harmless substances through some chemical action, or (*b*) by setting up an action in the body opposite to that of the poison.

First-aid and other antidotes are given under the various poisons, *e.g.* ACIDS, ALKALIES, ARSENIC, MERCURY, 'ANTI-FREEZE' (ethylene glycol), plant ALKALOIDS.

ANTIFEBRIN (*see* ANTIPYRINE).

'ANTIFREEZE'. Garages contain one poison which claims more cats and dogs as victims every year, namely ethylene glycol, or antifreeze. The symptoms are depression, ataxia and coma, sometimes with vomiting and convulsions. Ethylene glycol is oxidised in the body to oxalic acid, the actual toxic agent, and crystals of calcium oxalate may be found on post mortem examination in the kidneys and blood-vessels of the brain. Treatment attempts to swamp the enzyme systems which bring about this oxidation by offering ethanol as an alternative substrate. This is achieved by the intraperitoneal injection of 20 per cent ethanol and 5 per cent bicarbonate solution. (Prof. Clarke (1975), *Vet. Rec.*)

ANTIGEN is a substance which causes the formation of antibodies. (*See* IMMUNE RESPONSE, VACCINES, H-Y ANTIGEN.)

ANTIGLOBULIN. An antiserum against the globulin part of the serum, and used in the indirect fluorescent antibody test and Coombs' test.

ANTIHISTAMINES are drugs which neutralise the effects of histamine in excess in the tissues. They are useful in treating shock following burns and also allergic disorders, *e.g. some* cases of: laminitis, urticaria, azoturia, light sensitisation, bloat, acetonaemia, anaphylaxis, acne, etc. They include mepyramine maleate, promezathine hydrochloride, Anthisan, Benadryl, and Phenergan. They should not be used except under professional advice.

Recently, eosinophil cells have been found to be a rich source of an antihistamine factor. (*See* EOSINOPHIL.)

ANTIHORMONES. True antibodies formed consequent upon the injection of hormones.

ANTIKETOGENIC is the term applied to foods and remedies which prevent or decrease the formation of ketones.

ANTIMONY is a metallic element belonging to the class of heavy metals. Antimony salts are less used now in veterinary medicine than formerly, less toxic substitutes being preferable.
USES. Tartar-emetic, the double tartrate of antimony and potassium, used for intravenous injection against certain trypanosomes and other protozoon parasites. (*See* ANTIDOTES.)

ANTIOXIDANTS (*see* VITAMIN E).

ANTIPHLOGISTICS (*see* POULTICES AND FOMENTATIONS).

ANTIPYRETICS are drugs used to reduce temperature during fevers.

ANTIPYRINE, or PHENAZONUM, one of the coal-tar derivatives which is of crystalline form, possesses the following properties: It dulls pain, reduces temperature, produces profuse perspiration, in the horse especially. The principal of these drugs, in addition to antipyrine, are acetanilide or antifebrin, and phenacetin.

ANTISEPTICS. Agents which inhibit the growth of micro-organisms, and are suitable for application to wounds or the unbroken skin. Preparations designed to kill organisms are properly called 'disinfectants' or 'germicides'. Many substances may be either antiseptic or disinfectant according to the strength used.

Very strong antiseptic or disinfectant solutions should not be used for wounds because of the destruction of cells they cause. The dead cells may then retard healing, and in some cases are later cast off as a slough.

The chief of the chemical antiseptics which are of service in animal medicine are as follows:

Chlorine compounds in several different forms are used for cleansing wounds from the presence of organisms. During war they are extensively used for continuous irrigations of large septic shot-wounds and give good results. Among the class may be mentioned eusol, eupad, 'TCP',* 'Fecto', etc. They include sodium hypochlorite and chloramines, both also used as disinfectants.

Quaternary ammonium compounds (see under this heading), are widely used in dairy hygiene. They include cetrimide (see under separate heading) and benzalkonium chloride.

'Dettol',* **Liquor Chloroxylenolis, BP.** Powerful bactericides of low toxicity. Much used for skin cleansing, obstetrical work, and disinfecting premises. The bactericidal action is reduced in the presence of blood or serum.

Crystal violet. A 1 per cent solution forms a useful antiseptic for infected wounds, burns, fungal skin diseases, and chronic ulcers. Similarly, gentian violet.

Common salt (a teaspoonful to a pint of boiled water) is useful as a wound lotion and is usually easily obtainable when other antiseptics may be lacking.

Sulphonamides have proved of great use in wounds infected with streptococci and certain other organisms (see SULPHONAMIDE DRUGS).

Iodoform* is a powerful, poisonous but soothing antiseptic formerly often used for dusting on to wounds as a powder with boric acid.

Iodine* in an alcoholic solution is more penetrating and irritant, especially to delicate skins. For use on the unbroken skin *only*.

Alcohol is a very powerful antiseptic chiefly used for removing grease and septic matter from the hands of the surgeon and the skin of the patient. (Ether is used in this way also.)

Hydrogen peroxide (See under that heading.)

ANTISERUM. A serum for use against a specific condition is produced by inoculating a susceptible animal with a sub-lethal dose of the causal agent or antigen and gradually increasing the dosage until very large amounts are administered. The animal develops in its blood serum an antibody which can be made use of to confer a temporary protection in other animals against the bacterium or toxin.

The use of antiserum alone confers a temporary immunity, and in most cases this probably does not protect for longer than from 10 days to a maximum of about 21 days. Antisera are used in the treatment of existing disease, and also as a means of protecting animals exposed to infection. (*See* BLACK-QUARTER, TETANUS, JAUNDICE (Leptospiral) for examples of diseases where serum therapy may be useful.) (*See also* ANAPHYLAXIS, IMMUNITY.)

ANTISIALICS. Substances which reduce salivation; *e.g.* atropine.

ANTISPASMODICS are remedies which diminish spasm or 'cramp'. They mostly act upon the muscular tissues, causing them to relax, or soothing nerves which control the muscles involved.

Modern anti-convulsive drugs include CHLORPROMAZINE, PHENYTOIN SODIUM, PHENOBARBITONE, LARGACTIL and MYSOLINE (*see under those headings*).

ANTITETANIC SERUM is a serum used against tetanus. Nowadays the antitoxin is preferred. (*See* TETANUS.)

ANTITOXINS, or **ANTITOXIC SERA** are substances to neutralise the harmful effects of a toxin. (*See* SERUM THERAPY.)

ANTIVENINE is a substance produced by the injection of snake venom into animals in small but increasing doses. In course of time the animal becomes immune to the particular venom injected, and the antivenine prepared from its serum is highly effective in neutralising venom injected by the bite of a snake of the same species. To be of any use it must be administered within about one hour of the snake bite.

ANTIVIRAL. Used against viruses. (*See* INTERFERON.)

ANTIZYMOTIC. An agent which inhibits fermentation.

ANTRYCIDE. A synthetic drug used in the control of trypanosomiasis.

ANTS are of veterinary interest as intermediate hosts of the liver fluke *Dicroelium dendriticum*. This fluke, which is smaller than *Fasciola hepatica*, the common fluke, is found in sheep, goats, cattle, deer, hares, rabbits, pigs, dogs, donkeys, and occasionally man. In the British Isles, the fluke occurs only (it is believed) in the islands off the Scottish mainland.

The fluke's eggs are swallowed by a land-snail of the genus *Helicella*. From the snail, cercariae periodically escape and slimy clumps of them are eaten by ants (*Formica fusca* in the USA). Grazing animals, swallowing ants with the grass, then become infested.

* (Their injudicious use could lead to toxicity in **cats**, so for them other antiseptics are preferable.)

Ants also act as the intermediate host of a tapeworm of the fowl, guinea-fowl and pigeon, *Raillietina tetragona*.

Pharaoh's ants have been shown to be of considerable medical importance. They are much smaller than the common black ant; the worker, brownish-orange in colour, measuring only 2 mm in length. They are a tropical species and in a temperate climate survive where there is central heating or its equivalent.

Their nests have been found behind tiles, in light fittings, fuse-boxes, and even in hospital operating theatres! Small nests are sometime found between the folds of sheets and towels coming from laundries.

These ants eat meat, and also sweet foods. Unfortunately, in their quest for water, they visit sinks, drains, lavatories, etc. and can therefore contaminate food. They also, apparently, feed on the discharges from infected wounds.

Pharaoh's ants constitute a public health danger since, in nine hospitals, important disease-producing bacteria were isolated from them; and in the isolation unit of a school of veterinary medicine they ruined one experiment by carrying infection from known infected animals to the uninfected 'controls'.

In America a nationally advertised dry dog food was submitted to the Animal Diseases Diagnostic Laboratory, Oklahoma, after complaints that one bird and some rats had died after eating the food. These complaints were not borne out in the laboratory, but microscopical examination showed that black specks in the food were parts of insects – later identified as *Tapinoma sessile*, the 'odorous house ant'. USA regulations did not cover this type of contamination.

Fire ants (*Soleropsis invicta*) have become established in the S E states of the USA. They are very aggressive and masses of them will attack and eat quail fledglings, for example, and unweaned rabbits. People camping out near fire ant colonies have also been attacked; the ant 'venom' causing blurred vision, loss of consciousness, sometimes convulsions. (Joyce, J. R. (1983) *Veterinary Medicine/S A C* **7,** 1107.)

ANTU. Alphanaphthylthiourea, used to kill rodents. One gram may prove fatal to a 20 to 25 lb dog. The poison gives rise to oedema of the lungs. (*See alo* THIOUREA.) Antu is banned in the UK.

ANURIA is a condition in which little or no urine is excreted or voided for some time. (*See* URINE, KIDNEY.)

ANUS. In health it is kept closed by the *sphincter ani*, a ring of muscle fibres about 1 inch thick in the horse, which is kept in a state of constant contraction by certain special nerve fibres situated in the spinal cord. If this ring fails to relax, constipation may result, while in some forms of paralysis the muscle becomes unable to retain the faeces. (*See also* IMPERFORATE ANUS.)

Anal glands (sacs). There are two of these in the dog, situated below and to each side of the anus. They produce a fluid which possibly acts as a lub-

ricant to aid defaecation. Each gland has a duct opening just inside the anus. These ducts may become blocked by a grass seed or other foreign body, so that the secretions cannot escape and the glands swell; but more commonly there is infection. Irritation or pain then results.

Dr M. Tirgari described (*Veterinary Record* (1988) **123,** 365) a technique for impregnating the anal sacs with a dental mould material. After the latter has set the sacs can be more easily ablated surgically.

SIGNS include yelping on sitting down, tail-chasing, but more commonly the dog drags itself along the ground.

Perianal fistulae in dogs were treated by either cryosurgery (64 cases) or excision of diseased tissue (35). The success rate was high for both techniques in dogs with either mild or moderately severe lesions; neither method proved satisfactory when the dogs were seriously affected. The main postoperate complications with cryosurgery were stricture of the anal orifice and recurrence of the fistulae while with excision it was faecal incontinence. (Vasseur, P. B. (1981), *Journal of the American Animal Hospital Association* **17,** 177.)

Perianal furunculosis is sometimes a recurring problem in dogs. Surgical removal of the anal sacs has been recommended to prevent recurrence.

AORTA is the principal artery of the body. It leaves the base of the left ventricle and curves upwards and backwards, giving off branches to the head and neck and forelimbs. About the level of the 8th or 9th thoracic vertebra it reaches the lower surface of the spinal column, and from there it runs back into the abdominal cavity between the lungs, piercing the diaphragm. It ends about the 5th lumbar vertebra by dividing into the two internal iliacs and the middle sacral arteries. The internal iliacs supply the two hindlimbs and the muscles of the pelvis. At its commencement the aorta is about 1½ inches in diameter in the horse, and from there it gradually tapers as large branches leave it. It is customary to divide the aorta into *thoracic aorta* and *abdominal aorta*. (*See* ARTERIES, ANEURISM.)

AORTIC RUPTURE. This follows degenerative changes in the aorta, and is a not uncommon cause of death of male turkeys aged between 5 and 22 weeks. It was first reported in the USA and Canada. In Britain most cases occur between July and October. No symptoms are observed; the birds being found dead. 'In a flock of 500 turkeys, 30 or more may die from this disease over a period of 2 to 3 weeks' (BOCM Poultry Advisory Service). The use of Reserpine has been recommended in order to lower blood-pressure and so prevent further deaths in a flock.

AORTIC STENOSIS IN CATS. The clinical findings in six cats (four less than eight months old and the others three and four years old) included dyspnoea, and congestive heart failure. Congenital aortic stenosis was diagnosed and confirmed by angiographic imaging of a discrete, consistent subvalvular obstruction, Doppler-echocardiography, or by post mortem examination. (Stephen, R. L. & Bonagura, J. D. (1991) *Journal of Small Animal Practice* **32**, 341.)

APHTHA, MALIGNANT. This, and contagious aphtha, are other names for FOOT-AND-MOUTH DISEASE (which see).

APLASTIC. Relating to aplasia, the congenital absence of an organ. In aplastic anaemia, there is defective development or a cessation of regeneration of the red cells, etc. (*See* ANAEMIA.)

APNOEA means the stoppage of respiration which occurs when the blood is artificially supplied with too much oxygen; for instance, when several deep breaths are taken in quick succession. (*See* ASPHYXIA.)

APOMORPHINE is a derivative of morphine which has a marked emetic action in the dog and is used in that animal to induce vomiting when some poisonous or otherwise objectionable material has been taken into the stomach.

APONEUROSIS is a sheet of tendinous tissue providing an insertion or attachment for muscles, which is sometimes itself attached to a bone, and sometimes is merely a method of attaching one muscle to another.

APOPLEXY. The effect upon part of the brain of bleeding from a cerebral artery or of thrombosis of an artery – the equivalent of a 'stroke' in human medicine. There is usually a sudden loss of consciousness and there may be some degree of paralysis on one side of the body. (*See* BRAIN, DISEASES OF.)

APOPROTEINS are involved in the transport of LIPIDS throughout the body. Apoproteins are produced by cells in the liver or intestine. (*See* LIPOPROTEIN.)

APPALOOSA. The Appaloosa Horse Society of America and the British Spotted Horse Society are concerned with the breeding of this horse, which has some Arab blood and is characterised by a silky white coat with black (or chocolate-coloured) spots which can be felt with the finger.

APPETITE.

Pica ('depraved appetite'). A mineral or vitamin deficiency may account for some cases of animals eating rubbish such as coal, cinders, soil, plaster, stones, faeces, etc. Pica is often associated also with pregnancy; and is an important sign of rabies in dogs. It may result from worm infections.

In cats pica is a sign of anaemia. They will lick concrete or eat cat litter.

Excessive appetite may be a sign of dyspepsia or diabetes, of internal parasites, of tuberculosis, listeriosis, or of the early stages of cancer.

Diminished appetite. Anorexia, or a diminished appetite, is a sign usually present in most forms of dyspepsia, in gastritis and enteritis, in many fevers, and in abnormal conditions of the throat and the mouth, when the act of swallowing is difficult or painful. In other cases the appetite is in abeyance for no apparent reason. It may be merely an indication that a dog or cat or other animal has overeaten, and a rest from eating may be all that is needed. (*See* NURSING OF SICK ANIMALS, MINERALS, VITAMINS.)

AQUACULTURE (*see* FISH FARMING).

AQUEDUCT OF SYLVIUS, or the cerebral aqueduct, connects the third and fourth ventricles of the brain, and conveys cerebrospinal fluid.

AQUEOUS HUMOUR (*see* EYE).

ARACHNIDA is the name of the class of Arthropoda to which belong the mange mites, ticks, and spiders.

ARACHIDONIC ACID (*see* EICOSANOIDS).

ARACHNOID MEMBRANE is one of the membranes covering the brain and spinal cord. (*See* BRAIN.) Arachnoiditis is inflammation of this membrane.

ARBOVIRUSES. This is an abbreviation for arthropod-born viruses. They are responsible for diseases (such as louping-ill, equine encephalitis and yellow fever) transmitted by ticks, insects, etc. They are known as Togaviruses. (*See* VIRUSES table.)

ARC. The Agricultural Research Council, under whose control a number of U K veterinary research institutes function, was renamed the Agricultural & Food Research Council (A F R C).

AREOLA means a small space, and is the term applied to the red or dusky-brown coloured ring around the nipple in the human female and in the dog, or to an inflamed ring. In some breeds of toy dogs it is possible to distinguish a darkening of the areolae of the nipples in early pregnancy, but this feature is not so marked nor so reliable as it is in the human subject.

AREOLAR CONNECTIVE TISSUE is loose in character and occurs in the body wherever a cushioning effect, with flexibility, is needed; *e.g.* between skin and muscle, and surrounding blood vessels.

ARIZONA INFECTION in turkeys was reported for the first time in the U K in 1968. The infection is caused by the Arizona group of the enterobacteriaceae – closely related to the salmonellae and the coliform group. Young birds can be infected by contact or through the egg. Nervous symptoms and eye lesions are characteristic in birds surviving the initial illness.

Over 300 antigenically distinct serotypes of *Arizona* have been identified. One at least appears to be host adapted to sheep, and has been recovered from scouring sheep, from ewes which died in pregnancy and from aborted foetuses. Food-poisoning in man and diarrhoea in monkeys have been attributed in Arizona infection.

ARRHYTHMIA means that the heart-beat is not occurring regularly, or that a beat is being periodically missed. It may be only temporary and of little importance, or on the other hand it may be a symptom of some form of cardiac disease.

ARSANILIC ACID. One of the organic compounds of arsenic which has been used as a growth supplement for pigs and poultry.

It should not be given within 10 days of slaughter, nor should the recommended dosage rate be exceeded, as residues – especially in the liver – may prove harmful if consumed. The permitted maximum of arsenic in liver is 1 part per million. In a random survey (1969), 4 of 93 pig livers contained from 1·2 to 3·5 ppm of arsenic.

Blindness, a staggering gait, twisting of the neck, progressive weakness and paralysis are symptoms of chronic poisoning with arsanilic acid in the pig.

ARSENIC is a metal, but by the word as commonly used is meant the oxide, or arsenious acid. It is contained in a great variety of substances, among the most common of which are: Scheele's green and emerald green – the two arsenites of copper; Orpiment or King's yellow, and Realgar – sulphides of arsenic; Fowler's solution – the liquor arsenicalis of the *British Pharmacopoeia*, which contains arsenic trioxide; older varieties of sheep-dip, especially those sold as a powder; weed-killers, haulm destroyers, rat-poisons, fly-papers, wall-papers; and in lead shot as a hardening agent.

USES. Arsenic has been used in some compound animal feeds in order to improve growth rate. The disposal of dung containing arsenic residues from poultry-houses, etc., may accordingly be fraught with danger. (*See also* ARSANILIC ACID.)

Administered in small doses over a long period, arsenic may give rise to cancer.

ARSENIC, POISONING BY. Arsenic is an irritant poison producing in all animals gastroenteritis. The rapidity of its action depends on the amount that is taken, on the solubility of the compound, on the presence or otherwise of food in the digestive system, and on the susceptibility of the animal.

SIGNS include violent purging, severe colic, straining, a staggering gait, coldness of the extremities of the body, unconsciousness, and convulsions. When the poisoning is the result of the taking of small doses for a considerable period, cumulative symptoms are observed. These include an unthrifty condition of the body generally, swelling of the joints, indigestion, constant or intermittent diarrhoea, often with a foetid odour, thirst, emaciation, and distressed breathing and heart action on moderate exercise.

CAUSES

Cattle have died after straying into a field of potatoes sprayed with arsenites to destroy the haulm. Others have died following the application to their backs of an arsenical dressing, and of the use of arsenic-contaminated, old bins for feeding purposes.

Sheep. Probably most cases of arsenic poisoning in sheep occurred from the use of arsenical dips before BHC was introduced. The source of this poisoning is in many cases the herbage of the pastures which becomes contaminated either from the drippings from the wool of the sheep, or from the washing of the dip out of the fleece by a shower of rain on the second or third day after the dipping. Absorption through wounds or laceration of the skin may result in arsenic poisoning, and when dips are made up too strong absorption into the system may also occur. The obvious precautions, apart from care of the actual dipping, are to ensure that the sheep are kept in the draining pens long enough to ensure that their fleeces are reasonably dry (some 15 to 20 minutes) and subsequently are not allowed to remain for long thickly concentrated in small fields or paddocks. Where double dipping is carried out, the second immersion in an arsenic dip must be at half-strength.

Dogs and cats are particularly susceptible to poisoning by arsenic. The symptoms are nausea, vomiting, abdominal pain, dark fluid evacuations, and death preceded by convulsions.

ANTIDOTES. Sodium thiosulphate is a better antidote than ferric hydroxide, and a solution can be given intravenously. (*See* DIPPING, TONICS, etc.)

ARTERIES. With the exception of the pulmonary artery, which carries venous blood to the lungs, the arteries carry oxygenated blood; that is, blood which has recently been circulating in the lungs, has absorbed oxygen from the inspired air, and has become scarlet in colour. The pulmonary artery carries blood of a purple colour which has been circulating in the body and has been returned to the heart, to be sent to the lungs for oxygenation.

The arterial system begins at the left ventricle of the heart with the aorta (*see* AORTA). This is the largest artery of the body. It divides and subdivides until the final branches end in the capillaries which ramify throughout all the body tissues except cornea, hair, horn, and teeth. The larger of these branches are called *arteries*, the smaller ones are *arterioles*, and these end in the *capillaries*. The capillaries pervade the tissues like the pores of a sponge, and bathe the cells of the body in arterial blood. The blood is collected by the venous system and carried back to the heart.

STRUCTURE. The arteries are highly elastic tubes which are capable of great dilatation with each pulsation of the heart – a dilatation which is of considerable importance in the circulation of the blood. (*See* CIRCULATION.) Their walls are composed of three coats: (*a*) *adventitious coat*, consisting of ordinary strong fibrous tissue on the outside; (*b*) *middle coat*, composed of muscle fibres and elastic fibres, in separate layers in the great arteries; (*c*) *inner coat* or *intima*, consisting of a layer of yellow elastic tissue on whose inner-most surface rests a single continuous layer of smooth, plate-like *endothelial cells*, within which flows the blood-stream. The walls of the larger arteries have the muscles of their middle coat re-placed to a great extent by elastic fibres so that they are capable of much distension. When an artery is cut across, its muscular coat instantly shrinks, drawing the cut end within the fibrous sheath which surrounds all arteries, and bun-ching it up so that only a comparatively small hole is left for the escape of blood. This in a normal case soon becomes filled up with the blood-clot which is Nature's method of checking haemorrhage. (*See* HAEMORRHAGE; BLEEDING, ARREST OF.)

ARTERIES, DISEASES OF. These include:
(1) **Arteritis** during specific virus diseases such as African Swine Fever, Equine Viral Arteritis. Canine Viral Hepatitis; etc.
(2) **Chronic inflammation,** or **Arterio-sclerosis,** is a process of thickening of the arterial wall and subsequent degenerative changes, resulting in an abnormal rigidity of the tube and hindrance to the circulation.
(3) **Degenerative changes** include Atheroma – thickening and degeneration of the lining of the artery. Degeneration occurs in the arteries of pigs, especially, during the course of several diseases. Examples are haemorrhagic gas-tritis and Herztod disease.
(4) **Thrombosis.** This includes aortic-iliac thrombosis in horses (*see* THROMBOSIS), and femoral thrombosis in dogs and cats. (*See* PARAPLEGIA.)
(5) **Embolism.**
(6) **Aneurysm.**
(7) **Equine verminous arteritis.**
(8) **Heartworms.**
(9) **Aortic rupture** in turkeys.

ARTHRITIS. A common disease of all farm and pet animals.
CAUSES include trauma, rheumatism, a min-eral deficiency, and FLUOROSIS.
    Infections which cause arthritis include BRUCELLOSIS, TUBERCULOSIS, and SWINE ERYSIPELAS. (*See also* SYNOVITIS, BURSITIS, *and* JOINT-ILL.)

Rheumatoid arthritis. Examination of synovial fluid suggests that 'there are increased immune responses to canine distemper, and that these re-sponses may be due to the presence of the distem-per virus in affected joints.' (Bell, C.S. & others. *Research in Veterinary Science* (1991) **50,** 64.)

Open-joint injuries. Of 58 horses injured in this way, and examined within 24 hours, 53 developed septic arthritis. Fifty-four per cent of the treated horses recovered, aided by surgery and anti-biotics. (Gibson, K.T. & others. *Journal of the American Veterinary Medical Association* (1989) **194,** 398.)

ARTHROGRYPOSIS (*see* GENETIC DEFECTS under GENETICS).

ARTHROSCOPY. The application of endoscope techniques to the study of joint cavities.

ARTHROSIS. Degenerative disease of a joint, as opposed to inflammation. (The word can also mean an articulation.)

ARTIFACT. An apparent lesion in a histological or pathological specimen, not existing during life, but made accidentally in preparing the specimen.

ARTIFICIAL ABORTION (*see* STILBOESTROL MALUCIDIN. *See also* CAESAREAN SECTION).

ARTIFICIAL BONES. In racing greyhounds, badly fractured scaphoids have been removed and replaced with plastic replicas. (Hare Spy won a race on January 16, 1958, after such an opera-tion.) (*See also* IMPLANTS.)

ARTIFICIAL INDUCTION OF PARTURITION (*see* DRUG-INDUCED PARTURITION).

ARTIFICIAL INSEMINATION. The introduction of male germ cells (*spermatozoa*) into the female without actual service.
    The practice is a very old one. In the fourteenth century Arab horse-breeders were getting mares in foal by using semen-impregnated sponges. In Italy bitches were artificially inseminated as long ago as 1780, and at the close of the nineteenth century the practice was applied, to a very limited extent, to mares in Britain.
    It was the Russian scientist Ivanoff who saw in AI the possibilities of disease control, and in 1909, a laboratory was established in Russia for the development and improvement of existing techniques. By 1938 well over a million cattle and 15 million sheep had been inseminated in the USSR, where all the basic work was done. Den-mark began to take a practical interest in AI in 1936 (and within eleven years had a hundred cooperative breeding stations inseminating half a million head of cattle annually); the USA in 1937. The UK began to practise AI on a commer-cial basis in 1942, and by the end of 1950 had close on a hundred centres and sub-centres in opera-tion, serving over 60,000 farms. From the Milk Marketing Board's AI centres more than 2,000,000 cows were inseminated during 1972–3.
    In 1975 the Milk Marketing Board began offering reduced rates for **batch insemination,** fol-lowing the introduction of an ICI prostaglandin product – claimed to make practicable and econ-omic precisely scheduled AI programmes with-out the need for oestrus detection. (*See also* 'CON-TROLLED BREEDING', PROSTAGLANDINS.)
    By 1976 more than 50,000,000 calves had been bred in England and Wales by means of AI. In 1977–78 first inseminations totalled a little over 1,857,000.
    New regulations for AI in cattle were intro-duced in 1986 in the UK.
USES. The use of AI in commercial cattle breeding is dependent upon the fact that, in normal mating, a bull produces between 50 and 100 times as much semen as is required to enable

one cow to conceive. By collecting the semen, diluting it and if necessary, storing it in a refrigerator, the insemination of many cows from one ejaculate becomes possible.

A I reduces the spread of venereal disease, and hence greatly reduces the incidence of the latter. Farmers in a small way of business are able to dispense with the services of a communal bull – an animal seldom well bred and often infected with some transmissible disease. At the same time, the farmer has the advantage of the use of a healthy, pedigree bull without the considerable expense of buying, feeding, and looking after it. Owners of what are sometimes called commercial herds are enabled to grade these up to pedigree standard, with an increase in quality and milk yield. In many of the ranching areas overseas, where stock-raising is carried out on an *extensive*, rather than an *intensive*, scale, to achieve satisfactory production of animals for trade and commercial purposes, sires have to be imported at regular intervals from the essentially sire-producing countries – of which Britain is the chief. The method of artificially inseminating a large number of females from an imported sire enables bigger generations of progeny to be raised and consequently more rapid improvement to be achieved.

METHODS. Various methods are employed. Those which give best results involve the use of an artificial vagina in which to collect the semen from an ejaculation. This is used outside the female's body, being so arranged that the penis of the male enters it instead of entering the vagina. The full ejaculation is received without contamination from the female.

After the ejaculation has been collected it is either divided into fractions, each being injected by a special syringe into the cervix or uterus of another female in season, or – in commercial practice – it is diluted 20 times or more with a specially prepared 'sperm diluent', such as egg-yolk citrate buffer. Dilution rates of up to 1 in 100 have been successful, but it appears desirable to inseminate 12 or 13 million sperms into each cow.

The method requires skill to carry out successfully, and necessitates the employment of strict cleanliness throughout. (*See* CONCEPTION RATES.)

Artificial insemination has also been carried out in pigs (*see* FARROWING RATES), goats, dogs, turkeys and other birds, bees, etc.

Canine A I is now practised in many parts of the world. In the UK the Kennel Club reserves the right to decide whether to accept for registration puppies obtained by means of A I rather than by normal mating. Applications are usually made by the owner of the bitch. Those concerned with a newly imported breed, and who wish to widen the genetic pool, may not be able to find a suitable male for purchase and import. However if semen from a satisfactory dog can be obtained, and MAFF agree to its import under licence, A I may be a good way of increasing the available genes. Registrations will not be accepted where A I is requested because either the prospective sire or dam is unable to mate owing to disease. (Stockman, M. J. R. (1985) *Veterinary Record* **116**, 503.)

Storage of semen. Diluted semen may be stored at A I centres for a few days if kept at a temperature of 5°C. In practice, a good deal is wasted because its fertilising power has diminished before it is all required for use. Research work, carried out at Cambridge, has made it possible, however, to store semen for months and even years. In this technique, glycerol is added to the sperm diluent, and it is this addition which enables the spermatozoa to withstand a temperature of −79°C (110° below zero, Fahrenheit) without losing their power to fertilise when thawed. In practice the diluted semen was stored in special cabinets containing solid CO_2. Nowadays it is stored and transported at −196°C, using liquid nitrogen.

The advantages of this method are many. There is less wastage of semen, more can be stored, and the semen of any particular bull can be made available on any day. It is possible for several thousand cows to be got in calf by a given bull. In fact, a Hereford bull owned by the Milk Marketing Board, had by 1960 sired 50,000 calves. The disadvantages of using a given bull or bulls too widely must be borne in mind, but that is a matter of policy and not of technique.

The deep freezing of boar semen did not lead to conception until it was introduced directly into the sow's oviducts. By this method it is possible to inseminate a thousand sows with one ejaculate of a boar. A simple surgical operation is at present necessary but Agricultural Research Council work is continuing to find a surgery-free technique.

A two-step insemination technique for sows was described by K. Takeda and M. Sone of Japan (*Vet. Record* (1981) **108**, 146). They commented: 'Injected semen is likely to leak out through the vagina, because the cervical canal is curved and narrow.' Their apparatus is designed to overcome this difficulty.

Infected semen. Viruses (including that of foot-and-mouth) and mycoplasmas have, on occasion, been found in stored semen. (*See also* RABIES). (*See also* 'CONTROLLED' BREEDING.)

ARTIFICIAL REARING OF PIGLETS. Cows' colostrum makes a satisfactory substitute for sows' colostrum, and may be frozen and later thawed when required. Pig's serum as an addition enhances the value of cows' colostrum.

ARTIFICIAL RESPIRATION. This is resorted to in: (1) Cessation of respiration while under general anaesthesia; (2) cases of drowning when the animal has been rescued from the water – chiefly applicable to the small animals; (3) poisoning by narcotics or paralysants; (4) cases of asphyxia from fumes, smoke, gases, etc.

Horses and cattle. Release from all restraint except a loose halter or head-collar, extend the head and neck to allow a straight passage of the air into the lungs, open the mouth, and pull the tongue well out. Should the ground slope the horse must be placed with his head downhill. While such adjustments are being carried out one or two assistants should compress the elastic posterior ribs by alternately leaning the whole weight of the body on the hands pressed on the ribs, and then releasing the pressure about once every 4 or 5 seconds, in an endeavour to stimulate the normal movements of breathing. As an alternative in a larger animal a heavy person may sit himself with some vigour astride the ribs for about the same time, rise for a similar period, and then re-seat himself. If no response occurs, these measures should be carried out more rapidly.

The inhalation of strong solution of ammonia upon a piece of cotton-wool and held about a foot from the upper nostril often assists in inducing a gasp which is the first sign of the return to respiration, but care is needed not to allow the ammonia to come into contact with the skin or burning will occur. After 2 or 3 minutes' work the animal should be turned on to the opposite side to prevent stasis of the blood. Sometimes the mere act of turning will induce the premonitory gasp. So long as the heart continues to beat, no matter how feebly, the attempts at resuscitation should be pursued.

Proprietary calf resuscitators are available to give the 'kiss of life'.

Pigs and sheep. The outlines of procedure given for the larger animals are equally applicable. An ordinary domestic funnel can be used for giving pigs the 'kiss of life'.

In an American research station's herd they were getting in 1964 9 per cent of piglets 'born dead'. By 1975, the figure had been reduced to 3 per cent. This was achieved by recognising the fact that many of these so-called stillbirths were not really dead, and could be revived by mouth-to-mouth resuscitation.

The method of giving the 'kiss of life' to a piglet is to use a flexible polyethylene funnel, and fit this over the animal's mouth and nostrils. Air is then blown into the stem of the funnel, and passes down into the piglet's lungs.

For the method to be effective, the procedure is as follows: (1) Hold the piglet by its hind legs with head down in order to drain any fluid from its air passages; (2) turn the pig with its head upwards and apply the funnel; (3) blow forcefully into the funnel; (4) remove the funnel and allow the piglet to breathe out; (5) repeat the operation. After several repetitions, the piglet should kick or show other signs of life. Lay the animal on its side or stomach and massage its chest and mouth.

Piglets have been revived up to half an hour after treatment began. Of course, the heart must be beating and resuscitation started promptly to achieve success.

Dogs and cats. A modification of the Schafer system is to lay the dog on its side with the head at a lower level than the rest of the body, place one hand flat over the upper side of the abdomen and the other on the rib-cage, lean heavily on the hands, and in a second or two release the pressure.

The motions of artificial respiration should in all cases be a little faster than those of normal respiration, but a slight pause should always be observed before each rhythmic movement. Use less pressure for cats.

A respiratory stimulant may be given by injection. (*See* CORAMINE.) A carbon dioxide 'Resuscitator' may be used.

ASCARIDAE is the name of a class of worms belonging to the round variety or *Nemathelminthes*, which are found parasitic in the intestines of horses, pigs, dogs, and cats particularly, although they may affect other animals. They attain a size of 15 or 18 inches in the horse, but are small in other animals. (*See* ROUNDWORMS.)

ASCITES means oedema involving the abdomen; a very common complication of abdominal tuberculosis, of liver, kidney, or heart disease, as well as of some parasitic infestations. (*See* OEDEMA.)

ASCORBIC ACID. Synthetic vitamin C.

ASEPSIS. Aseptic surgery is the ideal, but among animals it may be difficult to attain if carried out under farm conditions; despite care in sterilising instruments and the use of sterilised dressings, rubber gloves, etc. Moreover, it is an exceptionally difficult matter to prevent accidental infection in a surgical wound after the operation, for the animal cannot be put to bed, and it may object to the dressings and do all in its power to remove them. (*See* ANTISEPTICS, SULPHONAMIDES, PENICILLIN.)

ASH POISONING has been reported in cattle. Symptoms include: drowsiness, oedema involving ribs and flanks, purple discoloration of perineum. The green leaves and fruits from a broken branch of a tree led to these symptoms. (Reeves, R. J. C. (1975), *Vet. Rec.*)

ASPERGILLOSIS is a disease of mammals and birds produced by the growth of the fungus *Aspergillus* in the tissues of the body.

Infection probably occurs chiefly through inhalation of the fungal spores, which may be abundant in hay or straw under conditions of dampness. Entry of the spores into the body may also be by way of the mouth; in herbivorous animals from contaminated fodder or bedding, and in cat and dog from the eating of infected birds or rodents.

Once in the animal's tissues, *hyphae* grow out from the spores, as happens also in ringworm; and from the branching filaments more spores are produced. Local necrosis and abscess formation are caused.

Numerous organs and tissues can become infected, including the nose and nasal sinuses, the lungs, brain, uterus, and mammary glands.

Cattle and horses. *Aspergillus* may cause abortion or pneumonia, and similar disease could occur in horses.

Dogs and cats. Aspergillosis is a common cause of chronic nasal disease, and should be suspected when there is a discharge from one nostril.

Poultry. Respiratory disease or enteritis may occur. In young turkey poults brain involvement has led to an unsteady gait, walking backwards, and turning the head to one side.

Pet parrots may die from aspergillosis, as well as wild birds.

Brain infection may occur in all species, and give rise to symptoms described under ENCEPHALITIS. Paresis and ataxia may, rarely, be caused by fungal infections of the spine.

Aspergillosis does not readily respond to treatment. In human medicine, local infusions of nystatin have been found helpful. Both thiabendazole and ketaconazole have been used in cases of canine nasal aspergillosis. (*See* Sharp, N. *JAVMA* (1989) 78.2).

ASPHODEL (*see* BOG ASPHODEL).

ASPHYXIA may occur during the administration of anaesthetics by inhalation, during the outbreak of fires in animal houses, where the fumes and the smoke present are responsible for oedema, and in cases of poisoning. (*See also* 'KITCHEN DEATHS'.)

In Africa, cattle have been deliberately strangled – a cause of asphyxia seldom encountered elsewhere in domestic animals.

SIGNS. The direct cause of death from asphyxia is an insufficiency of oxygen supplied to the tissues by the blood. The first signs are a rapid and full pulse, and a quickening of the respirations. The breathing soon changes to a series of gasps, and the blood-pressure rises, causing the visible membranes to become intensely injected and later blue in colour. Greater struggles for breath occur, and soon general convulsions supervene. The convulsions are followed by quietness, when the heart-beat may be almost imperceptible and respiratory movements practically cease. The actual time of death is unnoticed as a rule, since death takes place very quietly.

During the stage of convulsions, when the amount of carbon dioxide circulating in the blood is increased, the smaller arteries vigorously contract and cause an increase in the blood-pressure. This high blood-pressure produces an engorgement of the right side of the heart, which cannot totally expel its contents with each beat, and becomes more and more dilated until such time as the pressure in the ventricles overcomes the strength of the muscle fibres of the heart and the organ ceases to beat. During this stage immediate relief follows bleeding from a large vein.

TREATMENT. The first essential in all cases of asphyxia is to remove the cause by opening ventilators or windows; or by carrying the animal into the open air and adjusting the head and neck so that no pressure is placed on the air passages. So long as the heart is beating, recovery may be hoped for. (*See* ARTIFICIAL RESPIRATION.) If the breathing is shallow and the membranes livid, administration of OXYGEN is indicated.

PREVENTION. Ensure adequate ventilation in rooms where there is a gas or solid-fuel heating system. (Many dogs and cats have been found dead in the kitchen in the morning as a result of CARBON MONOXIDE poisoning.)

ASPIRATION means the withdrawal of fluid from the natural cavities of the body or from cavities produced by disease. It may be performed for either curative purposes, when a large quantity is usually removed, or for diagnostic purposes, when only a small amount is removed. (*See* PARACENTESIS.)

ASPIRIN is a preparation of acetylsalicylic acid. It is a mild analgesic. It must be used with extreme caution in cats; the dose not exceeding 25 mg/kg once daily.

In both cats and dogs, *overdosing* with aspirin may cause inflammation of the stomach, haemorrhage, some pain, and vomiting. The antidote is sodium bicarbonate which can be given in water by stomach tube; or, for first-aid purposes, by the cat-owner, in milk or water. (*See* SALICYLATE POISONING.)

ASTHENIA is another name for debility. *Asthenic* is applied to the exhausted state that precedes death during some fevers.

ASTHMA is a term somewhat loosely applied. Strictly speaking, the term should be reserved for those conditions where a true spasmodic expulsion of breath occurs without the effort of a cough. The so-called 'asthma' of birds is due in nearly every case to aspergillosis. (*See* ASPERGILLOSIS.) Asthma in horses may be difficult to differentiate from 'BROKEN WIND', and in all animals from simple BRONCHITIS.

CAUSES. These are obscure, but it is generally held that true spasmodic asthma is of nervous origin, and due to a sudden distressful contraction of the muscle fibres which lie around the smaller bronchioles. In some cases asthma may be an allergic phenomenon. In other cases a chronic inflammation of the lining mucous membrane of the small tubes is the cause.

Botanical and clinical studies have shown that the spores of fungi (*e.g.* cladosporium, botrytis, and alternaria) are potent allergens, and can account for many cases of asthma, especially recurrent summer asthma, in man. There are, however, a number of patients with seasonal (summer or autumn) asthma who are not sensitive to spores of any of the above nor to pollen. (*See* ALLERGY.)

Dog. Many cases that are really chronic bronchitis are spoken of as 'bronchial asthma' owing to their similarity to asthma in man, with which many owners of animals are familiar. In true asthma the attacks of dyspnoea (*i.e.* distressed respiration) occur at irregular intervals, and there are periods between them when the dog is to all appearances quite normal. The attacks occur suddenly, are very distressing to witness, last for from 10 minutes to half an hour, and then suddenly cease. The dog gasps for breath, makes violent inspiratory efforts without much success, exhibits a frightened, disturbed expression, and stands till the attack passes off.

The condition appears to be hereditary in some breeds, especially the Maltese terrier. Cardiac dysfunction also gives rise to 'asthma'. (*See also* ATOPIC.)

TREATMENT. Inhalations of amyl nitrite often serve to cut short an attack; internally antispasmodics. Antihistamines or heart tonics may be of service. Regulation of exercise and diet is necessary.

ASTRAGALUS, or TALUS, is the name of one of the bones of the tarsus (hock), with which the tibia forms the main joint. The articulation between these two bones is sometimes referred to as the 'true hock joint', the others being more or less secondary and less freely movable joints. (*See* BONES.)

ASTRINGENTS include sulphate of zinc, alum, tannic acid, witch-hazel.

ASTROCYTES. Supporting cells found in the central nervous system, and each consisting of a cell body and numerous branching processes. Astrocytes are thought to be concerned with the nutrition of neighbouring nerve cells.

ASTROVIRUS. Was first detected in the faeces of children in 1975, and has since been isolated from lambs, calves, turkeys, deer, etc. It is not regarded as a serious pathogen in veterinary medicine, but studies in gnotobiotic lambs indicates that the virus multiplies in the epithelial cells of the villi of the small intestine, producing some degree of atrophy of the villi, with diarrhoea.

ASYMMETRIC HINDQUARTER SYNDROME (AHQS). Outbreaks of a lop-sided condition of the hindquarters in the pig, technically known as Asymmetric Hindquarter Syndrome, or AHQS for short, have been described by J. T. Done and others. This condition has been seen in Germany, Belgium, and Britain.

AHQS, which would appear to have an hereditary basis, could become of economic importance since it affects carcase conformation, and could lead to carcase condemnation.

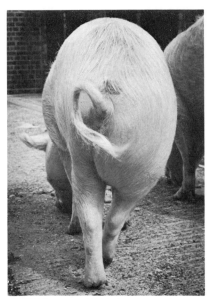

AHQS, asymmetric hindquarter syndrome.

The abnormality does not usually become obvious before pigs reach about 30 kg liveweight, when one thigh may be seen to be much smaller than the other though of the same length. Even in severe cases it was observed that the gait was normal.

The incidence of AHQS within litters of affected families varies from 0 to 80 per cent, and the breeds involved include Large White, Hampshire and Lacombe.

ASYSTOLE means a failure of the heart to contract, generally due to the walls having become so weak that they are unable to contract and expel the blood, with the result that the organ becomes distended – a feature found after death.

ATAXIA means the loss of the power of governing movements, although the necessary power for these movements is still present. A staggering gait results. Ataxia is a symptom which may be observed in many diverse conditions; for example, rabies, weakness or exhaustion; encephalitis; meningitis; poisoning; a brain tumour.

Cattle. A progressive form of ataxia of unknown origin has been found in French-bred Charolais heifers, with symptoms first appearing at 8 to 24 months of age: slight intermittent ataxia to recumbency over 1 to 2 years. Urine is passed in a continuous but uneven squirting flow. When excited affected heifers may show nodding of their heads.

Cats. Ataxia is seen in feline infectious peritonitis, poisoning by ethylene glycol ('anti-freeze') and streptomycin, for example, and before eclampsia (lactation tetany).

Horses. 'Cervical spinal compression continues to be the commonest problem'. (Animal Health Trust, 1983.)

ATHEROMA is a degenerative change in the inner and middle coats of the arteries. (*See* ARTERIES, DISEASES OF.)

ATHEROSCLEROSIS. A degenerative change in the inner lining (*intima*) of arteries, associated with changes in the middle coat also.

ATLAS is the name given to the first of the cervical vertebrae, which forms a double pivot joint with the occipital bone of the base of the skull on the one hand, and forms a single gliding pivot joint with the epistropheus – the second cervical vertebra – on the other hand. The freedom of movement of the head is due almost solely to these two joints.

ATONY means want of tone or vigour in muscles or other organs. (*See* TONICS.)

ATOPIC DISEASE. A hypersensitivity to pollens and other inhaled protein particles. (*See* ALLERGY.) Hay-fever-like symptoms may be produced in the dog; also intense itching affecting the feet, abdomen, and face. As well as sneezing, conjunctivitis, rhinitis and asthma, there may be some discoloration of the coat. In allergy tests on 208 dogs, about 40 per cent were found to be hypersensitive to human dandruff.

Atopic disease also occurs in cats and cattle (*see* BOVINE ATOPIC RHINITIS).

ATOXYL, or SODIUM ARSANILATE, is a white powder constituting an organic preparation of arsenic. It is used by intramuscular and intravenous injection for treatment of certain diseases due to the presence of trypanosomes in the blood. (*See also under* ADDITIVES.)

ATRESIA means the absence of a natural opening, or its obliteration by membrane. Atresia of the rectum is found in newly-born pigs, lambs, calves, and foals. Atresia is sometimes met with in the vaginae of heifers, when it constitutes that is known as 'white heifer disease'. (*See* WHITE HEIFER DISEASE.)

ATRIAL. Relating to the atrium or AURICLE (which see) of the heart.

ATROPHIC MYOSITIS (*see under* MUSCLES, DISEASES OF).

ATROPHIC RHINITIS. A disease of pigs. (*See under* RHINITIS.)

ATROPHY is a wasting of the tissues.

Following paralysis of a motor nerve, when the muscles supplied by it are no longer able to contract, atrophy of the area takes place. This is seen in paralysis of the radial nerve. (Cf. HYPERTROPHY.)

ATROPINE is the alkaloid contained in the leaves and root of the deadly nightshade (Atropa belladonna). Preparations of belladonna owe their actions to the presence of atropine, and are active in such proportions as the percentage of the alkaloid varies. It depresses sensory nerve-endings and thus relieves pain and spasm in parts to which it is applied. It checks secretion in all the glands of the body when given internally; and whether given by the mouth or rubbed on the skin it causes a dilatation of the pupil of the eye and paralysis of accommodation. In large doses it induces a general stimulation of the nervous system, but this action is rapidly followed by depression, and the primary effect is not noticed in the administration of ordinary doses. The action on the heart is one of stimulation, since the inhibition fibres are paralysed, while the accelerator nerves are not interfered with, except when large doses are given and paralysis of all motor fibres occurs.
USES. Atropine is the antidote to morphine poisoning, when it is given as the sulphate of atropine by hypodermic injection, and also to some of the organo-phosphorus compounds used as farm sprays. Atropine is also used to dilate the pupil in order to facilitate eye examinations, and to diminish secretions.

ATROPINE POISONING may occur as the result of the unintentional administration of too large amounts of the alkaloid or of the drug belladonna in one form or another, or it may be induced by feeding on the plant growing wild, and it may happen that after the application of a belladonna liniment or plaster the drug is absorbed into the circulation, or the animal may lick the area, and toxic symptoms result. (*See* BELLADONNA.)

The signs of poisoning shown are restlessness, delirium, dryness of the mouth, a rapid and weak pulse, quick, short respirations, an increase in temperature, and dilatation of the pupil. In addition there is sometimes seen a loss of power in the hind-limbs.
ANTIDOTES. To those animals that vomit, an emetic should be given at once if the poison has been taken by the mouth. Horses and cattle should have their stomachs emptied by the passage of the stomach-tube, in so far as that is possible. Stimulants such as ammonia should be given, and pilocarpine, by hypodermic injection, is the physiological antidote.

ATTENUATED (*see under* VACCINE).

AUDITORY NERVE, or ACOUSTIC NERVE, is the 8th of the cranial nerves, and is concerned with the special sense of hearing. It arises from the base of the hind-brain just behind and at the side of the pons. It is distributed to the middle and internal ears, and in addition to its acoustic function it is also concerned with the balance of the body. (*See* EAR.)

AUJESZKY'S DISEASE. Also known as Pseudo-rabies and Infectious Bulbar Paralysis, occurs in cattle, pigs, dogs, cats, and rats, and is caused by a virus. The disease has a very short incubation period, and is characterised by intense itching. It was first described in Hungary by Aujeszky in 1902, is not very common in the UK; and has been encountered in several parts of the USA, South America, Australia, the continent of Europe, etc. In the UK the disease is NOTIFIABLE. and an eradication campaign began in 1983. The infection may be windborne.
SIGNS.

Cattle. The first symptom to be observed is usually a persistent licking, rubbing or scratching of part of the hindquarters (or sometimes of the face) in an attempt to relieve the intense itching. The affected part soon becomes denuded of hair, and may be bitten and rubbed until it bleeds. Bellowing, salivation, and stamping with the hind-feet may be observed. Within 24 hours the animal is usually recumbent and unable to rise on account of paralysis. Death, preceded by convulsions, usually occurs within 36 to 48 hours of the onset of symptoms.

Goats. An outbreak recorded in Holland by C. H. Herweijer and colleagues resulted in the death of 13 out of 15 goats housed for a time with 40 pigs. One pig died, the remainder showing only loss of appetite and dullness for a couple of days. Some of the in-contact goats died without preliminary symptoms being observed; others were restless, sweated profusely, uttered cries, and had convulsions and paralysis. Pruritus was *not* a feature. Virus was isolated from the central nervous system of both the two goats subjected to autopsy. (Herweijer, C. H. and Jonge, W. K. De (1977). *Tijdschr. Diergeneesk.* **102**, 425.)

Pigs. In these animals the disease runs a milder course, with a mortality of 5 per cent or less. Signs may include, besides some evidence of pruritus, loss of appetite, vomiting, diarrhoea, convulsions, drooling of saliva, paralysis of the throat. Mummification of the fetuses may occur in pregnant sows affected with Aujeszky's disease. Such sows may show loss of appetite and constipation, or stiffness and muscular inco-ordination without itching at all. For the screening of pig serum samples, the ELISA test was found to be the most sensitive, speediest and cheapest of four methods for detecting antibodies to Aujeszky's disease virus. (Central Veterinary Laboratory.)

Prevention: Working with 10-week-old pigs, De Leeuw and Oirschot showed that intranasal vaccination with attenuated virus was more effective than parenteral vaccination with inactivated virus, as maternally derived antibodies interfered with the latter. (De Leeuw, P. W. & Van Oirschot, J. T. (1985) *Research in Vet. Sci.* **39**, 34.)

A vaccine is available (RMB Animal Health), and field trials involving over a million pigs are being (1991) conducted by Upjohn on the Continent.

Dogs and cats. Restlessness, loss of appetite, vomiting, salivation, signs of intense irritation (leading to biting or scratching) about the face or some other part, and occasionally moaning, groaning, or high-pitched screams are among the symptoms observed.

In one outbreak, 11 out of a pack of 51 harrier hounds died of the disease (apparently as a result of being fed raw carcase meat from a large pig unit). The characteristic skin irritation was shown by only four hounds. (R. Gore *et al.*, *Vet. Rec.* (1977) **101**, 93.)

The disease often occurs in the animals named above following an outbreak among rats, and may be spread by rat-bites. Cattle are often infected by pigs. Dogs have died after eating meat from carcases of cattle dead from Aujeszky's disease. Recent work has suggested that the rat may be an incidental rather than a reservoir host of the virus, and less important in the spread of the disease than was previously thought.

Poultry. About 10,000 out of a batch of 49,000 chicks died after being inoculated at one day old with a Marek's disease vaccine. 'It seems that Aujeszky's disease vaccine virus adapted to chicken cells was likely to have been the cause.' (B. Kouwenhoven and others, *Veterinary Quarterly* (1982), **4**, 145.)

Horses. The virus was isolated from the brain of a horse after showing the following signs: excessive sweating, muscle tremors, and 'periods of mania.' (Kinman, T.G. & others, *Veterinary Record* (1991) **128**, 103.)

Public health. Aujeszky's disease virus can infect people, but it seems that only laboratory workers, as opposed to pigmen, are likely to find this a health hazard.

AURAL. Relating to the ear.

AURAL CARTILAGES are the supporting structures of the ears. There are three chief cartilages in most animals, viz, the *conchal*, which gathers the sound waves and transmits them downwards into the cavity of the ear and gives the ear its characteristic shape; the *annular*, a cartilaginous ring below the former which is continuous internally with the bony acoustic canal; the *scutiform*, a small quadrilateral plate which lies in front of the others and serves for the attachment of muscles which move the ear.

Accidents and diseases of the cartilages of the ear are not common in animals, with the exception of dog/cat fights. Ulceration of the cartilages, chiefly the annular, occurs as a complication of ear inflammation in the dog. Laceration of the conchal cartilage is seen as the result of the application of a twitch to the ear in the horse.

AURICLE, or ATRIUM. The auricles, right and left, are the chambers at the base of the heart which receive the blood from the body generally, and from the lungs respectively. Opening into the right auricle are the cranial and caudal vena cavae, which carry the venous blood that has been circulating in the head and neck and the abdomen and thorax. This blood is pumped into the right ventricle through the tricuspid valve. Opening into the left auricle are the pulmonary veins which bring the arterial blood that has been purified in the lungs; when this auricle contracts the blood is driven into the left ventricle through the mitral valve. (*See* HEART, CIRCULATION.)

AUSCULTATION is a method of diagnosis by which the condition of some of the internal organs is determined by listening to the sounds they produce. Auscultation is practised by means of the stethoscope.

AUTOGENOUS means self-generated, and is the term applied especially to bacterial vaccines manufactured from the organisms found in discharges from the body and used for the treatment of the particular individual from which the bacteria were derived.

AUTO-IMMUNE DISEASE is due to a defect or failure of the bodily defence mechanisms in which antibodies become active against some of the host's own cells. An example is spontaneous auto-immune thyroiditis which occurs in dogs, poultry, monkeys and rats, and resembles Hashimoto's thyroiditis of man. Another example is auto-immune haemolytic disease, in which the blood's red cells are affected.

Auto-antibodies can be produced at any time by any individual, but in most they are eliminated by suppressor cells. However, auto-antibodies may persist if there is abnormal B-cell activation, or T-cell dysfunction.

Immune-mediate diseases are of two kinds: (1) *Primary*, an auto-immune reaction only against self; and (2) *secondary*, a similar reaction occurring when viruses, tumours, parasites, or drugs are involved.

Primary diseases are either organ-specific, *e.g.* auto-immune haemolytic anaemia, or systemic, *e.g.* lupus erythematosus. (Tony Venn, *Veterinary Times*). (*See* those two diseases, *also* THROMBO-CYTOPENIA, POLYARTHRITIS, PEMPHIGUS.) (*See also* BOVINE and CANINE AUTOIMMUNE HAEMOLYTIC ANAEMIA, DIABETES MELLITUS, LUPUS.)

AUTO-INFECTION. Infection of one part of the body, hitherto healthy, from another part that already is suffering from the disease. Thus, sheep suffering from 'orf' on their feet may bite the painful areas and convey the organisms to their mouth, where the disease becomes established.

AUTOLYSIS. Self-digestion.

AUTONOMIC NERVOUS SYSTEM is that part of the nervous system which governs the automatic or non-voluntary processes, such as the beating of the heart, movements of the intestines, secretions from various glands, etc. It is usually regarded as composed of two distinct but complementary portions: the *parasympathetic* and the *sympathetic* systems.

Organ	Stimulation by chemical or other means of	
	Parasympathetic	Sympathetic
Pupil	Contracts	Dilates
Heart	Slows	Accelerates
Salivary glands	Thin watery secretion	Thick glairy secretion
Stomach and Intestines	Causes movement	Inhibits movement
Pyloric, anal, and ileocaecal	No action	Causes constriction
Bladder	Contracts	Relaxes
Bronchial muscles	Causes contraction	Causes relaxation
Gastrointestinal and bronchial glands	Produces secretion	No action
Sweat glands	No action	Causes secretion

The parasympathetic system is composed of a central portion comprising certain fibres present in the following cranial nerves: Oculomotor, Facial and Glossopharyngeal; and the whole of the outgoing (efferent) nerves in the important Vagus nerve. There is also a sacral set of autonomic nerve fibres present in the ventral roots of some of the sacral nerves.

The sympathetic system is composed of nerve fibres present in the ventral roots of the spinal nerves lying between the cervical and lumbar regions.

The two systems are mutually antagonistic in that stimulation of each produces opposite effects. These effects are shown in the form of the now classic table.

Under normal circumstances there is a harmony preserved between the working of the two systems, which are flexible enough to provide for the ordinary exigencies of life.

AUTONOMIC POLYGANGLIONOPATHY (*see* KEY–GASKELL SYNDRONE).

AUTOPSY (from the Greek, seeing with one's own eyes) is the examination of the internal structures of the body performed after death. From a *post-mortem* examination much valuable information can be learned, especially when there has been doubt about the disease condition during life. It has been said that it is 'unfair to the living animals, as well as a handicap to the progress of veterinary science, for owners to prohibit an autopsy because of sentiment'.

An autopsy is obligatory where notifiable diseases, *e.g.* rabies, are involved, so that laboratory tests may be carried out to confirm or establish diagnosis. In the case of rabies, gloves and goggles must be worn, and every precaution taken, by the person carrying out the autopsy. With other communicable diseases (*see* ZOONOSES) similar precautions are necessary.

Valuable information can be obtained in slaughter-houses as to the extent of a disease, such as liver-fluke infestation in cattle and sheep, over a region or indeed throughout a whole country; and if suitably recorded and collated, the information can indicate the economic importance of diseases in farm animals and so lead to disease-control measures being taken as part of a regional or national campaign.

See under WOOL BALLS for an example of a layman's misinterpretation of *post mortem* findings.

AUTOSOMES are the chromosomes present in the nuclei of cells other than the sex-chromosomes. They are of the same type in both sexes in each species of animal, whereas the sex-chromosomes of the female are different from those of the male. (*See* CYTOGENETICS.)

AUTUMN FLY (*Musca autumnalis*). This is a non-biting fly which is a serious pest of grazing farm live-stock in the UK and elsewhere. They cause cattle to huddle together and to cease feeding. Large numbers may collect on the upper part of the body, feeding on secretions from nose, mouth, eyes and on discharges from any wounds. (*See* FLY CONTROL.)

AUXINS. Plant hormones. These include oestrogens in pasture plants.

AVERMECTINS. A group of chemical compounds, derived from a fungus discovered in Japan in 1975, effective in very low dosage against nematode parasites and also against external parasites. (*See* IVERMECTIN, which is the most useful of the group). The discovery of the fungus in a soil sample was part of Merck Sharp & Dohme's international screening programme.

Technically, the avermectins are a series of macrocyclic lactone derivatives produced by fermentation of the actinomycete *Streptomyces avermitilis*.

AVEYRON DISEASE (of sheep). (*See* BOVINE VIRUS DIARRHOEA.)

AVIAN CONTAGIOUS EPITHELIOMA (*see under* FOWL-POX).

AVIAN INFECTIOUS ENCEPHALOMYELITIS.
A disease of chicks and turkey poults.
CAUSE. A picornavirus. (Infection via the egg, as well as bird to bird.)
SIGNS. Leg weakness, followed by partial or complete paralysis of the legs. The chicks struggle to balance with the help of their wings. Trembling of the head and neck occurs in some cases.
DIAGNOSIS. An ELISA test.
MORTALITY. A 40 per cent rate is not unusual.
PREVENTION. Vaccination has proved very successful.

AVIAN INFECTIOUS LARYNGOTRACHEITIS
of poultry is caused by a Herpes virus, prevalent in NW England. Loss of appetite, sneezing and coughing, a discharge from the eyes, difficulty in breathing are the main symptoms. Birds of all ages are susceptible. Mortality averages about 15 per cent. No treatment is of value. Control is best achieved by depopulation and fumigation. A vaccine has been used.

AVIAN INFLUENZA (Fowl Plague) attacks domesticated fowl chiefly, but turkeys, geese, ducks, and most of the common wild birds, are sometimes affected. It is not known to affect the pigeon. The disease is found in Asia, Africa, the Americas and to a lesser extent in parts of the continent of Europe, and is always liable to be introduced to countries hitherto free from it through the migrations of wild birds. An outbreak occurred among turkeys in Norfolk in 1963. This was the first recorded outbreak in Britain since 1929. An outbreak occurred in the Republic of Ireland in 1983; a slaughter policy followed. Infection may have come from Pennsylvania, where a similar policy was adopted.
CAUSE. *Myxovirus influenzae.*
SIGNS. In some cases the number attacked is small, while on the same premises the next year 80 or 90 per cent of the total inhabitants of the runs die. The affected birds often die quite suddenly. In other instances the sick birds isolate themselves from the rest of the flock, preferring some dark out-of-the-way corner where they will be undisturbed. They are dull, disinclined to move, the tail and wings droop, the eyes are kept closed; the bird may squat on its breast with its head tucked under a wing or in amongst the shoulder feathers; food is refused, but thirst is often shown; the respirations are fast and laboured but not impeded by mucus; the temperature is very high at the commencement (110° to 112°), but falls shortly before death to below normal. (The normal temperature of birds is 106·5°F.) The comb and wattles become purple or blue, and oedema of the head and neck is common. The illness seldom lasts more than 24 to 36 hours, and often not more than 6.
CONTROL. Vaccines may be used.

AVIAN LISTERIOSIS. An infectious disease of poultry, occurring as an epidemic among young stock (often as an accompaniment of other diseases) or sporadically among adults.
CAUSE. *Listeria monocytogenes,* a Gram-positive motile rod-shaped organism.
SIGNS. In the epidemic type wasting occurs over a period of days or even weeks. For 48 hours before death birds refuse all food.
The sporadic type is characterised by sudden death without much loss of condition.
DIAGNOSIS. Depends upon bacteriological methods. (*See also* LISTERIOSIS.)

AVIAN LYMPHOID LEUKOSIS virus (L L V) infection is widespread among chickens in the UK, and causes mortality from tumours.
This disease, which has to be differentiated from Marek's disease, affects birds of 4 months upwards, is egg-transmitted, and is characterised by leukaemia, or cancer involving the liver and other organs.
Congenital infection occurs in the oviduct, and swabs can be tested for the presence of the virus; thereby identifying hens likely to transmit the infection to their progeny. The A F R C has found that it is possible to eliminate L L V from a commercial strain within two generations by this means.

AVIAN MALARIA (*see* PLASMODIUM).

AVIAN MONOCYTOSIS (*see* 'PULLET DISEASE').

AVIAN NEPHRITIS. 'This is a new problem in the UK,' stated the AFRC in 1988. They added that many commercial poultry and turkey flocks have antibodies to avian nephritis virus (ANV).
In chick embryos the latter causes stunting, haemorrhage, oedema – besides the nephritis.

AVIAN SEX DETERMINATION, by laparoscopy, has been widely used since 1976. Details of the technique will be found in the *Veterinary Record* (1983), **112,** 105.

AVIAN TUBERCULOSIS. TB was prevalent on general farms where birds were kept for several years, but is less so on the modern specialist poultry farm, where birds are seldom kept for more than 2 years.
However, avian TB does sometimes affect birds less than one year old and kept under good conditions.
CAUSE. *Mycobacterium tuberculosis* (avian).
SIGNS. Dullness, loss of appetite, a disinclination to move, and a tendency to squat on the breast with the head tucked under one wing.
Body temperature may reach 112°F (i.e. 6° above normal).
The comb and wattles become almost purple, and oedema of the head and neck is common.
Cattle. Avian tuberculosis rarely causes progressive disease, but quite commonly one or two lymph nodes become infected, and this will affect the interpretation of the tuberculin test. (*See* the COMPARATIVE TEST.)

Infection occurs following ingestion of food and water contaminated by the droppings of affected birds. Young birds are susceptible, but the disease is slow in progression. The comb and wattles become pale, and flesh is lost rapidly, the sternal muscles in some cases almost disappearing. Lameness is sometimes noticed. Inappetence may be seen, but other birds feed well till near the end, many being affected with diarrhoea.

POST-MORTEM. Emaciation is usually well marked, and whitish yellow nodules are present in the liver and spleen; also the intestines. The lungs are rarely affected in avian tuberculosis. In birds which have died suddenly death is often found to be due to rupture of the liver, which when affected with tuberculosis is often enlarged and friable.

With valuable pedigree birds the intradermal tuberculin test may be employed, but before applying this test all birds should be examined and all thin birds destroyed, since those in the advanced stages of the disease may fail to react. Birds which pass the test should be put in clean houses on fresh ground.

(*See* DISPOSAL OF CARCASES.)

'AVICALM'. A proprietary water-soluble tranquilliser for poultry based on Metoserpate hydrochloride. It is recommended for use before catching, handling or crating of birds, and is given in the drinking water.

AVITAMINOSIS is a term used to describe conditions produced by a deficiency or lack of a vitamin in the food. Thus 'avitaminosis A' means a deficiency of vitamin A. (*See* VITAMINS.)

AVOCADA POISONING in birds. (*See* CAGE BIRDS.)

AVOCADO LEAVES. *Persea americana* fed to goats and sheep, during a drought in South Africa, caused death within a few days from heart disease.

AWNS/GRASS SEEDS. A review by Kathleen E. Brennan and Peter J. Ihrke, School of Veterinary Medicine, University of California, of 182 cases in dogs and cats over a one-year period showed that grass awns comprised 61 per cent of all foreign body cases. The most common site is the ear canal (51 per cent), and rupture of the tympanum has been an occasional sequel. Other sites are the interdigital skin, conjunctiva, nose, lumbar region. Lumbar osteomyelitis has been caused. Perforation of a bronchus led to necrosis of a lung lobe. In a cat with chronic cystitis, two awns were found in the bladder; and in another cat several awns were found at autopsy to have caused peritonitis. (*JAVMA* (1983), **182,** 1201.)

AXILLA is the anatomical name for the region between the humerus and the chest wall, which corresponds to the arm pit in the human being.

AXON (*see* NERVES).

AZOTAEMIA. The presence of urea and other nitrogenous products in greater concentration than normal in the blood.

AZOTURIA (*see* EQUINE MYOGLOBINURIA).

B

B. CELLS. One of the two types of lymphocytes. They are important in the provision of immunity, and they respond to antigens by dividing and becoming plasma cells that can produce antibody that will bind with the antigen. Their source is the bone marrow. It is believed that the function of B. cells is assisted by a substance provided by T. CELLS (which see). With HAPTENS (which see) it is apparently the B. cells which recognise the protein carrier, and the T. cells which recognise the hapten. (*See also* LYMPHOCYTES, IMMUNE RESPONSE.)

B. VIRUS. This is a virus of the Herpes type, which gives rise in Man to a rare disease with an almost 100 per cent mortality. It may be transmitted to Man from monkeys – especially newly-imported Rhesus and Cynomolgus monkeys. Lesions on the face and lips of monkeys should arouse suspicion of this condition.

It is believed that B. virus, Herpes virus, and Aujeszky's disease virus have a common origin.

BABESIA is another name for piroplasm, one of the protozoan parasites belonging to the order Haemosporidia.

These are generally relatively large parasites within the red blood cells and are pear-shaped, round, or oval. Multiplication is by division into two or by budding. Infected cells frequently have two pyriform parasites joined at their pointed ends. Sexual multiplication takes place in the tick.

Babesiosis (Piroplasmosis). Nearly all the domestic mammals suffer from infection with some species of *Babesia*; sometimes more than one species may be present. The general symptoms are the appearance of fever in 8 to 10 days after infection, accompanied by haemoglobinuria, icterus, and, unless treated, 25 to 100 per cent of the cases are fatal. Red blood cells may be reduced in number by two-thirds. Convalescence is slow and animals may remain 'salted' for three to eight years.

TRANSMISSION. Development occurs in certain ticks which transmit the agent to their offspring. The various species are similar, but are specific to their various hosts. The ticks should probably be regarded as the true or definite hosts, while the mammal is the intermediate host. The following species are important:

B. divergens	British and European red-water in cattle.
B. major	(in Britain, but less pathogenic than *B. divergens.*)
B. bovis	(in Europe, South America, Africa, Australia and Asia.)
B. bigemina	Texas fever in cattle (not confined to America).
B. motasi	in sheep.
B. ovis	in sheep.
B. canis	Malignant jaundice in dogs.
B. gibsoni	in dogs.
B. vitalii	in dogs.
B. caballi	Biliary fever in horses.
B. equi	Biliary fever in horses.
B. felis	in cats.

Cattle. Babesiosis in cattle is due to:
(*a*) *B. divergens* and *B. major*, causing British Red-water.
(*b*) *B. bigemina*, causing Texas Fever.
(*See* RED-WATER and TEXAS FEVER.)

Sheep. Ovine babesiosis may be due to at least three species of *Babesia*. There is a relatively large form, *Babesia motasi*, which is comparable to *B. bigemina* of cattle, and which produces a disease, often severe, with high temperatures, much blood-cell destruction, icterus, and haemoglobinuria. This is the 'carceag' of Eastern and Southern Europe. The second parasite, of intermediate size and corresponding to *B. bovis* of cattle, is *Babesia ovis*. It produces a much milder disease with fever, jaundice, and anaemia, but recoveries generally occur. The small species is *Theileria ovis*, which appears to be similar to *T. mutans* of cattle, and is relatively harmless to its host.

B. motasi, *B. ovis*, and *T. ovis* are all transmitted by *Rhipicephalus bursa*.

Animals recovered from *T. ovis* infection apparently develop a permanent and sterile immunity. The disease occurs in Europe, Africa, Asia, and North America.

SIGNS. In acute cases the temperature may rise to 107°F, rumination ceases, there is paralysis of the hindquarters, the urine is brown, and death occurs in about a week. In benign cases there may only be a slight fever for a few days with anaemia.

Babesia

A theileriosis, caused by *T. hirci*, has been described from sheep in Africa and Europe. It causes an emaciation and small haemorrhages in the conjunctiva.

'BABY PIG DISEASE'. The provisional name for a condition associated with a fall in the level of blood sugar within 48 hours of birth. The piglets cease suckling and appear dull. Temperature is subnormal. Artificial rearing is indicated. Otherwise, piglets will die from the condition itself or as a result of overlying by the sow.

The causes are now considered to be: (*a*) failure of sow's milk supply; (*b*) failure – due to haemolytic disease or to one of several infections – of the piglet to suck.

BACILLARY WHITE DIARRHOEA (*see* PULLORUM DISEASE).

BACILLUS. This genus contains many species which are not regarded as pathogenic, and which are found in soil, water, and on plants. Spores formed by bacilli are resistant to heat and disinfectants, and this fact is important in connection with *B. anthracis*, the cause of ANTHRAX. Another pathogenic bacillus is *B. cereus*, a cause of food poisoning and also of bovine mastitis. (*See* BACTERIA.)

BACITRACIN. A feed antibiotic.

BACK-CROSS is the progeny resulting from mating a heterozygote offspring with either of its parental homozygotes. Characters in the backcrosses generally show a 1:1 ratio. Thus if a pure black bull is mated with pure red cows (all homozygous), black calves (heterozygotes) are produced. If the heifer calves are 'back-crossed' to their black father, their progeny will give one pure black to every one impure black. If a black heterozygous son of the original mating is mated to his red mother, the progeny will be one red to one black.

Back-crossing can be employed as a means of test-mating, or test-crossing to determine whether a stock of animals is homozygous, when it will never throw individuals of different type, or whether it is heterozygous, when it will give the two allelomorphic types. (*See* GENETICS AND HEREDITY.)

BACK-FENCE (*see* STRIP-GRAZING).

BACK MUSCLE NECROSIS. A disease of pigs first described in Belgium in 1960, and recognised eight years later in West Germany (where it is colloquially known as 'banana disease'), has recently been recorded in the UK; with 20 cases occurring in a single herd.
SIGNS. R. Bradley, of the Central Veterinary Laboratory, Weybridge, and colleagues, described it as a sudden and sporadic condition affecting pigs weighing over 50 kg. In the acute stage, the animal shows signs of pain, has difficulty in moving, becomes feverish, loses appetite and appears lethargic, and shows a characteristic swelling on one or both sides of the back. When only one side is affected, spinal curvature occurs with the convexity of the curve towards the swollen side.

The colloquial name 'banana disease' apparently arose from arching (as compared with lateral curvature) of the back, and all the cases which a British veterinary surgeon C. W. Furley, working in Germany saw there involved arched backs.

Some pigs die from acidosis and heart failure; some recover, apparently completely; while others are left with atrophy of the affected muscles resulting in a depression in the skin parallel to the spine. Some examples of BMN are discovered only in the slaughterhouse.
POST-MORTEM examination reveals necrosis and bleeding, especially in the *longissimus dorsi* muscle, as well as the widely recognised condition known as PSE or pale soft exudative muscle.
CAUSES. MAFF findings support the view that the disease is associated with stress, and they do not conflict with the German view that heredity also comes into the picture.
(C. W. Furley. *Vet. Record* (1979) **104**, 268.)

BACTERIA. According to peculiarities in shape and in group formation, certain names are applied: thus a single spherical bacterium is known as 'coccus'; organisms in pairs and of the same shape (*i.e.* spherical) are called 'diplococci'; when in the form of a chain they are known as 'streptococci'; when they are bunched together like a bunch of grapes the name 'staphylococcus' is applied. Bacteria in the form of long slender rods are known as 'bacilli', wavy or curved forms have other names.
REPRODUCTION. The mode of multiplication of most bacteria is exceedingly simple, consisting of a splitting into two of a single bacterium. Since the new forms may similarly divide within half an hour, multiplication is rapid. (*See* illustration of *Salmonella dublin* in the act of division.) (*See also under* PLASMIDS.)

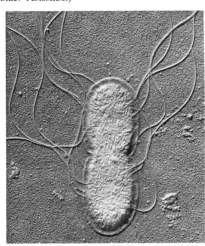

About to divide. *Salmonella dublin* in the process of division into two. Note also the flagellae. (AFRC photomicrograph)

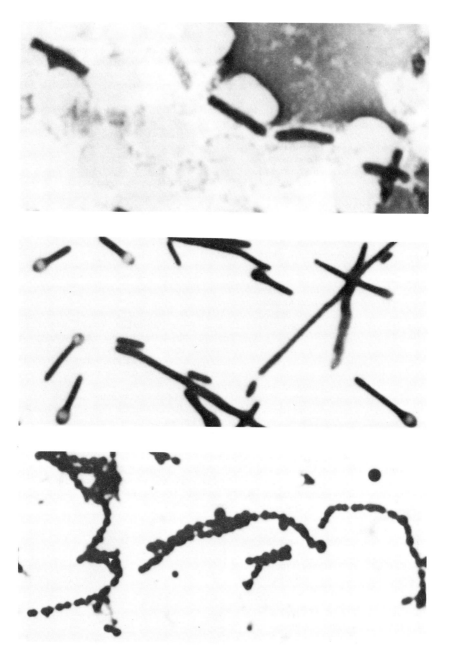

Photomicrographs of (1) *Bacillus anthracis* (×4200); (2) *Clostridium tetani* (×3250) (showing the characteristic drum-stick appearance; (3) *Streptococcus pyogenes* (×3000). (With acknowledgements to Burroughs Wellcome & Co., Veterinary Division).

Some bacteria of veterinary importance

Name	Associated or specific diseased conditions caused
Actinobacillus lignièresi	Actinobacillosis.
Actinomyces bovis	Actinomycosis.
Aeromonas shigelloides	Chronic diarrhoea in cats.
Bacillus anthracis	Anthrax in all susceptible animals.
Bacillus cereus	Bovine mastitis; food poisoning.
Bacillus lichenformis	Abortion in ewes
Bacillus piliformis	Tyzzer's disease.
Bacteroides species (including *Fusiformis*)	Foot infections in horses.
Bordetella bronchiseptica	Complicates distemper in the dog. Kennel cough. Atrophic rhinitis.
Brucella abortus	Brucellosis.
Brucella melitensis	Brucellosis in goats; undulant fever in man (in part).
Campylobacter fetus	Infertility, abortion.
Clostridium botulinum (five types – A to E)	Botulism in man and animals.
Cl. chauvoei	'Black-quarter' (and also pericarditis and meningitis in cattle) in cattle and partly in sheep.
Cl. difficile	Chronic diarrhoea in dogs and piglets.
Cl. novyi (oedematiens)	'Black-quarter' in cattle and pigs in part; 'black disease' in sheep; septicaemia in horses and pigs (wound infection).
Cl. septicum	Gas gangrene in man; black-quarter; braxy in sheep.
Cl. tetani	Tetanus in man and animals.
Cl. welchii (perfringens)	Lamb dysentery; present in many cases of gas gangrene.
Corynebacterium pseudotuberculosis	Caseous lymphadenitis in sheep; some cases of ulcerative lymphangitis and acne in horses.
C. pyogenes	Abscesses in liver, kidneys, lungs, or skin in sheep, cattle, and pigs especially; present as a secondary organism in many suppurative conditions; causes summer mastitis in cattle.
C. equi	A cause of pneumonia in the horse and of tuberculosis-like lesions in the pig.
Dermatophilus congolensis	Chronic dermatitis.
Group EF-4 bacteria	Pneumonia in dogs and cats, and isolated from human dog bite wound.
Erysipelothrix rhusiopathiae	Swine erysipelas.
Eschicheria coli (sub. types are many)	Always present in alimentary canal as commonest organism; becomes pathogenic at times, partly causing enteritis, dysentery (lambs), scour (calves and pigs), cystitis, abortion, mastitis, joint-ill, etc.
Fusiformis necrophorus	Associated with foot-rot; calf diphtheria; quittor, poll evil, and fistulous withers in horses; necrosis of the skin in dogs, pigs, and rabbits; navel ill in calves and lambs; various other conditions in bowel and skin.
F. nodosus	Foot-rot in sheep.
Haemophilus somnus	'Sleeper syndrome' in cattle
H. parainfluenzae *H. parasuis*	Chronic respiratory disease in pigs.
Klebsiella pneumoniae	Metritis in mares; pneumonia in dogs, etc.
Leptospira ictero-haemorrhagiae	Leptospiral jaundice, or enzoötic jaundice of dogs; Weil's disease in man.
Lept. canicola	Canicola fever in man, and nephritis in dogs.
Lept. hardjo	Bovine mastitis.
Listeria monocytogens	Listeriosis.
Mycobacterium johnei	Johne's disease of cattle.
Myc. tuberculosis (bovine, human, and avian types	Tuberculosis in man and animals.
Pasteurella multocida	Fowl cholera, Haemorrhagic septicaemia in cattle.
P. haemolytica	Pneumonia.
P. tularensis	Tularaemia in rodents.
Pseudomonas mallei	Glanders in equines and man.
P. pseudomallei	Melioidosis in rats and man; occasionally in dogs and cats.

(continued overleaf)

Some bacteria of veterinary importance (continued from previous page)

Name	Associated or specific diseases caused
P. aeruginosa	Mastitis in cattle.
P. pyocyanea	Suppuration in wounds, otitis in the dog.
Salmonella abortus equi	Contagious abortion of mares naturally, but capable of causing abortion in pregnant ewes, cows, and sows experimentally.
S. abortus ovis	Contagious abortion of ewes occurring naturally.
S. dublin	Causes enteritis, sometimes abortion. (*See* SALMONELLOSIS.
S. gallinarum	Klein's disease or fowl typhoid.
S. pullorum	Pullorum disease.
S. cholerae suis	Salmonellosis septicaemia in pigs.
S. typhimurium	Salmonellosis
Staphylococcus albus	Suppurative conditions in animals.
Staph. aureus	Suppurative conditions in animals and man, especially wound infections where other pus-producing organisms are also present. Present in various types of abscess, and in pyaemic and septicaemia conditions. Cause of mastitis in cows.
Staph. hyicus	A primary or secondary skin pathogen causing lesions in horses, cattle, and pigs. It may also cause bone and joint lesions.
Staph. pyogenes	Often associated with the other staphylococci in above conditions; causes mastitis in cows.
Streptococcus equi	Strangles in horses, partly responsible for joint-ill in foals, and sterility in mares.
Str. agalactiae	Mastitis in cows.
Str. pyogenes	Many suppurative conditions, wound infections, abscesses, etc.; joint-ill in foals. (In the above conditions various other streptococci are also frequently present.
Treponema hyodysenteriae	Swine dysentery.
Vibrio (*see Campylobacter*.)	
Yersinia enterocolitica	(*see* YERSINIOSIS.)
Y. pseudotuberculosis	(*see* YERSINIOSIS.)
Y. pestis	Plague in man and rats. In an often subclinical form this may also occur in cats and dogs.

For other, non-bacterial infective agents, *see* VIRUSES, RICKETTSIA, MYCOPLASMA, CHLAMYDIA.

SPORE-FORMATION. Some bacteria have the power of protecting themselves from unfavourable conditions by changing their form to that of a more resistant body known as a 'spore'. One bacillus gives rise to one spore.

SIZE. Bacteria vary in size from less than 1 micron (one thousandth of a millimetre) diameter, in the case of streptococci and staphylococci, up to a length of 8 microns, in the case of the anthrax bacillus.

MOBILITY. All bacteria do not possess the power of movement, but if a drop of fluid containing certain forms of organism which are called 'motile' be examined microscopically, it will be observed that they move actively in a definite direction. This is accomplished, in the motile organisms, by means of delicate whip-like processes which thrash backwards and forwards in the fluid and propel the body onwards. These processes are called 'flagella'.

Methods of diagnosis:

(1) MICROSCOPICAL. In order satisfactorily to examine bacteria microscopically a drop of the fluid containing the organisms is spread out in a thin film on a glass slide. The organisms are killed by heating the slide, and the details of their characteristics are made obvious by suitable staining with appropriate dyes. (*See under* separate heading GRAM-NEGATIVE. *See also* ACID-FAST.)

(2) CULTURAL CHARACTERS. By copying the conditions under which a particular bacterium grows naturally, it can be induced to grow artificially, and for this purpose various nutrient substances known as 'media' are used. (*See* CULTURE MEDIUM.)

After a period of incubation on the medium on previously sterilised Petri dishes or in tubes or flasks, the bacteria form masses or colonies, visible to the naked eye.

The appearance of the colony may be sufficient in some instances for identification of the organism.

(3) (*See* LABORATORY TESTS.)

(4) ANIMAL INOCULATION. This may be necessary for positive identification of the organism present in the culture. One or more laboratory animals are inoculated and, after time allowed for lesions to develop or symptoms to

appear, the animal is killed and a *post-mortem* examination made. The organisms recovered from the lesions may be re-examined or re-cultured.

BACTERIAL ADHESIVENESS aids some pathogenic bacteria to adhere to the mucous membrane lining the intestine, and may be an important criterion of virulence. Bacteria which possess this property include *E. coli, Salmonella typhimurium, Mycoplasma pneumoniae,* and *Moraxella bovis.*

Many strains of *E. coli* have a filamentous protein antigen called K88. This enables K88-positive *E. coli* to adhere to piglets' intestinal mucosa and to multiply there. (*See also* K88.)

BACTEROIDES. Species of this anaerobic bacterium, including *B. melaninogenicus,* are now being frequently isolated from equine foot lesions and wounds.

BACTERIOPHAGES are viruses which multiply in and destroy bacteria. Some bacteriophages have a 'tail' resembling a hypodermic syringe with which they attach themselves to bacteria and through which they 'inject' nucleic acid. 'Phages' have been photographed with the aid of the electron microscope. The growth of bacteriophages in bacteria results in the lysis of the latter, and the release of further bacteriophage. Phage-typing is a technique used for the identification of certain bacteria. Individual bacteriophages are mostly lethal only to a single bacterial species.

BACTERIOSTATIC. An agent which inhibits the growth of micro-organisms, as opposed to killing them.

BACULOVIRUSES. (*See under* CATERPILLARS.)

BADGERS. Tuberculosis in badgers caused by *Myobacterium bovis* was first described in Switzerland in 1957, and in England in 1971. Transmission of the infection to cattle led to their reinfection in the south-west of England mainly. Badgers are now regarded as a significant reservoir of *M. bovis* infection.

Piroplasmosis also occurs in badgers, which are of veterinary interest too in connection with rabies.

BAKERY WASTE. This must be regarded as a form of swill, since it may contain sausage and other meat. An outbreak of Swine Vesicular Disease in Scotland was attributed to it.

BALANITIS (*see* PENIS, ABNORMALITIES OF).

BALANTIDIUM. A ciliated, protozoan parasite. *Balantidium coli* is a ciliate which often occurs in the pig's intestines, where usually it produces no damage. Occasionally, however, in pigs that are debilitated for other reasons it causes a low-grade dysentery. It is pear-shaped about 80μ long by 60μ broad, and possesses a large sausage-shaped nucleus.

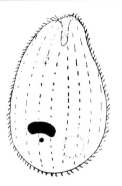

Balantidium coli.

BALD areas (*see* ALOPECIA).

'BALDY CALF SYNDROME'. A lethal disease, causing progressive loss of weight or failure to grow, in the descendants of a Canadian Holstein in Australia. (T. F. Jubb and others, *Australian Veterinary Journal* (1990) **67,** 16, who suggest that INHERITED EPIDERMAL DYSPLASIA would be a better name, and that a single autosomal recessive gene is involved.)

BALING WIRE. Discarded pieces of this are often eaten by cattle and give rise to traumatic pericarditis. (*See under* HEART DISEASES.)

BALLOTTEMENT. A technique of clinical examination in which the movement of any body or organ, suspended in a fluid, is detected.

'BANANA DISEASE' of pigs (*see* BACK MUSCLE NECROSIS).

BANDAGES and BANDAGING. The application of bandages to veterinary patients is much more difficult than in human practice, because not only must the bandage remain in position during the movement of the patient, but it must also be comfortable, or it will be removed by the teeth or feet, and it must be so adjusted that it will not become contaminated by either urine or the faeces.

Wounds often heal more readily if left uncovered, but bandaging may be necessary to give protection against flies and the infective agents which these carry. Much will depend upon the

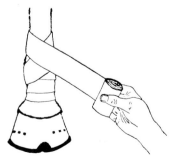

'Figure-of-eight' bandage (roller) for fetlock, also known as a 'spica'.

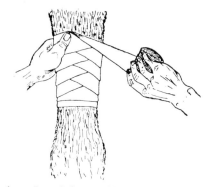

Ascending spiral-reversed bandage for fore-arm.

site of the wound, its nature, and the environment of the animal.

Bandages may be needed for support, and to reduce tension on the skin.

BARBITURATES are derivatives of barbituric acid (malonyl-urea). They include a wide range of very valuable sedative, hypnotic or anaesthetic agents. Several are used in veterinary practice, including Nembutal (pentobarbitone) and Luminal (phenobarbitone), and thiopentone.

In case of barbiturate poisoning, use a stomach tube, keep the animal warm, give picrotoxin, or leptazol, or strong coffee, caffeine.

(*See also under* EUTHANASIA, HORSE-MEAT.)

BARIUM POISONING sometimes takes place through the ingestion of rat-poison, which is frequently prepared with the chloride of barium as its active toxic agent.

The symptoms are excessive salivation, sweating (except in the dog), muscular convulsions, violent straining, palpitation of the heart, and finally general paralysis.
TREATMENT. As soon as the cause is established the stomach contents should be evacuated, either by inducing vomiting, or by means of the stomach-pump.

Doses of Epsom salts given by the mouth in a water solution act as antidotes by converting the chloride into the insoluble sulphate of barium, and the administration of demulcent fluids, such as milk, barley-water, white of egg, etc., should follow. Anaesthesia may be needed.

BARIUM SULPHATE being opaque to X-rays, is given by the mouth prior to a radiographic examination for diagnostic purposes. (*See* X-RAYS.)

BARIUM SULPHIDE is sometimes used as a depilatory for the site of surgical operations.

BARK. A change in the tone of a dog's bark occurs in many cases of rabies.

BARK EATING by cattle should be regarded as a symptom of a mineral deficiency, *e.g.* manganese and phosphorus. The remedy is use of an appropriate mineral supplement.

BARLEY POISONING. As with wheat (and to a much less extent, oats) an excess of barley can kill cattle and sheep not gradually accustomed to it.

During the severe weather of early 1963 trouble of this kind was experienced in several Pembrokeshire flocks fed in various ways, *e.g.* crushed barley 80 per cent, oats 20 per cent, with cake and hay; whole barley and hay; crushed barley and turnips. Owing to the continued hard frost there was no access to grass. In the first 2 types of feed, deaths occurred about the 10th day after commencement of the diet. In the third, deaths were seen on the 4th day. It was noted that the greedy feeders were the first to be affected. Symptoms comprised staggering and blindness, with subnormal or normal temperatures. This was followed in 24 to 48 hours by recumbency, and finally coma and death. A profuse yellowish diarrhoea was present. Milder cases recovered when the barley ration was discontinued. The flock mortality varied from 5 to 20 per cent.

Similar symptoms, with dullness and loss of appetite have been seen in young cattle the day after *ad lib.* feeding of an 85 per cent barley ration began, with deaths following in about 18 per cent of those affected.

The sudden introduction of cereal feeding is known to give rise to acidity in the rumen, and to acetonaemia. It has been suggested also that very acid conditions in the rumen may damage the lining mucous membrane, allowing bacteria to enter the blood-stream and reach the liver, injuring this.

Work at the Rowett Research Institute has shown that, even when cattle are adapted to complete cereal feeding, some problems remain, *e.g.* lesions on the rumen wall characterised by clumped papillae. In these, animal and vegetable hairs become trapped and some may penetrate, causing inflammation of the wall of the rumen – and also liver abscesses. (*AFRC Research Review* 1976 **2**, 37).

It is important that barley should not be fed in a fine, powdery form. To do so is to invite severe digestive upsets, which may lead to death. Especially if ventilation is poor, dusty food also contributes to coughing and may increase the risk of pneumonia. (*See also under* BEEF FROM BARLEY, MOULDY FOOD.)

'BARN ITCH'. The American name for sarcoptic mange in cattle.

BARRIER CREAM. A protective dressing for the hands and arms of veterinarians engaged in obstetrical work or rectal examinations.

BARROW. A castrated male pig.

BARS OF FOOT. At each of the heels of the horse's foot the wall turns inwards and forwards instead of ending abruptly. These 'reflected' portions are called the bars of the foot. They serve to strengthen the heels; they provide a gradual rather than an abrupt finish to the important wall; and they take a share in the formation of the bearing surface, on which rests the shoe.

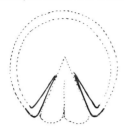

Diagram of the position of the bars of the horse's foot. The dotted line shows the outline of the wall and frog.

The bars are sometimes cut away by smiths or others, who hold the erroneous idea that by so doing they allow the heels of the foot to expand; what actually happens in such instances is that the union between the component parts of the foot is destroyed, and the resistance to contraction which they afford is lost. They should therefore be allowed to grow and maintain their natural prominence.

BARTONELLOSIS. Infection with *Bartonella* organisms, which occasionally occurs in dogs and cattle but is of most importance in laboratory rats. Symptoms are mainly those of anaemia.
TREATMENT. Neoarsphenamine has been used.

BASIC SLAG has caused poisoning in lambs, which should not be allowed access to treated fields until the slag has been well washed in to the soil. Adult sheep have also been poisoned in this way, scouring badly, and so have cattle. In these animals the symptoms include: dullness, reluctance to move, inappetence, grinding of the teeth, and profuse watery black faeces.

BASOPHIL. A type of white blood-cell. (*See under* BLOOD.)

BASOPHILIC. Blue-staining.

BATHS. Bathing of animals may be undertaken for the sake of cleanliness, for the cure of a parasitic skin disease, or for the reduction of the temperature.
Cattle, sheep (*see* DIPS AND DIPPING).
Dogs. For ordinary purposes the dog is bathed in warm water to which a pinch of soda has been added (about a dessert-spoonful to 2 gallons) contained in a tin or wooden bath. It is bad practice to bath the dog in human bath or in a sink, for obvious reasons. It is necessary to add derris, or a proprietary preparation containing BHC, to the water to ensure the destruction of fleas, lice, etc. The dog is firstly thoroughly soaked in the water (which should be about blood-heat) and then lathered with hard toilet soap. (Soft soap contains a certain amount of free alkali, and is apt to blister the more delicate parts of the skin.)
Dish-washing detergent liquid should not be used for shampooing puppies or even adult dogs. (*See* ETHANOL POISONING.) Hard toilet soap is suitable.
Cats. Because cats are fastidious creatures

which wash themselves nearly all over (they cannot reach the back of their necks or between their shoulder blades), the question of bathing them does not arise except in cases of a severe infestation with external parasites; very old cats which have ceased to wash themselves; entire tom cats which as a result of stress or illness have also ceased to look after themselves; as a first-aid treatment for heat stroke/stress; and in some cases where a cat has fallen into a noxious liquid.
Shampoos/flea-killers, etc., sold for use on dogs are not all safe for cats. Owners should read the small print on packets and look for 'Safe for cats' where a preparation has not been prescribed by a veterinary surgeon.

BATS (*see* RABIES, VAMPIRE BATS, HISTOPLASMOSIS). Bats are mammals, and usually produce one offspring in late spring or early summer. Fifteen species have been identified in Britain, where they are classified as protected creatures under the Wildlife & Countryside Act (1981). Their body temperature may vary by 15°C over a 24-hour period. They live up to 30 years. (Andrew Routh, *Veterinary Record* (1991) **128**, 316.)

BATTERY SYSTEM. A method of keeping pullets in cages; one, two, or even three birds per cage. Feeding and watering may be on the 'cafeteria' system, with food containers moving on an endless belt, electrically driven. Advantages: ease of culling, since it is easy to see which birds are laying well; labour-saving. Disadvantages: high capital cost, an unnatural system which is not much used for breeding stock.
The practice of keeping two or three birds in one cage, where they can hardly move, has been deplored by the BVA. 'If cannibalism occurs, the victim cannot escape.'
Caged hens show a strong preference for cages which have a large vertical space allowance. When filmed in cages with unrestricted headroom, nearly 25 per cent of hens' head movements occurred above 40 cm.
An EC Directive provides for a minimum space allowance of 450 sq cm per bird. (UK favoured a minimum of 600 sq cm). Applies to new cages from 1988 and for existing cages after 1995.
A space allowance of 450 sq cm per bird in battery cages 'is acceptable by the UK only as a first step towards more generous welfare provisions.' (Moss, R. (1986) MAFF.)
'Cage Layer Fatigue', a form of leg paralysis, is sometimes encountered in battery birds. Birds let out of their cages on to a solid floor usually recover. A bone-meal supplement may help. (*See* INTENSIVE LIVESTOCK PRODUCTION, EGG YIELD.)
The battery system has, in a somewhat different form, been applied to pig rearing. (*See* WEANING, EARLY.)

BCG VACCINE is the name given to a vaccine of the so-called *Bacillus Calmette-Guérin*. This was originally a strain of the *Mycobacterium tuberculosis* repeatedly cultivated upon a potato medium with glycerin and bile, so that the organisms lost their power to produce the disease.

BCG may be used for dogs and cats in Britain in households where the owner has tuberculosis. (*See* TUBERCULOSIS.)

In 1985 research in the UK on the possible use of BCG vaccine for the immunisation of badgers against bovine tuberculosis was instituted; and a trial was made of the vaccine for the treatment of equine SARCOIDS (which see.)

BEAK (*see* DE-BEAKING, 'SHOVEL BEAK').

BECQUEREL (*see* RADIATION).

BEDDING and BEDDING MATERIALS. Whenever animals are housed in buildings it is both necessary and economical to provide them with some form of bedding material. The reasons are as follows:

(1) All animals are able to rest more adequately in the recumbent position, and the temptation to lie is materially increased by the provision of some soft bedding upon which they may more comfortably repose than on the uncovered floor. Indeed, there are some which, in the event of the bedding being inadequate, or when it becomes scraped away, will not lie down at all.

(2) The provision of a sufficiency of some non-conductor of heat (which is one of the essentials of a good bedding) minimises the risk of chills.

(3) The protection afforded to prominent bony surfaces – such as the point of the hip, the points of the elbow and hock, the stifles and knees, etc. – is important, and if neglected leads to bruises and injuries of these parts.

(4) From the point of view of cleanliness, both of the shed or loose-box and of the animal's skin, the advantages of a plentiful supply of bedding are obvious.

(5) In the case of sick animals, the supply and management of the bedding can aid recovery. (*See also* SLATTED FLOORS.)

Horses:
Wheat straw. Wheat straw undoubtedly makes the best litter for either stall or loose-box, but on board ship it has certain disadvantages, the chief of which is its inflammability.

Wheat straw should be supplied loose or in hand-tied bundles for preference. Trussed or baled straw has been pressed and has lost some of its resilience or elasticity in the process. The individual straws should be long and unbroken, and the natural resistive varnish-like coating should be still preserved in a sample. The colour should be yellowish or a golden white; it should be clean-looking and free from dustiness. Straw should be free from thistles and other weeds, and should be crisp and firm to the touch.

Wheat straw has a particular advantage in that horses will not eat it unless kept very short of hay.

Oat straw. This straw is also very good for bedding purposes, but it possesses one or two disadvantages when compared with wheat straw. The straw is considerably softer, more easily broken and compressible than wheat, and being sweet to the taste, horses are often induced to eat it.

Barley straw is inferior to either of the two preceding for these reasons: it is only about half the length; it is very soft and easily compressed and therefore does not last so long as oat or wheat; more of it is required to bed the same-sized stall; and it possesses numbers of awns. The awns of barley are sharp and brittle.

Awns irritate the softer parts of the skin, cause scratches, and sometimes penetrate the soft tissues of the udder, lips, nose, or the region about the tail.

Rye straw. It has the same advantages as wheat straw, but it is a little harder and rougher.

Peat-moss is quite a useful litter for horses. It is recommended for town stables and for use on board ship, or other forms of transport. A good sample should not be powdery, but should consist of a matrix of fibres in which are entangled small lumps of pressed dry moss. It is of a brownish peaty colour, and therefore never looks clean, and it is very absorbent – taking up six or eight times its own weight of water. It has the disadvantage of clogging up horses' feet; and if there are covered drains in the building it works into the gratings over the traps and blocks them also. When it is used the drains should be of the open or 'surface' variety, or covered drains should be covered with old sacks, etc.

It should never be used in a loose-box in which there is an animal suffering from any respiratory disease, on account of its dusty nature.

Sawdust as a bedding must be renewed frequently for the dung and urine cause it to ferment. Pine sawdust is apt to mask the smell of any decomposition that may be taking place in the deeper layers.

Sand makes a fairly good bed when the sample does not contain any stones, shells, or other large particles. It is clean-looking, has a certain amount of scouring action on the coat, is cool in the summer, and comparatively easily managed. Sand should be obtained from a sand pit or the bed of a running stream; not from the sea-shore, because the latter is impregnated with salt, and likely to be licked by horses when they discover the salty taste, of which they are very fond. If this habit is acquired the particles of sand that are eaten collect in the colon or caecum of the horse and may set up a condition known as 'sand colic', which is often difficult to alleviate.

Ferns and bracken make a soft bed and are easily managed, but they always look dirty and untidy, do not last as long as straws, and are rather absorbent when stamped down. With horses that eat their bedding there is a risk of bracken poisoning.

Cattle. Wheat straw is the most satisfactory. Oat straw is used in parts where little or no wheat is grown. Barley straw is open to objection as a litter for cows on account of its awns, which may irritate the soft skin of the perineal region and of the udder. Sawdust has been found very convenient in cow cubicles, also shavings. Sand has been used on slippery floors below straw bedding, when it affords a good foothold for the cows and prevents accidents. (*See also* DEEP LITTER.) Special rubber mats have been found practicable and economic for use in cow cubicles.

A disadvantage of sawdust is that its use has led to coliform mastitis (sometimes fatal) in cattle. Sand may then be preferable.

In milk-fed calves, the ingestion of peat, sawdust or wood shavings may induce hypomagnesaemia. (*See Veterinary Journal*, October, 1970, **126**, 10.) (*See also* BRACKEN POISONING.)

Pigs. Many materials are used for the pig, but probably none possesses advantages over wheat straw, unless in the case of farrowing or suckling sows. These should be littered with some very short bedding which will not become entangled round the feet of the little pigs, and will not irritate the udder of the mother. For this purpose chaff, shavings, and even hay, may be used according to circumstances.

Piglets bedded on red African hardwood shavings have died, as explained under Bedding for dogs.

Slurry systems need not necessarily mean the total abandonment of bedding for pigs. Where vacuum tankers, as opposed to pipelines, are used for distributing the slurry on the land, moderate quantities of sawdust and shavings are not ruled out as bedding materials. Certainly, straw might well be thought of as the pig's best friend – and an ally of the farmer, too, despite its high handling costs.

For straw can make up for deficiencies in management and buildings as nothing else can. It serves the pig as a comfortable bed, as a blanket to burrow under, a plaything to avert boredom, and a source of roughage in meal-fed pigs which can help obviate digestive upsets and at least some of the scouring which reduces farmers' profits. Straw can mitigate the effects of poor floor insulation, of draughts, and of cold; and in buildings without straw ventilation, to quote David Sainsbury, 'becomes a much more critical factor'.

The Food & Agricultural Research Council pointed out that, as a new-born piglet spends so much of its time lying in direct contact with the floor of its pen, much body-heat can be lost through conduction. 'Depending on the type of floor, this effect could be large enough to affect the piglet's growth rate and be a potential threat to its survival.' Looking at it another way round, providing the straw was equivalent to raising the ambient temperature from $10°$ to $18°C$. Wooden and rubber floors were not as effective in reducing conductive heat loss as the straw.

Dogs and cats. Dogs have died as a result of the use for bedding of shavings of the red African hardwood (*Mansonia altissima*), which affects nose, mouth, and the feet, as well as the heart.

Fatal poisoning of cats has followed the use of sawdust, from timber treated with pentachlorophenol, used as bedding.

Poultry (*see* LITTER, OLD).

BEDSONIA (*see* CHLAMYDIA).

BEEF-BREEDS and CROSSES. The native British beef breeds are the Aberdeen Angus, Shorthorn, Hereford, Devon, South Devon, Sussex, Galloway, Highland and Lincoln Red. Recently continental breeds including the Charolais, Simmental, Limousin, Blonde d'Aquitaine, Gebvieh, Belgian Blue and Piedmontese have been imported for use in the United Kingdom. The continental breeds are more muscular, have higher mature weights and better performance than native beef breeds, the Meat & Livestock Commission has commented.

The beef breeds are generally used as terminal sires on cows not required for breeding dairy herd replacements and some beef cross heifers are used for suckler herd replacements. The cross-bred calves exhibit hybrid vigour and fetch a premium in the market over purebred dairy calves.

Recent enthusiasm for exotic breeds and crosses has led to the importation, not only of Charolais – now well established here – but of Limousins, Chianinas and other breeds referred to under CATTLE, BREEDS OF.

Beef which is acceptable to the butcher can be produced economically by crossing the Charolais bull with Guernsey and Jersey cows. In a trial conducted by Spillers Limited, Charolais × Guernsey steers reached 850 lb live-weight in 342 days – a performance equal to that of pure Friesian steers on a similar system. Daily liveweight gain was 2.24 lb. (*See* CHAROLAIS, LUING, *and* BEEVBILDE.)

Since the above was written, the Charolais has become the third most important beef-breed as judged by A I figures.

BEEF CATTLE HUSBANDRY in Britain. What follows is not a series of dogmatic statements but a summary of what farmers have been practising in beef herds recorded by the M LC.

Around 58 per cent of home produced beef is derived from the dairy herd, partly from dairy-bred calves reared for beef and partly from culled dairy cows. A further 34 per cent comes from the beef suckler herd, and 8 per cent from imported Irish stores. Irish stores are a declining source of UK beef production.

Development of beef production systems in Britain since 1960 has resulted in a reduction in the age and weight at which cattle are slaughtered. This has been associated with the development of production systems with higher rates of daily liveweight gain.

Other than the breeding herd itself, systems of beef production differ according to whether they utilise the dairy or beef-bred calf, and particularly with the length and the proportion of the complete production cycle which occur on a single farm. Complete systems are those where the full production cycle, both rearing and finishing, take place on the same farm. Partial systems are those where stores are purchased for either finishing or for re-sale as older, heavier stores. The latter represent the traditional basis of beef production and still predominate in Britain. The production of suckled calves is a distinct system, to which the finishing of the suckled calf may be added on the same farm as a separate system.

Store systems. Cattle are usually on one farm for less than a year, typically a winter (yard finished) or summer period (grass finished), but sometimes as short a period as three months.

Because only part of the production cycle takes place on a single farm the possibility for using a wide range of technical inputs is limited. The profitability is dominated by the relationship between buying and selling prices, and these systems are characterised by large year-to-year fluctuations in margins. As a generalisation the longer the cattle are on the farm the higher the margin, and less the year-to-year fluctuations.

Suckled calves are normally sold at the autumn sales, the heavier older calves are finished in their first winter at about 18 months of age, the lighter calves are overwintered, some are grass finished at about 20 months of age, some will be winter finished at about two years of age. The latter might change hands up to three times or more before slaughter. Dairy stores are generally sold on a less well defined seasonal pattern, but again the major transfers occur in the spring and autumn, with a traditional movement from west to east in the autumn and the reverse in the spring, *i.e.* from grassland farms to arable farms for the winter, and the reverse in the spring.

Complete beef production systems. Complete beef systems for utilising the by-product calf from the dairy herd differ markedly in the level of concentrates fed, and the age and weight at slaughter. They are characterised by having predetermined target levels of performance to achieve a fairly limited weight range at slaughter at a given age. Cereal and arable-product beef systems involve housed cattle which make no direct use of land and are mostly slaughtered between 11 and 15 months of age. In grass/cereal beef systems cattle make use to a varying extent of grass for both grazing and winter feed and are normally slaughtered between 15 and 24 months of age.

The term 'grass/cereal systems' embraces several methods for dairy-bred calves, depending upon season of birth of calf, level of concentrate feeding and whether one or two grazing seasons are involved. At one end of the range is 15 month grass/cereal beef which utilises winter- and spring-born calves finished on a high concentrate diet after one grazing season at 13–17 months of age. At the other end of the range is grass beef, also generally using winter- and spring-born calves, but with a growing ration during the second winter and cattle being slaughtered at heavier weights off grass during their second

grazing season at 20–24 months. For the most common method, 18 month grass/cereal beef, autumn- and winter-born calves are used. The aim is to finish the cattle out of yards at about 16–20 months of age. These systems are not absolutely rigid; they can be adapted to suit the time of calf purchase and individual farm resources.

Suckler herds. Under the traditional system, the average suckler cow produced a calf gaining less than 1½ lb per day, and took 3 acres to do it. The new concept calls for a cow with plenty of milk; able to over-winter on arable by-products such as potatoes, peahaulm silage, sugar-beet tops, straw and supplement; able to produce a calf gaining at least 2·5 lb per day; and needing only 1 acre to do it.

Winter feeding of winter/spring-calving herds should maintain cow bodyweight and condition until the last month of pregnancy. The feeding level is then gradually increased to provide for the rapid growth of the unborn calf and subsequent lactation. Generally, hay or silage is fed, supplemented with low levels of concentrate in late pregnancy. For a 550-kg cow, 25 to 30 kg medium quality silage per day should be sufficient to maintain weight. (Self-feeding of good quality silage, resulting in intakes above this level, is economically undesirable.) In the last month extra feed should be provided by 1 kg concentrates (in winter) to allow for growth of unborn calf and prepare for lactation. After calving, feed is increased to 2 kg as the calf takes more milk. It is important that the cow is in good body condition (score 2½–3) when bulled at 3 months to aid conception. Good grazing does not require concentrate supplements at any stage of the production cycle. Additional protein is required, states the MLC, only when cows are wintered on low-quality roughages. Some farmers use arable by-products; a typical daily ration being 7 to 9 kg straw and 2 to 3 kg barley, supplemented with urea, vitamins, and minerals. Autumn-calved cows need higher levels of winter feed to maintain milk production. A typical daily ration would be 28 kg of medium-quality silage and 2 kg of barley. (*See also* CREEP-FEEDING.)

Cereal beef production. Late-maturing breeds are best suited to this system. Most farmers favour Friesian steers, though there is an increasing use of bulls. Dairy-bred calves are weaned at 5–6

Targets for beef production systems using the dairy-bred calf*

	Age at slaughter (months	Liveweight at slaughter (kg)	Daily gain (kg)	Concentrate usage (kg)	Stocking rate head/*ha*
Cereal beef	11	400	1·1	1,770	—
Grass/cereal					
18 month	15	430	0·9	1,300	7·5
Grass 20 month	20	480	0·7	760	2·8
Grass 24 month	24	500	0·7	760	2·7

* Friesian steers

Each of these systems has very different implications for farm resources, both physical – feeds, grazing, labour and buildings; and financial – cash-flow and working capital

MLC Targets–grass beef

Period	Gain (kg/day)	Period	Stocking rate (beasts/hectare)
To turnout	0·7	Grazing:	
First summer	0·7	First summer	10·0
Winter	0·5	Second summer	3·5*
Second summer	1·0		3·0†
Overall	0·7	Overall (includes conservation)	3·0*
			2·5†

* Slaughter at 450 kg (H×F)
† Slaughter at 500 kg (F)

Systems of beef production		
Type	Age at slaughter	Weight at slaughter*
Intensive beef	10 to 14 months	700 to 900 lb.
Semi-intensive	15 to 20 months	850 to 1150 lb.
Extensive	24 to 29 months	900 to 1300 lb.

*The wide range depends upon whether the cattle are of late, early, or medium maturing breeds (MLC figures). (*See also* BULL-BEEF.)

weeks old on to a concentrate ration. At 10–12 weeks old (and weighing about 100 kg) they are introduced to *ad lib* feeding of a diet based on rolled barley with a protein, vitamin, mineral mix. The cattle are slaughtered at 385–410 kg when 10–12 months old. (Carcase weight 205–240 kg.) (*See* UREA, BEEF FROM BARLEY-FED CATTLE.)

18-Month grass/cereal beef. Friesian or Hereford × Friesian steers are generally preferred for this system; although there is a potential within it for bulls. The calves are early weaned and receive hay or silage, together with a ration of concentrates – about 1½ kg daily for 2–3 weeks after being turned out, until they are used to grazing; and with a maximum of 2¼ kg per day. About one-third of the grassland area is reserved for grazing in the first half of the season, with 5 or more paddocks rotationally grazed for best results. Topping of pasture is recommended. Two-thirds of the grassland area is cut for silage in late May. In mid-July the cattle are moved to fresh aftermath and an anthelmintic given if parasitic worms are troublesome. Regrowth of grass on the paddocks can be conserved.

From late August concentrate feeding is justified to maintain liveweight gains (if these fall, costs of winter feeding to retrieve the situation will be high). During the winter, barley is limited to about 2¾ kg for Hereford × Friesian cattle, but up to 5 kg for Friesians. The cattle are slaughtered when 16–20 months old and weighing 410–520 kg (carcase weight 180–270 kg).

20–24-Month grass beef. Early-maturing dairy-bred calves, such as Hereford × Friesian or Aberdeen Angus × Friesian are recommended for this system in preference to Friesians 'because they finish more easily'.

Calves are early weaned and turned out to grass in spring or as soon afterwards as possible. 'If the calves accept it, a barley supplement is fed throughout the grazing season, in order to achieve a daily liveweight gain of 0·7 kg.

In the autumn the cattle are yarded and fed good hay/silage plus 1½ kg concentrate, to achieve a daily gain of 0·5–0·6 kg. When turned out to grass in the following spring, cattle should make good growth off grass. Slaughter is at 20–24 months old in July to September, at a liveweight of 430–530 kg. (Carcase weight 230–290 kg.)

BEEF FROM BARLEY-FED CATTLE. Sudden and unexpected deaths among calves being fattened on barley have been reported from several parts of the country. Two entirely different causes account for many of these deaths. One is a failure on the part of the owner of the animals to make a gradual change from their previous diet to one mainly of barley. This brings about ill-effects in the rumen and is referred to under BARLEY POISONING.

The other health problem is the coughing which persists in some intensively reared cattle from a month or two after they are housed right through until they are slaughtered. For a few days, the calves may appear feverish and off their food, but then they usually rally and thrive reasonably well. From time to time, however – and this is the experience of several veterinary surgeons – complications occur with alarming suddenness, and there are deaths from what is technically known as Cuffing Pneumonia.

Such deaths have occurred under 'seemingly ideal conditions' to quote one report; but usually a predisposing cause is inadequate ventilation, and when this is improved health is found to improve, too. In one building, in an effort to increase warmth, sacks had been placed over wire netting above the calves, which became acutely ill – with constant coughing and distressed breathing – within 4 days; 3 dying after a further 2 days.

Liver abscess is a not uncommon condition in 'barley beef' animals. *See* LIVER, DISEASES OF.

Especially on slats, according to the MLC, bloat may be a problem – if so 1 kg hay may be fed daily. (*See* BLOAT.)

'BEEFALO.' A hybrid beef animal (⅜ bison, ⅜ Charolais, and ¼ Hereford.) It has been claimed that this American breed of cattle reach a market weight (1000–1100 lb) in 12 to 14 months on grass alone, 6 months or so faster than ordinary cattle fed on grain-based diets.

BEET TOPS (*see* FODDER POISONING *under* POISONING).

BEEVBILDE CATTLE. Breeding is based on 54 per cent polled Lincoln Red blood, 40 per cent polled Beef Shorthorn, and 6 per cent Aberdeen-Angus.

BELGIAN BLUE CATTLE. This is a beef breed noted for exceptional hindquarter muscling. The British name is a misnomer, and 'White-Blue' is said to be a better translation. Dystokia may be a problem, in breeds other than those of extreme dairy type, e.g. Holsteins. Maiden heifers should *not* be got in calf by a Belgian Blue bull.

BELLADONNA is another name for the deadly nightshade flower (*Atropa belladonna*). (*See* ATROPINE.)

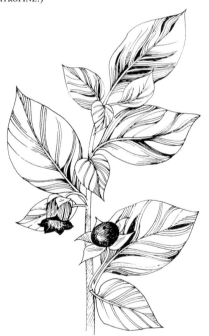

Belladonna (*Atropa belladonna*), also known as Deadly Nightshade, has thick, fleshy roots, dark green leaves, and purplish flowers. The berries change in colour from green to red, and then to black. The plant grows to a height of about 5 ft. All parts of the plant are poisonous. (*See* ATROPINE POISONING)

BENADRYL is the proprietary name of beta-dimethylamino-ethylbenz-hydryl ether hydro-chloride, which is of use as an antihistamine (which see) in treating certain allergic conditions.

BENZALKONIUM CHLORIDE. One of the qua-ternary ammonia compounds. (*See under* QUATERNARY.)

BENZENE HEXACHLORIDE. The gamma isomer of this is a highly effective and persistent parasiticide, of great value in destroying flies, lice, and fleas, ticks, and mange mites. It has a low toxicity for domestic animals except cats, and is the main ingredient of several well-known pro-prietary preparations, designed for use as dusting powder, spray, dip, etc.

B H C is the common abbreviation for the gam-mer isomer (*See* B H C POISONING.)

BENZOCAINE is a white powder, with soothing properties, used as a sedative for inflamed and painful surfaces. It is antagonistic to the sulphonamides.

Benzocaine poisoning. This has occurred in cats following use of either a benzocaine spray or ointment, and results in methaemoglobin ap-pearing in the blood.
SIGNS. In one case a cat showed signs of poisoning following an application of the cream to itchy areas. Cyanosis, open-mouth breathing, and vomiting occurred. Collapse followed within 15 minutes.

Improvement was noticed within ten minutes of giving methylene blue intravenously; and within 2 hours breathing had become normal again. The cat recovered.

BENZOIC ACID is an antiseptic substance used for inflammatory conditions of the urinary sys-tem. It is excreted as hippuric acid, and renders the urine acid. It is used in the treatment of ringworm, and as a food preservative.

Benzoic acid poisoning. Cases of this have been reported in the cat, giving rise to extreme aggressiveness, salivation, convulsions, and death. A curious symptom sometimes observed is jumping backwards and striking out with the fore-limbs 'as though catching imaginary mice'. The source of poisoning was meat prepared in slab form as a pet food and containing either an excess of, or badly mixed, benzoic acid as a preservative.

BENZYL BENZOATE is a useful drug for treating mange in dogs and horses. It is usually employed as an emulsion. It is prepared from balsam of Peru. It should not be used over the whole body surface at once.

BENZYLPENICILLIN. This antibiotic is a bacteriocide, active against Gram-positive bacteria, and given by parenteral or intramam-mary injection. It is inactivated by penicillinase.

BEPHENIUM EMBONATE. A drug which is used in sheep to kill nematodirus worms.

BERRICHON DU CHER. A French breed of heavy milking sheep. The breed contains some merino blood.

BESNOITA (*see* GLOBIDIOSIS).

BETA-BLOCKER (*see* AGONIST).

BETAMETHASONE. A corticosteroid.

BHC (an abbreviation for BENZENE HEXACHLORIDE).

BHC POISONING. This may arise, especially in kittens and puppies, from a single dose (*e.g.* licking of dusting powder). Symptoms include: twitching, muscular inco-ordination, anxiety, convulsions.

A farmer's wife became ill (she had a convulsion) after helping to dip calves, but recovered after treatment. Two of the calves died. This shows that even BHC must be regarded with respect, and precautions taken to avoid the use of too strong a dip or dressing, or of not washing all of the residue off one's own skin. (*See also* GAMEBIRDS.)

BHC is highly poisonous for fish; and must be used with great care on cats, for which other insecticides, such as selenium preparations are to be preferred.

The use of BHC sheep dips is no longer permitted in the UK.

BHS. Beta haemolytic streptococcus.

'BIG HEAD.' A condition associated with *Clostridium novyi* (Type A) infection in rams which have slightly injured their heads as a result of fighting. It occurs in Australia and South Africa. (*See also* HYDROCEPHALUS.)

BILE is a thick, bitter, golden-brown or greenish-yellow fluid secreted by the liver, and stored in the gall-bladder when that organ is present. The *Equidae* possess no gall-bladder, but it is present in the other domesticated mammals and birds. Bile is composed of water, mucus, brown or green pigments, cholesterol, and salts of taurocholic and glycocholic acids.

It has digestive functions, assisting the emulsification of the fat contents of the food. It has in addition some laxative action, stimulating peristalsis, and it aids not only absorption of fats but also of fat-soluble vitamins. (*See* CHOLECYSTOKININ.)

Jaundice, a symptom rather than a disease, may be caused when the flow of the bile is obstructed and does not reach the intestines, but remains circulating in the blood. As a result the pigments are deposited in the tissues and discolour them, while the visible mucous membranes show a yellowishness or even a brown coloration in bad cases. In addition, the appearance of the urine changes, due to some of the bile salts being excreted by the kidneys.

Vomiting of bile usually occurs when the normal passage through the intestines is obstructed, and during the course of certain digestive disorders. (*See also* GALLSTONES.)

BILHARZIOSIS is a disease produced by bilharziae or Schistosomes; these are parasites of about ¼ to 1 centimetre in length which are sometimes found in the bloodstream of cattle and sheep in Europe, and of horses, camels, cattle, sheep, and donkeys, in India, Japan, and the northern seaboard countries of Africa. (*See* SCHISTOMIASIS.) Dogs may also suffer from these flukes.

BILIARY FEVER (*see* CANINE BABESIOSIS, EQUINE BILIARY FEVER).

BINOVULAR TWINS are twins which result from the fertilisation of two ova, as distinct from 'monovular twins' which arise from a single ovum.

BIOPSY is a diagnostic method in which a small portion of living tissue is removed from the animal and examined by special means in the laboratory so that a diagnosis may be made.

BIOTECHNOLOGY. The application of biological knowledge, of micro-organisms, systems or processes to a wide range of activities, such as cheese-making, animal production, waste recycling, pollution control, and human and veterinary medicine. For the manipulation of genes, see 'Genetic Engineering' under GENETICS.

BIOTIN. A water soluble vitamin of the B group. (*See below.*)

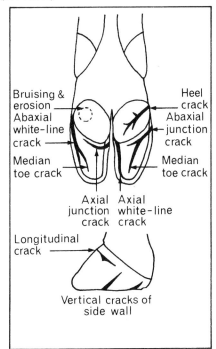

Bruising & erosion
Abaxial white-line crack
Median toe crack
Heel crack
Abaxial junction crack
Median toe crack
Axial junction crack
Axial white-line crack
Longitudinal crack
Vertical cracks of side wall

The position of foot lesions in pigs suffering from a biotin deficiency. (With acknowledgement to Dr Peter Brooks.)

However, the incidence of dermatitis, and soundness of feet and legs did not appear to be affected by adding biotin to the diet, according to Hamilton and Veum. They studied the effect of the supplement, added to the diet of sows, over a three-year period, using 160 sows and 414 litters.

Half the sows received a corn-soybean meal containing 0·55 ppm biotin; the control group received the same diet but without the biotin. (However, sows on the biotin supplement weaned more piglets per litter overall.) (Hamilton, C. R. & Veum, T. L. (1984) *Journal of Animal Science* **59**, 151.) The value of biotin remains controversial. Simmins, P. H. & Brooks, P. H. (*Veterinary Record* (1988) **122**, 431) concluded that supplementation of the diet of breeding sows with biotin from an early stage of development 'made a significant contribution to the maintenance of their horn integrity.'

BIOTYPE. The type species of a genus, or an organism's genetic constitution.

BIRD-FANCIER'S LUNG. 'Patients were regarded as having bird-fancier's lung if they satisfied all the following criteria: recent history of avian exposure; serum avian precipitins; diffuse shadowing on chest radiograph; a significant reduction (less than 70 per cent predicted value) of carbon-monoxide transfer factor (single breath); and improvement or no deterioration when exposure to birds and their excreta ceased.' (Berrill, W. T., *et al.* (1975) *Lancet.*)

In some cases there have been changes in the intestine (villous atrophy).

In the acute form, most often seen in pigeon fanciers after cleaning the loft, influenza-like symptoms, a shortness of breath and a cough occur after 4 to 6 hours. The disease in elderly patients has to be differentiated from bronchitis and emphysema. (D. Davies, *BMJ* (1983) **287**, 1239).

BIRD IMPORT CONTROLS were imposed in Great Britain in 1976, and a licence is required for all imports of captive birds and hatching eggs. All birds are subject to a period of quarantine, normally 35 days. (*See also* PIGEONS.)

BIRD LOUSE is a parasitic insect belonging to the order *Mallophaga*, which attacks most domesticated and many wild birds. The lice eat feathers and the shed cells from the surface of the skin, but they do not suck blood. Dusting with BHC or other parasiticide powder is an efficient remedy. (*See* LICE.)

BIRD MALARIA. A tropical disease of fowls and turkeys caused by *Plasmodium gallinaceum*, *P. durae* and other species, transmitted by mosquitoes.

It may run a rapidly fatal course, or a chronic one with anaemia and greenish diarrhoea.

BIRD REPELLENTS. Thiram and anthraquinone are examples. In the UK birds have avoided contact with the chemical by picking out the cotyledons after germination of the treated seed.

BIRDS (*see* CAGE BIRDS, FALCONS, GAMEBIRDS, TURKEYS, POULTRY, ORNITHOSIS, BOTULISM, and DUCK VIRUS HEPATITIS, also under AVIAN, and disease headings, and PETS; *also* RABIES; and OSTRICHES, RHEAS.)

BIRDS, BLOOD SAMPLING. The toenail clip method enables blood to be collected into a microhaematocrit tube or pipette. The bird can be held with its back against the palm of the hand; head between thumb and forefinger.

The alternative is jugular venepuncture. This too can be accomplished single-handedly. (Koob, M. D. & Van Alstine, W. G. *Modern Veterinary Practice* (1988) **69**, 68.)

BIRDS, HUMANE DESTRUCTION OF. For poultry and other birds a lidless wooden box or chamber (of a size to take a polypropylene poultry crate) and a cylinder of carbon dioxide with regulating valve are useful. The box has a ½-inch copper pipe, drilled with $^9/_{64}$-in. holes at 4-in. centres fitted at levels 2 in. and 2 ft 2 in. from the bottom and connected by plastic tubing to the regulator valve of the cylinder.

BIRDSVILLE DISEASE occurs in parts of Australia, is due to a poisonous plant *Indigofera enneaphylla*, and has to be differentiated from Kimberley Horse Disease. Symptoms: sleepiness and abnormal gait with front legs lifted high. Chronic cases drag the hind limbs.

BIRTH (*see* PARTURITION).

BISMUTH is one of the heavy metals.
USES. The carbonate, subnitrate, and the salicylate are used in irritable and painful conditions of the stomach and intestines to relieve diarrhoea and vomiting. The salts of bismuth are reputed to form a protective covering over any ulcerated areas used in these conditions.

The oxychloride and the subnitrate are used as bismuth meals prior to taking X-ray photographs of the abdominal organs for purposes of diagnosis. The massed bismuth salt forms a barrier to the passage of the rays; and the outline of the opaque bowel appears in the print. Bismuth compounds, when given in excess, give the faeces a dark smoky-black colour, which is rather alarming to the uninitiated.

BITES, STINGS and POISONED WOUNDS. The bites of animals, whether domesticated or otherwise, should always be looked upon as infected wounds. (*See* WOUNDS). In countries where rabies is present the spread of this disease is generally by means of a bite. (*See* RABIES.)

Bees, wasps, and hornets cause great irritation by the stings with which the females are provided. Death has been reported in pigs eating windfall apples in which wasps were feeding. The wasps stung the mucous membrane of the throat, causing great swelling and death from suffocation some hours later.

Anti-histamine preparations may be used in treatment if numerous stings make this necessary. (*See also* VENOM.)

Cat-bites are usually followed by some degree of suppuration. *Pasteurella multocida* infection of the bite wound is common. (*See also* RABIES, CAT-SCRATCH FEVER.)

Dog-bites are usually inflicted upon other dogs,

defenceless sheep or goats, and sometimes pigs; cattle may be bitten by the herd's dog and serious wounds result. The bite is generally a punctured wound, or large tear, depending upon the part that is bitten. Where an animal is bitten in numerous places, even though no individual bite is large, there is always a considerable degree of danger. Antibiotics should be given by injection. The wounds should be dressed with some suitable antiseptic, the hair or wool being first clipped from the area; and left open. (*See* WOUNDS, RABIES.)

In the USA about a million dog bites a year require medical treatment of people; and in the UK the figure has been estimated as about 99,000. Dog-bite wounds are often infected by *Pseudomonas* species, *Staphylococcus aureus*, *Streptococcus viridans*, *Pasteurella multocida*, and Group EF-4 bacteria.

Harvest-mites, fleas, lice, ticks, mosquitoes, etc., are dealt with under section on MITES.

Horse-bites. Actinobacillosis has been transmitted to a bitten person.

Monkey-bites can transmit encephalitis caused by *Herpes simiae*; human infectious hepatitis; also TB. (*Lancet* (1983), **2,** 553).

Snake bites (*see* separate entry under this heading).

Spider-bites (*see separate entry:* SPIDERS).

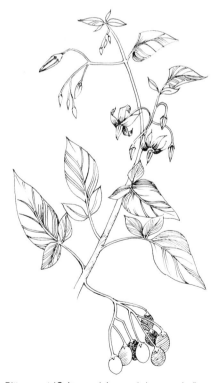

Bittersweet (*Solanum dulcamara*): has purple flowers with bright yellow anthers. The berries are first green, then yellow, finally turning to a brilliant red. This is a climbing plant and may reach a height of 6ft or so. Bittersweet is also known as Woody Nightshade.

BITTERSWEET POISONING. The common 'bittersweet' – *Solanum dulcamara* – is a frequent denizen of hedgerows and waste lands, and, although not likely to be eaten to a great extent by domesticated animals, cases of poisoning due to its ingestion have been recorded. All parts of the plant – stem, leaves, and berries – contain the toxic principle, which is an alkaloid similar to *Solanine* found in the potato, but it appears that in different seasons and in diverse parts of the country the toxicity varies. In addition to solanine the stems contain a glycoside called *Dulcamarin*, which imparts a bitter taste when chewed.

SIGNS. In cattle and sheep the symptoms are giddiness, quickening of the respiration, staggering gait, dilated pupil, greenish diarrhoea, and raised temperature.

BLACK DISEASE is the name given to infectious necrotic hepatitis of sheep and occasionally of cattle in Australia, New Zealand, Scotland, Wales, and NW England. It is typically caused by a combined attack of immature liver flukes and bacteria: a strain of *Clostridium oedematiens*, which is one of the so-called 'gas gangrene' group, and is capable of forming resistant spores.

In black disease these spores are apparently present in the liver in an inactive state until, with the migration of (perhaps) large numbers of young immature flukes (*Fasciola hepatica*) from the intestine, the liver substances become injured and the spores become active. The liver becomes necrotic and there is a rapid toxaemia.

SIGNS. The sheep are usually found dead in the early morning, death in some instances being so exceedingly rapid that the animal has food between the lips or teeth, indicating that death took place during feeding. Where affected sheep have been noticed ill, they are first seen to lag behind the others, then to lie down in the usual position on the sternum. Breathing becomes rapid and shallow and pulse-rate is greatly increased. The animal may yawn or gasp occasionally, and a little later respiration becomes distressed, stertorous, and death occurs quietly. The duration of illness in observed cases varies between a few minutes and 48 hours, most cases terminating within 20 to 30 minutes of having first been noticed ill.

On *post-mortem* examination the most striking feature is the rapidity with which sheep dead from this disease have undergone decomposition. Within only a few hours the carcase has decomposed so much that characteristic lesions are masked. In carcases of sheep recently dead or killed in the later stages, the skin is a dark bluish-black colour, and the underlying tissues are congested and oedematous. In the liver, where the most constant lesions are found, there are one or more necrotic areas about 1 inch in diameter, roughly circular in outline and yellowish-white in colour. In some cases they may be seen to be associated with a 'fluke burrow', in others young flukes may actually be found. Exudation of fluid into the pericardium is typical, and usually the peritoneal and thoracic cavities contain inflammatory exudate.

PREVENTION. An antiserum and a vaccine are

available. Eradication of flukes and the avoidance of fluke-infested land for grazing sheep serve to some extent to prevent loss. Carcases of dead sheep should be burned or buried so that infection in them may not spread.

BLACK FAECES are passed when either iron or bismuth salts are given to dogs and pigs. The most serious cause of black motions is haemorrhage into the early part of the digestive system, the blood mixing with the ingesta and becoming changed into a dark colour. Such conditions may result from ulceration of the stomach and haemorrhage, or from injury by a foreign body that has been eaten and passed into the stomach. A dark-coloured diarrhoea may be seen in the dog suffering from deficiency of the B vitamin complex.

BLACKHEAD OF TURKEYS is a very common and fatal disease of young turkeys (from 3 weeks to 4 months old), which is caused by a small protozoön parasite, *Histomonas meleagridis*, which passes part of its life in a worm (*Heterakis gallinae*); this acts as an intermediate host. The histomonas is found in adult worms and eggs, ingestion of the latter is the chief means of spread.

Though turkeys are chiefly affected, the disease has been seen in chickens, partridges, pheasants, grouse, quail and pea-fowl.
SIGNS. Loss of appetite and of condition. The droppings may be semi-liquid and bright yellow. Death, in 5 to 8 days, may occur in 70 to 90 per cent of young turkeys, in which the disease is very acute and prevalent in summer and autumn. In adults, mortality is lower, and the disease may persist in winter. An acute form of the disease may be seen in which death occurs without any previous symptoms of illness.
PREVENTION. This can be largely achieved by hygiene and (*a*) good management; (*b*) the use of certain preparations given regularly in the food.

A nitrothiazole compound, given in the food is effective; Furazolidone is also used but over long periods can cause leukopenia. It is necessary to feed from hoppers that are not readily fouled by faeces, and to keep the drinking water free from pollution.

BLACK-QUARTER, also called BLACK-LEG, QUARTER-ILL, etc., is an acute specific infectious disease of cattle, sometimes of sheep, and likewise of pigs, characterised by the presence of rapidly increasing swellings containing gas, and occurring in the region of the shoulder, neck, thigh, quarter, and sometimes on the trunk. Young cattle between the ages of 3 months and 2 years are most susceptible.

The disease has been seen in the reindeer, camel, and the buffalo.
CAUSES. *Clostridium chauvaei*, which lives in the soil until such time as it gains entry into the animal body either along with the food or else by abrasions of the skin (*see* TATTOOING). It remains at the seat of its lesions and does not invade the blood-stream.

On exposure to the air the organisms form spores which are resistant to extreme cold, or even

exposure to 100 degrees Centigrade of dry heat. The uncubative period is from a few hours to 5 days.
SIGNS. The finding of a dead animal may be the first indication of the disease; though sometimes lameness is observed, and part of the udder swollen and very painful. If seen in the early stages, the swelling is hot and pits on pressure, but, increasing rapidly, it becomes puffed up with gas (emphysematous), and if pressed it crackles as if filled with screwed-up tissue-paper. Death usually occurs within 24 hours. *Sheep* show somewhat similar symptoms, but they may be attacked at almost any age. There are often blood-stained discharges from both the nostrils and the rectum.
PREVENTION. Marshy ground that has been responsible for the loss of numerous animals in the past has often been rendered safe by the draining of the land and heavy liming.
Vaccine. A vaccine gives very good results.
Curative. There is generally no opportunity to treat cases, since death occurs after only a few hours' illness; otherwise penicillin and antiserum may be tried.

'BLACK TONGUE'. The counterpart of human pellagra. It is shown in the dog fed a diet deficient in nicotinic acid, and, experimentally, on jowar (*Sorghum vulgare*), a cereal. (*See also* SHEEPDOGS and 'BROWN MOUTH'.) Symptoms include discoloration of the tongue, a foul odour from the mouth, ulceration, loss of appetite, and sometimes blood-stained saliva and faeces. Death will occur in the absence of treatment.

BLACK VOMIT is due to the presence of blood in the stomach. The appearance of the vomit may be either that of black masses of clotted blood, or it may resemble coffee-grounds.

BLACK-WATER FEVER (*see* TEXAS FEVER).

BLADDER, DISEASES OF (*see under* URINARY BLADDER, DISEASES OF; *also* GALL-BLADDER).

BLASTOCYST is the name given to a very early stage in the development of the fetus, in which the mass of cells resulting from the fertilisation of the ovum, which is to become the new animal, assumes a hollow, spherical at first and then ellipsoidal, bladder-like form. This blastocyst stage is preceded by the **morula stage,** and is followed by the **differentiation stage,** when the *epi-, meso-,* and *hypoblast* are formed. (*See* EMBRYOLOGY.)

BLASTOMERE. A cell, or group of cells, forming the blastoderm; for example, a morula cell.

BLASTOMYCOSIS OF DOGS. A UK case of infection with *Blastomyces dermatitidis*, involving the liver and kidneys, was reported. The animal suddenly lost appetite and showed persistent vomiting.

The disease is fairly common in both man and dogs in North America. Diagnosis depends upon a laboratory demonstration of the fungus, which typically causes chronic debility often with a fatal outcome.

Infection is usually through inhalation. Bone lesions, resulting in lameness, often occur; sometimes the brain, nose, eyes, and prostate gland show lesions.

'BLEEDER' HORSES. (*See* RACEHORSES, PULMONARY HAEMORRHAGE IN.) Those which show blood at their nostrils after exercise such as racing.

BLEEDING, or HAEMORRHAGE may be classified according to the vessel or vessels from which it escapes: *e.g.* (*a*) *arterial*, in which the blood is of a bright scarlet colour and issues in jets or spurts corresponding in rate and rhythm to the heart-beats; (*b*) *venous* when it comes from veins, is of a dark colour, and wells up from the depth of a wound in a steady stream; and (*c*) *capillary*, when it gradually oozes from a slight injury to the network of capillaries of an area. (*See also under* CANINE HAEMOPHILIA, HAEMORRAGIC DIATHESIS, INTERNAL HAEMORRHAGE.)

NATURAL ARREST. When an artery with a small calibre is cut, the muscular fibres in its middle coat shrink, and the cut end is slightly retracted within the stiffer fibrous covering. This results in a diminution in the size of the cut end and in a lessened capacity for output of blood. In the space between the end of the muscular coat and at the end of the fibrous coat a tiny clot commences to form, which, later, is continued into the lumen of the vessel. This is added to by further coagulation of blood, until the whole of the open end of the vessel and of the cavity of the wound is sealed by a clot. A fall in blood-pressure, due to shock, and loss of blood, contributes to the natural arrest of bleeding. (*See* CLOTTING.)

Bleeding, external: First Aid for. When a vein is cut, crimson blood will *flow*. From a cut artery scarlet blood will *spurt*, issuing in jets corresponding with the heart beats.

When a large vessel is cut, pressure should be applied above the wound if the bleeding is from an artery, below it if bleeding is from a vein; but the first-aider should take precautions, *see* RESTRAINT.

Pressure with the fingers is a helpful preliminary while someone else is finding material to use as a pressure pad. For large animals a clean pillowslip, small towel, or piece of sheet will serve; for small animals a clean handkerchief may suffice. The pad is then placed over the wound, and held there; pressure being applied and maintained for a quarter of an hour.

If the wound is large, and the point from which the blood is coming can be seen, pressure by a washed thumb or fingers may be applied direct; and a pressure pad, moistened with clean water, then pressed into the wound and kept there by hand or bandaging.

TOURNIQUET. Only if these measures fail to stop serious haemorrhage should a tourniquet be used. A tourniquet can be improvised from a rolled handkerchief, its two ends knotted, slipped around the limb, and tightened with a pencil.

Tightening must be just sufficient to stop the bleeding, no more. For large animals a piece of rubber tubing or a *soft* rope may be used. **A tourniquet must never** be left on for more than 20 minutes, or permanent damage to the limb will result. When releasing the tourniquet, do so gradually. A tourniquet should not be used on cats, in which a pressure pad will suffice to control bleeding.

PROFESSIONAL HELP should be obtained as soon as possible. It may be necessary to deal with a small artery by means of artery forceps, and a larger artery may require application of a ligature.

Sometimes the actual point or points of bleeding cannot be located, especially when the wound is deep or ragged, and the blood issues in a

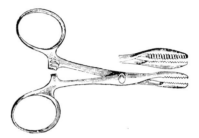

Artery forceps, with jaws shown enlarged.

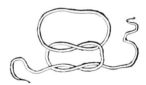

Surgeon's knot, or reef knot, used for ligaturing cut vessels.

more or less continuous stream showing no tendency to clot. In such cases it is necessary to resort to packing the wound with GELATIN SPONGE (which see).

Professional help will also be needed to counter SHOCK (which see). (*See also* BLOOD TRANSFUSION, DEXTRAN.)

Bleeding from special parts

(1) THE HORNS. The horns of cattle are sometimes broken by falls or blows, and severe bleeding follows. If the horn is broken completely off, the haemorrhage is to the outside from the stump, but it often happens that while the bony horn-core is fractured the horn itself holds the broken end in position and the escaping blood finds its way down into the frontal sinus and out by the nostril. Haemorrhage from a stump may be controlled by the application of a pad and a bandage and the temporary use of a tourniquet round the base of the horn.

(2) LEGS AND FEET. The tourniquet described earlier in this article may be applied, to the lower side of the injury if the bleeding is venous, and above it if it be arterial. When the upper parts of the limbs are injured and the haemorrhage is considerable, one of the methods of pressure is

adopted. If the attendant has a knowledge of the arteries that supply the bleeding part, and when these are near enough to the surface to be compressible, he may press his two thumbs firmly over the artery above the wound until more permanent measures can be taken.

(3) **STOMACH.** The vomiting of blood by dogs, cats, and pigs in considerable amounts is a very serious symptom of severe injury or disease in the stomach.

A dog may be offered ice cubes to lick. The animal should be kept as still as possible, and veterinary assistance obtained. Alcohol is not advisable, as it causes a dilatation of the vessels of the stomach wall and tends to promote the bleeding.

(4) **UTERUS AND VAGINA.** After parturition in all animals there is a certain risk of haemorrhage, especially in those which have a diffuse placenta, such as the mare and ass, and when the foetal membranes have been forcibly removed. If it is copious, it may prove fatal. Prompt veterinary attention is necessary.

Overseas, where professional attention is not quickly available, an attempt may be made to control the haemorrhage by packing the vagina with a clean sheet or towel (for the larger animals) preferably sterilised before use by boiling for 10 minutes and allowing to cool. Hands should be scrubbed with antiseptic solution and the nails trimmed before inserting the pack. For small animals, cottonwool swabs may be boiled, cooled, and used similarly. (*See also under* WOUNDS *and* INTERNAL HAEMORRHAGE.)

(5) **NAVEL** in piglets. *See* VITAMIN C for prevention.

Bleeding, internal (*see* INTERNAL HAEMORRHAGE).

BLEPHARITIS means inflammation of the eyelids. It is usually associated with conjunctivitis.

BLEPHAROSPASM is a spasm of the eyelids.

BLINDNESS (*see* EYE, DISEASE OF; VISION).

BLOAT is a condition of tympanites occurring in cattle, sheep, and goats. With the increased use of lucerne and clovers, bloat has become of more common occurrence among cattle and is now a matter of serious economic importance.

The rumen becomes distended with gas, and pressure is exerted upon the diaphragm.

The medium-sized cow's rumen has a capacity of some 35 gal, and fermentation within it gives rise to bubbles of gas. This comprises carbon dioxide (CO_2) and methane (CH_4) in surprisingly large quantities; cattle producing as much as 800 litres of CO_2 in 24 hours, and as much as 500 litres of CH_4. Some of this gas, perhaps a quarter, escapes via the bloodstream to the lungs and is breathed out but that still leaves a great deal which can be expelled only by belching. If something makes that impossible, then gas pressure builds up and is exerted on the diaphragm, heart and lungs, so that the cow becomes ill with bloat, is barely able to breathe, and is in considerable distress.

At a symposium organised by Smith Kline & French Laboratories, Dr Brian Bagnall listed three important factors interfering with the cow's ability to belch: physical obstruction of the oesophagus; paralysis of the muscular wall of the rumen; and foaming of the rumen contents.

The first diagram shows a healthy state of affairs in the rumen, with the cardia – a muscular valve at the junction of oesophagus and rumen – temporarily open so that gas can escape up the oesophagus. But when this tube is obstructed by a piece of turnip or a tumour or an abscess, the gas cannot get away or not in sufficient quantity, and 'gassy bloat' results. Paralysis of the muscular wall of the rumen has a similar effect, since expulsion of gas is aided by contraction of these muscles.

'The most common cause is ruminal acidosis due to attempted digestion of a high carbohydrate diet ('cereal bloat') with the low rumen pH producing paralysis of the rumen muscles,' Dr Bagnall said. 'But gassy bloat is occasionally seen in grazing cattle, indicating that the precise causal mechanisms are poorly understood and prevention difficult.'

Several hypotheses have been advanced in the past. For example, a suggestion that hydrocyanic acid may be liberated in the rumen during digestion of plants containing cyanogenetic glucosides and paralyse the rumen musculature; or that an allergy may cause shock in a cow already sensitised to some particular plant protein, leading to failure of the cardia to relax and open.

Returning to Dr Bagnall's paper, he said: 'If the underlying cause be ruminal acidosis, administration of an antacid drench may be indicated on veterinary advice'. He advocated use of a stomach tube as the best method of relieving gassy bloat. 'If there is an obstructing object, it can often be pushed along. Once the trapped gas is reached, it will rush out of the tube, providing relief'.

Frothy bloat. With the frothy type of bloat, puncturing the rumen with a trocar and cannula in an emergency may do more harm than good – not releasing gas and perhaps causing leakage of some solids into the abdominal cavity.

This frothy type of bloat is the more important from an economic point of view, as it can occur simultaneously in a number of animals, with a fatal outcome. The second diagram shows the rumen distended by foam, with bubbles of gas trapped and unable to escape.

Mr A. R. Austin, MRCVS, of the Grassland Research Institute, Hurley, pointed out that even when the cardia is open so that gas trapped in foam can enter the oesophagus, belching is not stimulated, because the foam induces reflex swallowing instead of the forward-moving waves of contraction which occur with belching. Once a strong foam has been produced, therefore, it means that gas in the rumen will be trapped there.

If a cow with frothy bloat is spotted in time, treatment with an anti-foam drench can, to quote Dr Bagnall, 'produce rapid dissolution of the foam', and a stomach tube may facilitate treatment.

What produces the foam? There is at present no universally accepted answer to this question. It

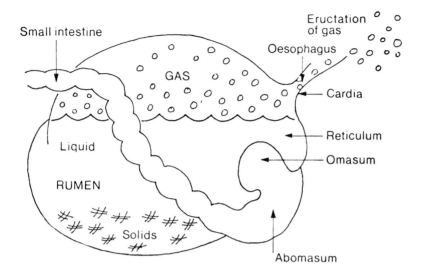

The normal rumen with gas able to escape.

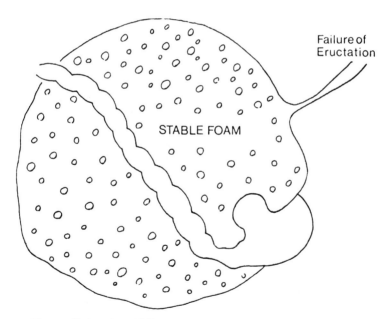

Gross distension of Rumen

Acute frothy bloat – stable foam fills the rumen.

was suggested in Wisconsin some years ago that the natural pectin present in herbage interacts with an enzyme released during rumination, producing pectic acid and alcohol – calcium salts in the plant food then resulting in a gelatinous honeycomb-like mass. Plant saponins have been suspected, too, but now it seems that the chief suspects are plant proteins. Genetic susceptibility to bloat comes into the picture too.

In intensively-fed cattle, high-grain diets may lead to frothy bloat, and Professor G. E. Lamming warned that finely chopped or ground roughage can provide a suitable medium in which this type of bloat can occur. He also suggested that use of urea, justified on economic grounds, to replace oilseed proteins has led to a decreased oil content of rations which has increased the risk of bloat. *Ad lib* feeding decreases the risk by avoiding high feed intakes by animals which are hungry.

PREVENTION. The use of anti-foaming substances of the type available in Britain, *e.g.*, poloxalene, manufactured by SKF and sold under the name 'Bloat Guard'. This can conveniently be used as a pre-mix given to dairy cows in their concentrates.

The experience of bloat and its prevention on the Elveden Estates, Thetford, Norfolk, was given by Mr W. M. Sloan, general manager and agent. In his paper he stated that it was his practice to include Bloat Guard in the ration of dairy cows grazing lucerne at the rate of about 7 kg/ tonne. Young stock and beef cows not receiving concentrates during the summer must be introduced to lucerne gradually – perhaps for half an hour the first day, having previously been fed straw. As they gradually become accustomed to the crop, bloat does not occur.

SIGNS. The left side of the body, between the last rib and the hip bone, is seen to be swollen; the whole abdomen gradually becoming tense and drum-like. There is obvious distress on the part of the animal which appears restless. Breathing is rapid. (*See* TYMPANITIC RESONANCE.)

BLOAT IN PIGS affects not the stomach but the small intestine, excluding the duodenum. It is sometimes referred to as 'colonic bloat' or 'whey bloat'. (*See* HAEMORRHAGIC GASTROENTERITIS.)

BLONDE d'AQUITAINE. A French breed of cattle, for which an English breed society has been formed. (*See* BEEF BREEDS.)

BLOOD is a red, slightly alkaline fluid which serves as a carrier of nutrients from the digestive system to the various tissues, transports oxygen from the lungs and carbon dioxide to the lungs, carries hormones from the endocrine glands, maintains a correct water balance in the body and assists with temperature control, carries waste products to the kidneys, and has an important role in the defence of the body against bacteria, viruses, etc. By its ability to clot, blood has its own built-in safety factor for use in the event of damage to the blood vessels. Blood also assists in the maintenance of the correct pH of tissues.

The blood is circulated through the body by a

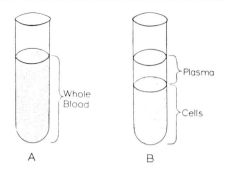

Diagram illustrating different physical states of blood. A unclotted blood, cells dispersed uniformly throughout; B blood treated with anticoagulant. Cells permitted to settle leaving clear plasma. (Frandson: *Anatomy and Physiology of Farm Animals*, 2nd edition, Lea & Febiger.)

system of arteries, capillaries, and veins, and it receives its propulsion by pulsations of the heart.

Composition. Blood consists of a fluid portion, or plasma, in which blood-cells are suspended. They are of three chief varieties: red blood-cells (or corpuscles), white blood-cells, and platelets.

PLASMA forms about 66 per cent of the total amount of the blood and contains three protein groups – *Fibrinogen, serum-globulin*, and *serum-albumin*. Fibrinogen is of great interest and importance, owing to its role in the coagulation of the blood.

When shed, plasma separates into two parts: a liquid, which is called *serum*, and a solid, which is the fibrin clot. Blood serum is therefore plasma which has lost its fibrinogen, the latter having gone to form the fibrin of the clot; but it contains two newly-formed proteins – *fibrino-globulin* and *nucleo-protein*. These are derivatives of fibrinogen which are split off from the fibrinogen when it forms the fibrin clot. (*See* GAMMA-GLOBULIN.)

Besides the proteins mentioned above, the plasma contains non-protein nitrogenous material such as amino acids; waste products such as urea; glucose; fats; inorganic salts of sodium, potassium, calcium, magnesium, etc.

RED BLOOD-CELLS constitute about 32 per cent of the total amount of the blood. Seen under the microscope they appear as biconcave discs, circular in shape, and they possess no nucleus; having lost it before entering the circulation. (*Note.*–The red blood-cells of birds, fish and reptiles possess a nucleus, and biconvex.)

Red cells are soft, flexible, elastic envelopes containing the red blood-pigment known as *haemoglobin*, which is held in position by a spongy lacework of threads called *stroma*. They are present in large numbers in the blood. In the horse they number about 7 to 9 million per cubic millimetre, and about 6 million in the ox, on an average.

The red blood-cells are destroyed after 3 or 4 months in the circulation. The red blood-cells are formed in the red marrow of the bones, and appear first of all as nucleated red cells, called *erythroblasts*.

PACKED CELL VOLUME. The height of the column of red cells, as a percentage of total height, of a sample of centrifuged blood in the tube. The red cells lie at the bottom; the middle layer consists of the white blood cells and platelets; and the top layer is the serum.

BLOOD PLATELETS, or thrombocytes, are oval discs of protoplasm which take many shapes when seen in smears. Their main function seems to be to reduce loss of blood from injured vessels by the formation of a white clot. (For a deficiency of platelets, *see under* THROMBOCYTOPENIA.)

HAEMOGLOBIN – a complex substance – has the power of absorbing oxygen in the lungs, parting with it to the tissues, receiving carbon dioxide in exchange, and finally, of yielding up this carbon dioxide in the lungs. When haemoglobin carries oxygen it is temporarily changed into a substance called *oxyhaemoglobin*, and when it is carrying carbon dioxide it is known as *carboxyhaemoglobin*. The process of oxidation and reduction proceeds with every respiratory cycle.

'Haemolysis' is a process by which the haemoglobin of the red blood-cells becomes dissolved and liberated from the cell-envelope. Anything which kills the cell or destroys the envelope can accomplish this. Natural serum of one animal can act as a haemolytic agent when injected into the body of another animal of a different species. The serum from a dog is haemolytic to the red blood-cells of a rabbit, but if this serum be heated to 135°F it loses its haemolytic powers. The heat has destroyed the agent which caused the haemolysis.

'Agglutination' is the process by which the red cells of the blood are collected together into clumps, under the action of an agent in the blood called an 'agglutinin'. It sometimes precedes haemolysis.

WHITE BLOOD-CELLS can be seen as colourless bodies in among the red cells when blood is examined by the microscope. They are larger and fewer than the red cells, and nucleated, and possess the power of spontaneous (*i.e.* 'amoeboid') movement. They are collectively called white blood-cells, but are divided into certain classes. They exist in a varying proportion to the red cells, from 1 to 300, to as few as 1 to 700, and their numbers are liable to great fluctuation in the same animal at different times.

White blood-cells or **leukocytes** comprise the following:

Neutrophils, in which the cytoplasm contains granules which – with stains containing eosin and methylene blue – are not coloured markedly red or blue. The nuclei are of many shapes, and the term *polymorphonuclear leukocyte* is applied to neutrophils. They can migrate from the blood-vessels into the tissues and engulf bacteria (phagocytosis), are found in pus and are very important in defence against infection.

Eosinophils have red-staining granules, contain hydrolytic enzymes, and have been observed to increase in numbers during the course of certain chronic diseases.

Basophils have blue-staining granules, containing histamine which is secreted during allergy. Basophils and mast cells have receptors for IgE antibodies, and when basophils with IgE

antibodies on their surfaces are stimulated by antigen (usually of parasitic origin) they release histamine, and in severe reactions the animal may die.

Monocytes have very few granules, engulf bacteria, and are important in less acute infections than those dealt with by neutrophils. When they migrate from blood-vessels into surrounding tissues, they increase in size and are called *macrophages*.

Lymphocytes also have few granules and are likewise formed in lymphoid tissue, *e.g.* lymph nodes, spleen, tonsils. B and T cells are concerned with antibody formation and form barriers against local disease. (*See* B CELLS.)

Coagulation (*see under* CLOTTING).

Temperature. The temperature of the blood is not uniform throughout the body. It is coolest near the surface, and hottest in the hepatic veins. It varies from 100° to 105°F.

BLOOD, DISEASES OF (*see* ANAEMIA, and the blood disorders given under that heading; *also* LEUKAEMIA, THROMBOCYTOPAENIA, HAEMOLYTIC disease in the foal, *also* THROMBASTHENIA, CANINE HAEMOPHILIA, LEUKOPENIA, HAEMOLYSIS, VIRAEMIA, PYAEMIA, TOXAEMIA, SEPTICAEMIA).

BLOOD ENZYMES (*see* CREATINE KINASE, for a reference to diagnosis). Other blood enzymes, now routinely used in diagnosis, include: aldolase, alkaline phosphatase, alanine aminotransferase, asparate aminotransferase, acetycholinesterase, gamma glutamyltransferase, glutathione peroxidase, α-hydroxybutyrate dehydrogenase, lactate dehydrogenase and superoxide dismutase.

For information on their activities in fresh serum, as compared with those in plasma containing anticoagulants and preservatives, see Jones, D. G. (1985) *Research in Veterinary Science* **38**, 301.

BLOOD GROUP. There is apt to be confusion over this term, since it is sometimes applied to single blood factors or agglutinogens, but usually to combinations of blood factors. It is preferable to speak of blood group systems, and the factors within these.

Cattle. The blood group systems of cattle, and the factors within each system, are as shown in the table, reproduced here by courtesy of Dr J. Moustgaard, Royal Veterinary and Agricultural College, Copenhagen.

Since the particular blood serum protein character on which the grouping is based, is inherited, examination of blood samples from within a breed might eventually prove a very useful means of selection. It might also indicate what matings could be expected to result in infertility.

Dogs. In dogs, eight major groups have been recognised in the USA, and they are referred to as in the Table on the next page.

Cats. In 1953 R. Holme found three blood groups in the UK, later designated A, B and AB.

Blood Groups of Cattle

Group systems	Group factors														
A	A_1,	A_2,	D,	H,	Z'										
B	B,	G,	K,	I_1,	I_2,	O_1,	O_2,	O_3,	P,	Q,	T_1,	T_2,	Y_1,	Y_2,	
	A_1',	A_2',	B',	D',	E_1',	E_2',	E_3',	I',	J',			K',	O',	P',	Y'
C	C_1,	C_2,	E,	R_1,	R_2,	W,	X_1,	X_2,	X_3,	L'					
FV	F_1,	F_2,	V_1,	V_2											
J	J														
L	L														
M	M_1,	M_2													
891	S_2,	U_1,	U_2,	U'											
Z	Z_1,	Z_2													
R'S'	R',	S'													

New nomenclature*	Common name	Incidence** (%)
DEA – 1.1	A_1	40
DEA – 1.2	A_2	20
DEA – 3	B	5
DEA – 4	C	98
DEA – 5	D	25
DEA – 6	F	98
DEA – 7	Tr	45
DEA – 8	He	40

*Dog erythrocyte antigen system; **in random dog population.
(With acknowledgements to Dr Jean Dodds and *In Practice*, March 1983.)

These same groups have been found in Australia, in the proportions of 73 per cent, 26 per cent, and less than 1 per cent. L. Auer and colleagues found that 60 per cent of cats with blood group B went into a state of shock within two minutes of being given a blood transfusion containing incompatible A cells. In order to avoid this, vets in Australia carry out blood typing and cross matching before giving a blood transfusion to a cat.

In America it was found by Kilrain and Gieger in 1987 that 99 per cent of cats were type A. Only one of the 100 cats tested, a Himalayan, had group B blood. This explained why USA vets rarely observed any transfusion reactions, and usually proceed without preliminary cross matching. (Dr Meredith S. Bird and colleagues at Tuft's University School of Veterinary Medicine, Massachusetts. *Companion Animal Practice*.)

For B phenogroups, *see under* PHENOGROUPS. (*See also* BLOOD TYPING *and under* ELECTROPHORESIS.)

BLOOD PARASITES OF BRITISH CATTLE:

Piroplasms	*Babesia divergens* (Redwater agent)
	B. major
	Theileria mutans
	T. sergenti
Rickettsiae	*Cytoectes* (= *Ehrlichia*) *phago-cytophilia*
	(Tick-borne fever agent)
	Haemobartonella bovis
	Eperythrozoon wenyoni
	E. tuomii
	E. teganodes
Flagellate	*Trypanosoma theileri*

BLOOD-POISONING is a popular name for 'septicaemia' or 'pyaemia'. (See these headings.)

BLOOD SPOTS IN EGGS. A vitamin A supplement for hens has been suggested as a means of ridding eggs of this unappetising but harmless defect.

BLOOD TRANSFUSION is used in veterinary practice in cases of haemorrhage and shock, and to a lesser extent as part of the treatment of certain infectious diseases. In cattle, donor and recipient are usually in the same herd, a fact which lessens the risk of introducing infection. Blood is collected from the jugular or other vein (after the skin has been cleaned and all precautions taken to achieve asepsis) by means of a suitable needle (*e.g.* 13 BWG) and syringe, and is allowed to flow into a sterilised bottle containing sodium citrate solution (10 grains of sodium citrate in a little sterile water for every 100 cc of blood collected). The bottle must be shaken during collection. The donor's blood, 400 cc or more, thus collected, is transferred to the recipient's vein.

Normal antibodies against the blood group factor J are sometimes found in cattle. Thus, if the donor's blood is J-positive, and the recipient's blood contains the normal antibody anti-J, so-called transfusion reactions might be expected immediately following blood transfusion, in the form of dyspnoea, muscular twitching, increased salivation, and circulatory disturbances (hypotension). In a very few cases, weak reactions of this kind do occur. If, however, an animal has been exposed to repeated blood transfusions, a different situation arises. The animal will now have formed antibodies against the blood group antigens it does not have itself. It is therefore by no means unlikely that the blood of donor and recipient are incompatible. If this is so, the blood transfusion will set off strong transfusion reactions. Such reactions can occur on the second or on subsequent blood transfusions, even though there are no serologically demonstrable amounts of antibody in the recipient's blood. (Dr J. Moustgaard.)

In dogs, if not in cattle, it is desirable to inject a little local anaesthetic at the site where the needle is to be introduced, after clipping the hair and cleaning the skin. The jugular, radial, or external saphena vein will serve. A 19 BW G needle is useful. Sodium citrate is used, as mentioned above. The blood is transferred to the recipient from the collecting bottle by the Simplex Apparatus or by means of a syringe.

For 1983 advice on canine blood transfusion, *see* paper by Dr Jean Dodds in *In Practice*.

In the new-born foal suffering from haemolytic disease, exchange transfusion has been the means of saving life. Up to 5500 ml of the foal's blood are removed, being replaced by up to 7000 ml of compatible donor's blood. This process takes some 3 hours and is only practicable with special apparatus. (*See also* BLOOD GROUPS, PLASMA SUBSTITUTES, FELINE INFECTIOUS ENTERITIS, DEHYDRATION.)

Single blood transfusions in domestic animals, without cross-matching or typing, are generally safe, and may be the means of saving life in a dog involved in an accident leading to severe haemorrhage; or in an unvaccinated cat with feline enteritis (to give two examples). In cats, blood groups A and B are present in the approximate proportions of three to one; less than 1 per cent are A B. In dogs there are nine known blood groups.

BLOOD TYPING. In Canada extensive use is made of blood typing in respect of cattle, and results of a blood test have been accepted as evidence in court in a case where a man was convicted of falsifying a pedigree. The basis of this evidence was that to prove parentage of an animal all the factors found in the blood of a calf must be present in the blood of either the sire or the dam. If certain factors found in the blood of the calf could not be found in the blood of either the sire or the dam, then that calf could not have been of that particular mating – as was proved in this case.

Blood typing is also used in the diagnosis of freemartins. In one series 228 freemartins were found out of 242 sets of twins.

Blood-typing has been used to decide the paternity issue in a heifer calf born to a cow inseminated twice in the same heat period with semen from two different bulls; to reveal discrepancies in pedigrees; and to allay or confirm suspicion on the part of a Breed Society asked to register a calf born following a very short or a very long gestation period.

The UK's first cattle blood typing service was established in 1967 and, by 1972, was at the Animal Breeding Research Organisation, Edinburgh, testing some 3,000 samples a year.

The work falls into two categories: commercial and research. In the former category there are routine pedigree parentage cases involving one bull, one cow, and one calf. Out of 403 such cases in 1972, 26 (or 6·5 per cent) were found to be incorrect. Checking the parentage of bulls to be used in AI as well as typing bulls being used in AI are carried out. Other applications include the diagnosis of freemartins, the control of egg transplantation, i.e. checking that the offspring is from the egg put in and not from the host cow's own egg.

Blood typing is of service in the policing of screening tests, *e.g.* for brucellosis. It is not unknown for lazy or unscrupulous people to fill several sample tubes with blood from the same animal and label them as coming from several animals. If several tubes are found to have identical types, fraud is virtually certain to have occurred, since the likelihood of two samples, other than from identical twins, having the same blood type is negligible.

On the research side, cattle blood grouping opened up many possibilities in the field of animal health. For example it has resulted in a diagnostic method for detecting abscesses deep in the body which cannot be seen, *e.g.* a liver abscess which is an all too common complication of barley beef production. (*See also* EQUINE BLOOD TYPES.)

THE PREPARATION OF TEST SERA containing antibodies, or blood group reagents, is based on the injection of blood corpuscles from one animal into another of the same species, or into one of a different species. The first procedure is called iso-immunisation, the second heteroimmunisation. As a result of both procedures, the recipient animal produces antibodies to the antigenic factors associated with the donor blood corpuscles, provided that these factors are not already present in the recipient animal. (No animal can produce both an antigen and its antibody.) The diagram (page 74) demonstrates the principle of iso-immunisation in cattle.

It shows that the donor possesses blood group factors A, B, and C while the recipient has only blood group factor A. On immunisation, the recipient will therefore form antibodies to blood group factors B and C. The antibodies thus formed are called anti-B and anti-C. A serum containing several blood group antibodies is known as a crude serum. This serum will react with red corpuscles not only from the donor, but also from all cattle with the blood group factor B or C.

To obtain a blood group reagent which reacts with only one blood group factor, for example B, the anti-C antibody must be removed. To do this, the prepared crude serum is mixed with blood corpuscles which are C-positive but B-negative. The anti-C is then bound to the blood corpuscles and can be removed by centrifuging, as illustrated. This procedure is called antibody absorption. As the figure indicates, a specific B-reagent prepared in this way can be used to decide whether the blood group factor B is or is not present in a cow or bull, provided that rabbit complement is also present.

To obtain sufficiently high concentration of antibodies, donor blood corpuscles are injected into the recipient once a week for 4 to 6 weeks. The antibody concentration of the recipient's blood serum, or its titre, is estimated by determining the power of the serum to react with donor blood corpuscles, or with blood corpuscles possessing a similar antigenic structure. In some cases, one single period of immunisation is inadequate to achieve a satisfactorily high antibody concentration in the recipient's blood. This can often be achieved, however, by repeating the immunisation a few months later (reimmunisation). (Dr J. Moustgaard.) (*See also* TRANSFERRIN, EQUINE

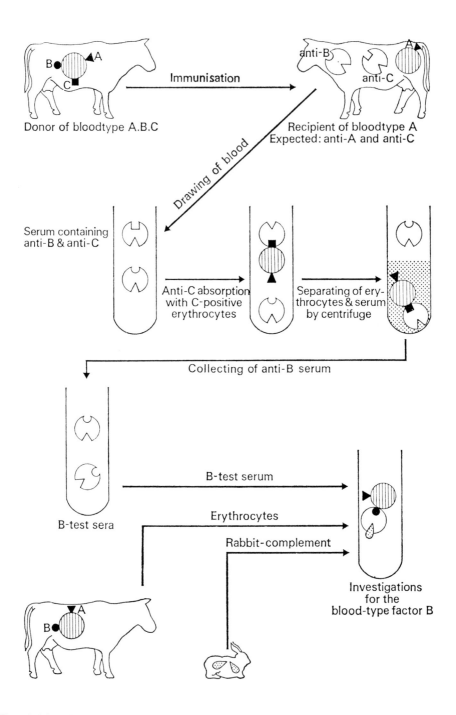

The principles of producing a test serum and its use in blood grouping (*with acknowledgements to Dr J. Moustgaard, Royal Veterinary and Agricultural College, Copenhagen*).

BLOOD TYPES, GENETIC ENGINEERING – monoclonal antibodies, ELECTROPHORESIS).

BLOUWILDEBEESOOG. A disease of sheep, cattle and horses, characterised by enlargement of the eyes leading to blindness. It occurs in Africa, and is apparently spread by blue-wildebeest. Cause: unknown.

BLOW-FLIES (*see* FLIES *and also under* 'STRIKE').

BLOWPIPE DARTS (*see* PROJECTILE SYRINGES).

'BLOWS'. Distention of the caecum in the rabbit as a result of excessive gas formation. The rabbit assumes a huddled posture.

BLUE COMB (*see* PULLET DISEASE).

'BLUE-EAR' DISEASE OF PIGS. (Also known as *porcine reproductive and respiratory syndrome.*)
This was first recognised in Germany. Up to the end of March 1991, there had been about 2,500 outbreaks in Germany, 1,100 in the Netherlands, twelve in Belgium, and several in the Humberside area of the UK.
It was made NOTIFIABLE in the UK in 1991, following outbreaks in Humberside, Norfolk and Lincolnshire.
CAUSE. This has been named the Lelystad agent; and there is evidence that the infection can be spread not only by the movement of pigs but also by the wind.
Extensive tests in several countries have failed to link the cause with any previously known infective agent.
SIGNS. Late abortions, stillbirths, premature farrowing; weakness, oedema and death of piglets.
A possibly identical disease, cause unknown, has been reported from the USA. ☞

'BLUE-EYE' (*see* CANINE VIRAL HEPATITIS).

BLUE-GRAY. The offspring of a Galloway or of an Aberdeen-Angus crossed with a Beef Shorthorn bull.

BLUE NOSE DISEASE is apparently a form of Light Sensitisation occurring in the horse, following the eating of some particular meadow plant. The name arises from the blue discolouration observed in some cases on the muzzle (but not, for example, on the same animal's white socks). Sloughing of the non-pigmented skin occurs, and there is often intense excitement amounting to frenzy – during which the horse may do itself a fatal injury. (*See* LIGHT SENSITISATION, ANTIHISTAMINES.)

BLUE-TONGUE. A disease formerly confined mainly to Africa but, of recent years, reported also in America, Portugal, Spain, and Cyprus, Israel, etc. In 1958 the Australian Government imposed a ban upon imports of cattle as well as of sheep on account of the risk of introducing the disease.
A clinical case of the disease was detected in a sheep in 1989. Quarantine is not an effective safeguard in the case of cattle, since if infected they rarely become ill with the disease.* Infection is carried by biting midges and probably the mosquito, and consequently outbreaks are commonest near the breeding haunts of such insects – damp, marshy regions.
In a survey of nearly 3,000 samples of blood sera from farm animals slaughtered in Iran and examined for the presence of blue-tongue virus precipitating antibodies, these were found in 7·6 per cent from sheep, 13·6 per cent from goats, 0·6 per cent from cattle, 5·9 per cent from camels, and 4·5 per cent from pigs.
A survey of 6250 sera from cattle, sheep and goats in seven Caribbean and two South American countries showed that antibody to Blue-tongue virus was widely distributed in each species. Overall prevalences of antibody were 70 per cent in cattle, 67 per cent in sheep, and 76 per cent in goats – as assessed by a laboratory test. *Yet no clinical cases* had been confirmed in the area, and no virus isolates were available to indicate which serotype(s) was/were causing the infection. (Gibbs, E. P. J. & others. (1983) *Veterinary Record* **113**, 446.)
CAUSE: An orbivirus.
SIGNS. A rise in temperature up to 107°, and after a week or 10 days eruptions on the tongue, lips, and dental pads with a swelling and blueness of these parts, mark the typical appearance of an attack. Both the mouth and nose show a discharge, and there is an accompanying smacking of the lips. In spite of the soreness of the mouth the sheep are inclined to feed, but loss of flesh is very rapid, particularly when diarrhoea sets in. Thirst is usually great during the fever stage. In from 3 to 5 days, the mouth lesions begin to heal, and the disease is seen in the feet. These become sore; sheep are stiff in their movements, and feed from the kneeling or recumbent positions. In bad cases the hoofs may be shed.
In both cattle and sheep the disease may be subclinical.
TREATMENT. Isolation of the affected into shady paddocks, sheds, or orchards, where they are immune from disturbance, antiseptic mouth washes, good feeding of a soft, succulent quality, the provision of a clean water-supply and salt-licks.
It should be noted that if the sheep can be kraaled at night, so that they have a roof over their heads, the number affected will be greatly reduced, or even, in many cases, the disease will never appear. Dipping has given good results.

---

* At least one strain of virus (identical with a Californian strain) is stated to have caused an outbreak involving cattle in 1959–60. An interesting feature is that 10 per cent of the cattle died but that sheep were not affected at all. Death was mostly a result of thirst and starvation due to the difficulty of swallowing. Similar effects have been recorded in South Africa.

PREVENTION. A quadrivalent vaccine is available.

BOARDING KENNELS (*see* ANIMAL BOARDING ESTABLISHMENTS ACT).

BODY-SCANNER (*see under* X-RAYS).

BOG ASPHODEL (*Narthecium ossifragum*) is a cause of light sensitisation in sheep. Ears, face, and legs of white lambs may all be affected. Skin necrosis may follow the inflammation. In severe cases, jaundice may be a complication.

In Ireland the loss of lambs' ears and blindness are attributed by farmers to this plant.

BOG SPAVIN. An old name for osteitis and arthritis of the hock (*tarsus*) of horses. Deposition of new bone may result in lameness. However, bony enlargements do not invariably accompany the condition; the hock appearing normal to the touch, when therm 'occult spavin' is used. (*See also* BONE SPAVIN.)

Bog spavin is technically known as *tarsal hydrarthrosis* and probably starts with a synovitis. It seldom causes lameness.

BOLLINGER, BODIES (*see* FOWL POX).

BOLUS. A roughly spherical mass of food, which has been chewed and mixed with saliva, ready for swallowing. Bolus also means a cylindrical mass, 1½ to 3 inches long, and up to ½ inch in diameter, of a medicine in paste form for administration to horses and cattle. It is also known as a 'ball' – hence BALLING GUN. A slow-release bolus

for the administration of anthelmintics or trace elements is a modern development.

A bolus of slow dissolving soluble glass containing copper, selenium and cobalt for trace element supplementation in cattle and sheep was introduced by the Wellcome Foundation.

Cosecure contains 13·4 per cent w/w copper, 0·3 per cent selenium and 0·5 per cent cobalt in a glass bolus made of sodium, phosphorus, calcium and magnesium oxides. It is claimed to give a controlled supply of these elements for 12 months.

(*See* WORMS, FARM TREATMENT AGAINST.)

BONE is composed partly of fibrous tissue, partly of phosphate and carbonate of lime. Since the bones of a young animal are composed of about 60 per cent fibrous tissue, and those of an old animal of more than 60 per cent of lime salts, one readily understands the toughness of the former and the brittleness of the latter. Two kinds of bone are noteworthy: *dense bone*, such as forms the shafts of the long bones of the limbs, and *cancellous* or *spongy bone*, such as is found in the short bones and at the ends of the long bones. Dense bone is found in a tube-like form, with a central cavity in which normally *yellow marrow* is found, composed mainly of fatty substances; the walls of the tube are stout and strong, and the outer surface is covered by 'bone membrane' or *periosteum*. Cancellous bone has a more open framework, is irregular in shape, and, instead of possessing a cavity, its centre is divided into innumerable tiny spaces by a fine network of bony threads, which support the important *red marrow*. (*See* MARROW.)

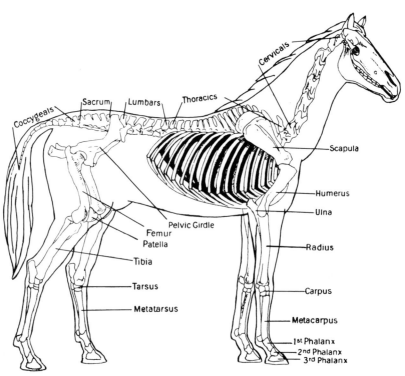

Skeleton of horse

All bone is penetrated by a series of fine canals (Haversian canals), in which run blood-vessels, nerves, lymph-vessels, etc., for the growth, maintenance, and repair of the bone.

VARIETIES OF BONE. Apart from their structural classification, bones are arranged according to their external shape into: (*a*) *long bones*, like those of the limbs; (*b*) *short bones*, such as those of the 'knee' and hock; (*c*) *flat bones*, such as those of the skull and the shoulder-blade; (*d*) *irregular bones*, such as those of the vertebral column; and (*e*) the *'spongy' bones* of the feet of horses and cattle and the claws of other animals. This last type of bone is really extraordinarily dense in structure, but multitudes of both large and small blood-vessels penetrate into its depth from the outside and give it the appearance of being soft and spongy.

THE SKELETON is composed of a varying number of bones in the different animals, and the number varies even among individuals of the same species and breed. These variations are due to age in some cases – the younger animals having certain bones separate that fuse together later; sex may alter the number – the male dog has a bone in its penis that the female does not possess; while in the tails of all animals the number of bones is likely to differ according to the varying length of that structure in animals of the same breed and size. The skeleton is divided into: (1) an *axial* part, consisting of the skull, the vertebrae, the ribs with their cartilages, and the sternum or breast-bone; and (2) an *appendicular* portion, consisting of the four limbs. In addition to these divisions, certain parts of the skeleton are embedded in the substance of organs, and are described as the *visceral* skeleton, *e.g.* the bones in the tongue, that in the heart of the ox, the snout of the pig, the penis of the dog, etc.

BONE, DISEASES OF. Since bones are deeply seated and not richly supplied with blood-vessels diseases of bone are apt to be overlooked for a much longer time than in the case of other tissues similarly affected.

Growth-plate. A layer of cartilage between the diaphysis and the epiphysis of a long bone **GROWTH-PLATE DISORDERS.** 'Failure of chondrogenesis leading to cessation of growth is commonly the result of trauma to the plate, occasioned by a fracture or crush injury, or of the interruption of the vascular supply to the germinal cells. Diseases such as scurvy, rickets, osteomyelitis and endocrine disorders make the plate more vulnerable to injury and predipose to epiphyseal separation.'

Epiphyseal injury in the foal, for example, may be of two types:

Type 1. Separation without fracture. After re-alignment healing is rapid and the prognosis is good. Femoral head detachment is the exception because if the epiphyseal vessels are damaged avascular necrosis of the head follows.

Type 2. The most common, involving fracture of a triangular piece of metaphysis. With accurate reduction the prognosis is good.

Such injuries 'usually involve the epiphyses in the distal radius, distal metacarpus and proximal first phalanx. These cases often have the appearance of acute joint sprains but epiphyseal damage should always be suspected because at this age growth plates are weaker than collateral ligaments. Radiography is essential to identify the type of defect present.

Prompt and accurate replacement of the epiphysis is required followed by external support with a cast or splint to maintain alignment. In certain instances fixation of the fragments with a compression screw may offer greater security.' (Professor L. C. Vaughan). (*See* VALGUS for picture.)

Acute inflammation of bone is divided into acute *periostitis*, or inflammation of the surface of the bone and its covering membrane, the periosteum; acute *osteitis* or *ostitis*, inflammation of the bone substance itself; and acute *osteomyelitis*, inflammation in the bone and the central marrow cavity. These three conditions are grades in severity; the deeper the inflammation extends the more serious is the condition. It is seldom that the three can be differentiated from each other except after death.

Acute inflammation of the bone surface almost always results from external violence. Osteomyelitis is usually due to bacteria gaining access either through the blood- or lymph-streams, or through the broken tissues resulting from a deep wound. The mildest types are often due to an inflammation in a ligament or tendon spreading to the periosteum in the near vicinity and causing it to become inflamed as a consequence. (*See also* RHEUMATISM.)

Symptoms vary according to the bones affected. In all cases there are signs of pain when the affected part is handled, and if it be a limb bone, as is often the case, there is lameness. In very severe instances, where the bone tissue has become infected, there is fever; dullness and a disinclination for movement; and there are signs of severe general debility. If the bone is near the surface, such as in the case of 'sore shins', a condition that affects the cannon bones of young thoroughbreds when their training has been too severe or when the ground is very hard, the bone seems to be swollen and hot to touch during the first few days; and later, when the acuteness of the symptoms gets less, the bone is found to be still more swollen, but the pain and heat are less. This thickening of the bone often remains for long periods and in some animals never wholly disappears.

Complete rest from work is essential: in fact work, or even walking, is often impossible. Hot fomentations, soothing and cooling liniments or applications, are usually sufficient to cut short mild attacks. For this purpose 'Antiphlogistine', a preparation of glycerine and kaolin with other agents, is very useful. The severer cases, in which infection has reached the bone, call in the first place for penicillin or the sulphonamides, or immediate opening up of the area and the elimination of any pus that has collected. After that, any pieces of dead bone that are present are removed, and the wound treated as an infected open wound.

Chronic inflammation includes several diverse conditions, *e.g.* tuberculosis, actinomycosis, etc.

Generally speaking, when a chronic suppurative inflammation affects a bone, sooner or later the pus and debris of a liquid nature will burrow through the surrounding tissues and burst on to the surface of the skin. A discharging sinus results which proves intractable to treatment. At the bottom of this sinus lies the dead piece of bone, and until it has been removed or absorbed the leakage of purulent material will continue in spite of antiseptic injections and other surface treatment.

The offending dead portion of bone must be removed in the first instance, and the whole sinus tract must be laid open. This is not always an easy matter, and much depends upon the situation of the 'sequestrum', as well as on the mouth of the sinus. The area afterwards is treated as an open wound, and if all the necrotic parts have been removed, recovery generally takes place.

Exostosis is an outgrowth of rarefied bone tissue upon the surface of a bone. Among the commonest forms of exostoses are the following: certain forms of splints, ring-bones, bone spavins, some side-bones. (*See also* ACROPACHIA.)

Tumours of bone are sometimes met with. The commonest of these is the osteosarcoma of the limb-bones of dogs. The bony tissue is invaded by the cells that are characteristic of the tumour, and there is swelling and pain.

Rickets is a disease of young animals in which the bones of the limbs are affected, and often small pea-like swellings are found at the junction of each of the ribs with its cartilage. (*See* RICHETS.)

Osteomalacia is the equivalent of rickets occurring in the adult animal, especially during pregnancy. (*See* OSTEOMALACIA.)

Osteodystrophic diseases are a group of diseases which are due to errors in feeding owing to an incorrect calcium:phosphorus ratio in the diet, or to lack of one or more of the minerals – calcium, phosphorus, magnesium, and sometimes manganese – and if vitamin D has been inadequate in amount in the food eaten for some considerable time (*e.g. see* OSTEOFIBROSIS, FELINE JUVENILE OSTEODYSTROPHY).

Porphyria is a rare disease, hereditary in origin, occurring in man, cattle, and pigs. It is characterised by brown or pinkish discoloration of the bones and teeth, and by changes in the urine. In cattle a hairless, scabby condition of the skin is also a symptom. (*See also under* HEXA-CHLOROBENZENE.)

BONE GRAFTS (*see* section at the end of FRACTURES).

BONE MARROW (*see* MARROW, ANAEMIA, HAEMOGLOBIN, RED BLOOD CELLS).

BONE PINNING. A method of treating fractures. In medullary pinning, a pointed stainless steel 'pin' is driven down the marrow cavity of the bone concerned; in ordinary pinning transverse 'pins' are used, driven through the bone at right angles to its length, and the pins held in position by a special adjustable metal splint.

These methods obviate the use of cumbersome plaster casts, and they also enable cases of serious

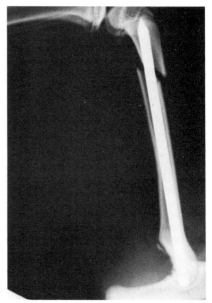

The insertion of a metal pin down the marrow cavity of the bone.

and multiple fracture (*e.g.* as caused in a dog or cat knocked down by a car) to be successfully treated – a result often impossible of achievement by older methods. These techniques require a high degree of specialised skill and strict asepsis and, of course, the use of a general anaesthetic.

BONE SPAVIN. An old name for osteitis and arthritis of the hock (*tarsus*) of horses. Deposition of new bone may result in lameness. However, bony enlargements do not invariably accompany the condition; the hock appearing normal to the touch, when the term 'occult spavin' is used. (*See also* BOG SPAVIN.)

Faulty conformation, probably inherited, accounts for some cases of spavin; local stress or trauma for others; while in some, malnutrition may be a factor.

TREATMENT may include injection of prednisolone into the joint.

BONES thrown to pigs, or given raw to dogs and carried by them to ground to which pigs have access, have caused outbreaks of foot-and-mouth disease in pigs; the bones having come from imported beef carcases infected with virus.

For troubles caused in dogs by unsuitable bones, *see under* CHOKING and INTESTINES, DISEASES OF.

BORACIC, or BORIC ACID, is found in volcanic districts, or is prepared from borax.

USES. Boracic acid is a popular but inefficient antiseptic. In solution, it was widely used as an eye-lotion. In human medicine, babies have died as a result of topical applications of boracic acid. In poultry boric acid poisoning gives rise to loss of appetite, diarrhoea, depression, and progressive weakness, coma, and death.

BORAN. An East African type of Zebu cattle.

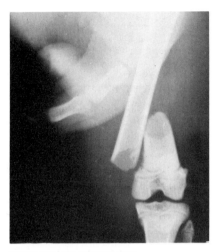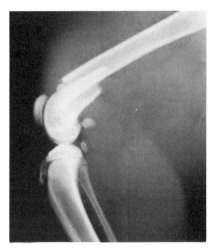

INTRA-MEDULLARY PINNING
(Above) Two views of the fracture of the femur in a dog. (Beaumont Animals' Hospital.)

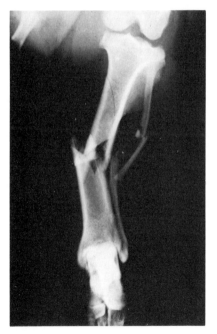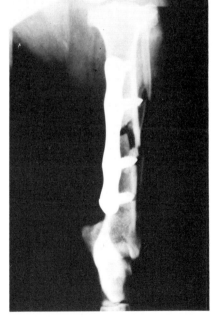

PLATING
This is another technique used in veterinary practice. The radiographs show a fracture of the tibia of a dog and the use of a metal plate screwed into the bone. (Beaumont Animals' Hospital.)

BORBORYGMUS means flatulence in the bowels.

'BORDER DISEASE' OF SHEEP. A disease occurring on the English–Welsh border, and first described in 1959.

CAUSE: The virus which causes the disease in lambs is classified as belonging to the family Togaviridae, genus Pestivirus.

SIGNS. The birth-coat is altered; the amount of hair in the fleece being increased. Lambs are smaller than normal, and grow more slowly. The shape of the head is slightly abnormal – likewise the gait which, however, shows only a slight swaying motion. Mortality is very high; most lambs dying during their first few weeks.

The disease has been recognised in New Zealand, the USA, Switzerland.

A feature of the disease is acute necrosis of the placenta associated with abortion.

It appears that there is an immunological relationship between Border disease, mucosal disease, and swine fever. Possibly all three are caused by closely related viruses. In-contact piglets may be infected by sheep with Border disease.

BORDETELLA (*see under* BACTERIA). *B. bronchiseptica* is a secondary invader complicating cases of canine distemper, and may also produce respiratory disease (*see* KENNEL COUGH) in the dog independently of viruses. This bacterium is also the cause of chronic respiratory disease in many other animals. (*See under* RHINITIS.)

BOREDOM. Among housed stock, this can undoubtedly have a serious effect upon health and consequently upon the farmer's profits. Boredom is regarded by many people as one cause of TAIL-BITING (which see) in intensively reared pigs. In laying batteries, it is one cause of egg-eating. In horses, it is a cause of weaving, windsucking, and crib-biting.

BORNA DISEASE A disease of horses mainly, but also of ruminants, in Europe and elsewhere.

CAUSE. A virus which is closely related to those causing EQUINE ENCEPHALOMYELITIS (which see) occurring in various tropical, subtropical and temperate regions; the diseases bearing such names as Near Eastern Encephalitis, Venezuelan, Eastern, Western, and Japanese B. Encephalitis.

TRANSMISSION. Mosquitoes, midges, and ticks can transmit the virus, of which birds are also hosts.

SIGNS. Depression and fever. Recovery may follow without involvement of the central nervous system, but probably in most cases such involvement does occur. Signs then include walking in circles, or pressing the head against a fixed object, a facial twitch, hanging of the head, ataxia, and paralysis.

DIAGNOSIS depends upon a fluorescent antibody test or the detection of Joest-Degen antibodies. A differential diagnosis of Borna disease in sheep must take into account louping-ill, maedia-visna, rabies, listeriosis, scrapie, cerebro-cortical necrosis, poisons, etc.

BOROGLUCONATE. The salt of calcium used in solution for intravenous or subcutaneous injection in cases of hypocalcaemia ('Milk Fever').

BORRELIA. A species of SPIROCHAETES (which see), causing disease in fowls in the tropics, and also human tick-borne relapsing fever. The distribution of the latter is, with the exception of Australia, almost world-wide. The signs include fever, erythema, sometimes jaundice. In the USA the name Lyme disease is given to a children's illness characterised by arthritis, headache, lethargy, and sometimes meningitis or encephalitis. (*See* LYME DISEASE.)

BOSS COWS (*see* BUNT ORDER).

BOT-FLIES belong to the Oestrus family, and their maggot forms are parasitic upon various of the domestic animals, chiefly the horse, sheep, and deer. (*See* FLIES.)

BOTHRIOCEPHALUS is one of the parasitic tapeworms.

BOTRYOMYCOSIS (*see* Staphylococcus auresus *under* BACTERIA; *also* GRANULOMA).

'BOTTLE-JAW' (*see* illustration).

BOTULISM. A form of food poisoning, often fatal, caused by *Clostridium botulinum* toxins, which produce paralysis. Botulism occurs world-wide, but is especially common in the tropics.

Cattle and sheep. Large numbers may die in regions where they suffer from mineral deficiencies (especially phosphorus) and are driven to eating the bones of dead animals to obtain the minerals they need.

C. botulinum may inhabit the alimentary tract of a healthy animal without ill effect. However in a decaying carcase, rapid multiplication of the bacterium, with toxin production, occurs. Carrion is therefore the main source of botulism in animals, but proliferation can also occur in decaying vegetable matter. Carcases may pollute well water or forage, and in Britain botulism in cattle has been associated with the use of broiler litter on grazing land; such waste containing a few carcases.

SIGNS. Large doses of toxin may result in sudden death, but often the illness lasts a few days; the animal becoming first stiff and dejected, and then recumbent, lying on the sternum with the cow's head turned to one side. Salivation may be profuse, swallowing difficult or impossible, so that botulism has to be differentiated from rabies when making a diagnosis.

CONTROL. The use of mineral supplements where osteophagia occurs (*see* LAMZIEKTE), or of vaccines.

Horses: the signs are ataxia, difficulty in swallowing, and posterior paralysis; or sudden death. In the UK cases have occurred in horses fed big-bale silage.

Smith and Young found that 5 per cent of 174 samples of British soil contained *Cl. botulinum* type B, and soil contamination of big-bale silage (as well as contained rodent carcases) has been suggested as one source of botulism in horses.

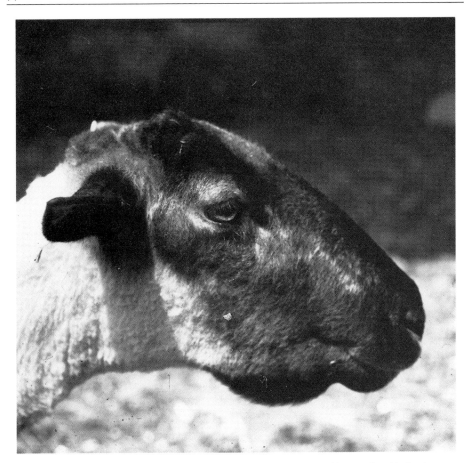

'Bottle-Jaw'. Oedema of the lower jaw caused by *Haemonchus contortus*, a parasitic worm found in the abomasum of sheep and goats. It is also a cause of severe anaemia. (Photo reproduced by permission of Dr M. A. Taylor BVMS, PhD, of the Central Veterinary Laboratory, Weybridge; Crown Copyright Reserved.)

(Ricketts, S. W. & Frape, D. L. (1986) *Veterinary Record* **118**, 55.)

Progressive symmetrical muscle weakness in eight horses on an American farm was linked to the presence of *Cl. botulinum* in the alfalfa hay which they were receiving. Two of the horses became recumbent within 24 hours of the onset of clinical signs.

One horse was found dead, euthanasia was resorted to in six of the cases, and one recovered. (J. J. Wichtel and others. *JAVMA* (1991) **199**, 471.)

Dogs. Botulism was almost certainly the cause of an outbreak of paralysis in a pack of foxhounds. Some were unable to stand and, in response to calls, could lift only their heads and tails. There were two deaths. *Cl. botulinum* was isolated from the remains of meat which had been fed. (Darke, P. G. G. *et al. Vet. Rec.* (1976) **99**, 98.)

In another outbreak of botulism among foxhounds, intoxication by *Cl. botulinum* type C was confirmed by laboratory means. The source was probably a dead calf. (W. F. Blakemore *et al. Vet. Rec.* (1977) **100**, 57.)

Birds. Type C botulism has been reported in Britain among both chickens and waterfowl also pheasants. (*See also under* MAGGOTS.)

Symptoms of botulism in an outbreak among captive birds included a characteristic statuesque behaviour; some individuals stood motionless for over one hour despite activity of other birds around them; paralysis, ranging from a single dropped wing to bilateral leg paralysis; inability to swallow; and terminal gasping.

For botulism in mink, *see under* MINK. For botulism in South African cattle, *see* LAMZIEKTE.

Public health. Human (and also animal) botulism may occur as the result of imperfectly preserved food or when cooked food is allowed to stand and later re-heated. An example of this was the outbreak in Germany in 1971 among people who had eaten smoked trout. *Cl. botulinum* Type E was found to be the cause. Although there have been very few cases of human botulism in Britain, recent investigations have shown that a high proportion of trout in fish farms are contaminated with this Type E, which can multiply at temperatures as low as 5°C, whereas the more common types A and B will not normally multiply at temperatures below 10°C. (*See also* MEAT, CURED.)

BOUTONNEUSE FEVER. A zoonosis which is transmissible from dogs to people. The cause is *Rickettsia conori*. There is a rash. Wrists, ankles, and then other parts of the body may be affected. The dog tick *Rhipicephalus sanguineus* is the vector.

BOVINE ATOPIC RHINITIS was stated (1982) by Dr A. Wiseman and colleagues at the University of Glasgow to have been diagnosed during three successive grazing periods. Recovery followed soon after housing. A discharge from eyes and nose, with some ulceration of nasal mucosa (and formation of granuloma) are symptoms in common with those of Bovine Infectious Rhinitis.

BOVINE AUTO-IMMUNE HAEMOLYTIC ANAEMIA. A heifer died within two days of showing anaemia and dyspnoea, and the diagnosis was as above and based on auto-agglutination (which increased on Coombs' testing) and the presence of anti-bovine IgG on red blood cell surfaces.

'Acute haemolytic anaemia could be due to many causes, including water intoxication, delayed copper toxicity, brassica poisoning, babesiosis, leptospirosis, and bacillary haemoglobinuria.' (P. M. Dixon and others, *Vet. Record* (1978), **103**, 155.)

BOVINE ENCEPHALOMYELITIS. (Buss disease) occurs in the USA, Australia, and Japan. In the USA it is a disease mainly of the summer and autumn months, and cattle under two years old are mainly susceptible.
CAUSE. *Chlamydia psittaci.*
SIGNS. A fever, which lasts a week or more. With loss of appetite, the animal loses condition and becomes weak. A nasal discharge or diarrhoea may be seen. Pushing the head against a wall, walking in a circle, hyperaesthesia, and convulsions are symptoms of which one or two may be seen. Economically the disease has a low incidence and generally a low mortality, but in some herds losses may be serious.

Autopsy findings include pleurisy, pericarditis and peritonitis, apart from any brain lesions.
Public health. Man is susceptible.

BOVINE ENZOOTIC LEUKOSIS. A virus-produced form of cancer, characterised by multiple malignant growths as well as, in some cases, leukaemia. The disease was first recorded in Britain in 1978, is fairly common on the European mainland, and is covered by EC legislation. Occasionally cattle show symptoms before they are 2 years old, but 4–8 years is a more common age. Digestive disturbance, anaemia and loss of condition result.

The virus is a Type C oncornavirus of the retravirus family.

In Britain the Enzootic Bovine Leukosis attested herds scheme was introduced by MAFF in January 1982 to encourage the establishment of EBL-free herds, as a first step towards eradication of the disease. To be registered as EBL-free two negative blood tests must be achieved; these being carried out with an interval of at least four months. Any reactors must be notified to the MAFF divisional veterinary officer, and must not be removed from the farm except for licensed slaughter. The disease is NOTIFIABLE.

BOVINE EPHEMERAL FEVER (*see* EPHEMERAL FEVER).

BOVINE HERPES MAMMILLITIS. An ulcerative disease of the cow's teats and udder, caused by herpes virus. (*See* VIRUS INFECTIONS OF COWS' TEATS.)

BOVINE IMMUNODEFICIENCY VIRUS (BIV). This causes a progressive wasting condition of cattle.

In 1989 there were no reports of this potentially important pathogen in the UK; but tests were being developed for the screening of cattle and BIV products. The project was being partly funded by the Medical Research Council's AIDS directed Programme.

BOVINE INFECTIOUS PETECHIAL FEVER. Also known as Ondiri disease, this affects cattle in Kenya, and is characterised by haemorrhages of the visible mucous membranes, fever, and diarrhoea. There may be severe conjunctivitis and protrusion of the eyeball. Death within 1 to 3 days is not uncommon, though some animals survive for longer, a few recovering. The cause is a rickettsia, believed to be spread by a biting insect, or a tick, and known as *Ehrlichia ondiri*. Symptoms are seen only in imported cattle as a rule. The bushbuck provides a reservoir of infection.

BOVINE MALIGNANT CATARRHAL FEVER. This infection may occur not only in cattle but also in sheep, farmed deer, and antelopes. It is most common in Africa, but cases have been recorded in the UK, EC countries, Australasia, and North America.
CAUSE: a herpesvirus.
SIGNS: Inflammation of the mucous membrane of the mouth, drooling of saliva, gastro-enteritis, keratitis (followed in some cases by blindness, and sometimes ENCEPHALITIS (which see)).

BOVINE PAPULAR STOMATITIS. This pox was first described in Germany and during recent years has been reported in the United Kingdom, Australia, East Africa, etc. The disease is not accompanied by fever or systemic upset. Slightly excessive salivation may occur.

Characteristically, early lesions are rounded areas of intensive congestion up to 1·5 cm in diameter, which in pigmented mucous membrane are visible as roughened areas with greyish discoloration. The centre of such areas becomes necrotic and in a later stage shows a depressed centre. Removal of the caseous material leaves a raw granulating ulcer but normally epithelial regeneration occurs in 3 to 4 days. A feature of the disease is the occurrence of concentric rings of necrosis and congestion. Secondary lesions of mouth, muzzle or nostril may prolong the disease over a period of months.
CAUSE: the parapox virus.

BOVINE PARALYTIC MYOGLOBINURIA (*see under* MUSCLES, DISEASES OF).

BOVINE PARVOVIRUS. A cause of diarrhoea in calves.

BOVINE PULMONARY EMPHYSEMA (*see* FOG FEVER).

BOVINE RESPIRATORY DISEASE COMPLEX (*see* SHIPPING FEVER).

BOVINE RHINOTRACHEITIS, INFECTIOUS (*see* RHINOTRACHEITIS).

BOVINE SPONGIFORM ENCEPHALOPATHY (BSE). This type of Scrapie-like brain disease of cattle was first recognised in 1986.
INCIDENCE. By October 1990, 17,817 cases had been recorded in the UK; and the 1990–1991 annual incidence was 3·9 cases per thousand cows. ☞
CAUSE: a PRION (a self-replicating infectious protein.)
SIGNS: Cattle become nervous and often aggressive. Their gait is a high-stepping one. The head is lowered. They may go down and be unable to get up again.

It is now thought that a proportion of 'Downer-cow syndrome' cases, both in the USA and the UK, have in fact been BSE.
DIFFERENTIAL DIAGNOSIS: BSE has to be differentiated from other disorders such as acetonaemia (in which short periods of delirium may occur); from listeriosis (in which cattle may become violent in the terminal stages); and from hypomagnesaemia and hypocalcaemia.

BSE is a NOTIFIABLE disease, and the policy is one of compulsory slaughter.
PREVENTION. In August 1990 the British Veterinary Association advised against breeding from the calves of cows diagnosed as having BSE.

Two months earlier Mr N. H. Christensen of the department of veterinary pathology and public health, Massey University, New Zealand, had raised the questions: 'If the scrapie-like agent of

BSE survives such temperatures as are used during continuous rendering, is it not possible for such an agent to survive the pelleting process used in poultry feed production, pass through the birds' intestines, and then be spread on pastures on which cattle are grazed?'

In November 1990 various European countries imposed a ban on the import of beef cattle from the UK.

No link had, by the end of 1990, been established between BSE in cattle and FELINE SPONGIFORM ENCEPHALITIS (FSE).

BSE is experimentally transmissible to mice, and has been diagnosed in several species of animals. (See SCRAPIE.)

The Rendering Industry. The European Commission (EC) is to contribute towards the cost of introducing safe procedures to ensure that processed material is free from infective levels of the agents of SCRAPIE and BOVINE SPONGIFORM ENCEPHALOPATHY.

In March 1990 BSE was diagnosed in five bulls at UK artificial insemination centres.

The processed material refers to brain, spinal cord, thymus, spleen, tonsils, and intestines.

By March 1991 one case of BSE had been reported in France, and two in Switzerland.

BOVINE SYNCYTIAL VIRUS. A member of the Paramyxovirus group (*see* VIRUSES), and an important cause of respiratory disease in cattle in many parts of the world. (*See* PNEUMONIA.)

BOVINE VIRUS DIARRHOEA/MUCOSAL DISEASE (BVD/MD). This has caused many outbreaks of illness in both housed and grazing cattle in Britain.

'Bovine virus diarrhoea (BVD) and mucosal

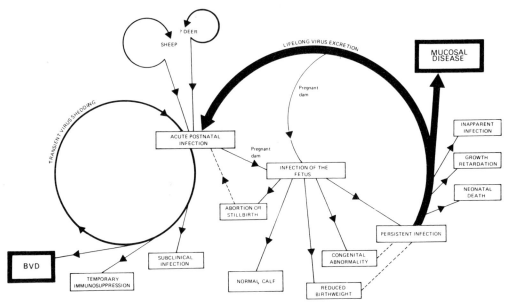

Bovine virus diarrhoea and mucosal disease: infection cycles.
Reproduced with permission from *Veterinary Record* (1985) **117**, 245, MAFF/HMSO. © Crown copyright 1985.
Relabelled for legibility on this page size.

disease (MD) are two clinically dissimilar conditions caused by the same virus.'

'BVD is the result of an acute infection in susceptible cattle which may occur at any age in post-natal life, and is usually a trivial illness of a few days' duration and negligible mortality.'

'By contrast, MD is almost invariably fatal but of low morbidity. It occurs in cattle which have a persistent BVD-MD virus infection acquired as fetuses, characterised by a specific immune tolerance to the infecting virus strain and consequent lack of antibody to it.'

'In Britain BVD-MD virus is widespread. More than 60 per cent of adult cattle have significant levels of serum neutralising antibody, and less than 10 per cent of herds are without serological evidence of past infection,' stated S. J. Duffel and J. W. Harkness (*Veterinary Record* (1985) **117**, 245.)

Dr. J. Brownlie and colleagues at the Institute for Research on Animal Diseases, Compton, stated (1984): Mucosal disease develops following an early *in utero* infection with non-cytopathic BVD virus which results in a persistent viraemia, and a later superinfection with cytopathic BVD virus in post-natal life.

'The implications are that any purchased developing mucosal disease must have been sold when persistently viraemic with non-cytopathic virus. Furthermore these persistently viraemic animals, often clinically normal, may act as a reservoir BVD virus and infect other cattle on the new premises.'

Should there be cows in early pregnancy on the farm, then their infection could result in **abortion**, resorption of the fetus, or the birth of more persistently viraemic calves.

Pigs can become infected with BOVINE VIRAL DIARRHOEA (q.v.) and show signs very similar to those of SWINE FEVER. (Terpstra, C. & Wensvoort, G. (1988) *Research in Veterinary Science* **45**, 137).

CAUSE. The BVD-MD virus belongs to the Pestivirus genus, and is a small RNA virus of the Togavirus family. The virus can survive storage at 4°C for at least 16 months; also repeated freezing and thawing.

SIGNS. in the very mildest cases, there may be a few ulcers in the mouth, perhaps also in the nostrils, but little else. More often, however, the animal runs a temperature of 104° or 105°F with loss of appetite, scouring, and a drop in milk yield. There may be ulcers in the cleft of the foot, and lameness can be a prominent feature of the disease. On some farms there have been outbreaks of an acute illness, on others it has taken a chronic course. Severe cases have been seen in many parts of England and Scotland, among both housed and grazing stock. On one farm 21 out of 50 calves died, and in other outbreaks mortality has been high.

As regards BVD/MD **abortion**, 1980 research findings of Dr J. T. Done and colleagues at the Central Veterinary Laboratory, Weybridge, are that when non-immune cows are, in the middle of their pregnancy, infected with the BVD/MD virus the latter is likely to cross the placenta and infect also the calf. The fetus may die, with abortion following; or alternatively the fetus may mummify. Moreover, those calves born alive may be stunted. Some may have under-developed brains, lungs, or thymus glands.

Dr Done and his colleagues have stated that if, as it is assumed, some 39 per cent of British cows become infected with BVD/MD virus during their first three pregnancies, and that they have vulnerable fetuses for about 180 days of each year, then approximately one in 16 of such calves can be expected to be at risk. This implies that of the viruses which may attack the unborn calf, BVD/MD is possibly the most important in Britain at the present time.

DIAGNOSIS. BVD/MD has to be differentiated from foot-and-mouth disease, Johne's disease, Cattle Plague, and other conditions. An ELISA test is available.

TREATMENT. There is no antiserum or other specific treatment available.

The virus can survive storage at a temperature of 4°C for at least 16 months; also repeated freezing and thawing.

BOW-LEGS obtain normally in some breeds of dogs, such as the pug and bulldog, but in other breeds they are usually the sign of rickets. The shafts of the long bones become softened and bend outwards under the weight of the body, so that the fore-limbs especially become curved outwards. (*See* RICKETS.)

BOWEL, OEDEMA OF THE. This disease affects mainly piglets of 8 to 14 weeks old, though occasionally it is seen in the new-born and in pigs of up to 5 months. In most cases a gelatinous fluid is found in the thickness of the stomach wall and other parts. The disease can be experimentally transmitted by inoculation of this fluid.
CAUSE. *E. coli.*
SIGNS. The finding of a dead pig – often the best in the litter – is usually the first indication. Puffy eyelids, from which there may be a discharge, and puffiness of snout and throat may be observed; together with leg weakness and convulsions.
TREATMENT. This is seldom practicable; diuretics have been tried in affected pigs. (*See* E. COLI.)

BOWELS (*see* INTESTINE).

'BOWIE'. A disease of unweaned lambs, resembling rickets, in New Zealand. A supplement of phosphates appears to be effective.

BOWMAN'S CAPSULE. A part of the nephron – the unit of structure of the kidney. Fluid passes from the glomerulus into the capsule as the first stage of filtration and urine formation.

BOXWOOD POISONING may sometimes occur through farm animals gaining access to gardens where the plant grows, or by eating the trimmings from box hedges along with other green food taken from the garden. The plant, known botanically as *Buxus sempervirens*, contains several toxic alkaloids, the chief of which is *buxine*. When large quantities have been taken, or if the beast is not able to vomit, nervous symptoms, lameness, muscular twitching, dizziness, diarrhoea, and acute abdominal pains are seen. In very severe cases there is the passage of blood-stained motions, great straining, convulsions, delirium, unconsciousness, and death. Pigs are the most susceptible of the farm animals.

BRACHIAL is a word meaning 'belonging to the upper arm', *e.g.* brachial plexus and brachial paralysis. A tumour, sometimes malignant, involving or pressing upon the brachial plexus is not uncommon in the dog and may cause a progressive lameness of one fore-limb together with atrophy of the muscles; also signs of pain which cannot be localised. (*See* NERVES.)

BRACHYCEPHALIC. The word is applied to the short skulls of such dogs as the bulldog, toy spaniel, or pug. In such the forehead is high, the skull broad, and the face foreshortened.

BRACKEN POISONING. The eating of bracken (*Pteris aquilina*) by horses, cattle or sheep may lead to serious illness and death; symptoms appearing a month or two after the first meal of the plant.
CAUSE. Bracken contains an enzyme, thiaminase, which in the horse and pig causes a thiamine deficiency. In cattle and sheep this vitamin is produced in abundance in the rumen, and bracken poisoning is due not to thiaminase but to the 'radiomimetic factor' also present in bracken. (Professor E. G. Clarke, *Vet. Rec.* 1976 **98** 215.) There are complex changes in the blood and bone-marrow. Poisoning is more prevalent in dry seasons than in wet weather, and young store stock are more often affected than adult cattle. The rhizomes are said to be five times as poisonous as the fronds – a fact of importance where the plough is being used for reclamation.
SIGNS. In the horse these take the form of a general loss of condition and an unsteady gait; with later on loss of appetite (but no rise in temperature), nervous spasms, and death. Affected cattle, on the other hand, run a high temperature. They segregate themselves from the rest of the herd and cease grazing. The visible mucous membranes are pale in colour, and numerous small red spots (petechial haemorrhages) are found scattered over the lining of the nose, eyes, and vagina. Diarrhoea, passed without straining, is usually blood-stained. Respirations are accelerated, and on the slightest exertion the animals fall and have some difficulty in rising. In many cases a knuckling of the fetlocks, especially of the hind-limbs, is noticeable. In some cases the throat becomes swollen, so that there is difficulty in breathing. The illness lasts from 1 to 6 days. In other cases, death may occur much sooner, and be accompanied by bleeding from nose and anus, when the carcases have some similarity to deaths from anthrax. Onset of symptoms may be delayed for up to two months.
TREATMENT. DL-Batyl alcohol injections have been recommended for cattle in the early stages of bracken poisoning. For the horse, injections of thiamine are usually successful if the illness is tackled in time.
PREVENTION. Avoid the use of green bracken as bedding, and avoid the situation in which animals turn to bracken out of sheer hunger or

thirst – semistarvation of live-stock is ever a false economy. Especially where the grazing is poor, it is essential to move animals to bracken-free land every three weeks. (*See also* BRIGHT DISEASE of sheep.)
Bracken and cancer. During the investigation of acute bracken poisoning in cattle, it was found that certain constituents of the plant were cancer-producing in rats and mice. In 1975 one of at least two bracken carcinogens was identified as shikimic acid, a constituent of many other plants also, and it has been shown to cause lethal mutations and to be a very potent cancer-producer in mice.
Both in the UK and in Japan young bracken shoots have been eaten by people as a vegetable. 'In Japan a link has been established between long-term bracken fern ingestion and stomach cancer.' (B. Widdop, Consultant Biochemist, Poison Unit, New Cross Hospital.)
In some parts of the world cancer of the bladder is an endemic condition in cattle, and in most places – states the World Health Organisation – it is associated with bracken. There is a suspicion, states *WHO Chronicle*, that drinking milk from cattle feeding on bracken may lead to cancer in man. (*See also* 'BRIGHT BLINDNESS' of sheep.)

BRADYCARDIA means slowness in the beating of the heart, with corresponding slowness of the pulse-rate. (*See* HEART, PULSE.)

BRADYKININ. Damaged tissue releases bradykinin, which stimulates nerve endings. Prostaglandins are also released and these increase the stimulus, resulting in the feeling of pain.

BRAFORD. A breed of cattle formed by crossing the Brahman and the Hereford.

BRAHMAN. Cattle of this name in the south of the USA were developed from a mixture of several zebu breeds (*Bos indicus*) plus some Shorthorn or Hereford content.

BRAILING. A means of temporarily preventing flight in pheasant poults, etc., by means of leather straps.

BRAIN. The brain and the spinal cord together form what is called the *central nervous system.*
Parts of the brain. In the domestic animals, as in man, the principal parts of the brain (front to back) are as follows:
(1) The **cerebrum.** This is by far the largest part, and consists of two hemispheres separated by a deep cleft. The surface of the cerebrum is increased by numerous ridges or *gyri* and by furrows called *sulci.* The hemispheres are joined by the fibres of the *corpus callosum.*
Each hemisphere is divided into sections or lobes, and its surface has a layer of grey matter – the *cortex.* At the front of each hemisphere is the *olfactory bulb*, which relays impulses from the olfactory nerves of the nose to the brain, and is concerned with the sense of smell.
The *thalamus* is concerned with relaying all sensory nerve impulses (except those concerned

with smell) to the cerebral cortex. Below is the *hypothalamus*, containing nerve centres for the control of body temperature, and connected by a stalk or pedicle with the *pituitary gland.*

Near the thalamus in the centre of the cerebral hemispheres are masses of grey matter called *basal ganglia* or nuclei.

The lateral *ventricles* are located within the corresponding hemispheres and are spaces filled with cerebro-spinal fluid, and communicating with the third and fourth ventricles.

(2) The **brain-stem** consists of nerve tissue at the base of the brain and includes the **mid-brain**, (of which the largest structures are the two *cerebral peduncles* and four *quadrigeminal bodies*), the *pons*, and the *medulla oblongata.*

(3) The **cerebellum**, which has two hemispheres and a middle ridge – the *vermis.* The cerebellum, with the pons, and the *medulla oblongata* are often spoken of as the **hind-brain.** the pons is a bridge of nerve fibres from one hemisphere of the cerebellum to the other. The medulla continues backwards as the spinal cord.

Structure. The brain is composed of white and grey matter. In the cerebrum and cerebellum the grey matter is arranged mainly as a layer on the surface, though both have grey areas imbedded in the white matter. In other parts the grey matter is found in definite masses called 'nuclei'.

The cells vary in size and shape in different parts of the brain, but all of them give off a number of processes, some of which form nerve-fibres. The cells on the surface of the cerebral hemispheres, for instance, are roughly pyramidal in shape, and each one gives off numbers of nerve-cell projections, called 'dendrites', from one end, and a single long process, called an 'axon', from the other. The white matter is made up of a large number of nerve-fibres, each of which is connected to a cell in the grey matter.

In both the grey and the white matter there is a framework of fibrous tissue cells, extremely fine and delicate, which acts as a supportive structure for the fibres and nerve cells, to which the name 'neuroglia' is applied. Permeating the grey matter is a complex system of blood-vessels, and in the white matter there are also vessels but to a less extent.

MENINGES. The brain proper is covered over by a thin membrane called the 'pia mater', the bones of the cranium are lined by a thick membrane called the 'dura mater', and between these is an irregular network called 'the arachnoid'. Between the arachnoid and the pia mater is a small amount of fluid, which serves as a kind of water-bed in which the brain floats.

Size. The brain varies very much in different animals and in different breeds, but the following table gives the average relation of the weight of the brain to the weight of the body:

Cat	1 to 99
Dog	1 to 235
Sheep	1 to 317
Pig	1 to 369
Horse	1 to 593
Ox	1 to 682

From this it will be seen that the cat has proportionately to the size of its body the largest brain.

Nerves. The nerves which leave the surface of the brain are twelve in number in the domesticated animals:

1. Olfactory, to the nose (smell).
2. Optic, to the eye (sight).
3. Oculomotor
4. Trochlear ⎬ to the muscles of the eyes.
5. Abducent
6. Trigeminal, to the skin of the face, etc.
7. Facial, to the muscles of the face.
8. Auditory, to the ear (hearing).
9. Glossopharyngeal, to the tongue (taste).
10. Vagus, to heart, larynx, lungs, and stomach.
11. Spinal accessory, to muscles in the neck.
12. Hypoglossal, to the muscles of the tongue.

Blood-vessels. The brain obtains its blood-supply from four main sources: two internal carotids and two occipital arteries. These branch and unite to form an irregular circle under the brain within the skull, called the 'circle of Willis'. From this numerous smaller branches leave to supply the whole of the brain substance. By such an arrangement any possibility of deficiency of blood is obviated, for should one of the main branches become cut or occluded, the others enlarge and the same amount of blood is still supplied. The blood leaves the organ by means of large venous sinuses situated in the membranes covering the brain, and finally finds its way into the jugular veins of the neck. (*See also* CENTRAL NERVOUS SYSTEM.)

Functions. *The Cerebrum* is concerned with memory, initiative, volition, intelligence, and, as well as these, it is the receiving station of the impulses that originate from the organs of sight, smell, taste, hearing, and touch. Fear, anger, and other emotions originate in the grey nerve cells of the cerebrum, which is also concerned with voluntary control of the skeletal muscles.

Sensations on the right side of the body, and muscular control in the right side, are dealt with by the left cerebral hemisphere; the right hemisphere being concerned with the left side of the body.

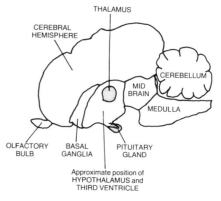

Brain of dog.

The Cerebellum is concerned with unconscious control, with balance, and with co-ordination of complex muscular movements. Each half of the cerebellum controls the muscular system of its own side of the body, and is in communication with the opposite side of the cerebrum. It closely communicates with the nerves, internal ear, and with certain nerves of muscle-sense that bear message dealing with the state of contraction that is in process in any particular skeletal muscle.

The *hypothalamus* controls body temperature, and influences blood circulation, urinary secretion, and appetite.

The *thalamus* functions as a 'relay centre' for sensory information as already described.

The *basal ganglia* are in control of posture and movement.

The *medulla* contains nerve centres for the control of involuntary, or reflex, actions such as respiration and heart-beat rates, coughing, vomiting, and the reflex part of swallowing.

BRAIN DISEASES include the following:

Abscess. The organisms may enter through an injury to the bone, through the medium of the ear (especially in the pig and dog), or may arrive by the blood-stream. Sometimes a foreign body, such as a needle that has become lodged in the throat, may pass upwards into the brain and set up an abscess. The condition may be produced during the course of pneumonia, metritis, endocarditis, etc., when the bacteria invade the blood-stream and get carried to the brain among other tissues.

For symptoms and first-aid, *see under* MENINGITIS, ENCEPHALITIS.

Cerebral haemorrhage. Formerly the name apoplexy was commonly applied to this condition, referred to in human medicine as a 'Stroke'.

Concussion means literally a violent shaking of the brain, but also the temporary loss of consciousness resulting from a head injury. Temporary blindness may occur after the animal has regained consciousness.

In domestic animals long-term effects include changes in behaviour, such as aggressiveness and excessive libido. Fits (epileptiform convulsions) may be a sequel to a head injury in dogs. (*See* EPILEPSY.)

Encephalomalacia (which see).

Inflammation (*see* ENCEPHALITIS; MENINGITIS).

Oedema of the brain is seen in salt poisoning in pigs, and in Polioencephalomalacia. Blindness and convulsions are produced.

(*See also* sections on 'DAFT LAMBS, HEATSTROKE, LIGHTNING STROKE, HYDROCEPHALUS, SWAYBACK, EPILEPSY, ECLAMPSIA, CHOREA, CEREBROCORTICAL NECROSIS, RABIES, EQUINE ENCEPHALITIS, 'SLEEPER' SYNDROME of cattle, etc.)

Parasites of the *human* brain include nematodes, such as larval hookworms, *Strongyloides*, ascarid worms (*Toxocara*), filarial worms, rat lungworm (*Angiostrongylus cantonensis*), and *Gnathostoma* spp.; trematodes, such as *Fasciola hepatica* (liver fluke), *Schistosoma japonicum,* and *Paragonimus*

spp. (lung fluke); the cestodes of hydatid disease, cysticercosis, and sparganosis; and fly maggots such as Tumbu fly of East and Central Africa (*Cordylobia anthropophaga*), tropical warble fly of South America (*Dermatobia hominis*), sheep botfly of the USSR and Mediterranean (*Rhinooestrus purpureus*), and cattle bots and warble fly in Europe (*Hypoderma bovis* and *lineata* of cattle and *H. diana* of deer) (*Lancet*). Such parasites may similarly occur in the brains of farm and domestic animals. (*See* COENURIASIS and HEARTWORMS; the latter being especially important in cats.)

Tuberculosis of brain (*see* TUBERCULOSIS).

Tumours of brain may cause circling movements, a staggering gait, frenzy, etc. Decreased activity, drowsiness, and blindness in cats are seen as a result of a meningioma.

BRAIN SURGERY. In veterinary practice this is performed to treat COENURIASIS. (See under this heading for the technique of the operation in sheep, and for the signs suggestive of this disease.)

Secondly, the cranial cavity is opened to relieve pressure on the brain caused by a tumour. For example, a 12-year-old cat referred to the Ohio State University's teaching hospital, had been walking in circles, aimlessly pacing, and Dr James Fingeroth noticed, purring almost continuously; however the cat was only intermittently responsive to human attention, and kept his tongue protruded from his mouth.

Under a general anaesthetic, after computerised tomography of the skull, to indicate the exact site of the lesion, a hole was drilled and through it the tumour (a meningioma) gradually removed. The cat made a perfect recovery.

BRAMBELL COMMITTEE REPORT. This was published in Britain in 1965 by HMSO under the full title *Report of the Technical Committee to inquire into the Welfare of Animals Kept Under Intensive Livestock Husbandry Systems*, under the chairmanship of Professor F. W. R. Brambell, a distinguished zoologist.

(*See* WELFARE.)

BRAN (*see* HORSES, FEEDING OF; OSTEOFIBROSIS).

BRAN MASH (*see under* NURSING).

BRANDING can be achieved with the minimum of pain by the technique of freeze-branding developed in the USA by Dr R. K. Farrell, a veterinarian.

When the branded area thaws the hair falls out. The new hair which grows in 2 or 3 weeks is white, and therefore shows up well on a darkish animal. For a white animal, the brand has to be left on longer to kill the hair roots. The brand-mark then resembles a hot-iron brand, but the hide damage may be less. (Early claims that 'there is no damage to the hide' have been disproved.)

A copper branding 'iron', cooled to −70°C with dry ice and alcohol, is applied to a clipped or shaved area for about 27 seconds; this is not a final recommendation.

Laser beams have been used for branding cattle

in the USA. It is claimed that 'with the 5000°C temperature of the branding beam, the speed of branding is faster than the pain reflex of an animal'.

Where a permanent brand is not necessary it is a simple matter to apply black hair dye or hair bleach, according to whether the animal is light or dark in colour. The gloved index finger is dipped in the liquid and applied to the animal's coat. The peroxide bleach will, it has been stated, last for a year; the black dye for several months. The method has been used with some success by New Zealand farmers.

BRANDY (*see* ALCOHOL).

BRASSICAE SPECIES. Illness may occur in cattle fed excessive amounts of kale, cabbage, Brussels sprouts, and rape, especially if other foods are not available or if the kale is frosted. Anaemia, haemoglobinuria, and death may result. (*See under* KALE.)

BRAXY is a disease of sheep characterised by a very short period of illness, by a seasonal and regional incidence, and, in the natural state, by a high mortality. It occurs in various parts of Scotland, Ireland, the north of England, Scandinavia, etc., chiefly on hilly land. It attacks young sheep under the age of two years, weaned lambs being very susceptible; the best members of the flock are more liable to become attacked than poorly nourished sheep, and it is most frequently seen during a spell of cold, severe weather with hoar frosts at night.
CAUSES. *Clostridium septicum.* It affects the mucous membrane of the 4th stomach of sheep and from there invades the tissues. It gains entrance to the alimentary canal by way of the mouth along with the grass from a 'braxy pasture'.

Infection with *C. septicum* is characterised by gas gangrene, and may occur in animals other than sheep – including man.
SIGNS. These – loss of appetite, abdominal pain, diarrhoea, with a high temperature and laboured breathing – are seldom in evidence for more than 5 or 6 hours; death being sudden. A characteristic odour is perceptible from the breath and body fluids. Decomposition is very rapid. The lesions are those of a gastritis in the 4th stomach (abomasum).
PREVENTION. Vaccination at the beginning of September, so that the animals have time to establish an immunity before the frosts begin, has given good results. On farms where the losses have been very heavy a second vaccination 14 days later may be needed. (*See* VACCINATION.)

BREATHING (*see under* RESPIRATION).

BREATHLESSNESS may be due to any condition that hinders the thorough oxygenation of the blood.
Tachypnoea is the name for an increase in the *rate* of respiration. This may arise from such diverse causes as anaemia, heat stress, heart disease, pneumonia, bronchitis, and paraquat poisoning.

Dyspnoea means laboured breathing, or breathing accompanied by pain or distress, such as may occur with oedema of the lungs, pneumonia, bronchitis, pleurisy, emphysema, and paraquat poisoning.

BREDA virus. A cause of diarrhoea in calves in the USA, and of respiratory disease in two-day-old calves which very soon died.

BREECH PRESENTATION (*see* PARTURITION).

BREEDING, 'CONTROLLED' (*see under* 'CONTROLLED', with reference to cattle and sheep).

BREEDING OF DOGS ACT, 1973, makes it unlawful for anyone to keep a dog breeding establishment unless it has been licensed by the local authority. A breeding establishment is defined as 'any premises (including a private dwelling) where more than two bitches are kept for the purpose of breeding for sale'.

BREEDING OF LIVESTOCK. Information about animals coming 'on heat' or being 'in season' is given under OESTRUS. Other information is given under PREGNANCY and PARTURITION.

Number of females per male varies. The stallion when he is four years old and upwards and in good condition will serve from 80 to 120 mares during a season. A 3 year old can take up to about 50 or 60, and from 15 to 20 are enough for a 2 year old. From 60 to 80 cows are sufficient for an average adult bull, but he should not serve more than 35 or 40 between 1 and 2 years of age. Twenty to 30 ewes are as many as the ram lamb will successfully serve, but shearlings may have as many as 40 to 50. Adult rams may successfully impregnate 80 ewes or more. The year-old boar should not be allowed more than 20 sows during a season, but when he is older he may have up to 30 or 35. In this connection it must be remembered that when a large number of females are served by a male, those served at the later stages are not so likely to prove fruitful as those served earlier.

In old age. There is little reliable data, but mares have bred foals when over 30 years, cattle and sheep up to 20 years, and cats till 14 years old. These, however, were all animals that had bred regularly in their younger days. It is difficult to breed from an aged female that has not previously been used for stud purposes. (*See also under* REPRODUCTION, ARTIFICIAL INSEMINATION.)

BREEDS OF STOCK. British breeds of livestock are not only of local interest, since they have been exported to many parts of the world. A list of the breeds is given under the headings HORSES, CATTLE, BEEF BREEDS, SHEEP, etc.

BREWER'S GRAINS are used both in the wet state and dry. They are a by-product of brewing, and consist of the malted barley after it has been exhausted. In both forms they are used for feeding cattle, while dry grains are sometimes fed to folded sheep. If stored in the wet state for any length of time they become mouldy and fermented unless packed tightly so as to exclude air. In the dry they can be kept for a considerable length of time without harm. They are rich in proteins and carbohydrates, but must not be fed to excess.

Some samples become infected with BACILLUS cereus (which see).

BRIDLE INJURIES. They take the form of: 1, injuries to the poll; 2, injuries to the chin, caused by the curb-chain; and 3, injuries of the mouth from the bit. Injuries to the poll are produced by outside agencies generally, and are aggravated by the poll-strap rubbing or chafing the skin. The damage is generally only superficial, but in a few cases pus forms and may burrow down into the ligamentous tissue of the poll and produce 'poll evil'. (*See* POLL EVIL.) In ordinary cases it suffices to protect the damaged skin by winding a piece of sheep-skin round the strap that is causing the injury, and dressing the abraded areas with, *e.g.* sulphanilamide powder each night. Those injuries to the chin that are caused by the curb-chain are usually only slight, and mainly affect young horses when they are being broken in. When they learn to answer the reins and acquire what is called a 'soft mouth', the chafed skin is allowed to heal and the condition passes off. In older horses that have 'hard mouths' and that constantly require the use of the curb-chain, the skin becomes thickened and calloused, and the surface of the bone may become irritated with a resulting deposition of new bone in the groove of the chin. Injury may be obviated by using a leather curb for young horses that have very tender skins, and by changing the bit for older animals. Care in driving of the horse, avoiding all sudden or severe pulls on the reins, will often do more to 'soften' a horse's mouth than the use of more drastic measures. Bit injuries consist of the abrasion of the mucous membrane of the lower jaw, just opposite the corners of the lips, where the bit crosses. Sometimes the membrane becomes actually ulcerated and a foul-smelling discharge escapes, but in the majority of cases the injuries are slight and heal in a few days.

BRIGHT BLINDNESS. This, a prevalent condition in Yorkshire hill sheep, was first described in 1965, and is characterised by progressive degeneration of the retina. The disease is of considerable economic importance in some flocks.
CAUSE: Bright blindness has been found in several breeds of sheep, in Scotland and Wales as well as in Northern England. In some flocks the incidence may be 5–8 per cent among the ewes, with a peak incidence in those 2 to 4 years old. The blindness is permanent. Bracken is the cause.

In ewes moved to bracken-free grazing before the disease is well advanced the condition will not progress further.

BRISKET DISEASE (*see* MOUNTAIN SICKNESS).

BRITISH DANE. A breed established by the Red Poll Cattle Society in the UK following the import of Danish Red cattle.

BRITISH VETERINARY ASSOCIATION. Its principal objects are the advancement of veterinary science in all its branches, the publication of scientific and clinical material, and the promotion of the welfare of the profession. It is intimately concerned with all matters of professional policy, and maintains contact with many outside bodies and Government Departments. (*See* BVA.)

BRITISH VETERINARY PROFESSION (*see* VETERINARY PROFESSION).

BROILERS. Good quality table chickens of either sex, about 10 to 12 weeks old, and weighing 2½ to 4 lbs (liveweight).
MORTALITY. If the chicks and their management are good, the total mortality for a broiler crop should be less than 5 per cent, frequently only 3 per cent. Most of these deaths will take place during the first fortnight. In fact, a 1½ per cent mortality is normal and to be expected during the early period.

For commercial reasons there is often the temptation to overcrowd broilers in their houses, and this practice will inevitably increase stress and hence the liability of disease – the effects of which may be the more severe. (*See also under* NEWCASTLE DISEASE; POULTRY, DISEASES OF.)
BROILER ASCITES, and colisepticaemia lesions in the pericardium and liver, are causes of carcase rejection at processing plants; as is 'swollen head syndrome' (subcutaneous oedema). Both are caused by *E. coli.*

'BROKEN MOUTH' is the name given to the mouths of old sheep that have lost some of their teeth. Loss of incisor teeth is not uncommon in hill sheep and is of economic importance because a ewe needs her incisors if she is to support herself and a lamb on the hill.

The condition involves resorption of bone from the jaw following premature loss of the incisor teeth. It does not respond to mineral supplementation, and it is now thought that the reason could be that the hill ewe is liable to suffer from a protein deficiency during the winter. It is already known that, in the rat, demineralisation of the skeleton can result from protein or mineral deficiency. Work is now continuing at the Moredun Institute and on Scottish hill farms to find a solution to the problem.

Broken incisors were seen in six- to eight-month-old sheep wintered for six to 12 weeks on swedes or turnips. Towards the end of this period up to two-thirds of the hoggets were in poor condition. The crowns of several incisors had fractured leaving short irregular brown stumps. The enamel was normal but there was softening and loss of dentine between the apical end of the enamel and the gum margin. It is suggested that this resulted from the effects of acids produced by bacterial action on the carbohydrates in the turnips and swedes. (Orr, M. B. & Suckling, G. (1985) *New Zealand Veterinary Journal* **33**, 104.)
SIGNS. Difficulty in feeding, dropping some of the food back into the trough, and 'quidding'.

'BROKEN WIND', or 'heaves', are outdated expressions applied to horses with long-standing respiratory diseases in which double expiratory effort is a feature. This particular symptom may arise from several different pathological processes in the lungs, not all of which are chronic or irreversible; *e.g.* allergic reactions, such as immediate-type hypersensitivity (as in bronchial asthma) and extrinsic allergic alveolitis (as in 'farmer's lung'), chronic bronchiolitis following bacterial or viral infections and, very rarely, lung tumours. In every case there is widespread bronchiolitis which initially gives rise to generalised over-inflation of alveoli (so-called 'functional emphysema'). This lesion is reversible but eventually there is destructive emphysema in which there is an increase beyond normal in the size of the air-spaces with destructive changes in the alveolar walls. Due to loss of alveolar tissue there is a decreased surface area for gas exchange, reduction of the pulmonary vascular bed, and loss of elasticity of the lung. These changes are irreversible and lead to progressive respiratory disability and eventual failure.

SIGNS. The clinical sign of double expiratory effort consists of an initial passive normal expiratory movement followed by an active contraction of the chest and abdominal muscles to expel the remaining air. In advanced cases this leads to hypertrophy of the *rectus abdominis* muscles, and the formation of a 'heaves line' beneath the posterior aspect of the rib cage – a feature characteristic of long-standing obstructive pulmonary disease in the horse.

A cough – typically dry, short, hollow and low-pitched – sometimes becomes paroxysmal after stabling or exercise, faster breathing, audible wheezing, nasal discharge, and intolerance of exercise.

DIFFERENTIAL DIAGNOSIS of these chronic respiratory disorders with a double expiratory effort depends upon detailed clinical evaluation, responses to corticosteroids and other drugs, the results of serological tests with appropriate antigens and, ultimately, autopsy. (*Eq. Vet. J.* (1973) **5** 26.) Infestation with the equine lungworm *Dictyocaulus arnfieldii*, tuberculosis, and hydatid cysts should also be considered.

CONTROL. Maintaining a dust-free environment helps; so does vaccination against equine influenza, since many cases appear to originate from an episode of acute respiratory disease.

(*See also* EMPHYSEMA.)

BROMOCRIPTIN. An ergot alkaloid. (*See* PSEUDOPREGNANCY.)

BRONCHIECTASIS means dilatation of the walls of the bronchioles due to weakening through excessive coughing. The condition is often met with in chronic bronchitis, and the cavities produced are often filled with pus.

BRONCHIOLITIS. Inflammation of very small bronchial tubes (bronchioles).

BRONCHITIS is inflammation of the lining mucous membrane of the bronchioles. It is a very common disease of all animals in temperate or cold climates. It may occur as an extension of inflammation of the trachea (tracheitis), and it may be followed by pneumonia or pleurisy, or both. An acute and a chronic type are recognised.

(*a*) **Acute bronchitis.** This may follow exposure to smoke from a burning building, or be the result of careless administration of liquid medicines which then 'go the wrong way'. More commonly acute bronchitis may occur during the course of some virus infections, following colds and chills, and may affect farm animals housed in badly ventilated buildings. In the dog, bronchitis often occurs during the course of distemper, and in the horse it may be associated with influenza or strangles. Acute bronchitis in cattle and sheep may be parasitic. (*See* PARASITIC BRONCHITIS; WORMS, TREATMENT AGAINST.) In pigs, too, parasitic worms may cause bronchitis. (*See also under* COUGH.)

SIGNS. A rise in temperature, accompanied by faster respiration, loss of appetite, a cough, and nasal discharge, are seen. The cough is at first hard and dry, but becomes softer and easier in the later stages. The breathing may often be heard to be wheezing and bubbling in the later stages.

TREATMENT. Attention to hygienic conditions is of first importance. The horse should be removed to a loose-box, provided with a plentiful supply of bedding, rugged if the weather demands, given plenty of clean water to drink, and fed on soft foods. It must on no account be drenched, for there is nearly always difficulty in swallowing, and a great risk of some of the medicine entering the trachea and complicating an already serious case. In animals suffering from bronchitis due to parasitic worms, suitable anthelmintics must be used. Where the cause is bacterial – secondary, very often to a virus infection – the use of antibiotics and/or sulphonamides is indicated. Liquid medicines should not be given. In housed livestock, attention must be paid to the ventilation. For the dog, a jacket of flannel or similar material may be made. In all animals, good, easily digested food is necessary. (*See* NURSING OF SICK ANIMALS, KENNEL COUGH.)

(*b*) **Chronic bronchitis.** This may follow the acute form, or it may arise as a primary condition. The smaller capillary bronchial tubes are affected and not the larger passages.

Chronic bronchitis is often seen in the old dog, occasionally in association with tuberculosis. The latter may also cause chronic bronchitis in cattle and other animals. In the horse, chronic bronchitis may lead to emphysema. (*See under that heading and* 'BROKEN WIND'.) Parasitic worms may be associated with some long-standing cases of bronchitis in animals.

SIGNS. A loud, hard cough, often appearing in spasms, respiratory distress on the least exertion, an intermittent, white, clotted, or pus-containing nasal discharge, which is most in evidence after coughing or exercise, and a gradual loss of condition, characterises this form of bronchitis; except that in the dog chronic bronchitis often occurs in the rather fat, middle-aged dog which has a cough persisting over weeks or months, with excessive secretion of mucus in the trachea and bronchi, but often no nasal discharge. (*See also* COUGH.)

TREATMENT should be along the lines indicated under ACUTE BRONCHITIS.

(*c*) **Bronchitis in chickens.** (*See under* INFECTIOUS BRONCHITIS).

BRONCHO-PNEUMONIA (*see* PNEUMONIA).

BRONCHOSCOPY. A bronchoscope was used in 209 dogs with a persistent disease of the tracheobronchial tree and in which clinical and radiological examinations failed to provide a diagnosis. The results included the following: normal, 6 per cent; abnormal morphology of the trachea, 17 per cent; laryngitis, tracheitis and bronchitis either singly or in combination, 62 per cent; bronchopneumonia, 6 per cent; foreign bodies or foreign material, 3 per cent; and neoplasia 2 per cent. Nineteen cats were also examined with inflammatory lesions and foreign bodies accounting for 12 and 3 cases, respectively. (Venker-van Kaagen, A. J. & others, (1985) *Journal of the American Animal Hospital Association* **21,** 521.)

BRONCHUS or bronchial tube, is the name applied to tubes into which the windpipe (trachea) divides, one going to either lung. The name is also applied to the later divisions of these tubes distributed throughout the lungs.

'BROWN MOUTH'. A syndrome characterised mainly by gum necrosis and dysentery, occurring as a complication of virus diseases in the dog. It appears to be infectious and yields to penicillin.

'BROWN NOSE'. A form of light sensitisation (which see) in cattle.

BROWN SWISS. A breed of cattle, now established in the UK.

BRUCELLOSIS is an infection with *Brucella.* Five species of this genus of bacteria are important, namely: *B. abortus* (the main cause of abortion in cattle); *B. melitensis*; *B. suis*; *B. ovis* and *B. canis.*

Public health. Human brucellosis may be caused by any of the five species of *Brucella*, as mentioned below. It often takes the form of 'undulant fever', with characteristic undulating fluctuations of the temperature. Human infection with *B. abortus* may follow the drinking of raw milk or the handling of infected fetal membranes. Accidental self-inoculation with S19 vaccine is another cause. Infected uterine discharge drying on the cow's skin may be inhaled.

For symptoms, *see* UNDULANT FEVER.

Serial Brucella agglutination tests were carried out on veterinary students at Bristol University between 1962 and 1968. A steady rise in the number of those with a significant positive titre was demonstrated in undergraduates and this was related to an increased exposure to farm livestock as their course progressed. A much larger proportion of individuals showed a significant titre in the period following graduation. While only 8·9 per cent of students in the first year of their course showed a significant titre, 49·5 per cent gave a serological response at 1/80 dilution or greater, within five years of graduation and of those in predominantly large animal practice almost 60 per cent showed this response. Only 7 per cent of those with a significant rise in titre reported symptoms suggestive of clinical disease.' (Cayton, H. R. *et al. Vet. Rec.* (1975), **97,** 447.)

A few herds (0·1 per cent, 162 herds) still had active *Brucella abortus* infection in 1983. Many of these breakdowns occurred in areas which were the last to be subject to eradication procedures: north east England, Devon, Cornwall and Wales. The number of human infections presumed to have been contracted in Britain has fallen from over 600 a year in the early 1970s to 20 in 1983. Relevant occupation or likely source of infection was mentioned for 325 of the 671 cases presumed to have been infected in Britain in 1976–1983; 207 were farm workers or dwellers, 46 were veterinary surgeons or nurses and 40 were slaughter house workers or butchers. (Public Health Laboratory Service, Communicable Disease Surveillance Centre (Scotland) (1984) *British Medical Journal* **289,** 817.)

What was formerly known as Malta Fever in man is due to *B. melitensis*, an infection of goats and sheep, occasionally cattle. Its occurrence in the UK was limited to one outbreak resulting from imported infected cheese.

The American strain of *B. suis* (found in pigs and hares) is pathogenic for man, causing undulant fever and arthritis.

B. canis, which infects dogs, can also cause illness in people.

B. ovis, which infects sheep, rarely causes human illness.

Horses. *B. abortus* may cause fistulous withers and lameness due to infection of other ligaments. In the mare, abortion may (rarely) occur (*see Vet. Record*, Feb. 4, 1967). A Coombs test may prove useful in diagnosis.

Cattle (*see* BRUCELLOSIS IN CATTLE).

Dogs. In the UK, *B. abortus* was isolated from the urine of a dog which had shown symptoms of stiffness and orchitis. At autopsy, cystitis and an abscess of the prostate were found. Such a dog would be a public health risk, and a danger to cattle. Abortion is another symptom. The infection has been found in kennels, following the feeding of meat from stillborn calves. Brucellosis in dogs is probably more common than generally realised. In Chile a survey showed that 40 per cent of dogs, on farms where the dairy herds were infected with *B. abortus*, were infected.

B. canis was first isolated in 1966. In the USA it has caused outbreaks of severe illness in laboratory beagles; it causes also illness in man.

'A unique feature of *B. canis* infection is lack of fever. Another feature is the duration of bacteraemia, which usually lasts for several months, but can last three or four years.'

'In males epididymitis, scrotal dermatitis, and testicular degeneration may occur, although it is not uncommon for male dogs to be "silent" carriers.' (Meyer, Margaret E. (1983) *Modern Veterinary Practice* **64**, 987.)

An outbreak of this infection in Germany was reported in 1980, and serological evidence for its existence in the UK was also reported in that year.

In Mexico City 203 **human** sera and 500 dog sera were tested for canine brucellosis, and a positive result was obtained for 13 per cent of the human samples and 28 per cent of the dog sera. (*Cornell Vet.* (1976) **66** 347.)

Sheep. Formerly, brucellosis was an important disease of sheep in the UK.

B. ovis gives rise (in Australasia, USA, and Europe) to infertility and scrotal oedema in rams. Abortion may occur in infected ewes. (*See also* RAM EPIDIDYMITIS.)

Goats. In Britain, brucellosis is not a serious problem in goats.

Pigs. In Britain, brucellosis does not occur. Overseas, abortion in pigs is caused by *B. abortus suis*.

Deer. There is no evidence that deer, infected with *B abortus*, have infected cattle grazing the same pasture.

Poultry. Chickens are susceptible to *B. abortus* infection, which they have transmitted to cattle.

Wild animals. Overseas, hares have commonly been found to harbour *B. suis* which caused orchitis in them.

In parts of Africa *Brucella* agglutinins have been recorded in wild animals, and *B. abortus* has been isolated from a waterbuck, and from rodents.

In Argentina **foxes** are commonly infected with *B. abortus.*

(See also FISTULOUS WITHERS, 'POLL EVIL', BUMBLEFOOT, RAM EPIDIDIMYTIS.)

BRUCELLOSIS IN CATTLE. (*B. melitensis* causes disease in some countries.) 'Contagious Abortion' is a specific contagious disease due to the *Brucella abortus.* Since the infection may exist and persist in the genital system of the bull, *Brucellosis* is to be preferred as a name for the disease. In females it is characterised by a chronic inflammation of the uterus (especially of the mucous membrane); usually, but not invariably, followed by abortion between the fifth and eighth months of pregnancy.

It is important to note that not all infected animals abort. Indeed, in over half of them pregnancy runs to full term. 'Any animal that has aborted once may be almost as dangerous at its next and subsequent calvings – which are generally at full term – as on the occasion it aborted.' (A. C. L. Brown.)

Infection may occur by the mouth or through the vagina during service, when a bull which has served an infected cow is called upon to serve a clean one afterwards, or when the bull is a 'carrier'. Contamination of litter with discharges from a previous case is an important factor in the spread of the disease in a herd. The hand and arm of the man who handles an aborted fetus may also transmit infection.

In the pregnant cow a low-grade chronic inflammatory reaction is set up in the uterus with the result that an exudate accumulates between the fetal membranes and the uterine mucous membranes, especially around the cotyledons. The cotyledons may appear necrotic, owing to the presence of fibrinous adherent masses upon their surfaces, and the fetal membranes may show similar areas after they have been expelled. Quite commonly in cattle the membranes are thickened and tough. The fetus may be normal or may show a dropsical condition of the muscles and the subcutaneous tissues, and there may be fluid present in the cavities of chest, abdomen, and cranium. In some cases the fetus undergoes a process of mummification, and when it is discharged it is almost unrecognisable as a fetus.

Cows at pasture may become infected by older 'carrier' cows (which are liable to harbour the organisms in their udders) or by wild animals (*e.g.* foxes), dogs or birds, which have eaten or been in contact with infected membranes or discharges upon other farms near by where the disease already exists.

SIGNS. Abortion may occur without any preliminary symptoms, and except that the calf is not a full-term one, may be practically the same as normal calving. Most cows which have aborted once will carry their next calf to full term, or practically to full term; while only very few cows will abort a calf three times.

As a rule if abortion occurs early in pregnancy the fetal membranes are expelled along with the fetus, but if towards the end of the period there is almost always retention of these. A continuous reddish-brown or brownish-grey discharge follows, and persists for about 10 to 20 days (often for about 2 weeks). In some instances it slowly collects in the cavity of the uterus, little or nothing being seen at the vulva, and then it is discharged periodically, often in large amounts at a time.

In the bull symptoms of infection may be very slight or absent, and laboratory methods are usually necessary to establish a diagnosis.

Brucellosis is not the only cause of abortion in cattle due to an infective agent, and in arriving at a diagnosis it must be differentiated from infections listed under ABORTION.

IMMUNITY. Infected animals gradually produce an immunity in themselves against further abortions. The organisms may persist in the system for long periods, and a cow which does not herself subsequently abort may spread infection to other cows in the herd. This natural immunity, however, is wasteful, both in the matter of calves and milk supply, so that methods have been adopted in which an effort is made to provide animals with an artificial immunity.

AGGLUTINATION TEST. This indicates that the antibodies are still present in the cow's bloodstream. (*See also* MILK RING TEST, ROSE BENGAL TEST, COOMBS TEST.)

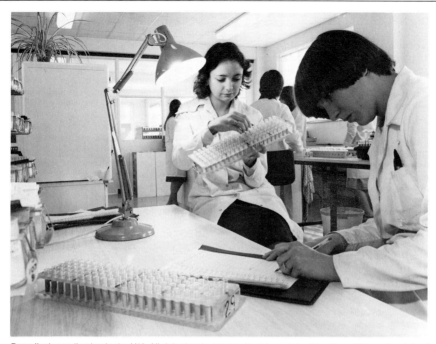

Brucellosis eradication in the UK. All dairy herds are monitored monthly. After the addition of a stained antigen, and incubation, herd milk samples are checked for a blue ring indicating Brucella antibodies. The picture shows this work in progress at the Milk Marketing Board's veterinary laboratory near Worcester.

ERADICATION. In October 1985 Great Britain was declared 'officially brucellosis-free' under an EC Directive governing intra-Community cattle trade, as a result of approved monitoring. Brucellosis has been successfully eradicated from many overseas countries, including Denmark, Sweden, Norway, Finland, Czechoslovakia, and Eire. Farmers' co-operation and discipline played an important part.

PRECAUTIONS. The greatest care must be taken in handling and disposing of an aborted fetus, fetal membranes, discharges, etc., both in the interests of human health and in order to prevent the spread of the disease among cattle. It is worth having a veterinary surgeon examine the cause of *any* abortion. There can be danger from the infected cow that has carried a calf to full term. Avoid buying in replacements from non-Accredited herds. Infected farm dogs can spread infection. A survey in Chile (*Vet. Rec.* (1980) **107** 22) showed that the incidence of brucella infection in dogs associated with dairy herds was 40 per cent. Many of these dogs were excreting brucella in their urine.

BRUCELLOSIS in SHEEP (*see* RAM EPIDIDYMITIS).

BRUISED SOLE is a condition of bruising of the sensitive sole of the foot, due to a badly fitting shoe, or the result of the horse having stood upon a projection, such as a stone, etc. Its character and its treatment do not differ from what is given under 'CORNS', except that while the corn has a more or less definite position in the foot, bruising of the sole may occur anywhere. (*See* CORNS.)

BRUIT and MURMUR are words used to describe several abnormal sounds heard in connection with the heart and arteries on auscultation.

BRUSH BORDER. On the free surface of some cells, the wall may be modified to provide finger-like projections: the brush border. This is seen, for example, in the convoluted tubule of the kidney and in the alimentary canal.

BRUSHING and CUTTING are injuries caused by the inside of the fetlock joint or coronet being struck by the hoof or shoe of the opposite limb; although bad shoeing may be responsible in a few instances, the cause is usually faulty conformation.

A brushing boot should be fitted, and an attempt made to avoid the future occurrence of brushing by skilful shoeing. (*See* SPEEDYCUT.)

BRUSSELS SPROUTS. Cattle strip-grazing these for 6 weeks, without other food, became ill with anaemia and haemoglobinuria. The illness caused by members of the *Brassicae* species is said to be always more serious near to the time of calving.

BSE (*see* BOVINE SPONGIFORM ENCEPHALOPATHY).

BUBONIC PLAGUE is an infectious disease of man and rats and mice, caused by *Yersinia pestis*.

More than half the cases of plague in America have occurred in New Mexico, where the disease was first recorded in 1949. Since then over 100 human cases have been reported, with several domestic cats involved – usually infected by the rock squirrel's flea. At least one veterinarian has become ill with plague after treating an infected cat.

'Dogs provide the best indications of a current or recent presence of plague in an area', stated P. Taylor and others in *Annals of Tropical Medicine & Parasitology* (1981), **75**, 165. Dogs develop a transient bacteraemia and a rapid serological response lasting for at least 300 days. The authors were referring to plague in Zimbabwe, first recorded there in 1974.

In man *bubonic plague* takes one of two forms: (1) After an incubation period of 2 to 7 days, the usual symptoms include the sudden onset of fever, rigors, muscular pain, headache and prostration. Within a few days the characteristic *buboes* (swelling of the lymph nodes in the groin and armpits) usually appear. These are accompanied by oedema, erythema, and great pain. (2) *pulmonary plague* has an incubation period of two or three days. Besides the sudden onset of fever there is a cough (usually with bloody sputum), headache, rigors, and prostration. When untreated this form of plague usually results in death within 2 to 5 days.

Various antibiotics are effective in treatment if given early enough.

A small outbreak of plague occurred in Glasgow in 1900, but was quickly suppressed.

The intermediate link between the infected rat and man is the rat flea. In South America at least 50 different species of rodents are believed to harbour the plague organism, *Yersinia (Pasteurella) pestis,* and nearly 5000 human cases were reported between 1960–69. The total number of cases of plague in man reported in 1974 was 2654, of which 155 were fatal (World Health Organisation). Asia, South America, and Africa all had outbreaks.

BUCCOSTOMY. An operation for the creation of buccal fistulae in order to prevent windsucking.

BUDGERIGARS (*see* CAGE BIRDS).

BUFFALO. The Asiatic water buffalo is named *Bubalus bubalis*; the African buffalo *Syncerus caffer*. (*See* WATER BUFFALO.)

BUFFALO FLY. This is *Lyperosia exigua*, a parasite of importance in Australia and in India and Malaya. It causes great irritation and even anaemia. (*See* FLIES.)

BUFFALO GNAT. Swarms of these, which breed in running water, attack cattle, often causing them to stampede, and producing serious bites which may lead to death. Man is also attacked. They are also known as Black Flies (*Simulium* species).

BUFFALO POX. A contagious disease of buffaloes which is of considerable economic importance. The infective agent is distinct from cowpox virus. (*See* POX.)

BUFFER. A substance which, when added to a solution, causes resistance to any change of hydrogen-ion concentration when either acid or alkali is added.

BUFFING is a term applied to the striking of the inside of one hoof at the quarter with some part of the opposite one. It is due to the same causes as BRUSHING (which see), but it occurs in horses that do not lift their feet very high. Less damage is done than in brushing, and it is not so likely to cause stumbling or lameness.

BUFOTALIN. The principal poisonous substance present in the skin and saliva of the common European toad, *Bufo vulgaris*. Very small quantities will cause vomiting in dogs and cats, and ·00917 mg per kg bodyweight has caused death from heart-failure in the cat. (*See* TOADS.)

BUIATRICS. The study of cattle and their diseases.

BUILDINGS (*see* HOUSING OF ANIMALS).

BULBAR PARALYSIS, INFECTIOUS (*see* AUJESZKY'S DISEASE). The term 'bulbar' relates to the *medulla oblongata* or the prolongation of the spinal cord into the brain.

BULL BEEF. This is beef from the entire animal as opposed to the castrate. (*See under* CASTRATION.)

There is no question that bull beef is a more economic proposition, the carcase providing more lean meat than a steer's, satisfying the export market, and bringing a better return for the producer.

In Italy 53 per cent of all beef came in 1972 from bulls, and in West Germany the percentage was 44, with only 2 per cent derived from steers. In the Netherlands and in parts of France bull beef is also popular.

'BULL-DOGS'. A small metal appliance used temporarily for the restraint of cattle. They are applied to the inside of the nose for holding an animal steady.

BULL-DOG CALVES. In Dexter cattle commonly, and in other breeds occasionally, a hereditary condition, which is scientifically known as *achondroplasia*, occurs. Calves are born in a deformed condition in which the short limbs, dropsical swollen abdominal and thoracic cavities, and a marked foreshortening of the upper and lower jaws give the calf an appearance resembling a bull-dog. Such calves are usually dead when born. The condition is governed by a semidominant gene.

BULL HOUSING. Ministry of Agriculture advice is as follows: The best system of housing is where a bull is kept loose and has constant access to an uncovered exercise yard or pen. The house may be a loose-box, at least 12 feet × 10 feet; the door which leads into the pen should be kept open during the day. An open fronted shelter, from 12 feet to 15 feet deep, across one end of the pen, and with a short baffle wall to shelter the sleeping area, is satisfactory also.

The yard or pen should be up to 30 feet long, if sufficient space is available, and at least 12 feet wide. The walls of the pen or exercising yard should be built to a height of 3½ feet and thereafter continued to a height of 6 feet with stout tubular steel rails. This allows the bull a good view of his surroundings and helps to prevent boredom, which can be one cause of viciousness in an animal. There should be a fodder rack and feeding trough, at the end away from the shelter, provided with just sufficient cover to give protection to the fodder and concentrates during rain and snow, and also to the animal whilst feeding. This arrangement encourages the bull to stay out in the open rather than in the box or shelter and is considered beneficial. The entrance to the pen should be convenient to the feeding area.

The feeding trough should be about 2 feet above ground level and should be fitted with a tubular tying arrangement which can be closed on the bull's neck when he puts his head through to the trough, if it is required to catch him. This equipment is very desirable as an added safety measure, as it permits the bull to be securely held before the attendant enters the pen. It is stocked by merchants specialising in cowshed fittings.

An arrangement which is very useful for dealing with vicious bulls is the provision of a strong overhead wire cable running from inside the house or shelter to the opposite end of the pen. This cable is threaded through a strong ring, about 2½ inches in diameter. This ring, which slides along the cable, is attached to a chain which passes up through the bull's nose ring, then around the back of the horns and is hooked to the upright chain in front of the forehead. In this way, the weight of the chain is carried by the head instead of by the nose ring and considerable discomfort to the animal thereby avoided. The chain should be just sufficiently long to allow the animal to lie down comfortably. The advantage of this arrangement is that a cow can be brought into the pen for service without the necessity of having to release the bull from his tying.

Another safety device which should be provided, where possible, in the walls or railings surrounding the pen, is escape slits. These are upright openings about 15 to 18 inches wide, sufficient to allow the attendant to pass through in case of emergency, but through which a bull could not pass. If, due to the location of the pen, it is not possible to provide these escape slits, the blind corners of the pen should be fenced off by means of sturdy upright steel rails set 15 to 18 inches apart, behind which an attendant could seek refuge.

BULL MANAGEMENT includes good feeding so that a youngster may be well grown and fit for service when 10 to 11 months old; exercise to keep him healthy, active, and with good hoofs; grooming to keep the skin clean and to keep him used to handling; service according to his age – not more than 1 per week or 3 in 2 weeks until 15 to 16 months old – and firm treatment always without either petting or teasing. Bulls should not be turned loose in a field with a herd of cows; the defects of this practice are that accurate records of dates of service cannot be kept, the fecundity of the bull may be impaired by unnecessary service, and there is a risk of breaking out of the field, especially if cows and heifers are in adjacent fields. Owners should realise that the bull is 'half the herd' and take care that in selection and management this 'half' is in no way neglected. Bulls should never be kept shut up in dark quarters – a cause of infertility. (*See* BULL HOUSING, *also* PROGENY TESTING.)

'BULLETS'. These are administered to cattle and sheep by means of a special dosing 'gun', and are used as a means of supplying the animal with a long-lasting supply of *e.g.* magnesium or cobalt, in order to prevent hypomagnesaemia or cobalt deficiency. Bullets can be somewhat costly and not always retained, but they are widely used and have proved successful in preventing deficiency disease in sheep. (*See* COBALT, BOLUS.)

BULLING (*see under* OESTRUS, *in the paragraph headed Cow*).

BULLS, DISEASES OF (*see* CATTLE, DISEASES OF; diseases listed under the word BOVINE; PENIS and PREPUCE).

BUMBLE-FOOT is a condition of the feet of poultry in which an abscess forms in the softer parts of the foot between the toes. It may be caused by the penetration of some sharp object, such as a piece of glass, thorn, stone, etc., or by bruising of the tender tissues below the hard cuticle. An abscess slowly forms, accompanied by distinct lameness. Usually *Staphylococcus aureus* is involved. *Brucella abortus* has been isolated from a case of bumble-foot in Germany. Experimentally infected fowls excreted this organism.
TREATMENT. It is necessary to open the pus-containing cavity and evacuate every small piece of the cheese-like contents.

BUN. Blood urea nitrogen. (*See* KIDNEYS, DISEASES OF.)

BUNOSTOMIASIS. Infestation with hookworms of the genus *Bunostomum.*

BUNT ORDER. Equivalent to the 'peck order' among poultry, this is the order of precedence established by cattle and pigs. With a newly mixed group of these animals there will be aggressiveness or actual fighting, until the dominant ones (usually the largest) establish their position in the social order. Once this is established, fighting will cease and the group will settle down, with the top animal being accorded precedence without having to fight for it. The second animal will be submissive to the first, but will take precedence over the rest; and so on down through the herd, with the bottom animal submissive to all. Occasionally two animals will be of equal rank, or there may be a somewhat complicated relationship between a small group as in the 'dominance circle'.

The bunt order can be important from a health point of view, and it can affect the farmer's profits. If, in large units, the batching of animals to ease management means frequent mixing or addition to established groups, stress will arise, and productive performance will decline. Stress will be *reduced* in the system whereby pigs occupy the same pen from birth to slaughter time. The health factor – as well as daily liveweight gains and feed conversion ratios – will be involved when there is, for example, insufficient trough space, and those animals at the bottom of the social scale may go hungry or thirsty. Similarly, the dominant animals will be able to choose more sheltered, less draughty places, while their inferiors may be cold and wet. (*See* STRESS.)

BUNYAVIRIDAE. This group of viruses includes the HANTAVIRUS (which see).

BUPRENORPHINE HYDROCHLORIDE. An analgesic used for dogs and cats, and as a premedicant for surgery, radiography, etc.

BURNS and SCALDS. Though the former is caused by dry heat and the latter by moist heat their lesions and the treatment of these are similar.

In animals a burn is usually easily recognised by singeing of the hair, or its destruction, but with a scald there may be little to be seen for several hours or even days. Moreover, a scalded area may remain concealed by a scab.

Burns and scalds are extremely painful and will give rise to shock unless they are slight. After a few hours the absorption of poisonous breakdown products from the damaged tissues may give rise to toxaemia; while destruction of skin affords means of entry for pathogenic bacteria, against which the burned tissues can offer little or no resistance. Death is a frequent sequel to extensive burns – the result of shock, toxaemia, or secondary infection.

FIRST AID. Scalds are mainly suffered by dogs and cats, as a result of mishaps in the home. Placing the animal *immediately* under cold, running water will reduce the temperature of the affected area, and is likely to reduce also the pain and subsequent skin damage. This applies to burns also.

TREATMENT. Where the burn or scald is at all extensive, no time should be lost in calling in the veterinary surgeon, who will have to administer an analgesic or anaesthetic before local treatment can be attempted (and in order to relieve pain, and lessen shock).

In an emergency occurring where no first-aid kit is available, a *clean* handkerchief (or piece of linen) either dry or soaked in strong tea may be applied as a first-aid dressing to a burn. The part

should be covered, the animal kept warm and offered water to drink.

The object of treatment, besides reducing pain, is to form rapidly a coagulum of protein on the surface of the burned area and diminish absorption of those altered proteins, from the damaged tissue, which give rise to toxaemia; and also to prevent infection – to which the damaged tissue is so susceptible. Tannic acid (the useful constituent of the strong tea mentioned above) forms the desired coagulum. A tube or two of tannic acid jelly should be included in every first-aid kit for dealing with small burns. It should not be applied over large areas.

In remote areas overseas, where the animal-owner cannot obtain professional assistance, subsequent treatment must aim at avoiding sepsis; the damaged tissues being very prone to infection. Sulphathiozole or sulphanilamide powder may be dusted lightly on to the area before a first or second application of tannic acid jelly. Subsequent irrigation of the part may be carried out with a hypochlorite solution, *e.g.* 'TCP'.

For burns caused by caustic alkalis use vinegar or dilute acids; for phenol and cresol burns, swab with cotton-wool soaked in alcohol and then smear with Vaseline, oil, or fat.

Blood transfusion and the use of normal saline may be indicated in all serious burns.

BURNT SOLE is a condition which results from the fitting of a hot shoe to the horse's foot when the horn has been reduced to too great an extent, or when the hot shoe has been held to the foot for too long a time. It is most likely to occur when the horn is naturally thin, and when the sole is flat or convex. The heat penetrates through the thickness of the horn, and burns or blisters the sensitive structures below. It causes great pain and lameness, and may result in the production of a piece of dead sensitive tissue, with resultant separation of the horn and the production of pus. Professional advice should be sought.

BURSA OF FABRICIUS. A lymphoid organ in birds having a similar role in immunity to that of the thymus of mammals. (*See* T-LYMPHOCYTES.)

BURSAE are natural small cavities interposed between soft parts of the structure of the body where unusual pressure is likely to occur. They are found between a tendon or muscle, and some underlying harder structure, often a bony prominence, between fascia and harder tissue, and some are interposed between the skin and the underlying fascia. They are lined by smooth cells which secrete a small quantity of lubricating fluid. (*See* BURSITIS.)

BURSAL DISEASE (*see* INFECTIOUS BURSAL DISEASE of poultry).

'BURSATI' (*see* ROUNDWORMS – Horse, stomach).

BURSITIS. Inflammation within a bursa.

Acute bursitis is generally due to external violence. It commonly occurs after runaway accidents, falls, continued slipping when driven at fast paces, and after kicks in the shoulder, where the bursa of the biceps tendon is involved.

Chronic bursitis. The blemishes resulting are very commonly seen in all the domestic and many wild animals. The walls of the bursa increase in thickness, more fluid than usual is poured out, leading to a soft, almost painless swelling. Later this becomes hard, and fibrous tissue invades the clotted material. 'Capped elbow' and 'capped hock' in the horse are instances of the condition due to lying on hard floors for a long period, or in the case of the elbow to the calkins of the shoe; 'lumpy withers' are of the same nature, due to the pressure of a badly fitting saddle, and often lead to fistulous withers; hygromata or 'big knees'.in cattle result either from a shortage of bedding at the front of the stall, or from the animals continually striking their knees on a too high feeding trough when rising; in dogs the same conditions are often seen both on the knees, hocks, sternum, and stifles, particularly in old and very lean individuals which lie a lot; monkeys, both in captivity and in a free state, develop similar lumps on the points of their buttocks.

'BUSH FOOT' is a severe lesion associated with foot-rot in pigs in New Zealand, Australia, the UK, etc. The infection involves *Fusiformis necrophorus* and spirochaetes in the UK. (See *Vet. Record* September 18, 1965.) (*See* FOOTROT IN PIGS.)

BUSH SICKNESS. A cobalt deficiency disease occurring in certain sheep-rearing districts of North Island, New Zealand. It is characterised by inability to thrive, emaciation, anaemia, and ultimate prostration, and affects probably all herbivorous animals, although sheep and cattle suffer most. One of the greatest sources of loss is the difficulty experienced in getting females to breed in a bush sick area.

The type of soil is usually blown coarse sand, coarse-textured gravelly sand, or 'sandy silt', and the disease is always worst on land that has been recently cleared and burnt. With time, especially if cultivation is undertaken, the severity of the condition decreases, and it may entirely disappear.

The cause is a deficiency in the soil, and consequently in the herbage, of the small amounts of cobalt, which is the trace element needed to enable the body to utilise iron needed for the formation of the haemoglobin of the red blood cells. In this respect, bush sickness is very similar to conditions which are called by other names in various parts of the world such as 'Pining', 'Vanquish' or 'Vinquish' in Scotland; 'Nakuruitis' in Kenya; 'Coast disease' in Tasmania; and 'Salt sickness' in Florida.

Earlier it was shown in New Zealand that the oxide of iron deposit known as 'limonite' may be used on bush sick holdings as a lick, and will prevent or cure the disease very effectively. It contains very small amounts of copper and cobalt as impurities. Various medicinal compounds may be administered to ailing animals by hand. A mineral lick in which small amounts of the essential trace elements are incorporated is used for preventing illness in deficient areas; also cobalt pellets which disintegrate slowly in the (usually 4th) stomach, giving protection for 9 months or so. (*See* 'BULLETS').

BUSS DISEASE (*see* BOVINE ENCEPHALO-MYELITIS).

'BUTCHER'S JELLY' (*see* 'LICKED' BEEF).

BUTENOLIDE. A fungal toxin which can cause gangrene of the feet in cattle. (*See* FESCUE.)

BUTTERCUP POISONING. The common buttercups seldom cause poisoning, although all contain a poisonous oil, protoanemonin, to a greater or lesser degree. Species most likely to cause poisoning include *Ranunculus sceleratus* and *R. acris.*
SIGNS. Stomatitis, gastroenteritis, abdominal pain; faeces are blackish. Eyelids, lips and ears may show tremors; with convulsions (and rarely death) following. (*See also* WEEDKILLERS.)

BUTTERFAT (*see* Fibre under DIET *and also* MILK).

BUTYRIC ACID. This is a fatty acid and a product of digestion in the rumen by micro-organisms. Butyric acid is also a fermentation product in silage making. (*See* SILAGE.)

BVA. The British Veterinary Association, of 7 Mansfield Street, Portland Place, London W1M 0AT.

C

C-REACTIVE PROTEIN. This stimulates PHAGOCYTOSIS. A greatly increased quantity of the protein in the blood is found after trauma, inflammation, infection, necrosis, and surgical operations.

CABBAGE contains a goitrogenic factor and may cause goitre if it forms too large a proportion of the diet over a period.

Excessive quantities of cabbage fed to cattle may lead to anaemia, haemoglobinuria and death.

CADERAS, MAL DE (*see* MAL DE CADERAS).

CADMIUM. Experiments at the Rowett Research Institute have shown that as little as three parts per million of cadmium in the diet of young lambs causes an 80 per cent reduction in the copper stored in the liver within 2 months.

CADMIUM ANTHRANILATE was used in America against ascarid worms in the pig, the dose being given mixed in the food. The Food and Drug Administration, however, insisted that it must be used only once during the store pig's lifetime owing to the danger to human consumers. Acute cadmium poisoning results in vomiting. In the rat, chronic poisoning is characterised by bleaching of the incisor teeth, anaemia, hypertrophy of the heart, and hyperplasia of the bone-marrow.

CAECUM is the blind end of the large intestine. (*See* INTESTINES.) For rupture of the caecum in brood mares, *see* INTESTINES, DISEASES OF. Dilatation of the caecum is usually an acute illness. **DIAGNOSIS.** On rectal examination it was possible to palpate the distended, displaced, or twisted organ in 95 per cent of 111 heifers and cows. (Braun, U. and others, *Veterinary Record* (1989) **125**, 265.)

CAESAREAN SECTION. This major operation is chiefly performed in bitches, sows, cows, and ewes; occasionally in the mare – when the pelvic passage is for some reason unable to accommodate and discharge the fetus; when the fetus has become jammed in such a position that it cannot pass through the pelvis, and its delivery cannot be effected; when the value of the progeny is greater than the value of the dam; and when the dam is *in extremis* and it is believed that the young is or are still alive. (In this latter case the dam is usually killed and the abdomen and uterus are opened at once. There is a possibility of saving the fetus in the mare and the cow by this method, provided that not more than 2 minutes elapse between the time when the dam ceases to breathe and when the young animal commences. The foal or calf will die from lack of oxygen if this period be exceeded.)

Other indications for Caesarean section are: cases of physical immaturity of the dam, failure of the cervix to dilate, torsion of the uterus, the presence of a monster and, perhaps, pregnancy toxaemia.

CAESIUM (*see* RADIATION).

CAFFEINE is a white crystalline substance obtained from the coffee plant, of which it is the active principle. It is almost identical with *theine*, the alkaloid of tea. Caffeine is used as a heart stimulant for cases of collapse. It can be given either hypodermically or by mouth.

The use of caffeine as a stimulant in greyhound racing is an offence under the UK's NGRC rules.

CAGE BIRDS, DISEASES OF. Budgerigars, canaries, parrots, and other birds commonly kept in cages are subject to a wide range of diseases, including PSITTACOSIS which is easily communicable to man. Other diseases include: rickets (common in young budgerigars and to be suspected if the wings are powerless and the legs stunted), osteomalacia and osteodystrophy, 'feather cysts' (hard, yellow swellings under the skin of back and wings in the canary), fatty tumours and malignant growths.

Feather picking. 'The difference in life-style between the wild, gregarious parrot, and the singly caged pet parrot accounts for behavioural problems including feather-picking.'

Other causes include infestation with the depluming mite, or lice, but 'these are rare in caged birds.' (Lawton, M. *You and Your Vet* (1989).)

The crop may be impacted, and if medicinal liquid paraffin has no effect, it may have to be opened surgically. A torn crop is a common condition, and requires sutures. Persistent vomiting may indicate 'sour crop'; for which 0·1 per cent gentian violet solution, given by eyed-dropper into the mouth, may be tried, and the diet varied. Prolapse of the rectum may be due to, or simulated by, a tumour. Rupture of the abdomen may follow fatty degeneration of the abdominal muscles. An ill bird with a soft swelling of the abdomen may have a ruptured oviduct and peritonitis. Prolapse of the oviduct may occur.

Laboured breathing, associated with rhythmical dipping of the tail, and closing of the eyes while on the perch, suggests heart disease and oedema of the lungs. Gape-worms, mucus, or aspirated food material may block the upper air passages. Air-sacs may be punctured by the claws of cats, and if infected, or filled with blood or exudate, pneumonia is to be expected as a sequel.

So-called 'going light' in show budgerigars is a chronic and eventually fatal disease, due to either *Trichomonas gallinae* or bacteria. (Henderson, G. M. & others. *Veterinary Record* (1988) **123**, 492.) (*See also under* TRICHOMONIASIS.). The birds lose weight, though eating well, over a period of weeks or months. Diarrhoea is seen in a few birds; vomiting may also occur. At autopsy an enteritis is found.

Ascarids are the most common nematodes of birds of the parrot family.

Capillaria worms may cause anaemia and diarrhoea.

Worms in the gizzard and proventriculus may cause peritonitis, airsacculitis and sudden death from visceral perforation.

Tapeworms usually cause diarrhoea and weight loss only in heavily infected birds. Niclosamide or praziquantel can be used for treatment.

Eyeworms can be manually removed. (Stauber, Erik & Schussman, Sheri. (1985) *Modern Veterinary Practice* **66**, 457.)

Faulty diet, infestation by mites, and injury are among the causes of beak abnormalities, which need correcting at an early stage with scissors. In the female budgerigar especially, the nostrils may become blocked by sebaceous or other material. Horn-like excrescences near the eyes may be associated with mite infestation.

Dry gangrene of the feet may follow a fracture of the limb or the presence of ergot in the seed. Fractures of the legs result from their being caught in the wires of the cage. Dislocation of the hip is not rare. Overgrown and twisted claws are common. (*See also* PSITTACOSIS, TUBERCULOSIS.)

Coccidiosis and Giardiasis have caused heavy mortality in budgerigar nestlings. (J A V M A (1981) **179**, 575)

Canary-pox is an example of the pox diseases (*see* POX).

The causes of infertility were investigated in 23 male and 46 female budgerigars. Many of the infertile males had small and inactive testes, with no evidence of spermatogenesis and no semen in the vas deferens or seminal glomerulae. This condition was often associated with diseases which did not affect the reproductive system directly; the most common was mycotic infection of the proventriculus. Three male birds behaved abnormally, attempting to copulate with their perch and showing no interest in females; abnormal behaviour also occurred in two female budgerigars. However, the most common conditions which caused infertility in females were perineal hernias, non-reproductive disease, salpingitis, cystic oviduct and abnormal ovarian follicles, which together accounted for 31 of the 46 cases. (Baker, J. R. (1991) *Journal of Small Animal Practice* **32**, 6.)

The over-heating of 'non-stick' frying pans in kitchens gives rise to vapour which was shown in 1969 to kill budgerigars and other small birds within half an hour. The substance involved is polytetrafluorethylene.

Over-heated fat in an ordinary frying pan may also prove lethal (*see* 'FRYING PAN DEATHS'). Birds have died after being taken into a newly painted room.

(*See also under* ORNITHOSIS, BIRD-FANCIER'S LUNG, and PETS.)

Pseudotuberculosis (caused by *Yersinia pseudotuberculosis*) causes sporadic deaths of birds in aviaries – sometimes an acute outbreak, especially in overcrowded conditions. Death may occur from a bacteraemia, or follow chronic caseous lesions in lungs, air sacs, spleen, and pectoral muscles. (N. H. Harcourt-Brown, *Vet. Rec.* (1978), **102**, 315.)

For information on handling and anaesthetising, see *In Practice* (1983) **5**, 29 for an article by John E. Cooper, and also under ANAESTHESIA.

'CAGE LAYER FATIGUE'. A form of leg paralysis in poultry attributed to insufficient exercise during the rearing period. (*See* BATTERY SYSTEM.) Most birds recover within a week if removed from the cage or if a piece of cardboard is placed over the floor of the cage.

The long bones are found to be very fragile. The precise cause is obscure. A bone-meal supplement may prove helpful.

CAGE REARING OF PIGLETS. This system of pig management is briefly described under WEANING EARLY.

CAKE POISONING (*see* LINSEED, GOSSYPOL *and* CASTOR SEED POISONING).

CALAMINE, or CARBONATE OF ZINC, is a mild astringent used to protect and soothe the irritated skin in cases of wet or weeping eczema, and is used in the form of calamine lotion.

CALCIFEROL is a crystalline substance extracted from irradiated ergosterol. (*See* VITAMIN D and under RAT POISONS.)

CALCIFICATION is a term used in pathology to indicate that condition of a tissue in which there is a deposit of calcium carbonate laid down as a sequel to an inflammatory reaction (*e.g.* following caseation in chronic tuberculosis).

Calcification in the lungs of puppies, has led to death at 10 to 20 days old.

CALCINED MAGNESITE contains 87 to 90 per cent magnesium oxide, and being cheaper than pure magnesium oxide is used for top-dressing pastures (10 cwt per acre), and for supplementary feeding of cattle in the prevention of hypomagnesaemia. In the powder form, much is apt to get wasted, but if the granular kind is well mixed with damp sugarbeet pulp or cake, the manger is usually licked clean.

CALCINOSIS (*see under* GOUT, CALCIUM).

CALCITONIN. A hormone. (*See under* THYROID GLAND and CALCIUM, BLOOD.)

CALCIUM, BLOOD. Levels of calcium in the blood are controlled by the *parathyroid hormone* and by the hormone *calcitonin* (*see* table under PARATHYROID GLANDS). For an insufficiency of blood calcium, *see* HYPOCALCAEMIA. The calcium/ phosphorus ratio is extremely important for health (*see, for example,* CANINE and FELINE JUVENILE OSTEODYSTROPHY). Resistance to infection is reduced if calcium levels are inadequate.

CALCIUM SUPPLEMENTS. These may consist of bone meal, bone flour, ground limestone, or chalk.

Such supplements must be used with care, for an excess of calcium in the diet may interfere with the body's absorption or employment of other elements. A high calcium to phosphorous ratio will depress the growth rate in heifers. The late Dr Ruth Allcroft pointed out that: 'This effect of excess dietary calcium on absorption of magnesium and on growth rate make it pertinent to consider that many modern rations for cattle and sheep supply very high intakes of calcium. For example, the majority of proprietary pelleted rations for cows, calves, and sheep contain from 1 to 4 per cent of a mineral supplement consisting of limestone, bone flour and salt. These concentrate rations are frequently fed as well as grass, hay, and silage. Legume hays, and to some extent, grass-clover hays are very high in calcium. In addition most stock are offered *ad lib.* compound mineral mixtures which may contain a high percentage of calcium as limestone, bone flour or dicalcium phosphate and often contain limestone as well as either of the other calcium-phosphorus compounds. Thus, the heavily yielding dairy cow, or the calf which is being 'done extra well', may be ingesting excessive amounts of calcium in relation to magnesium and other essential minerals, thereby causing conditioned deficiencies.

'For many years now there have been indications that too much calcium is a contributory cause of goitre.

'The inter-relationship of zinc and calcium in the development of parakeratosis in pigs is well known', and a calcium carbonate supplement in excess can increase the risk of Piglet Anaemia. Calcium without phosphorus will not prevent rickets; both minerals being required for healthy bone.

The calcium: phosphorus ratio is also of great importance in dogs and cats. (*See* CANINE/FELINE JUVENILE OSTEODYSTROPHY.)

Calcium alginate, derived from seaweed, has been used as a wound dressing.

CALCULI are stones or concretions containing salts found in various parts of the body, such as the bowels, kidneys, bladder, gall-bladder, urethra, bile and pancreatic ducts, etc. They are either the result of the ingestion of a piece of foreign material, such as a small piece of metal or a stone (in the case of the bowels), or they originate through some one or other of the body secretions being too rich in salts of potash, calcium, sodium, or magnesium.

Urinary calculi, found in the pelvis of the kidney, in the ureters, urinary bladder, and often in the male urethra, are collections of urates, oxolates, carbonates, or phosphates, of calcium and magnesium. (*See* struvite *under* FELINE UROLOGICAL SYNDROME.)

Urinary calculi associated with high grain rations, and the use of oestrogen implants, produce heavy losses among fattening cattle and sheep in the feed-lots of the United States and Canada. 'However, this condition does not seem to present the same problem in the barley beef units in this country, although outbreaks do occur in sheep fed high grain rations. Udall found that the inclusion of 4 per cent NaCl in the diet decreased the incidence of urinary calculi.' – H. C. Wilson. (*See also* UROLITHIASIS.)

Calcium carbonate in the form of calcite plus substituted vaterite was the major component of 18 **equine** urinary calculi examined by X-ray diffraction crystallography from 14 geldings, two stallions, and one mare. In 14 of the cases the calculi were in the bladder. Calcium carbonate crystals were also demonstrated in the urine of two normal horses. (Mair, T. & Osborn, R. R. (1986) *Research in Veterinary Science* **40**, 288.)

Intestinal calculi (enteroliths) are found in the large intestines of horses particularly. They are usually formed of phosphates and may reach enormous sizes, weighing as much as 22 lb in some instances. In many cases they are formed around a nucleus of metal or stone which has been accidentally taken in with the food, and in other instances they are deposited upon the surfaces of already existing oat-hair balls. (*See* WOOL BALLS.)

Salivary calculi, found in the duct of the parotid gland (Stenson's duct), along the side of the face of the horse. A hard swelling can usually be both seen and felt, and the horse resents handling of this part. They are rarely seen in cattle and dogs.

Biliary calculi are found either in the bile-ducts of the liver or in the gall-bladder. (*Note.* There is no gall-bladder in animals of the horse tribe.) They may result either from bile which has undergone concentration and 'inspissation', or they may be salts deposited from it in the same way as with urine. They are combinations of carbonates, calcium, and phosphates, along with the bile pigments, and have, accordingly, many colours; they may be yellow, brown, red, green, or chalk-white in colour.

Pancreatic calculi in the ducts of the pancreas have been observed, but are rare.

Lacteal calculi, either in the milk sinus of the cow's udder or in the teat canal, are formed from calcium phosphate from the milk deposited around a piece of shed epithelial tissue. They may give rise to obstruction in milking.

CALF DIPHTHERIA is a disease of calves generally under 6 weeks of age, in which greyish patches appear on the mucous membrane of the mouth and throat, and less often on the nose, caused by the *Fusiformis (Bacteroides) necrophorus.*

SIGNS. Affected calves cease to suck or feed, salivate profusely, have difficulty in swallowing, become feverish, and may be affected with diarrhoea. The mouth is painful, the tongue swollen, and yellowish or greyish patches are seen on the surface of the mucous membrane of the cheeks, gums, tongue, and throat. On removal of one of these thickish, easily detached, membranous deposits, the underlying tissues are seen reddened and inflamed, and are very painful to the touch. In the course of 3 or 4 days the weaker or more seriously affected calves die, and others may die after 2 or 3 weeks. Some recover.

CONTROL. Isolate affected calves. Antibiotics are helpful if used early in an outbreak.

CALF HOUSING. Important but neglected aspects of this were raised by P. Davidson who commented: 'When we talk about housing calves, this should immediately make us act very carefully, for we are attempting something completely alien to this young animal.

'We are preparing to force upon it our ideas as to what is a fit substitute for the cow and her choice of surroundings. We are trying to substitute a house for a herd and a trough for a teat.'

The calf often lies in contact with the cow (back-to-back or between her legs), and receives both shelter from the wind and warmth from the cow.

'This substitute for careful mothering, nourishment and behaviour adjusted to seasonal conditions can be disastrous when added to the stresses of separation from the cow, exhausting transportation and re-location. These last three strains are seldom recognised as such by the farmer, but they rapidly promote disease and set the scene for yet another dead calf.' (*See also under* COLOSTRUM.)

Housing for calves must be warm but not stuffy (well ventilated), dry, well lit by windows, and easy to clean and disinfect. Individual pens prevent navel-sucking.

Calf hutches. These are widely used in the USA, and said to be healthier and cheaper than rearing calves in large sheds. An English version is now being marketed by Mr P. Padfield, Hayleys Manor Farm, Thornwood, Epping. The hutches, made of heavy-duty polyethylene, measure 7 ft × 6 ft, and are easily movable to 'clean' sites. The calf can lie on straw bedding inside the hutch or go outside into its own small enclosure, which is wire-netted. The idea is to use them for the first 8 weeks or so of life, and to reduce the risk of pneumonia.

CALF PNEUMONIA. Virus pneumonia of calves occurs in Britain, the rest of Europe, and North America. It is a disease of housing, and the practice of good hygiene and the avoidance of damp, dark, cold surroundings will go a long way towards preventing it. Scours are often associated, probably the result of secondary bacterial infections.

Viral infections include the following: –

Parainfluenza 3 – a myxovirus
Bovine adenovirus 1 – an adenovirus
Bovine adenovirus 2 – an adenovirus
Bovine adenovirus 3 – an adenovirus
Infectious bovine rhinotracheitis – a herpes virus
Mucosal disease virus – a pestivirus
Bovine reovirus(es) – reovirus
Bovine syncytial virus
Herpes virus

Mycoplasma and chlamydia are other infective agents which may cause calf pneumonia. A F R C research has confirmed a synergism between *Mycoplasma bovis* and *Pasteurella haemolytica* (an important bacterial cause of calf pneumonia.) In calves housed in groups an almost subclinical pneumonia may persist; a harsh cough being the only obvious symptom, and although growth rate is reduced, there may be little or no loss of appetite or dullness. Often this type is a CUFFING PNEUMONIA caused by *M. dispar*. However, this mild, chronic pneumonia can suddenly develop into an acute form with increased coughing, loss of appetite, fever, and faster breathing. This change for the worse often occurs following stress resulting from sale, transport, and mixing with other calves. Mortality may vary from under 5 per cent to up to 10 per cent. (Source: Drs Alasdair Wiseman & Hugh Pirie, *In Practice*).

In very young calves, abscesses may form in the lungs during the course of a septicaemia arising from infection at the navel ('Navel-ill'). Also in individual calves, an acute exudative, lobular pneumonia may affect calves under a month old; with, in the worst cases, areas of consolidation. (*See also* PNEUMONIA.)

CALF-REARING. *In dairy herds,* as a rule, only bull calves being kept for breeding are ever allowed to suckle for the normal period or are pail-fed with whole milk throughout.

Otherwise, calves are either removed at birth, or are allowed to suckle the dam for 3 or 4 days before being removed; in the latter case, they receive the colostrum at the normal temperature. (*See* COLOSTRUM, CALF HOUSING.)

After colostrum, the calves receive ordinary whole milk (which should be fed warm 3 or 4 times a day for the first 3 weeks); or more often they are given a proprietary milk substitute. (*See* EARLY WEANING, *and also* SALMONELLOSIS.)

Clean water should be offered *ad lib.* from 3 weeks of age. The use of skim milk or whey may, where convenient, be introduced as variants of the systems given above.

In beef herds, single suckling is the rule in typical beef-producing areas where only beef animals are bred; but multiple suckling on nurse cows is common practice in beef-rearing herds where calves are bought in for the purpose. Under this system a cow suckles 2 or more calves at a time for at least 9 to 10 weeks and these are then weaned and replaced by another two which suckle for a similar period. Another 2 calves, or perhaps only one, may follow these and then, as a rule, one more calf is suckled. Thus, one cow, according to her milk-yielding capacity, may suckle from 3 to 10 calves in the course of the lactation. (*See* NURSE COWS.)

Professor M. M. Cooper commented: 'Except where it is a means of utilising an otherwise idle cow, multiple suckling is not advocated. It is expensive in terms of milk usage, it is a "messy job", and it results in uneven lots of cattle which are not easily bunched. Quite the best method is the new method of early weaning, using a high-quality dry food. Provided the calf has had colostrum, it can go on to a reputable proprietary milk substitute until about a month old. Meanwhile, it has been offered, and will be eating the palatable dry food which need not be expensive proprietary pencils. At Cockle Park we have reared many calves very successfully on the following type of home mix:

45 parts of flaked maize.
25 ,, ,, rolled oats.
10 ,, ,, dried skim milk.
10 ,, ,, Molassine meal.
10 ,, ,, soya bean or linseed meal.

Plus vitamins and minerals.

'This is fed, along with good hay *ad lib.*, up to a maximum of 5 lb daily, till the calves are 10 weeks old, when they are switched to a cheaper mix, such as the following:

35 parts of rolled oats.
30 ,, ,, crushed barley.
20 ,, ,, flaked maize.
15 ,, ,, soya bean meal.

'This is fed at 3 to 4 lb per day along with hay and silage to appetite.

'The system is an economical one, in terms of both food and labour; and once calves are weaned from milk, which is best done abruptly, there is a virtual absence of scouring. By the time the calves are four months old they will have attained their normal weight for age.'

(*See also* BEEF-BREEDS AND CROSSES.)

The bought-in calf often arrives, from market or dealer, suffering from exposure, exhausted by a long journey, or nearing starvation. Often the calf has been exposed to infection on the way; and it should be remembered that antibodies received from its dam in the colostrum protect only against infections current in its original environment – not necessarily against infections present on another farm. Liquid feeding for the first day may consist of 3 feeds of 2 pints warm water into which has been dissolved 2 tablespoons of glucose. An early-weaning concentrate should be on offer *ad lib.*

Feedlot calves. The injection of the antibiotic tilmicosin, either on arrival at a feedlot or 72 hours later, was evaluated in a group of 308 calves. The medicated group had an improved daily liveweight gain as compared with the non-medicated calves.

From France came the report of a new diarrhoeic syndrome in calves one to two weeks old. Dehydration was absent, but nervous signs such as ataxia or paresis were shown. (Espinasse, J. & others. *Veterinary Record* (1991) **128**, 422.)

Ventilation is of prime importance in calf houses, and warmth may have to be sacrificed if efforts to attain both result in a warm, damp atmosphere. The critical temperature for a calf during the first week of life has been quoted as 55°F. J. Walker-Love has stated: 'Insulation and, at the very early stages, supplementary heat, will allow adequate ventilation without a serious drop in temperature on the one hand or condensation on the other.' (*See* CALF PNEUMONIA.)

CALF SCOURS (*see* DIARRHOEA).

CALICIVIRUSES are members of the picorna virus group, and have been isolated from cats, pigs, and man. (*See under* FELINE.)

CALIFORNIA MASTITIS TEST (CMT). Using Teepol as a reagent, this test may be carried out in the cowshed for the detection of cows with subclinical mastitis. The test can also be used as a rough screening test of bulk milk.

CALKINS are the portions of the heels of horses' shoes which are turned down to form projections on the ground surface of the shoe, which will obtain a grip upon the surface of paved or cobbled streets. Upon modern roads and on the land, they serve no useful purpose and may do harm. If they are too high they lead to atrophy of the frog and induce contracted heels unless the shoe possesses a bar.

CALLOSITY means thickening of the skin, usually accompanied by loss of hair and a dulling of sensation. Callosities are generally found on those parts of the bodies of old animals that are exposed to continued contact with the ground, such as the elbows, hocks, stifles, and the knees of cattle and dogs. (*See* HYGROMA.)

CALLUS is the lump of new bone that is laid down during the first 2 or 3 weeks after fracture, around the broken ends of the bone, and which holds these in position. (*See* FRACTURES.)

CALOMEL, or MERCURIC SUBSCHLORIDE, should not be confused with the much more active and poisonous *perchloride*. Calomel is a laxative having a special action on the bile-mechanism of the liver. (*See* MERCURY.)

CALORIE. A unit of measurement, used for calculating the amount of energy produced by various foods. A calorie is defined as the amount of heat needed to raise the temperature of 1 g of water by 1°C. A kilo-calorie, or Calorie, equals 1,000 calories. (*See also* cross-references under ENERGY.)

CALVES, DISEASES OF. These include DIARRHOEA, JOINT-ILL, CALF DIPHTHERIA, TUBERCULOSIS, JOHNE'S DISEASE, PARASITIC GASTROENTERITIS, PNEUMONIA, RINGWORM, MUSCULAR DYSTROPHY, GASTRIC ULCERS, RICKETS, SALMONELLOSIS, HYPOMAGNESAEMIA, PARASITIC BRONCHITIS. (*See also* CATTLE, DISEASES OF.)

CALVING (*see* PARTURITION and TEMPERATURE).

CALVING, DIFFICULT. Safety rules for the cowman are: (1) Never interfere so long as progress is being achieved by the cow; (2) do not apply traction until the passage is fully open and it has been established that the calf is in a normal presentation; (3) time the traction carefully to coincide with maternal efforts; and (4) *never* apply that long, steady pull often favoured by the inexperienced.

The force exerted by the cow herself through her abdominal muscles and those of her uterus, in a normal calving, and the forces exerted by mechanical traction in cases of assisted calving, were discussed in a paper presented by Mr. J. C. Hindson, who used a dynamometer to measure these forces. He gave a figure of 150 lb for bovine maternal effort in a natural calving. Manual traction by one man was found to exert a force not much greater. However, three men pulling on calving ropes can exert a force of 600 lb. If mechanical aids are used, the forces become much greater. For example, one man using a calf-puller can exert a force of up to 900 lb; while with a pocket pulley-block he can apply a force of 960 or so lb.

The danger to the cow and calf are therefore very real. Obvious risks include tearing of the soft tissues, causing paralysis in the cow, and damaging the joints and muscles of the calf. The latter's brain may also be damaged, so that what appears to be a healthy calf will never breathe.

The diagram shows the cow's pelvis and various directions of traction with the cow in a standing position. (Her failure to lie down may be due to stress, and in itself complicates delivery. Other causes of difficulty in calving include not only a large calf, an abnormal calf (monster), and an awkward presentation, but also a lack of lubrication due to loss of fluid or to death of the fetus, and inertia of the uterine and abdominal muscles – due to stress, subclinical 'milk fever', or exhaustion.)

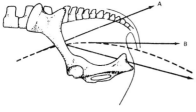

In the diagram, line A indicates the direction of pull which would be the ideal were it not impossible because of the sacrum and vertebrae closing the roof of the pelvis. Line B is a good direction but again one usually impossible to achieve. Line C indicates the actual direction of pull, which will vary a little according to the height of the man doing the pulling, and also according to the space available in the calving area. The broken curved line indicates the direction taken by the calf.

The veterinary surgeon will not, of course, rely on traction alone. He will correct, if practicable, not only any malpresentation, but will endeavour to make good any fluid loss, treat any suspected subclinical 'milk fever', and endeavour to overcome the inertia if such be present. He will also form an opinion as to whether it is physically possible for that calf to pass through that pelvis; if it is not, he will probably recommend a Caesarean operation. (J. C. Hindson, *Veterinary Record* (1978), **102**, 327).

Dystocia, Prevention of. To minimise risks heifers should not be served at a body-weight of less than 260 kg and bulls should only be selected if their records revealed less than 2·5 per cent dystocias, their offspring had a below average gestation length and they were the sons of an 'easy calving' bull.

Management of body condition at calving was also important. At calving cows should have a body score of 2 to 2·5 and it might be necessary therefore to restrict energy intake during the last two months of pregnancy. It was also worthwhile supplementing magnesium and checking for iodine and selenium deficiencies.

Frequent observation around calving, at least five checks a day, and the provision of exercise facilities should be considered as the incidence of dystocias is lower for cows kept in yards and paddocks than in pens. (Mrs Bridget Drew from ADAS speaking at a British Cattle Veterinary Association meeting.)

CALVING EARLIER. The Institute of Animal Science in Copenhagen has carried out experiments with groups of Danish Red identical twins, one reared on a special diet designed to give optimum growth rate and inseminated to calve when 18 months old, and the other group at an age of 30 months, and fed at a standard level.

These experiments showed that a heifer's breeding ability depends on her weight rather than on her age. The two groups came into heat for the first time when they reached a weight of between 570 and 595 lbs. In the case of the more generously reared twins this corresponded to an age of 275 days, and with the standard fed twins 305 days. More than 50 per cent of the heifers conceived at the first service.

However, other work suggests that breeding too early may lead to infertility in later life. Although very early calving (i.e. at less than 22 months of age) cannot yet be recommended for farmers, early calving at around two years can greatly reduce heifer costs and *is* recommended. This was the joint view of the Milk Marketing Board and the Meat & Livestock Commission in 1977.

CALVING INDEX, INTERVAL. In England and Wales in 1968 the average calving interval was about 13 months, but farmers' profits could be higher if it were 12 months.

In order to achieve a calving index of 365 days, it is necessary to get a cow in calf between the eighth and twelfth week after calving. This entails regarding the period up to 7 or 8 weeks after calving as a 'preparation period', during which all heat periods, and expected subsequent heat periods, should be recorded on a wall chart or breeding calendar.

Cows that do not come into season regularly generally have cysts or other infertility disorders which, when spotted at an early stage, can be treated by the veterinary surgeon so that they are cycling regularly again before they have been calved more than eight weeks, thus improving their chances of holding to the first service to calve within the year.

Mr F. J. Willis, of ADAS, commented (1973): 'A "calving index" of 365 days is not necessarily anything to boast about. It may indicate that a herd has no breeding problems – but it may not. It all depends on how many cows have been sold in-calf because they had lost a lot of time and would be "mis-fits" if retained. We should remember, too, that barreners do not figure at all in the calving index calculation. Similarly, in herds which cull empty cows the moment they are dry, the "percentage dry cow" figure can be equally misleading.

'If a dairy farmer needs a reliable guide to his herdman's breeding operations, he should calculate at the year end the "average number of days open" (*i.e.* not in calf) for the herd as a whole. Better still, perhaps, he can pay a bonus on every cow, on a sliding scale, at the time of calving; the size of the bonus to depend on the time lapse since the previous calving. Otherwise, by the time a herd owner has established that he has a measurable degree of infertility, the problem may already have shown up on the debit side of the balance sheet.' Synchronisation of calving, using a prostaglandin, was achieved at the University of Utrecht. (Dutton, J. *Veterinary Times*, January 1991.)

CAMBOROUGH. A hybrid female developed from Large White and Landrace pigs. Litter size consistently averages 10 or more.

CAMELIDAE. This genus includes the llama, alpaca, vicuna, guanaco, and camel. South American camelids comprise four closely related species; all of which can interbreed and produce fertile offspring.

Poisoning. Camels are susceptible to poison-by the trypanocidal drugs diminazine aceturate and isometamidium chloride, at doses harmless to other ruminants. (Ali, B. H. *Veterinary Record* (1987) **120,** 119.)

Anatomy. For camel anatomy, see *The Anatomy of the Dromedary* by N. M. S. Smuts and A. J. Bezuidenhout, Oxford University Press, priced at £90 in 1987.

Anaesthesia. A mixture of xylazine and ketamine has been recommended as superior to either drug used separately: administered by intra-muscular injection in the neck. (White, R. J. and others. Institute for Desert Research, Israel.)

CAMELS. There are two species: the one-humped Dromedary (Arabian), and the two-humped Bactrian (its head carried low). The former are found mainly in the deserts of North Africa, the Middle East, Asia, and Australia. Bactrian camels inhabit rocky, mountainous regions, including those of Turkey, the USSR, and China.

Cross breeding occurs, and mating the Dromedary to the Bactrian male produces a superior animal.

Dromedaries: Body temperature varies in summer between 36° and 39°C, according to time of day. Gestation period: about 13 months. Birthweight: 26 to 52 kg. Puberty occurs in males at 4 or 5 years; in females when 3 or 4 years old. Life span: up to 40 years (but usually slaughtered for food long before such an age is reached).

In the Sahara camels often go without drinking for a week; and in the cooler months for much longer periods if grazing freely plants with a high water content. For further information see *The Camel* by Hilde Gauthier-Pilters & Anne Innis Dagg (published by the University of Chicago Press, 1981).

Diseases. Camel pox is the commonest viral disease diagnosed. The camel is also important as a carrier of rinderpest, foot-and-mouth disease and Rift Valley fever, although cases of the clinical diseases are rare. Among the bacterial diseases anthrax, brucellosis, salmonellosis, pasteurellosis and tetanus are not uncommon but contagious skin necrosis appears to be declining in incidence with the use of extensive management systems. Tuberculosis is an important disease of Bactrian camels farmed for milk production. Ringworm is the only fungal agent believed to be important and it is widely diagnosed in young animals. (McGrane J. J. & Higgins, A. J. (1985) *British Veterinary Journal* **141,** 529.)

Sarcoptic mange is also an important and debilitating disease of camels. The cause is *Sarcoptes scabiei* var *cameli*. Other external parasites include fleas, lice, and ticks. (Higgins, A. J. (1985) *British Veterinary Journal* **141,** 197.) (*See also* POX, SURRA, HAEMORRHAGIC SEPTICAEMIA, RABIES, BLUETONGUE, BLACK-QUARTER, BILHARZIOSIS, URETHRAL OBSTRUCTION, SPEEDS OF ANIMALS.)

CAMPYLOBACTER INFECTIONS.

Cattle. C. *fetus* is an important cause of infertility in dairy herds.

The disease is a venereal one, transmitted either at natural service or by artificial insemination. Many cows served by a particular bull fail to conceive, although usually a few become pregnant at the first mating. The genital organs of the bull, and his semen, appear normal. Following service the cows may have a slight redness of the vagina near the cervix, which is usually slightly swollen with an increase of mucous secretion – appearances not very different from those of a cow on heat. In a cow which has been infected for some time these appearances are altogether absent.

One infected bull was brought into an AI centre in the Netherlands, and of 49 animals inseminated with his semen only three became pregnant. Of these three, two aborted and C. *fetus* infection was diagnosed in them. Of the remaining 46 cows, 44 were inseminated with semen from a healthy, fertile bull; and it required six or seven inseminations per cow before pregnancy was achieved. These and many other experiences have led to the conclusion that infertility from this cause is temporary – cows developing an immunity some three months after the initial infection. Bulls, on the other hand, do not appear to develop any immunity and may remain 'carriers' for years. On the average, abortion due to C. *fetus* seems to occur earlier than that due to brucellosis, but later than that due to *Trichomonas.*

In an infected herd investigated in England, infertility was associated with retained afterbirth, vaginal discharges after calving, still-births, weak calves which later died, and a low conception rate. It was also found that abortions occurred between the fifth and eighth month of pregnancy – and not during the first months of pregnancy as quoted above.

In Scotland in 1977 the infection was detected in 12 herds, with 44 bulls involved. Movement of bulls, part ownership, and movement of cows for service were regarded as causes of spread of infection.

Confirmation of diagnosis is difficult, and at present entirely dependent upon laboratory methods. A mucus agglutination test devised at Weybridge is of service except when the animal is on heat.

CONTROL. A period of sexual rest, use of A I, and treatment of infected bulls by means of repeated irrigations of the prepuce with antibiotic suspensions.

Campylobacter fecalis may also cause enteritis in calves. (R. R. Al-Mashat & D. L. Taylor. *Vet. Rec.* (1981) **109**, 97.)

Ewes. *C. fetus* may cause infertility and abortion.

Dogs. Species of Campylobacter have been isolated from dogs suffering from diarrhoea or dysentery, and in some instances people in contact with those dogs were also ill with acute enteritis. Did the human illness arise from the canine infection? This question has not been completely answered, but in medical circles canine Campylobacter infection tends to be regarded as a zoonosis. Investigation by Mr B. D. Hosie (*Vet. Rec.* (1979) **105** 80) suggested that Campylobacter species are not primary pathogens of dogs. Two questions remain to be answered: Are all Campylobacter strains in the dog pathogenic for human beings? Does human infection cause illness in the dog?

One of the species involved is *C. jejuni*, isolated in one survey from almost 54 per cent of dogs with diarrhoea, but only from 8 per cent without diarrhoea. (*British Veterinary Journal.*)

Pigs. *Campylobacter sputorum,* subspecies *mucosalis,* has been linked with PORCINE INTESTINAL ADENOMATOSIS (which see), and *Campylobacter coli* with diarrhoea in piglets.

Public health. Campylobacters were isolated from 259 (31 per cent) of 846 faecal specimens collected from domestic animals. The highest isolation rate was found in pigs (66 per cent); lower rates were recorded for cattle (24 per cent) and sheep (22 per cent). All porcine isolates were *Campylobacter coli* while about 75 per cent of isolates from ruminants were *C jejuni*. The results indicate that farm mammals constitute a large potential source of campylobacter infection for man. (Manser, P. A. & Dalziel, R. W. (1985) *Journal of Hygiene* **95**, 15.)

CANALICULUS means a small channel, and is applied to the minute passage leading from the lacrimal pore on each eyelid to the lacrimal sac in the nostril.

CANCELLOUS. (*See* BONE.)

CANCER is perhaps best thought of as a group of diseases rather than as a single disease entity. The term refers both to malignant tumours and to leukaemia (sometimes colloquially referred to as 'Cancer of the blood').

Cancer is far from rare in domestic animals and farm livestock. In the latter, however, the incidence of cancer tends to be less, because cattle, sheep, and pigs are mostly slaughtered when comparatively young. Nevertheless bovine enzootic leukosis may appear in a clinical form in cattle under two years old; and cancer of the liver is seen in piglets – to give but two examples.

In the old grey horse a melanoma is a common tumour. In dogs the incidence of tumours generally (including non-malignant ones) is said to be higher than in any other animal species, including the human. (*See* CANINE TUMOURS.) An osteosarcoma is a not uncommon form of cancer affecting a limb bone in young dogs. LEUKAEMIA provides another example of cancer. In cats, a survey of 132 with mammary gland tumours showed the ratio of malignant to benign growths to be 9:1. (*See* FELINE CANCER.) The relative risk in spayed cats is said to be significantly less than in intact females.

Malignant tumours can be defined as non-inflammatory, non-encapsulated new growths; multiplication of the cancer cells not being under normal control.

Cancerous growths differ from benign ones in that the latter's cells do not infiltrate and destroy normal tissue at the site (though sometimes a benign tumour exerts pressure on a nerve or other tissue). Again, benign tumours do not give rise to secondary growths in other parts of the body.

Any secondary growths are termed *metastases,* and their method of spread as *metastasis.* Metastases may occur in various organs and tissues.

Two important types of malignant growth are Sarcomas and Carcinomas. There are several subtypes of each, classified according to the nature of their cells or the tissues affected. *Sarcomas* are, as primary growths, often found in bones, cartilage, and in the connective tissue supporting various organs. Common sarcomas include osteosarcoma, fibrosarcoma, and lymphosarcoma.

Carcinomas are composed of modified epithelial tissue, and are often associated with advancing age. Primary carcinomas affect the skin and mucous membranes, for example, and the junction between the two, such as lips, conjunctiva, etc.

A 'rodent ulcer' is a carcinoma of the skin; less malignant than most in that, while it tends to spread and destroy much surface tissue, it does not as a rule form metastases.

The structure of some carcinomas resembles that of glands; the growth being named an adenocarcinoma. This may occur in the liver for example. Carcinomas may involve a wide variety or organs.

CAUSES OF CANCER. As has been demonstrated experimentally, several different factors can lead to the production of cancer.

One of the factors is *repeated irritation* of a part. This idea was propounded by Virchow. His theory was supported by the fact that cancer of the scrotum was common in chimney sweeps, cancer of the horns common in bullocks yoked for draught purposes. Cancer of the lips was common in clay-pipe smokers, and in users of early X-ray apparatus there was a high incidence of cancer, too.

Soot was probably the earliest recognised *carcinogen*, (though that word was not then in use.) Japanese research workers later showed that by repeatedly painting the skin of the mouse with tar or paraffin oil, cancer often resulted. Later, carcinogenic compounds were isolated from the tar or paraffin and gave less variable results.

It was found too that there is a chemical relationship between one of the carcinogens in tar and the hormone oestrin. This suggested that hormones were associated with the production of some tumours: a view currently accepted. (*See* CANINE TUMOURS.) (For other carcinogens, *see* AFLATXOXINS, BRACKEN, HORMONES IN MEAT PRODUCTION, NITROSAMINES.)

Oncogenic viruses. Moving forward now, by 1971 it was accepted that 'a wide variety of animal tumours are caused by viruses. Several oncogenic RNA viruses have been isolated: the Rous chicken sarcoma virus, the Bittner mouse mammary carcinoma virus, the Gosse mouse leukaemia virus and, more recently, the Jarrett cat lympho-sarcoma virus and possibly the Northern European bovine leukosis virus. Of the DNA viruses, several oncogenic viruses have been isolated, but of special importance are the herpes viruses causing Marek's disease in chickens and, recently, a fatal lymphoreticular tumour in monkeys.' (*Lancet*)

DIVERSITY OF CAUSES EXPLAINED. Recent research has provided an answer to the question: how is it possible for cancer to have such diverse causes as oncogenic viruses, X-rays, tar, or hormones? The answer is that 'all carcinogens act upon DNA. Radiation may break it or cause adjacent units to fuse; chemicals bind tightly to it and alter its functions; viruses join into it.' (Professor W. F. H. Jarrett FRS, 1982).

IMMUNOLOGY OF CANCER. Some light has been thrown on this by studying the development of immunity towards further tumour implants in experimental animals. H. Rinderknecht, Los Angeles, has reported in *The Lancet*:

'In 93 per cent of the mice bearing Ehrlich's adenocarcinoma, when treated with mycetin from the culture medium of *S. felis*, complete regression of the tumour was observed and the animals became resistant to further implants of this tumour. Transplanted lymphomas in mice, treated with colchicine, permanently regressed, and immunity towards this tumour developed. Seventy per cent of rats bearing Flexner-Jobling carcinoma when treated with triethyleneimino-s-triazine responded with complete destruction of the tumour and development of resistance to further implants of the same tumour.

When chickens with metastasising lymphomatosis were infected with Russian summer and spring encephalitis, louping-ill, and Japanese encephalitis, the tumour quickly regressed and immunity developed.

Ligation of the methylcholanthrene-induced tumours in mice produced regression and immunity to further implants. Spontaneous tumours, however, when destroyed by ligation, did not produce immunity to later implants of the same tumour. When tumour tissue mixed with adrenaline was implanted, the implants were resorbed and resistance to the same type of tumour developed. Complete regression of leukaemia in mice under treatment with polycarbonyl compounds was accompanied by immunity to further implants.'

In 1971 it was reported that the growth of Walker sarcoma was entirely suppressed or greatly enhanced in *Nippostrongylus brasiliensis* infected rats depending on the timing of the tumour-cell inoculum in relation to the parasitic infection. Early in the immune response to the parasite, the tumour did not grow, but, once the immune response had developed, tumour growth was enhanced. The enhancing effect could be transferred with antiserum from animals immune to the parasite only, suggesting that the tumour and parasite share antigens. (Keller, R.; Ogilvie, B. M. and Simpson, E., *Lancet*, April 3, 1971.)

ONCOGENES. In the July 1982 issue of the BVA's *In Practice* Professor W. F. H. Jarrett FRS gave a review of recent research under the title 'Cancer: New horizons'.

'A major discovery', he wrote, 'was that when most tumour viruses infect and enter a cell, they have mechanisms for inserting their genes into the DNA of the host cell. This means that, for all practical purposes, the host has acquired a new set of genes, and when the host cell divides and all of its genes are replicated, so are those of virus.'

'This offers an explanation of another main attribute of cancer; i.e. it is heritable at cell level. When a transformed cell divides, all of its daughter cells inherit the new genes. It is this family or *clone* of cells which grows up to form the cancer as seen clinically.'

'This integration of viral genes into the host genome means that the virus can produce copies of itself without destroying the host cell, and this is the main difference between a tumour virus and a destructive or lytic virus such as canine distemper or foot-and-mouth disease virus'.

'When leukaemia viruses such as avian leukosis or feline leukaemia viruses were studied, it was found that they inserted three genes into the host genome.' However, none of the proteins specified had anything to do with cell division; they were all concerned with virus mechanisms.

'The Rous sarcoma virus was found to have a fourth gene. If this were knocked out of action in the virus, sarcomas did not appear in an injected fowl; although the virus proliferated normally. Therefore this fourth gene was not necessary for virus replication, but was required for the transformation of the cell to malignancy.' It was the long sought *oncogene* or tumour-producing gene.

Further research led to the discovery of the also long sought 'transforming protein' – the presence of which in a cell led to malignancy. 'The protein was an enzyme of a previously unknown type, present in Rous sarcoma cells, but apparently not present in any quantity in any other cells.'

The question then arose: how do the leukaemia viruses produce malignancy when they do not have a *src* (from sarcoma) or *onc* gene?

Techniques of DNA hybridisation and the use of radioactive tracers led to the discovery that the Rous sarcoma virus contains a gene almost identical with a host gene, and concerned with cell multiplication.

'Where did the virus get it? Almost certainly the Rous sarcoma virus started off as a leukaemia virus, and inserted itself by chance into the host DNA immediately in front of the multiplication gene. When the virus was replicating it must have packaged the host gene along with the three virus genes into the virus envelope; so creating a sarcoma virus from a leukaemia one.'

'This gene is therefore host and not virus in origin, and has now been demonstrated to be present in an almost identical form in the normal genome of cats, monkeys, and humans.'

'The cancer cell has 100 times more *src* protein than a normal dividing cell. Why does it go on producing this protein and hence keep the cell permanently malignant?'

In the diagram a small box is shown at both ends of the virus genes. This is a piece of DNA which does not code for any protein but contains the control mechanism for the genes. Generally, two types of control are thought to occur: one consisting of 'switch-on' and the other 'keep going'. The latter means that a lot of protein will be produced when it is in action. The virus needs its own controls so that it can keep multiplying when the host is 'switched off.'

'Note that the virus has two control boxes, one at each end. Only the one on the left is used by the virus as the genes are switched on from left to right ... However, the box at the right can become active if, by chance, the virus integrates precisely in front of one of the cell's oncogenes. It is thought that it might switch this on permanently, giving rise to a tumour clone from that cell.'

'This would explain how the leukaemia viruses cause malignancy when they have no *src* gene, and why they take so long to induce leukaemia' (as compared with the Rous sarcoma virus which, when injected into fowls, produces cancer very quickly). The length of time 'is explained by the fact that the viruses integrate at any place in the cell DNA, and it is a completely chance occurrence, as a function of time, that one should integrate next to a host *onc* gene.'

'This theory was originally worked out using fowl leukosis as a model, but it probably applies to other species such as the cat, cow, and human being.'

Further research has shown that 'if only a small part of the right end of the virus genome is taken and coupled up to the *onc* gene, this is enough to transform a cell. Once that cell is transformed and its gene switched on, pieces of DNA without the virus part can be transferred to normal cells and cause them to become malignant. These genes appear therefore to have been permanently switched on by the virus, but once they have been affected they do not appear to need the continued presence of the virus. It is conceivable therefore that chemical and physical carcinogens may cause similar effects as viruses, but this is at present unknown.'

'What is clear is that we all have oncogenes, and that these are normally repressed. In cell division, such genes may be switched on to pro-

duce small amounts of the protein which does the job. When this is used up, cell division stops. In the forms of cancer described above, the genes get switched on but, in addition, they produce much larger amounts of the transforming protein and, being unable to switch this off, they go on dividing. But the cancer change is at the gene level, each daughter cell inherits these changed genes and goes on dividing. Thus a cancer arises.'

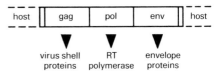

Leukaemia virus genes in cell DNA

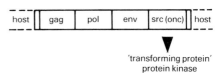

Rous sarcoma virus genes in cell DNA

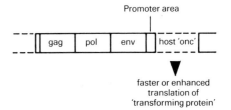

Leukaemia virus and cell oncogene

There is reciprocal translocation between two chromosomes and this results in the placing of the *myc* gene into the active immunoglobulin transcribing genes of the lymphocytes. (This would happen in the herpes virus-induced Burkitt's lymphoma.)

TREATMENT. Surgical removal of a malignant growth is more difficult than removal of a benign tumour, which normally has a line of demarcation to guide the surgeon. Moreover removal of a primary cancer may be followed by cancer elsewhere, as a result of metastases.

Radium treatment: seldom used in veterinary medicine, not only because of the prohibitive cost but also on the grounds that euthanasia will be preferable on humane grounds.

Interferon is expensive and scarce, and hardly likely to be more successful in veterinary medicine that it has been in human medicine (*see* INTERFERON).

Progress in human cancer control has been achieved in certain cases by the use of stilboestrol or hexoestrol, especially for cancer of the prostate gland. Some success has also attended its use in old dogs.

The heat treatment of skin cancer in the dog and cat appears promising. With the animal anaesthetised, the tumour is heated to 50°C by means of radiofrequency current. Dr R. L. Grier reported that of 19 squamous-celled carcinomata in cats, 13 regressed completely. Combining complete and partial tumour reduction, a 89 per cent favourable response was claimed. The tumour-heating method, in which R F current is applied for 15 to 30 seconds, was successful also with perianal tumours in the dog. (R. L. Grier *JAVMA* (1980) **177**, 277.)

Local current field radiofrequency (LCF-RF) heat treatment was used to treat 38 superficial skin tumours (predominantly squamous cell carcinomas) of the nose, face and ears in 35 cats. The LCF-RF apparatus comprises a battery, a radio frequency generator and a surface probe which consists of two 20 mm long electrodes fixed 5 mm apart. The device heats a local area of tissue by the passage of a radiofrequency current between the two electrodes. LCF-RF hyperthermia was applied at 50°C for 60 seconds at single or multiple sites depending on the tumour size. Each cat was observed over a four month period after treatment and 14 out of 35 cases were also available for re-evaulation eight months after treatment. Tumours which had not resolved completely within one month after the initial treatment were retreated. LCF-RF treatment is most suited for the treatment of superficial skin tumours less than 5 mm diameter and 2 mm deep. Ninety-two per cent of tumours of this dimension showed some regression and 60 per cent completely resolved. Fifty-seven per cent of larger tumours regressed after treatment but only 14 per cent resolved. LCF-RF treatment is not recommended for tumours of the pinnae as five out of six tumours at this site failed to respond. (Kabay, M. J. & Jones, B. R. (1983) *New Zealand Veterinary Journal* **31**, 173).

(*See also* DOXORUBICIN.)

Chemotherapy has a place in human medicine. CONTROL. 'The recent development of highly effective vaccines against Marek's disease constitutes a most exciting advance in the realm of control of a cancer by vaccination. Indeed, Marek's disease vaccines represent the first and only effective vaccines for the control of a naturally occurring malignant neoplasia in any species.' (Victor J. Cabasso, *Vet. Rec.* (1975), **96**, 563.)

Professor W. F. H. Jarrett F R S and colleagues developed an experimental vaccine against the FELINE LEUKAEMIA VIRUS (which he discovered), and a commercial vaccine was, in the USA, marketed in 1986.

(*See also* CYTOKINES.)

CANDIDA ALBICANS is a fungus which gives rise to the disease MONILIASIS or CANDIDIASIS; both in humans and in farm livestock.

CANICOLA FEVER. The disease in man caused by the parasite *Leptospira canicola*, which is excreted in the urine of infected dogs. Paresis may occur and some few cases of this disease may resemble poliomyelitis. 'Mild conjunctivitis and nephritis accompanying symptoms of meningitis are suggestive of Canicola fever.' The parasite may be harboured by pigs and the disease has been recorded among workers on pig farms and milkers in dairy units. (*See* LEPTOSPIROSIS.)

CANINE ADENOVIRUS INFECTION (*see* CANINE VIRUS HEPATITIS).

CANINE AUTOIMMUNE HAEMOLYTIC ANAEMIA. A progressive disease caused by a dog forming antibodies against its own red blood cells. A deficiency of platelets may occur simultaneously.

SIGNS: pale mucous membranes, lethargy, weakness, and collapse.

DIAGNOSIS. A commercial Coombs' antiglobulin test.

TREATMENT. Prednisolone is stated to be successful in many cases. (D. Bennett & others. *Vet. Record.* (1981) **109**, 150.)

CANINE BABESIOSIS (PIROPLASMOSIS), which is also called tick fever, malignant jaundice, and biliary fever, is a disease of the dog occurring in South Africa, India, many countries in the Far East, Italy, and France.

CAUSES. It is due to a blood parasite, *Babesia canis*, which is carried from an infected dog to a healthy one by means of a tick, and causes the breakdown of red blood cells and anaemia. *B. gibsoni* is another cause of the disease in Asia, Africa and America.

B. canis is transmitted by:

Haemaphysalis leachi (South Africa).

Dermacentor reticulatus and *D. venustus* (Europe).

Rhipicephalus sanguineus (many countries).

Another form of canine babaesiosis, due to *Babesia gibsoni*, is found in India. The parasite is smaller than *B. canis* and also differs from it in the absence of the characteristic pairs of pear-shaped forms. The disease it causes has an insidious start, is chronic with severe anaemia and emaciation, but without haemoglobinuria. *Rhipicephalus sanguineus* and *Haemaphysalis bispinosa* are the tick vectors.

SIGNS. In 5 to 20 days after inoculation there is a rise in temperature to 107°F with emaciation, anaemia, and icterus. Haemoglobinuria is not constant. Cerebral symptoms may be seen. The disease may be chronic, but the disease is frequently fatal particularly in imported dogs.

TREATMENT. Trypanblue has been replaced by the more specific diamino-diphenyl ether compounds, *e.g.* Acapron, Phenamidine. In addition, it is necessary to attend to the nursing of the dog.

CANINE BRUCELLOSIS (*see* BRUCELLOSIS).

CANINE DISTEMPER (*see* DISTEMPER).

CANINE DYSAUTONOMIA. A syndrome resembling the Key–Gaskell syndrome in cats has been reported in dogs, and has been tentatively linked with canine parvovirus.

CANINE EHRLICHIOSIS (*see* CANINE TROPICAL PANCYTOPAENIA).

CANINE FERTILITY. It has been suggested that a total output of 200 million sperms per ejaculate is necessary if a dog is to be regarded as sound for breeding. Individual progressive motility of less than 70 per cent of sperms, and sperm head and midpiece abnormalities in more than 40 per cent of sperms, are associated with infertility. (Wong, W. T. & Dhaliwal (1985) *Veterinary Record* **116**, 310.)

CANINE FILARIASIS (*see* HEART WORM and TRACHEAL WORMS).

CANINE HAEMOPHILIA. This is an uncommon disease of male dogs of virtually all breeds, characterised by an inherited defect causing abnormally slow clotting of the blood, so that bleeding may occur and continue following only a minor injury.
CAUSE. A sex-linked recessive (*see* GENETICS). Should the dam carry this, then 50 per cent of her dog pups are likely to be affected and show symptoms. Bitches, though carriers of the gene, seldom show symptoms themselves.
SIGNS. These may sometimes be vague and misleading, in that a temporary swelling on the forehead, for example, or transient lameness, may be attributed solely to violence of some kind. The first time that a haematoma is found in the animal, violence may again be thought to be the only cause of the bleeding, and even after repeated episodes it may be thought the animal is suffering from warfarin poisoning. In some cases the abnormally slow clotting of the blood gives rise to excessive bleeding at teething, or if the toenails are inadvertently trimmed too close.
DIAGNOSIS. Proof depends upon costly laboratory tests.
PRECAUTIONS. Affected dogs cannot lead a rough-and-tumble life without bleeding occurring, so the owner must try to prevent knocks and bumps occurring; or agree to euthanasia. A bitch which is known to be a carrier should not, of course, be bred from.
Dr J. G. Golden and colleagues have stated that vaccines, aspirin, penicillin, sulfa drugs, local anaesthetics, and antihistamines are all to be avoided in the treatment of a haemophiliac dog. (J. G. Golden *et al, Mod. Vet. Prac.* (1980), **61**, 671.)

CANINE HERPESVIRUS. A virus isolated from vesicles affecting the genital system of the bitch and associated with infertility, abortion, and stillbirths.

CANINE JUVENILE OSTEODYSTROPHY. This is known also by other names, e.g. nutritional secondary parathyroidism. It arises from a calcium deficiency which stimulates the release of parathyroid hormone (*see the Table under* PARATHYROID GLANDS.) Resorption of bone follows.
CAUSE. The main cause of this disease is feeding the dog a (muscle) meat-rich diet containing little calcium but much phosphorus. (*See* DOG'S DIET.)
SIGNS include pain, and the animal may cry out in anticipation of being forced to move. Short, hesitant steps may be taken. Splaying of the toes is sometimes seen; also swelling at the elbow or carpi – which, in severe cases, may deviate laterally.

CANINE LEISHMANIASIS (*see* LEISHMANIA).

CANINE MYASTHENIA GRAVIS (*see* MYASTHENIA).

CANINE NASAL MITES. A white mite, *Pneumonyssoides caninum*, is an uncommon inhabitant of the nose and nasal sinuses of dogs; and has also been found in the bronchi, and in the fat near the pelvis of the kidney.
Rubbing the nose on the ground and shaking the head are symptoms of this infestation, which has been reported from Scandinavia, America, Australia, and South Africa.
Breathing dichlorvos vapour from a polythene bag is stated to be effective in killing the mites. (L. Blagburn & others. VM/SAC (1982) **77**, 768.)

CANINE PANOSTEITIS. A rarely diagnosed condition, of unknown origin, affecting the shafts of the long bones, mainly of the larger breeds. It may be a cause of sudden lameness in the young dog.

CANINE PARVOVIRUS (CPV) infection appeared as a new disease entity in 1978–79 in Europe, Australia, and America. Not having encountered this virus previously, dogs naturally proved highly susceptible, and serious outbreaks of the illness occurred with numerous deaths. By 1981 many dogs had acquired a useful degree of immunity against the virus, following either recovery from a naturally occurring attack or vaccination; with puppies protected for up to 16 weeks by the antibodies received in the colostrum of their dams, assuming that the latter were themselves resistant.
CAUSE. A parvovirus, possibly a mutation of the feline enteritis or the mink enteritis virus.
'Although canine parvovirus (CPV-2), feline panleucopenia virus (FPV), and mink enteritis virus share common antigens, CPV-2 has at least one specific antigen which is not present in the other viruses.' (Wallace, B. L. & others. (1985) *Veterinary Medicine* **78**, 41.)
SIGNS. The illness takes the form of a severe gastro-enteritis, and diarrhoea is the main symptom. In the early outbreaks many dogs died within 48 hours. Puppies may die suddenly, within minutes of eating or playing, as a result of the virus having infected the heart muscle and caused myocarditis.
TREATMENT. This must include measures to overcome the severe DEHYDRATION (which see) resulting from the diarrhoea. Treatment of the myocarditis is seldom effective.
PREVENTION. A feline enteritis vaccine, using the Snow Leopard strain of the virus, called Felocell, (Smith Kline Animal Health Ltd), previously licensed for use in cats was licensed also for dogs in 1980. A combined vaccine to give protection against canine parvovirus, canine hepatitis virus, and leptospirosis (Duphar Veterinary Ltd.) was licensed in 1981. In 1982 the Wellcome Foundation announced the introduction of their inactivated canine parvovirus vaccine, Epivax P.
Since then a number of other vaccines have appeared on the market. In 1984 Smith Kline

Animal Health introduced two new vaccines: 'Enduracell Parvo L' for immunisation against canine parvovirus and leptospirosis; and 'Enduracell 7' which is a polyvalent vaccine to protect against canine parvovirus, distemper, leptospirosis (both canine forms), infectious virus hepatitus (using CAV-2 antigen), and respiratory infections caused by adenovirus and parainfluenza virus.

These vaccines were the first in the UK to contain live canine parvovirus.

Cooper Animal Health has introduced Vaxitas Parvo, a live attenuated vaccine against canine parvovirus; and Vaxitas DA2, which protects against distemper, hepatitis and parvovirus.

Coopers stated that the vaccines have no immunosuppressive activity, offer a year's protection, produce no clinical signs, no pyrexia or lymphocytopenia and no shedding of challenge virus. Coopers Animal Health, Crewe.

Smith Kline are recommending vaccination at 8, 12 and 16 or, preferably, 18 weeks of age. Hoechst are recommending vaccination at 12 weeks and again at *not less* than 16 weeks for their Maxavac vaccine, which contains inactivated virus grown in fetal feline cell line.

It should be added that apart from the effect of persisting MATERNAL ANTIBODIES, vaccination may fail in some individuals which have a defective immune system and cannot produce adequate antibodies. This occurs with all vaccines.

CANINE PASTEURELLOSIS. (For this infection, *see under* BITES.)

CANINE RESPIRATORY DISEASE (*see* DISTEMPER, 'KENNEL COUGH', KLEBSIELLA).

CANINE RICKETTSIOSIS (*see* CANINE TROPICAL PANCYTOPENIA below; *also* ROCKY MOUNTAIN FEVER).

CANINE STAPHYLOCOCCAL DERMATITIS. This is seen in Irish setters, collies and shelties. The lesions appear on the fine skin with few hairs on abdomen or between the thighs. The condition is itchy, and causes the dog to scratch or lick the part. The lesions consist of roughly circular areas of reddened skin, some with a ring of blackish or greyish crust, having papules or pustules at the edge. The appearance may suggest ringworm at first glance.

The *Staphylococcus aureus* involved has penicillinase, so some other antibiotic must be used. An autogenous vaccine may be needed if antibiotics do not succeed.

CANINE TEETH are the so-called 'eye-teeth', which are such prominent features of the mouths of carnivorous animals. In different animals they are known by different names, *e.g.* 'tusks' in the pig, and 'tushes' in the horse and ass. (*See* DENTITION, TEETH.)

CANINE TRANSMISSIBLE VENEREAL TUMOURS affect mainly the mucous membrane of the vagina or that of the prepuce; occasionally the lips of both sexes. The lesions resemble warts, and can result in infertility.

CANINE TROPICAL PANCYTOPENIA (TCP) is a tick-borne rickettsial disease of dogs, also known as canine ehrlichiosis. The disease occurs in many parts of Africa, the Middle East, SE Asia, the Caribbean, and the USA and the Mediterranean area.

It has been suggested that the distribution of the disease coincides with the prevalence locally of the tick *Rhipicephalus sanguineus*.

CAUSE. The rickettsia causing TCP is known as *Ehrlichia canis* or *Rickettsia canis*.

SIGNS include high fever, sometimes haemorrhage from the nose, sometimes vomiting and dysentery. A brown deposit may form on teeth and gums. Ascites is present in some cases. Excitement, convulsions, and partial paralysis also sometimes occur. Death may occur within a week, or later after a period of wasting.

DIAGNOSIS. A feature of the disease is a marked reduction in the number of blood platelets or thrombocytes. A fluorescent antibody test may be used.

TREATMENT. Tetracycline hydrochloride. It seems that the infection may sometimes remain subclinical; heat stress triggering an outbreak. Dogs which have recovered may become carriers.

CANINE TUMOURS. These are common. 'It is arguable that the incidence of neoplasia in the dog is higher than in any other animal species including man. In fact, the age-adjusted incidence rate for mammary neoplasia is three times larger in the bitch than in women. Tumours arising in the mammary glands of the bitch and the perianal glands of the dog together may account for almost 30 per cent of all canine neoplasms. The predilection of these tumours for one sex or the other and their responsiveness, in some cases, to endocrine ablation or hormone therapy has promoted their designation as hormone-dependent. (Evans, C. R. and Pierrepoint, C. G., *Vet. Rec.* (1975), **97**, 464.) (*See also* TUMOURS, CANCER.)

CANINE VIRAL HEPATITIS is also known as Rubarth's disease or *Hepatitis contagiosa canis*, or CVH, or Infectious Canine Hepatitis (ICH).

Dogs of all ages may be affected – even puppies a few days old – but perhaps the disease occurs most frequently in young dogs of 3 to 9 months. Canine Virus Hepatitis may occur simultaneously with Distemper (which see).

A 'new' canine hepatitis infection. A new transmissible agent, causing acute hepatitis, chronic hepatitis, and cirrhosis of the liver, was discovered at the University of Glasgow. (Professor W. F. H. Jarrett FRS and B. W. O'Neill (1985) *Vet Rec* **116**, 629.)

CAUSE. A canine adenovirus (CAV). CAV–1 is associated with liver, eye, kidney, and respiratory disease. (CAV–2 is implicated only in respiratory disease.)

SIGNS. Infection may exist without symptoms, and in such cases it can be recognised only by means of laboratory methods. In the very acute form of the disease a dog, apparently well the night before, may be found dead in the morning. In less acute cases the dog may behave strangely and have convulsions. A high temperature, wasting, anaemia, lethargy, and coma are other symptoms observed in some cases. A thin, thready pulse is characteristic.

Vomiting, diarrhoea, and dullness may persist for 5 or 6 days, and be followed by jaundice. Such cases may be thought to be leptospiral jaundice.

Puppies may show symptoms of severe internal haemorrhage, and have blood or blood-stained fluid in the peritoneal cavity, with petechial haemorrhages from several organs. Haemorrhages, including subcutaneous ones, may also occur in older dogs. More commonly, there is fever, dullness, some vomiting, tenderness of the abdomen. Of those that survive 5 days or so, many recover. Keratitis ('blue-eye') occurs a week or two after the beginning of the illness in some cases. In older dogs, restlessness, convulsions, and coma are common.

Antiserum is useful in treatment. Glucose and vitamin K are also recommended.

Dogs which have recovered may continue to harbour the virus and act as 'carriers', spreading the disease to other dogs via the urine. (*See also under* GLOBULIN.)

DIAGNOSIS. A gel diffusion test is useful at *post-mortem* examination, especially where decomposition of the animal's body has involved cell disintegration.

PREVENTION. Vaccines are available. A strain of CAV–2 has been developed to provide a vaccine giving protection against acute canine viral hepatitis, caused by CAV–1 and also against the respiratory illness caused by CAV–2. This vaccine can form part of a quadruple one. It is claimed to have all the advantages of a live vaccine but without the 'blue-eye' risk. (Smith Kline Animal Health Ltd.) (*see under* DISTEMPER).

'CANKER' OF THE EAR is a colloquial and somewhat misleading term used by dog-owners, since it often includes both uncomplicated Ear Mange and also painful and suppurative conditions which may follow untreated Ear Mange or may arise from another cause (*see* EAR, DISEASES OF.)

CANNABIS (*see* MARIJUANA).

CANNIBALISM.
Poultry. Cannibalism may follow feather-picking – especially if blood is drawn – or a case of prolapse. The crowding together of housed birds is a common cause; and boredom (no scratching for insects as out-of-doors) is a factor, too. Occasionally a nutritional deficiency may be involved. In broiler plants, debeaking or subdued red lighting has been resorted to. (*See also* SPECTACLES.)

Pigs. Tail-biting is a serious vice. (*See under* TAIL-SORES. These can lead to death.) Cannibalism, where sows eat piglets mainly at birth or shortly afterwards, has been seen increasingly among farrowing sows kept on free range, chiefly on arable farms. The cannibal sow does not eat her own litter but guards it fiercely against other predatory sows. Thus this vice is entirely different from the occasional savaging of a litter by an hysterical sow or (more commonly) gilt in intensively kept pig herds.

CANNON of the horse. (*See* METACARPAL.)

CANTHARIDES is a powder made from the dried bodies and wings of the Spanish fly *Cantharis vesicatoria*, or *Lytta vesicatoria*, and in some cases the Chinese blister fly *Mylabris phalerata*, although this latter is generally used as an adulterant.

Cantharadin poisoning has been reported in a horse and a mule, which died after eating hay contaminated by beetles (*Epicanta vittata*) which contain cantharadin.

ACTIONS. Cantharidin has an irritant action on the genital and urinary organs by which it is eliminated from the body. Cantharides was sometimes employed to stimulate the sexual appetite, but the risk of setting up acute inflammation of kidneys or bladder – leading to very serious illness or death – is very great.

CANTHUS is the angle at either end of the aperture between the eyelids.

CAPILLARIASIS. Infestation with Capillaria worms. *Capillaria obsignata* has been increasingly recognised as of economic importance in intensely reared poultry in Britain. Haloxon, given in the drinking water, has been recommended as treatment. (*See also* URINARY BLADDER, DISEASES OF.)

CAPILLARIES are the very minute vessels that join the ultimate arteries (or arterioles) to the commencement of the veins. Their walls consist of a single layer of fine, flat, transparent cells, joined together at their edges, and the vessels form an intricate mesh-work throughout the tissues of the body, bathing them in blood, with only the thin walls interposed, and allowing free exchange of gases and fluids. These vessels are less than 1/1000th of an inch in diameter. (*See* BLOOD CIRCULATION.)

CAPILLARY REFILL TIME. A means of obtaining a rough assessment of the state of the peripheral circulation. The time should normally be less than two seconds.

CAPONISATION. The castration of cockerels, carried out in order to provide a more tender carcase, and also to obviate crowing and fighting. Surgical caponisation has now been largely superseded by chemical methods – the implantation of pellets of stilboestrol or hexoestrol. This is done under the skin high up the neck, about 4 to 6 weeks before killing at 12 to 16 weeks of age. Older birds may need 2 injections, one 6 and one 12 weeks before killing.

It is important that offals or residues from the chemically caponised birds should not be fed to mink or to pet animals, as sterility or abortion may result.

CAPPED ELBOW (*see* BURSITIS).

CAPPED HOCK is a term loosely applied to any swelling over the point of the hock. At this point there are two bursae: the first, a false bursa, distention of which constitutes true 'capped hock', lies between the skin and the tendon which plays over the bone, and the second, the true bursa, separates the tendon from the bone.

The lesion is virtually identical with that of capped elbow, and treatment is practically the same.

Since the condition may be brought about in the mare by continual kicking at the heel posts of the stall (*e.g.* in cases of nymphomania), it is necessary to pad the heel posts or to house the horse in a loose-box.

'CAPPIE', a disease of sheep. (*See under* 'DOUBLE SCALP'.)

CAPRINE ARTHRITIS–ENCEPHALITIS. In Kenya, where in 1983 there was an increasing demand for dairy goats, this disease new to Africa was recognised. It is caused by a virus, antigenically related to the maedi-visna virus of sheep.

SIGNS. A lowered milk yield, due to mastitis, is sometimes the first sign noticed; and transmission of the virus is thought to be mainly via colostrum and milk.

The main sign however is arthritis. Lameness does not always accompany swelling of the joints.

A chronic interstitial pneumonia occurs in some goats.

The encephalitis affects mainly kids two to four months old. Lesions may occur in the spinal cord also. Head-tilting and trembling may be seen, together with an unsteady gait. Opisthotonus may occur. Partial paralysis may lead to recumbency and often death. (Dawson, M. and Wilesmith, J. W. (1985) *Veterinary Record* **117**, 86.)

The disease is present in Britain, Switzerland, France, Norway, the USA and Canada. It was following import of goats from Switzerland and the USA into Kenya that the disease reached Africa in 1983. In Australia a retrovirus was isolated from goats which caused a clinical disease similar to caprine arthritis-encephalitis, and produced antibodies in goats similar to those caused by maedi-visna virus, which has never been recorded in that continent.

It follows that the caprine arthritis-encephalitis and the maedi-visna viruses are antigenically related. (Smith, V. W. and others (1985) *Veterinary Record* **117**, 61.)

Subclinical infections may occur.

Dr R. Oliver and colleagues at the Central Animal Health Laboratory, New Zealand, showed that the virus could be transmitted experimentally to sheep and, more recently, that lambs could be infected by feeding them milk from infected goats.

CAPRIPOX VIRUSES (*see* LUMPY SKIN DISEASE AND POX).

CAPSULE is a term used in several senses. The term is applied to a soluble case, either of gelatine which dissolves in the stomach, or keratin which only dissolves in the small intestine, for enclosing small doses of medicine. The term is also applied to the fibrous or membranous envelope of various organs, as of the spleen, liver, or kidney. It is also applied to a 'joint capsule'.

CAR EXHAUST FUMES. These may be used for the humane destruction of mink, and have been used to destroy – on public health grounds – a large flock of turkeys. (*See under* BIRDS, HUMANE DESTRUCTION OF; EUTHANASIA FOR CATS.)

CAR, PARKED IN THE SUN. It should be borne in mind that the temperature inside a car parked in the sun, even with two windows opened to the extent of one inch, can within three hours reach 92°F., when the shade temperature outside the car is only 65°F. (J. A. Rohrbach. *Vet. Record* (1976) **102**, 534.) With only one window opened one inch, or all windows closed, a dangerously high temperature would obviously be reached much sooner. A dog left in a car parked not in the shade is in danger of HEAT-STROKE; a cat similarly. (*See under* that heading; *also* HYPERTHERMIA).

CAR SICKNESS (*see under* TRAVEL SICKNESS).

CARBAMATES. These compounds are used as agricultural insecticides and sometimes cause accidental poisoning in animals. Carbamates inhibit cholinesterase.

Symptoms of **poisoning** include profuse salivation, muscular tremors. Atropine is used in treatment. (*See* ORGANOPHOSPHATE POISONING.)

CARBOHYDRATE is a term used to include organic compounds containing carbon, hydrogen, and oxygen, the two latter being in the same proportions as they are present in water, viz., two parts of hydrogen to every one part of oxygen. The simplest carbohydrates are the monosaccharid sugars (*e.g.* glucose), then come disaccharid sugars (*e.g.* cane sugar), and the various higher compounds. The complex carbohydrates, *e.g.* such as the starches, celluloses, and lignified compounds in hay, must be broken down into simpler sugars by both bacterial and protozoa action and by the processes of digestion before they can be absorbed and made use of in the system.

CARBOLIC ACID (*see* PHENOL).

CARBOLIC ACID POISONING may occur from the application of dressings to the skin; from the internal administration of the drug by mistake; and cases have been recorded from the use of strong carbolic disinfecting powders sprinkled on to the floors of animal buildings. (*See* PHENOL.)

CARBON DIOXIDE is formed by the tissues, taken up by the blood, exchanged for oxygen in the lungs, and expired from them with each breath. In a building, the ventilation must be such as will get rid of it rapidly so that it does not accumulate in the atmosphere. (*See* VENTIL-ATION.) In the air it is present to the extent of about 0·03 per cent by volume, although this amount varies. CO_2 is used as a respiratory stimulant by anaesthetists.

CARBON DIOXIDE ANAESTHESIA. CO_2 derived from dry ice, has been widely used for anaesthetising pigs prior to slaughter. The pigs are driven in single file through a tunnel and in-hale the CO_2 for less than a minute, after which a very brief period of unconsciousness follows – long enough, however, for shackling and 'sticking' to be accomplished without causing pain. There is no adverse effect upon the carcase. CO_2 has also been used, instead of chloroform, in lethal chambers or cabinets for the euthanasia of cats, but if it is to be humane the technique must be correct.

CARBON DIOXIDE SNOW is formed when CO_2 is first compressed in a cylinder to a liquid and then released through a small nozzle. The tem-perature falls to about $-70°C$ and the CO_2 solidifies as a snow. This is then compressed into solid blocks, which are used for a variety of pur-poses where a low temperature is required for a considerable time, such as to cool meat, milk, or fish in transit by rail, to preserve tissues, bacteria, or foods, so that normal enzyme action is arrested, and sometimes to produce local anaesthesia by freezing or to cauterise a surface growth on the skin.

A piece of 'dry ice' or carbon dioxide 'snow' placed on the floor of an infested building will act as a bait for ticks which will gather round it and can then be collected and destroyed.

CARBON FIBRE IMPLANTS. These have been used in the surgical repair of tendons in race-horses, and dogs, and have generally given good results.

CARBON MONOXIDE poisoning may result from gas and solid-fuel heating systems in the home when there is an inadequate supply of air. Many dogs and cats have been found dead in the kitchen in the morning.

In Britain, until the late 1960s, town gas (derived from coal) contained 10–20 per cent of carbon monoxide. Natural and oil-based gas contain less than 1 per cent. However, where there is inadequate ventilation, incomplete combustion may occur leaving not carbon dioxide and water but carbon monoxide.

Stillbirths have been reported by MAFF vet-erinary investigation centres in sows, 'associated with incomplete combustion in propane gas heaters and inadequate ventilation during cold weather'. In one herd when poor ventilation and faulty heaters were corrected, the stillbirth rate dropped from 28 to 6·7 per cent. Mr. E. N. Wood emphasised that the pig fetus is very susceptible to this form of poisoning, and dies in the uterus or at farrowing, without clinical signs of ill health being shown by the sow.

Car exhaust fumes have been used for the humane destruction of mink and turkeys.

DIAGNOSIS. Cherry-red tissues and body fluids are suggestive of poisoning. Analysis of blood samples for carboxy-haemaglobin can be used for confirmation.

Abortion may be caused by carbon monoxide even at levels too low to cause signs in adult pigs.

CARCASES, DISPOSAL OF (*see under* DIS-POSAL).

CARCINOGENS are oncogenic viruses or sub-stances which give rise to cancer. (*See* NITROSAMINES, BRACKEN, AFLATOXINS, HORMONES IN MEAT, and substances mentioned under CANCER.) 'All carcinogens act upon DNA'. (Prof. W. F. H Jarrett FRS.)

CARCINOMA is a type of malignant growth – described under CANCER.

CARDIA is the upper opening of the stomach at which the oesophagus terminates. It lies close behind the heart.

CARDIAC DISEASE (*see* HEART DISEASES).

CARDIAC PACEMAKERS (see PACEMAKERS).

CARDIOGRAPHY is the process by which graphic records can be made of the heart's action. Auricular and ventricular pressures can be recorded, the sounds of the heart-beat can be con-verted into waves of movement and recorded on paper, and the changes in electric potential that occur can be similarly recorded. (*See* ELECTRO-CARDIOGRAPH.)

CARDIOLOGY is the name given to a study of the heart and heart diseases.

CARIES (*see* TEETH, DISEASES OF).

CARMINATIVES are substances which relieve TYMPANY. Almost all the aromatic oils are carminatives.

CARNASSIAL TOOTH (*see* drawing of dog's skull under SKULL).

CAROTENE is a pigment, present in carrots among many other foodstuffs, which is a precur-sor of vitamin A and can be converted into this vitamin in the liver and stored there. (*See* VITAMINS.)

CARPITIS. Arthritis affecting the carpus.

CARPUS is the wrist in man, or the 'knee' of the fore-limbs of animals.

'CARRIER' is an animal recovered from a dis-ease, or not showing symptoms, but capable of passing on the infection to another animal. For example, a bull may be a carrier of brucellosis; dogs may be carriers of *leptospirae*; a cow may be a carrier of *Salmonella dublin*.

CARRYING INJURED dogs and cats. (*See illustration under* ACCIDENTS.)

CARTILAGE is a hard but pliant tissue forming parts of the skeleton, *e.g.* the rib cartilages, the cartilages of the larynx and ears, and the lateral cartilages of the foot, as well as the cartilages of the trachea. Microscopically it consists of cells arranged in pairs or in rows, embedded in a clear homogeneous tissue devoid of blood-vessels and nerves. The surfaces of the bones that form a joint are covered with *articular cartilages*, which provide smooth surfaces of contact and minimise shock and friction. In some parts of the body there are discs of cartilage interposed between bones forming a joint, *e.g.* between the femur and tibia and fibula there are the cartilages of the stifle joint, and between most of the adjacent vertebrae there are similar discs. When a bone is still growing, there are layers of cartilage interposed between the shaft and its extremities; these are called *epiphyseal cartilages* (*see* BONE, Growth of).
Diseases of cartilage. Two chief diseases affect cartilages in animals. *Necrosis*, or death of the cells of the cartilage, results from accident, injury, or in some cases from pressure. The treatment is wholly surgical, and consists in the removal of the dead piece or pieces and the provision of drainage for discharges.
Ossification. Many of the cartilaginous structures of the body become ossified into bone in the normal course, especially in old age; but as the result of a single mild or many slight injuries to a cartilage the formation of bone may take place prematurely, and interference with function results.

CARUNCLE. A small fleshy protuberance, which may be a normal anatomical part. In the uterus of ruminants, for example, mushroom shaped caruncles project from the inner surface to give attachment to the cotyledons of the fetal membranes.

CASEATION is a process which takes place in the tissues in tuberculosis and some other chronic diseases. The part changes into a firm, cheese-like mass, which may later calcify. (*See* CALCIFICATION.)

CASEIN. A protein of milk and an important constituent of 'Solids-not-fat'.

CASEOUS LYMPHADENITIS is a chronic disease of the sheep and goat, characterised by the formation of nodules containing a cheesy pus occurring in the lymph nodes, lungs, skin, or other organs; exhibiting a tendency to produce a chronic pneumonia or pleurisy.
Amongst the domesticated animals it occurs in the sheep and the goat, but can be produced in the rabbit, the guinea-pig, and the rat by artificial means. An outbreak occurred in the UK in 1990, involving a herd of goats.
CAUSE. *Corynebacterium pseudotuberculosis.* Faeces of affected sheep contain the organisms

and so aid in spreading the disease. Wound infection is a common source.
TREATMENT. This is difficult as the lesions become encapsulated and so inaccessible to antibiotics. Veterinary advice should be sought.

CASSAVA (*Manihot esculenta*) is a widely grown crop for human food in the tropics, and is the source of tapioca. The potato-like tubers, however, if eaten raw cause cyanide poisoning. Moreover, when used for people on an iodine-deficient diet as a staple crop instead of a standby, goitre becomes a serious problem. Livestock in the tropics have died from cyanide poisoning due to this crop.

CASTOR SEED POISONING has occurred overseas through animals being accidentally fed either with the seeds themselves or with some residue from them. The seeds of the castor plant (*Ricinus communis*) contain an oil which is used not only as a medicinal agent, but also for lubricating. Processing leaves behind in the press-cakes the toxin *ricine*, and renders these 'castor-cakes' unsuitable as a food-stuff for all live-stock. Overseas, however, unscrupulous cattle cake merchants sometimes sell them for feeding cattle after treating the residual press-cakes with steam, but with the result that the ricine is not all destroyed and poisoning may occur.
SIGNS. These consist of dullness, loss of appetite, elevation of the temperature, severe abdominal pain, and usually constipation. The heart's action is tumultuous, the surface of the body is cold; there may be a watery cold sweat, and the respiration is distressed. In cattle there is often a blood-stained diarrhoea, especially if comparatively small amounts have been taken. Where large amounts have been eaten the faeces are usually hard, dry, and brown in colour. Upon *post-mortem* examination there is an intense inflammation of the stomach and intestines, with 'false membrane' formation in the small bowel particularly.
FIRST-AID. Give milk or oatmeal gruel pending veterinary advice.

CASTRATION.
In Britain, it is illegal to castrate horse, ass, mule, dog, or cat without the use of an anaesthetic. For other animals, an age limit is in force. (*See* ANAESTHETICS, LEGAL REQUIREMENTS.)

Reasons for castration. To the humanitarian who has not an extensive acquaintance with animals the necessity for this operation may not be obvious, and it is advisable at the outset that the reasons for castration should be given.
Bullocks are able to be housed along with heifers without the disturbance which would otherwise occur during the oestral periods of the female, and they live together without fighting, and without becoming a risk to man. The uncertainty of the temper of an entire male animal, especially of the larger species, and the risk of injury to attendants, are well known. The same remarks apply to horses, asses and mules.

Another reason for castration of domesticated animals living under artificial conditions is that breeds and strains can be more easily kept 'pure', desirable types can be encouraged and retained and undesirable types eliminated.

It used to be held that meat from uncastrated animals was greatly inferior to that from castrated ones. In fact, apart from such considerations as obtaining docility and avoiding promiscuous breeding, meat-quality was the main reason advanced for doing the operation. Nowadays that phrase 'greatly inferior' has tended to become 'slightly inferior'.

Some disadvantages of castration. The growing practice of early slaughter of meat-producing animals, so that the majority never fully mature, has posed the question: is castration still necessary or, for efficient meat production, even advisable?

In all species, the entire male grows more quickly and produces a leaner carcase than that of the castrate. Since rapid and economic production of lean flesh is essential in modern meat production, the principle of male castration may seem to be becoming out of date.

The problem differs from one species of farm animal to another. Veal calves are not castrated. They have a better food conversion ratio than castrated calves. In 1963 a trial with up to 500 'beef bulls' was authorised by the Ministry of Agriculture. Between January–August 1972, 8159 young bulls were slaughtered for beef. (Young bulls tend to be obstreperous rather than bad-tempered.)

With pigs, a change may come. At the 6th BOCM Boar Performance Test, the average boar took only 151 days to reach bacon weight (200 lb), and had a food conversion ratio of 2·87 between 70 and 200 lb liveweight. If the animals in the test had been castrated they would each have required about ¾ cwt more food to reach 200 lb liveweight. (*See also under* STRESS, BULL BEEF.)

Methods. The operation consists of opening the scrotum and coverings of the testicle by a linear incision, separating the organ itself from these structures, and dividing the spermatic cord well above the epididymis which lies on the testicle, in such a way that haemorrhage from the spermatic artery does not occur. In very many cases the larger animals are operated upon in the standing position, but lambs and young pigs are usually held by an assistant. There are also the 'bloodless' methods of the emasculator and rubber rings.

Among possible future methods of castration is an **immuno-castration** technique, which could possibly replace surgical methods. Complex in itself, but involving merely subcutaneous injections to apply, it prevents the release of *gonadotrophins* – hormones secreted by the pituitary gland – which in turn results in the testis ceasing to grow, prevention of secretion of the male sex hormone *testosterone*, and prevention of sperm production. 'Although immuno-castration has been successfully achieved, the possibility remains that the effect may be temporary.' This could be an advantage, however, in allowing

phased management of beef cattle, for example, while finishing at grass, before returning to an intensive finishing period as bulls. (I. S. Robertson, J. C. Wilson & H. M. Fraser, *Vet. Rec.* (1979), **105**, 556.)

Immuno-castration was successfully used in a **cryptorchid stallion** which – following removal surgically of an inguinal testicle – had subsequently shown sexual aggression.

The technique involved active immunisation against the hypothalmic neuropeptide luteinising hormone releasing hormone (LHRH). This was administered intramuscularly in two sites over the shoulders. The stallion was rendered docile and easy to handle. However, repeated booster doses were needed. (Sabacher, B. D. & Pratt, B. R. (1985) *Veterinary Record* **116**, 74.)

So-called **'chemical castration'**, using scar-forming substances, has also been the subject of experimental work in several countries and in rats, goats, pigs – and even man. (M. D. Freeman & D. S. Coffey, *Fertil and Steril* (1973) **24**, 884.) (T. A. Bowman and others. *J. of Animal Science* (1978) **46**, 1063.)

Horses. Entire colts are usually castrated when one year old, *i.e.* in early spring of the year following their birth, but they may preferably be castrated as foals, at an age of 5 months or younger. The colt may be caught with a long neck rope, have a canvas anaesthetic mask applied. When the foal can no longer stand as a result of the anaesthetic, a hind-leg is pulled forward to expose the operation site, and castration performed with the foal lying on its side. By this method,* 6 colts can be castrated in an hour; less assistance is required; the gelding is not frightened when handled later, as occurs when the 2-year-olds are castrated. Owners have been well pleased with the results of this early castration, which is more humane.

Instruments used. (*See* ECRASEUR, *and* EMASCULATOR.)

After castration the colt is either turned out into a well-strawed yard or put into a roomy loose-box and given a feed; or, if climatic conditions are favourable, it may be turned out to grass again. It is always advisable to see the colt at intervals during the 24 hours after castration, to ensure that there is no bleeding, that hernia has not developed, or that no other untoward accident has happened. Cryptorchid castration is briefly mentioned under the heading RIG.

Cattle. Bull calves are usually castrated between the ages of 2 and 8 months, but in some districts it is quite usual to leave them until they are somewhat older than this. A number of male calves are also left in the expectation that they will materialise into animals which may be fit for breeding purposes, but some of these must be castrated later on when they are between 12 and 15 months old. In very young calves – *i.e.* those between a month and 6 weeks old – castration is very often carried out by merely opening the scrotum and scraping the spermatic cord through with the edge of the knife. An alternative method

*Recommended in the *Veterinary Record* of March 3, 1960.

of castrating cattle is to use a 'Burdizzo emasculator'. The instrument is placed with the jaws over the neck of the scrotum in such a way that when closed they will crush the spermatic cord through the skin of the scrotum. An assistant presses the handles together while the operator holds the cord from moving away from the closing jaws. The skin of the scrotum is not severed, there is no haemorrhage and very little danger of infection, and the method is expeditious and clean. The disadvantages of the Burdizzo emasculator are that the cord is liable to slip away from between the jaws of the instrument and so escape crushing, and that, even when the cord is properly crushed in the larger young bulls, the blood-supply of the testicle may not be completely cut off, and a certain amount of its function remains. To avoid these disadvantages as much as possible the majority of practitioners make a point of crushing each cord separately in two places about an inch apart, the testicle gradually shrinks and atrophies, until in a month's time it is but little larger than a walnut. This method is not ideal, may cause painful swelling, and requires skill.

The rubber-ring method (see 'ELASTRATOR') causes pain immediately after the application of the ring; and also, in a proportion of cases, after 2 or 3 weeks when ulceration occurs.

Sheep. The most convenient age at which lambs are castrated is when they are between a week and a month old, the operation usually being carried out at the same time as docking. The point of the scrotum is cut off transversely and each testicle exposed by the one incision. They are then held alternately by a pair of rubber-jawed forceps, turned round and round so as to twist the cord, and then pulled off, or the cord may be scraped through with a knife. Special small emasculators are also used.

The rubber-ring method (see 'ELASTRATOR') is also used, and the Department of Agriculture, New Zealand, has stated that there was no significant difference in the fat quality of lambs castrated at 3 weeks of age by (*a*) rubber ring, (*b*) knife, and (*c*) emasculator. Lambs castrated at birth by the rubber-ring method were, however, lighter and smaller.

This method is not ideal. Pain immediately following application may be severe, and subsequent ulceration of the skin may also be painful and conducive to tetanus infection.

For the castration of adult rams the Burdizzo emasculator is probably the best instrument. Any method of castration of adult rams which involves opening the scrotum is usually attended by a percentage of deaths, no matter with how much care and asepsis the operation is performed.

Pigs. Young male pigs are usually castrated at the time they are weaned or a little before it, *i.e.* between 7 and 9 weeks old, although a number are operated upon when only about 5 weeks old. Many people consider that the earlier period is not to be recommended because it entails placing the newly castrated pigs back with the sow; with a fractious gilt, or with an irritable old sow, the small amount of bleeding which may occur is apt to induce the mother to attack and perhaps kill her unfortunate offspring. At the same time many other owners prefer to have the pigs castrated before they are weaned, so that the check to their growth which always follows weaning does not coincide with the check they receive from the operation. Probably the best arrangement is to leave the piglets with the sow until they are about 8 weeks old, and then to castrate them and wean them at the same time, giving extra good feeding for a short while afterwards.

In the United States it is becoming common practice for piglets to be castrated when they are between 4 and 7 days old. Instead of the conventional incising of the scrotum, small incisions are made at different sites and, by means of a surgical hook, the spermatic cords are withdrawn and severed. The testicles may be left in position. It is claimed that this method reduces the danger of subsequent wound infection.

Dogs and cats. Dr Ian Fraser Dunbar, of the Department of Psychology, University of California, commented (*Vet. Rec.* (1975), **96,** 92): 'The main reason for castrating cats and dogs is to render them infertile. However, in clinical practice they are often castrated at the request of the owner, in the hope of reducing or abolishing 'objectionable behaviour' such as mounting and onanism, urine and scent-marking, fighting and roaming.'

A study of male cats following castration showed that there was 'a post-operative decline in fighting, roaming and urine-spraying in 88 per cent, 94 per cent, and 88 per cent, respectively'. Improvement – especially as regards urine-spraying – was obtained in most cases within a fortnight.

Castration of dogs seems to produce no reliable effect on either aggressive or scent-marking behaviour.

There are significant species differences between cats and dogs as regards the effects of castration, but 'the major effect of castration in either species is reflected by an overall reduction in the frequency of intromissions sometimes followed by a decrease in mounting behaviour. Nevertheless, some individuals retain the ability to copulate for a substantial period of time. Castration is likely to have a more pronounced effect on the mating behaviour of male cats than on that of male dogs.' (*See also* SPAYING *and* VASECTOMY.)

Castration accidents or complications following the operation. *Haemorrhage* may occur either immediately following the operation or at any time afterwards up to the sixth or seventh day (usually within the first 24 hours). As a rule the small amount of haemorrhage which nearly always occurs immediately after the operation can be disregarded, since it comes from the vessels in the skin of the scrotum. When bleeding is alarming it is necessary to pack the scrotum with sterilised cottonwool or gauze or to search for the cut end of the cord, and apply a ligature. This is a task for a veterinary surgeon. (*See* BLEEDING, ARREST OF.)

Hernia of bowel or of omentum may occur where

there is a very wide inguinal ring. The replacement or amputation of any tissue that has been protruded from the abdomen requires the services of a veterinary surgeon. All that the owner should do until he arrives is to secure the animal, pass underneath its abdomen a clean sheet that has been soaked in a weak solution of an antiseptic, and fix this sheet over the loins in such a way that it will support the protruded portions and prevent further prolapse.

Peritonitis, which is almost always fatal in the horse, may follow the use of unclean instruments, or may be contracted through contamination from the bedding, or by attack by flies subsequent to the operation.

Tetanus may arise as a complication following castration in horses and lambs particularly. Sometimes there is a considerable loss among lambs from this cause. (*See* TETANUS.) In districts where tetanus is common, colts should be given a dose of tetanus anti-toxin before castration, which will protect them until the wounds have healed.

Severance of a calf's urethra by a farm worker using a Burdizzo castrator was reported by Mr. J. S. Steward. It was the third such death on that farm.

CAT BITES/SCRATCHES. These may sometimes give rise in man to CAT-SCRATCH FEVER (which see), and also yersiniosis, rabies, etc., should the cat be infected with organisms causing these diseases.

'CAT 'FLU'. An inaccurate but convenient term widely used by owners for illness caused by FELINE VIRAL RHINOTRACHEITIS and FELINE CALICIVIRUS INFECTION.

CAT FOODS. A diet of heart is injurious and if fed exclusively can lead to paralysis within a matter of weeks.

An all-liver diet is also dangerous since it gives rise to an excess of vitamin A, which in turn can lead to ankylosis of the cervical vertebrae. The 'angry cat' position may be observed by the veterinary surgeon called in to examine the animal. An exclusive diet of all-muscle meat, e.g. minced beef, can also cause deformity of the skeleton. (*See* FELINE JUVENILE OSTEODYSTROPHY.) (*See also* CHASTEK PARALYSIS, STEATITIS, TAURINE.)

In general, cats need more protein in their diet than do dogs.

Canned cat foods from reputable manufacturers are both palatable and nutritious, and carefully formulated so as to provide a balanced meal. However, it is wise to alternate them with fresh food.

CAT LEPROSY. A skin disease in which granuloma formation occurs and ulcers may appear on the head and legs. Forty-four cases of feline leprosy were reviewed; the majority of cats being between one and three years old. The condition is a non-tuberculosis granulomatous skin disease associated with acid-fast bacilli. The main differences between the human and feline condition, on histological grounds, are the areas of caseous necrosis and the consistent lack of nerve involvement observed in cats.

CAUSE. *Mycobacterium lepraemurium*, which is believed to be transmitted by mice and rats.

DIFFERENTIAL DIAGNOSIS: Cat leprosy needs to be distinguished from tuberculosis, neoplasia, foreign body granuloma, mycotic infection, nodular panniculitis, pansteatitis, and chronic abscesses secondary to feline leukaemia virus infection. (Stephen D. White & others *JAVMA* (1983) **182**.)

CAT LUNGWORM. *Aleurostrongylus abstrusus* can give rise to symptoms such as coughing, sneezing, and a discharge from the nostrils. Recent research has disclosed a relationship between infestation with this lung-worm and abnormality of the pulmonary arteries. Often it is only when the cat is subjected to stress or to some other infection that lungworms cause serious illness.

CAT-SCRATCH FEVER is a disease of man. The main symptom is a swelling of the lymph nodes nearest the scratch; sometimes fever, and a rash; occasionally encephalitis. The cause is a bacillus, for the identification of which the Warthin-Starry stain is used.

CATS, BREEDING DIFFICULTIES OF, summarised. For the novice breeder and others, the following facts and figures may be of interest.

Dystokia. In a survey of 4,007 cats, Dystokia occurred in only 134; that is to say 3·3 per cent. An oversize kitten is seldom a cause, unless the queen has had a fracture of the pelvis. Occasionally a malpresentation such as a turning of the foetal head may render normal birth impossible and necessitate a Caesarean operation.

Prolapse of the uterus is rare. In one case, four kittens were born at 4 a.m., but at breakfast time the queen had a Y-shaped protrusion from her vulva. Veterinary treatment put matters right.

Ectopic pregnancy. This occurs when a fertilised egg, instead of passing down one of the Fallopian tubes towards the uterus, is released from the hind end of the tube, and develops outside the uterus. Another cause is violence of some sort leading to rupture of the uterus. Mummified foetuses have been found alongside the stomach, for example.

Uterine inertia is rare. So is torsion of the uterus. In a case of the former, veterinary advice was sought concerning a 9-month-old queen in her 70th day of gestation. Following injections, a dead kitten was born. Ninety minutes later three live ones followed.

Pyometra. In 183 queens the signs were distension of the abdomen, feverishness, and – in some cases – a vaginal discharge. A complete recovery followed surgery in 168 cats. Any postoperative complications in 20 per cent of the patients cleared up within a fortnight after being returned home. Euthanasia or natural death accounted for 15.

CATS, DISEASES OF (*see* diseases beginning with the word FELINE; also under CAT FOODS and succeeding paragraphs. For other diseases see ALOPECIA, ASPERGILLOSIS, AUJESZKY'S DISEASE, BUBONIC PLAGUE, CANCER, CHLAMYDIA infection, POX, CRYPTOCOCCOSIS, DIABETES, DIARRHOEA, ECLAMPSIA, EOSINOPHILIC GRANULOMA, GINGIVITIS, GLOSSITIS, FELINE DYSAUTONOMIA, NOCARDIOSIS, PYOTHORAX, RABIES, SALMONELLOSIS, STEATITIS, TGE of pigs, TOXOCARIASIS, TUBERCULOSIS, TYZZER'S DISEASE, YERSINIOSIS, SPOROTRICHOSIS, FELINE SPONGIFORM ENCEPHALOPATHY, ACROMEGALY, POTOMAC HORSE FEVER, THROMBOSIS OF FEMORAL ARTERIES.)

CATS, FALLING. They have an astonishing capacity for survival after falling from great heights. In New York Drs W. O. Whitney and C. J. Mehlhaff recorded the injuries suffered by 132 cats which had fallen from a height of between two and 32 storeys on to concrete pavements below. Ninety per cent of the cats which they treated survived.

Injuries increased, as would be expected, in proportion to the distance fallen – up to about seven storeys. However, the number of fractures decreased with falls from a greater height than that.

The two veterinarians suggested that this was because the cats then extended their legs to an almost horizontal position, like flying squirrels, making the impact more evenly distributed. This resulted in more chest injuries than fractured ribs, however.

Emergency treatment was required in 37 per cent of the cats, non-emergency treatment in 30 per cent.

What causes them to fall? In a few instances, it seems, they lose their balance while turning on a narrow window-ledge. More often it happens while trying to catch a bird or insect. It has also been known for a cat to panic, and leap off the ledge, when threatened by a strange dog let into the room behind. (Whitney, W. O. & Mehlhaff, C. J. *Journal of the American Veterinary Medical Association* (1987) **191**, 1300.)

CATS, WORMS IN. In a survey of 110 cats autopsied in the University of Sheffield, *Toxocara cati* were found in 35·4 per cent, the tapeworm *Dipylidium caninum* in 44·5 per cent, *Taenia taeniaeformis* in 4·5 per cent. In another survey made in the London area, and based on the microscopic examination of faecal samples over an 18-month period, it was found that of the 947 cats, 11.5 per cent were infected with *Toxocara cati*, 1.9 per cent with *Isospora felis*, 1.2 per cent with *Dypilidium caninum*, 1.2 per cent with *Taenia taeniaeformis*, 0.8 per cent with *I. rivolta*, and 0.2 per cent with *Toxascaris leonina*. (S. Nichol & others. *Vet. Record* (1981) **109**, 252.) (*See also above,* 'LIZARD POISONING' and WORMS.)

CATAPHORESIS is a method of treatment by introduction of medicine through the unbroken skin by means of electric current. (*See also* IONIC MEDICATION, IONTOPHORESIS.)

CATAPLASM is another name for a poultice.

CATAPLEXY. Human patients suffering from NARCOLEPSY (which see) may also have attacks of cataplexy; this is true also of the dog. A case in a bull was reported in which the animal would periodically, for no apparent reason, collapse on to its knees; getting to its feet again very soon afterwards. Apart from a 'sleepy demeanour', the bull seemed otherwise normal. There was a sudden snatch of a foreleg before attacks, which could be provoked by loud noise. (A. C. Palmer and others. *Vet. Rec.* (1980) **106**, 421.)

CATARACT is an opacity of the crystalline lens of the eye. (*See under* EYE, DISEASES OF.)

CATARRH. Inflammation of mucous membranes, particularly those of the air passages, associated with a copious secretion of mucus.

CATERPILLARS. Those of the brown-tailed moth (*Euproctis chrysorrhoea*) were extremely numerous in the Portsmouth area in two successive years, and 30 cats and one dog had lesions attributed to the caterpillars' hairs, or *setae*, which are barbed and also contain an enzyme. Loss of appetite, excessive salivation, wet patches on their flanks (probably the result of persistent licking) and redness of the under-lying skin was observed. The dog developed a red rash under one eye, and later an excoriated area there which took three weeks to heal. (Cunningham, W. D. & Machon, F. J. (1985) *Veterinary Record* **116**, 71.)

Several other caterpillars have setae which can cause an urticarial rash; and also SPIDERS (which see).

CATHARTICS (*See* LAXATIVES.)

CATHETERS. Long, slender, flexible tubes for insertion into veins, the heart, body cavities.

The range of catheters includes cardiac, endotracheal, eustachian, and urethral instruments.

Catheter embolus. During the catheterisation of a dog's vein, part of the 18-gauge catheter was accidentally severed. Radiographs showed this unusual foreign body lodged in the right atrium and ventricle of the heart.

Dr Foah and colleagues had ready a 'cobra-shaped polyethylene end-hole catheter, which they turned into a loop snare by passing through it wire folded in half – forming a loop extending from the hole at the end of the catheter. With the guidance of a fluoroscope, they introduced the catheter with its loop snare into the right ventricle.

'The loop was enlarged by feeding one end of the doubled guide wire through the catheter loop, and the loop then passed over the foreign body, and tightened. It was safely removed, and the dog showed no ill-effects.'

Dr Foa and colleagues referred in their paper to 42 human patients in whom catheter emboli were *not* removed. Fourteen had potentially life-threatening complications; and sixteen died.

CATIONIC PROTEINS (*see* ORIFICES, IMMUNITY AT).

CATTLE: Names given according to age, sex, etc. Different localities have their own names for particular cattle at particular ages, periods of life, etc., and these names vary somewhat. The following is a list of the most usual names:

Bobby or slink calves. Immature or unborn calves used for human food, and often removed from the uteri of cows when the latter are killed. The flesh of slink calves is often called **slink veal.**

Freemartin. (*See separate heading.*)

Calf. A young ox from birth to 6 or 9 months old; if a male, a *bull calf*; if a female, a *cow* or *heifer calf.*

Stag. A male castrated late in life.

Steer or stot. A young male ox, usually castrated, and between the ages of 6 and 24 months.

Stirk. A young female of 6 to 12 months old, sometimes a male of the same age, especially in Scotland.

Bullock. A two-year-old (or more) castrated ox.

Heifer or quey. A year-old female up to the first calving.

Maiden heifer. An adult female that has not been allowed to breed.

Cow-heifer is a female that has calved once only.

Bull. An uncastrated male.

Cow. A female having had more than one calf.

CATTLE, BREEDS OF. There are now in the world nearly 1000 breeds of cattle, including 250 major breeds. 'If,' commented Dr St C. S. Taylor, of the Animal Breeding Research Organisation, Edinburgh, 'we believe in crossbreds, the above figures mean that we have 1 million crossbreds to choose from or, with triple crosses, 100 million.'

European breeds stem from *Bos taurus*, thought to have originated in temperate or western Asia. *Bos indicus* (literally, Indian cattle) or zebus, have spread to S E Asia, China, Africa, the U S A, and Australia. In Africa there have been many crosses between *Bos indicus* and *Bos taurus* groups, *e.g.* Africander. (Professor J. Francis.)

(*See also* COWS, BULL MANAGEMENT, BEEF-BREEDS AND CROSSES, CALF-REARING, HOUSING OF ANIMALS, MILK YIELDS, and CATTLE HUSBANDRY.)

CATTLE CRUSH (*see* CRUSH).

CATTLE, DAIRY herd management. (*See under* DAIRY HERD.)

CATTLE, DISEASES OF. Surgical conditions include displaced abomasum, bloat, gastric ulcers, traumatic pericarditis, foul-in-the-foot. Other diseases include: ACTINOBACILLOSIS, ACTINOMYCOSIS, ANTHRAX, BLACKQUARTER, BLOU-WILDEBEESOOG, BLUETONGUE, BOVINE ENCE-PHALOMYELITIS, BRUCELLOSIS, CAMPYLOBACTER (Vibrio) infection, CATTLE PLAGUE, CEREBROCOR-TICAL NECROSIS, CLOSTRIDIAL ENTERITIS, COCCI-DIOSIS, CONTAGIOUS PLEURO-PNEUMONIA, ENTEQUE SECO, FOOT-AND-MOUTH DISEASE, HUSK, HYPOCU-PRAEMIA, HYPOMAGNESAEMIA, INFECTIOUS OPH-THALMIA, JOHNE'S DISEASE, LEPTOSPIROSIS, MALIGNANT CATARRH, MASTITIS, MILK FEVER, MUCOSAL DISEASE, MUCORMYCOSIS, PARASITIC

GASTRO-ENTERITIS, PASTEURELLOSIS, POLIOEN-CEPHALOMALACIA, POST-PARTURIENT HAEMO-GLOBINURIA, PYELONEPHRITIS, RABIES, REDWATER, RHINOSPORIDIOSIS, RHINOTRACHEITIS, SALMONEL-LOSIS, 'SKIN TUBERCULOSIS', TICK-BORNE FEVER, TRICHOMONIASIS, TUBERCULOSIS, VIRAL ENTERITIS, VIRUS INFECTIONS OF COWS' TEATS, VULVO-VAGINITIS. (*See also* CALVES, DISEASES OF and BOVINE ENZOOTIC LEUKOSIS, 'SLEEPER' SYNDROME, EYE, DISEASES OF.)

CATTLE HANDLING (*see* COWS, CRUSH, VET-ERINARY FACILITIES ON THE FARM).

CATTLE HUSBANDRY. For information on this and related health and disease problems which can cause economic loss to farmers, and for preventive measures, see under the following headings:

ABORTION, ARTIFICIAL INSEMINATION (AI), BARLEY-POISONING, BEDDING, BEEF from BARLEY-FED CATTLE, BEEF CATTLE HUSBANDRY, BEEF BREEDS and CROSSES, BRACKEN, BULL BEEF, BULL HOUSING, BULL MANAGEMENT, BUNT ORDER, CALF HOUSING, CALF REARING; CALVING DIFFICULT; CASTRATION, CLOTHING, COBALT, COLOSTRUM, COW KENNELS, COWS, 'CONTROLLED BREEDING', CREEP FEEDING, CULLING, DAIRY HERD MANAGEMENT, DIARRHOEA, DIET, DISINFECTANTS, DRIED GRASS, ELECTRO-CUTION, EXPOSURE, FLY CONTROL, FOOT BATHS, GENETICS, GRAZING BEHAVIOUR, HORMONES IN BEEF PRODUCTION, HOUSING OF ANIMALS, INFECTION, IN-FERTILITY, INTENSIVE LIVESTOCK PRODUCTION, ISOLATION, LAMENESS, 'LICKING SYNDROME', LIGHTING, MILK YIELDS, MILKING, MILKING MACHINES, NOTIFIABLE DISEASES, OESTRUS, OESTRUS DETECTION, PARASITES, PREGNANCY, PARTURITION; PARTURITION, DRUG-INDUCED; PASTURE CONTAM-INATION, PASTURE MANAGEMENT, POISONING, PRO-GENY TESTING, RATIONS, SEAWEED, SILAGE, SLAT-TED FLOORS, SLURRY, 'STEAMING-UP', STOCKING RATES, STRAW, STRIP-GRAZING, TRACE ELEMENTS, TRANSPLANTATION of MAMMALIAN OVA, TROPICS, UREA, VENTILATION, VETERINARY FACILITIES OF THE FARM, VITAMINS, WATER, WEANING; WORMS, FARM TREATMENT AGAINST; YARDED CATTLE.

CATTLE PLAGUE (*see* RINDERPEST).

CATTLE, Reasons for emergency slaughter. A Swiss survey covered 44,704 cattle; the losses representing 1·83 of insured animals. Major causes were dystocia (8·84 per cent, 3950 cattle), BLOAT (8·44 per cent; 62 per cent of this group were aged two months to three years), respiratory diseases (6·49 per cent; 72 per cent were two months to three years old), joint disease (5·78 per cent), reticular foreign bodies (5·16 per cent), circulatory disease (5·14 per cent), enteritis (4·65 per cent), fractures unrelated to parturition (4·43 per cent; 60 per cent were two months to three years old), recumbency (4·10 per cent), claw disease (3·46 per cent; 35 per cent aged six to nine years, 27 per cent were nine years old or more) and abortion (3·39 per cent); poisoning (1·07 per cent) and spastic paresis (1·02 per cent). (Wyss, U., Martig, J. & Gerber, H. (1984) *Schweizer Archiv für Tierheilkunde* **126**, 339.)

ARTIFICIAL INSEMINATION: NUMBER OF INSEMINATIONS BY BREED

Breed of Bull	England and Wales a		Scotland b		Northern Ireland c	
	1988–9	1989–90	1988–9	1989–90	1988–89	1989–90
	thousands		number			
Dairy						
Ayrshire	13	13	7,626	7,279	471	892
Dairy Shorthorn	5	5	360	304	2,810	2,333
Friesian/Holstein	1,047	1,079	68,706	71,595	57,807	61,815
Guernsey	12	12	44	51	–	–
Jersey	21	22	536	720	167	257
All Dairy	**1,099**	**1,131**	**77,272**	**79,949**	**61,255**	**65,297**
Beef						
Aberdeen Angus	68	63	8,591	8,691	16,581	13,007
Beef Shorthorn	...	...	789	770	–	–
Belgian Blue	112	86	7,260	4,072	1,655	4,248
Blonde d'Aquitaine	31	30	2,662	2,082	21,387	18,225
Charolais	222	206	12,373	12,884	24,973	23,150
Chianina	...	...	13	4	–	–
Devon	4	3	–	–	–	–
Hereford	143	117	2,185	1,776	5,896	4,237
Limousin	281	223	19,265	15,616	39,714	23,809
Murray Grey	7	6	83	66	–	–
Piedmontese	4	23	758	1,489	–	–
Romagnola	...	...	1,055	608	557	900
Simmental	98	106	12,326	14,027	59,844	48,924
South Devon	4	4	87	25	–	–
Sussex	4	4	–	1	–	–
Welsh Black	8	9	52	16	–	–
Other Beef	1	1	708	2,049	–	2,556
All Beef	**988**	**880**	**68,207**	**64,176**	**170,607**	**139,056**
Other Breeds	4	6	324	623	484	–
All Breeds	**2,091**	**2,016**	**145,803**	**144,748**	**232,346**	**204,353**

a *Actual Inseminations: Board Centres only.*
b *Actual inseminations: Scottish and North of Scotland Board Centres. First inseminations: Aberdeen Board Centres.*
c *Actual Inseminations: AI Services (NI) Ltd.*
(*Dairy Farming* copyright. Reproduced with the Editor's permission.)

CAUDA EQUINA, meaning 'tail of a horse', is the termination of the spinal cord in the sacral and coccygeal regions where it splits up into a large number of nerve fibres giving the appearance of a 'horse's tail', whence the name.

CAUDAL. Relating to the tail. The caudal end of any part of the body means the posterior end.

CAUSTICS. The chemical caustics in veterinary use are pure acetic, carbolic acids, caustic potash and soda, silver nitrate, copper sulphate, zinc chloride, and caustic collodion.
USES. Caustics are used to destroy small warts or tumours on the surface of the skin, etc.

CELL COUNT SERVICE. A service operated by the Milk Marketing Board (and by other commercial organisations also) for the detection of sub-clinical mastitis in a dairy herd. (*See under* MASTITIS.)

CELL-MEDIATED IMMUNITY (*see under* IMMUNE RESPONSE).

CELLS are the microscopic units of which all the tissues of the animal and plant kingdoms are composed.
Every cell consists essentially of a *nucleus*, a cell wall or membrane, and the jelly-like *cytoplasm* (protoplasm) contained within the cell membrane. The cytoplasm consists of water, protein, lipids, inorganic salts, etc.
(The circulating red blood corpuscles have in mammals no nucleus, and although commonly referred to as red *cells* are not typical cells, their nucleus having been lost.)
Classical descriptions of the cell (before the introduction of the electron microscope) referred to *organelles* (presumed living) and non-living *inclusions*.
Organelles include the nucleus which controls the activities of the cell and contains its genetic

material (*chromatin* in the non-dividing cell; *chromosomes* in the dividing cell), *Golgi apparatus*; *mitochondria* (containing enzymes); *ribosomes* (granules containing R N A); and others.

The nucleus is bounded by the *nuclear membrane* and contains a *nucleolus* or two or more nucleoli. D N A and R N A are both present in the nucleus.

Cells vary very much in size, the smallest being about 1/10000th of an inch in diameter, and the largest being the egg of a bird, which is still a simple cell, although much distended with food.

It is estimated that mammalian cells contain about 10,000 genes, but only a small proportion of these will be active at any one time, Professor W. H. F. Jarrett F R S has stated. 'All cells contain all genes, so that the function of a cell is determined by which genes are "expressed" and which are "repressed".' (*In Practice*, July 1982). (*See* CANCER.)

(*See* TISSUES OF THE BODY; BLASTOCYST; GIANT CELLS; BLOOD; LYMPHOCYTES. *See also* GENETIC ENGINEERING; B CELLS; T CELLS.)

CELLULITIS. A diffuse area of inflammation and suppuration, as compared with an abscess which is localised. Whereas an acute abscess tends to come to a head, or 'point' and then burst, this does not happen with cellulitis which, if untreated, is liable to spread beneath the skin.

CAUSE. Pasteurella organisms are mainly involved. (*See* PASTEURELLA.) In New Zealand injuries inflicted by DRENCHING GUNS during the 'bloat season' have been suggested as a likely means of infection, with the possibility that antibloat compounds have entered the wound and caused initial tissue reaction.

TREATMENT. Antibiotics are used. If however treatment has been delayed, it may be necessary to lance the lowest part of the area.

Cattle. The term Necrotic Cellulitis has been applied to cases of diffuse swelling beginning under the jaw and then, if untreated, extending down the neck to the brisket.

Horses. Cellulitis occurs in a form referred to also as ULCERATIVE LYMPHANGITIS.

Cats. Cellulitis is more common than an abscess which is localised and comes to a head.

Animals in the tropics. For a form of cellulitis occurring in many species, *see under* HAEMORRHAGIC SEPTICAEMIA (Pasteurellosis).

CENTRAL NERVOUS SYSTEM (CNS). This comprises the brain and spinal cord, each with its grey and white matter. The 12 pairs of cranial nerves from the brain and the 42 pairs of spinal nerves carry between them all the messages to and from the brain.

For descriptive purposes the CNS is divided into two further systems: (1) Somatic, and (2) Autonomic.

Somatic. This system is concerned with the control of voluntary muscles, and with nerve impulses from the skin, eyes, ears, and other sense organs. Accordingly this system includes both *motor* and *sensory* nerves.

Autonomic. This system of the CNS maintains the correct internal environment of the body (*e.g. see* HOMEOSTASIS), and its functions lie outside voluntary control. This system regulates breathing and heart rates, for example, and likewise the activity of the liver, digestive tract, kidneys, bladder, etc. This autonomic system comprises *sympathetic* and *parasympathetic* nerves. Most organs receive nerve impulses from both these, and they have opposite effects. For example, sympathetic nerves increase heart rate, while parasympathetic nerves slow heart action.

The *sympathetic* nervous system prepares the body for 'flight or fright'; *i.e.* for emergency action. Accordingly, under its influence breathing becomes more rapid, the heart's action faster, and blood is diverted from the digestive organs to heart, C N S, and voluntary muscles; while the liver releases glucose for extra muscular activity.

The *parasympathetic* system restores the situation after the emergency, slows the heart, and relaxes the body generally, as it also does during sleep. (*See also* BRAIN, SPINAL CORD, and NERVES.)

CENTROSOME (*see* EMBRYOLOGY).

CEPHALOSPORIN ANTIBIOTICS. One of these, Cephaloridine, is bacteriocidal to both Gram-positive and Gram-negative bacteria. It is used as an intramammary preparation against *E. coli* mastitis. Cephalexin is another example.

CERCARIA is an intermediate stage in the life-history of the liver fluke, viz., the tadpole-like form, which is produced in the body of the freshwater snail *Limnoea truncatula*, bores its way out of the snail, and attaches itself to a suitable blade of grass to wait for the arrival of a sheep which will eat it. In the sheep's stomach and intestines further development takes place. (*See* FLUKES.)

CEREALS, such as wheat, barley, oats, rye, maize, millets, and rice are all rich in starch and comparatively poor in proteins and minerals, and mostly poor in calcium but richer in phosphorus. Some dangers of cereal feeding for cattle are referred to under BARLEY POISONING (*see also* MOIST GRAIN STORAGE, DIET; HORSES, FEEDING OF.)

CEREBELLUM and CEREBRUM (*see* BRAIN).

CEREBRAL HAEMORRHAGE is, in human medicine, referred to as a *stroke*. An older name was *apoplexy*. It is characterised by loss of consciousness, and may arise from bleeding from an artery in the brain or following embolism or thrombosis.

CEREBROCORTICAL NECROSIS. A condition first reported in ewes and calves in Britain in 1959. The cause is a thiamin deficiency. Symptoms include: circling movements, a staggering gait, excitement, and convulsions. Only a few animals in a flock or group become affected; but nearly all of those die.

A differential diagnosis has to be made between CCN and bacterial meningitis, gid, listeriosis, and lead poisoning – each of which can give rise to similar symptoms.

R. Jackman and Dr E. E. Edwin, of the Central

Veterinary Laboratory, MAFF, described a rapid and relatively simple method: autofluorescence is seen when the CCN-affected brain is examined under ultra-violet light.

Another name for CCN is POLIOENCEPHALOMALACIA (which see).

The lesions consist of multiple foci of necrosis of the cerebral neurones.

CEREBROSPINAL FLUID SAMPLING in the dog. Indications include the following:

Encephalitis	Intracerebral
Meningitis	haemorrhage
Myelitis	Subarachnoid
Toxoplasmosis	haemorrhage
Brain neoplasia	Spinal cord
Spinal cord neoplasia	compression caused
	by epidural abscess

(Jayne A. Wright (1984) *In Practice* January 1984 – the technique is described.)

CEROIDOSIS. A form of liver degeneration characterised by deposition of a pink/golden, fat-insoluble material within cells. It is associated with the use of rancid or vitamin-E deficient feeds. (*See* FISH, DISEASES OF, *also* LYOSOMES.)

CERVICAL means anything pertaining to the neck.

CERVICAL SPONDYLOPATHY (*see under* SPINE, DISEASES OF).

CERVICITIS is inflammation of the *cervix uteri*. (*See* UTERUS.)

CETAVLON (*see* CETRIMIDE).

CETRIMIDE. An antiseptic of value in wound treatment and for cleaning cows' udders and teats; a 0·1 per cent solution being effective against *Streptococcus agalactiae*, a cause of mastitis. A 1 per cent solution acts as a detergent. It is also recommended as an application to wounds caused by rabid animals. (*See* RABIES.)

CHAGAS' DISEASE. This is an infection with *Trypanosoma cruzi*, mainly occurring in wild mammals (such as opossums, armadillos, and wood rats) of Central and South America, but also infecting man, dogs, cats, and pigs. (*See* TRYPANOSOMES – American trypanosomiasis.)

CHALAZION is a small swelling of the eyelid caused by a distended Meibomian gland. It is commonly seen in dogs.

CHANCRE. In human medicine this term is reserved for the ulcer or hard 'sore' which is the primary lesion of syphilis. In a veterinary context it means the local skin reaction at the sites of bites by tsetse flies carrying trypanosomes. The chancre – the first sign of trypanosome infection – begins as a small nodule, developing into a hard, hot, painful swelling measuring up to three or four inches across.

CHAPERONES. 'A diverse group of proteins' involved in protein synthesis 'to prevent incorrect folding and assembly – even though they do not form part of the protein's final structure.' (Professor John Ellis FRS, University of Warwick.)
Chaperonins. A group closely related to the above, found in bacteria, mitochondria, and cells of the respiratory tract. Their study could aid genetic engineering strategies. (AFRC and University of Warwick.)

CHARLOCK POISONING. The common charlock *Brassica sinapis* (wild mustard) is dangerous to livestock after its seeds have formed in the pods, and then only when eaten in large amounts. The seeds contain the volatile oil of mustard and also a glycoside.
SIGNS are those of abdominal pain, loss of appetite, a yellowish frothy liquid at mouth and nostrils, diarrhoea. There is nephritis, and the urine may be blood-stained.
FIRST-AID. Give milk and strong tea.

CHAROLAIS CATTLE. This is the second (numerically) largest breed of cattle in France, and they have been exported throughout Europe and the USA. The Charolais, white, is an excellent beef animal, a most efficient grazer, with a rapid growth-rate and a quiet disposition. The loin and thigh muscles are exceptionally well developed. The bulls are colour-marking and highly prized for crossing purposes. UK trials of this breed for crossing purposes were approved in 1961, and the British Charolais is now the third most important beef breed.

CHAROLAIS SHEEP. This breed was developed in the 19th century by crossing Dishley Leicester with the local sheep of Central France, and has been recognized as a breed since 1974. Mature ewes weight up to 79 kg and rams up to 109 kg. Both sexes are polled.

'CHASTEK PARALYSIS'. A condition of secondary vitamin B_1 deficiency, seen in foxes and mink on fur farms as a result of feeding raw fish. An enzyme in the latter has the property of destroying the vitamin, also known as THIAMIN (which see). The condition is seen also in cats.

CHECK LIGAMENT. This is joined to the Perforans tendon, and acts as a check on the movement of the pastern joint. The check ligaments are often strained in the racehorse.

CHEESE. A high proportion of all cheese is made from raw milk. *Brucella* organisms may live in such cheese for 2 years. (*See* BRUCELLOSIS.)

CHELATING AGENTS are substances which have the property of binding divalent metal ions to form stable, soluble complexes which are non-ionised and so virtually lacking in the toxicity of the metal concerned. Derivatives of ethylene-diamine-tetra-acetic acid (EDTA) afford examples. EDTA itself is poisonous, as it removes calcium; but the calcium-EDTA complex has been recommended in the treatment of acute lead poisoning, being given repeatedly for several days. It would possibly be of service in mercury, copper, and iron poisoning.

CHEMOSIS means swelling of the conjunctival membrane that covers the white of the eye, leaving the cornea depressed.

CHEMOTHERAPY means the treatment of disease by chemical substances. Modern chemotherapeutics generally denotes the use of antibiotics, sulphonamides, and the aromatic diamidines which are so useful in the trypanosome diseases, to give but a few examples.

CHERNOBYL disaster (*see* RADIATION).

CHEST, or THORAX, is a conical cavity, with the apex directed forwards. The base is formed by the diaphragm, while the sides are formed by the ribs, sternum, and vertebrae. Lying between adjacent ribs on the same side there are two layers of intercostal muscles, those on the outside running almost at right angles to those on the inside. The intercostal muscles fill up the spaces between the ribs and their cartilages, and are active agents in moving the ribs during respiration. The outsides of the chest walls are covered with the masses of the shoulder muscles, and the shoulder-blades or scapula lie one on either side, anteriorly over the rib-cage, but not attached to it by bony connections.
Contents. These include the termination of the trachea, the bronchial tubes, and the lungs. Between the lungs, but projecting towards the left more than to the right, lies the heart and its associated vessels. The oesophagus or gullet, runs through the chest, passing for the greater distance between the upper parts of the lungs, and enters the abdomen through an opening in the diaphragm. The thoracic duct, which carries lymph from the abdomen, runs forwards immediately below the bodies of the vertebrae and ends by opening into one of the large veins in the apex of the cavity. Various important nerves, such as the two vagi which control the abdominal organs, the phrenics, which supply the muscles of the diaphragm, and sympathetics, etc., pass through the chest in particular situations. The thymus gland lies in the anterior portion of the chest. Lining each of the two divisions of the chest cavity is the pleura, a fold of which also covers the surface of the lung, and the heart is enclosed in a special sac or pericardium. (*See* HEART, LUNGS, PLEURA, PERICARDIUM.)

CHEST INJURIES/DISEASES. Injuries to the chest wall are often the result of dogs or cats being struck by a car; or of falls leading to fractured ribs and closed PNEUMOTHORAX. Puncture-type wounds from animal bites are less common and seldom lead to pneumothorax as they are self-sealing; but some subcutaneous emphysema may occur. Infection may lead to PLEURISY.
(*See* THORACOTOMY, PNEUMOTHORAX, DIAPHRAGM (ruptured), HYDROTHORAX, 'FLAIL' CHEST, PYOTHORAX; also BRONCHITIS, PLEURISY, PNEUMONIA, HEART diseases, PARASITIC BRONCHITIS, 'BROKEN WIND', LUNGS, diseases of.)

CHESTNUTS (*see under* POINTS OF THE HORSE).

'CHEWING DISEASE'. The colloquial name in the USA for a type of encephalomalacia in the horse caused by yellow star thistle (*Centaurea solstitialis*).

CHEYLETIELLA PARASITOVORAX. A mite which infests dogs, cats, birds, rabbits, squirrels, etc. It gives rise to itching and scurfiness of the skin. In man Cheyletiella species (including *C. yusguri*) may cause urticarial weals of trunk and arms, together with intense itching.
C. blakei infests cats; *C. parasitovorax*, rabbits; *C. yasguri*, dogs.

CHEYNE-STOKES' RESPIRATION is an abnormal form of breathing in which the respirations become gradually less and less until they almost die away; after remaining almost imperceptible for a short time they gradually increase in depth and volume until they are exaggerated; after attaining a maximum they again decrease until nearly imperceptible. This alternation proceeds with considerable regularity.
Cheyne-Stokes' breathing is always a very serious condition, which is generally associated with severe nervous disturbance, shock, and collapse, or with heart or kidney disease. It is most obvious in the dog and horse after they have sustained very severe injury but without internal haemorrhage (which induces what is generally known as 'sobbing respiration').

CHIANINA. These Italian cattle are named after their place of origin, the Chiana valley. Probably the largest cattle in the world, a mature bull can weigh over 1¾ tons and be 6 feet tall at the withers. Formerly used as draught animals, they are an excellent beef breed, now present in the UK.

CHICK OEDEMA (*see* 'TOXIC FAT SYNDROME').

CHICKS. Hover temperature should be 90°F, and the room temperature must be kept above 60°F during the first 5 weeks or so of life. Chilling is one of the commonest causes of pullet chick mortality. Chicks require artificial heat for 3 to 8 weeks, depending upon the type of house, weather, etc. (*See* Chick feeding under POULTRY.)

CHILBLAIN SYNDROME in dogs. This was first described by Major P. G. H. Jepson, Royal Army Veterinary Corps, as affecting several Service dogs in Northern Ireland. These dogs had previously thrived in unheated, outdoor kennels, but were affected during March 1981. The first sign was biting of the tip of the tail – found to be red, swollen, warm and intensely itchy. Ulceration, infection, and necrosis of the tail tip occurred in a few cases, necessitating amputation of the tip. 'It is not unknown for a dog to eat the affected part of its tail.' Elizabethan collars, protective tail covering, and anti-inflammatory drugs were used in treatment.

CHILLING (*see under* CHICKS and HYPOTHERMIA).

CHIMERA. An animal having in its body cell populations with different KARYOTYPES (which see) which have originated from two or more zygotes with different karyotypes. A freemartin is, technically, an example of XX:XY chimerism. This is secondary chimerism. Primary chimerism occurs if two sperms fertilise the same ovum. (*See* CYTOGENETICS.)

In China a fertile female mule, Red Dragon, 'appears to have inherited a mixture of both horse and donkey chromosomes, and is phenotypically a chimera rather than a hybrid.' ('Totaliser' (1985) *Veterinary Record* **117**, 676.) ☞

CHINCHILLA. In domestication the average litter-size is two: in the wild state it is believed to be four. In their natural surroundings, chinchillas live at 10,000 feet above sea-level in the Andes. Those at lower levels are said to have poorer coats. There are two species.

The period of gestation is about 111 days. The life span may be over 7 years. Composition of the urine and faeces is such as to make this an odourless animal. A favourite diet in captivity is dried bread and hay.

CHINCHILLA, DISEASES OF. Enteritis sufficiently severe to cause death is common in chinchillas, judging by the sparse literature on the subject. Out of a series of 1000 post-mortem examinations made in the USA, 'epidemic gastro-enteritis' was found in 23 per cent of the chinchillas, as against 25 per cent with pneumonia, and 12 per cent with impaction (blockage of the intestine). In a further series of 1000 examinations, the figures were: impaction, 20 per cent; pneumonia, 22 per cent; and enteritis, 24 per cent.

An important cause of pneumonia is *Klebsiella pneumoniae*. This may also produce loss of appetite, diarrhoea, and death within about 5 days. The infection can also prove fatal in people too.

Acute and fatal gastro-enteritis may be caused by *Yersinia enterocolitica*. (*See* YERSINIOSIS.)

Lying on one side and stretching the legs are said to be symptoms of impaction. The feeding of too many pellets with too little roughage is believed to be a cause, and clearly the means of prevention lies largely in the breeder's hands.

Intussusception is not uncommon and sometimes follows enteritis.

Fur-chewing – that bane of the North American chinchilla industry – has been attributed to 'environmental stress' – the frustration and depression associated with captivity. Of course, the wrong diet may enter into it, too; so a little more freedom, combined with some fresh greenstuff, is always worth an immediate trial – with a little apple and a raisin or two now and then for good measure.

Gastro-enteritis due to *Y. enterocolitica* has caused severe losses among chinchillas on farms in California, and also in Europe.

CHITIN This is found in some fungi, and is the main constituent of the body covering of insects, ticks, mites, spiders, etc.

CHLAMYDIA. Round or ovoid micro-organisms. The genus comprises two species: *C. trachomatis* which includes the human strains causing trachoma, inclusion conjunctivitis and *lympho-*

granuloma venereum; and *C. psittaci* which includes the strains associated with PSITTACOSIS (and ORNITHOSIS); with ENZOOTIC ABORTION in ewes and polyarthritis ('joint-ill') in lambs and calves; and with conjunctivitis and pneumonia in cats.

Psittacosis. Illness in people and in birds of the parrot family (including budgerigars and cockatiels).

Imported birds may have a latent infection which, under the stress of transport, overcrowding or underfeeding, becomes overt, giving rise to symptoms.

Ornithosis is the name given to the same infection in birds other than those of the parrot family. In the UK ornithosis is common in pigeons, and in commercial duckling flocks – with conjunctivitis and rhinitis in evidence.

SIGNS. Affected parrots may not show any symptoms for some considerable time after contracting the infection, but once the symptoms have appeared illness becomes marked, and death occurs in a very few days. The birds are listless and dull; a haemorrhagic diarrhoea is often seen, and a catarrhal condition of the nasal passages and eyes may be shown in the later stages of the disease.

In one Edinburgh outbreak, 100 out of about 300 budgerigars in an aviary died. Human cases followed and a dog was found to be excreting *Chlamydia* organisms and to have a lung infection. In cats, especially in boarding or breeding catteries, pneumonia is a common sequel to infection.

POST-MORTEM findings include enlargement of liver and spleen, together with pneumonia. Confirmation of diagnosis is largely dependent on inoculation of chick embryos or laboratory mammals.

TREATMENT and CONTROL. Millet and oat pellets medicated with chlortetracycline, fed to the birds, are effective. The use of such medicated food for imported psittacine birds is a requirement for commercial imports under USA quarantine regulations. In Britain it has been suggested from time to time that the sale of imported birds should be restricted to a few registered dealers, who would have to keep records of sources, incontact birds, and purchases.

The Ministry of Agriculture is responsible for safeguarding the UK's poultry against psittacosis infection from abroad, under the Importation of Birds, Poultry and Hatching Eggs Order 1979. All diagnoses of the disease in imported birds are notified by the State Veterinary Service to medical officers of environmental health.

Thirteen of 15 **cats** in a cattery developed conjunctivitis at various times over nine months. The condition was severe and prolonged (two weeks) treatment with tetracycline was required to effect clinical recovery. Nine of 14 cats developed significant complement fixing antibody titres. By comparison, only 17 (13 per cent) sera samples collected from 134 randomly selected cats aged one month to 16 years contained complement fixing antibodies to chlamydia group antigen. (Studdert, M. J., Studdert, V. P. & Wirth, H. J. (1981) *Australian Veterinary Journal* **57**, 515.)

Public health. Human psittacosis in its milder forms resembles influenza. In children the symptoms are slight or absent altogether, but in older people the illness is more likely to be severe. Symptoms include shivering, headache, backache. Death from pneumonia may follow. Acute kidney failure has been recorded; also heart disease. Human infection comes through handling infected birds; but two cases in pregnant women who had assisted at lambing were also recorded. Pregnancy was complicated, and one patient died. (R. J. S. Beer and others. *British Medical Journal* (1982) **284**, 1156.)

A farmer's wife who aborted spontaneously in early March after a short febrile illness, in the 28th week of pregnancy, had helped with difficult lambings in January and February. Five of 200 ewes had aborted and a serum sample had shown high antibody titres to chlamydia. Elementary bodies of *Chlamydia psittaci* were detected in smears of liver, lung and placenta from the human fetus, and sections of the placenta showed many chlamydial inclusions. This circumstantial evidence strongly suggests that the organism was transmitted from the sheep and was probably an ovine strain associated with enzootic abortion on the farm. Veterinary surgeons and doctors should be aware of the risk to pregnant women from chlamydial infections of farm animals. (Johnson, F. W. A. & others (1985) *British Medical Journal* **290**, 592.)

Person-to-person transmission appears likely.

CHLORAL HYDRATE is a clear, crystalline substance with a sweetish taste and dissolves rapidly in water.
ACTIONS. Internally, chloral acts as a hypnotic. (*See also under* ANAESTHETICS, TRANQUILLISERS, EUTHANASIA.)

CHLORAL HYDRATE POISONING. In the dog, poisoning has occurred after eating from horses humanely euthanased by means of chloral hydrate.

CHLORAMINES are widely used as a disinfectant. Their activity depends upon the amount of available chlorine.

CHLORAMPHENICOL. An antibiotic which has a similar range of activity to the tetracyclines. It can be given orally (except to ruminants), by intravenous injection, and by local application. Because of its importance in the treatment of human typhoid and the avoidance of resistant strains, its use in veterinary medicine should be confined to the treatment of respiratory infections in calves, feline leukaemia, Moraxella infections of the eye, and possibly salmonellosis in cattle.

In human medicine poisoning by chloramphenicol has led to aplastic anaemia, skin eruptions, and moniliasis. There are three side-effects 'about which specific warnings should be given': allergy or hypersensitivity to the drug; damage to the blood or bone-marrow; and gastro-intestinal upsets. (*Lancet*, Oct. 6, 1973.)

Intramuscular injections of chloramphenicol are painful, in the dog at least. The toxicity and high cost of this antibiotic limited its use and its use in veterinary medicine in the UK has been greatly restricted following the recommendations of the Swann Committee.

CHLORATE POISONING. In acute cases cattle may die after showing symptoms suggestive of anthrax. In subacute cases, a staggering gait, purgation, signs of abdominal pain, and red-coloured urine may be seen. Cyanosis and respiratory distress are also symptoms.
TREATMENT. Gastric lavage. If cyanosis is present, methylene blue should be given intravenously.

CHLORDANE. A highly toxic insecticide of the chlorinated hydrocarbon group. It is volatile and poisoning through inhalation may occur.

CHLORFENVINPHOS. An organophosphorus acaricide and insecticide, used in sheep dips, etc.

CHLORINATED HYDROCARBONS. These insecticides include: DDT, DDD, methoxychlor, benzene hexachloride, toxaphene, aldrin, dieldrin, isodrin, and endrin plus a range of others less well known. Ingested at toxic levels, or absorbed through the skin, they act primarily on the central nervous system causing excitement/frenzy at the outset followed by muscular tremors leading to convulsions in acute cases. Species capable of vomiting do so. Loss of appetite with marked loss of body weight is usual in subacute poisoning. Cats are especially susceptible. Wash off any residues from the skin. Give a barbiturate.

Most compounds – methoxychlor is an exception – can be stored in the body fat and excreted in the milk and so may constitute a public health problem. It is interesting to note in passing that out of 901 samples of market milk collected throughout the USA in the autumn of 1955, 62 per cent contained residues of chlorinated organic parasiticides, some samples containing up to 1·5 parts per million.

CHLOROFORM is a colourless, mobile, non-inflammable liquid, half as heavy again as water. It is less used now than formerly as a general anaesthetic. (*See* ANAESTHETICS, EUTHANASIA.)

Four stages of chloroform anaesthesia are recognised:

(1) *The stage of excitement* begins immediately the drug is administered. Vigorous animals struggle violently, and when in the standing position may rear or strike out with their forefeet and shake their heads in an endeavour to dislodge the mask. In the recumbent position there is in nearly all horses an attempt to get their heads doubled down towards their fore-feet; a position which should be prevented in all cases, for there is a risk that in such positions the spinal column will be fractured. (*See* CASTING.) Deep breaths are taken often in a gasping manner, and in from 3 to 6 or 7 minutes the second stage follows.

(2) *The stage of depression* follows the stimulation stage, and is marked by a quieting of the movements of the voluntary muscles, by a lessening of the force and volume of the pulse, and by slower and deeper breathing. Pain is still felt, and if inflicted induces reflex movement.

(3) *The stage of anaesthesia* produces complete muscular relaxation and unconsciousness. This is the safe or operating stage; all the centres of the brain are subdued except those that govern respiration and heart action.

(4) *The stage of paralysis* occurs when the anaesthetic is pushed beyond the safe stage. The centres of respiration and heart action, in common with all the other nervous centres, become paralysed. It consists of two phases: firstly, the cessation of the respiration; and secondly, the cessation of the heart-beat. The heart stops beating about 2 minutes after respiration ceases, and it is owing to this fact that any attempts at artificial respiration must be prompt. (*See* ARTIFICIAL RESPIRATION.)

CHOCOLATE POISONING. The feeding of waste chocolate bars to cattle has led to fatal poisoning in calves in the UK. The animals showed excitement, stared about in all directions, walked with exaggerated strides, and had convulsions.

It was suggested that the caffeine content would account for the excitement; the theobromine content may have caused heart failure in the calf which died.

In dogs, the signs include panting, vomiting, thirst, diarrhoea, excitement, fits, coma.

TREATMENT. Use of an emetic or gastric lavage. (Activated charcoal is used in human medicine.) For control of the convulsions, diazepam is recommended.

AUTOPSY findings include cyanotic mucous membranes, swollen and reddened gastric mucosa. (Hornfeldt, C. S. *Modern Veterinary Practice* (1987) **68**, 552.)

(*See also* COCOA POISONING.)

'CHOKING' (Obstruction of Pharynx or Oesophagus). The word 'choking' is, by dictionary definition, an obstruction to respiration, but in a farming context the word has been misused to denote an obstruction to the passage of food through the pharynx and oesophagus, either partial or complete. (*See also* OBSTRUCTION TO RESPIRATION.)

The domesticated animals, especially cattle and dogs, are very prone to attempt to swallow either foreign bodies or masses of food material too large to pass down the oesophagus (gullet), with the result that they often become jammed. Such substances hinder the free passage of solid or fluid food, give rise to pain and discomfort, and are very often attended by serious and even fatal consequences. Choking in cattle, dogs, and cats is usually due to a hard, large, sharp-pointed, or irregularly shaped object; while in the horse it is most often due to a mass of dry impacted food material, or to a portion of a mangold or turnip.

Cattle. Choking is of comparatively common occurrence, particularly in districts where roots are fed whole to the animals, and where there is a quantity of rubbish scattered about the pastures.

SIGNS. The animal immediately stops feeding, and becomes uneasy. It coughs and gasps, and may lower the head and attempt to vomit. In a few minutes there is a profuse flow of saliva from the mouth, particularly when the object is lodged in the pharynx or high up in the oesophagus. A remarkable feature of nearly all cases of choking in cattle is the rapidity with which gas formation occurs in the rumen. (*See* BLOAT.)

When the object is lodged in the upper part of the oesophagus, it usually causes a swelling which can be seen or felt from the outside, but if it is situated in the part of the gullet which passes through the chest its presence can only be suspected. The careful passage of a probang down the oesophagus will, of course, definitely establish the presence or absence of an obstruction.

In a number of cases of choking relief occurs quite spontaneously after the lapse of from ½ to 2 or 3 hours from the origin of the symptoms. This is because the muscles of the gullet, which have been tightly gripping the obstruction, gradually become fatigued and relax, thereby allowing the object to pass down into the stomach. Naturally, such a satisfactory termination cannot occur wherever there is a sharp projecting point on the object causing the obstruction, but it frequently happens with eggs, apples, potatoes, and other smooth bodies.

FIRST-AID. In all cases of choking, no matter how simple they appear to be, the owner should seek veterinary assistance as soon as possible.

PROFESSIONAL TREATMENT involves the passage of a probang or stomach-tube down the oesophagus.

Horses. Fortunately, the horse is less often choked than the cow, but owing to the long and narrow equine oesophagus, the accident is more serious.

TREATMENT. Avoid raising the head or giving drenches, lubricating or otherwise. It is imperative to secure professional assistance at once.

Dogs and cats.

SIGNS. At first there is usually a sudden pain, which causes the animal to cry out. If it has been feeding it immediately ceases, and becomes very restless. It may paw at its mouth. Salivation is often profuse.

When a threaded needle has become fixed in the throat or below it, the end of the thread may often be seen.

TREATMENT. Swallowed objects which become jammed in a dog's oesophagus can be treated in one of two ways: surgically or conservatively. The latter includes the use of an endoscope, passed into the oesophagus and enabling the foreign body to be grasped with forceps and drawn out or, alternatively, pushed down into the stomach, whence it can, if necessary, be removed.

In a series of 90 cases treated by J. E. F. Houlton and others at the University of Cambridge, 85 of the foreign bodies were pieces of bone, and two were composed mainly of gristle. A potato, a fish-hook, and a ball were also found. The success rate of treatment by surgical and conservative means was 82 per cent.

CHOLAGOGUES are substances reputed to act on the liver, increasing the secretion of the bile.

CHOLANGIOHEPATITIS. Inflammation of bile ducts and associated liver parenchyma.

CHOLANGITIS. Inflammation of the intra-hepatic bile ducts.

CHOLECYSTITIS. Inflammation of the gall-bladder.

CHOLECYSTOGRAPHY is the term used for X-ray examination of the gall-bladder after its contents have been rendered opaque by administration of lipiodol or pheniodol compounds.

CHOLECYSTOKININ. A hormone produced in the small intestine and causing emptying of the gall-bladder.

CHOLERA, FOWL (see FOWL CHOLERA).

CHOLESTEATOMA. An epidermoid cyst within the middle ear cavity of dogs, complicating simple otitis. (Little, C. J. L. & others. *Veterinary Record* (1991) **128,** 319)

CHOLESTEROL. A sterol present in blood, brain and other tissues, in bile, and in many foods. It is produced in the liver and adrenal glands.

A high cholesterol level can be a precursor to high blood pressure, ATHEROMA, and THROMBOSIS (which see.)

CHOLESTHIASIS (see GALLSTONES).

CHOLINE is found in egg-yolk, liver, and muscle, and is a member of the vitamin B complex. Acetyl choline is essential for the transmission of an impulse from nerve to muscle and choline chloride is used as a drug in veterinary medicine for certain cases of acetonaemia.

CHONDRITIS. Inflammation of cartilage.

CHONDROCYTES. Cartilage-forming cells.

CHOLINESTERASE is an enzyme which inactivates acetylcholine. Some poisons, such as carbamates and organophosphates, cause cholinesterase inhibition, and it is inactivated by a substance isolated from white clover S.100.

CHONDROGENESIS (see Growth Plate. Disorders under BONE, DISEASES OF).

CHONDROMA A rare tumour, composed of cartilage-like cells, which has been seen in dogs, rats, and mink. (Allison, N. & Rakich, P. *Journal of Comparative Pathology* (1988) **98,** 371.)

CHOREA is characterised by a succession of involuntary spasmodic contractions (clonic spasms) affecting one or more of the voluntary muscles. The spasm is of a rhythmic nature, occurring at fairly regular intervals, and between the individual contractions relaxation of the affected muscle takes place.

The condition affects dogs almost exclusively, although muscular spasms of a similar nature have been seen in horses, cattle, and pigs. In lambs, congenital chorea is described under BORDER DISEASE. (*See* TREMBLING.)

CAUSES. In dogs chorea generally follows a mild attack of distemper. It may appear within a few days after apparent recovery, or its appearance may be delayed. All dog owners would be well advised to regard cases of distemper as not cured until the lapse of at least 10 days after *apparent recovery,* and during this period to continue to treat the animal as though it were still sick, so far as exercise is concerned.

SIGNS. Twitchings usually begin about the lips and face, or in the extremities of one or more limbs. Later, perhaps the whole head is seen continually nodding or jerking backwards and forwards, quite irrespective of the pose or position of the animal. As the condition progresses, there comes a time when it is unable to rest, loss of condition and weakness result; and the dog becomes exhausted. Ulceration of the affected limb, as the result of continual friction with surrounding objects, the ground, etc., is not uncommon. Chorea is always a serious condition.

TREATMENT. (*See* ANTISPASMODICS.)

CHORION is the outermost of the three foetal membranes, the others being the amnion and the allantois. The chorion is a strong fibrous membrane, whose outer surface is closely moulded to the inner surface of the uterus. Chorionic villi are the vascular projections from the chorion which are inserted into the crypts of the uterine mucous membrane. (*See also* PARTURITION.)

CHORIONIC GONADOTROPHIN (*see* HORMONE THERAPY).

CHOROID, or CHORIOID is the middle of the three coats of the eye, and consists chiefly of the blood-vessels which effect nourishment of the organ. (*See* EYE.)
Choroiditis. Inflammation of the choroid.

CHRISTMAS FACTOR (*see under* CLOTTING of the blood *and* CANINE HAEMOPHILIA).

CHRISTMAS ROSE (*see* HELLEBORE).

CHROMOBACTER VIOLACEUM. An organism, often regarded as non-pathogenic, which has caused a fatal pneumonia in pigs in the USA.

CHROMOSOMES. Minute bodies, within the nucleus of cells, which carry the genes (*see* GENETICS), and are composed largely of DNA. The number of chromosomes is constant for any given species. (*See under* GENETICS.) The haploid number (n) represents the basic set found in the gametes, *i.e.* egg and sperm. The diploid number (2n) represents paired basic sets, one set from the sire, the others from the dam, and this number is found in all somatic cells.

(*See also under* CYTOGENETICS for chromosome abnormalities; and PLASMIDS.)

CHRONIC OBSTRUCTIVE PULMONARY DISEASE (COPD). A provisional name for a disease of horses affecting principally the small airways. It seems that *Micropolysporum faeni,* hay dust, and food mites are all possibly involved in causing COPD, which – in one survey – was found to have a higher incidence in stables with much ammonia and dust particles in the air. Dyspnoea is worse at night, as is the case with human asthma. (Dixon, P. M. (1986) *Veterinary Record* **118**, 224.)

CHYLE The milky fluid which is absorbed by the lymphatic vessels of the intestine. The fluid mixes with the lymph and is discharged into the thoracic duct. (*See* LYMPH, DIGESTION.)

CHYLOTHORAX. The presence of pleural fluid identifiable as chyle, following injury to, or a tumour of, the thoracic duct. Treatment consists of repeated drainage. The condition has been recorded in cats and dogs.

CHYME is the partly digested food passed from the stomach into the first part of the small intestine. It is very acid in nature, contains salts and sugars in solution, and the animal constituents in a semi-liquid state.

CICATRIX is a scar.

CILIA. This term covers both the eyelashes, and the microscopic hair-like projections from mucous membranes lining the larynx and trachea. (*See* AIR PASSAGES.)

CILIATA. Ciliated protozoa are found in the alimentary canal of animals. (*See* BALANTIDIUM.)

CIRCLING MOVEMENTS. These may be a symptom of meningitis or encephalitis. (*See* BRAIN, DISEASES OF.)

CIRCULATION OF BLOOD. The veins of the whole body – head, trunk, limbs, and organs in the abdomen – with the exception of those in the thorax, pour their blood into one of the three great terminal radicles which open into the right atrium of the heart. This contracts and drives the blood into the right ventricle, which then forces the blood into the lungs by way of the pulmonary artery. In the lungs it is contained in very thin-walled capillaries, over which the inspired air plays freely, and through which the exchange of gases can easily take place. The blood is consequently oxygenated (*see* RESPIRATION), and passes on by the pulmonary veins to the left atrium of the heart. This left atrium expels it into the left ventricle, which forces it on into the aorta, by which it is distributed all over the body. Passing through the capillaries in the various organs and tissues it eventually again enters the lesser veins, and is collected into the cranial and caudal vena cava and the vena azygos (*see* VEINS), from where it passes to the right atrium once more.

In one part of the body there is, however, a further complication. The veins coming from the stomach, intestines, spleen, and pancreas, charged with food materials and other products, unite into the large 'portal vein' which enters the porta of the liver and splits up into a second capillary system in the liver tissue. Here it is relieved of some of its food content, and passes to the caudal vena cava by a second series of veins, joining with the rest of the blood coming from the hind parts of the body, and so goes on to the right atrium. This is known as the 'portal circulation'.

The circuit is maintained always in one direction by four valves, situated one at the outlet from each cavity of the heart (*see* HEART), and by the presence of valves situated along the course of the larger veins.

The blood in the arteries going to the body generally (*i.e.* to the systemic circulation) is a bright red in colour, while that in the veins is a dull red; this is owing to the oxygen content of arterial blood being much greater than that of venous blood, which latter is charged with carbon dioxide (*see* RESPIRATION). For the same reason the blood in the pulmonary artery going to the lungs is dark, while in the pulmonary veins it is bright red.

There is normally no connection between the blood in the right side of the heart and that in the left; the blood from the right ventricle must pass through the lungs before it can reach the left atrium. In the fetus, two large arteries pass out from the umbilicus (navel), and convey blood which is to circulate in close proximity to the maternal blood in the placenta, and to receive from it both the oxygen and the nourishment necessary for the needs of the fetus, while one large vein brings back this blood into the fetal body through the umbilicus again. There are also communications between the right and the left atria (the *foramen ovale*) and between the aorta and the pulmonary artery (the *ductus arteriosus*), which serve to 'short-circuit' the blood from passing through the lungs in any quantity. At birth these extra communications rapidly close and shrivel up, leaving mere vestiges of their presence in adult life. There are rare instances, however, in which one or more of the passages may persist throughout life.

CIRCULATION OF LYMPH (*see* LYMPH).

CIRRHOSIS, or FIBROSIS, is a condition of various internal organs, in which some of the non-parenchymatous cells of the organ are replaced by fibrous tissue. The name 'cirrhosis' was first used for the disease as it occurs in the liver, because of the yellow colour, but it has been applied to fibrosis in the lung, kidney, etc. Classic instances of cirrhosis are seen in the liver in chronic ragwort poisoning in cattle, in chronic alcoholism in man, and in old dogs.

CITRULLINAEMIA. This disease occurs in some Australian Friesian cattle; also in dogs. It is hereditary in origin, and due to a deficiency of the amino-acid Citrulline. In calves depression, recumbency, and convulsions result.

CLAVICEPS. A fungus (*see* ERGOT).

CLAVICLE is another name for the 'collar-bone' in man. This bone is not present in the domesticated mammals (except sometimes in a very rudimentary form in the cat), but is present in the fowl.

CLAWS (*see* NAILS).

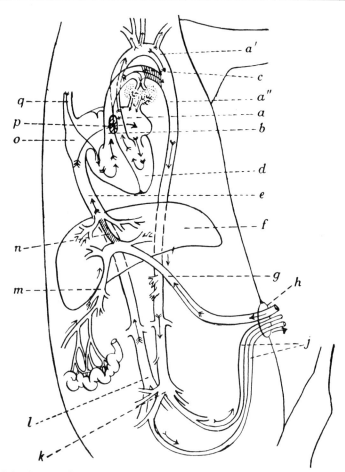

Diagram of fetal circulation. *a*, Origin of aorta; *a'*, arch of aorta; *a"*, posterior aorta; *b*, origin of pulmonary artery; *c*, the ductus arteriosus (shaded); *d*, left ventricle; *e*, caudal vena cava; *f*, liver; *g*, umbilical vein; *h*, the umbilicus; *j*, umbilical arteries; *k*, bifurcation of aorta; *l*, origin of caudal vena cava; *m*, portal vein; *n*, ductus venosus, which short-circuits blood from umbilical vein to vena cava without passing through liver; *o*, right atrium; *p*, foramen ovale (shaded); *q*, crania vena cava. (After Bradley's *Thorax and Abdomen of the Horse*.)

CLAY PIGEONS. Eating of these has led to fatal poisoning in pigs. (*See* PITCH POISONING, LEAD POISONING.)

'CLEAN' PASTURE (*see* PASTURE).

'CLEANSING' (*see* PLACENTA).

CLEFT PALATE is a hereditary defect of the roof of the mouth, generally seen in puppies of the toy breeds that have been in-bred. It consists of a gap in the structures forming the palate, often so extensive as to allow of communication between the mouth and the nasal passages. Puppies so affected are usually unable to suck, and die soon after birth unless given artificial feeding; others are able to obtain some small amount of nourishment, but never thrive as the rest of the litter. The condition of 'hare-lip', or 'split-lip', is often associated with cleft palate. The palate may also be cleft as the result of violence; for example, it is commonly seen in the cat which has fallen from a considerable height. (*See* HARE-LIP.)

Cleft palate in cattle is referred to under GENETICS – defects.

CLENBUTEROL HYDROCHLORIDE. A specific β_2 antagonist, used as a bronchodilater in coughing horses; and to suppress contractions of the uterus in cows to aid obstetrics.

Clenbuterol has also a metabolic effect, and is an effective growth-promoter in beef cattle; increasing the volume of skeletal muscle (as well as heart muscle) and decreasing fat. The size of other organs is not increased, as is the case with anabolic steroids such as trenbolone acetate. (AFRC).

CLIMATE IN RELATION TO DISEASE (*see* ENVIRONMENT, TROPICS).

CLINICAL means literally 'belonging to a bed', but the word is used to denote anything associated with the practical study of a sick person or animal, such as clinical medicine, clinical thermometer. (*See also* SUBCLINICAL.)

CLIPPING OF HORSES. The covering of hair over the body of certain of the domesticated animals is liable at times to interfere with health if allowed to grow unchecked, and accordingly it is customary to remove it at certain periods of the year; in horses the long winter coat, if left to grow, hinders efficient grooming and drying, prevents the skin from excreting waste products, and causes the horse to perspire more. (*See also* SHEARING.)

Methods. Clippers work best when used against the flow of the hair, and should be thoroughly and frequently lubricated. It is of course essential that the blades should be sharp. For racehorses, carriage-horses, ponies, etc., it is usual to clip 'down to the ground', as it is called, *i.e.* all the hair is clipped from the body, legs, and face, the mane is 'hogged' (clipped short), and the tail is thinned. For saddle-horses a 'hunter's clip' is preferred; in this the hair is taken from the body, except for a patch on the back which corresponds with the outline of the saddle ('saddle-patch'), and the legs, which are left covered with hair below the level of an oblique line running across the middles of the fore-arms and gaskins. The mane is hogged, and the tail is thinned and cut straight across about a hand's-breadth above the level of the points of the hocks.

Times for clipping. The time for clipping horses varies according to the weather, but should take place as soon as the winter coat has 'set', *i.e.* as soon as the summer coat has been fully cast off and the winter coat is well grown. It usually happens that in an ordinary autumn this condition is fulfilled about the end of October and the beginning of November, but in some years it is earlier and in some later. Sometimes horses are clipped twice during the winter, once before Christmas and once some time after; but this is only necessary in animals which have a luxuriant growth of hair.

Precautions. Never clip a horse suffering from a cold or other respiratory trouble. Never clip during excessively severe weather. Always provide a rug when standing outside for the first week or ten days to allow the heat-regulating mechanism to become accustomed to the more rapid radiation of heat from the body surface. Thoroughly dry a newly clipped horse after coming into the stable in wet or snowy weather, by means of straw or hay wisps. Do not allow newly clipped horses to stand in draughty places in a stable without protection. Give extra bedding for a few days after clipping. Give an extra ration of hay and oats to recently clipped horses to make good the loss of heat occasioned.

CLIPPING OF DOGS. These animals are usually clipped for medical reasons, such as to allow better dressing of the skin during treatment of mange. There are some owners, however, who have their dogs regularly clipped at the beginning of the summer to rid them of long matted, or thick winter, coats. In addition to this, certain breeds are clipped for show purposes, such as the French poodle and the Bedlington terrier.

CLIPPING OF SHEEP (*see* SHEARING, CLOTHING OF ANIMALS).

CLITORIS: the small organ composed of erectile tissue, situated just within the lower commissure of the vulva. It is the homologue of the penis.

Clitoral sinusectomy. The RCVS has ruled

that veterinary surgeons who are asked to carry out clitoral sinusectomies on mares which are destined for export to the United States can be clear that they will not be held to be acting unethically, even if, at the time of the performance of the operation, there is no evidence that the mare is infected with the CEM organism.

It is contended by the United States Department of Agriculture that clitoral sinusectomy:

(a) could show up, on the subsequent culturing of the excised material, that CEM was present when swabbing proved negative;

(b) when accompanied by the prescribed follow-up treatments would eliminate the CEM organism if it was present; and

(c) was the method by which the CEM outbreaks in Kentucky had been eliminated. (*See* EQUINE CONTAGIOUS MERITIS.)

Enlargement of the clitoris may occur in bitches treated with androgens for the suppression of oestrus.

CLOACA (*see* 'VENT GLEET').

CLONES. A group of cells derived from a single cell by mitosis.

CLONIC is a word applied to spasmodic movements of muscles lasting for a short time only.

CLOPROSTENOL. An ICI prostaglandin analogue, used to cause regression of the *corpus luteum* in cattle. It has been used in cows showing no visible signs of oestrus; for removal of a mummified fetus; in cases of misalliance and unwanted pregnancies; and in the treatment of pyometra. (*See* 'CONTROLLED BREEDING'.)

CLOSTRIDIAL ENTERITIS. This is a cause of sudden death in cattle. The deaths usually, though not invariably, occur shortly after calving. The animal, usually one, is found dead. Where death is not immediate, 'milk fever' may be suspected, but the elevated temperature at once rules this out. The cow may be in considerable pain before succumbing. On post-mortem examination, acute inflammation of the intestine is found – such as might be expected with some types of poisoning. This enteritis is associated with the presence of a toxin, difficult to demonstrate in the laboratory, produced by the organism *Clostridium welchii* Type A. The same condition may account for the sudden death of pigs. *Clostridium oedematiens* may likewise be a cause of sudden death in sheep, pigs, and cattle.

CLOSTRIDIAL MYOSITIS (*see* BLACKLEG and GAS GANGRENE).

CLOSTRIDIUM. A genus of anaerobe spore-bearing bacteria of ovoid, spindle, or club shape. They include *Cl. tetani*, *Cl. perfringens*, (welchii), *Cl. oedematiens*, *Cl. septicum*, *Cl. botulini* and *Cl. difficile* (a possible pathogen of piglets, especially if receiving antibiotics, and associated with enteritis. *Cl. chauvoei* may cause pericarditis and meningitis, as well as BLACK-QUARTER in cattle (and

sheep). (*See above, and* TETANUS, LAMB DYSEN-
TERY, BRAXY, BOTULISM.)

Clostridium perfringens caused the sudden
death from enterotoxaemia of 18 cats, aged 2
months to 3 years, in Saudi Arabia. They died
within a few hours of scavenging on chicken
remains, which caused vomiting and diarrhoea.
(El Sanousi & others, of King Faisal University.
Veterinary Record (1991) **129**, 334.)

CLOTHING OF ANIMALS. As a general rule,
only cow, horse, and dog, of the domesticated
animals are supplied with clothing. Sheep
already possess protection in the form of wool
sufficient except in severe weather on the uplands;
while pigs carry a deep layer of subcutaneous fat.

Horses. Horses require clothing for the following reasons: (1) to provide protection against
cold, chills, draughts, and sudden lowering of the
temperature; (2) to protect parts of the body from
bruises and abrasions, such as might occur while
travelling by road, rail or on board ship; (3) to
afford protection from sudden showers of rain or
snow when at work in the open. For the latter
purposes waterproof sheets lined with woollen
fabric on the inside are usually used.

Cattle. Formerly, it was only for sick cattle, and
for use at agricultural shows and upon similar
occasions, that clothing was provided for cattle,
but of recent years Jersey, etc., cows often wear
coats. A large quarter-sheet, kept in position by a
surcingle, and sometimes provided with fillet-
strings, is most commonly employed. An ordinary
horse-rug serves the purpose, but the buckle at the
neck should never be fastened for cattle.

Sheep. Jute coats are now on the market for
ewes. They were designed and introduced by Mr
William Wilson, a Carlisle farmer, who found
them economic in his flock in severe weather on
the Pennines. The idea is for the coats to be worn
from mating to lambing. Five stitches secure the
coat. Rugs or coats of man-made fibre have been
used in Australia to protect the fleeces of sheep,
and have proved economic, since wool buyers
have paid more. Plastic coats have been used for
lambs in the UK.

In Australia an estimated 800,000 sheep die
each year during the first fortnight after shearing.
Many of the deaths are associated with cold, wet,
windy weather. The use of plastic coats during
this period has saved many lives.

Head caps have been found to give good and
sometimes complete protection against the Headfly in the UK.

Dogs. For the dog a coat made of woollen fabrics which wraps round the body and buttons or
straps together is often used. Dog-coats or rugs are
made according to various patterns, but whatever
variety is selected should provide protection for
the front and under part of the chest, as well as for
the sides of the body. The elaborate garments
which are used for coursing greyhounds and whip-
pets are excellent articles of clothing, and may be
copied with advantage for other breeds of dog.

CLOTTING OF BLOOD. This is a very complex
process, and an obviously important one since on
it depends the natural arrest of haemorrhage.

The jelly-like clot consists of minute threads or
filaments or *fibrin*, in which are enmeshed red
blood corpuscles, white blood-cells, and
platelets.

When the injury giving rise to the bleeding
occurs, *thromboplastin* is released from the damaged tissue and from the platelets, and reacts with
circulating *prothrombin* and calcium to form
thrombin. This reacts in turn with circulating
fibrinogen to produce the fibrin.

The above, however, is only a part of the story,
for several other factors are now known to
operate first. They include the Hageman Factor,
Plasma Thromboplastin Antecedent, Christmas
Factor, Factor V, and Stewart-Power Factor.

Clotting time varies in different species and
under different degrees of health, but normally it
takes between 2½ and 11 minutes after the blood is
shed. After some hours the fibrin contracts and
blood serum is squeezed out from the clot.

For clotting to take place, adequate vitamin K
is necessary; prothrombin supply being, it seems,
dependent on this vitamin.

Clotting may be inhibited by anticoagulants,
such as heparin, dicoumarol, warfarin. In cases of
haemophilia, a disease from which some dogs suffer, clotting is also inhibited. (*See* CANINE HAEMO-
PHILIA.)

'CLOUDBURST' is a colloquial name for false
pregnancy in the goat which, after an apparently
normal gestation, suddenly voids from the vulva
a large quantity of cloudy fluid – after which the
size of the abdomen returns to normal. 'Cloudburst' is a fairly common condition.

CLOVER (*see* INFERTILITY, BLOAT, SILAGE, HAEMO-
RRHAGIC SYNDROME OF CATTLE, HAY and mouldy
hay, LEYS, SILAGE, PASTURE MANAGEMENT).

COAT COLOUR CHANGE. (*see* CUSHING'S
SYNDROME).

COB is a short-legged horse, suitable for saddle
work of a prolonged but not rapid nature; also
used for light trade-carts. Cobs generally stand
from 13½ to 14½ hands high.

The word 'cob' is also used for cubes made
from *unmilled* dried grass.

COBALT is one of the mineral elements known
to be essential to normal health, but only
required in minute amounts. Because of this, cobalt is said to be one of the 'trace elements'. Its
function is to act as a catalyst in the assimilation
of iron into haemoglobin in the red blood corpuscles. (*See* BUSH SICKNESS; PINING; ANAEMIA;
TRACE ELEMENTS; MOLYBDENUM.)

Cobalt deficiency occurs in parts of Scotland,
Northumbria, Devon, and North Wales.
Affected sheep may show symptoms such as progressive debility, anaemia, emaciation, stunted
growth, a lustreless fleece, and sunken eyes from
which there is often a discharge, with a mortality
of up to 20 per cent.

However, symptoms are seldom as definite and
clear cut as the above description might suggest,
and in many flocks a 'failure to thrive' is all that is

observed or suspected. Sometimes poor performance comes to be accepted as normal, and yet could be remedied by preventive measures after soil analyses had indicated a cobalt deficiency.

Nowadays, according to the Hill Farming Research Organisation, 0·25 part per million of cobalt in the soil is regarded as an acceptable level; and 0·17 ppm as constituting a deficiency.

Two methods of treatment were compared – the administration of a single cobalt 'bullet', and two doses of cobalt chloride. Dr. A. J. F. Russel and colleagues at HFRO reported that these two methods appeared to have been equally effective in alleviating the deficiency as judged from the liveweight response of the lambs. 'Treatment by cobalt bullet was, however, more effective in increasing and, more importantly, in maintaining serum vitamin B_{12} [closely related to cobalt] than was the cobalt dosing régime.' Under their conditions, dosing would have had to be carried out at frequent intervals of probably not more than three weeks to be effective.

Prevention may be attempted by dressing cobalt-deficient land with a mixture of cobalt chloride and cobalt sulphate at the rate of 4 lb/acre.

Poisoning. Overdosage must be avoided. Twelve beef stores on cobalt-deficient land died when they were not only offered a cobalt supplement in boxes, but drenched as well with cobalt sulphate 'measured' by the handful.

(*See also under* SELENIUM.)

COCAINE, or COCA. Coca leaves are obtained from two South American plants, *Erythroxylon coca*, and *Erythroxylon bolivianum*, and contain the alkaloid *cocaine*. This acts as a local anaesthetic by paralysing the nerves of sensation in the region to which it is applied. It has now been largely displaced by synthetic local anaesthetic agents which are less toxic and do not come under the Dangerous Drugs Act regulations.

COCCIDIAN PARASITES/DISEASES (*see* COCCIDIOSIS, HAMMONDIA, SARCOSPORIDIOSIS, TOXOPLASMOSIS).

Coccidian life cycle. The oocyst is passed in the faeces. It consists of the zygote, which results from the union of the male and female elements, enclosed within a protective membrane or cyst wall. On the ground and in the presence of moisture, oxygen, and a suitable temperature development proceeds. The zygote splits into two or four sporoblasts (depending upon the genus), each of which becomes enclosed in a capsule to form oval sporocysts. The contents of each sporocyst divide into four (or two) sporozoites. Once this process of sporulation is completed the oocyst is 'ripe' and capable of infecting a host, unsporulated oocysts are not infective. When ripe oocysts are swallowed by a suitable host, the action of the digestive juices on the cyst walls allows the motile sporozoites to escape and each penetrates an epithelial cell. Here each parasite increases in size and finally becomes a large rounded schizont. This divides into a number of small elongated merozoites which, escaping from the epithelial cell into the gut, attack new cells, and

the process is repeated. The massive feeding stage in the cell before it starts dividing is called a trophozoite, and is usually a young schizont. Under certain conditions, however, some trophozoites develop into large female forms or macrogametocytes which, when mature, become macrogametes. Meanwhile certain other trophozoites develop into male cells or microgametocytes, which divide into a number of small microgametes. One of these unites with each macrogamete, and the resulting cell is called the zygote. The fertilised macrogamete, or zygote, then secretes a thick capsule around itself, forming an oocyst which is discharged into the lumen of the organ intestine or bile-duct and thus escapes from the host in the faeces.

(a) *Isospora* – the mature oocyst contains *two* sporocysts, each with four sporozoites.

(b) *Eimera* – the mature oocyst contains *four* sporocysts, each with two sporozoites.

COCCIDIOMYCOSIS is a fungal disease, involving chiefly the lymph nodes, and giving rise to tumour-like (granulomatous) lesions. It occurs in cattle, sheep, dogs, cats, and certain wild rodents, caused by infection with a fungus, called *Coccidioides immitis*. It has been recognised in many parts of the USA and Canada. It is seen in animals with immuno-suppression; especially young dogs.

SIGNS. Loss of appetite, fever, weight loss, cough, enlarged lymph nodes.

Chiefly recognised in abattoirs during the inspection of meat for human consumption, or in other animals at post-mortem examination. The lesions are sometimes confused with those of actinomycosis or actinobacillosis. In the dog, the disease may involve several internal organs and also bone.

In 1981 a case was reported in a recently imported baboon, with skin lesions on muzzle and tail consisting of raised, plaque-like ulcers. M. D. Welshman and others, *Vet. Rec.* stated that the lesions can resemble those of *Mycobacterium tuberculosis* and *Yersinia pseudotuberculosis*. Coccidiomycosis is communicable to man.

COCCIDIOSIS. A disease affecting many species of farm and domestic mammals; also people and birds.

CAUSE. Eimeria, a group of protozoan parasites. For the life-history of the parasites causing this disease, *see under* COCCIDIAN.

Cattle: Red dysentery.

CAUSAL AGENT: *Eimeria zürnii*.

This is believed to be the most important species affecting cattle. Developmental forms occur wholly in the large intestine and caecum where considerable denudation of epithelium occurs, resulting in extensive haemorrhage. The oocysts are nearly spherical, and sporulation, under favourable conditions, takes place in from 48 to 72 hours. It is found in Europe, Africa, and N. America. It is prevalent during the warm season, and attacks especially animals of 2 months to 2 years.

SIGNS are first seen in 1 to 8 weeks after infection. There is a persistent diarrhoea which becomes haemorrhagic. After about a week emaciation is evident, the temperature rises, and there are digestive disturbances. Milk is diminished or stopped. Passage of faeces is attended by straining or even eversion of the rectum. Convalescence is slow. The lesions are mainly in the large intestine. Mortality varies between 2 per cent and 10 per cent of affected, and, generally speaking, the younger the animal the more likely is it to succumb.

TREATMENT consists of isolation of all sick animals and careful nursing, with the use of sulphamezathine or sulphaquinoxaline or dapsone.

Sheep and Goats.

CAUSAL AGENTS: At least seven species of *Eimeria* occurs in these animals, and mixed infections with two or more species is the rule rather than the exception. The various species are widely distributed and as a rule the clinical disease is seen in lambs and kids, seldom in the old animals which, however, may harbour coccidia.

SIGNS are those of a pernicious anaemia accompanied by diarrhoea and emaciation. There is no fever. The course of the disease may be very quick or may last several weeks. The lesions are mainly in the small intestine.

Lambs reared indoors apparently suffer less from coccidiosis if reared on expanded metal floors without bedding than when bedded on straw.

Pigs. Coccidiosis is seldom reported as a serious disease in the UK, and its importance is debatable. However, reports of increasing losses from it in the USA led to a re-appraisal. In 1980 MAFF's veterinary investigation centre at Norwich identified *Eimeria debleicka* – one of the species associated with piglet diarrhoea in the USA – in material taken at autopsy. In Scotland Dr. L. Roberts and E. J. Walker reported finding a mixed infection of rotavirus and *Isospora suis* in scouring piglets. 'Substantial' benefit followed control measures, which consisted of feeding amprolium or monensin premixes in the feed for one week before farrowing; together with thorough cleaning of farrowing pens between one occupant and another.

Horses. Diarrhoea, emaciation and death have occurred following infection. (*See also* GLOBIDIOSIS.)

Rabbits. There are two forms of the disease; one attacking the intestines, and the other the liver. Young rabbits may have acute enteritis, leading to death. The hepatic form often takes a chronic course, with diarrhoea developing later. Affected livers show whitish spots at autopsy.

Dogs and Cats. The following species are known:

Isospora felis
I. rivolta
I. bigemina
Eimeria canis and *E. felina*

Most of these parasites have been isolated from healthy animals. The majority of coccidial infections of dogs and cats are light, and there is little evidence of serious damage to the hosts. In some cases, however, there is diarrhoea and occasionally fatal dysentery.

Coccidiosis in carnivores is commoner than was once believed, especially in young cats, where the parasite is *Isospora felis*. The disease causes no symptoms except diarrhoea where a heavy infestation has occurred. Death is rare. The rabbit parasite may be found in faeces when diseased rabbits have been eaten.

Isospora canis was isolated from 4 per cent of 481 faecal samples from dogs in North Island, New Zealand; *I. ohioensis* from 9 per cent.

Fowls. At least seven species of *Eimeria* have been implicated. The disease commonly affects chicks 5 to 7 weeks old, as well as older growing birds. In the former the mortality may be high. Diarrhoea, often with blood in the faeces, is seen. Lack of activity, weakness, and emaciation are other signs.

CONTROL of coccidiosis in poultry can now be achieved by means of a live, attenuated vaccine produced by the AFRC's Institute of Animal Health in the UK.

Before the introduction of this vaccine, control was dependent upon antibiotics such as MONENSIN and SALINOMYCIN, or upon AMPROLIUM.

Turkeys. Six species of *Eimeria* cause disease.

Ducks. Coccidiosis occurs, but is of little economic importance.

Geese. Three species of *Eimeria* occur in the intestine. Rather severe outbreaks have been ascribed to *E. anseris*. A fourth, important species is *E. truncata*, which causes a severe form of renal coccidiosis. The disease affects goslings from 3 weeks to 3 months of age, and in heavy infections goslings may die within 2 or 3 days after symptoms are first seen. The mortality is often very high.

COCCYGEAL vertebrae are the tail bones. One or more may fracture if a dog, cat, etc. becomes caught by a closing door or gate. (*See* BONE – Skeleton.)

COCOA POISONING. Poisoning of pigs and poultry, as a result of feeding cocoa residues or waste, was recorded in the UK during the 1939–45 war. (*See also* CHOCOLATE POISONING.)

CODEINE is one of the active principles of opium, and is used as the phosphate of codeine to check severe coughing in bronchitis, common cold, and in some cases of laryngitis. (*See* OPIUM.)

COD-LIVER OIL. A valuable source of vitamin A and D supplements for animal feeding. It should be purchased on a guarantee basis. The best varieties contain about 1000 to 1200 International Units of vitamin A, and 80 to 100 Units of D, per gramme. It should be stored in a dark-coloured container preferably in a cool place, and if air can be excluded until it is to be used, this will enable it to be kept longer. Both strong sunlight and oxygen cause a destruction of vitamin A. (*See* VITAMINS.)

USES. It has a particularly beneficial action in warding off rickets in young animals, and if this trouble has already started it may be checked, or cured, by the administration of cod-liver oil. Synthetic vitamins have largely replaced cod-liver oil.

Swabs of cod-liver oil are also useful in eye injuries and in simple burns.

'COD-LIVER OIL POISONING'. This may occur through the use of oil which has been allowed to oxidise or become rancid. One result may be Muscular Dystrophy in cattle (which see).

COENURIASIS. Infestation of the sheep's brain with cysts of the dog (and fox) tapeworm *Taenia multiceps*. (*See under* TAPEWORMS.)

COGGINS TEST. The agar-gel immunodiffusion test. Useful in the diagnosis of, *e.g.*, equine infectious anaemia.

COIT, MAL DU (*see* DOURINE).

COITAL EXANTHEMA (*see* VULVOVAGINITIS; *also* RHINOTRACHEITIS).

COITUS (*see* REPRODUCTION).

COLBRED. A cross between the East Friesland and 3 British breeds of sheep (Border Leicester, Clun Forest, and Dorset Horn). The aim of Mr Oscar Colburn, their breeder, was to produce ewes with a consistent 200 per cent lambing average and a sufficiency of milk for this.

COLCHICINE. The alkaloid obtained from Meadow Saffron (*Colchicum autumnale*). It is used in plant and experimental animal breeding as 'a multiplier of chromosomes'. It has been possible to produce triploid rabbits, pigs, etc., by exposing semen to a solution of colchicine prior to artificial insemination. (*See* TRIPLOID.)

COLCHICUM POISONING (*see* MEADOW SAFFRON POISONING).

COLD (*see* HYPOTHERMIA, EXPOSURE, FROSTBITE, SHEARING).

COLIC is a vague term applied to symptoms of abdominal pain, especially in horses. In order to emphasise the large number of different conditions which may produce abdominal pain **in the horse**, the following list is included:

1. *Acute indigestion*, resulting from the feeding of unsuitable food, the presence of gas (flatulent colic).

2. Severe *organic disorders*, such as impaction of the colon, intussusception, volvulus, or strangulation of the bowel, rupture of the stomach, enteritis, and peritonitis, are among the serious causes.

3. The presence of large numbers of *parasitic worms, horse bots*, etc. (*See under* EQUINE VERMINOUS ARTERITIS.)

4. *Calculi* present in the kidney, urinary bladder, or urethra in the male, causing irritation of these organs.

5. *Anthrax*, where one of the common symptoms is abdominal pain.

6. Approaching *parturition* in the pregnant mare.

7. *Grass Sickness.*

8. (*See also* HYMEN, IMPERFORATE.)

9. Uterine rupture.

10. Nephritis.

11. Various poisons (*see* POISONING).

12. In addition, in countries where RABIES is endemic, this disease should be borne in mind when presented with a horse which appears to have colic.

The horse has a peculiarity in the arrangement of its alimentary canal, in that while the stomach is comparatively small, the intestines, and especially the large intestines, are of great bulk and capacity. In addition to this, the stomach itself has the peculiarity that its entrance and exit are small; the former only allows escape of gas into the gullet under exceptional circumstances, and the latter, owing to the S-shaped bend of the pylorus and first part of the small intestine, is very liable to become occluded when there is any considerable pressure of gas within the stomach. These two facts combine to make it difficult or impossible for gas collected in the stomach, as the result of fermentation, either to escape by the mouth or to pass on into the intestines. Fermenting or otherwise bad food may cause tympany of the stomach; while an excess of good food may lead to *impaction* of the stomach; and occasionally to its rupture.

Inflammation or *volvulus* may affect the small intestine, but most cases of colic involve the large intestine. *Impaction* of the *caecum* or *colon* may occur; likewise *tympany*.

The ileum, supplied only by a single artery, appears to be particularly vulnerable to ischaemia, following thrombosis often caused by *Strongylus vulgaris* worms.

Anaerobic bacteria and their toxins may exacerbate the situation after circulation defects have occurred.

(*See also* INTUSSUSCEPTION, another cause of colic.)

SIGNS. (1) *Spasmodic colic* is typified by sudden and severe attacks of pain, usually of an intermittent character. Breathing is blowing and faster than usual; there is an anxious expression about the face; and the pulse is accelerated and hard. In a few minutes the attack may pass off and the horse becomes easier, or the pain may continue. In the latter case the horse lies down and rolls, after having first walked round about the box. In some cases rolling appears to afford some measures of relief, but in others the horse rises again almost at once. During an attack the horse may kick at its belly, or may turn and gaze at its flank.

In another form, *ileus*, often called *flatulent colic*, the pain begins suddenly, but there are not such distinct periods of ease. The horse walks round and round the box, kicks at the abdomen, gazes at its sides, breaks out into patchy sweating, and breathes heavily. The horse frequently crouches as if to lie down, but only actually lies in the less severe cases, and seldom or never remains lying for any length of time. Attempts at passing urine are noticed, but, as in the truly spasmodic colic, they are seldom successful. Faeces may be passed in small quantities, and are usually accompanied by flatus.

(2) *Obstructive colic* may arise through impaction of the bowel with dry, fibrous, partly digested food material. Symptoms develop slowly, commencing with dullness and depression, irregularity in feeding, and abdominal discomfort. In 12 hours or so signs of abdominal pain appear. The horse looks round at its flank, paws with the fore-feet, and kicks at the abdomen. When on the ground it usually stretches out on one side, very often the off, and appears to derive some ease from lying in this position. Considerable grunting and groaning usually accompany recumbency, and breathing is often long and 'sighing'. In some cases acute pain is shown, the horse rolling on the ground in agony. Small amounts of faeces are passed with considerable frequency at first, but when an attack is well established the passage of both urine and dung ceases. An attitude to which some importance may be attached, since it is very strongly suggestive of impaction of the colon, is one in which the horse backs against the manger or other projection, and appears to sit upon it, sometimes with the hind-feet off the ground. In other cases a horse with obstruction in the colon or caecum may sit with the hindquarters on the ground, but retains an upright position with the fore-legs – somewhat similar to the position assumed by a dog. (*See* CALCULI for another cause of obstruction.)

(3) *Colic due to a twist* (*volvulus*). There is great pain, during which the horse may become restless and violent. Sometimes the pain passes off, and sweating occurs, before a further period of pain. The temperature may be 105 or 106°, becoming subnormal in the last stages. Pulse-rate may rise to 120. Death is usually preceded by convulsions.

Expert assistance should be sought whenever an attack of colic persists for longer than 3 hours. The simpler cases seldom last as long as 6 hours, and when symptoms are continued for longer than that it should be an indication that the case has passed beyond the simple stage, and the sooner skilled assistance is sought the less likely is it that complications will arise. Many colics end fatally, and it is certain that many horses might have been saved if a veterinary surgeon had been summoned at the outset.

A SURVEY OF 134 CASES of colic, seen at the veterinary clinic, University of Zurich, in 1980, included 34 which were symptomless on arrival, required no treatment, and were regarded as cases of *spasmodic* colic. Thirty-three horses had *impaction* of the pelvic flexure of the colon and were treated conservatively; as were 14 with impaction of the ampulla coli (4), caecum (1). There were seven cases of *tympany of the stomach* and two of *impaction*. Of 53 cases of *ileus*, the prognosis was hopeless in seven which were destroyed, and owners refused surgery in another six cases. Forty underwent laparotomy, and 24 were discharged. Surgical success rate was 60 per cent; overall success of treatment was 68 per cent. Suggestions included maintenance of a nasal stomach tube to eliminate possibly lethal consequences of secondary gastric distension by fluid and gas during journey to the clinic; and 1 to litres of 5 per cent sodium bicarbonate solution intravenously to help control the start of acidosis. (Stohler. T &

Fricker C. (1982) *Schweizer Archiv für Tierheilkunde* **124,** 133) (*See also* HORSES, COMMON CAUSES OF DEATH IN.)

PREVENTION. Regular feeding; good quality foods, neither too bulky nor too concentrated, and with succulents when available; clean water in plentiful supply, and watering before feeding for working horses; regular worming.

COLIFORM. A convenient term used to describe several species of lactose fermenting bacilli which inhabit the gut. The most commonly encountered is *Escherichia coli* and approximately 80 per cent of coliform isolates tested at the National Institute for Research in Dairying are *E. coli*. Other coliform species implicated in bovine mastitis include *Klebsiella pneumoniae, K. oxytoca, Enterobacter cloacae, E. aerogenes* and *Citrobacter freundii*. All are 'gut associated' but some, notably *K. pneumoniae* and Enterobacters, may be free-living in forest environments or soil and be introduced into a dairy herd with wood products used for cattle litter. (Eric Jackson & John Bramley *In Practice* July '83.)

COLIFORM INFECTIONS. Examination of cattle carcases at slaughter-houses showed that coliform organisms were isolated from surface swabbings from 208 out of 400 head of cattle (52 per cent); 81 of these being resistant to one or more antibiotics. Of 400 pig carcase swabs, 331 (83 per cent) were positive for coliforms; 246 being resistant to one or more antibiotics. Chloramphenicol resistance was present in 19 pig isolates and 1 cattle isolate. (John R. Walton, MRCVS, *Lancet*, Sept. 12, 1970.) (*See E. coli*; SAWDUST; MASTITIS, ANTIBIOTIC-RESISTANCE.)

COLITIS means inflammation of the colon, or first part of the large intestine. (*See* INTESTINES.)

COLLAGEN (*see* FIBROUS TISSUE; *also* CUTANEOUS ASTHENIA).

COLLATERAL CIRCULATION (*see* ANASTOMOSIS).

COLLICULUS SEMINALIS. This protrudes into the lumen of the urethra, and at its centre is a minute opening into a tiny tube (the *uterus masculinus*) which runs into the prostate gland.

COLLIE EYE ANOMALY. A congenital disease occurring in some rough collies, smooth collies, and Shetland sheepdogs. In the worst cases, blindness may follow detachment of the retina or haemorrhage within the eye.

COLLODION is a thick, colourless, syrupy liquid, made by dissolving gun-cotton in a mixture of ether and alcohol. When painted on to the skin, the ether and alcohol evaporate, and leave a tough film behind. *Flexible collodion*, made by adding castor oil and Canada balsam, is more elastic and does not crack with the movements of the part, and is eminently suitable for application to regions around joints. Medicated collodion contains substances such as salicylic acid and iodoform. A collodion preparation containing a caustic is used for destroying the horn-buds of calves. (*See* DISHORNING.)

COLLOID is matter in which the individual particles either of single large molecules, such as proteins, or aggregates of smaller molecules, more or less uniformly distributed in a dispersion medium, *e.g.* water, oil. Examples: colloidal silver (used for eye infections), and colloidal manganese.

COLLUNARIUM is a nose wash.

COLLUTORIUM, or COLLUTORY is a mouth wash.

COLLYRIUM means an eye wash.

COLOBOMA. A congenital eye defect. (*See under* EYE, DISEASES OF.)

COLON (*see* COLITIS, INTESTINE).

COLOSTRUM is the milk secreted by the udder immediately after parturition and for the following 3 to 4 days. It contains 20 per cent or more protein, a little more fat than normal milk, and may be tinged pink due to blood corpuscles. It coagulates at about 80° to 85°C, and cannot therefore be boiled. This is sometimes used as a test. It is normally rich in vitamins A and D provided the dam has not been deprived of these in her food. It acts as a natural purgative for the young animal, clearing from its intestines the accumulated faecal matter known as 'meconium', which is often of a dry, putty-like nature. Of much greater importance, it is through the medium of the colostrum that the young animal obtains its first supply of antibodies which protect it against various bacteria and viruses.

Research findings concerning the immunoglobulins (antibodies) which give colostrum its protective effect for the calf were the subject of a paper (*Brit. Vet. J.* (1974), **130,** 406) by Dr E. F. Logan, of the Veterinary Research Laboratories, Stormont.

Before the cow calves, her udder selectively withdraws these immunoglobulins from her blood into the colostrum. In the suckling calf, the immunoglobulins become active in the blood serum after absorption, and they also have a local protective action within the small intestine. 'If the calf is to survive, both the serum and intestinal immunoglobulins must be present in adequate quantities'; for the serum immunoglobulin will protect against septicaemia, but not against the enteritis which leads to scouring and dehydration.

The importance of the calf receiving colostrum early has for long been emphasised, and it is well known that the calf's intestine becomes impermeable to immunoglobulins within hours of birth. To say that, however, is to over-simplify. Some immunoglobulins can be absorbed through the gut faster than others, but for practical farm purposes it can be taken that colostrum must be fed within 6 hours of the calf's birth.

Dr I. E. Selman, and research colleagues carried out a survey and found that beef suckler cows suckled their calf within 1½ hours of birth whereas, on average, dairy cows suckled their calves after 4 hours.

Research workers at the A F R C Institute of Animal Physiology, Babraham, have shown that immunoglobulin – a complex protein – is absorbed very poorly – except in the presence of catalytic factors, which they identified. It has also been demonstrated that 'the physical presence of the dam with the calf, in some unknown way, facilitated absorption of immunoglobulin'.

Hookworm larvae have been found in a bitch's colostrum (10 were recovered by experimental milking before whelping), and larvae of *Strongyloides ransomi* in a sow's milk.

Colostrum has been given by means of a catheter to newborn lambs, in order to reduce neonatal mortality. However, there have been cases of a severe and sometimes fatal anaemia in lambs after they had received cow's colostrum. Dr P. Franken, Veterinary Health Service officer in the Netherlands, has suggested that bovine colostra which might produce anaemia be identified by a gel precipitation test on colostral whey after this trouble has occurred on a farm. (*See also* TOXOCARIASIS.)

COLOSUSPENSION. A method of treatment for urinary incontinence in the bitch when the sole cause is incompetence of the urethral sphincter. In 150 cases the treatment was completely successful; in 40 there was no improvement. The technique was described by Dr P. E. Holt (*J. Small Animal Practice* (1985) **26** 237.)

COLOUR-MARKING BULLS, *e.g.* Hereford, Aberdeen-Angus, Charolais, and Galloway, for mating with cows in dairy herds which are of dual-purpose type and moderate to poor milkers, in order to increase the number of store cattle suitable for fattening for beef production. (*See also* BEEF-BREEDS AND CROSSES.)

COLT. A young male horse.

COMA is a state of profound unconsciousness in which the patient not only cannot be roused, but there are no reflex movements when the skin is pinched or pricked, or when the eyeballs are touched, etc. The cause is generally an excessively high temperature, brain injury, cerebral haemorrhage, some poisons, or too much or too little insulin in cases of diabetes, or the terminal stage of a fatal illness.

A collie bitch recovered from a coma lasting seven weeks after its owner had asked a non-veterinarian to inject it with ivermectin (which is not licensed for use in dogs in Britain). (*See* IVERMECTIN.)

COMB. In healthy poultry, this should be bright red and well developed. When birds go out of lay or are caponised, the comb becomes smaller and paler. Anaemia may also cause this. A pale comb of normal size suggests internal haemorrhage. Scurfiness is suggestive of favus, yellow scabs of fowl-pox.

COMENY'S INFECTIOUS PARALYSIS OF HORSES. This was first described in French army horses by Comény. A suspected outbreak of this at the Evans Biological Institute, Runcorn, in 1961 was described in the *Veterinary Record* of April 3, 1965.

SIGNS. A sudden rise in temperature to 104° or 105°F, persisting for 5 days, and followed in some cases by paralysis after a period of hind-limb inco-ordination and difficulty in turning.

COMMENSALISM is the association of two species in which one alone benefits, but the other does not suffer. Commensals are found on the skin surface, for example, and do not produce disease.

COMMISSURE means a joining, and is a term applied to strands of nerve fibres that join one side of the brain to the other, to the band joining one optic nerve to the other, to the junction of the lips at the corners of the mouth, etc.

COMMUNICABLE DISEASES. For diseases communicable *to* man, *see under* ZOONOSES. For diseases communicable *from* man to farm live-stock, etc., *see* ANTHROPONOSES.

COMPARATIVE TEST (*see* TUBERCULIN TEST).

COMPENSATION is the term applied to the method by which the body makes good a defect of form or function in an organ which is abnormal in these respects.

COMPLEMENT. This is a constituent of serum and plays an essential part in the production of immunity. Bacteria are killed by the specific antibody developed in an animal's serum only in the presence of complement. Complement is also necessary for haemolysis.

An immune serum may contain antibodies which, together with the antigen, absorb or fix complement and are hence called *complement-fixing antibodies*. These form the basis for the Complement Fixation Test, which is used in the diagnosis of certain diseases, *e.g.* Johne's. As an indicator for the test, red blood corpuscles plus their specific antibody are used, *i.e.* the corpuscles plus the antiserum heated at 55°C to inactivate or destroy the complement. In the test, on adding the indicator, haemolysis will not occur if the complement has been fixed.

COMPOUND FEEDS. A number of different ingredients (including major minerals, trace elements, vitamins and other additives) mixed and blended in appropriate proportions, to provide properly balanced diets for all types of stock at every stage of growth and development. (*See* DIET, FLUOROSIS.)

COMPULSIVE POLYDIPSIA. The urge to drink excessive quantities of water, due to some psychological disturbance, is a recognised syndrome in human medicine, and it probably occurs in dogs as a result of stress; leading to urinary incontinence. (*See also* DIABETES INSIPIDUS.)

CONALBUMIN. A constituent of egg-white. (*See* IRON-BINDING PROTEINS.)

CONCENTRATES. The bulk of these in Britain today come from highly reputable compound feeding-stuffs manufacturers, and are expert formulations related not only to the current price of various ingredients but also to the proper balancing of these ingredients. Computers are often used in the formulations. The inclusion of trace elements, minerals, and vitamins makes these compound feeding-stuffs foods complete in themselves. Suitable mixes are obtainable for every class of farm live-stock.

Farm-mixed concentrates are commonly used on large arable farms, using home-grown barley, oats, beans, etc. Very small-scale mixing is apt to be inefficient and result in a less bulky ingredient being unequally distributed. The expertise required for formulation may also be lacking, so that on the smaller farm proprietary concentrates are often to be preferred. (*See* DIET, CUBES; *also* ADDITIVES, COMPOUND FEEDS, SUPPLEMENTS.)

CONCEPTION RATES following artificial insemination of cattle are stated to be in the region of 65 per cent in dairy breeds, and over 70 per cent in beef breeds. In the UK, the conception rate is usually based upon the number of animals which, on a 3-month period, do not return to the first insemination. In Denmark, the conception rate is based on the evidence of a physical pregnancy diagnosis carried out 3 months after insemination.

Conception rates are influenced by many factors. The best time for insemination is between 2 and 20 hours after 'heat' is observed; after that delay will mean a lower conception rate. Health of male and female, and inseminator's skill also influence the rate. (*See also* FARROWING RATES.)

CONCEPTUS. The product of conception: initially a fertilised egg, later an embryo which develops into a fetus plus fetal membranes.

CONCRETE. The precise nature of the ingredients of this may prove important where floor feeding is practised. Suspected iron poisoning from the licking of concrete made with sand rich in iron has been described in fattening pigs. Concrete floors of piggeries, etc., should be made with integral air spaces in order to have some insulating effect, and should not be abrasive. If they are, they can lead to injuries, followed by staphylococcal or other infection which may cause severe illness or death *even in a new pig pen*. (*See under* FOOTROT OF PIGS, HOUSING OF ANIMALS, *and* BEDDING.)

CONCUSSION (*see* BRAIN).

CONDENSATION IN BUILDINGS (*see* NITRITE POISONING, CALF REARING, PNEUMONIA, SWEAT HOUSE, YORKSHIRE BOARDING, VENTILATION).

CONDITION (*see under* MUSCLE).

CONDYLE is the rounded prominence at the end of a bone; for instance, the condyles of the humerus are the two prominences on either side of the elbow-joint in animals, while the condyles of the femur enter into the formation of the stifle joint.

CONFORMATION ASSESSMENT in the **COW** (*see last part of* PROGENY TESTING).

CONGENITAL deformities, diseases, etc., are those which are either present at birth, or which, being transmitted direct from the parents, show themselves some time after birth. (*See* Genetic Defects under GENETICS.)

CONGESTIVE HEART FAILURE (*see under* HEART, DISEASES OF).

CONIINE (*see* HEMLOCK).

CONJUNCTIVA is the membrane which covers the front of the eye. It lines the insides of the eye-lids of all animals, both upper and lower, and from each of these places it is reflected on to the front of the eyeball. The membrane is transparent in its central portion, where it is specialised to form the covering to the cornea, which admits light into the cavity of the eye.

CONJUNCTIVITIS means inflammation of the conjunctiva. (*See* EYE, DISEASES OF.)

A veterinary surgeon with an ulcerating nodule on one eyelid, and conjunctivitis, was found to be infected with cowpox.

CONNECTIVE TISSUES. These include (1) white fibrous (collagenous) tissue, having fibres of collagen produced by fibroblasts; *e.g.* in tendons, ligaments. (2) yellow elastic tissue, composed of kinked fibres. (3) reticular tissue, composed of fine fibres which form a framework for bone-marrow. (4) adipose tissue or fat. (5) cartilage or gristle. (6) bone.

CONSOLIDATION is a term applied to solidification of an organ, especially of a lung. The consolidation may be of a permanent nature due to formation of fibrous tissue or tumour cells, or temporary, as in acute pneumonia.

CONSTIPATION. The faeces are passed in a variety of ways among the domestic animals. In the horse, cow, and sheep, the excreta appears to be evacuated with very little or even no effort. The horse can defaecate perfectly and naturally when galloping in harness, and seems only partly aware of the process. In the case of the dog and pig, on the other hand, the process involves a cessation of all other occupation, the assumption of a special position of the body, and an obviously conscious effort. This attitude towards the process is more nearly that of human beings, and it is easy to understand that the more involved and particular the process, the more likely is it to become upset when circumstances arise which alter the animal's mode of living. Consequently it is found that while dogs and pigs are liable to suffer from the true form of constipation, especially after exposure to some unusual factor, horses, cattle, and sheep, although they are liable to suffer from acute obstruction of the bowels, are seldom affected with true constipation.

CAUSES. Anything which is likely to interfere with the normal peristaltic movements of the bowels, such as the use of too dry, bulky, or concentrated foods, overloading of the alimentary tract with unsuitable foods, tumours in the abdomen, pain originating from an enlarged prostate gland, or from obstructed anal glands, will at any rate predispose to constipation if not actually cause it. Inadequate exercise and too much food is a common cause. Changes from one owner to another, or from one district to another, or stress in the case of nervous individuals, are said to be a cause.

TREATMENT. (*See* LAXATIVES, ENEMA.)

Cats. It is important that owners do not mistake what may at first appear to be constipation for difficulty in, or inability to, pass urine owing to UROLITHIASIS (which see).

CONTAGIOUS ABORTION OF CATTLE (*see* BRUCELLOSIS IN CATTLE).

CONTAGIOUS AGALACTIA (*see* AGALACTIA).

CONTAGIOUS BOVINE PLEURO-PNEU-MONIA. This disease has decimated herds throughout Europe and in other parts of the world on several occasions, and probably has been directly responsible for the death of more cattle than any other single disease with the possible exception of cattle plague (rinderpest).

In the year 1860 alone, 187,000 cattle were lost from this disease in Great Britain, and between 1869 and 1894, 103,000 more. From 1891 onwards the disease rapidly decreased, only one case being recorded in 1898, since when Great Britain has been entirely free; as are most countries in Europe. It is present in Asia and Africa, while in recent years outbreaks have occurred in Australia and South America. No case has been seen in the United States of America since 1892.

Cattle, buffaloes, and related species, such as reindeer, yak, and bison, are susceptible. Other animals, including man, are immune. Housed cattle are always more susceptible than those in the open.

CAUSE. *Mycoplasma mycoides.* (*See under* MYCOPLASMOSIS.)

Infection may occur by direct contact. Buildings which have housed infected cattle may remain infective for long periods.

INCUBATION PERIOD. 3 weeks to 6 months.

SIGNS. The first sign of illness is a rise of temperature to 103° or 105°F. In the acute disease this rise of temperature is soon followed by signs of general illness, such as dull coat, debility, loss of appetite, cessation of rumination. Shortly afterwards a dry, short, painful cough makes its appearance.

Pregnant cows are liable to abort.

Death usually follows in 2 or 3 weeks after the symptoms have become pronounced and acute. Recovery is frequently more apparent than real, for a chronic cough remains, and the disease may again become acute and even end fatally.

POST-MORTEM APPEARANCES. Large or small areas of pneumonia in the lungs, which are often of a marbled appearance. The lesion is primarily one of interstitial pneumonia, with thickened septa dividing the lung up into lobules; some lobules show acute congestion, some are in a stage of red or grey hepatisation, while others consist of dead encapsulated tissue, known as 'sequestra'. Evidence of pleurisy with often much fibrinous deposit around the lungs is usual.

DIAGNOSIS. The slaughter of suspected animals may be essential for this. Corroboration may be obtained by laboratory methods.

TREATMENT is not allowed in most countries, but neoarsphenamine has proved useful elsewhere.

IMMUNISATION. There are four methods which have been practised to immunise cattle against this disease.

CONTAGIOUS CAPRINE PLEURO-PNEUMONIA. A disease of goats, caused by a mycoplasma and occurring in Europe, Asia, and Africa. Acute, peracute, and chronic forms occur. Mortality may be 60 to 100 per cent. Antibiotics are useful for treatment where a slaughter policy is not in force.

CONTAGIOUS DISEASES. Certain of these are notifiable. (*See under* NOTIFIABLE DISEASES.) The responsibilities of animal owners are discussed under DISEASES OF ANIMALS ACT, 1950.

CONTAGIOUS ECTHYMA OF SHEEP is another name for ORF.

CONTAGIOUS EPITHELIOMA OF BIRDS (*see* AVIAN CONTAGIOUS EPITHELIOMA).

CONTAGIOUS EQUINE METRITIS (*see under* EQUINE). This is a NOTIFIABLE disease in the UK, under the Infectious Diseases of Horses Order 1987.

CONTAGIOUS PUSTULAR DERMATITIS in sheep. (*See* ORF.)

CONTAGIOUS STOMATITIS (*see* FOOT-AND-MOUTH DISEASE; *also* VESICULAR STOMATITIS).

CONTRACEPTIVES (*see under* STILBOESTROL). (For preventing cats, etc., coming on heat, *see under* OESTRUS, SUPPRESSION OF.) Contraceptives have been used in limited but successful trials as a means of rabies control. (*See also* STILBENES, GOSSYPOL.)

CONTRACTED FOOT, or CONTRACTED HOOF. A condition of the horse in which some part of the foot, very often a quarter or heel, becomes contracted and shrunken to less than its usual size. It is brought about by anything which favours rapid evaporation of the moisture in the horn, such as rasping away the outer surface of the wall; or by conditions which prevent expansion of the hoof, such as paring away the frog so that it does not come into contact with the ground, cutting the bars, allowing the wall at the heels to fall inwards, shoeing with high calkins, etc.

PREVENTION consists in leaving the frogs as large and well developed as possible; reducing the overgrowth at the heels and bars to the same extent as at the toe and other parts of the foot, shoeing with shoes which allow the frog to come into contact with the ground.

TREATMENT. In severe cases a run at grass with tips on the affected feet, and leaving the heels bare, is advisable. (*See also* HOOF REPAIR.)

CONTROL, CONTROLLED EXPERIMENT. In any scientifically conducted experiment or field trial, the results of treatment of one group of animals are compared with results in another, untreated, group. Animals in the untreated group are known as 'the controls'.

'CONTROLLED BREEDING'. 'Manipulation of oestrus in sheep is a very practical proposition ... the problems with cattle and pigs are far greater', commented Dr J. M. Chesworth at the Aberdeen School of Agriculture's 1975 symposium on the detection and control of breeding activity in farm animals.

He listed the factors which need to be taken into account when developing techniques for the control of breeding: (1) the procedures must be reasonably cheap, simple, and require a minimum of labour; (2) they should have identical effects upon all normal animals; (3) they must not reduce fertility or fecundity; (4) with pharmaceutical compounds there must be no side-effects upon the animal, its progeny, or the ultimate consumer of the animal or its products; and (5) if it is proposed to use natural service, then there must be no interference with the appearance of behavioural oestrus, or with the timing of oestrus relative to ovulation.

Although the words 'oestrus' and 'ovulation' are often used as though they were synonymous, Dr Chesworth emphasised that a very careful distinction must be made in the context of manipulation. 'The behavioural signs of oestrus can be produced in the absence of ovulation; and there is a trend in the development of control procedures towards systems in which fertilisation does not depend upon oestrus.' (Fertilisation in the absence of oestrus is only of value when AI is used.)

Synchronisation in ewes. Professor I. Gordon, University College, Dublin, described the results of 10 years' research in Eire. About 20,000 ewes have been treated with FGA-impregnated intravaginal sponges and PMSG in more than 500 flocks.

In the summer of 1973 sheep farmers in many parts of Eire could call on their local AI station for treatment of their sheep with intravaginal sponges and PMSG for early lamb production. The charge, equivalent to £0·60 per ewe (35p of this for the sponge and PMSG), covered two visits by a technician – the first to insert the sponge and the second, 14 days later, to remove the sponge and inject the ewe with serum gonadotrophin (PMSG).

Professor Gordon emphasised that his paper dealt with results only from dry sheep treated in the period July–December. 'Nevertheless, the induction of pregnancy in the *post-partum* ewe in the spring months has been done with great success at the Rowett, and the French are using oestrus synchronisation and sheep AI on a very considerable scale during all months of the year. The number of treated ewes in that country was in the region of 300,000 in 1974.'

(FGA is described under PROGESTOGENS.)

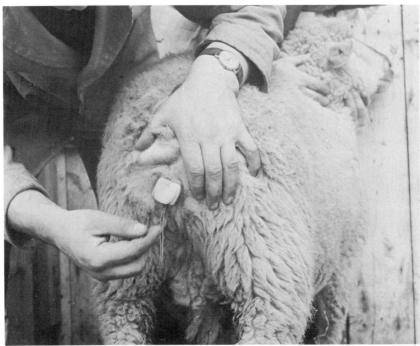

About to withdraw the progestogen-impregnated sponge at the end of the 2-week treatment period. At this time, the ewe receives a single intramuscular injection of PMSG – to complete the controlled breeding treatment.

The potential with cattle. Difficulty in detecting oestrus at present deters some farmers from using AI on maiden heifers and on beef suckler cows. This means, of course, that the potential advantages of using top-quality bulls – better liveweight gains and shorter time to slaughter weight – are forfeited, to the detriment of profit margins. Controlled breeding could in many instances overcome this, and also ease management by facilitating batch inseminations and calvings.

There are currently available for synchronisation of oestrus in cattle two methods: (1) administration of a progestogen – but progestogen-induced timing of oestrus has proved far more difficult in cattle than in sheep; many attempts have been made to synchronise oestrus with progestogens given in the feed, injected, or applied as intravaginal tampons; or (2) injection of a synthetic analogue of the naturally occurring prostaglandin $F2_\infty$.

There are indications that ovulation may occur independent of oestrus in prostaglandin-treated animals. 'If this is proved to occur on a large scale, it would render prostaglandin treatment much more useful for AI than for natural service, as insemination could merely be performed at a set time from prostaglandin injection,' said Dr Chesworth.

Prostaglandins have been administered by the intra-uterine route, but the preferred route appears to be intramuscular. 'The only disadvantage with prostaglandins appears to be associated with inadvertently injecting them into a pregnant animal, as this leads to very rapid abortion.'

A prostaglandin for cattle. Precisely scheduled artificial insemination programmes without need for oestrus detection are, it is claimed, made practicable and economic by an ICI prostaglandin product, Cloprostenol, introduced in 1975. Two intramuscular injections, 11 days apart, bring a cow on heat 3 to 4 days after the second injection. Then two inseminations are given, 24 hours apart (72 and 96 hours after the second injection), to maximise the likelihood of pregnancy.

ICI is marketing the product as part of a planned breeding concept involving the veterinary surgeon, the AI service and, of course, the farmer.

Mr R. W. Plenderleith, of Glasgow University, described the advent of prostaglandins as a great step forward in dairy herd fertility schemes. In dairy and beef herds, the calving to conception interval had been reduced by 15 days in animals treated with prostaglandins. However, he said, good results depended very much on maturity and nutrition. Ideally, heifers should be served when they had attained a weight of about 350 kg at 15–18 months of age. Good feeding was necessary before service with, for example, 4–6 lb barley per day for at least six weeks previously and for four weeks afterwards. Mr Plenderleith also recommended grass nuts, and commented that prostaglandins were additionally useful in tackling the problem of 'no visible oestrus'. (It should be added, however, that pregnancy is a common cause of the latter and that, to quote Mr T. S. Anderson, an injection of prostaglandin is just as effective in getting rid of 'wanted pregnancy' as an 'unwanted pregnancy', so that care is necessary).

Progesterone and *oestradiol* (natural hormones) form the basis of Prid (Ceva Ltd) for controlled breeding in cows.

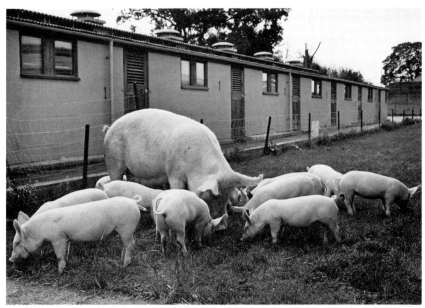

This Large White sow (on the farm of the AFRC's Institute of Animal Physiology, Babraham, Cambridge) produced 138 viable piglets in 12 litters between May 1974 and July 1979. All her farrowings were induced by prostaglandins to facilitate daytime supervision.

Prostaglandins for sows. In large pig units farrowing can be induced to take place at a time when stockmen are normally available, Mr D. W. Marriott stated at an Upjohn symposium. This meant that losses of newborn piglets through overlying, the savaging of litters, obstruction to breathing fetal membranes, and agalactia could be minimised. With an average gestation period of 115 days, the prostaglandin would be given on day 112, for the sow to farrow on day 113 or 114, he stated; but the injection should be given only when the sow had plenty of milk.

CONTROLLED ENVIRONMENT HOUSING. Temperature, ventilation, and humidity are controlled within narrow limits by means of electric fans, heaters, etc., and good insulation. Poultry, for example, are protected in this way from sudden changes in temperature, rearing can be carried out with the minimum loss throughout the year, and increased egg yields and decreased food intake can effect a considerable saving in costs of production. Some of these houses are windowless; artificial lighting being provided. Respiratory disease may occur through overcrowding or ventilation defects.

FAILURE OF AUTOMATIC CONTROL.

A thunderstorm blew the fuse in the fan circuit of a controlled environment house, and unfortunately 'fail-safe' ventilation flaps did not work. As a result 520 fattening pigs died of heat-stroke. (MAFF report.)

In another incident the heating system continued to function in a house containing 82 pigs. The fans failed, and minimal natural ventilation resulted in the temperature reaching 46°C, and the death of 65 pigs. (VI Service report 1985).

CONVEX SOLE, or DROPPED SOLE. The sole of the horse's foot, instead of being arched (concave) when viewed from the ground surface, is convex and projects to a lower level than does the outer rim of the wall in many cases. (*See* LAMINITIS.)

CONVOLVULUS POISONING (*see under* MORN-ING GLORY).

CONVULSIONS are powerful involuntary contractions (alternating with relaxation) of muscles, producing aimless movement and contortion of the body, and accompanied by loss of consciousness. (*See* SPASM, FITS.)

COOMBS (antiglobulin) TEST is a valuable laboratory aid in the diagnosis of brucellosis in, for example, people and horses.

COOPWORTH. A breed of New Zealand sheep derived from the 'Border-Romney' cross.

COPD (*see* CHRONIC OBSTRUCTIVE PULMONARY DISEASE of horses).

COPPER is used in veterinary medicine in the form of various salts, notably the sulphate (other examples below). Copper sulphate is used in cases of copper deficiency, phosphorus poisoning, as a growth promoter in pigs, and to stimulate closure of the OESOPHAGEAL GROOVE.

Copper is also one of the trace elements which is essential in the nutrition of animals. It acts as a catalyst in the assimilation of iron, which is needed in the production of haemoglobin in the liver. Its absence from the foodstuffs eaten in some areas leads to a form of anaemia.

In several parts of the world a deficiency of copper in the herbage has been a major obstacle to livestock production, and appropriate dressings of the land have permitted dramatic increases in production.

In several parts of Britain copper deficiency is a serious condition. In cattle, it may be more widespread than was previously thought and may account for a reduced growth rate in calves in areas where copper deficiency has not hitherto been suspected. (*See* HYPOCUPRAEMIA.)

Two types of copper deficiency are recognised: primary and secondary. The former arises from an inadequate intake of copper and, while herbage levels of copper below 5 ppm are uncommon in Britain, a 1974 survey showed that over 50 per cent of 1078 beef herds in mid-Wales had low blood copper levels, probably associated with low intake.

Secondary copper deficiency is the more common form in the UK and occurs where absorption or storage within the animal body of copper is adversely affected by a high sulphate or molybdenum intake, even though there is adequate copper in the diet.

An excess of molybdenum in the 'teart' soils and pastures of central Somerset, and of areas in Gloucestershire, Warwickshire, Derbyshire and East Anglia, has long been recognised, giving rise to scouring (especially from May to October), a greyness of the hair around the eyes, staring coats and a marked loss of condition.

However, analysis of sediments from stream beds in many counties shows that herbage may contain excessively high concentrations of molybdenum.

Copper supplements given in the feed will not all contain sufficient copper to close the oesophageal groove, and so they will reach the rumen where molybdenum and/or sulphates may interfere with copper utilisation.

Work at the Animal Diseases Research Association and the Hill Farming Research Organisation has provided a new treatment for copper deficiency in cattle and sheep. Four conventional injections of copper can now be replaced by a single dose given by mouth.

The preparation used for this purpose consists of large, brittle particles of cupric oxide, administered to the animal in capsules. The cupric oxide is in the form of what the AFRC calls **'needles'**, obtained by oxidising copper wire, and their effectiveness is because 'large oral doses are tolerated and retained in the abomasum, where they slowly release absorbable copper.'

However, a single oral dose of cupric oxide needles can supplement sheep with copper for several months. But north Ronaldsay sheep absorb copper more efficiently than other breeds and are, therefore, more susceptible to copper poisoning. Two north Ronaldsay sheep dosed with 2 g of needles (the manufacturer's recommended dose) remained healthy but a third, dosed with 4 g, died of acute copper poisoning 19 days after dosing. It is important to use only the correct dose of cupric oxide needles in sheep known to be susceptible to copper poisoning and in the offspring from cross-breeding such animals. (Britt, D. P. and Yeoman, G. H. (1985) *Veterinary Research* **9**, 57.)

Molybdenum. Under field conditions at the Hill Farming Research Organisation a single dose given to ewes at lambing time, or to lambs when five weeks old, prevented the severe blood-copper deficiency which occurred in control animals grazing improved pastures containing high molybdenum and sulphur concentrations in the herbage.

Under experimental conditions at the Animal Diseases Research Association, a single dose effectively raised the liver copper reserves of steers and heifers to a satisfactory level. In ewes a small fraction of the known tolerable dose alleviated hypocupraemia in those kept on a copper-deficient diet for 286 days when the diet was low in molybdenum and sulphur, and for 117 days when these two elements were added to the diet.

The above treatment has the advantage that it does not involve injections – a consideration of some importance in relation to the spread of diseases such as scrapie and maedi/visna in sheep.

The same is true of the 'sustained release' capsules for oral dosage of ewes and lambs. (*See also* BOLUS.)

Caution – Sheep. Indiscriminate dressing of pasture with copper salts is likely to cause poisoning in sheep if the quantities used are too large, or if sheep are re-admitted to dressed pasture before there has been sufficient rain to wash the copper salts off the herbage.

Copper sulphate for pigs.

Copper sulphate, added to the fattening ration at the rate of 150–180 parts per million, has produced an improvement in the growth rate in pigs. (*See* SWAYBACK; *also* MOLYBDENUM.)

COPPER, POISONING BY. With the exception of sheep, which may be given an overdose to expel worms, animals are not likely to be poisoned through internal administration of copper sulphate *as a medicine.* Poisoning has occurred, however, in sheep given a copper-rich supplement, intended for pigs, over a 3½ months' period; in a heifer similarly, also in pigs given too strong a copper supplement. Poisoning also occurs when animals are grazed in the vicinity of copper-smelting works, where the herbage gradually becomes contaminated with copper, in orchards where fruit-trees have been sprayed with copper salts and also in sheep grazing land treated with copper sulphate (either crystals mixed with sand, or as a sprayed solution) as a snail-killer in the control of liver-fluke or as a preventative of swayback.

SIGNS are those of an irritant poison – pain, diarrhoea (or perhaps constipation), and weakness; staggering and muscular twitchings are seen in chronic cases. A fatal chronic copper poisoning may occur in pigs fed a copper supplement of 250 parts per million.

Failure to achieve accurate mixing of small quantities of copper sulphate into farm-mixed rations has led to fatal poisoning of pigs.

Mr R. M. Loosemore has pointed out that copper poisoning is almost specific to the housing of sheep. It occurs even on diets ostensibly containing no copper supplement. 'The capacity of the sheep for storing copper from the normal constituents of the diet is higher than that of other animals, and markedly higher in housed sheep.'

And it is a remarkable fact that lambs reared indoors have died because their hay was made from grass contaminated by slurry from pigs on a copper-supplemented diet.

It is dangerous to exceed 10 ppm of copper in dry feeds for sheep over a long period.

AFRC research has shown that the sheep's physiological response to copper is influenced by heredity, and that there are significant breed differences as regards SWAYBACK and copper poisoning. (*See also under* **needles** in the preceding section.)

TREATMENT. Following some Australian research, it was shown at the Rowett Research Institute that three subcutaneous injections of tetrathiomolybdate (on alternate days) can remove copper from the livers of both sheep and goats without causing any apparent ill-effects. (AFRC).

COPPERBOTTLE. *Lucilia cuprina*, the strike fly which attacks sheep in Australia and South Africa.

'COPPER NOSE'. A form of Light Sensitisation (which see) occurring in cattle.

COPROPHAGY. The eating of its faeces by an animal. In rabbits this is a normal practice. Within 3 weeks of birth, foals will eat their dams' faeces and thereby acquire the various bacteria needed for digestive purposes in their own intestines. Overnight coprophagy has also been reported in adult horses in adjusting to 'complete-diet' cubes when no hay is on offer.

It was further suggested that foals may obtain nutrients, and that coprophagy may be a response to a maternal pheromone signalling the presence of deoxycholic acid which may be required for gut 'immuno-competence' and myelination of the nervous system. (Crowell-Davis, S. L. & Houpt, K. A. (1985) *Equine Veterinary Journal* **17**, 17.)

COPULATION (*see* REPRODUCTION).

CORAMINE. Proprietary name of a solution of nikethamide; a valuable respiratory and circulatory stimulant, given by injection.

CORIUM. (*See* SKIN.)

'CORKSCREW PENIS' (*see* PENIS, DEVIATION OF).

CORN COCKLE POISONING. The plant *Lychnis* (or *Agrostemma*) *githago*, a weed of corn fields, is usually avoided by livestock; but they may be poisoned through eating wheat or barley meal contaminated with the seeds. The latter contain SAPONINS (which see).

Dogs and young animals are most susceptible to poisoning; the signs of which are restlessness, frothing at the mouth, colic, paralysis and loss of consciousness.

FIRST AID. Large amounts of white of egg, starch paste, and milk may be given to calves and dog as a drench.

CORNS. A bruise of the sensitive part of the horse's foot occurring in the angle formed between the wall of the hoof at the heel and the bar of the foot.

SIGNS. In the majority of cases the horse goes very lame either gradually or suddenly. When made to walk he does so by using the toe of the affected foot, keeping the heels raised. Sometimes the pain is so great that he refuses to place the affected foot on the ground at all, but hops on the sound foot of the other side.

TREATMENT. The shoe should be removed as in all cases of lameness, and the hard dry outer horn pared away. Particular attention should always be paid to the region of the heels, for stones often become lodged there. If a corn is present the horse will show pain whenever the knife is applied to the affected part, and efficient paring will necessitate an analgesic.

Mild cases take about 5 days to a week to recover, while horses with severe suppurating corns may be as long as 6 or 7 weeks before they are fit to work. (*See also* FOOT OF HORSE.)

CORNEA is the clear part of the front of the eye through which the rays of light pass to the retina. (*See* EYE.)

CORONARY is a term applied to several structures in the body encircling an organ in the manner of a crown. The coronary arteries are the arteries of supply to the heart which arise from the aorta, just beyond the aortic valve; through them blood is delivered with great pressure to the heart muscle.

CORONARY BAND, or CORONARY CUSHION, is the part of the sensitive matrix of the horse's foot from which grows the wall. It runs round the foot at the coronet, lying in a groove in the upper edge of the wall. Its more correct name is the *coronary matrix*. (*See* FOOT OF HORSE.)

CORONARY THROMBOSIS, associated with *Strongylus vulgaris*, is a cause of sudden death in yearling and 2-year-old horses. (*See* ARTERITIS, VERMINOUS.)

CORONAVIRUSES cause diarrhoea in calves, foals, dogs, cats, turkeys, sheep, and pigs (*see* TRANSMISSIBLE GASTRO-ENTERITIS OF PIGS); infectious bronchitis in chickens; hepatitis in mice, respiratory disease in mice; feline infectious peritonitis; and encephalomyelitis in pigs.

CORONET (*see* FOOT OF THE HORSE).

CORONOID PROCESSES. One of these is present on the MANDIBLE (lower jaw); the other on the ULNA.

CORPORA QUADRIGEMINA form a division of the brain. (*See* BRAIN.)

CORPUS LUTEUM. Also known as the *yellow body*, this is formed by the cells lining the empty follicular cavity, under the influence of the luteinising hormone, as explained under OVARY.

CORRIDOR DISEASE. This affects the African buffalo and also cattle, and is caused by the protozoan parasite *Theileria lawrencei*, transmitted by ticks. It resembles East Coast Fever, and has a 60 to 80 per cent mortality in cattle.

CORTICOSTEROIDS. These comprise the *natural* glucocorticoids, cortisone, and hydrocortisone – hormones from the adrenal gland; and the *synthetic* equivalents, *e.g.* prednisone, prednisolone, and fluoroprednisolone. (For the dangers of corticosteroid therapy, see *Vet. Record*, April 23, 1966.)

In veterinary medicine, corticosteroids are used in the treatment of inflammatory conditions, shock, stress, ketosis.

A corticosteroid given intravenously in late pregnancy is likely to induce abortion.

Referring to their use in human medicine, the *Lancet* commented in 1970: 'Controversy about the relative merits of corticosteroids and corticotrophins continues, particularly in the treatment of asthma and rheumatoid arthritis. There seems little evidence that one is more effective than the other, but no agreement can be reached on the question of whether one causes more pituitary suppression than the other. It is accepted that natural or synthetic corticosteroids may cause suppression of pituitary function and, in turn, adrenal atrophy. This serious complication may be especially dangerous in the presence of infection or after an operation.' (*See also* CORTISONE, ADRENAL GLANDS, DIABETES.)

Corticosteroids are immunosuppressive and contra-indicated when treating heartworm disease, *Filaroides hirthi* infestation, Catpox, etc.

CORTICOTROPHIN. The hormone from the anterior lobe of the pituitary gland which controls the secretion by the adrenal gland of corticoid hormones. These corticosteroids, or steroid hormones, are of three kinds: (1) those concerned with carbohydrate metabolism and which also allay inflammation; (2) those concerned with maintaining the correct proportion of electrolytes; (3) the sex corticoids.

CORTISOL. A steroid hormone from the adrenal gland.

CORTISONE. A hormone from the cortex of the adrenal gland. In medicine the acetate of cortisone is used, prepared from extracts of the adrenal cortex or partly synthetically. It is a white or cream-coloured crystalline powder almost insoluble in water.

Actions. Cortisone raises the sugar content of the blood and the glycogen content of the liver, among other actions.

Uses. Cortisone has been used with success in the temporary relief of rheumatoid arthritis, but when the drug is discontinued symptoms return. In human medicine, it has been concluded that long-continued cortisone treatment is not to be recommended. It has been used in the relief of navicular disease in the horse and of other forms of lameness, being given by injection into the joint involved. (*See Vet. Record*, Dec. 16, 1961.)

Cortisone has also been used in the treatment of acetonaemia in cattle, and successful results have been claimed.

The healing of wounds may be delayed in animals receiving cortisone. Over-dosage may give rise to wasting and diabetes. Cortisone has, when given by injection, a suppressive effect on antibody production and may increase an animal's susceptibility to viral infection. (*See* CORTICOSTEROIDS.)

CORYNEBACTERIUM. A genus of slender, Gram-positive bacteria which includes the cause of diphtheria in man. In veterinary medicine *C. pyogenes* is of importance, causing 'summer mastitis' and 'foul-in-the-foot' in cattle. A generalised infection has been reported, giving rise in cattle to lameness, slight fever, leg-swellings, lachrymation, and later emaciation and death.

C. suis is responsible for infectious cystitis and pyelonephritis in pigs.

C. ovis causes caseous lymphadenitis in sheep and some cases of ulcerative lymphangitis and acne in horses.

C. equi causes pneumonia in the horse and tuberculosis-like lesions in the pig.

COTTON-SEED CAKE or MEAL may, if undecorticated, contain up to 25 per cent of indigestible fibre, and lead to intestinal impaction if fed to calves or pigs. Gossypol poisoning may also result. (*See* GOSSYPOL.)

COTYLEDONS (*see* PLACENTA and PREGNANCY).

COUGHING.

Horses. Where coughing occurs with a normal temperature, horses may prove to be infested with the lung-worm *Dictyocaulus arnfieldi*. More common causes of coughing in horses include equine influenza; other virus infections; laryngitis and bronchitis from other causes; an allergic or asthmatic cough often heard in the autumn; strangles; and 'broken wind'.

(For a list of viruses which cause coughing (and also other symptoms) in the horse, *see* EQUINE RESPIRATORY VIRUSES.)

Clenbuterol is widely used for treatment.

Pigs. Coughing may be due to dusty meal or to enzootic pneumonia.

Dog. A sporadic yet persistent cough, noticed especially after exercise or excitement, may be a symptom of infestation with the common tracheal worm *Oslerus osleri*. Mortality among puppies of 4 to 8 months has been as high as 75 per cent in some litters, following emaciation. Less serious is infestation with *Capillaria aerophilia*, which may give rise to a mild cough. Far more commonly, however, a cough is a symptom of acute or chronic bronchitis. In the dog – often fat and middle-aged – chronic bronchitis may result in a cough persisting for weeks or months at a time and recurring in subsequent years, and is due to excessive secretion of mucus in the trachea and bronchi. It may follow an attack of pneumonia. A cough is also a symptom of valvular disease of the heart; *and see* KENNEL COUGH.

Cats. Coughing is (in addition to sneezing) one symptom of viral diseases such as Feline Viral Rhinotracheitis and Feline Calicivirus Infection; tonsillitis; as the result of grass seeds lodged in the pharynx; infestation by the cat lungworm; pleurisy; bronchitis; pneumonia; tuberculosis; and some cases of Feline Leukaemia. (*See under* separate headings).

Cattle. (*See* TUBERCULOSIS, PARASITIC BRONCHITIS.)

COUMARIN. A chemical compound present in sweet vernal grass, in sweet clovers, and other plants. Although harmless in itself, coumarin may be converted to DICOUMAROL (which see) if hay containing such plants becomes mouldy or overheated.

COW KENNELS. These have become popular as a cheaper (first cost) alternative to cubicle houses, though some have been developed to the point where they are almost cubicle houses, with the wood or metal partitions forming an integral part of the structure. Slurry can be a problem, and sometimes exposure to draughts and rain requires protection with straw bales or hardboard at the ends. (*See also* CUBICLES FOR COWS.)

COW-POX (*see* POX).

COW-POX, PSEUDO- (*see* MILKER'S NODULE).

COW'S MILK, ABSENCE OF. In a newly calved cow giving virtually no milk, the cause may be a second calf in the uterus, and a rectal examination is accordingly advised. A normal milk yield can be expected, in such cases, to follow the birth of the second calf which may occur a few months later. (*See* SUPERFOETATION, *also* AGALACTIA.)

COWS. Gentle treatment. Cows should at all times be quietly and gently treated. Hurried driving in and out of gates and doors, chasing by dogs, beating with sticks should not be tolerated. A cow in milk must have time to eat, chew, and digest her food in comfort, and rough treatment will not only interfere with digestion but will also disturb the nervous system which more or less controls the action of the milk-making glands, and thus lessens the milk yield. (*See* STRESS.)

Gentle treatment should begin with the calf, and be continued with the yearling, 2-year-old, and in-calf heifer; where it is customary to approach and handle young stock at all ages there will be no difficulty in the management and milking of the newly-calved heifer; her milk-yield will be increased, and much time will be saved. (*See* MILKING, *also* VETERINARY FACILITIES ON THE FARM.)

Comfort and fresh air. The housing provided should ensure comfort. In winter sufficient bedding should be provided to keep the cows warm and clean. (*See* HOUSING OF ANIMALS, RATIONS.)

COWBANE POISONING (*see* WATER HEMLOCK).

COWMEN. Occupational hazards include BRUCELLOSIS, LEPTOSPIROSIS, Q FEVER, TUBERCULOSIS, COWPOX, MILKER'S NODULE, SALMONELLA, SPOROTRICHOSIS, BUBONIC PLAGUE (not in the UK).

COWPER'S GLAND (*see* SEMEN).

COXALGIA means pain in the hip-joint.

COXIELLA (*see under* Q FEVER).

COYOTES are rabies-vectors in the USA.

CRAB LICE (*Phthirus pubis*) occasionally infest dogs, but this happens only in a household where people are infested.

CRACKED HEELS IN HORSES (*see under* NECROSIS, BACILLARY).

CRAMP. Painful involuntary contraction of a muscle. Cramp is of importance in the racing greyhound, which is observed to slow down and drag both hind-legs, or – in severe cases – may collapse and struggle on the ground. The animal's gait and appearance are 'wooden'. The muscles of the hindquarters are hard to the touch. Cyanosis may be present. Recovery usually takes place within a quarter of an hour, aided by rest and massage. Possible causes include: fatigue, defective heart action, bacterial or chemical toxins, sexual repression, a dietary deficiency, poor exercise, and cold. (*See also* SCOTTIE CRAMP.)

CRANIAL NERVES are those large and important nerves that originate from the brain. They are twelve in number, as follows:

1. Olfactory — Sensory (smell)
2. Optic — Sensory (sight)
3. Oculomotor — Motor
4. Trochlear or pathetic — Motor
5. Trigeminal or trifacial — Mixed
6. Abducent — Motor
7. Facial — Mixed
8. Auditory — Sensory (hearing and equilibration)
9. Glossopharyngeal — Mixed
10. Vagus or pneumo-gastric — Mixed
11. Spinal accessory or accessory — Motor
12. Hypoglossal — Motor

(*See also under* BRAIN.)

'CRAZY CHICK' DISEASE occurs in the USA, and also in the UK. It is associated with a diet too rich in fats, or containing food which has gone rancid, and Vitamin E has been used in its prevention. 'Crazy Chick' Disease has included not only this Nutritional Encephalomacia but also a virus disease of chicks under 6 weeks of age known as avian encephalomyelitis. Symptoms in each case include falling over and paralysis.

CREATINE (*see* MUSCLES, Action of).

CREATINE KINASE is an enzyme found mainly in muscle. The activity of this enzyme in serum or plasma is used as an aid to the diagnosis of skeletal or heart muscle lesions.

Early detection of intestinal necrosis 'remains difficult because there are few diagnostic tests' to detect it, but G. M. Greaber and colleagues found experimentally that creatinine kinase is a better indicator of mesenteric infarction in dogs than alkaline phosphatase, because serum levels of the former increase more and at a faster rate. (Graeber, G. M. & others (1984) *Journal of Surgical Research* **37**, 25.) (*See* ENZYMES.)

CREEP-FEEDING. The feeding of un-weaned piglets in the creep – a portion of the farrowing house or ark inaccessible to the sow and usually provided with artificial warmth. Creep-feeding often begins with a little flaked maize being put under a turf, and is followed by a proprietary or home-mixed meal from 3 to 8 weeks. Creep-feeding of in-wintered lambs and calves is also good practice.

Housed calves usually creep-feed hay or silage plus concentrates from a few weeks of age. Excessive creep feeding with concentrates before turn-out of autumn-born calves depresses gains at grass.

Creep feeding at grass from the late summer can improve calf performance. With autumn-born calves, creep feeding a total of up to 100 kg barley will improve weaning weights by up to 23 kg. But as the calves grow larger it is difficult to allow them access to a creep while excluding smaller cows. Some producers wean early, graze the calves on high-quality aftermaths and use the cows to eat down rougher areas. Because milk contributes more to the growth of spring-born calves, creep feeding can be delayed until later in the season. But in the last few weeks before weaning, a total of 40 kg barley can be expected to increase weaning weights by up to 15 kg.

Creep feeding of calves prior to weaning also has the advantage of conditioning them for future diets and guarding against any check in growth rate that may occur as a result of weaning. (*See* MLC figures.)

Effects of creep feeding on calf weaning weight

	Supplementary feed (kg)	Extra calf weaning wt. (kg)
Autumn-born calves	76	19
Spring-born calves	30	10

CREEP-GRAZING is a method of pasture management, enabling lambs to gain access to certain areas of pasture in advance of their dams.

CREOSOTED TIMBER may give rise to poisoning in young pigs where the wood is freshly treated. For disease in cattle from this cause *see under* HYPERKERATOSIS.

Cats are prone to creosote poisoning. Contaminated paws may be cleaned by coating them with cooking oil, and then washing this off with a mild detergent.

CREPITUS means the grating sound of fractured bones when handled.

CRESOL SOLUTIONS (*see* DISINFECTANTS).

CRETINISM. Dwarfism caused by an insufficiency of the hormone THYROXIN. (*See* THYROID GLAND.)

CREUTZFELDT-JAKOB DISEASE, which has a world-wide distribution, is characterised by spongiform degeneration of the brain. 'Once symptoms appear it is invariably fatal.' Transmission through a corneal transplant has occurred. (*British Medical Journal* (1988) **296**, 1581.)

CRIB-BITING and WIND-SUCKING are different varieties of the same vice, which are learned chiefly by young horses. In each case the horse swallows air. A 'crib-biter' effects this by grasping the edge of the manger or some other convenient fixture with the incisor teeth; it then raises the floor of the mouth; the soft palate is forced open; a swallowing movement occurs; and a gulp of air is passed down the gullet into the stomach. A 'wind-sucker' achieves the same end, but it does not require a resting-place for the teeth. Air is swallowed by firmly closing the mouth, arching the neck, and gulping down air in much the same way.

In crib-biters the incisor teeth of both jaws show signs of excessive wear.

Remedial measures are not always satisfactory. Crib-biters may cease the habit if housed in a bare loose-box, being fed from a trough which is removed as soon as the feed is finished.

Proprietary preparation, with an unpleasant taste, are available for treating woodwork.

Surgical methods have been tried – Forssell's operation and, for wind-sucking, buccostomy – with success, it is claimed.

Ten horses underwent myectomy of the sternothyroid, sternohyoid and omohyoid muscles together with denervation of the sternomandibular muscles (neurectomy of the ventral branches of accessory nerves) to correct crib-biting. The claimed advantages are a smaller wound, faster healing and a better cosmetic result. Eight horses were cured.

Fricker, C. & Hugelhofer, J. (1981) *Schweizer Archiv für Tierheilkunde* **123**, 219.)

CROP, of birds, is a dilatation of the gullet at the base of the neck, just at the entrance to the thorax. In it the food is stored for a time and softened with fluids. It acts as a reservoir from which the food can be passed downwards into the stomach, gizzard, etc., in small amounts.

CROP, DISEASES OF. By far the commonest trouble affecting the crop of the bird is that known as 'crop-bound', in which food material collects in the crop through the swallowing of bodies which cannot pass on to the stomach and gizzard, such as feathers, wool, straw, small pieces of stick, etc. Other cases are due to a lack of vitality in the walls of the crop, which become too weak to force the contents onwards.

The dilated crop can often be noticed pendulous and distended. Death occurs from exhaustion unless relief is obtained. Massage of the impacted food material from the outside, along with the introduction of warm liquid in small amounts through a rubber tube, may be sufficient to dispel mild impactions, but usually surgical opening is required. (*See under* CAGE BIRDS.)

CROSS-IMMUNITY. Immunity resulting from infection with one disease-producing organism against another. For example, rinderpest virus infection in dogs gives rise to a degree of immunity against canine distemper virus.

CROSS PREGNANCY. Development of a fetus in the opposite horn of the uterus to that side on which ovulation occurred. Migration from one horn to the other may occur.

CROUP of the horse is that part of the hind-quarters lying immediately behind the loins. The 'point of the croup' is the highest part of the croup, and corresponds to the internal angles of the ilia. The crupper of the harness passes over the croup, and derives its name from it.

CROWS. Carrion crows often cause injury to ewes and lambs, sometimes death, and in addition they may transmit CAMPYLOBACTER infection.

In India house crows (*Corvus splendens*), which live in close contact with people and domestic animals, can be important in the transmission of Newcastle disease to domestic poultry. The crows themselves may show no symptoms, but can excrete highly virulent virus over a short period.

CRUCIATE LIGAMENTS are two strong ligaments in the stifle-joint which prevent any possibility of over-extension of the joint. They are arranged in the form of the limbs of the letter X. Degenerative changes leading to rupture of one or both ligaments in dogs engaged in strenuous exercise (*e.g.* police dogs, gun dogs, sheepdogs) is common among all breeds and gives rise to lameness. If both ligaments are ruptured, instability of the joint follows, and surgery may be necessary if lameness is severe. However, strict rest for 8 weeks, is often successful in itself, especially when only one ligament is involved. (J. R. Campbell, *Vet. Rec.* (77), **101**, 318.)

CRUELTY, AVOIDANCE OF (*see* LAW; ANAESTHESIA, LEGAL REQUIREMENTS; CASTRATION; TRANSPORT; WATER; EUTHANASIA; DOCKING; NICKING; WELFARE CODES; NUTRITION, FAULTY; STRESS; TETHERING; OVERSTOCKING).

CRURAL. Relating to the leg.

CRUSH. An appliance constructed of wood or tubular steel, and used for holding cattle, etc., in order to facilitate tuberculin testing, inoculations, the taking of blood samples, etc.

A wooden crush is better than a metal one because it involves less noise; clanging metalwork can be alarming to cattle. Collecting cattle in darkened pens or boxes an hour before testing is due to begin makes for better behaviour in the crushes.

One of the best crushes described in the *Vet. Record* 'is in a building through which the cows always come on leaving the parlour. The two ends are solid and fixed in concrete. The sides consist of iron gates hinged one on the front and the other on the back of the crush. Before an animal enters, the gate hinged on the front is opened back against the wall. This provides a wide space and she is not asked to enter a narrow confine. When she is in, the gate is shut and the neck secured with a rope. The other gate may now be opened and testing done without reaching through the side of the crush'.

A funnel-shaped pen for filling the crush is useful, and if the crush is big enough to hold two animals, the second will enter more readily. Fast working can be achieved with a race to hold 7 or 8 cows; there being 2 men each with a rope on the side opposite to the veterinary surgeon. The whole batch is tested before release.

For testing purposes, as opposed to dehorning, the use of a rope – preferably fitted with a steel eye or ring – is far better than a yoke. Indeed, some yokes with a narrow 'V' at the bottom, are dangerous. Cattle tend to lean on them, and may lose consciousness in a matter of seconds and even die in the crush. Covering in the sides and end of a crush at the bottom tends to make cattle keep their heads up.

The conventional neck-yoking feature of cattle crushes was abandoned in a design announced by MAFF in 1982. The animal is restrained by pressure from the sides of the crush moving together. Cattle were said to enter it more readily and to stand more quietly in it.

It is generally agreed that behaviour in crushes is partly dependent upon breed. For example, Dairy Shorthorns are generally docile, Ayrshires easily alarmed, and Friesians often more angry than frightened. Angus and Galloways seem to resent the crush rather than be alarmed by it.

Much also depends, of course, upon gentle treatment and avoiding the indiscriminate use of sticks. Some farm workers never learn to hold cattle properly by their noses, but push a thumb into one nostril and try and cram all their fingers into the other – naturally the animal struggles for breath! Even when it is done properly, Angus and Galloways seem to dislike this form of restraint intensely.

It may save a lot of time in the end if animals are *accustomed* to being put into a crush. An experiment at the Ministry's central veterinary laboratory involved weekly weighings of 60 adult heifers, which were obstreperous in the extreme. Each was led (with a head-collar, not a halter) from its standing in a cowshed to a crate mounted on the low platform of a large weighing machine in a yard. The first weighing occupied two strenuous periods totalling 135 minutes. The thirty-seventh weighing was accomplished in 38 minutes! The heifers not only learnt what was expected of them but seemed to relish this break in their routine; trotting into the crate, coming to a dead stop, and standing stock still while the weighing machine beam was adjusted. (*See also* VETERINARY FACILITIES ON FARMS.)

'CRUTCHING' means shearing of wool from sheep's breech, tail, and back of hind-legs. It is done before May and in autumn as an aid to controlling 'Strike'.

CRYOSURGERY. Destruction of unwanted tissue (*e.g.* of a tumour) by the use of very low temperatures. For example, a metal rod, cooled in liquid nitrogen to $-196°C$, may be applied to the tumour.

Dogs. Cryotherapy has been found useful in several conditions, including intractable inter-digital cysts and 'lick granuloma'.

Cats. It has been used for the relief of highly irritant eczema, and also eosinophilic granulomatous lesions; especially those involving the lips and hard palate. Trevor Turner has used it with success in cats suffering from chronic gingivitis/stomatitis; employing for this purpose a spray of liquid nitrogen for about 15 seconds, repeated for three freeze/thaw cycles. 'Following reduction of the initial oedema, all (14) cats have shown an improvement in appetite and a reduction in signs of pain when eating.'

The treatment may need repeating at 8-month intervals. (Turner, T. (1986) *Veterinary Record* **118**, 251.)

Horses. Cryosurgery is valuable in the treatment of sarcoids, squamous cell carcinoma and other neoplastic conditions of the skin, and for the removal of excessive granulation tissue. In ophthalmology it can be used for the treatment of retinal detachments, iris prolapse, glaucoma and the extraction of cataracts. Cryoneurectomy has been reported, particularly in the treatment of navicular disease. (Munroe, G. A. (1986) *Equine Veterinary Journal* **18**, 14.)

CRYPTOCOCCOSIS. Infection with the yeast *Cryptococcus neoformans* occurs occasionally in all species. Lungs, udder, brain, etc., may be involved. It has been described as the least rare of fungal infections in the cat – in which it may give rise to sneezing, a discharge from the eyes, and sometimes to a nasal granuloma. Other signs include cough, dyspnoea.

Bone and eye lesions may be produced. (*See also* EPIZOOTIC LYMPHANGITIS.)

CRYPTORCHID. An animal in which one or both testicles have not descended into the scrotum from the abdominal cavity at the usual time. The condition may cause some irritability in the animal. The retained testicle(s) may be defective. (*See also under* GELDING.)

In several breeds of pigs it has been shown that some individual males start with two apparently normal testicles in the scrotum at birth, but that within a few weeks or months one testicle may decrease in size and then may disappear from the scrotum, ascending back into the inguinal canal inside the abdomen. Absorption of this testicle may occur, so that by the time the animal is 6 months old there may be no remains, or virtually none, of the missing testicle to be found.

The name 'late cryptorchids' has been given to such animals which have two testicles in the scrotum at birth, but subsequently only one. A research worker at the Central Veterinary Laboratory, Weybridge, has referred to the finding of 44 such late cryptorchids out of 110 cryptorchid Lacombe boars. (*See also under* MONORCHID *and*, re equine cryptorchids, IMMUNO-CASTRATION.)

CRYPTOSPORIDIOSIS. Disease caused by protozoan parasites of the genus *Cryptosporidium* and of the order Coccidia. *Cryptosporidia* are not host-specific like other coccidia.

Transmission is via an oocyst stage. The parasites cause diarrhoea in calves, piglets, kittens, etc., and respiratory disease in poultry.

Cattle. In Norway Henriksen and colleagues examined samples from over 4,000 **cattle**. Diagnosis was based on the detection of oocysts in smears from small intestine mucosa, colon contents, or faeces. The highest prevalence was found in calves aged 4 to 30 days, with a peak figure in the age group 8 to 14 days (25 per cent positive). Adult pigs may be carriers.

Cats. The disease was found after euthanasia of a 6-month-old **cat** with an eight weeks' history of diarrhoea, inappetance, and weight loss.

In a second case described by M. Bennett & others, cryptosporidium oocysts were found in the faeces of a kitten, following diagnosis of the disease in its owner, a 5-year-old boy undergoing treatment for leukaemia. This kitten had no diarrhoea.

Public health. Person-to-person and cattle-to-person infection can occur. Possible transmission from a cat to its owner has also been reported. (Bennett, M. (1985) *Veterinary Record* **116**, 73.) Pigmen, abattoir workers, and vets need to take precautions. ☞

TREATMENT. There is as yet no specific treatment, but *see* COCCIDIOSIS, Control.

CUBES and PELLETS. A cow takes about 10 minutes to eat 8 lb of cubes: a fact of some importance in the milking parlour where time may not permit of a high-yielder receiving her entire concentrate ration. (The figure for meal is about 6 lb in 10 minutes.) (Compare also with LIQUID FEEDING.)

It is sometimes suggested that cubes can replace hay for horses on pasture in winter, or for rabbits, chinchilla, etc., which are not out at grass. However, roughage is needed in addition for peristalsis and the health of the digestive system. (*See also* HORSES, FEEDING OF, DRIED GRASS.)

The type of lubricant used in cubing and pelleting machines is important; hyperkeratosis can

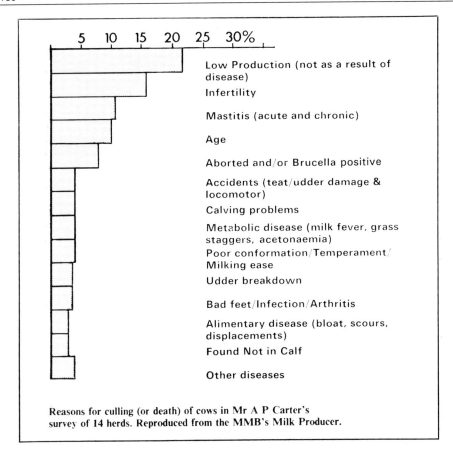

5   10   15   20   25   30%

Low Production (not as a result of disease)

Infertility

Mastitis (acute and chronic)

Age

Aborted and/or Brucella positive

Accidents (teat/udder damage & locomotor)

Calving problems

Metabolic disease (milk fever, grass staggers, acetonaemia)

Poor conformation/Temperament/Milking ease

Udder breakdown

Bad feet/Infection/Arthritis

Alimentary disease (bloat, scours, displacements)

Found Not in Calf

Other diseases

Reasons for culling (or death) of cows in Mr A P Carter's survey of 14 herds. Reproduced from the MMB's Milk Producer.

arise in cattle if an unsuitable one is used. (*See* LUBRICANTS.)

CUBICLES FOR COWS. These leave the cows free to come and go between the silage face and the cubicles, which have a concave floor (to retain sawdust) sloping slightly backwards away from the wall. For larger breeds of cows the cubicles are made about 6 ft 9 in long by 3 ft 9 in. Two horizontal rails, the lower one not less than 15 in high, divide the cubicles. The cubicles are raised 6 to 12 in, to prevent a cow backing in and soiling the litter. Where sawdust is used, about 10 lb is required per cow, per week, and the system is much cheaper than with straw used in conventional housing.

There are now several types of cubicle. It appears that the type of heelstones, floor, and the width are important factors in determining whether cows take to cubicles or not. (*See also* COW KENNELS.) Bad design can lead to injury and lameness.

CUBONI TEST for pregnancy involves a single urine sample. It is an alternative to rectal palpation in the mare.

CUD and CUDDING (*see* RUMINATION).

CUFFING PNEUMONIA. A pneumonia of calves caused by a virus or mycoplasma. A chronic cough is the usual symptom. It is so called because a 'cuff' or sheath of lymphocytes forms around the bronchioles.

CULLING diseased, infertile or low-yielding animals, or those of poor conformation is a necessary process in herd improvement.

The histogram (above) illustrates the reasons for culling or death of cows in 14 herds, totalling 1350 animals, as revealed by a survey carried out by Mr A. P. Carter, the Milk Marketing Board's veterinary officer at Chippenham. Altogether, 240 cows were culled or died during the 12 months' period – or 17·7 per cent.

CULTURE MEDIUM. That substance in or upon which bacteria and other pathogenic organisms are grown in the laboratory. Such media include nutrient agar, broths, nutrient gelatin, sugar media, and many special ones adapted to the requirements of particular organisms. Viruses cannot be grown in such media but require living cells, *e.g.* of chick embryos.

CURARE is a dark-coloured extract from trees of the *Strychnos* family, used by the South American

---

Indians as an arrow poison. Such arrow-heads were used by a veterinary surgeon in 1835 in treating tetanus in a horse and a donkey.

Curare, when injected under the skin, is one of the most powerful and deadly poisons known, but by the mouth it is harmless, since the kidneys are able to excrete it as rapidly as it is absorbed, and it does not collect in the system. Its action depends on the presence of an alkaloid, *curarine*, which paralyses the motor nerve-endings in muscle, and so throws the muscular system out of action yet leaving the sensory nervous system unaffected. Consequently an animal into which the drug is injected lies incapable of the slightest action, but fully conscious of its surroundings. Finally, death results. A standardised preparation of tubocurarine is now available and is of use to ensure full muscular relaxation during anaesthesia. (*See also under* MUSCULAR RELAXANTS.)

CURB is a swelling which occurs about a hand's-breadth below the point of the hock, due to sprain, or local thickening of the calcaneocuboid ligament, or to similar conditions affecting the superficial flexor tendon. Lameness is usually present at first.

'CURLED TONGUE'. A deformity occurring in turkey poults, due to feeding an all-mash diet, composed of very small particles in a dry state, during the first few weeks of life. If a change is made to wet feeding many of the poults will become normal.

CUSHING'S SYNDROME. This has been recognised and treated in the dog, and occurs usually after the age of 5 years, and cat.
CAUSE. Excessive production of corticosteroids by the adrenal cortex. In some cases there is a tumour affecting the adrenal gland or the pituitary; in others merely excessive growth of the adrenal cortex.

'Pituitary tumours are thought to account for at least 80 per cent of cases of the syndrome.' (Gruffyd-Jones, T. J. *Veterinary Record* (1989) **124**, 317.)
SIGNS. These include lethargy, premature ageing, baldness, skin eruptions, thirst, 'pot belly', and an appetite which at times could be described as ravenous. Wasting of the temporal muscles may be seen. Skin changes may not occur until up to a year after thirst becomes noticeable.

There may also be a change of coat colour. This was seen in a 6-year-old male poodle. The dog had been clipped eight months previously. On each side of the trunk the coat was now sparse and fluffy, and instead of being an apricot colour was now pure white, *Veterinary Practice* stated.

The dog was drinking over 800 ml of water per day, and scavenging for food. A diagnosis of Cushing's disease was confirmed by means of the adrenocorticotrophic hormone (ACTH) test.
TREATMENT with mitotane (Lysodren; Bristol-Myers) given orally completely restored this miniature poodle's health and, with a weekly maintenance dose, there was no recurrence of the disease at the end of three years. The coat colour reverted to apricot.

This treatment is a preferable alternative to surgery, but success has followed surgical removal of both adrenal glands where intensive care has been provided both before and after the operation. Salt supplementation and implants of desoxycorticosterone acetate (DOCA) are necessary following the adrenalectomy.

CUTANEOUS means belonging or pertaining to the skin. (*See* SKIN.)

CUTANEOUS ASTHENIA is associated with defects in the formation and maturing of collagen fibres. The skin becomes fragile and more elastic than normal, and a dog's skin may appear 'too big for its body'. (The human equivalent is the Ehlers-Danlos syndrome.)

CUTTER. A pork pig weighing 140–190 lb (liveweight) or 100–140 lb (dead-weight).

CUTTING (*see* BRUSHING.)

CVH. Canine Virus Hepatitis.

CYANIDES are salts of hydrocyanic or prussic acid. They are all highly poisonous. (*See* GLYCERIDES, HYDROCYANIC ACID.)

CYANOBACTERIA (blue-green algae) are micro-organisms able to convert nitrogen from the air to ammonia, using the enzyme nitrogenase and sunlight as the energy source; water providing the necessary reductant. Cyanobacteria contribute fixed nitrogen to soils; aiding agriculture and especially rice crops.

(For **Cyanobacterial poisoning,** *see* ALGAE POISONING.)

CYANO-COBALAMIN. This is the water-soluble vitamin B_{12} which contains cobalt. Hydroxo-cobalamin, vitamin B_{12a}, is in mice an antidote to cyanide poisoning.

CYANOSIS. A blue or purple discolouration of the tongue, lips, gums when there is a shortage of oxygen in the blood. It sometimes results when excessive strain is put upon the heart, in animals that have been hunted or chased. It is a symptom of nitrite poisoning, and also occurs in a few cases of feline pyothorax, and in ASPHYXIA.)

CYCLONITE POISONING. A plastic explosive, known as PE4, has as its active ingredient cyclonite, and this has caused poisoning in a police dog trained to detect explosives. In both dogs and man the poison causes epileptiform convulsions, best controlled by diazepam given intravenously, plus barbiturates if necessary. In the above case, the dog bit into some of the PE4 which had been concealed for a training exercise.

CYCLOPHOSPHAMIDE. This has been used (not in the UK) as a chemical means of defleecing sheep, and of treating mycotic dermatitis.

CYCLOPROPANE-OXYGEN ANAESTHESIA.
A costly but otherwise useful form of anaesthesia for dogs and cats. It has also been used for horses and goats. Cyclopropane is an inflammable gas.

CYCLOPS. This genus of minute crustaceans act as intermediate hosts of the broad tapeworm of man, dog, and cat.

CYPRESS POISONING. This is rare. A 1962 report refers to the death of two yearling heifers. They had been in a field where several cypress trees (*Cupressus sempervirens*) were felled one morning. One heifer was dead by the afternoon; the other two nights later.

CYSTIC CALCULI (*see* CALCULI).

CYSTIC OVARIES (*see* OVARIES).

CYSTICERCOSIS (*see* TAPEWORMS).

CYSTINE. An amino acid (and a constituent of some urinary calculi).

CYSTITIS means inflammation of the bladder. (*See* URINARY BLADDER, DISEASES OF.)

CYSTOPEXIA. Surgical fixture of the urinary bladder to the wall of the abdomen.

CYSTS. This term is applied to swellings containing fluid or soft material, other than pus, and to hollow tumours – usually non-malignant.

Varieties.
(*a*) *Retention cyst.* This may be no more than a swollen sebaceous gland, filled with its normal secretion which has been unable to reach the skin surface owing to blockage of its duct. Retention cysts of other glands arise similarly.
(*b*) *Ovarian cysts* are formed when some disturbance of the normal function of the ovary occurs. They are formed from failure of a Graäfian follicle to burst and release its ovum. They may grow to a large size or may become multiple. They generally give rise to symptoms of nymphomania in mares and cows, and lead to temporary or permanent infertility. (*See* OVARIES, DISEASES OF.)

(*c*) *Developmental cysts.* The most important of these are dermoid cysts. (*See* DERMOID CYST.)
(*d*) *Hydatid cysts* are produced in internal organs through the ingestion of the eggs of tapeworms from other animals. They occur in the peritoneal cavity, liver, spleen, brain, etc.
(*e*) *Hard tumour cysts* sometimes occur in tumours growing in connection with glands, such as the adeno-carcinomata, which may occur in the mammary gland.
(*f*) *'Interdigital cysts'* in between the toes of dogs are in reality often granulomas or abscesses. (*See* INTERDIGITAL ABSCESSES IN DOGS.)

CYTOECTES (*see* EHRLICHIOSIS, BLOOD PARASITES of British cattle).

CYTOGENETICS, or the study of chromosomes, received a great stimulus when it was found in 1959 that Mongolism and various other congenital abnormalities in man were associated with abnormal chromosomes.

Veterinary cytogenetics, as a science, has advanced more slowly, due to lack of facilities and 'the great difference in attitude to congenital abnormalities between those responsible for babies and those responsible for domestic animals', to quote Dr J. A. Harvey, MRCVS, speaking at the 1975 BVA Congress. Nevertheless, in recent years several 'chromosomal aberrations' have been detected; and the chromosome screening of bulls has become standard practice in several countries.

Chromosome analysis. Usually white blood-cells are used, and these are inoculated into a liquid tissue culture medium, supplemented with serum and antibiotics. Phytohaemaglutinin, a plant extract which stimulates the white cells to divide, is added. The cultures are incubated for two days at 38°C. Then colchicine is added to arrest the dividing cells at the metaphase stage. Hypotonic solutions are used to swell the cells and spread out the chromosomes. The cells are then fixed, dropped on to slides, and stained.

Suitable cells containing well-spread chromosomes are selected on the slides after examining them under the microscope at 1000 magnifications. Some of the cells are then photographed, and the individual chromosomes cut out from the prints, paired and stuck on to a card. This is called the *karyotype*.

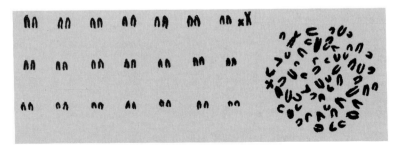

Left: the karyotype. (With acknowledgements to Dr C. R. E. Halnan and to the *Veterinary Record*.)
Right: a bull's lymphocyte in metaphase of mitosis.

Examples of chromosome abnormalities in cattle are: the freemartin. Whereas the normal heifer calf has a karyotype 60, XX, the freemartin has a proportion of XY cells. The condition is technically known as *XX:XY Chimerism*.

CENTRIC FUSIONS (Robertsonian translocations) are the result of two chromosomes fusing to form one, so that the total number of chromosomes in the cells is reduced. The *1/29 translocation* was discovered by Gustavsson in about 1 in 7 of the Swedish Red and White breed of cattle, and has since been found in many other breeds. This autosomal abnormality, involving a member of each of pairs 1 and 29, has been found to be inherited through both the male and the female in Red Poll and Charolais cattle in Britain, and appears to be associated with lowered fertility in the female.

Another common centric fusion is the *13/21 translocation,* first found in 1973 in a New Zealand bull of the Swiss Simmental breed, and in 1974 in that bull's sire in Scotland.

Many other chromosomal abnormalities have been found. (*See* MOSAIC, TRISOMY, TRANSLOCATION, POLYPLOIDY.)

Cytogenetics has also proved useful in confirming or detecting the origins of some breeds of cattle. For example, in Australia Dr C. R. E. Halnan and Professor J. Francis have stated: 'The Africander has anatomical and other characteristics of an animal of approximately 3/4 *Bos indicus* heredity. The fact that these cattle carry the *Bos taurus* Y chromosome supports this view and indicates that the local cattle in South Africa would have been crossed with one or more *Bos*

taurus bulls. Droughtmaster and Braford cattle retain the *Bos indicus* Y chromosome because *Bos indicus* instead of *Bos taurus* bulls were used to establish these *taurindicus* breeds.' (*Vet. Rec.* (1976), **98**, 88–90.)

Chromosome abnormalities have also been detected in infertile mares. One, which had never shown oestrus, was found to have the karyotype 63, X; *i.e.* lacking an X chromosome. Another mare, which had shown irregular oestrus, had the karyotype 63, X/64, X; *i.e.* containing both the abnormal cell line and normal cells.

(*See also* 'Sex chromosome mosaicism and infertility in mares'. Halnan, C. R. E. (1985) *Veterinary Record* **116**, 542.)

CYTOKINES. Naturally occurring compounds which cause tumours either to grow more slowly, or to destroy the malignant cells. (*See* INTERFERON, the first to be discovered.) Genetic engineering has made possible large-scale production of cytokines.

CYTOTOXIC DRUGS have been used in human medicine for the treatment of cancer. Some use of them has also been made of them in veterinary practice in the USA; for example, in the treatment of canine lymphosarcoma. A side-effect of cyclophosphamide is haemorrhagic cystitis.

HAZARDS. Use of these drugs presents serious risks to health from residue disposal, spillage, etc. Miscarriage in nurses was twice as frequent in those who had been exposed to anti-cancer drugs, according to a study in Finland at 17 hospitals, as compared with unexposed nurses.

D

D-VALUE. This is the percentage of digestible organic matter in the dry matter of the feed.

D-value is used to assess or describe the digestibility of animal feeds, such as dried grass, hay, silage, etc.

DF-2. A Gram-negative bacillus commonly present in the mouths of healthy dogs. It has caused death in immunosuppressed people and alcoholics, and those who have had a splenectomy. (McCarthy, M. & Zumla, A. *BMJ* (1988) **26**, 1355.)

'DAFT LAMBS'. Those affected with cerebellar atrophy – a condition associated with incoordination of head and leg movements. AFRC research has shown it to be due to a recessive gene. (*See* Genetic Defects under GENETICS.)

'DAGGING'. Removal of soiled wool by shepherd from sheep's hindquarters as an aid to preventing 'Strike'.

DAIRY HERD MANAGEMENT. Even in 1970 herd size averaged only 30 in the UK, and 80 per cent of cows were still tied up in cowsheds. There was, however, a growing movement towards larger herds, and many of those which formerly were 50 to 70 cows became 90 to 120 in size, while there are several 300-cow units, and a few larger still.

Increase in size became accompanied by other changes: notably, milking in a parlour and housing in a cubicle house instead of in a cowshed. (*See* CUBICLES FOR COWS, COW KENNELS.) There has been a tendency to replace the tandem parlour by the herringbone. Parlour feeding is now, in some very up-to-date units related automatically to milk yield; and this both makes for economy and avoids the problem of cow identification in the big herd, so far as the milker is concerned. Identification is still necessary, however, for use in conjunction with herd records and in the parlour where the milker or relief milker (who will rarely know all the cows) must feed according to yield in the absence of automated equipment. Plastic numbered collars, anklets, discs on chain or nylon, freeze branding and even udder tattooing are the methods currently used.

Feeding outside the parlour has been mechanised in many large units by means of auger feeders delivering direct from tower silos. In others, side-delivery trucks are drawn by tractor down the feeding passages and deliver into the long mangers. Self-feed silage, with the clamp face in or near the cubicle house, is another labour-saver. Group feeding (*e.g.* of dry cows, high yielders, and low yielders) is convenient management practice but may give rise to stress (*see* BUNT ORDER). (*See also under* 'STEAMING UP' and the advice on feeding given under ACETONAEMIA – prevention.)

ADAS advice stresses the need for adequate feeding in early lactation. 'Since appetite is often limited at this stage, only the highest quality food should be fed: whether it is good hay, early cut silage, or 3½ lb per gallon cake. This will allow optimum intake of nutrients at the responsive stage of the lactation – weeks 1–12 after calving.'

Zero-grazing is practised on some farms where poaching is a serious problem in wet weather, or where the movement of a large number of cows is involved. With a very large herd on a very small acreage (such as an American 550-cow herd on under 5 acres) zero-grazing obviously becomes essential.

Paddock grazing now forms an important part of dairy herd management, and includes the two-sward system in which separate areas are used for grazing and for conservation.

Dung disposal presents difficulties with large herds. There are two ways: treat it as a solid or a liquid? Straw bedding lends itself to solid muck handling, with the liquid (urine, washing-down water, rainwater) being taken separately to a lagoon or to an underground tank. Slatted floors can be used in a cubicle house, either over a dung cellar which is cleared out once a year, or over a channel leading to an underground tank. With the semi-solid method, dung may be spread on the land by tanker, or the slurry may pass to a lagoon or be pumped through an organic irrigation pipeline system.

Where this is used, cows must not be expected to graze pasture until there has been time for rain to wash the slurry off the herbage. The use of organic irrigation is not entirely free from the risk of spreading infectious diseases.

Poaching must be avoided by the use of concrete aprons at gateways, by mobile drinking troughs, by wide corridors between paddocks with an electric fence dividing the 'corridor' so that one half can be kept in reserve, or by moveable ramps as used in New Zealand.

In the large herd one of the biggest problems is spotting the bulling heifer or the cow on heat. Properly kept herd records can be a help in alerting cowmen to the approximate dates. (*See* CALVING INTERVAL; OESTRUS, DETECTION OF; CONTROLLED BREEDING.)

On several large units regular weekly visits by veterinary surgeons help in the detection and treatment of infertility and the application of veterinary preventive medicine. (*See* HEALTH SCHEMES, CULLING, and VETERINARY FACILITIES ON FARMS; CALF HOUSING; *also* 'CONTROLLED BREEDING' *and* CATTLE HUSBANDRY.)

DANGEROUS DOGS ACT 1991 (*see* LAW, THE).

DANGEROUS WILD ANIMALS ACT 1976.
This requires people keeping lions, tigers, poisonous snakes, certain monkeys and other unusual

pets, such as crocodiles and bears, to obtain a licence – authorised by a veterinary surgeon.

Local authorities have power to refuse licences, on the advice of an authorised veterinary surgeon, on such grounds as safety, nuisance or inadequate or unsuitable accommodation.

Before a licence is granted local authorities must be satisfied about arrangements for the animal's food, exercise and general comfort, fire precautions, and precautions against infectious diseases.

People with such animals will have to take out insurance.

Conviction for the keeping of an animal without a licence or contravening a condition of one could result in a fine of up to £400 and a ban from holding a licence.

Zoos, circuses, pet shops and research workers are exempted under the Act. (*See* LICENSING ACT 1981.)

DANISH RED CATTLE. More than half the cattle in Jutland, and 97 per cent of those in the Islands, belong to this breed, which is a very old one, though its official name (meaning Red Danish Milk breed) dates from 1878.

Danish Reds are strong, dual-purpose animals with a good 'barrel', teats and udders, and weigh between 1100 and 1700 lb. In 1955 a Danish Red gave over 2850 gallons. (*See also* BRITISH DANE *under* CATTLE, BREEDS OF.)

DANOFLOXACIN. A fluoroquinalone which has proved successful in the treatment of acute bacterial pneumonia in cattle.

DAPSONE. A bacteriostatic given by injection into the udder in cases of mastitis due to *Streptococcus agalactiae*; and by mouth in the treatment of coccidiosis in cattle.

DARNEL POISONING. The grass known as 'Darnel' (*Lolium temelentum*). It is a common weed in cereal crops and in pastures in some parts, but it does no harm when eaten before the seeds are ripe (or almost so). Many instances are on record where harmful results to man and animals have followed the use of meal or flour which contained ground-up darnel seeds, and there are numerous references in classic literature to the harmful effect produced upon the eyes as the result of eating bread made from flour containing darnel.

TOXIC PRINCIPLE is a narcotic alkaloid, called *temuline*, which is said to be present to the extent of about 0·66 per cent, but some authorities assert that a substance called *loliine*, and others that *pricrotoxin*, should be considered responsible. A fungus called *Endoconidium temulentum* is very often found present in the seeds of darnel, living a life that is to a great extent one of symbiosis; and the poisonous alkaloid *temuline* is found in the fungus.

SIGNS. Darnel produces giddiness and a staggering gait, drowsiness and stupefaction, dilatation of the pupils in the horse, and interference with vision in almost all animals. Vomiting, loss of sensation, convulsive seizures, and death follow when it is eaten by animals in large amounts. In some cases tremblings of the surface muscles are seen, and the extremities of the body become cold. Death usually occurs within 30 hours of eating the darnel seeds.

FIRST-AID. Strong black tea or coffee at once.

DARROW'S SOLUTION is used for fluid replacement therapy in cases of a potassium deficiency, and contains potassium chloride, sodium chloride and sodium lactate. It is useful in calf scours. (*See under* DEHYDRATION.)

DART GUNS/SYRINGES (*see under* PROJECTILE SYRINGES).

DATURINE. An alkaloid. (*See under* STRAMOMIUM.)

DAY-OLD CHICKS (*see* CHICKS).

DDT. The common abbreviation for dichloro-diphenyl-trichlorethane, a potent parasiticide, lethal to fleas, lice, flies, etc. DDT was once used incorporated in dusting powders, for applying to animals; and dissolved in solvents for use as a fly-spray. DDT-resistant insects are now found in nearly all countries, unfortunately, and the dangers of DDT residues in human and animal tissues has led to its abandonment in the UK and elsewhere.

DDT preparations should not be applied to animals, owing to the risk of poisoning. The use of DDT with oils or fats enhances its toxic effects, and should be avoided. Symptoms of poisoning include coldness, diarrhoea, and hyperaesthesia. Minute doses over a period result in complete loss of appetite. DDT sprays may contaminate milk if used in the dairy; and may lead to poisonous residues in food animals when applied in live-stock buildings, with consequent danger to human beings eating the contaminated meat. DDT can also contaminate streams and rivers, and prove harmful to fish.

However, in the control of human trypanosomiases in Africa both DDT and dieldrin have been extensively used for ground spraying, often by aircraft.

DEAD ANIMALS, DISPOSAL OF (*see* DISPOSAL OF CARCASES).

DEADLY NIGHTSHADE is the popular name of *Atropa belladonna*, from which the alkaloid *atropine* is obtained. It is a deadly poison, and parts of the plant are sometimes eaten by stock. (*See* ATROPINE and BELLADONNA.)

DEAFNESS.

Congenital deafness is common in **white bull terriers** and also in **blue-eyed white cats.** In the USA the Dalmatian breed is reported to have the highest prevalence of deafness of all breeds of dogs, with a risk factor of 40–50 per cent. One or both ears may be affected.

Conductive deafness is that caused by interference with the transmission of sound waves from the external ear to the Organ of Corti in the inner ear. Such interference may be due to: (1) excess of wax in the ear canal; (2) perforation of, or infection involving, the eardrum. (In human medicine otosclerosis is another cause; being a loss of flexibility between the bones of the middle ear and the membrane connecting them with the inner ear, possibly due to hardening or ossification.)

Nerve deafness results from pressure upon, or damage to, the auditory nerve; it can also be a side-effect of antibiotics such as streptomycin and neomycin, and possibly chloramphenicol.

Deafness is or may be also a symptom of santonin poisoning, coal-gas poisoning, of a vitamin deficiency, and in human medicine, a side-effect of streptomycin, aspirin. Other causes include damage to the internal ear, to the Eustachian tube, nervous system, etc.

DEATH, CAUSES OF SUDDEN. In the majority of cases either failure of the heart or damage to a blood-vessel (*e.g.* in cattle caused by a nail or a piece of wire from the reticulum) is the direct cause, but nervous shock following an accident or injury, cerebral haemorrhage, anthrax, blackquarter, lightning-stroke, braxy, and over-eating of green succulent fodder in young cattle, are all capable of producing sudden death. In the case of pigs, sudden death has sometimes been met with from 'heat stroke'. (*See also* OEDEMA OF THE BOWEL.) In both cattle and pigs sudden death due to *Clostridium welchii* Type A has been reported. In cattle, hypomagnesaemia is a cause. In countries bordering the Red Sea, horses that have not been bred locally are sometimes attacked by a form of heatstroke with fatal results. (*See also* POISONING *and* (*with reference to dogs*) CANINE PARVOVIRUS INFECTION and CANINE VIRUS HEPATITIS.) Sudden death, without obvious preliminary symptoms, may occasionally occur in cases of rabies, botulism, foot-and-mouth disease. (*See also* ELECTRIC SHOCK.)

DEATH, SIGNS OF. The physical signs of death are well known, but there are occasions when it is difficult to state whether an animal is dead or not. In deep coma an animal may have all the superficial appearances of being dead, and yet recovery is possible if effective measures are taken. In the later stage of milk fever a cow has been mistaken for dead, has been dragged out of the byre preparatory to removal to the slaughterer's, has been examined by a practitioner, found to be living, has been suitably treated, and within 2 hours has been up on her feet again looking well. Foals have been discarded soon after being born and considered dead, have been removed to the outside of the loosebox while attention was paid to the dam, and later have been found living, the fresh cold air having revived respiration and stimulated the circulation, etc.

When an animal dies, the essential sign of the cessation of life is said to be the stopping of the heart. This, however, is not strictly correct, for it is possible by massage to resuscitate an already stopped heart, and to recover an apparently dead creature. Strictly speaking, it is almost impossible to say exactly when death takes place, but it

is considered that when heart and respiration have ceased, when the eyelids do not flicker if a finger be applied to the eyeballs, when a cut artery no longer bleeds, and when the tissues lose their natural elasticity, life is extinct. A few of the common tests that are applied in uncertain cases are as follows: The animal is dead when (1) a piece of cold glass held to the nostrils for 3 minutes comes away without any condensed moisture upon it; (2) when a superficial incision in the skin does not gape open; and (3) the natural elastic tension of the tissues disappears. Changes that follow death in a variable period depending upon the species of animal, and upon the weather at the time, are: (1) the clotting of the blood in the vessels; (2) the onset of *rigor mortis* – the stiffness of death; and (3) the commencement of decomposition of the carcase, usually first evident along the lower surface of the abdomen.

DE-BEAKING is done by poultry-keepers either when feather-picking or cannibalism begins, or as a routine method of prevention when the pullets are about to be put in the laying houses. Some trim the tip of the beak; but most cut back a third of the upper beak, which gives rise to bleeding. Electro-cautery is an alternative. Infectious sinusitis is sometimes a sequel of de-beaking, especially in turkeys. On some farms de-beaking may be so badly done that deformity or fatal haemorrhage results. De-beaking wastes feed. (*See* WELFARE.)

DE-FLEECING (*see under* CYCLOPHOSPHAMIDE).

DE-HORNING (*see under* DISHORNING).

DE-SNOODING. The removal of a turkey poult's snood, which may be pinched out or removed with a suitable instrument. De-snooding is done by turkey owners in order to reduce the risk of cannibalism.

DE-WATTLING. The removal of a fowl's wattles. (*See also* DUBBING.)

DEBRIDEMENT. Removal of infected tissue from a wound surface. This may be done by enzymes. (*See* STREPTODORNASE.) Maggots also have been used in human medicine.

DECUBITUS is the recumbent position assumed by animals suffering from certain diseases.

DECUSSATION is a term applied to any place in the nervous system at which nerve fibres cross from one side to the other, *e.g.* the decussation of the pyramids in the medulla, where the motor fibres from one side of the brain cross to the other side of the spinal cord.

DEEP-FREEZE (*see* ARTIFICIAL INSEMINATION, SEMEN, STORAGE OF; FROZEN EMBRYOS).

DEEP LITTER FOR CATTLE. This is a very satisfactory system if well managed. Straw, shavings, and sawdust can be used. Warmth given off as a result of the fermentation taking place in the litter makes for cow-comfort; and there is, of course, the added advantage of a thick layer of insulation between the cows and the concrete of a covered yard. In the 'Bed-and-breakfast' system, cows were bedded on top of a self-feed silage clamp in a covered yard.

A considerable depth – 2 or 3 feet – is often attained, and the cost is much less than that of conventional straw litter as bedding.

DEEP LITTER FOR POULTRY. Chopped straw, shavings, and sawdust are commonly used. Musty straw could cause an outbreak of Aspergillosis. Peat-moss is apt to be too dusty. Oak sawdust should not be used as it may discolour the egg-yolks. The depth should be at least 4 inches. The litter should be forked over, and added to from time to time. If it gets damp, the ventilation should be attended to. Many coccidia larvae get buried in the litter, and this is an advantage. After each crop of birds, the litter should be removed and heaped, so that enough heat will be generated to kill parasites. If deep litter is returned to a house, the succeeding batch of birds *sometimes* suffer from ammonia fumes, which may cause serious eye troubles and even blindness.

DEEP-ROOTING PLANTS are valuable in a pasture for the sake of the minerals they provide. Examples of such plants are: chicory, yarrow, tall fescue.

DEER, DISEASES OF. Deer are susceptible to the following infections: BRUCELLOSIS, BOVINE VIRUS DIARRHOEA, ELAPHASTRONGYLUS, EPIZOOTIC HAEMORRHAGIC DISEASE, FOOT-AND-MOUTH DISEASE, JOHNE'S DISEASE, LISTERIOSIS, LOUPING-ILL, MALIGNANT CATARRHAL FEVER, MENINGOENCEPHALITIS (caused by *Streptococcus zooepidemicus*), PARASITIC BRONCHITIS, TICK-BORNE FEVER, TUBERCULOSIS, WARBLES, YERSINIOSIS, and also an enzootic ataxia resembling Swayback in lambs.

T.B. in deer. In County Wicklow, Eire, tissues from 130 deer shot during 1983–84 were examined for evidence of tuberculosis, and gross lesions of the disease were found in five deer (3·8 per cent). This was a pilot study, carried out because of repeated assertions by farmers that deer might be responsible for the persistence of tuberculosis in their cattle.

'It is a moot point,' stated Dr K. Dodd, of the faculty of veterinary medicine, University College, Dublin, 'whether the deer infected local cattle, or vice versa, or whether there is a separate cycle within the deer population. The role of other wild life is also a possibility. Tuberculosis in badgers has been reported in Ireland, and in Switzerland deer are regarded as a possible source of the disease in badgers.'

Dr Dodd warned that people casually hand-recognise only severe cases of the disease. Indeed, he suggested that compulsory veterinary examination of deer carcases before sale might be advisable. (Dodd, K. (1984) *Veterinary Record* **115**, 592.)

In the U K a compulsory slaughter policy is in force for tuberculous deer.

The **Tuberculosis (Deer) Order 1989** provides for the individual marking of farmed or transported deer, and can be used for enforcing movement restrictions on affected or suspect animals.

Farmed deer research. In the U K the A F R C has been conducting research aimed at improving venison production. In 1984, at the Rowett Research Institute's low-ground red deer unit, two events were regarded as promising. One was the arrival of the first calf of the year on April 18th – six to eight weeks ahead of normal; and the second was the birth of the first induced set of twins.

Whereas, stated the A F R C, June calving is suitable on the hill, the lowground hind would benefit from an April calving as the high nutritional demands of lactation would then coincide with the spring flush of pasture; so improving milk yields and calf liveweight gains. Also, early-born calves might then attain marketable weights before Christmas at seven to eight months of age. This would avoid overwintering feed and housing costs, and give the producer a higher return.

The research programme, besides including manipulation of the hind's reproductive cycle, is also concerned with induced twinning.

In Britain there were in 1985 an estimated 150 deer farms, mostly in Scotland; annual production totalling about 5,000 carcases. Virtually all are red deer; fallow deer being more difficult to manage, and roe deer extremely so.

In Britain the harvesting of antlers velvet from live stags is illegal.

In New Zealand yersiniosis has become a serious disease of farmed red deer. It appears to be triggered off by stress, and most cases occur during the winter. An investigation in Invermay, South. Island, resulted in *Yersinia pseudotuberculosis* being isolated from 675 apparently healthy small mammals and birds. In descending order of prevalence were feral cats (27·8 per cent), Norway rats (8·6 per cent), mice, hares, rabbits, ducks, sparrows, seagulls and starlings. (Mackintosh, C. G. & Henderson, T. (1984) *New Zealand Veterinary Journal.*

The incidence of malignant catarrhal fever (MCF) in red deer herds in Canterbury, New Zealand, ranges from 0·2 to 10 per cent a year. In 1984/85 about 20 Père David's deer (*Elaphurus davidianus*) were imported to five properties and within a year about half the deer on each property had died of MCF. In April 1985 Invermay Agricultural Centre imported two two-year-old stags, four yearling stags and 18 yearling hinds from the Woburn Estate herd in England. Within a year five of the six stags and eight of the 18 hinds had died of MCF. The clinical illness lasted between one and 33 days, and the most common clinical signs were depression, a hunched stance and diarrhoea. At post mortem examination most of the deer showed recent localised haemorrhages, often into the large intestine, and in all of them there was histological vasculitis, especially in the brain. It seems, therefore, that Père David's deer are particularly susceptible to MCF. (Orr, M. B. & Mackintosh, C. G. (1988) *New Zealand Veterinary Journal* **36**, 19.)

Meningoencephalitis, caused by *Streptococcus zooepidemicus*, resulted in the death of farmed red deer exported from the UK and Denmark to New Zealand. Autopsy findings were congestion of lungs and liver, the presence of frothy fluid in trachea and bronchi, and acute meningoencephalitis. (de Lisle, G. W. & others. *Veterinary Record* (1988) **122**, 186.)

Dictyocaulus viviparous is the most important parasite of red deer in New Zealand and frequent drenching with oxfendazole is used to control it. Eight yearling deer, housed and used to handling, were drenched with 4·53 mg oxfendazole/kg bodyweight and, later, four of them had the treatment repeated while they were at pasture. Blood examinations showed that oxfendazole was rapidly metabolised and excreted. The authors concluded that the recommended dose rate for red deer is too low and may lead to development of resistant species of *D. viviparous*. (Watson, T. G. & Manley, T. R. (1985) *Research in Veterinary Science* **38**, 231.)

Another parasitic worm of importance in deer is *Elaphostrongylus cervi*. It is pale and thread-like, 4 to 6 cm long, and found in the intramuscular fascia and also in the meninges of the brain. This parasite occurs in Scotland, the mainland of Europe, and Australasia.

Eggs reach the lungs via the bloodstream and hatch in the alveolar capillaries, causing slight pneumonia. Nervous signs appear when the brain is involved. (Hollands, R. D. (1985) *Veterinary Record* **116**, 584).

A cause of eye disease in Red Deer, both farmed and wild, has been found to be a 'new' herpes virus; provisionally called HVC-1 (herpesvirus of *Cervidae* type 1). The latter can be differentiated from bovine herpesvirus 1. (Nettleton, P. F. & others. (1986) **118**, 267.)

DEFAECATION is very differently performed in the various animals, and some diagnostic importance is attached to the manner of its performance. (*See* CONSTIPATION, DIARRHOEA.)

DEFICIENCY DISEASES. These form a group of diseases bearing no clinical resemblance to each other, but having the common feature that in each some substance or element essential for normal health and nutrition has been absent from the diet for a longer or shorter period. The essential element may be one of the inorganic mineral substances, such as calcium, phosphorus, magnesium, manganese, iron, copper, cobalt, iodine, or more than one of these; it may be a protein or an amino acid; or it may be a vitamin. In the latter case the condition is often referred to as an 'Avitaminosis', and the particular vitamin is specified, *e.g.* A, B, or D. Starvation through inadequacy of general nutritive food intake, is not classed as a deficiency disease. Some deficiency diseases are simple, such as iron deficiency in young pigs, others are more complex, such as phosphate deficiency in South Africa, which is associated with botulism through the gnawing of bones of dead animals contaminated with *C. botulinus*. (*See* VITAMINS; TRACE ELEMENTS; NUTRITION, FAULTY.)

DEFINITIVE HOST. This is the host in which an adult parasite with an indirect life-history lives and produces its eggs. A definitive host is the final host, as compared with the intermediate host or hosts. For example, an ant is one of the intermediate hosts of one species of liverfluke (*see* ANTS); the definitive host is a sheep or other grazing animal.

DEFORMITIES of cattle and sheep, etc., are mentioned under GENETICS – Defects. (*See also* HARE-LIP; MOUTH, DISEASES OF; MONSTERS.)

DEGLUTITION means the act of swallowing. (*See* CHOKING.)

DEHISCENCE. A breakdown in the union of a suture of adjoining bones of the skull. The condition can be treated successfully by surgery.

An example of this is a breakdown of the suture line in mandibular fractures. It can be corrected by minor surgery. The term is also applied to the re-opening of wounds.

DEHYDRATION. Loss of water from the tissues, such as occurs during various illnesses, especially those producing vomiting or diarrhoea; in impaction of the rumen and as a result of serious burns.

'Measurement of faecal volume shows that by this route a scouring calf may lose as much as 100 ml of water from each kilogramme bodyweight in a period of 12 hours. Most of the water loss is into the intestine but some is lost by respiration and minimal urine formation. Because urine formation is reduced to minimal levels in an attempt to conserve body fluids there is a marked increase in metabolic waste material in the plasma. In a calf which has diarrhoea, but has kept its plasma volume within normal limits by movement of water from the intracellular fluid phase, the blood urea concentration will usually increase from a normal 10 to 20 mg per 100 ml to 30 to 45 mg per 100 ml but, as dehydration progresses beyond the point of compensation, this accumulation of urea increases rapidly to levels as high as 120 mg per 100 ml.

'Irrespective of the causes of diarrhoea, several factors are common to all cases. Some degree of inanition and dehydration occurs due to the upset absorption of food; in addition to this losses of specific electrolytes occur due to the continuation of gastro-intestinal secretion. The main electrolytes secreted in the abomasum are sodium and chloride while those secreted in the intestinal tract are principally bicarbonate, sodium, and potassium. Losses into the gut of a diarrhoeic calf are water, bicarbonate, potassium, sodium, and chloride in order of magnitude.

'Diarrhoea is accompanied by a metabolic acidosis; this is related to losses of bicarbonate in the faeces and ketone body accumulation due to starvation.

'TREATMENT. Homologous plasma is the first recommendation, although dextran solutions can be used as an alternative. The object of infusing homologous plasma in the early part of fluid replacement therapy is so that the circulatory defects produced by high blood viscosity, higher than normal plasma potassium levels and lowered blood pH are reduced rapidly and effectively to nearer normal limits.

'Initially the rate at which the fluid is administered should be carefully supervised, lest acute venous congestion occur with the danger of producing pulmonary oedema. The flow-rate should be increased gradually to about 6 ml per minute (90 drops from standard drip set) but, at the first sign of respiratory distress, if necessary this rate of flow may have to be drastically curtailed. Once 150 to 200 ml have been infused the flow-rate can be increased to the maximum capable of delivery by the apparatus under gravity flow. After 400 to 600 ml have been infused the rate should be reduced to 2 to 3 ml per minute and kept at this rate or slightly slower throughout the remainder of the infusion. The amount of plasma usually sufficient to return the circulation of the animal to reasonable efficiency is 400 to 800 ml.

'Having achieved the first stage of repair the remaining problem is to hydrate the tissues and replace some of the electrolyte losses which have occurred. The simplest method of achieving this is to alternate the fluids (*e.g.* 500 ml Darrows solution followed by 500 ml glucose solution) from the end of the infusion of plasma and continued for 24 hours. The majority of calves do not require further fluid therapy after 24 hours' continuous drip but a few individuals are still recumbent or slow to respond at the end of this period. In these cases the procedure is simply to repeat the whole course of therapy as for the first day, having first re-assessed and re-calculated the fluid requirements.

'The effects of infusion of plasma plus electrolyte solutions appear to be considerably greater than the effects of replacement of electrolytes alone. The reason for the increased benefit may, in part, be due to the more rapid and efficient repair of the circulation which is a feature of plasma administration. The infusion of plasma gives better perfusion of the tissues without the development of hypertension in the major bloodvessels which tends to occur when crystalloids are administered intravenously. Such hypertensions increase secretion of urine and the passage of fluid into the intestine so that a considerable part of the benefit of the infusion may be lost to the animal. It is important to promote renal function in order to eliminate the metabolic waste material which tends to accumulate in tissues of the calf but this will be more beneficial if it is accompanied by adequate tissue rehydration.

'The plasma used, being the pooled product of groups of at least 10 healthy young adult animals, contains most of the substances normally present in the plasma of such animals; in addition it contains some 3 per cent of dextrose which is added to the collected blood as a preservative. Thus it has nutritive properties. Also, it contains the gamma-globulin fraction of the plasma proteins of these donor animals. As yet there is little knowledge of the standard of survival of these proteins during the processing of the plasma to the freeze-dried state but there is increasing evidence that some of their immunological properties are retained.'

(Source: J. G. Watt, *Vet. Record*, Dec. 4, 1965.)

With untreated scouring calves' death probably results from acidosis and the high plasma potassium levels.

In a horse suffering from intestinal obstruction, up to 10 l of whole blood or plasma may be required to restore the blood volume, while the total fluid deficit may be much greater.

For first-aid purposes, glucose-saline may be given by mouth to all animals. UNICEF's 'Oral Rehydration Salts', intended for infants and children, may be used; the sachet contents being dissolved in 1 litre of water (which must not be boiled thereafter). The formula is:

Sodium chloride	3·5 g
Potassium chloride	1·5 g
Sodium bicarbonate	2·5 g
Glucose	20·0 g

Rehydration with glucose-saline can be lifesaving in pigs suffering from streptococcal meningitis or 'salt poisoning', and administration of 10 to 25 ml by enema is recommended (P. W. Balckburn. *Vet Record* (1983) **113**, 4), in non-scouring pigs.

Glucose-saline can also be administered to other animals per rectum, or subcutaneously.

DELIVERY (*see* PARTURITION).

DEMEPHION. An organophosphorous preparation used as an insecticide and acaricide. Livestock should be kept out of treated areas for at least a fortnight.

DEMODECOSIS. Another name for Demodectic Mange.

DEMODECTIC MANGE, or FOLLICULAR MANGE is caused by the *demodectic* parasite *Demodex folliculorum*. This parasite, microscopic and cigar-shaped in appearance, with very short stumpy legs, lives deep down in the hair follicles, and is accordingly difficult to eradicate by dressings. (*See* MITES.)

In cattle *Demodex bovis* is in the UK responsible for mild and infrequently reported cases of demodectic mange, but in some parts of the world the disease may be severe. Fatal, generalised cases have been reported from Africa.

D. caprae infestation of goats may also be severe in the tropics.

The parasites have been recovered from the eyelids of cattle, sheep, horses, dogs, and man. (*See* IONTOPHORESIS.)

DEMULCENTS are substances which exert a soothing influence upon the skin or the mucous membranes of the alimentary canal, and in addition afford some protection when these are inflamed. Examples of demulcents for internal use are arrowroot, glycerin, bismuth subnitrate, bismuth carbonate.

DEMYELINATION. Destruction of the myelin, a semi-fluid which surrounds the axis-cylinder of a medullated nerve fibre.

DENDRITES (*see* NERVES).

DENGUE (*see* EPHEMERAL FEVER).

DENTAL PLAQUE (*see* TARTAR).

DENTINE is the dense yellow or yellowish white material of which the greater part of the teeth is composed, and which in elephants, etc. constitutes ivory. The dentine is pierced by numberless fine tubules which communicate with the sensitive pulp in the hollow of the tooth-root, along each of which run tiny vessels and nerves which nourish its structure. In the young newly-erupted tooth the dentine is covered over with a layer of enamel, hard, dense, and brittle, which prevents too rapid wear of the softer dentine. (*See* TEETH.)

DENTITION

Dentition is the study of the configuration and conformation of the teeth, with special reference to their periods of eruption through the gums.

Among domesticated stock it is possible within certain limits to estimate the age of an animal by an examination of the appearance of its teeth; but while such an estimation is reasonably reliable, it is by no means always accurate. Numerous factors influence the dates of eruption of both temporary and permanent teeth, and it is not always possible to take these factors into consideration in any given case, for they may not be known. Artificial methods of management, forced feeding upon concentrated food-stuffs and the selection of early maturing breeding types, have combined to produce earlier and earlier eruption of the teeth, so that very considerable variations now exist between breeds of stock which are managed under an intensive system and those that are kept under more natural conditions.

In the following description the periods of eruption given are those considered to be average for each species of animal in Great Britain, and while variations from them will certainly be met with, the majority of animals will be observed to cut their teeth at the periods stated, or within a narrow margin of time before or after.

Horses. The full permanent dentition of the horse consists of the following teeth:

	Incisors	Canines	Molars
Upper jaws	6	2	12, 13, or 14
Lower jaws	6	2	12, 13, or 14

The variation in the number of molars depends upon whether '*wolf teeth*' are or are not present. These are small rudimentary teeth situated in front of the first molar; one, two, three, or four 'wolf teeth' may be present in an adult horse, but in the majority of cases there are none. One other variation must be mentioned: in the mare canine teeth may be either absent or they may be small and rudimentary.

The permanent teeth are not, however, present in the young foal; the majority of them are preceded by *milk, temporary,* or *deciduous* representatives. The temporary dentition consists of the following teeth:

	Incisors	Canines	Molars
Upper jaws	6	0	6
Lower jaws	6	0	6

Some authorities distinguish between molars and premolars in the permanent dentition; those teeth which are represented in the temporary dentition (*i.e.* the first *three* in either jaw, right and left, and upper and lower) being called *premolars*; while those which have no such representatives are known as *molars*. This may lead to some confusion, however, and all the cheek teeth will be called 'molars' in this section, and will be designated by a number (*i.e.* from No. 1 to No. 6) to avoid confusion.

Incisor teeth, 'nippers' or 'pincers', are six in number in the upper and lower jaws; they are found in the front of the mouth in each jaw, and reference is made to them almost exclusively for the purpose of estimating the ages of animals; the molars are only examined when irregularities or abnormalities are present in the incisor region. The temporary incisors differ from the permanents in that while each of the former possesses a definite crown, neck, and root, the latter do not. Moreover, the temporaries are smoother, whiter, and smaller, and to some extent resemble the incisors of cattle. When there are both temporaries and permanents present in the mouth it is not usually difficult to differentiate between them, but inexperienced persons sometimes confuse temporaries and permanents in yearlings and 5-year-olds, or in 2-year-olds and 6-year-olds. A typical unworn permanent incisor tooth from a horse possesses an *infundibulum,* or 'tucking-in' from its free edge or crown (*see* TEETH), and since this results in an infolding of the enamel, two rings of enamel, an outer and an inner, are seen in the partly worn tooth. However, as wear proceeds there comes a time when the inner ring of enamel disappears, since the level of wear has passed the depth of the infundibulum. In addition to the disappearance of the infundibulum the outline of the tooth changes from an oval to a quadrilateral, and eventually to a triangle, since the tooth is tapered from crown to root. It is upon an examination of these factors that the estimation of the age of an adult horse is based.

The incisors are named *centrals, laterals* or *intermediaries,* and *corners,* according to their situation in the mouth.

Canines. 'Tushes', 'eye-teeth', or 'dog-teeth' number two in each of the jaws – one on the right and one on the left side. In the horse tribe canines are only typically present in male animals, although they may be found in mares upon occasion. As a rule, if present in the mare they are either small or rudimentary. They are situated in a position between the last incisor and the first molar, one on either side, being nearer to the incisors than to the molars. The spaces between the canines and the molars are spoken of as the *bars* of the mouth, and across the bars runs the bit in the bridled horse. The canine teeth are comparatively simple, showing no folding of enamel.

Molars. 'Grinders', or 'cheek teeth', number six or seven in each of the four jaws, according to whether 'wolf teeth' are or are not present. The first three permanent molars are represented in the milk dentition and are therefore sometimes called *premolars.* Each tooth has a complicated folding of the enamel which bears some resemblance to the capital letter 'B'. The roots of the molars are long, and there is but little tapering from the crown downwards – an arrangement which allows maximum wear.

ERUPTION. The 'eruption' means the time when the tooth cuts through the gums, and not when it comes into wear. It will be convenient to consider the eruption of the horse's teeth in tabular form. It must be remembered that in the following table allowance has to be made for the time of foaling. All thoroughbreds are dated as having their birthdays on the 1st of January each year, and all other breeds of horses on the 1st of May, so that with an early foal the teeth will appear sooner than the corresponding periods subsequent to 1st May or 1st January in any year, and with a late foal later. Allowance must also be made for the system under which horses are kept; in the case of New Forest ponies or those reared on rough pasturage, for example, the teeth are slower in erupting than in animals that are bred under an intensive system.

Time of Eruption	Incisors	Canines	Molars
Birth to 1 week	2 temporary centrals	—	—
2 to 4 weeks	2 temporary laterals	—	Nos. 1, 2 and 3 temporary molars
7 to 9 months	2 temporary corners	—	No. 4 permanent molar
1 year 6 months to 1 year 8 months	—	—	No. 5 permanent molar
2 years 6 months	2 permanent centrals	—	Nos. 1 and 2 permanent molars
3 years 6 months	2 permanent laterals	—	No. 3 permanent molar
4 years	—	All 4 canines	No. 6 permanent molar
4 years 6 months	2 permanent corners	—	—

It should be also noted that as a rule the teeth in the upper jaw erupt sooner than those in the lower jaw, although there are many exceptions to this rule.

APPEARANCE OF TEETH AT VARIOUS AGES. To facilitate reference, although it entails some repetition, the appearance of the horse's teeth at various definite periods of its life will be described.

At birth the foal usually has the two central temporary incisors in each jaw through the gums, or just appearing. They are placed somewhat obliquely in the small mouth. In a few cases the laterals may also be showing, especially in foals carried longer than the usual gestation period. The first three molars can be felt below the gums, but they have not yet cut.

At 1 month, or soon after, the two temporary laterals erupt, whilst the two centrals are in wear and placed more nearly parellel in the mouth. At about this time the first three temporary molars cut through the gums.

At 6 months the foal's mouth has a neat, compact appearance, the centrals and laterals being well developed and in wear upon their anterior edges, although they are not all usually wearing along their posterior edges.

At 9 months the colt has the two temporary corners through the gums, but these are only touching along their anterior edges. The appearance of the mouth in profile shows an angular space between the upper and lower corner incisors. The centrals and laterals are well in wear. At about this time the 4th molars (permanent) cut through the gums, but do not yet come into wear.

At 1 year old the 4th molar is in wear. The corner incisors are still shell-like and only touching along their anterior edges.

At 1 year 6 months the corner incisors are now wearing all along their edges, and the centrals and laterals have become large and well-formed. At about this time the 5th molars (permanent) erupt, coming into wear at about 2 years.

At 2 years the corner incisors are well in wear, and all the incisor teeth have well-formed tables. There is as yet no sign of the displacement of the centrals.

At 2 years off, i.e. about 2 years and 3 months, the central incisors are often loose and the gums are receding from their necks. The teeth are only held in position by a short portion of fang or root.

At 2 years 6 months the two central temporary incisors fall out and their places are taken by the permanent centrals. At the same time the first two temporary molars (nos 1 and 2) in each jaw are shed, and the corresponding permanent molars are erupted.

At rising 3 years, i.e. about 2 years 9 months the two centrals have come well through the gums, but they do not quite meet each other until a little later. Nos 1 and 2 permanent molars in each jaw are well up and in wear.

At 3 years old the two central permanent incisors have met their fellows of the opposite jaw, but only a slight amount of wear is showing on their tables. The infundibula are only slightly worn and the 'tucked in' appearance can be well seen. In most cases there is a little wear showing on the anterior edges, but the tables are not yet well-formed.

At 3 years off the tables of the permanent central incisors are formed and show an appreciable amount of wear. There is some indication of replacement of the laterals, such as was noticed at 2 years off in connection with the centrals.

At 3 years 6 months some or perhaps all four of the permanent laterals have erupted, pushing out the corresponding temporaries in the process. Very shortly after this age the 3rd permanent molars are cut, the '3rd temporary molars making way for them by falling out.

At rising 4 years the permanent laterals are coming into wear. They may be touching, but an examination of their tables shows no appreciable wear. The centrals are well in wear and their tables are formed. About this time the canines or 'tushes', in the male, are beginning to show signs of eruption, the mucous membrane over them becoming bulged, white in colour, and painful on pressure. The 6th and last permanent molars are cutting through the gums, or may be already partly through, but they are not yet level with the other molars.

At 4 years the picture is similar to that at rising 4 years, but the laterals are now in wear, and the 6th molars are level or are nearly level with the other teeth.

At 4 years 6 months, or about that time the temporary corner incisors fall out and the last permanent corner teeth to erupt – the corners – cut through the gums. The molars are all well in wear and level. The horse has now a 'full mouth', all teeth being cut, although they are not all in wear.

At 5 years the corner incisors have met their fellows of the other jaw along their anterior edges, but their posterior corners are still rounded off and unworn. At this stage an angular space is visible when the mouth is looked at in profile with the jaws shut.

At 5 years off the corner incisors are showing more wear but they do not accurately meet until the horse is rising six years.

From this time onwards the age of the horse is estimated by a consideration of the appearance of the wear on the tables of the *lower incisor teeth*, by the changes in their outlines, and by the gradual lessening of the angle at which they meet the upper incisors.

At 6 years the corner teeth have lost their shell-like appearance and are in wear along both sides of their central cavity or 'mark'. In some cases the inner edge of the tooth is indented (especially the upper tooth), and a small part of the margin may not be quite in wear, but this is not a uniform feature. The laterals present cavities more shallow than those of the centrals, but still easily recognisable as such. Both the rings of enamel (outer and inner) are intact, and the outline of the centrals and laterals is distinctly oval, with the long axis in line with the rest of the teeth. In the central incisors the cavity is almost worn out, but the rings of enamel are distinct. The tushes are usually well developed and are prominent features of the male animal's mouth; their points are sharp.

At 7 years the tables of the lower corner teeth are well formed and the infundibulum in each is shallow. The central rings of enamel in both the central and lateral teeth are nearer to the poster-ior edge of the tooth than the anterior edge, and in the centrals though the ring is present it has lost its cavity. A shallow cavity is present in the laterals. The outline of the centrals is now much broader (anteroposteriorly) than at 6 years old, and also broader than is that of either the laterals or corners. In fact, the outline of the central teeth is becoming triangular (with the innermost angle rounded), while the outlines of their central enamel rings are broader ovals than formerly. In addition there is formed at this age what is often known as the '7-year-old hook'. This is seen when the jaws are examined in profile. It is due to the fact that the lower corner incisor is placed somewhat farther forward in the jaw than the corresponding upper tooth, and it is not so large. There results an imperfect apposition, and the posterior corner of the upper tooth develops a notch where wear occurs, and a slight projection where there is none. Some horses with badly aligned jaws do not develop this hook.

At 8 years the central teeth are more distinctly triangular than they were, and the central ring of enamel is also becoming triangular. The cavities in the centrals and laterals are either wholly obliterated or are nearly so, but in each case the inner ring of enamel is still perfect. A shallow true cavity is generally present in the corners. If the tables of the centrals are carefully examined a brownish or yellowish-brown linear streak will be seen running transversely across the tooth between the inner and outer rings of enamel and situated just behind the anterior edge of the tooth. This is called the 'dental star', and though it may be found in all six incisor teeth at 8 years, it is usually confined to the centrals, or to these and the laterals. The teeth are meeting each other at an angle considerably less than 180° when viewed in profile. The 7-year-old hook has worn out from the upper corner teeth, or is almost gone.

Beyond 8 years the teeth of horses vary to such an extent that, while a rough estimate is possible, it is very easy to make considerable mistakes. Much depends upon the management, rate of development, quality of the food, wear of the teeth as determined by their softness or hardness, and upon other factors. The subsequent notes must therefore be understood to apply only to average horses, and to be suggestions rather than rules.

At 9 years the central and lateral teeth are no longer triangular in outline but are becoming rounded – their angles disappearing. The outline of the corner teeth is never very definite. A small irregular enamel ring still persists, which encloses about one-fifth of the area of the table surface. The cavity has disappeared from the corner teeth, and these as well as the centrals and laterals show a fairly definite dental star occupying practically the centre of the table surface. There is more of each tooth exposed from the gums, which appear to have receded. The teeth are more oblique in their incidence, and are less fresh-looking than at 8 years.

At 10 years the central tables are almost as broad antero-posteriorly as they are long transversely, and there only remains a small inner ring of enamel, almost circular in outline and possessing no central depression. The inner rings in the laterals and corners are, however, still irregularly oval. The dental star is distinct in all the lower incisor teeth and occupies a central position. At this age 'Galvayne's groove', which is seen as a groove just protruding from under the gum on the outer surface of each of the upper corner teeth, appears. This groove appears at 10 years, has grown about halfway down the tooth at 15 or 16 years, reaches the free edge of each tooth at about 21, and by 25 has started to disappear, the upper part of the tooth becoming once more smooth. By about 30 years the groove has quite disappeared.

At 11 to 13 years all the teeth appear longer on account of the receding of the gums. The tables of each of them gradually assume distinctly round and then square outlines. By the time 12 years is reached only a very small indistinct inner ring of enamel remains, and when the horse is 13-years-old, it has typically disappeared from the centrals and laterals, but in the corners it may persist very close to the inner margin. A distinct dental star remains in all the teeth; this is small, rounded in outline, and occupies the centre of the table. The slope of the teeth in each jaw is now such that they meet at a much more acute angle when viewed in profile. A hook often appears in the upper corner teeth, similar to the 7-year-old hook but less regular.

At 15 or 16 years the tables of the teeth are becoming broader antero-posteriorly than they are long, and in the centre of the dental star a cleft or depression usually appears, due to the softer consistence of the tissue there. Galvayne's groove has grown about half-way down to the free edge in the upper corner teeth.

At 18 to 20 years the angle formed between the teeth of the two jaws is almost a right angle, and the tables of teeth are getting much smaller. In outline they are triangular, or are like quadrilaterals which have been flattened from side to side. A distinct depression appears in the centre of the dental star. Galvayne's groove has almost reached the free border.

From 20 to 30 years the teeth gradually appear older and more worn. They become smaller, and occupy a line along the gum which is no longer a definite arc, but gradually gets flatter until at about 30 years it is almost straight across, and the teeth are huddled together with no spaces between them.

As can be understood, an estimate of the horse's age can only be approximate in later life. Galvayne's groove is practically the only definite guide, and even it may be indistinct or absent.

Cattle. The *permanent dentition* of cattle consists of the following teeth:

	Incisors	Canines	Molars
Upper jaws	0	0	12
Lower jaws	8	0	12

In the upper jaw there are neither incisors nor canines, while in the lower jaw there are 8 teeth

present in the incisor region. The most posterior of these (*i.e.* one on either side) are supposed to be in reality modified canines, which have moved forward in the gums and have assumed the shape and the functions of incisors.

The *temporary* or *milk dentition* is as follows:

	Incisors	Canines	Molars
Upper jaws	0	0	6
Lower jaws	8	0	6

Incisors are absent from the upper jaw of cattle, their place being taken by the 'dental pad', a hard, dense mass of fibrous tissue developed in the upper incisor region, against which the 8 lower incisor teeth bite. Each is a simple tooth possessing a spatulate (spade-shaped) crown, a constricted neck, and a tapered root or fang. The teeth are loosely embedded in the jaw so that a slight amount of movement is normally possible. They are named *centrals, first intermediates* or *medials, second intermediates* or *laterals*, and *corners*; but it is perhaps more convenient to enumerate them from the central pair as 1st pair, 2nd pair, etc. The temporary incisors are small, brittle, and little or no trouble is likely to be met with in differentiating them from permanents.

Canines are absent unless the corner incisors are considered as modified canines.

Molars are like those of the horse in number and arrangement, except that they are smaller and progressively increase in size from first to last, so that the first is quite small, and the length of gum which accommodates the first three is only about half that occupied by the last three. One or more 'wolf teeth' may be present in rare cases.

ERUPTION. In ruminants – whether domesticated or not – the eruption of the permanent teeth is subject to very considerable variations. As in the horse, but even more so, the eruption of the teeth is influenced by domestication, methods of management, and nature of the food, and what applies to the more highly specialised improved breeds does not apply to commonly-bred cattle, and what applies to these latter does not hold good for ranch cattle. It is therefore necessary to give average figures for each of these classes, and to emphasise that while in any particular type of cattle the times given are about the average for that type, individual animals will be met with whose teeth are cut at periods very much earlier or later than the times given.

Sheep. The terms which were used as applied to cattle, and the description of the various teeth, may be taken to hold good for sheep as well. The sheep has 8 lower incisor teeth but none in the upper jaw. There are 24 molar teeth, 12 in each jaw, of which half these numbers are represented in the temporary dentition.

ERUPTION. The following is given as an average eruption table for improved breeds of sheep in Great Britain.

Time of Eruption	Incisors	Molars
Birth to 1 month	All 8 temporaries	All 12 temporaries
3 months	—	4th permanent
9 months	—	5th permanent
1 year to 1 year 3 months	1st pair permanent	—
1 year 6 months	—	6th permanent
1 year 9 months	2nd pair permanent	1st and 2nd permanents
2 years	—	3rd permanent
2 years 3 months	3rd pair permanent	—
2 years 9 months	4th pair to 3 years	— permanent

Pigs. There is probably no farm animal which shows such variation in the eruption of its teeth as the pig, but because of the demand for young pigs for killing by weight and size rather than by age, and because of the intractability of older breeding animals – sows and boars – the actual age of the pig is not of such very great importance, except perhaps for fat stock show purposes.

When the *permanent teeth* have all erupted they are distributed as follows:

	Incisors	Canines	Molars
Upper jaws	6	2	14 (*i.e.* 8 and 6)
Lower jaws	6	2	14 (*i.e.* 8 and 6)

In the molar region there is one little tooth in each of the four jaws, erupting at about 5 to 6 months, which is permanent from the very beginning. It is sometimes called *the premolar*, and in some cases is never developed. The next 3 teeth behind it are represented in the temporary dentition, the permanents replacing them in the usual way. The last three teeth are true molars; *i.e.* permanents only.

The *temporary dentition* is as follows:

	Incisors	Canines	Molars
Upper jaws	6	2	6
Lower jaws	6	2	6

Incisors. The upper incisors are small, and are separated from each other by spaces. The 1st pair (centrals) are the largest, and converge together. The 2nd pair are narrower and smaller; while the corner pair are very small and laterally flattened. The lower incisors are arranged in a convergent manner, and point forwards horizontally in the jaw. The 1st two pairs are large prismatic teeth deeply implanted in the jaw-bones and are used for 'rooting' purposes. The corner pair are smaller, and possess a distinct neck.

Canines, or *Tusks*, are greatly developed in the entire male, and both upper and lower tusks project out of the mouth. The upper canines of a boar may be 3 to 4 inches long, while the lower ones may reach as much as 8 inches in an aged animal. Each has a large permanent pulp cavity from which the tooth continues to grow throughout the animal's life.

SMITHFIELD RULES

1. Pigs having their *corner permanent incisors cut* will be considered as exceeding 6 months.

2. Pigs having their *permanent tusks more than half-up* will be considered as exceeding 9 months.

3. Pigs having their *central permanent incisors up*, and any of the *first three permanent molars cut*, will be considered as exceeding 12 months.

4. Pigs having their *lateral temporary incisors shed* and the *permanents appearing* will be considered as exceeding 15 months.

5. Pigs having their *lateral permanent incisors up* will be considered as exceeding 18 months.

In spite of the above, many pigs will be encountered in which, for some reason not well understood, the teeth are cut at times widely different from those given.

APPEARANCE OF TEETH AT VARIOUS AGES.

At birth the little pig has two pairs of sharp-pointed teeth in each jaw, top and bottom, placed so that there is a distinct space between each pair. These are the two temporary tusks and the 2 temporary corner incisors. These are the only teeth present in the gums, though the temporary molars, Nos. 2, 3, and 4, can be felt below the gums.

At 1 month, or sometimes a little sooner, the two central incisors, which are broader than the laterals and tusks, are cut, and the three molars above mentioned come through the gums.

At 2 months the temporary central incisors are fully up and there are signs of the eruption of the laterals.

Time of eruption	Incisors	Canines	Molars
At birth	Corner temporaries	All 4 temporaries	—
1 month	Central temporaries	—	Nos. 2, 3 and 4 temporaries
2 months	Lateral	—	—
5–6 months	—	—	No. 1, which remains through life and No. 5 permanent
8 months	Corner permanents	—	—
9 months	—	All 4 permanents	—
10–12 months	— permanent	—	No. 6
12–13 months	Central permanents	—	Nos. 2, 3 and 4 permanents
17–18 months	Lateral permanents	—	No. 7 permanent

At 3 months the lateral temporary incisors are well up, and the temporary molars are well in wear.

At 5 months there are signs of the cutting of the premolars (*i.e.* the No. 1 molars), and the 5th molar (a permanent) is seen behind the temporaries. It is, however, not yet in wear.

At 6 months the premolars are cut and the 5th permanent molar is in wear.

At 7 to 8 months there are signs of the cutting of the corner permanent incisors, or they may already be through the gums. The permanent tusks are also often cutting through the gums at this age in forward animals.

At 9 months the corner permanent incisors are well up and the permanent tusks are through the gums, although in many cases there may be still one or two of the small temporary tusks in position. Where they are cut they are not far through the gums.

At 1 year it is generally held that the central permanent incisors cut through the gums, but there are a large number of animals which do not cut these teeth till about 13 months old. The 6th permanent molar cuts at this time, and is more reliable than the incisors for reference.

Shortly after 1 year the 3 temporary molars fall out and their places are taken by the permanents. They are into line with the other molar teeth 3 months later.

At 17 to 18 months, when the final changes occur, the 7th molar, the last permanent molar tooth, and the lateral permanent incisors, are cut through the gums. By this time the pig has obtained its full permanent dentition, and the succeeding changes are not sufficiently reliable to warrant estimations of age being based upon them.

Dogs. Many attempts have been made to draw up a table which will roughly indicate the age of the dog as evidenced by its teeth, but owing to the very great variations in the size, rate of maturity, and shape of the skulls of present-day breeds of dogs there is no method of judging the age with accuracy. At birth the jaws of the puppy contain no teeth. From 3 to 4 weeks the temporary canines erupt and at 4 to 5 weeks the temporary incisors and the first 3 temporary cheek teeth erupt. About 4 months of age will generally show the eruption of the permanent premolar, and soon afterwards the fourth cheek tooth erupts. In the toy breeds, the permanent canines may appear at this time and sometimes they show before the premolar. In other dogs, the permanent canines appear at about 5 to 6 months and the corner incisors as well as the first three permanent cheek teeth erupt. The fifth cheek tooth shows very soon afterwards, and the sixth, often absent in the top jaw, shows at 6 to 8 months.

At 1 year the incisors are all in wear but they still retain their triple crown (called the 'fleur-de-lys'). By 2 years this is wearing off, or may have already disappeared. At about 4 years the cutting edges of the incisors in upper and lower jaws show a line of wear but the amount of wear depends on the shape of the jaws and the kind of food eaten.

The average adult dog has 42 teeth. The upper jaw contains 6 incisors, 2 canines, 8 premolars, and 6 molars. The lower jaw has 6 incisors, 2 canines, 8 premolars, and 6 molars. (There is some breed and individual variation in the number of permanent teeth, short-skulled breeds, e.g. Pekingese, Boxer, and Bulldog, having fewer teeth.)

Cats. The number of teeth in the adult cat averages 30. In the upper jaw there are 6 incisors, 2 canines, 6 premolars and 2 molars; while the lower jaw has 6 incisors, 2 canines, 4 premolars, and 2 molars. Some cats have only 28 permanent teeth; lacking 2 premolars.

DEOXYRIBONUCLEIC ACID (*see under* DNA).

DEPILATION the process of the destruction of hair that takes place during certain skin or other diseases, or after the application of chemical or thermal substances to the surface of the body. (*See* MANGE, RINGWORM, BALDNESS, BURNS, CYCLOPHOSPHAMIDE, ALOPECIA, etc.)

DEPLUMING SCABIES is a form of parasitic mange affecting the fowl, in which the feathers are eaten through close to the skin surface and fall off or break off. It is best treated with a Gammexane preparation. (*See* MITES.)

'DEPRAVED APPETITE' (*see under* APPETITE).

DERMATITIS means any inflammation of the skin. (*See* SKIN, ECZEMA, ALLERGY.)

DERMATOPHILUS infection results in a chronic dermatitis, in which the hairs stand erect and matted in tufts, like a wet paint brush. Many species of animals are susceptible, e.g. horses, cattle, sheep (also dog and cat).

CAUSE. *Dermatophilus congolensis*, which is a Gram-positive bacterium having some fungus-like characteristics, e.g. the production of branching filaments.

The disease, also known as cutaneous streptothricosis, follows the prolonged wetting of an animal, is widespread in the tropics, but occurs also in temperate climates, such as Ireland, Britain, etc. For examples in horses, *see* 'GREASY HEEL', 'RAIN SCALD', 'MUD FEVER'.

Predisposing causes, other than wetting, include tick and insect bites, wounds from thorns, etc. Fly transmission is recognised. The bacterium can resist drying, but under wet conditions it invades the epidermis, with effects mentioned under 'GREASY HEEL', where first-aid and precautionary measures are given. Antibiotics are helpful in treatment.

In the tropics dipping to control ticks is regarded as important, and acaricide preparations used in sheep dips are effective against *Dermatophilus*. (*See also* SENKOBO, STREPTOTHRICOSIS.)

DERMATOSIS VEGETANS. A hereditary disease of young pigs characterised by raised skin lesions, abnormalities of the hooves, and pneumonia. The semi-lethal recessive gene probably originated in the Danish Landrace. UK outbreaks occurred in 1958, 1964.

DERMATOSPARAXIS. A rare feline disease, resembling the human Ehlers-Danlos syndrome, and characterised by abnormal elasticity of the skin. The latter and its blood vessels also become fragile. Any wound healing takes longer than normal. The disease is inherited.

DERMIS (*see* SKIN).

DERMOID CYST is one of the commonest of the teratomatous tumours. It consists usually of a spherical mass with a surrounding envelope of skin. In this there are sebaceous glands and hair follicles from which grow long hairs. These, together with shed cells, sebaceous material, form the central part of the mass.

They develop subcutaneously in various situations, and are also found in ovary or testicle. They arise through the inclusion in other tissues of a piece of embryonic skin, which continues to grow and produces hair, etc., just as does skin on the surface of the body. Owing to the cystic structure (*i.e.* the cavity being a closed one) there is no means of getting rid of shed hair, debris, etc., and these substances accumulating in the centre cause the cyst to continue slowly increasing in size.

A dermoid sinus is a common congenital abnormality of the Rhodesian Ridgeback dog.
TREATMENT. No local treatment is of benefit. Surgical removal of the cyst wall and its contents, with the necessary means to obliterate the cavity, is desirable with subcutaneous dermoid cysts.

DERRENGUE. A paralysis of cattle occurring in El Salvador, and attributed to the ingestion of a weed, *Melochia pyramidata*, during periods of drought when scrub is the only available fodder. The symptoms resemble vampire-bat transmitted rabies (Derriengue) and include a paralysis first of the hind legs, with knuckling of the fetlocks. Death 'from inanition' occurs within a fortnight. (Palmer, A. C. and Woodham, C. B. (1975), *Vet. Rec.*)

DERRIENGUE. The Mexican name for vampire-bat rabies. (*See* VAMPIRE-BAT RABIES.)

DERRIS. The powder, obtained by grinding the root of a South American plant, is a valuable parasiticide, useful against warbles, fleas, and lice. It will not kill the nits of the latter, however, and hence the dressing must be repeated. Against fleas and lice it can be used as a constituent of a dusting powder, or with soap and warm water as a wet shampoo. It is safe for cats (compare D DT) provided the normal precautions against licking are taken – *i.e.* the bulk of the powder is brushed out of the coat after 10 minutes or so, during which licking is prevented – but must be used with caution on young kittens.

Derris is highly poisonous to fish – a fact which must be borne in mind when disposing of the powder or solutions in circumstances which could lead to river pollution.

DERZSY'S DISEASE. This can cause a high mortality among goslings. The cause is the goose parvovirus strain B. A mutant virus is used to immunise layers and so protect their goslings.

DESQUAMATION means the scaling off of the superficial layers of the skin, and is applied to the peeling process that accompanies some forms of mange and ringworm, as well as to the state of the skin in dry eczema.

DESTRUCTION (HUMANE) OF ANIMALS (*see* EUTHANASIA).

DETERGENTS are substances which cleanse, and many are among the best wetting agents (*i.e.* substances which lower the surface tension of water and cause it to spread over a surface rather than remain in droplet form). Detergents include soap, washing soda, and many new synthetic compounds analogous to soap but derived from alkalies and petroleum rather than from alkalies and vegetable or mineral oils. Disinfection of food vessels, milk pails, etc., requires the use of detergents as well as disinfectant solutions or the application of steam. Examples of detergents are cetrimide and sodium lauryl sulphate.

DETERGENT RESIDUE in syringes used for spinal injections have caused serious demyelinating complications in humans. Similarly, an unrinsed 'spinal outfit' has led to paraplegia in a dog.

DETOMIDINE (Domosedan). Given by intravenous injection, this drug has been found useful for the sedation of horses during radiography, endoscopy, etc. Sedation lasts for 20 to 30 minutes. An analgesic is needed in addition.

DEW CLAWS in cattle are sometimes torn off or injured by slatted floors. For dew claws in dogs *see* NAILS.

DEXTRAN. A plasma substitute, for use in transfusion instead of whole blood in cases of severe haemorrhage, etc.

DEXTRAN SULPHATE. An alternative anticoagulant to Heparin, longer lasting in its effects.

DEXTRIN is a soluble carbohydrate substance into which starch is converted by diastatic enzymes or by dilute acids. It is a white or yellowish powder which, dissolved in water, forms mucilage. Animal dextrin, or glycogen, is a carbohydrate stored in the liver.

DEXTROSE is another name for purified grape sugar or glucose.

DHREK. An Asiatic tree of which the leaves and fruits are poisonous to farm animals. (*See* MELIA.)

DIABETES INSIPIDUS, or POLYURIA, is a condition in which there is secreted an excessively large quantity of urine of low specific gravity. It results from a deficiency in the blood-stream of the anti-diuretic hormone (ADH). (*See* PITUITARY GLAND.) It may occur in dogs as a result of fright; symptoms including poor appetite, dull coat, and frequent urinating in the house. This may persist and require treatment, *e.g.* with pitressin tannate in oil. Feeding in the mornings only may prevent urine being passed in the house at night. (*See Vet. Record*, April 25, 1964.) (*See* URINE, sub-heading 'Polyuria'.)

DIABETES MELLITUS is a state of chronic hyperglycaemia (i.e., the state of having an excessive concentration of glucose in the blood), which may result from many environmental and genetic factors, often acting jointly . . . The major effects of diabetes include characteristic symptoms: ketoacidosis (diabetic 'coma'), the progressive development of disease of the capillaries of the kidney and retina, damage to the peripheral nerves, and excessive arteriosclerosis.

From: WHO Technical Report Series, No. 646, 1980 (*WHO Expert Committee on Diabetes Mellitus*).

In human medicine, diabetes is no longer regarded as a single entity, but rather as a group of diseases.

CAUSE. Pancreatic disease in which insulin (a hormone produced by the islets of Langerhans) is deficient. Disease may be due not necessarily to a deficiency of insulin but to an excess of insulin-antagonist circulating in the blood-stream. (*See also under* KETOSIS.)

PREDISPOSING FACTORS include:
(1) Inflammation of the pancreas (this pancreatitis being associated with a transient or permanent hyperglycaemia, as the result of a hormonal imbalance and loss of functional beta-cells in the islets of Langerhans); (2) Glucocorticoids can exhaust the beta-cell insulin reserve because of the combined effects of increased glucagon production and peripheral insulin antagonism; (3) MEGESTROL ACETATE (which see) treatment for oestrus suppression stimulates the effects of GLUCOCORTICOIDS and thereby antagonises the effects of insulin. (Michael Schaer (1984) *Carnation Research Digest* **20**, 3.)

SIGNS. These are vague at first. The diabetic animal develops an excessive thirst, and passes more urine than formerly. Appetite remains good, and sometimes becomes almost ravenous. Loss of weight occurs over a period of weeks or months. A previously active animal tends to become sluggish. A cataract may develop in one or both eyes. The urine contains an abnormal amount of sugar. Sometimes the liver becomes enlarged.

These signs may progress to sudden depression and vomiting, which alert the cat- or dog-owner to the illness. Great weakness, a fall in blood pressure, prostration, and diabetic coma may ensue as the result of keto-acidosis.

In 43 cases of **canine** diabetes, Doxey and others found that the major presenting signs included thirst and polyuria (95 per cent), weight loss (38), polyphagia (26), cataracts (26), vomiting (12) and anorexia (12). Doxey, D. L., Milne, M. M. & Mackenzie, C. P. (1985) *Journal of Small Animal Practice* **26**, 555.)

The function of insulin, whether produced normally from the pancreas or injected subcutaneously, is to enable proper use to be made of the sugar circulating in the blood-stream and to prevent its passage into the urine, whereby it is wasted. The chemical details involved are very complex.

Diabetes is commoner in females than in males, and in hot countries than in temperate or cold countries.

Treatment with an excessive dosage of cortisone or other steroids may give rise to diabetes.

In human medicine, viruses are now believed to be among the causes of damage to the islets of Langerhans. It was pointed out in the *Lancet* (Oct. 9, 1971) that mumps is a well recognised cause of inflammation of the pancreas, and that it may be followed by diabetes. 'However, mumps pancreatitis is rare and diabetes is relatively common. Other viruses have come under suspicion, especially some of the picorna viruses. These include foot-and-mouth disease virus, but of the picornaviruses commonly infecting man the Coxsackie group, and in particular Coxsackie-B4, appears to be linked with inflammation of the pancreas leading to diabetes.'

Again in human medicine, 'for several years circumstantial evidence has been accumulating that insulin-dependent diabetes is associated with disorders of the immune mechanisms. A statistical association between insulin-dependent diabetes and the organ-specific "autoimmune" diseases, Hashimoto's disease, pernicious anaemia, and idiopathic adrenal atrophy, has been detected, and serological work has revealed high prevalence of humoral, organ-specific autoantibodies in insulin-dependent diabetes. Schmidt's syndrome, a combination of adrenalitis and thyroiditis, has been reported associated with insulin-dependent diabetes in nearly 200 cases. There are also accounts of families with multiple disorders affecting the immune mechanisms and associated with insulin-dependent diabetes.' (*Lancet*, Nov. 20, 1976.)

(It should be mentioned that a temporary presence of sugar in the urine, due to a metabolic disorder, involving liver and other tissues, is encountered from time to time in the course of fever, some forms of poisoning or overdosage with chloroform, chloral or morphine, and when excessive amounts of sugars or starchy foods have been eaten. These cases return to normal with recovery from the exciting cause.)

TREATMENT. The only effective method of treatment is injection of *insulin*, at regular intervals for the rest of the animal's life, and attention to the diet. This is a matter which must be undertaken with expert supervision.

Cats. They tolerate the daily injections unexpectedly well and owners find the routine easy. 'The proper dose of insulin does *not* depend on the cat's weight,' N.S. Moise & T.J. Reimers commented (*JAVMA* (1983) **182**, 158). They advised beginning regulation with a dose of 1 unit. 'The dose is increased by 1-unit increments until hyperglycaemia is controlled. Most cats will require administration of NPH insulin twice daily; and of PZ insulin once daily. It is important that the cat be fed at dosing time and just before the insulin action peaks.' Long-acting insulins are prone to cause hypoglycaemic crises hence zinc suspension insulin or protamine zinc insulin are recommended. Prognosis is more favourable than in dogs. Survival periods of 6 to 7 years are known in patients which became diabetic at 9–10 years of age.

In the cat the onset and peak action times can occur as early as a few hours after the insulin injection, thereby predisposing the animal to severe episodes of hypoglycaemia.

'In households where the cat is receiving only one dose of insulin per day, the clinician should suspect this adverse reaction when symptoms of hypoglycaemia occur in the late morning or early afternoon.' To help prevent this complication, Dr Schaer recommends reducing the total dose of insulin per day by about 25 per cent, and then evenly dividing the remaining amount into morning and evening injections. This split-dose method provides the patient's total insulin requirement, yet lessens the risk of hypoglycaemia.

Hypoglycaemia must be treated as soon as possible in order to avoid irreversible brain damage. If the cat is having fits or coma, the owner can use ¼ to ½ an ampoule of glucagon, and give carbohydrate when the cat has regained consciousness.

In the **emergency situation**, when ketoacidosis is approaching the coma stage, dehydration must be countered by intravenous injections.

Nowadays insulin does not necessarily have to be given by injection; it, or sulphonylureas or other drugs, can be given in tablet form and is satisfactory in some cases.

Records of 333 cats with diabetes mellitus were related to the records of 135,651 cats from the same population. Breed had no detectable effect on the risk of a cat developing diabetes, but body-weight, age, sex and neutering had significant effects. Cats weighing more than 6·8 kg had a 2·2-fold higher risk, even after adjustment for the effects of age and sex. More than half the affected cats were more than 10 years old, and there was a 14·4-fold increase in risk for these cats. Male cats were 1·5 times more likely to develop diabetes than females, and neutered cats were nearly twice as likely to develop the disease as entire cats. (Panciera, D. L. & others. (1990) *Journal of the American Veterinary Medical Association* **197**, 1504.)

DIAGNOSTIC IMAGING. (*See* X-RAYS, RADIO-ISOTOPES.) **Diagnostic Tests.** (*See* LABORATORY TESTS.)

DIAPHORESIS is another name for PERS-PIRATION.)

DIAPHORETICS are remedies which promote perspiration.

DIAPHRAGM is the muscular and tendinous structure which separates the chest from the abdominal cavity in mammals. It is an important organ in respiration. (*See* MUSCLES.)

DIAPHRAGMATOCELE means a rupture in the diaphragm through which some of the abdominal organs, often the small intestine, stomach, and perhaps spleen and liver, have obtruded themselves, so that they become situated actually within the chest cavity. It occurs during falls, when jumping from a great height, and sometimes in cats and dogs hit by a car. The breathing becomes very much disturbed and the animal usually shows an inclination to assume an upright position, whereby the organs are encouraged to return to the abdominal cavity and pressure on

the lungs is relieved. Treatment by surgical means has occasionally been effected in the dog and cat. (*See* THORACOTOMY.)

DIARRHOEA is not, of course, a disease in itself, but merely a symptom, which may indicate nothing more than the result of an 'error of diet', or a 'chill'. A sudden change of diet, or the feeding of unsuitable, mouldy, rancid, or fermenting material will give rise to diarrhoea – a symptom of enteritis, and also of specific diseases in which enteritis is one symptom.

Continuing diarrhoea is always serious because not only are the digestive processes and the absorption of nutrients impaired, but the loss of fluid gives rise to DEHYDRATION – a frequent cause of death unless treatment is undertaken in time. If diarrhoea persists for 48 hours or more, veterinary advice should be sought by livestock-owners.

Other causes include poisons such as lead, arsenic and mercury, infection with tuberculosis in some part of the bowel wall; the presence of parasites such as worms, flukes, or coccidiae; infection with specific diseases, such as Johne's disease, salmonellosis, lamb dysentery, white scour, etc.; or the excessive action of purgatives given in too large doses. In all of these instances there are other symptoms which help in the diagnosis of the condition, and examination of the diarrhoeic material will often show the presence of the agent responsible (*see* SALMONELLOSIS).

TREATMENT. The treatment of diarrhoea from causes which are specific, is dealt with under these headings. (*See also* WORMS, FARM TREATMENT.)

If diarrhoea persists, the mere withdrawal of large amounts of fluid from the body may itself become serious, and it becomes essential to replace this fluid. (*See under* DEHYDRATION.)

Various antiseptics such as sulphaguanidine, salol, salicylate and bismuth, carbonate of bismuth, dimol, or brilliant green may be given. Irrigation of the bowel with warm saline is useful in some cases of severe diarrhoea in puppies.

Adult cattle. The best first-aid measure is to feed hay only. If 'scouring' persists beyond 48 hours, obtain veterinary advice. Specific diseases in which diarrhoea is a symptom include COC-CIDIOSIS, JOHNE'S DISEASE, MUCOSAL DISEASE, SAL-MONELLOSIS, PARASITIC GASTROENTERITIS, TUBERCULOSIS, CRYPTOSPORIDIOSIS, BOVINE VIRUS DIARRHOEA.

Calves. Neonatal diarrhoea is still regarded as the most important disease of young calves in both dairy and beef herds. Mortality varies widely from 0 to 80 per cent, and in non-fatal cases the resultant poor growth rate and the cost of life-saving treatment can be a source of considerable loss to the farmer.

The causes are various. 'Although', stated (1975) G. N. Woode of the A F R C's Institute for Research on Animal Diseases, Compton, 'pathogenic strains of *E. coli* are important in the septicaemic and enterotoxaemic forms of the disease, there is doubt concerning the role of *E. coli* in all outbreaks of typical calf scours.'

Of the many other bacteria which have been *associated* with the disease few – with the exception of Salmonella – can be shown to be the *cause*.

For viruses associated with diarrhoea in calves *see* ROTAVIRUS, CORONAVIRUS, REOVIRUS.

The second coronavirus was originally isolated from scouring calves in Nebraska, USA, and shown to be present also in the UK. This virus resembles the virus causing transmissible gastro-enteritis of pigs (TGE). (*See also* WHITE SCOURS, SALMONELLOSIS, COLOSTRUM.)

From France came the report of a new diarrhoeic syndrome in calves one to two weeks old. 'Dehydration was absent,' but nervous signs such as ataxia or paresis were seen. (Espinasse, J. & others. *Veterinary Record* (1991) **128**, 422.)

Sheep. Lamb dysentery, *E. coli* infection, coccidiosis, parasitic gastro-enteritis, salmonellosis, poisoning, and a sudden change to grain feeding are among the causes of diarrhoea. (*See also* JOHNE'S DISEASE; WORMS, FARM TREATMENT AGAINST; SOIL-CONTAMINATED HERBAGE, CAMPYLOBACTER, COCCIDIOSIS, COPPER POISONING, ROTAVIRUS.)

Pigs. The causes are numerous and include: iron deficiency; high fat content of sow's milk at about third week; stress, caused by, *e.g.*, long journeys; cold, damp surroundings; change of diet; vitamin deficiencies; poisons; viruses, *e.g.* TGE; rotavirus; bacteria, *e.g. E. coli* (some strains), *Campylobacter, Salmonella cholerae suis, Salmonella dublin, Clostridium welchii, Erysipelothrix rhusiopathiae* (the cause of erysipelas); protozoa, *e.g. Balantidium coli, coccidia;* fungi; yeasts; worms.

E. coli is regarded as being associated with a high proportion of outbreaks of scouring, though it can be obtained from the gut of virtually any healthy pig. Its precise importance and roles are explained under E. COLI. *E. coli* vaccines have been administered to sows before farrowing on farms where scouring is a problem. (*See also* K.88.)

Scouring piglets need plenty of drinking water, for there is always danger of DEHYDRATION. (*See also* SWINE DYSENTERY, ANTIBIOTIC SUPPLEMENTS, SOW'S MILK, SWINE FEVER, ILEUM, NECROTIC ENTERITIS.)

Dogs. Diarrhoea may be associated with distemper, toxoplasmosis, tuberculosis, nocardiosis; occasionally with pyometra; with allergies; tumours; and poisoning.

Diarrhoea may also result from an infestation of dog biscuits or meal, stored in large bins, by FLOUR/FORAGE MITES (which see). (*See also* SALMONELLOSIS, E. COLI, STRESS, PANCREAS, WORMS, CANINE PARVOVIRUS, LYMPHOSARCOMA, CAMPYLOBACTER, ROTAVIRUS, YERSINIA, GIARDIASIS.)

Chronic diarrhoea is sometimes caused by *Clostridium difficile*. Metronidazole has proved useful in treatment, though relapses may occur.

Cats. Similar causes (except Distemper) apply, and *see also* FELINE INFECTIOUS ENTERITIS, FELINE INFECTIOUS PERITONITIS, COCCIDIOSIS, AEROMONAS, CORONAVIRUS.)

Horses. Clinical evidence has suggested a possible association between diarrhoea, stress, and antibiotic therapy. For example, a horse which is undergoing stress and happens to be a salmonella carrier may develop diarrhoea; and this may be exacerbated by tetracycline therapy which removes normal bacterial antagonists of the salmonella (R. Owen, 1975). Diarrhoea may, of course, be unassociated with stress, and among the many other causes is ulceration of the colon and caecum – probably caused by the thromboembolism associated with migrating larvae of the worm *Strongylus vulgaris*. In a study of 91 cases at the Royal Veterinary College, Dr J. C. Greatorex found that clinically the cases could be grouped as: (*a*) sudden onset of profuse and persistent diarrhoea accompanied by shock and sometimes leading to death within a few hours (10 cases); (*b*) sudden onset of profuse and persistent diarrhoea which lasted for weeks or months and caused dehydration and rapid emaciation (56 cases); (*c*) faeces like 'cow-pats' for a few days, alternating with bouts of diarrhoea which eventually became profuse and continuous and caused progressive emaciation (25 cases). (*Vet. Rec.* (1975), **97**, 221.)

Thirty-three species of bacteria were isolated from the gastrointestinal mucosa of 23 adult horses and two foals. The bacteria isolated could be related to gross and microscopical lesions in some cases. *Clostridium perfringens* type A, *Actinobacillus equuli, Salmonella typhimurium* and *Campylobacter coli* biotype 1 could all be associated with gastrointestinal lesions. *C. jejuni* biotype 1 and *Aeromonas hydrophila* were both recovered in this study and have been identified as causes of enteritis in horses or in other species. The case of *C. coli* enteritis appears to be the first such report. (Al-Mashat, R. R. & Taylor, D. J. *Veterinary Record* (1986) 453.) (*See also* FOALS, DISEASES OF, CHRONIC CATARRHAL ENTERITIS; SALMONELLOSIS; EQUINE INFECTIOUS ANAEMIA; EQUINE VIRAL ENTERITIS, HORSES, WORMS IN; GLOBIDIOSIS; CANCER; *and* POTOMAC HORSE FEVER.)

Whenever an apparently simple diarrhoea lasts for more than 1 or 2 days in an animal it is wise to seek professional advice rather than attempt what must at best be only empirical treatment. The temperature is a useful guide to the severity of the condition, especially in young animals such as foals and puppies, and in all cases where it is high it is an indication that there is some serious condition complicating the diarrhoea which demands immediate attention. (*See also under* ANTIBIOTIC SUPPLEMENTS.)

DIASTASIS is a term applied to separation of the end of a growing bone from the shaft.

DIASTOLE means the relaxation of a hollow organ. The term is applied in particular to the heart, to indicate the resting period that occurs between the beats (systoles) while the blood is flowing into the organ.

DIATHERMY is a process by which electric currents can be passed into the deeper parts of the body so as to produce internal warmth and relieve pain, or, by using powerful currents, to destroy tumours and diseased parts bloodlessly. The use of short-wave therapy is gaining ground in the treatment of muscle, tendon, and ligament strains. In horses with, *e.g.*, flexor tendon trouble, 20-minute treatments over a period of a week are often effective – more so that the old blistering and firing which are thereby obviated.

DIAZEPAM. A tranquilliser. Valium is a proprietary name.

DIAZINON. An anti-tick organo-phosphorus compound.

Diazinon granules are used for the control of wireworms on lawns and larger areas of grassland. If applied too liberally there is a risk of poisoning to birds, and also to young cattle.

In a case involving ornamental peafowl adult birds fell forward on to their chests, with legs stretched out behind, when attempting to walk. Some could not walk at all. Diarrhoea and dyspnoea were evident. Sick birds remained alert but refused food. Two young birds were found dead; but the ill adults all recovered without treatment.

DICHLOROPHEN. A drug of value against tapeworms in the dog. Dichlorophen ointment and a spray preparation have been used in the treatment of ringworm in cattle.

DICHLORVOS. A parasiticide used against fowl mites on laying hens and turkeys. Strips of resin impregnated with dichlorvos have been used successfully for the control of dog and cat fleas, over a period of three months or so. (*See* 'FLEA-COLLARS'.)

Poultry have died after gaining access to the faeces of horses dosed with dichlorvos for anthelmintic purposes. Dichlorvos is effective against horse bots as well as round worms.

Dichlorvos (an organophosphate) is effective against ascarid worms. *Trichuris suis*, and Oesophagostomum in pigs.

DICOUMAROL which is chemically related to WARFARIN, is an anti-coagulant and a cause of internal haemorrhage (*see* HAEMORRHAGIC SYNDROME IN CATTLE). The latter condition may develop after cattle have eaten mouldy hay containing sweet vernal or sweet clovers; the COUMARIN content of which has been converted to Dicoumarol.

DICROELIUM (*see* LIVER-FLUKES).

DICROTIC pulse is one in which at each heartbeat two impulses are felt by the finger that is taking the pulse. A dicrotic wave is normally present in a tracing of a pulse as recorded by special instruments for the purpose, but in health it is imperceptible to the finger.

DICTYOCAULUS VIVIPARUS (*see* PARASITIC BRONCHITIS).

DIELDRIN. An insecticide formerly used against the maggot-fly of sheep. Dieldrin is highly poisonous to birds, and fish. The symptoms of Dieldrin poisoning in foxes (which have eaten poisoned birds) are stated to resemble closely those of Fox Encephalitis. Dogs and cats have been poisoned similarly. (*See also* DOG KENNELS.) Dieldrin has been suspected as a cause of infertility in sheep, and residues in the fat may be a danger to people eating the mutton or lamb. The use of dieldrin sheep dips was banned in the UK in 1965, following similar bans in Australia and New Zealand. Dieldrin was also banned as a dressing for winter wheat early in 1975, but cases of dieldrin poisoning continued to occur among wild and domestic pigeons, and in kestrels, etc., fed on pigeons, during that year. Dieldrin is still used for ground spraying in Africa (*see under* DDT; *and* CHLORINATED HYDROCARBONS.).

DIESEL OIL POISONING. Thirsty cattle have drunk diesel oil with fatal results.

Symptoms include loss of appetite, depression, vomiting, tympany of the rumen, emaciation. Death (sometimes from lung damage) may occur after several weeks.

Poisoning has also been recorded in a ewe after eating grass contaminated by oil from a fuel tank sited in a field. (Susan F. Ranger, *Vet. Rec.* (1976) **99,** 508.) Breath, urine and faeces all smelt strongly of the oil. Treatment with olive oil brought no improvement, but recovery followed rumenotomy and replacement of rumen contents by 2 litres of fresh slaughterhouse material.

DIET AND DIETETICS

The most important part of animal husbandry is sound feeding of the animals. This is not by any means, as might be supposed, a simple matter.

In order fully to understand rational feeding, the stock-owner must be conversant with the various food constituents and what part they play in the body, he must have an idea of the composition of the many foods that are available to him, and he must know how to make the best use of them. He should never under-rate *the importance of palatability*.

Composition of foods. By ordinary chemical analysis foods can be split up and separated into: water, proteins, fats or oils, soluble carbohydrates, crude fibre or insoluble carbohydrates, minerals, and trace elements. In addition to these there are vitamins.

WATER. Water, as an essential need for live-stock, has been discussed under the appropriate heading (*see* WATER). All foods contain a certain percentage of water. It is found in greatest amount in roots, succulents such as cabbages and kale, wet brewer's grains, silage, and pasture grasses, which contain from 75 to 90 per cent. Cereal grains, such as wheat, oats, barley, etc., average 11 per cent. Meadow grass yields from 70 to 80 per cent of water, but when it is air-dried and made into hay under favourable circumstances, this is reduced to 12 to 14 per cent.

CARBOHYDRATES. The carbohydrates in foods are divisible into two groups, the *crude fibre*, and the *soluble carbohydrates*. The crude fibre is the less digestible part of the carbo-hydrate.

Oats contain 10 per cent of fibre, and hay and wheat-straw 25 per cent and 40 per cent respec-tively.

Crude fibre is a mixture of celluloses, lignin, cutin, and some pentosans, etc. While it is cheapest of all food materials, it is nevertheless an indispensable constituent of all properly balanced rations. Cellulose is the material that forms the cell-wall of plants. In its simplest form it is easily digested, but with the growth of the plant cellulose becomes associated with *lignin*, which gives stiffness to the parts of the plant requiring support, and also *cutin*, which is a waterproofing material.

The carbohydrates are made up of carbon, hydrogen, and oxygen. Food containing much carbohydrate are called carbonaceous foods; for example, the cereal grains, potatoes, molasses, etc. The cereals contain from 60 to 70 per cent of carbohydrate. The simplest of the carbohydrates, such as the simple sugars, are absorbed directly from the gut, while the more complex sugars, and still more complex starches, have to be reduced by processes of digestion to more simple forms before they can be absorbed and be of use to the body. Starch is one of the chief forms in which food is given to animals.

FATS OR OILS. Fat is present in all foods, but the quantity varies greatly; thus in hay there is 3 per cent, in turnips there is 0·2 per cent, in cereals from 2 to 6 per cent, and in linseed as much as 40 per cent, while linseed cake, from which most of the fat has been expressed, contains on an average rather less than 10 per cent. In meals produced from fat rich foods such as cotton seed or linseed, by extraction with a solvent, all the oil except some 1 or 2 per cent is removed.

Cakes and other foods in which the fat has gone rancid are dangerous for animals, and often cause diarrhoea. (*See* UNSATURATED FATS, COD-LIVER OIL POISONING.)

PROTEINS. The proteins or albuminoids in a food differ from the other constituents we have considered, in that in addition to having carbon, hydrogen, and oxygen in their composition, they also contain nitrogen and usually sulphur and sometimes phosphorus. They are very complex substances, and are made up of a number of much simpler bodies called *amino acids*. (*See under that heading.*) The practical importance of all this to the stockowner is that he feeds his animals on a mixed diet, so making sure that the animals will get the amino acids from the various proteins that they may require.

MINERAL MATTER OR ASH. The mineral matter in a food is sometimes called its *inorganic* constituent, to distinguish it from the foregoing organic constituents. The mineral matter, like the other constituents, is taken into the plant through the roots from the soil; and as the soil differs in its mineral character in different localities, so will the mineral content of the herbage vary in charac-ter and quantity. Individual plants also have their own mineral peculiarities; for example, the leguminous plants are rich in calcium which is so necessary for animals; other foods, such as maize, are deficient in calcium, but contains phosphorus; while others again, such as the wheat offals, have an unbalanced mineral content.

VITAMINS (*see under that heading*).

Function of food constituents. All the consti-tuents of foods above mentioned play an impor-tant part in nourishing the animal, and the secret of success in animal rearing and feeding lies in giving these substances not only in sufficient quantity but also in proper proportion. It is important that the stock-owner should know of what use these food elements are to the body.

CARBOHYDRATES. The carbohydrates are chiefly utilised for the production of energy and heat, and what is not required for immediate use is stored as fat, which is to be regarded as a reserve story of energy. It is the carbohydrates which are mainly used for the deposition of fat when animals are fattened.

FIBRE. A certain amount of crude fibre is necess-ary in the diet of all animals except those under 3½ weeks of age, when all young domesticated animals are on a fluid diet and most are supported solely by suckling. If animals, especially herbivorous animals, are given insufficient fibre they fail to thrive, are restless and uncomfort-able, and every cattle-feeder knows that without 'bulk' to the ration the animals do not do well.

Adequate fibre is necessary to cattle for proper muscular activity of the whole digestive system. Secondly, the proportion of fibre in the diet has an important bearing upon the actual digestion done by living organisms within the rumen. Thirdly, a high-protein and low-fibre intake may lead to bloat. Fourthly, adequate fibre is necessary in the cow's rations if she is to give a high yield of butterfat and solids-not-fat.

On the other hand, if too much fibre is given in the ration the animals cannot digest enough food to get sufficient nutriment. This is the reason why wheat straw would be a very bad food for hard-working horses. Ruminants make the most use of fibre, then horses, pigs, and dogs, in the order given. Fattening pigs, though requiring a certain amount of fibre, must have the allowance strictly limited, though sows and boars can do with more.

FAT. The fat that is digested and absorbed may be oxidised to form energy direct, or it may be built up to form body fat. Speaking generally, fat has two and a half times the value of carbohydrates or protein as energy producer. While a certain amount of fat is desirable, indeed necessary, in the daily diet of animals, an excessive amount does harm. For proper utilisation by the body, the fats have to oxidise fully; where too much fat is taken in the food, this oxidation does not proceed fully and a series of harmful substances, called ketones, accumulate in the system. The quality of fat is obviously important. Some calf starters have been found to contain tallow infected with Salmonella organisms.

Certain polyunsaturated fats are dietary essentials for all animals (Milk is particularly poor in these, and has been criticised as a human food for this reason.)

PROTEIN. It is, of course, now accepted that it is not only the amount of protein in the ration which is important, but also the quality of that protein.

Cereal protein is of poor quality, being deficient in lysine and methionine; and wheat is worse in this respect than barley. Accordingly, herring, (other) fish, and soya bean meals being relatively good sources of the desirable amino acids – the building blocks, so to speak, for proteins – are incorporated in animal feeds. (The importance of selecting feed ingredients containing the most valuable and, indeed, essential amino acids, is referred to in the separate section headed AMINO-ACIDS.)

For substitution of *some* of the protein in a ration or diet, *see under* UREA.

For health in all animals, adequate protein of good quality is essential in the diet. Failure to provide it can result in economic loss to farmers; losses often being far higher than the cost of the 'extra' necessary protein. Excess protein, on the other hand, can bring its own problems. (*See under* ACETONAEMIA for example.)

MINERALS, TRACE ELEMENTS. These are essential for bone formation and maintenance, milk production, fertility, and for the metabolism as a whole. The essential minerals and trace elements are phosphorus, calcium, sodium, potassium, magnesium, iron, manganese, copper, zinc, sulphur, iodine and cobalt. Not only are they essential, but the balance is important, too: the ratio of one to another. For example, as explained under CALCIUM SUPPLEMENTS, the ratio of this mineral to phosphorus can mean the difference between health and ill health.

Proprietary concentrates from reputable manufacturers ensure a feed for farm animals with well balanced minerals and trace elements as a rule, and this is something which cannot always be achieved in a farm mix unless a proprietary minerals premix is used.

On some soils, deficiencies of certain trace elements may occur – resulting in similar deficiencies in plants grown on those soils – so that special supplements may be needed.

Further information will be found under METABOLIC PROFILES, TRACE ELEMENTS, CONCENTRATES, OSTEOFIBROSIS, FELINE JUVENILE OSTEODYSTROPHY, PIGLET ANAEMIA, IODINE DEFICIENCY, COBALT, SALT, etc.

VITAMINS are discussed elsewhere; for information on these important substances, see therefore, VITAMINS.

Antibiotic supplements (*see under* ADDITIVES).

General principles of feeding. A well-balanced ration is one that contains all the nutriments, and these in proper ratio the one to the other, that the particular animal may require. Each class of animal, and each animal in particular, requires its own particular diet; there is no such thing as a well-balanced ration suitable for all animals and all needs.

Sudden changes, involving a major proportion of the ration, are to be avoided in all stock. Changes should be made gradually or involve only one or two out of several ingredients. In ruminants a sudden change on to a predominantly cereal diet can prove fatal. (*See* BARLEY POISONING.)

Standards of feeding and published figures of digestible constituents in foods should be used rather as guides than as definite formulae.

Work at the Hannah Dairy Research Institute by Sir Kenneth Blaxter and his colleagues suggests that long-accepted standards (based on work more than half a century old) need revision. **'We tend to overfeed the low-producing cow, and underfeed the high yielder.'**

Regularity in the times of feeding is essential for success. Only good quality food should be used; there is no economy in feeding with inferior or damaged fodder; on the contrary, the use of such food has been the cause of much illness. There should not be long intervals between meals; with horses this is one of the common causes of colic. When compounding a ration it should be remembered that a mixture of foods gives a better result than the use of one or two foods. The ration should contain a sufficiency of energy-producing constituents, sufficient protein, fibre, and mineral matter, and an adequate allowance of the various constituents the one to the other has also to be studied. (*See* CONCENTRATES.)

The digestibility of foods. Only that part of a food which is digested is of value to an animal. The digestibility of foods varies greatly, some being easily and completely digested, while others, especially those containing much fibre, are digested imperfectly and with difficulty; and, of course, some animals will digest a particular food better than other animals will. The method of feeding is important; if it is erratic instead of at regular intervals the food will not be well digested as when the feeding hours are regular. (*See* D-VALUE.)

Preparation of foods. Some foods are fed to animals in the natural state, while others are prepared in some such way as by grinding, bruising, cutting, chaffing, boiling, steaming, or soaking in water. The object of preparing a food before giving it to an animal is to increase its digestibility. Oats may be bruised for hard-working horses, for colts changing their teeth, and for calves; there is undoubtedly a slight increase in the digestibility of bruised over whole grain, but for an economic advantage the total cost of bruising should be less than 10 per cent of the whole grain. Beans should be split or 'kibbled' for horses, as the tough seed-coat makes them difficult to masticate. Maize also is more easily eaten if it is cracked.

Grinding grains to a meal is advisable for pigs, **but it is important that the particle size is not too small.** Absence of milk in the recently farrowed sow and bowel oedema may, it has been suggested (*Veterinary Record*, April 3, 1971), be associated with too fine meal particles.

Deterioration with storage. It is important to remember that bruised or kibbled seeds do not keep well, especially if exposed to a damp atmosphere, and are liable to turn musty, owing to fermentation changes. So long as the grain is whole and intact it is essentially still a living entity. When crushed, etc., it is killed, and the normal processes of deterioration and decomposition commence.

All feeds tend to deteriorate, and to become less palatable, on storage. With whole cereals this deterioration will be very slight, but with maize meal it can be rapid. The Ministry recommends that the following storage periods should not be exceeded.

Maximum safe storage periods	
Vegetable proteins	3 months
Animal proteins	1 month
Molassine meal	2 weeks
Ground cereals	1 week
Mixed feed	1 week

FLOUR MITE INFESTATION. At the National Institute for Research in Dairying it was suspected that infestation with flour mites of an experimental feed, during prolonged storage, was the cause of reduced performance of growing pigs in a diet trial. The help of MAFF's Slough laboratory was sought, and a comparison made between deliberately infested feed and control samples. It was demonstrated that, as the mite infestation increased, there was a considerable loss of dry matter, carbohydrate, and amino acids. Subsequent growth trials showed that the daily liveweight gain and feed: gain ratio were significantly reduced in the pigs on the mite-infested diet. Dr R. Braude and his colleagues commented: 'Under the conditions of this test about one-fifth of the nutritive value of the diet was lost to the pig through progressive infestation with flour mites,' and consider that their findings may be on considerable significance for efficient production.

Palatability. It is important that foods offered to animals should be palatable and appetising. Some foods are not very palatable, such as palm kernel cake or meal, but may be made more palatable by mixing with some molasses or locust bean meal. On the other hand, foods which are naturally palatable may become very unappetising if they have been allowed to get damp and musty. The inclusion of even a small quantity of musty food – such as foxy oats and mouldy hay – in a ration spoils the whole food. The greatest care should be taken to see that the food is fresh and wholesome and that food-troughs and water-troughs are kept clean.

For dangers of poisoning by mouldy food, *see* AFLATOXINS and MYCOTOXICOSIS.)

Variety and mixtures. Animals benefit from variety in their rations. It is often found that while a given ration may give excellent results for a time, there is a tendency for animals to eat their food without zest. This applies less to pigs and horses than to cattle, sheep, poultry, dogs, and cats. A change, which may be quite simple, results in a return of the normal zest.

Also, as a rule, mixtures of several different foods are more palatable and are better digested than single food-stuffs. This is partly because during digestion foods of different origins actually assist to digest each other, and partly because if there is any deficiency in a particular food substance in one food, it may be made good to the animal by being present in another one of the mixture.

Maintenance and production rations. Rations given to animals can be divided into two parts, a maintenance and a production part. A maintenance ration may be described as that which will maintain an animal that is in a resting and nonproducing condition and in good health, in the same condition and at the same weight for an indefinite period.

A production ration is that part of the daily diet which is given in excess of maintenance requirements, and which is available for being converted into energy, as in working horses, or into milk, or into fat or wool, or is used for growth.

It will be clear that a maintenance ration by itself is uneconomical, since it gives no return.

In devising a maintenance ration it should be clearly understood that any food will not do; wheat straw does not contain sufficient protein for the maintenance of health in yearling bullocks, but wheat straw in combination with good quality hay will do so. (*See* RATIONS, WINTER DIET.)

The most practical application of maintenance and production rations is in use where the cows are fed according to their milk yield.

Substitutional dieting. A farmer having fixed a daily ration for, let us say, his dairy cows, desires to change some of the constituents in the diet by substituting other foods. If foods are merely changed haphazardly pound for pound it is almost certain that the diet will be altered appreciably. For example, if 5 lb of maize is substituted for 5 lb of oats in a horse's ration the animal will be getting more nutriment than formerly, as 80 lb of oats are equal to 60 lb of maize. Again, oat straw, pound for pound, has rather less than half the nutriment found in meadow hay, and so on. Most stockowners have a general idea of the relative values of foods, but it is only by studying them on the basis of their starch equivalent and protein content that a real idea of their energy value can be obtained and that substitution can be effected in an economical manner. (*See* STARCH EQUIVALENT, PROTEIN EQUIVALENT, RATIONS, DRIED GRASS, SILAGE, UREA.)

When substituting one food for another it is important that the change be made gradually. Disastrous results have followed the sudden change of a diet. (*See also* NUTRITION, FAULTY; VITAMINS; HORSES, FEEDING OF; DOG'S DIET; CAT FOODS.)

DIET DURING ILLNESS or convalescence. (*See* NURSING.)

DIGESTIBILITY (*see* DIET).

DIGESTION, ABSORPTION, and ASSIMILATION are the three processes by which food is incorporated into the body.

Salivary digestion begins as soon as the food enters the mouth and becomes mixed with saliva secreted by the salivary glands. It is not very thorough in animals, such as the dog, which bolt their food without careful chewing, but in the horse during feeding, and in the ox and sheep while rumination is proceeding, it reaches a greater state of perfection, especially when starchy foods are eaten. Raw starches, which are very often enclosed in a matrix of cellulose or woody material, are not acted upon to any great extent until the cellulose covering has been dissolved, through the action of bacteria, in other parts of the system. Saliva has no digestive action upon proteins. In the domesticated dog, however, there seems little doubt that when given dry biscuits, which necessitate a certain amount of chewing, some salivary digestion does occur.

There is found in the dog's saliva an enzyme called *ptyalin*, which actively changes the insoluble starch of carbohydrate foods into partly soluble sugars, but the process requires consummation by the enzymes of the small intestines. Ptyalin is only able to act in an alkaline medium, and its action therefore ceases as soon as the food has become permeated with acid gastric juice in the stomach. The saliva has one other very important function: it is incorporated and mixed with dry or mealy foods by the process of chewing, so that these may be formed into little coherent masses known as 'boli' and be more easily swallowed.

Stomach digestion begins shortly after the food enters the true stomach and continues till it leaves this organ. There are great differences in the domesticated animals, due to the fact that some – *e.g.* ruminants – have a compound stomach, and these must receive separate consideration.

In the horse, pig, and dog, when food enters the stomach, 'gastric juice' is secreted from the digestive glands situated in its walls. This juice contains the enzyme *pepsin*, which, in the presence of dilute hydrochloric, also elaborated by these glands, acts upon the protein constituents. Before any action occurs, however, the stomach actively engages in a vigorous churning movement which has the effect of thoroughly mixing the gastric juice with the contained food, and of breaking up the latter. Actually the stomach does not prepare the food for absorption, but rather warms it up, incorporates with it the gastric juice, softens it, and converts the whole mass into a greyish-white (in pig and dog) or brownish (horse) mass of uniform consistency, in which particles of the various foods taken can be easily recognised.

Gastric lipase is another enzyme, present in both ruminants and simple-stomached animals, which is concerned with preliminary digestion of fats.

In the horse, food stays in the stomach till it is about two-thirds full, and is then hurried through to the small intestine to make room for further amounts entering from the mouth, and yet in spite of this the stomach is practically never found empty after death – unless the horse has been starved. In this way the stomach of the horse may allow an amount of food two or even three times greater than its maximum capacity to pass through it during a feed, but when no more food is taken the stomach retains the last portions and only allows them to pass slowly out into the intestines. In the pig and dog food is retained in the stomach for a variable time according to the state in which it was swallowed, and is thoroughly churned and mixed with gastric juice. During this time the softer portions along with fluids and semi-fluids are squeezed through the pylorus into the intestine. As soon as any solid hard material comes into contact with the walls near the pylorus, the latter immediately closes tightly and retains the hard substance.

In the ruminating farm animals – cattle and sheep – stomach digestion is complicated by the presence of three compartments before the true stomach is reached. These may briefly be said to be concerned in the preparation of the food before it enters the abomasum for true digestion. Although the rumen possesses no true digestive glands, yet a very considerable amount of digestion (if we term as digestion the splitting up of complex into simple products) takes place in it through the activity of cellulose-splitting and other organisms, which are normally present in enormous numbers. (*See also* RUMINAL DIGESTION.)

In the unweaned calf, the act of sucking apparently stimulates reflex closure of the oesophageal groove, so that the dam's milk by-passes the rumen (where it could not be effectively digested).

After the food has been subjected to the action of the organisms in the rumen, and has been chewed for a second time as 'cud', it is sent on into the third stomach or omasum for further breaking up by trituration, and then into the true stomach or abomasum, where digestive glands are present, and where a form of digestion similar to what occurs in the stomach of other animals takes place. The main function of the second stomach or reticulum is to act as a fluid reservoir from whence a supply of fluid can be sent into any compartment where it is needed for normal digestion.

Intestinal digestion. The softened semi-fluid material which leaves the stomach is commonly known as 'chyme'; it has an acid reaction, since it has been well mixed with the hydrochloric or lactic acid in the stomach. Shortly after entering the small intestine it meets with alkaline fluids and its acidity is neutralised. This occurs through the action of the bile from the liver and of the pancreatic juice from the pancreas. These fluids are similar in that they are both alkaline, but they differ greatly in their functions. The bile is partly composed of complex salts and pigments (*see* BILE). Its function is fourfold: it aids the emulsification of fats, dividing large droplets into tiny globules which are more easily split into their component parts by other enzymes prior to absorption; it assists in keeping the intestinal contents fluid and preventing undue fermentation and putrefaction through its slight antiseptic action against putrefactive organisms; it stimulates peristalsis to some extent, and it gives the faeces their characteristic colour. The pancreatic juice possesses at least three powerful enzymes which are probably sufficient in themselves to ensure complete digestion of a food without other assistance. The first of these is called *trypsin*, and is concerned in the further splitting up of protein substances which have been partly acted upon by the pepsin of the stomach. It completes the work of the pepsin, so to speak. After proteins have been acted upon for a period by trypsin they are capable of being absorbed and made use of in the body. The next pancreatic enzyme is called *amylopsin*. It acts on carbohydrate constituents, splitting them up into sugars and other substances, but not carrying the process far enough to allow of complete absorption. Amylopsin has an action similar to that of the ptyalin of saliva, but it is more powerful, and it can act upon raw starch which is not able to be split up by the latter. *Lipase*, or *steapsin*, is the name of the fat-splitting enzyme of the pancreatic fluid. It acts upon the tiny globules of fat which have been emulsified by the bile, etc., and splits them into their compounds – glycerol and a fatty acid, the latter depending upon the origin of the fat.

Now, it will be obvious that there must be occasions when some of the food constituents escape action by these enzymes. But any such food is dealt with by the intestinal juice. This is produced by the intestinal glands, and is of very complex composition. It contains a number of enzymes of which the most important are: *erepsin, enterokinase, maltase, lactase*, and *invertase*. The first of these completes the breaking up of any protein which may have escaped the action of the pepsin and trypsin. Enterokinase is concerned with the formation of trypsin from its fore-runner trypsinogen, and the last three complete the splitting up of carbohydrates into soluble sugars. Bacteria also have a most important digestive function in the intestines. In the large intestines of herbivorous animals they have a cellulose splitting action, which is somewhat allied to fermentation, and is similar to the activity of the organisms present in the first stomachs of ruminants. They act upon fats in a similar manner to the pancreatic juice; they form certain volatile obnoxious substances (indol and skatol) from proteins, which give the faeces their characteristic odour; they produce lactic acid in certain cases; and they may even destroy alkaloidal poisons which have been formed during other stages of digestion.

Absorption. Water passes through the stomach into the intestines almost immediately. But it is only after subjection to digestion in the intestines for some hours that the bulk of the food is taken up into the system. The chyme which leaves the stomach is converted by the action of the bile and pancreatic fluids into a yellowish-grey or a brownish-green fluid of creamy consistency called 'chyle', containing in the herbivorous animals particles of hay, oats, grass, etc. From this the fats are absorbed (after emulsification and breakdown) by the lymph vessels or 'lacteals' which occupy the centre of each of the 'villi' of the small intestines. The villi are small finger-like processes which project from the wall of the small intestine into its lumen, and are therefore continually in contact with the food passing through it. In the lacteals the fat globules are re-formed and from these they are collected by the lymph vessels of the intestines and are ultimately passed into the blood-stream. Sugar, salts, and soluble proteins pass directly into the small blood-vessels in the walls of the intestines, and are thence carried to the liver and so enter the general circulation.

The food is passed onwards through the various folds and coils of the intestines, each particular part of the bowel wall removing some portions of the food, and the residual, unabsorbable, useless constituents are eventually discharged from the rectum and anus during the process of defaecation, constituting the dung.

Assimilation takes place slowly. After the products of digestion have been absorbed into the blood- and lymph-streams they are carried round the body, ultimately reaching every organ and tissue, and the body cells extract from the blood in the capillaries whatever nutritive products they may require for growth or repair. For instance, cells in bony tissues extract lime salts, muscles take proteins and sugars, etc. When the supply of food is much in excess of immediate requirements the surplus is stored up, perhaps as glycogen in liver or muscle, perhaps as fat deposited in the looser areas of the body, *e.g.* in the peritoneal cavity, or around various organs, or under the skin and among the muscle fibres.

DIGITALIS is a preparation from the leaf of the wild Foxglove, *Digitalis purpurea*, gathered when the flowers are at a certain stage.

The leaves contain glycosides, including digitoxin, gitoxin, and gitalin; the seeds contain another glycoside, digitalin.

Digitalis is used in the treatment of chronic heart disease, in dogs mainly. The action of the heart is slowed down, the drug increasing the length of diastole, and at the same time it is strengthened.

Digitalis must be used with care, as the digitoxin is excreted only slowly and there is a cumulative effect which can readily lead to poisoning. Its use in cats is inadvisable, and liable to cause vomiting. This, together with loss of appetite, depression, and bradycardia may occur in some dogs even with normal dosage.

Digitalis Poisoning may occur from a single, large dose or from prolonged administration. The heart's action may become irregular. Diarrhoea may occur.

In grazing animals poisoning may result from the eating of the plant rosettes. Foxgloves included in hay have also caused poisoning.

DIHYDROTACHYSTEROL. An oil-soluble steroid used to raise the calcium level of the blood, and so treat or prevent hypocalcaemia.

DIHYDROXYANTHRAQUINONE. A nontoxic laxative, acting chiefly on the large intestine, effective in all the domestic animals, including horses. It may be given in the food, when it acts in about 24 hours.

DIMIDIUM BROMIDE. A trypanocide effective against *T. congolense*.

DIOCTOPHYMOSIS. Infestation with the kidney worm *Dioctophyma renale* a parasite of dogs encountered in Europe, America, and Asia. A survey of 500 dogs in Iran revealed an incidence of 1·3 per cent. Stray dogs and jackals have been found infested. Man may become infested through the eating of fish. (*See also under* ROUND-WORMS.)

DIODONE. A contrast medium used in radiography of the kidneys.

DIOESTRUS. During this stage of the sexual cycle in the female, progesterone is secreted by the *corpus luteum*. This causes the mare, for example, to reject the stallion and induces changes in the reproductive tract designed to provide a suitable environment for development of the embryo. In the mare dioestrus 'normally lasts 15–16 days and is terminated by the release of one or more luteolytic factors from the endometrium which induce(s) regression of the *corpus luteum*'. (Dr W. R. Allen, *Vet. Rec.* (1977), **100**, 68.) (*See* OESTRUS.)

DIOXIN is formed as an impurity during the synthesis of trichlorophenol and its derivatives, and with them it was involved in the disaster at Seveso in Italy. Exposure in such industrial accidents may lead to cancer, skin, eye, blood and liver damage; and also to abortion, foetal malformation and chromosomal aberrations.

Dioxin contaminated milk on a farm near a toxic waste disposal plant in the Netherlands. The dioxin was emitted during the destruction of polyvinyl plastic (PVC).

DIPHTHERIA, Calf (*see* CALF, DIPHTHERIA).

DIPHTHERIA, GUTTURAL POUCH, of horses. (*See under* GUTTURAL.)

DIPLEGIA means extensive paralysis on both sides of the body.

DIPROSOPUS. Duplication of the face. This is a congenital defect, and a type of conjoined twinning.

DIPS and DIPPING. In Britain mostly sheep are dipped, but beef cattle may also be dipped with advantage. Dipping is an important means of tick control in cattle, and is widely practised in the tropics.

Sheep are dipped in order: (1) to eradicate the commoner parasitic agents, such as keds, lice, ticks, etc.; (2) to act as a check upon the spread of mange in the sheep, commonly called 'sheep scab', and where that disease has broken out, to cure it; and (3) to prevent attack by the sheep-blowflies and consequent infestation with maggots.

In different districts there are different times for dipping according to the breeds kept and the climate. On farms in the south of England the sheep are sometimes dipped three times a year: once before clipping, once soon after clipping, and again in the autumn. In mountain districts dipping ordinarily takes place twice a year, the early spring dipping being missed. In addition to local custom, special dipping orders can still be enforced in Britain by the Ministry of Agriculture for the purpose of keeping in check such diseases as sheep scab, and for the eradication of ticks.

PRECAUTIONS. Owners should ensure that any dips they purchase carry on their labels the statement that the dip has been approved by the Ministry of Agriculture and Fisheries. The following precautions should be observed when sheep are dipped:

1. For 1 month or 5 weeks after service ewes should not be dipped lest abortion result. Pregnant ewes require careful handling to avoid injury, but with care they may be dipped almost up to the time they lamb, provided weather is favourable.

2. Early spring washing or dipping must be carried out with a solution which does not harm the wool, making the fibres brittle or stained.

3. Summer dipping should take place when there is a sufficiency of fleece to carry and hold the dip, and when parasites may most easily be destroyed, *i.e.* at from 3 to 5 weeks after clipping.

4. Autumn dipping should be finished before the first frosts of the season begin, and when the weather is so much settled that rain is not expected during the next 24 hours. This is of more importance in autumn dipping than otherwise, because the dip has to remain in the fleece during the winter, and it is more easily washed out before it has dried than afterwards.

5. Sheep should be offered a drink of water before being dipped in hot weather, as there is some risk of thirsty animals drinking the dip, with fatal results if it is a poisonous variety.

6. Sheep should be rested before actual immersion, especially if recently brought in from a hill, or when they have walked a distance to the dipper. This is particularly important in hot weather.

7. Sheep with open wounds or sores, and those that have recently been attacked with maggots or have been ill, should not be dipped until the skin is whole and until they have otherwise recovered. This is another reason why dipping should not immediately follow shearing.

8. Sheep must not be turned out on to grazing land immediately after being dipped, for the drainage from the fleeces contaminates the herbage, and the sheep being hungry may eat sufficient dip-sodden grass to produce poisoning. They should be allowed about 15 minutes in the draining pens.

9. Each sheep should be immersed in the dipper for the requisite length of time according to the instructions that are furnished with each kind of dip by the makers.

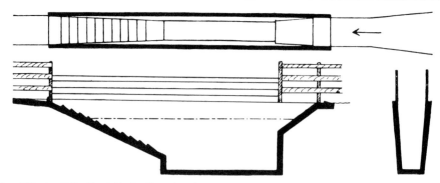

Plan of Dipping Bath. (See table for dimensions.)

10. The dip must be carefully made up according to instructions, and fresh dipping powder and fluid added to make up the loss that occurs from the removal of a small amount upon the fleece of each sheep. It is not sufficient to add water.

11. After dipping operations are finished the dip should be disposed of in such a way that there is no danger of it contaminating water-supplies, ponds, streams, etc. (*See* FISH, POISONING OF.)

Local regulations may require the use of a specific type of dip. It is important to get the dip from a good firm of known reputation, and it is essential to make it up strictly according to the accompanying instructions and to the exact strength stated.

In Britain. The ban on the use of dieldrin and aldrin-based sheep dips came into force at the end of 1965. With a view to replacing those organo-chlorine dips, a range of organo-phosphorous ones came on to the market. One good point is that, like dieldrin, an organo-phosphorus compound diffuses down the wool as it grows, so that no unprotected layer – vulnerable to the green-bottle's maggots – is left. The concentrated liquid must not be allowed to come into contact with human skin. There is, too, a prescribed period, varying with the chemical, to be observed between dipping and slaughter: usually 14 or 21 days.

In Britain dips containing **BHC** (benzene hexa-chloride) or **HCH** (hexachlorocyclohexane) have been **officially banned**.

BATHS AND THEIR USE. The bath to be used depends on many circumstances, such as numbers to be dipped, land and materials available, and so on. The best material to use is concrete, and the most popular shape is that shown. The dimensions for the various animals are as shown in table below.

	Horse	Cattle	Sheep	Pigs
	ft in	ft in	ft in	ft in
Breadth at top	5 9	5 2	3 3	3 3
Breadth at bottom	3 3	3 3	2 6	2 6
Depth	8 5	7 6	5 9	5 9
Length at top	55 0	50 0	45 0	35 0
Length of well	30 0	30 0	30 0	20 0
Entrance slope	7 3	6 6	5 0	5 0
Exit slope	16 3	13 0	10 0	10 0
Depth of dip from bottom	6 6	5 6	4 0	4 0

These figures are only given as a general guide.

In order to avoid waste of dip, the farmer needs to know exactly how much liquid the bath will hold, and he also needs a calibrated stick or side-marking to indicate the volume of liquid still in the bath at all stages of dipping. What is sometimes overlooked is the fact that a sheep with wool 1 to 1½ inches long will not merely remove permanently at least ½ gallon of liquid, but will strain off additional insecticide. This necessitates 'topping up' of the dip wash at double strength as compared with the liquid used for the first filling of the bath. Obviously, the number, size, and dirtiness of the sheep will determine the number of times that topping up is necessary for a given size of bath.

It is a false economy not to top up before the last 20 or 30 sheep are put through the dip, since any saving of money thereby could later be more than offset by those animals becoming victims of strike. Disappointing results of any dip can also follow if sheep are immersed for far short of 30 seconds; or if they are soaking wet when they enter the bath, for then their fleeces can carry much less than the normal quantity of wash.

A sheep with a short growth of wool (1 to 1½ inches) will emerge from the bath carrying 4 or 5 gallons of wash, and will retain ½ gallon. If there is not to be an expensive waste of dip, it is important that the floor of the draining pens should be such as to allow the maximum run-back of liquid to the bath.

Arsenic-dipped animals should never be allowed on to pasturage until there is no risk of contamination of grass.

In all cases the animal should be totally immersed at least once (hence the abrupt commencement of the bath), and special attention should be paid to the ears and tail. Dipping must be thorough.

One dipping will seldom (if ever) be effective in ridding an animal of parasites, as the dip may not affect the eggs. The dip must accordingly be repeated at suitable intervals. Against keds, dips require to be repeated in 3 to 4 weeks, and against mange in about 7 to 10 days.

LAMENESS. Especially in warm climates, where the dip has been allowed to remain in the tank and has become dirty, there is a danger of sheep becoming lame after dipping. This results from infection with *Erysipelothrix rhusiospathiae* (*see* under SWINE ERYSIPELAS) through any cuts or abrasions. Such lameness does not follow the use of a freshly prepared dip. It has been obviated by the addition to the dip of tetramethyl thiuram disulphide. This controls any bacteria which contaminate the dip liquid. Non-phenolic sheep dips have little or no action against bacteria.

SPRAYING. Dipping of all animals involves considerable trouble, expensive equipment, and in most cases is static so that animals must come to the dipper. The use of modern sprays and jets, whereby the chemical agent is directed on to the animal's skin with considerable force, has some advantages over dipping and is partly replacing dipping in some countries (see SPRAY-RACE.) (See also JETTING.) In Britain, those who practise spraying, as opposed to dipping, would be unwise to rely on more than 3 weeks' protection against strike. This is partly because less insecticide remains in the fleece after spraying; also, the organo-phosphorus insecticides move down the wool but, apparently, not sideways, so that if a patch is left unsprayed it remains vulnerable to strike.

For tick control in Africa see under TICKS.

DIQUAT. This herbicide has caused fatal poisoning in cattle, four years after the discarding of a container.

DIROFILARIASIS (see HEARTWORMS).

DISBUDDING is the removal of, or the prevention of growth in, the horn buds in calves, kids, and sometimes in lambs. (See under GOATS.)

DISC, INTERVERTEBRAL (see under SPINE).

DISCOSPONDYLOSIS. Inflammation of the inter-vertebral discs of the spinal column.

'DISEASE-FREE' ANIMALS. Piglet mortality is one of the main sources of economic loss to the pig industry, and it is in the study of these very important piglet diseases that special laboratory pigs are necessary. Without such animals research work may not only be hampered or even brought to a standstill by natural infections, but complications may arise.

From the moment the piglet leaves the security of the uterus and enters the birth-canal it becomes exposed to an infected environment. Under natural conditions it is protected against this environment, to a greater or lesser degree by the wide range of antibodies received from its dam in the first milk, the colostrum. When deprived of colostrum piglets almost always die. But the research worker wishes to avoid the feeding of colostrum, since this substance may well contain antibodies against the disease under investigation.

The problem is, then, to rear piglets which are both disease-free and devoid of antibodies. In principle, the solution to the problem is a simple one. All that needs to be done is to obtain the piglets before they reach the infected environment and to rear them away from possible infection, so that colostrum is unnecessary. In practice, these requirements are not easily met. However, by using a technique developed in the USA at the University of Nebraska, 'disease-free', antibody-devoid pigs have been produced at the School of Veterinary Medicine, University of Cambridge, and elsewhere.

The piglets are taken direct from the sow's uterus a day or two before the estimated farrowing date. The sow is anaesthetised, the whole uterus carefully but rapidly removed and passed through a bath of disinfectant, which forms an antiseptic lock, into a sterilised hood. The sow is immediately slaughtered. The hood is supplied with warm, filtered air under slight pressure and the two operators work through long-sleeved rubber gloves. In the hood the piglets are taken from the uterus, their navel cords are tied off, and they are dried with sterile towels. The piglets are then transferred, by means of a sealed carrying case, to sterile incubator units kept in a heated isolation room. The incubators, each of which holds one pig, are equipped with filter pads so that both the air entering the unit and that passing out into the exhaust system is filtered.

During the first few days of their independent existence, great care is necessary to protect the young animals from bacteria in general. The attendant wears mask and cap in addition to rubber gloves and overalls. Subsequently, masks and caps are unnecessary. The diet, which consists of pasteurised milk, eggs and minerals, is sterilised by heat for the first three days of life, but not thereafter. The piglets are fed from flat-bottomed trays 3 times daily – morning, midday and late afternoon. There are no night feeds. After some 10 days in the incubator units the young pigs are transferred to individual open cages in another isolation pen. There they are rapidly weaned to solid food. Later, the pigs are mixed together and treated as ordinary ones except that, of course, precautions are taken to prevent accidental infection.

Pigs reared by this technique are in a state of minimal disease: they are not germ-free. In fact, non-pathogenic bacteria are deliberately introduced by feeding pasteurised, instead of sterilised, milk from the fourth day of life onwards. These pigs are not, therefore, in the same category as the germ-free animals produced with the aid of elaborate and expensive equipment by Dr Reyniers at the University of Notre Dame in Indiana. (See GNOTOBIOTICS.) Production of 'disease-free' pigs was begun at Cambridge primarily to permit the critical investigation of pig diseases, particularly diseases of suckling pigs, but such pigs have obvious advantages for nutritional and genetic studies because the technique does eliminate that unpredictable variable, disease.

Another possible use for this technique, which may be of more immediate interest to pig farmers, is in ridding valuable blood lines of such maladies as rhinitis, pneumonia, enteritis, and aparasitic infection. When the salvage value of the sow is taken into account the procedure comes into the realms of practical economics. (See also SPF.)

DISEASES (see NOSOCOMIAL, IATROGENIC, and STOCKMEN).

DISEASES OF ANIMALS ACT, 1950. This Act (and Orders relating to it) is administered by the Animal Health Division of the Ministry of Agriculture of Great Britain.

It covers the diseases listed under NOTIFIABLE DISEASES.

The Act and Orders provide for the compulsory notification of the existence or suspected existence of these diseases; for the immediate isolation or segregation of diseased or suspected animals; for the diagnosis of suspected disease by specially trained persons; for the slaughter of diseased or in-contact animals where necessary, and for the safe disposal of their carcases; for the payment of compensation to owners in certain cases; for the apprehension and punishment of offenders; for the systematic inspection of markets, fairs, sales, and exhibitions, etc., and for the seizure of diseased or suspected animals therein; for regulating the transit and transport of animals by land or water, both within the country and in the home waters; for controlling the importation of animals and things which may introduce one or other of these diseases from abroad; and for inspection at the ports and quarantine or slaughter where necessary.

The following regulations have a general application to all scheduled diseases, but in practically every case there is at least one Order applicable to the particular disease, in which there is set out more fully regulations dealing with that disease. These Orders can be obtained from Her Majesty's Stationery Offices, and must be consulted individually if complete information is required.

Notification of diseases or suspected disease must always be made by the owner of an animal, or by the occupier or person in charge, and by the veterinary surgeon in attendance, to an inspector of the Local Authority or to a police constable, and that without undue delay.

Presumption of knowledge of disease. A person required to give notice if charged with failure to carry out his obligation shall be presumed to have known of the existence of the disease, unless and until he shows, to the satisfaction of the Court, that he had not knowledge thereof and could not with reasonable care have obtained that knowledge.

Separation of diseased animals. Every person having a diseased animal shall, as far as is practicable, keep it separate from animals not so diseased.

Facilities and assistance to be given for inspection, cleansing, and disinfection. Persons in charge of diseased animals are required to give every facility for the execution of the above, and must not obstruct or in any way hinder inspectors or other officers in doing their duty.

Prohibition of exposure of diseased animals. It is unlawful to expose a diseased or suspected animal in a market, sale-yard, fair, or other public or private place where such animals are commonly exposed for sale; to place an affected animal in a lair or other place adjacent to or connected with a market, sale-yard, etc., or where such animals are commonly exposed for sale; to send a diseased animal on a railway, or on any canal, inland navigation or coasting vessels; or to allow one on a highway or thoroughfare, or on any common or unenclosed land or in any insufficiently fenced field; or to graze one on the sides of a highway; or to allow one to stray on a highway or thoroughfare or on the sides thereof, etc.

Digging up carcases. No person may dig up the carcase of an animal that has been buried, without permission from the Ministry of Agriculture. (*See also* under each main heading of the scheduled diseases, *e.g.* ANTHRAX.)

DISEASES OF ANIMALS (WASTE FOOD) ORDER 1973 replaced the 1957 Order and strengthens the regulations concerning the handling, processing and distribution of swill.

DISHORNING OF CATTLE. It has been found advisable to remove the horns from dairy cows housed in yards and from fattening beef cattle in yards or pens, because there is usually one that obtained mastery over the others, and if it possesses horns it is liable to inflict wounds upon others or upon the attendants.

The most satisfactory method is that known as 'disbudding'. This consists of painting the young buds of the horns, when they first appear in calves, with caustic compound. It is best to disbud at one week of age and certainly not later than 10 days. A little Vaseline or thick grease may be rubbed on the hair around the base of the bud and care is needed to ensure that no caustic gets into the eyes. The bud of the horn is first cleaned with spirit to remove grease – an essential preliminary – and a second coating of the caustic is given after the first has dried. A scab will form over the bud and drop off, carrying with it the cells which would have produced horn. Little or no pain is occasioned to the calf by caustic collodion (whereas caustic potash sticks, now largely superseded, do cause much pain) and the horn is effectively prevented from growing.

In Great Britain the operation of dishorning cattle requires the administration of an anaesthetic. (*See* ANAESTHETICS, LEGAL REQUIREMENTS.) A saw, an electric saw, cutting wire or special horn shears may be used.

Bleeding from the matrix and horn core can usually be controlled by using a figure-of-eight tourniquet round the roots of the horns.

DISHORNING OF GOATS (*see* DISBUDDING).

DISINFECTANTS may be either physical or chemical. Among the former are heat, sunlight and electricity; while among the latter are solids, liquids, and gases. Steam may be used.

Chemical disinfectants. At the present time these are numerous and diverse. The Ministry of Agriculture and Fisheries test them from time to time and issues its approval only to those that are maintained up to standard. Consequently, owners should examine the labels on containers and use only those that carry the official approval since this is a guarantee of potency.

The Diseases of Animals (Approved Disinfectants) Order 1970 governs the uses of disinfectants in the UK, and specifies those approved for use in connection with foot-and-mouth disease, tuberculosis, fowl pest, and general orders relating to disease control. Dilution rates are also specified.

A full list of disinfectants approved for use in outbreaks of foot-and-mouth disease is given under that subject entry.

Disinfectants act in one of three ways: (1) as oxidising agents or as reducing agents; (2) as corrosives or coagulants acting upon the protoplasm of bacterial life; or (3) as bacterial poisons.

Most chemical disinfectants are supplied in a concentrated form and must be diluted with water before use. The water should be clean, preferably soft, and if it can be used warm the efficiency of the disinfectant is increased. After the active agent has been added the whole should be well stirred for a few moments to ensure thorough mixing. The solution must be applied so that it remains in contact with the offending material for a sufficiently long time to kill the bacterial life therein; generally ten minutes to half an hour should elapse before disinfecting solutions are rinsed away.

When two or more disinfectants are mixed together, instead of an increased disinfecting power in the mixture they often enter into chemical combination with each other and useless compound results. (See also ANTISEPTICS.)

Quaternary Ammonia Compounds (see under this heading).

Cresol Solutions. There are many of these, e.g. the cresol and soap solution of the BP, the compound cresol solution of the USAP, lysol, isal, cyllin, creolin, cresylin, Jeyes' fluid, or one of the proprietary preparations. These are used as 3 per cent to 5 per cent solutions for practically all purposes of disinfection about a farm premises, and very often as antiseptics also. Their action is enhanced by the use of hot water instead of cold. None of them are suitable for use in connection with food, for all are to a greater or lesser degree poisonous. Cresols are not very effective against many viruses or bacterial spores. The cresols are related to PHENOL (which see).

Formalin is sometimes used as a solution for disinfecting floors, about 5 per cent strength being necessary.

Formaldehyde gas may be used for fumigation of live-stock buildings where virus or other diseases have occurred. (See under DISINFECTION.)

DISINFECTION of buildings cannot be achieved by applying a disinfectant solution to walls and floors which are heavily contaminated with dirt. There are two reasons for this: (1) the disinfectant cannot reach most of the microorganisms, which will be protected by layers of dirt; and (2) the latter may alter the nature of the disinfectant solution chemically, rendering it ineffective.

Preliminary cleaning is therefore essential. The building must first be thoroughly scraped, brushed, and cleansed. Concrete floors may be power-hosed, scraped free from all dirt and debris. A hot detergent solution of 2½ to 4 per cent washing-soda is then thoroughly scrubbed onto floors, walls, stall partitions, mangers, troughs, or other fittings.

Disinfectants. To be effective, the application of disinfectants is the *second stage* of the process of disinfection, cleaning being the first stage.

In certain cases it may be desirable to fumigate the building. All air entrances and exits are securely closed, the inside of the walls and roof is soaked with water, and formaldehyde gas generated (e.g. by pouring on to 250 gm of potassium permanganate 500 ml of formalin per 1000 cu ft of air space.) All doors and windows are left shut for a day, and the building is then flushed out with clean water under pressure from a hose-pipe.

Steam cleaning may be carried out as part of a disinfection process.

MOVABLE OBJECTS. All pails, grooming tools, wheelbarrows, shovels, forks, etc., which have been used for the infected animals must also be disinfected before they can be considered safe for further use.

DISLOCATION is a displacement of a bone from its normal position in relation to a joint. Deformity is produced, and there may be intense pain if the part is interfered with. As well as displacement there is also bruising of the soft tissues around the joints, and tearing of the ligaments which bind the bones together.

Probably the most common dislocation is that of the patella which becomes lodged on the uppermost part of the outer ridge of the patellar surface of the femur and is unable to extricate itself from this position. In the dog, dislocation of the shoulder joint is by no means rare.

The causes of dislocations are similar to those which produce fracture. Violence applied in such a manner that the structures around the joint are unable to withstand the stress. (For inherited abnormality in dogs, see under PATELLA.)

SIGNS. The injured limb is useless, and as a rule is held off the ground in an unnatural attitude. There is generally little or no pain so long as the parts are not forcibly moved; but if a nerve trunk is pressed upon, the animal may perspire with the pain. When the limb is compared with that of the opposite side there is seen a marked difference in its contours or outline – the joint affected shows hollows or prominences where none are seen in the normal limb. There is a loss of the power of movement, but there is no grating sound heard when the joint or the whole limb is passively moved, such as occurs when a fracture exists.

TREATMENT. The reduction of most dislocations necessitates the use of anaesthesia.

DISPLACED ABOMASUM. A condition encountered in cattle some weeks after calving and leading to a complete lack of appetite. (See under STOMACH, DISEASES OF.)

DISPOSAL OF CARCASES. Carcases of animals may be disposed of by sending them to a knackery or destructor, or by burial or burning. It is most important that they should not be left lying for any length of time in summer weather, for within a few hours after death they are usually selected by female flies for the deposition of their eggs, and within 24 to 36 hours they are swarming with maggots. Moreover, where the cause of death has been a contagious disease there is always the risk of healthy animals becoming directly or indirectly affected, and of the disease spreading accordingly.

In most progressive countries there are Government regulations which provide for the safe disposal of the carcases of animals that have died from any one of the notifiable contagious diseases, such as anthrax, foot-and-mouth disease, cattle plague, etc., but it is important that *all* carcases should be safely and efficiently disposed of, no matter what has been the cause of death.

The safest and most expeditious manner of disposal is for the carcase to be digested in a special destructor, either by heat (burning, or by live steam) or by chemical agents. In country districts, however, such plants as these are seldom available, and it is necessary to bury or burn the carcases.

Burial of carcases. A suitable site should be selected where there will be no danger of pollution of streams, rivers, canals, or other water-supplies, and where there is a sufficiency of subsoil to allow a depth of 6 clear feet of soil above the carcase. A pit is dug, about 8 or 9 feet deep, in such a manner that the surface soil and the subsoil are not mixed, and a clear approach is left to its edge. Roughly, about 2½ to 3 square yards of surface are required for a horse, 1½ to 2½ square yards for an ox, and about 1 square yard for each pig or sheep. The dead animal should be arranged upon its back with the feet upwards, and if these rigidly project too far upwards, the hocks may be 'hamstringed' and the tendons round the knee divided. This allows the limbs to be folded into a more compact space. It is advisable to slash the skin after the carcase has been placed within the pit, to prevent its disinterment by unscrupulous persons desiring to salve the hide. Where the cause of death has been accidental there are no objections to the removal of the skin previously, but where a contagious disease has been the cause of death the removal of the skin is an instance of a 'penny wise, pound foolish' policy. The carcase is next covered with quicklime or a powerful disinfectant, and the pit filled in with the soil – subsoil first and surface soil last. If the weather is very wet, or if the soil is naturally loose and soft, the surface of the ground should be fenced off to prevent horses and cattle from passing over it and perhaps sinking into the loose soil. It is not safe to plough over a large burial pit for 6 months after it has been closed, nor should heavy implements or vehicles be allowed to pass over it.

Cremation of carcases. Where a large coal boiler or furnace is used for heating supplies of water, there is no reason why the carcases of small animals that have died should not be burned in it (but *see* PACEMAKERS).

Dead horses and cattle, and large sheep and pigs, should not be dismembered and destroyed in such a manner; they must be burned in a specially constructed cremation pit.

There are three methods of cremation: (1) The Crossed Trench; (2) The Bostock Pit; and (3) The Surface Burning Method.

In the first of these – the *crossed trench*– two trenches 7 feet long are dug so that they form a cross. Each is about 15 inches wide and 18 inches deep in the centre, becoming shallower towards the extremities of the limbs. The soil is thrown on to the surface in the angles of the cross, and upon the mounds so made two or three stout pieces of iron, beams of wood, or branches from a tree, are placed. Straw and faggots are piled in the trenches to the level of the surface of the ground, the carcase is placed across the centre of the trenches, and more wood or coal is piled around and above it. Two gallons of paraffin oil are poured over the whole, and the straw is lighted.

In the *Bostock pit*, an oval pit 7 feet long and 4 feet wide is dug to a depth of 3 feet to 4 feet, and a crossed trench 9 inches by 9 inches is dug in its floor. Upon the windward side of the pit a ventilation trench 4 feet long and 1 foot 6 inches wide, and a foot deeper than the main pit, and at right angles to it, is dug. A field drain-pape is placed in a tunnel connecting the trench with the pit, and this pipe is stuffed with straw. Straw is laid in the bottom of the main pit, wood or coal is piled above it so that about three-quarters of the pit is filled, and the carcase is next rolled into the pit. More wood or coal is piled around and above it, and paraffin oil is poured over the whole. The straw is finally lighted in the bottom of the ventilation trench. A carcase cremated by this method takes about 8 to 10 hours to burn away, and requires little or no attention. When burning is complete the soil is replaced and the ground levelled.

The *surface burning method* is mainly used where there are numbers of animals to be burned. One long trench is dug about 1 foot 6 inches deep and 1 foot wide, and about 3 feet length is allowed for each cattle carcase. At intervals along each side there are placed side flues to coincide with each carcase. Fuel (straw, wood, and coal) is placed around the central trench and the carcases are drawn across it. More fuel is heaped around and between them, and paraffin oil or petrol is sprayed over the whole. The straw is lighted. More fuel requires to be added at intervals.

Instead of the trench and side flues battens of stout wood are sometimes laid upon the ground, and the carcases are pulled over them. Fuel is piled around them and lighted, and more is added as required. This latter method is specially applicable where the ground is very wet, or where there is rock immediately below the soil and digging is impossible.

Precautions. Where the carcase of an animal that has died from a contagious disease is being disposed of in one of the above ways, it is very necessary to ensure that blood or discharges are not spilled upon the ground in the process of removal. An efficient method of preventing this is to stuff tow saturated with some strong disinfectant into all the natural orifices – nostrils, mouth, anus, etc. – and to cover the surface of the improvised sleigh (door or gate) with pieces of old sacking which have been soaked with disinfectant, so that parts of the carcase do not become chafed through friction with the ground and so leave behind bloodstains. Everything that has come into contact with the carcase must be carefully disinfected before it is removed. Old ropes, sacking, and other objects used for handling the dead animal may be burned. The surface of the soil around the edge of the pit, upon which the carcase rests, should be scraped off and thrown into the fire or pit so that any blood or discharges may be rendered harmless. Finally, all attendants should be impressed with the risks they run in handling diseased carcases, and with the risks there are of contaminating other healthy cattle, and each one of them should be made to wash his hands and arms, and to dip his feet into a pailful of disinfectant, before he leaves the place of disposal.

Disposal in the tropics (*see last entry under* TROPICS).

DISPOSAL OF VETERINARY CLINICAL WASTE (UK). Such waste is defined by the Health & Safety Commission as including animal tissue and execretions, drugs or medicinal products, sharp instruments, or similar materials or substances.

Clinical waste must be separated from other waste in accordance with the system agreed by the local authority, e.g. yellow sacks and reinforced containers. (The Collection & Disposal of Waste Regulations, 1989.)

DISTEMPER is a name applied to a specific virus disease. As a rule, all members of the Canidae and Mustelidae are susceptible to canine distemper. These classes contain all those animals which do not have retractable claws (as opposed to the Felidae), and include: dog, fox, wolf, ferret, mink, weasel, ermine, marten, otter, and badger.

Injection of dogs with measles or rinderpest virus confers immunity against distemper.

Canine distemper is an infectious disease mainly of young dogs, characterised usually by a rise in temperature, dullness, and loss of appetite, and in the later stages by a catarrhal discharge from the eyes and nostrils. The disease is often complicated by broncho-pneumonia, and in some cases nervous symptoms develop, either when the febrile conditions subside, or before this happens. The incubation period of the disease is stated to be from 4 to 21 days, though it may be longer.
CAUSE. A virus of which there is **only one antigenic type**, though various syndromes (including 'Hard Pad') may be associated with various strains; some of which can suppress or impair the body's natural defence systems, and this has a bearing upon possible complications due to secondary bacterial infections.

Certain bacteria are responsible for secondary lesions; for example *Bordetella* is often responsible for bronchitis.

Cases of Distemper may be complicated by the coexistence of other infections such as CANINE VIRUS HEPATITIS, LEPTOSPIROSIS and TOXOPLASMOSIS.

Although it is chiefly in young dogs that the disease is met with, older dogs are often affected; as a general rule, however, young animals between the ages of 3 and 12 months are the most susceptible.

KLEBSIELLA infection gives rise to symptoms similar to some of those of distemper.
SIGNS AND COMPLICATIONS. In typical cases the dog becomes feverish, has a discharge from eyes and nose, and a cough. In some cases the eye inflammation become severe. (*See* KERATITIS.)

Complications include broncho-pneumonia with a hacking cough. (*See* BORDETELLA.)

Gastro-enteritis, and mouth ulcers, complicate other cases.

Sometimes the first sign of the disease (apart from the fact that the dog has seemed unwell) to alarm the dog-owner is a fit. (*See* ENCEPHALITIS.) A change in temperament, with a tendency to viciousness, may occasionally be the first sign.

Paralysis of face muscles, or of a limb, may occur, and sometimes hindquarter paralysis (*see* PARAPLEGIA) accompanied by incontinence indicate that the dog is unlikely to recover.

HARD PAD DISEASE may cause a dog to make a tapping sound as it walks, and this manifestation of distemper may be accompanied by pneumonia and/or diarrhoea.
DIAGNOSIS AND TREATMENT. An early diagnosis is important, and a veterinary surgeon should be consulted as soon as any of the above symptoms appear, and will advise on the use of serum, sulphonamides, antibiotics, vitamin preparations, etc., as the situation demands. (*See also* NURSING.)
Convalescence. After recovery from distemper it is important to remember that, unless the dog is looked after with great care, relapses are liable to occur. For a week or 10 days after all symptoms have *apparently* subsided the dog should be given only a limited amount of exercise. A tonic or vitamin preparation may be prescribed.
AFTER-EFFECTS. CHOREA (which see) may occur when the dog appears to be making a good recovery, and often after an otherwise mild illness. Dr Alan Parker has described a syndrome 'Old dog encephalitis' in which, several months after being ill with distemper, even a young dog may become senile and forget its house training.
PREVENTION. Various vaccines have long been available and have included:

1. *Live, egg-adapted distemper virus*
   (a) obtained from embryonated hens' eggs
   (b) obtained from cultures of avian fibroblastic tissues.
2. *Live distemper virus adapted to homologous tissue tissue culture*
       obtained from cultures of dog kidney cells.

Combined vaccines against distemper, infectious canine hepatitis, and canine parvovirus are on the market, for example, various combinations are available in Wellcome's Epivax series and Hoechst's Maxavac range; while Smith Kline Animal Health's polyvalent Enduracell 7 offers protection against distemper, canine parvovirus, leptospirosis (both canine forms), infectious

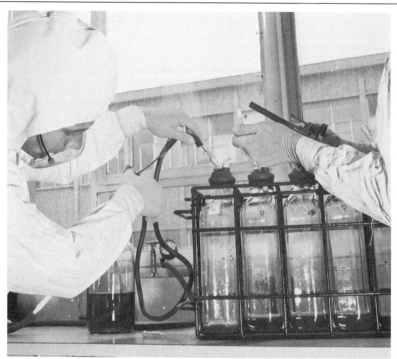

Technicians preparing cell cultures in which the distemper virus is grown during the manufacture of Epivax-TC.

canine hepatitis (using CAV-2 antigen), and respiratory infections caused by adenovirus and parainfluenza virus.

The timing of vaccination is crucial. Assuming an adequate intake of colostrum, puppies born to bitches immunised against distemper should have sufficient antibody to protect them during their first weeks of life. The immunity provided by the antibody wanes. 'At 7 to 9 weeks of age between 10 and 30 per cent of puppies'* may still, however, possess enough maternal antibody to prevent adequate response to distemper vaccination. By the time the puppy is 12 weeks old, the level of maternal antibody is negligible. It will no longer protect against naturally occurring virus; equally it will not interfere with distemper vaccination.

Puppies inoculated when between 7 and 9 weeks old should therefore receive a second dose of vaccine at 12 weeks of age.

A booster dose is often advisable when the dog is two years old.

(*See also* COLOSTRUM, GAMMA GLOBULIN, ANTISERUM, MEASLES VACCINE, MATERNAL ANTIBODIES.)

DISTICHIASIS is the presence of a double row of eyelashes, of which one or both rows are turned in against the eyeball, causing inflammation. It may lead in dogs to EPIPHORA (which see).

DISTILLER'S GRAINS. A feed for dairy cattle. For hazards of storage, *see* BREWER'S GRAINS.

DISTOMIASIS. Infestation with liver flukes.

DISH-WASHING DETERGENT (*see* ETHANOL POISONING).

*Hoechst Animal Health Division.

DIURETICS. Drugs which increase the amount of urine excreted. They act by inhibiting the reabsorption of sodium and chloride from the Loop of Henle (*See* KIDNEYS: Structure.)

They are used mainly in the treatment of oedema (dropsy). They act by causing the kidneys to excrete more urine. Thiazide diuretics, notably Hydrochlorothiazide, have been introduced and found useful in treating oedema whether of kidney, heart, or liver origin. Thiazides inhibit reabsorption of sodium and chloride and increase excretion of potassium.

For pulmonary oedema, frusemide may be used.

Diuretics may, of course, fail where serious heart or kidney disease is present. At best they can help, not overcome the condition which has given rise to the oedema.

DIVERTICULUM is a small pouch formed in connection with a hollow organ. There are certain diverticula which are normally present in the body, *e.g.* the *diverticulum of the duodenum*, which is found at the point of entrance of the bile and pancreatic ducts, or the *post-urethral diverticulum*, a little pouch behind the opening of the female urethra into the posterior genital tract in the sow and cow; while there are others which are found as the result of injury or disease, *e.g.* in the oesophagus, in the rectum, and sometimes in the intestines.

DNA. Deoxyribonucleic acid. This is found in the nucleus of every cell and carries coded information/instructions for reproducing other cells 'DNA can be visualised as a long coded tape, divided into segments. These segments are individual genes, and each carries information for the assembly of a specific protein. The genes issue the instructions for the cell; the proteins execute the orders. Some genes code for structural proteins such as hair, horn, etc, but most code for enzymes which perform tasks in the cell, such as motility, metabolism, and secretion.' (Professor W. F. H. Jarrett FRS.)

A chromosome is composed of a giant molecule of DNA, plus supporting protein, and it is the DNA which is the very basis of heredity. (*See* CELLS, GENES, CHROMOSOMES, 'GENETIC ENGINEERING'.) Bacteria, viruses, and plasmids contain DNA. (*See also* CANCER.)

DNA 'finger-printing' of human beings was first described by Dr Alec Jeffreys of Leicester University in 1935; and has since been used to prove the identification of sires of many different animal species.

The first case concerned a pack of Siberian huskies, and proving the true identity of puppies born to one of them, prior to registration with the Kennel Club.

Other applications of the technique are positive identification of thoroughbred horses, and of laboratory animals.

Genetic 'fingerprinting', to use another name, can also provide an effective means of tracing the source of microbial contamination as it differentiates between closely related microorganisms, making possible precise identification of individual strains.

DNOC. Dinitro-*ortho*-cresol, a yellow crystalline substance employed in agriculture as a weed-killer spray solution, acts as a powerful cumulative poison. In man the symptoms are excessive sweating, thirst, and loss of weight. Poisoning in domestic animals might well be encountered following contamination by the spray or residue.

DNP. A product somewhat similar to DNOC (which see).

DOCKING is removal of the tail or a part of that organ.

In Great Britain, docking of the **horse** (excluding amputation of the tail by a veterinary surgeon for reasons of disease) is illegal. (*See also* NICKING.)

Regulations introduced in the UK in 1983 prohibit very short docking. Enough tail must be left to cover the vulva, or anus in the case of the male. The use of rubber rings without anaesthetic is restricted to the first week of life.

The operation is performed as follows: a local anaesthetic solution is injected under the skin at the root of the tail, after first cleansing the part. The hair is clipped (or shaved in dogs) from about 1½ inches over the part that will become the end of the tail after docking, and a tape ligature is applied above this. The skin is rendered aseptic (or nearly so), by painting with surgical spirit, and when this is dry the preparations are complete. After the tail is severed the wound is closed by drawing the skin together by means of two or more stiches which are removed in 4 or 5 days' time.

(*See* ANAESTHETICS, LEGAL REQUIREMENTS.)

Dogs. Certain breeds are docked under Kennel Club rules. Docking of puppies is usually carried out when they are 3–5 days old. It can legally be done without anaesthesia by a layman up to the time the eyes open. Late docking should be done under anaesthesia by a veterinary surgeon.

Veterinary and public opinion is now beginning to turn against the docking of dogs, which is usually no more nor less than mutilation for the sake of fashion.

Sheep.
It is customary for **sheep** of lowland breeds to be docked, for if the tail is left long it accumulates dirt and faeces, and these predispose to the attacks of blow-flies. Many mountain breeds of sheep are left undocked; the long woolly tail helps to keep the hind part protected from frost and wind.

Lambs are usually docked by the use of a long sharp knife, the bleeding being negligible if the lambs are not more than a month old. The rubber-ring method is also used sometimes within 48 hours of birth.

DOCKS, POISONING BY. Although poisoning by docks is not at all common, yet there have been a few cases of it recorded, and losses of sheep have been occasionally ascribed to eating either the common Sorrel dock (*Rumex acetona*) or to Sheep's Sorrel (*Rumex acetosella*), both of which contain oxalates. A condition of staggering with dilated pupils, muscular tremors, and later, convulsions and prostration, has been noticed in horses which have eaten large quantities of sheep's sorrel. In sheep, there is a loss of appetite, rapid breathing, exhaustion, sometimes constipation and at other times diarrhoea, with an uncertain, drunken gait and occasionally death. The milk of cows that have eaten docks is made into butter only with difficulty.

DOG BITES. *Pasteurella septica* infection in man can result from these. (*See also* RABIES, BITES.)

DOG, FEMINISATION OF. (*See* SERTOLICELL TUMOUR *also* INTER-SEX.)

DOG, KENNELS. Former kennels should not, unless they have been thoroughly cleaned and disinfected, be used for the temporary housing of lambs or goatlings; as, in both, deaths have followed from cysticercosis of the liver. (*See* TAPEWORMS; *also* BEDDING, HOOKWORMS.)

Two sheep dogs died from dieldrin poisoning; their kennel having been washed weekly with old sheep dip.

DOG-SITTING POSITION. In pigs this may be a symptom of pantothenic acid (Vitamin B) deficiency, or lameness due to *mycoplasma hyosynoviae*. In the horse this position may be adopted during severe COLIC. With reference to the newborn Galloway calf, *see* Genetic Defects under GENETICS. Re lambs, *see* SWAYBACK.

DOG TICKS. In Britain these include *Ixodes hexagonus* (common on suburban dogs and cats); *I. ricinus* (the sheep tick, commonly found on country dogs; *I. canisuga* ('the British dog tick'); and *Dermacentor reticulatus* (which may infest also cattle and horses). *I. canisuga* may establish itself in buildings, as may *Rhipicephalus sanguineus*, which has infested houses in Denmark as well as quarantine stations. Modern central heating may facilitate the survival of this tick in northern latitudes. In a house in England, a sitting-room sofa, and a bedroom chair used by a dog, were infested. This tick may arrive in travellers' luggage. Hedgehogs are a source of *I. hexagonus*.

DOGS, BREEDS OF. The reader is advised to consult text-books on this subject (*see also* WILD DOGS.)

DOGS' DIET. Most owners wisely feed their animals on a mixed diet, offering some variety and at the same time providing the essential nutrients. However, some owners appear to believe that red (muscle) meat, cooked or raw, is a complete food for dogs and cats. It is not, since it does not provide enough calcium.

At the 1976 BVA congress, Dr R. S. Anderson stated that a dietary history of unsupplemented raw meat was found at two university veterinary hospitals to be the main factor responsible for bone diseases in young dogs, particularly of the large and giant breeds. (*See* CANINE JUVENILE OSTEODYSTROPHY.)

Referring to the calcium and phosphorus content of muscle meat in relation to dietary requirements, Dr Anderson said: 'thus a 22 lb puppy would require 1 cwt of muscle meat per day to supply its recommended calcium requirements.'

On the same subject, Dr D. W. Holme commented: 'Muscle meat is an excellent source of good-quality protein, and usually contains appreciable quantities of fat. It is better cooked than raw because it is very acceptable and less likely to cause digestive upsets or to carry risk of infection. Most meat, other than liver, is deficient in vitamin A, and all meats are particularly deficient in calcium. This is of great importance, because although meats do not have a high phosphorus content, it is high enough to give a very adverse calcium phosphorus ratio.

'Meat is a good source of most other minerals and of the B vitamins. However, it does not have any miraculous properties which confer benefits on dogs.'

'We have compared dogs maintained for over a year on biscuit plus raw meat, supplemented with minerals and vitamins, and dogs maintained on other foods, and could not detect differences in health and appearance, blood chemistry, or health of the teeth.'

Offal meats are also good sources of protein and fats, as well as vitamins. (It is, of course, the misfortune of some *cats* to be fed almost entirely on liver, and as a result they suffer from an excess of vitamin A which causes the vertebrae of the neck to become ankylosed (fused). (*See* FELINE JUVENILE OSTEODYSTROPHY.)

Eggs, cheese, and milk are all excellent items for the dog's diet. Canned foods are, said Dr Holme, 'usually very attractive, but only one or two products are suitable for feeding as the *only* food to dogs. Most canned foods should be mixed with biscuits or meals to provide a totally balanced diet.' (*See also* PET FOODS.)

DOGS, DISEASES OF. Several are listed under the prefix **CANINE**. Others include bacterial diseases such as brucellosis, 'kennel cough', salmonellosis, leptospirosis, tetanus, and tuberculosis. For skin diseases see eczema, mange, ringworm, hookworms, atopic disease. Other canine diseases are referred to under RABIES, PARALYSIS, PYOMETRA, FUNGAL DISEASES, BLACK TONGUE, CANCER, LYMPHOSARCOMA, CANINE PARVOVIRUS, CAMPYLOBACTER, ANAEMIA, ANTHRAX, AUJESZKY'S, BOTULISM, ORF, CHLAMYDIA, CHOREA, CRAMP, CUSHING'S DISEASE, DIABETES, DIARRHOEA, HIP DYSPLASIA, HYDATID DISEASE, HYSTERIA, MYASTHENIA GRAVIS, PARASITES, TGE of pigs, TOXOPLASMOSIS, YERSINIOSIS, SPOROTRICHOSIS, COCCIDIOSIS. (*See also* under the various organs and tissues, e.g. HEART, EYE, PANCREAS, PROSTATE, KIDNEY.)

Dogs' pharyngeal injuries are often caused during retrieving, or playing with, sticks thrown by the dog's owner. These injuries can be avoided if a rubber 'bone' or ring is substituted for the sticks. (A rubber ball can also be used, provided that it is too big for the dog to swallow.)

DOGS (Protection of Livestock) Act 1953 provides that the owner, and also the person at the time in charge of a dog, worrying livestock on agricultural land are guilty of an offence. The owner will not, however, be convicted if he proves that the dog was, at the time, in the charge of a fit and proper person other than himself. The maximum penalty for offences was increased to £200 by the Criminal Law Act 1977.

Amendments to the 1953 Act made by the **Wildlife and Countryside Act 1981,** now make it an offence for a dog to be at large in a field or enclosure where there are sheep unless it is on a lead or otherwise under close control. The maximum fine is £200. There are *exceptions* for a dog owned by, or in the charge of, the occupier of the field or the owner of the sheep or a person authorised by either of these; or a police dog, guide dog, trained sheep dog, working gun dog or a pack of hounds. This requirement applies only to fields or enclosures where there are sheep and not, therefore, to open hill areas.

DOGS, TRANSPORT BY AIR. This is governed by the Live Animal Board Regulations of the International Air Transport Association (IATA) 1989.

Greyhounds are usually transported by air between Ireland and England in wooden kennels similar in size to greyhound racing starting traps.

A study of 12 greyhounds showed that stress varied greatly as between individuals. They were transported either in the wooden kennels or in wider perspex kennels. These were stowed either in the belly hold or in the main cargo hold of jet freighter aircraft. Stress was greater in the belly hold. (Leadon, D. P. & Mullins, E. *Veterinary Record* (1991) **129,** 70.)

DOGS, WORMS IN (*see* WORMS).

DOLICHOCEPHALIC SKULL is one which is long and narrow, as distinct from one which is short and broad. Examples of the former are skulls of the greyhound and collie, and of the latter (*brachycephalic*), those of the pug and bulldog.

DOMINANT. That member of an allelic pair of genes which asserts its effects over the other dissimilar member (recessive) of a gene pair.

DONKEYS. Their life-span in Turkey, Egypt, Tunisia, Ecuador and Peru is only 11 years. In the UK the figure is 37 years. (The Donkey Trust, Sidmouth, Devon.)

They are spared many of the leg and joint troubles common in the horse, but they are very prone to lungworm infestations. This may not give rise to symptoms such as coughing, but Dr A. C. Fraser suggested (1971) that the lungworms may lower the donkey's resistance to strangles and equine influenza, from which more young donkeys die than young horses. Donkeys often constitute a source from which horses become infested with lungworms. (*See* PARASITES.)

For gestation period, *see under* PREGNANCY. (*See also* JENNY, HINNY, MULE.)

DOPPLER (*see* ULTRASOUND).

DOPAMINE. Early-weaned piglets which develop the 'vice' of nose-rubbing show evidence of decreased dopamine production in the brain.
Dopamine hydrochloride can be useful in overcoming the effects of anaesthesia with halothane, which depresses the cardiopulmonary system of horses.

DOSING INJURIES (*see* 'DRENCHING'; *also* radiograph *under* X-RAYS).

DOUBLE PREGNANCY. A term applied to the existence of two sets of fetuses, of different ages and born with a corresponding interval between litters, in the sow, cow, etc. (*See* SUPER-FETATION for further information.)

'DOUBLE SCALP'. A condition seen in older lambs and young sheep, mainly on hill grazings, in autumn and winter. There is unthriftiness associated with a thinning of the bones of the skull. In advanced cases the animal cannot eat or close its mouth. The cause is believed to be related to phosphorus-deficient pastures, but feeding bone-meal will not prevent the disease.

DOURINE is a venereal disease of horses due to a trypanosome called the *Trypanosoma equiperdum*, which is transmitted by sexual intercourse among breeding horses, asses, and mules. It occurs in Africa, Asia, parts of Europe, and in areas in both North and South America. (*See* TRYPANOSOMES.)

Transmission appears to be by coitus only, and is spread by 'carriers' which themselves show no symptoms.

A discharge from vulva or penis may be the first symptom, followed by oedema of the genital organs, with the swellings extending forward along the abdomen. Fever, loss of condition, and painful micturition may be observed. A few weeks later chancres may be seen on the flanks and elsewhere, lasting for a few hours or sometimes

days. Later still the horse becomes weak, loses weight, may be lame or have paraplegia, and dies.

Identification of 'carrier' animals is of the greater importance in controlling and eradicating the disease, and depends on the complement fixation test (though this presents difficulties in areas where other trypanosomiases occur). In most countries slaughter is obligatory.
TREATMENT. 'Berenil' is effective against trypanosomes.
CONTROL (*see also* TSETSE FLIES.)

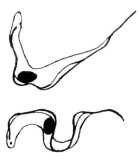

T. equiperdum.

'DOWNER COW' SYNDROME. Sometimes in cases of 'milk fever' (parturient paresis, hypocalcaemia) a cow goes down and never gets up again; even though the 'milk fever' itself is treated successfully. The critical factor may be the length of time the cow is recumbent with one hind leg (usually the right) underneath her body. If that time extends to six hours or more, there is often permanent muscle or nerve damage to that leg.

These were the main conclusions of Dr V. S. Cox, of the University of Minnesota, as stated at the BVA's 1981 annual congress.

Dr Cox's own experimental work suggested that 'because recovered and downer cows appeared to have similar degrees of muscle damage but markedly different degrees of sciatic nerve function,' nerve damage was the factor determining whether a recumbent cow became a downer. He suggested that slight differences in body position probably accounted for nerve damage in some animals but not in others.

Soon after the cows in his experiments recovered from the anaesthetic, they moved the right hind leg from under the body. This leg was extended and stiff. When the cow tried to lift her hind-quarters, she could not position this leg under her body. With only the left leg available for lifting, the pelvis tilted towards the disabled right side; throwing the animal off balance, with a resulting fall.

Dr Cox suggested that if, before going to bed, farmers or stockmen checked their cows, rather than leaving them unseen from the afternoon milking until the next morning's milking, the number of downer cows could be reduced. 'Some progressive farmers now have video monitors in their new calving barns, so that cows may be checked without leaving the comforts of home.'

Once a cow is found recumbent and showing signs of milk fever, it is important – Dr Cox emphasised – to change the animal's position so that tissue damage can be minimised while veterinary aid is awaited. When the veterinarian arrives, adequate help should be available to assist the cow into a standing position after she has recovered from the milk fever. If the cow is in close, cramped quarters, with a floor not providing a good grip, she should be moved to a better place. This can be achieved by sliding her on to a large piece of plywood, which can be used as a sledge for a considerable distance.

An inflatable bag, attached to a rigid base, and inflated by a 240-volt or 12-volt compressor, is marketed for lifting a cow on to its feet. (Alfred Cox [Surgical] of Coulsdon, Surrey).

Dr T. Andrews listed (*In Practice*, September 1986 188) some 30 possible causes of the syndrome, including *metabolic disorders*, such as hypocalcaemia, hypomagnesaemia, hypophosphataemia, hypokalaemia, and bloat; *toxaemia*, associated with mastitis, metritis, peritonitis, aspiration pneumonia; rupture of uterus, reticulum, abomasum, and traumatic pericarditis; *other injuries*, such as a fractured pelvis, displacement of the sacrum, obturator or sciatic nerve paralysis, dislocation of the hip, and rupture of muscles (e.g. adductor, gastrocnemius).

'About half of all downer cows get up within 4 days. After 10 days the prognosis is poor, but there have been cases of cows rising to their feet after two or three weeks, or even a month!'

A proportion of 'downer' cows are, in fact, cases of BOVINE SPONGIFORM ENCEPHALOPATHY (BSE).

DOXORUBICIN. An anthracycline anti-tumour antibiotic which has caused some canine malignant tumours to regress. (Ogilvie, G. K. & others. (*JAVMA* (1989) **195**, 1580.)

DRACUNCULIASIS (*see* GUINEA WORM).

'DRENCHING'. The giving of liquid medicine to animals. It must be done slowly, and with care, especially in the pig and horse – and in all animals suffering from bronchitis and consequently liable to cough. Pneumonia is a common sequel to liquid medicines 'going the wrong way'.

Another danger is associated with the use on pigs of a drenching gun intended for sheep. Unless these appliances are used with care, severe injury may result. In a series of cases reported in Australia, 24 pigs suffered rupture of the pharyngeal diverticulum – part of the throat – and 12 died. In sheep, rupture of the oesophagus has been caused.

DRESSED SEED CORN. Any surplus should *not* be fed to farm live-stock owing to the danger of poisoning. Pigs have been accidentally killed in this way after being given corn treated with mercury dressing. Dieldrin dressings kill birds.

DRIED GRASS has for long been incorporated by compounders into feeding-stuffs for poultry and pigs, but now an increasing quantity is being fed to dairy cows as part of a ration together with some roughage (straw, hay, silage) and some other concentrate feed, such as barley. Dried green crops are also being fed on a small scale to sheep and beef cattle.

The dried grass can either be milled and made into pellets or cubes; or left unmilled and pressed into cobs or wafers, which saves the high cost of hammer-milling. Unmilled material may have other advantages, too, for it has been shown that hammer-milling and pelleting decreases the digestibility of the product and, while increasing the efficiency with which digested nutrients are used by non-lactating animals, depress butterfat production of those in milk.

The hardness of the pellets and cobs is an important factor; if too hard, they can give disappointing results. Particle size is also important.

Minimum protein of dried grass for use without supplementary protein is considered to be 18 per cent; minimum digestibility figure about 60 per cent. A D A S work has shown that crude protein analysis is of little help in indicating digestibility. This (and hence energy equivalent) mainly determines milk production, not protein.

Work at the Grassland Research Institute and in Northern Ireland suggests that dried grass is as good as, or slightly better than, barley as a supplement for silage.

Fed with cereals and minerals, dried grass has successfully provided a standard feed for M L C Bull Performance Tests, giving an average daily liveweight gain of 3·3 lb over the 200-day test, with individual gains well over 4 lb.

DRINKING WATER (*see* WATER).

DRONCIT. The trade name of a Bayer preparation used in dogs and cats against tapeworms, and chosen for official Echinococcus eradication schemes. It contains praziquantel. Preparations are available for oral dosing and also for subcutaneous and intramuscular injections.

DROPPED ELBOW (*see* RADIAL PARALYSIS).

DROPPED SOLE (*see* LAMINITIS).

DROPSY (*see* OEDEMA).

DROPWORT POISONING (*see* WATER DROPWORT POISONING).

DROUGHTMASTER. A breed of cattle developed in Australia from Brahman and British (mainly Shorthorn) ancestors. It is claimed to be 10 times more tick-resistant than British breeds, and a more efficient beef producer under the relatively harsh grazing conditions of North Australia.

DROWNING. *Submersion* in water for a period of about 4 minutes is sufficient to cause asphyxia and death, but shorter periods, while they may cause apparent death, usually only produce a collapse from which recovery is possible. Practically all animals, even the very young, are able to swim naturally, so that *immersion* in water for this period does not necessarily result in drowning. Animals falling into water are drowned from one of several causes: they may be exhausted by struggling in mud; they may be carried away by a swift current, *e.g.* during floods; they may be hindered by harness or other tackle from keeping their nostrils above the level of the water; or they may become panic-stricken and swim away from shore. Remarkable instances of the powers of swimming that are naturally possessed by animals are on record; one example being that of a heifer, which, becoming excited and frightened on the southern banks of the Solway Firth, entered the water and swam across to the Scottish side, a distance of over seven miles, and was brought back the next day none the worse!

RECOVERY FROM DROWNING. As soon as the animal has been rescued from the water, it should be placed in a position which will allow water which has been taken into the lungs to run out by the mouth and nostrils. Small animals may be held up by the hind-legs and swung from side to side, and larger ones should be laid on their sides with the hindquarters elevated at a higher level than their heads. If they can be placed with their heads downhill, so much the better. Pressure should be brought to bear on the chest, by one man throwing all his weight on to the upper part of the chest wall, or kneeling on this part. When no more fluid runs from the mouth, the animal should be turned over on to the opposite side and the process repeated. No time should be lost in so doing, especially if the animal has been in the water for some time. (*See* ARTIFICIAL RESPIRATION.)

AFTER-TREATMENT. As soon as possible the animal should be removed to warm surroundings and dried by wisping or by vigorous rubbing with a rough towel. Clothing should be applied, and the smaller animals may be provided with one or more hot-water bottles. The danger that has to be remembered is that of pneumonia, either from the water in the lungs or the general chilling of the body, and the chest should be specially well covered. Sometimes the ingestion of salt water leads to salt poisoning in dogs, or to a disturbance of the digestive functions, and appropriate treatment is necessary.

DRUG INTERACTIONS. For those in which one drug enhances the action of another, see SYNERGISM. Veterinary readers will find a list of adverse drug interactions in the *Veterinary Record* (1983) **112**, 29.

DRUG RESIDUES (*see* HORMONES IN MEAT PRODUCTION, MILK (antibiotics in), SLAUGHTER).

DRUG RESISTANCE (*see under* ANTIBIOTIC RESISTANCE, DIPPING, FLY CONTROL).

DRUGS, DISEASE CAUSED BY (*see* IATROGENIC DISEASE).

DRUGS, METHODS OF ADMINISTERING (*see* BOLUS, 'BULLETS', 'DRENCHING', INJECTIONS, COPPER, WARBLES – dressing against, ELECTUARY, POWDERS, PILLS, TABLETS; and GLASS, SOLUBLE.)

'DRY EYE' (*see* EYE, DISEASES OF).

DRY FEEDING of meal may give rise to PARAKERATOSIS in pigs; to 'curled tongue' in turkey poults; and to 'shovel beak' in chicks. (*See under these headings*.)

DRY PERIOD. In cattle it is considered advisable on health grounds that the body should have a rest from lactation for about 8 weeks.

DRYING-OFF COWS. After milking out completely, the teats should be washed and a cloxacillin preparation inserted in each teat. Do not milk again unless it becomes necessary. The cows should be inspected daily.

If possible, keep the cows on dry food or very short pasture for 3 days after drying off.

DRYSDALE. A sheep with a very good fleece bred only in New Zealand. A natural mutation of the Romney, it was identified and developed by Dr F. W. Dry of Massey University.

DUBBING is performed with scissors by poultry-keepers, and involves removal of a crescent of comb – about $\frac{1}{16}$-inch deep – in day-old chicks. It is credited with increasing egg production by 3 to 4 per cent per year. It is also advocated in intensive rearing, where a floppy comb may be a disadvantage if pecking and cannibalism are rife; and in order to reduce the risk of frost-bite. Dubbing cannot be recommended from a veterinary point of view; being a cause of stress and an unnecessary mutilation.

DUCK VIRUS ENTERITIS (Duck plague). The disease appeared for the first time (so far as is known) in the UK in 1972 among birds on ornamental waters, not on commercial duck farms. One entire group of 72 Muscovy ducks died within 16 days.

Symptoms, which may not be observed before death occurs, include listlessness and very severe diarrhoea, drooping of wings, and a disinclination to take to water. Adult mortality may be high.

DUCK VIRUS HEPATITIS causes up to 90 per cent mortality among ducklings under 3 weeks of age, but in ducklings a month or more old losses are slight. Resistant ducks can be bred. A vaccine has proved successful. A notifiable disease, which should be suspected in cases of sudden death, especially if the birds, heads are stretched upwards and backwards.

Research by Animal Health Trust staff has shown that the **fatty kidney syndrome** can be reproduced in ducklings following infection with virulent duck hepatitis virus alone. Only birds which are dying or dead show the accumulation of lipid in the convulted tubules of the kidneys.

DUCKS, SEPTICAEMIA IN. Two forms occur, one due to *E. coli* and one due to *Pasteurella anatipestifer.*

The former may occur in ducklings 4–8 weeks of age. The latter infection causes losses in ducklings under 4 weeks old. Vaccines may prove to be the most effective method of control.

DUCTLESS GLANDS (*see* ENDOCRINE GLANDS).

DUCTUS ARTERIOSUS. This connects the left pulmonary artery to the arch of the aorta. (See the diagram of the fetal circulation on page 119.) If the duct remains open after birth, it is regarded as a congenital abnormality. (*See* HEART, DISEASES OF.) (*See also* LIGAMENTUM ARTERIOSUM for the remains of the duct in the normal animal.)

DULAA. A reddish, balloon-like organ arising from the soft palate of male camels, it fills with air from the trachea when the nostrils are closed. The dulaa is blown out of the mouth during rutting.

DUNG-FOULED PASTURE (*see* PASTURE MANAGEMENT).

DUNG HEAPS. Blades of grass growing near these often harbour large numbers of Husk worm larvae. (*See* HUSK.) Dung heaps are best fenced in. Care should be taken over the disposal of pig manure, as otherwise trichomoniasis might be spread from pigs to cattle.

DUODENUM is the first part of the small intestine immediately following the stomach. Into it open the bile and pancreatic ducts. (*See* INTESTINE.)

DURA MATER is the outermost and the strongest of the three membranes or meninges which envelope the brain and spinal cord. In it also are found the blood-vessels that nourish the inner surface of the skull. (*See* BRAIN.)

DURAZNILLO BLANCO. A poisonous plant of South America. (*See* ENTEQUE SECO.)

DUROC. A breed of pig, varying in colour from a light golden-yellow to a very dark red, originating from the eastern states of the USA.

DUSTING POWDERS form most convenient applications for wounds in animals. They may be used for an antiseptic effect, to control infection, or for astringent and protective effects to dry up superficial lesions and encourage scab formation.

Dusting powders containing parasiticides are used to destroy fleas and lice on animals.
Varieties. Some of the most satisfactory for animal treatment are compounds of sulphathiazole and amino-acridines, such as 'Flavazole' powder. Formerly iodoform was much used.

Parasitic dusting powders contain derris or BHC, for example, or pyrethrum.

DUSTY ATMOSPHERE. In piggeries, this can be a cause of coughing, etc., simulating Pneumonia. (*See* MEAL FEEDING.) Inoculations should not be carried out in a dusty shed. (*See* ANTHRAX.) Material in dust may give rise to an allergy (*see*

BROKEN WIND) and to abortion if fungi are present. (*See* UTERINE INFECTIONS.)

'DWARF TAPEWORM' (*Hymenolepis nana*). This parasite sometimes completes its life cycle in a single host (*e.g.* man or rodent), and sometimes the eggs are ingested by fleas or flour-beetles. Human infestation may follow eating of contaminated food or, accidentally, a flea.

DYNAMITE. Poisoning from this has occurred in cattle and sheep in the USA, after they have found mislaid or discarded sticks of the explosive. They apparently relish its taste. Poisoning is due to its nitrate content. (Gelignite, a type of dynamite, could be expected to be similarly toxic).

DYS is a prefix meaning painful or difficult.

DYSAUTONOMIA (*see under* FELINE DYSAUTONOMIA).

DYSCRASIA. A disease or disorder associated with faulty tissue development or a metabolic disturbance.

DYSENTERY is a condition in which blood is discharged from the bowels with or without diarrhoea. Dysentery is most commonly encountered in certain specific diseases such as anthrax, cattle plague, haemorrhagic septicaemia, purpura haemorrhagica, lamb dysentery, swine fever, and swine dysentery, although it may occur when there are large numbers of strongyle worms or coccidiae present in the bowels. Dysentery in young pigs may be due to *Clostridium welchii* infection, which causes death within 36 hours of birth. (*See also* SWINE DYSENTERY HAEMORRHAGIC GASTRO-ENTERITIS, and CANINE TROPICAL PANCYTOPAENIA.)

DYSPHAGIA means a difficulty in swallowing. (*See* 'CHOKING', BOTULISM, RABIES, MYASTHENA GRAVIS, and for one cause in horses, *see under* GUTTERAL POUCH DIPHTHERIA.) (*See also* GRASS SICKNESS, DOGS' PHARYNGEAL INJURIES, ABSCESS, FOREIGN BODIES, ACHALASIA.)

DYSPLASIA. Absence of some part of the body.

DYSPNOEA means a difficulty or pain in breathing (*see* BREATHLESSNESS, RESPIRATORY DIFFICULTY.)

DYSTOCIA or DYSTOKIA means difficulty during parturition. (*See* PARTURITION and CALVING, DIFFICULT.)

DYSTROPHY means defective or faulty nutrition, and is a term generally applied to some developmental change in the muscles occurring independently of the nervous system. (*See* MUSCULAR DYSTROPHY.)

DYSURIA means an absence of urine.

E

E. COLI. This is an abbreviation for *Escherichia coli*, formerly known as *Bacillus coli* – a normal inhabitant of the alimentary canal in most mammals. This bacterial family is a large one, comprising many differing serotypes which can be differentiated in the laboratory by means of the agglutination test. Only a few serotypes cause disease. (*See also* DIARRHOEA, JOINT-ILL, COLIFORM INFECTIONS.)

Sheep. E. coli scours and septicaemia are common in new-born lambs and often fatal. A vaccine, introduced by Hoechst, is available for protection.

Pigs. One serotype gives rise to oedema of the bowel, another to the death of piglets within a few days of birth.

An oral vaccine for use against *E. coli* has been developed at the Unilever Research Centre, Bedford, and is now on the market as an ingredient of piglet feeds. The vaccine, called Intagen, is claimed to be effective in the control of scouring due to *E. coli* especially in the early weaned pig where the withdrawal of the sow's milk means the loss of antibodies at a critical time.

Those strains of *E. coli* which cause diarrhoea in piglets only a few days old are able to do so because they are covered with an adhesive coat known as the K88 antigen. This enables them to adhere to the wall of the intestine where they induce disease by means of toxins, causing diarrhoea, dehydration, and death.

E. coli toxins. These are classified as (*a*) heat labile (LT), which may cause severe diarrhoea, dehydration and death of piglets; and (*b*) heat stable (ST) toxins associated with only a mild enteritis. A new vaccine was introduced by Smith Kline Animal Health Ltd, in 1984 to give protection against the LT toxins.

Scouring in older pigs may often be caused by strains of *E. coli* having no K88 antigen, and able to attach themselves by means at present unknown.

It has been shown that the K88 antigen can be prepared in the form of a vaccine. This, when injected into the mammary gland of the pig, is effective in conferring immunity to the suckling piglets as can be demonstrated in two ways. Firstly, the colostrum prevents K88 coated *E. coli* from adhering to the intestinal wall. Secondly, the vaccine confers demonstrable immunity in that the piglets are protected against challenge with pathogenic *E. coli*. (ARC research at Compton.)

A vaccine, Hoechst's Porcovac AT, is based on this research, and takes into account K99 and other more recently discovered antigens e.g. F41, 987P, CFAI and CFAII.

Another method of inducing resistance is based on the discovery that certain individual piglets were distinguishable in that their intestinal walls were not susceptible to adhesion with the K88 antigen. It now seems likely that this property is heritable, being genetically controlled by a single gene which is dominant. It may therefore be possible to breed resistant pigs.

Cattle. E. coli is an important cause of enteritis and of mastitis.

Poultry. Coliform septicaemia is a frequent cause of loss, and one difficult to control since infected birds are disinclined to eat or drink, which hinders drug administration.

Dogs. E. coli is perhaps the most important pathogen of the bladder and urethra; and also causes enteritis.

Horse (*see* FOALS, DISEASES OF.)

EAR. Sound is appreciated through the mechanism of the outer, middle, and internal ears. Sound waves are collected by the funnel-like external ear (*pinna*) and transmitted down into an external canal, across the bottom of which is stretched the ear-drum or *tympanum*, and against which these waves strike. Their impact causes a vibration of the tympanum, and the sound-wave becomes transformed into a wave of movement. This movement is transmitted through a chain of tiny bones, called *auditory ossicles*, in the middle ear, and then to fluid contained in canals excavated in the bone of the internal ear. The vibration of this fluid stimulates the delicate hair-like nerve-endings which are found in the membranous walls of the canals, and impulses pass to the brain, whereby an animal is able to appreciate external sounds literally by *feeling* them.

Structure. The middle and inner ears are essentially the same in all animals, but the external ears present certain differences in different species, and each merits a separate consideration here. (*See also* AURAL CARTILAGE.)

EXTERNAL EAR
Horses. The ears serves to some extent as an indication of the state of the horse's emotions – anger or viciousness being shown by laying the ears flat back against the head, and surprise, anticipation, or pleasure being indicated by 'pricking' the ears. At the base of the ear a complete cartilaginous tube is formed, and this leads into the bony canal or *external auditory meatus*.

MIDDLE EAR. The tympanic membrane, forming the 'drum', is stretched completely across the outer passage at its innermost extremity.

The cavity of the middle ear is a compartment excavated in the hard mass of the petrous part of the temporal bone which lodges the ossicles. These are the small auditory bones which carry impulses across its cavity and are called the *malleus* (hammer), *incus* (anvil), and *stapes* (stirrup). The Eustachian tube admits air from the throat, and so keeps the pressure on both sides of the tympanum equal.

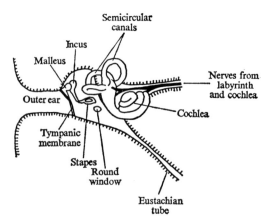

Outline of the structure of the ear. Reproduced from David Horrobin: *Medical Physiology and Biochemistry*, Edward Arnold, 1968, by kind permission of the author.

Horses have a diverticulum (guttural pouch) of the Eustachian tube. (*See* GUTTURAL POUCH *and* GUTTURAL POUCH DIPHTHERIA.)

INTERNAL EAR. This consists of a complex system of hollows in the substance of the temporal bone enclosing a membranous duplicate. Between the membrane and the bone is a fluid known as *perilymph*, while the membrane is distended by another collection of fluid known as *endolymph*. This *membranous labyrinth*, as it is called consists of two parts. The posterior part, comprising a sac, called the *utricle*, and three *semicircular canals* opening at each end into it, is the part concerned with the preservation of balance; the anterior part consists of another small pouch, the *saccule*, and of a still more important part, the *cochlea*, and is the part concerned in hearing. In the cochlea there are three tubes, known as the *scala tympani, scala media,* and *scala vestibuli*, placed side by side (the middle one being part of the membranous labyrinth), which take two and a half spiral turns round a central stem, somewhat after the manner of a snail's shell. In the central one (*scala media*) is placed the apparatus known as the *organ of Corti*, by which the sound impulses are finally received, and by which they are communicated to the auditory nerve, which ends in filaments to the organ of Corti. The essential parts of the organ are a double row of rods and several rows of cells furnished with hairs of varying length.

The act of hearing. The main function of the movement of the ears is that of efficiently collecting sound-waves emanating from different directions, without the necessity of turning the whole head, although in some animals the ears may be flicked to dislodge flies.

When sound waves reach the ear drum, the latter is alternately pressed in and pulled out; the movements being communicated to the *auditory ossicles.*

These movements are then transferred the perilymph in the scala tympani, by which in turn the fluid in the scala media is set in motion. Finally these motions reach the delicate filaments placed in the organ of Corti, and so affect the nerve of hearing, which conveys the sensations to the auditory centre in the brain.

EAR, DISEASES OF. Diseases of the ears of animals should never be neglected, for although in the early stages most are amenable to treatment, in the later stages treatment is likely to be more difficult.

SIGNS.

Shaking the head is often performed persistently for a few moments at a time. This behaviour is occasioned by some irritation in the ear, such as the presence of parasites, a foreign body (in one instance a grasshopper), wax, or inflammation (otitis).

Scratching the ears is a symptom of ear-mange mite (*Otodectes*) infection of the external ear canal. (*See* MITES-otodectic for first-aid and treatment.)

Other forms of mange may start at the ears and involve the *pinna*; e.g. psoroptic mange, notoedric mange.

Discharge from the ear, or the presence of pus within, is a sequel to a neglected case of parasitic otitis in the dog and cat and due to secondary infection by bacteria and/or moulds.

Excessive wax in the ear often leads to disease later. It is especially common in dogs which have large pendulous ear flaps, when ventilation is poor.

In some cases, dressing the inner parts of the ear is difficult or impossible because of the thickening and perhaps distortion. For these an operation, in which the cartilages at the lower parts are opened or resected, has been devised. Operation may also be needed where deep-seated ulceration of one or other of the aural cartilages has occurred, and even the mere initial cleaning of a very inflamed and painful ear must be done under an anaesthetic.

Foreign bodies, such as hay seeds, sand, pieces of glass, wood, peas, or parasites may become lodged in the ears of animals and give rise to irritation occurring very suddenly.

Haematoma is common in dogs and in cats which are affected with ear mange, but it may occur in almost any animal. A large fluctuating swelling appears upon the flap of the ear and causes the animal to hang its head towards the same side. In many cases little or no pain is experienced once the swelling has appeared, and, in fact, a small swelling becomes larger in many cases through the continued shaking of the head even after its original formation. The swelling is caused by bruising of the skin and the blood-vessels which lie between it and the cartilage, with a consequent extravasation of blood or serum under the skin. The condition is treated by opening the haematoma under conditions of surgical cleanliness, evacuating the fluid contents, and suturing the skin in such a way that the collection of more fluid is prevented.

Wounds of the flaps of the ears are usually caused by bites, or from barbed wire, etc., in the larger animals. The comparatively poor blood supply to the AURAL CARTILAGES means that, if torn or lacerated, necrosis may occur. In dogs it may be necessary to secure the ear-flaps by means of Elastoplast, or a head-cap improvised to give several 'tails' which can be tied.

Deafness (*see under separate heading*).

Middle-ear infection is always serious as it may lead to MENINGITIS.

Tumours are occasionally found. Warts are not uncommon in horses and cattle. In cats a polyp is occasionally found, and in white cats a squamous-celled carcinoma may affect the tip of the pinna.

Mange. Psoroptic and notoedric mange often begin on the pinna of the ear; auricular or oto-dectic mange involves the presence of mites (otodectes) within the ear canal. (*See* MITES.)

Fly strike. A dog brought to a veterinary surgeon in Cornwall was found to have a badly infected left ear, from which came a profuse purulent discharge. On auroscopic examination, Mr D. S. Penny BVet Med, who practises in Cornwall, was surprised to see three faces staring back at him! Under anaesthesia 18 large maggots were removed.

EAR TAGS (*see* FLIES).

EAR TIPPING of feral cats has been advocated by animal welfare organisations and practised in America and Denmark, for example. The idea is to identify those cats which have been spayed, and prevent any 'rescued' cat from being subjected to unnecessary anaesthesia and laparotomy.

In Australia ear tattooing is practised for the same purpose, but has the disadvantage that the spayed feral cat cannot be identified from a distance.

EARLY WEANING (*see under* WEANING).

EARS AS FOOD. Ears from beef-cattle which had been receiving sex hormones have been fed in breeding kennels with disastrous results.

EARTHING of electrical apparatus on farms, and especially in the dairy, is occasionally faultily carried out in such a way that in the event of a short-circuit, the water-pipes supplying the

cows' drinking-bowls become 'live' – leading to the electrocution of the cows. (*See* ELECTRIC SHOCK.)

EARTHWORMS are of veterinary interest in that they act as intermediate hosts to stages in the life-history of the gape-worm of poultry (*see* GAPES) and of lung-worm in pigs. Indirectly, they may also harbour viruses which cause disease in pigs. Earthworms can live for as long as 10 years. Earthworms can often be found at night in drains outside piggeries, and in crevices and cracks in the cement inside piggeries. (*See also* INFLUENZA.) An ARC research team at the Rothamsted Experimental Station found that earthworms, bred in cow manure, can provide a high-quality protein supplement for pigs, poultry, and especially fish.

EAST COAST FEVER (Theileriosis). An acute specific disease of cattle enzoötic in certain parts of Africa, especially in the eastern provinces of South Africa, in Kenya and in Zimbabwe. In these areas the native cattle attain a certain amount of natural immunity, and only imported animals are affected. Animals which recover are commonly known as 'salted', but the mortality is very high (*e.g.* 90 per cent) in new outbreaks of the disease. Buffaloes are also susceptible.

CAUSE. *Theileria parva*, which spends part of its life-history in cattle and part in ticks (*Rhipicephalus appendiculatus*).

SIGNS. After an incubation period of a fortnight or so, the animal becomes dull, listless, loses appetite, and runs a high fever. Lymph nodes become enlarged. There may be a discharge from eyes and nose. Laboured breathing and diarrhoea may be seen.

PREVENTION AND TREATMENT. East Coast Fever may be to a great extent prevented by systematic dipping of all newly purchased cattle, and quarantining them for at least 5 weeks before they are mixed with the rest of the stock.

Where the disease has broken out on a farm the 'short-interval' dipping system first devised by Watkins-Pitchford has proved of immense benefit in eradicating it. (*See under* TICK CONTROL.)

Since ticks responsible for the spread of East Coast Fever can live for some time on other domesticated animals, it is advisable to dip sheep, goats, and horses at suitable intervals.

The Wellcome Foundation introduced Parvaquone for the treatment of the disease.

EAST FRIESLAND MILK SHEEP. This breed comes from NW Germany, and in England has been used to produce the COLBRED (which see). East Friesland ewes average 120 gallons at 6 per cent butterfat in a lactation, rearing their lambs, and a yield of 220 gallons is not unknown. The lambs have a high growth rate and early maturity.

'EASTRIP SPECIAL BLEND'. A cross between Bluefaced Leicester and Poll Dorset sheep. A high lambing percentage is claimed.

EBOLA VIRUS. This, together with the Marburg virus, is a member of the filoviridae.

It is, in appearance, indistinguishable from Marburg virus, but antigenically distinct. It was found in 1976 in Zaire and Sudan, 500 people became ill; 350 died. (*See* MARBURG.)

An outbreak of disease caused by an Ebola-related filovirus, and by simian haemorrhagic fever, occurred at an American quarantine station among cynomolgus monkeys imported from the Philippines. Dr Peter B. Jahrling and colleagues commented that this was the first case in which 'a filovirus had been isolated from non-human primates without deliberate infection'. (Jahrling, P. B. *Lancet* (1990) **335**, 502.)

EC (*see* the EUROPEAN COMMUNITY).

ECBOLICS are drugs which cause contraction of the muscle fibres of the uterus, such as ergot, pituitrin, etc. They are used in cases of inertia at parturition.

ECCHYMOSIS means the collection beneath the skin of blood which has escaped from the vessels in the neighbourhood, as in a bruise.

ECHINOCOCCOSIS (*see* HYDATID DISEASE, TAPEWORMS).

ECHIUM PLANTAGINEUM. A poisonous plant, also known as Paterson's Curse, or Salvation Jane, which has caused the death of many sheep from copper poisoning in South Australia. In a 1983–84 outbreak 1,259 sheep died out of a total of 29,715 at risk. On one farm 500 of 3,000 ewes died. Merino × Border Leicester crosses appear to be especially susceptible. At autopsy, jaundice is evident; livers being friable and enlarged or, less frequently, shrunken and fibrotic. Kidneys are swollen, soft and blackish.

The plant contains up to 10 alkaloids, and is the first to show growth after a prolonged drought. (*Australian Veterinary Journal* **62**, 247.)

ECLAMPSIA is a disease occurring during the later stages of pregnancy or after parturition, and characterised by loss of consciousness or convulsions, or both. It occurs in the bitch, and cat. A preferable name is Lactational Tetany. It is associated with HYPOCALCAEMIA. (*See also* MILK FEVER, FITS.)

ECRASEUR. A surgical instrument used for castration of the larger domestic animals. Haemorrhage is largely prevented by crushing of the blood-vessels of the spermatic cord.

ECTASIS means a dilatation of a hollow organ, such as an artery or the stomach.

ECTHYMA is a localised inflammation of the skin characterised by the formation of pustules. (*See* ACNE, IMPETIGO.)

ECTO is a prefix meaning on the outside.

ECTOPIC means out of the usual place. Ectopic pregnancy is one in which a fetus is present outside the uterus. (*See* PREGNANCY, ECTOPIC.)

Ectopia Cordis Thoracoabdominalis. A very rare congenital abnormality characterised by protrusion of the heart to the outside of the body through a ventral body-wall fissure. A case in a piglet, which was able to suck, was described and illustrated. (Freeman, L. E. & McGovern, P. T. *Veterinary Record* (1984) **115**, 431.)

ECTROMELIA means literally absence of a limb or limbs. The word is also used to describe a contagious disease caused by a pox virus, which affects laboratory mice, and in the sub-acute form causes necrosis of a whole limb, toe, tail or ear. Outbreaks are usually very severe at the outset, killing many of the affected mice, but later on the mortality becomes less, and the outbreak gradually fades and disappears; though a latent infection may persist.

ECTROPION is a condition of the eyelids, in which the skin is so contracted as to turn the mucous membrane lining of the lid to the outside.

ECZEMA. An inflammation of the skin (dermatitis), occurring in both farm and domestic animals. Intense irritation or itchiness may accompany the acute form, and frantic licking of the affected area may exacerbate the condition. In chronic eczema there may be very little irritation.

Cats. Eczema is often referred to as *feline miliary dermatitis.* Symptoms include reddening of the skin, with the appearance of papules (small blister-like spots) and, later, scabs. These may be easier to feel than to see. The area of skin involved may be small or large. Neck, shoulders, and back are common eczema sites. Occasionally a bacterial infection is a complication.

The most common cause is considered to be hypersensitivity to flea bites. Once a cat (seldom a young one) has become sensitised to flea saliva, the presence of only a single flea on the cat's body is sufficient to cause the allergic reaction.

Miliary eczema occuring after spaying is too often assumed by owners to be the result of neutering and consequent hormone deficiency or imbalance. People tend to forget that the spayed cat is as liable to eczema from other causes as is the entire animal. Moreover, veterinary skin specialists on both sides of the Atlantic now regard the cat's hormone status as largely irrelevant so far as eczema is concerned.

Other allergies may produce eczema; for example, a 'hay-fever' type (*see* ATOPIC DISEASE), or a food allergy of some kind. Years ago much was heard of 'fish eczema' in cats and dogs, and while an excess of fish in the diet is no longer regarded by most veterinarians as a cause of eczema, an allergy to a particular type of fish is a possibility in some individuals. It has been suggested that cat foods containing colouring agents or preservatives are sometimes involved. Skin contact with some chemicals should also be considered. It is likely that among some breeds or strains there is a family pre-disposition to eczema. TREATMENT involves flea removal; and the veterinarian may prescribe a change of diet, a vitamin supplement, megestrol acetate (whose mode of action is not understood as regards relief of eczema), or an antihistamine, etc.

Dogs. The causes, symptoms and treatment of eczema are similar to those described above. The disease is more common in dogs, however, and an acute form often involves the skin between the toes, resulting in constant licking. Other sites are around the eyes, and the scrotum.

FIRST-AID. Calamine lotion may be applied if precautions can be taken to prevent its being immediately licked off.

In a few cases what a dog-owner assumes to be eczema may prove to be mange; so a professional diagnosis should always be obtained.

Horses. A common cause of eczema is sensitisation to midge-bites. *See* 'SWEET ITCH' for preventive measures.

Cattle and sheep. Some cases of eczema affecting white-haired areas of skin are the result of LIGHT SENSITISATION (which see). Overseas this condition is often referred to as 'Facial eczema' and follows sensitisation to sunlight following the eating of certain plants.

EDEMA is another spelling of oedema.

EFFERENT is the term applied to vessels which convey away blood or a secretion from a part, or of nerves which carry nerve impulses outwards from the nerve-centres.

EFFLUENT (*see* SLURRY, DAIRY HERD MANAGEMENT).

EGG-BOUND is the condition in laying poultry in which an egg (or eggs) may be formed in the oviduct, but, owing to weakness or overwork, the hen is unable to discharge it. The bird shows obvious discomfort, stands straining and pressing, and the abdomen is usually markedly dropped.

A 2-ml dose of liquid paraffin may be tried.

EGG EATING. Among intensively housed poultry, this may be a sign either of boredom or of pain.

EGG TRANSFER/TRANSPLANT (*see* TRANSPLANTATION OF MAMMALIAN OVA).

EGG YIELD. In Britain, the average is approximately 130 eggs per bird per year. An annual yield of 200 is obtained in well-managed batteries; about 190 on deep litter; 170 in fold units. A Honegger has laid 305 in 350 days.

EHLERS-DANLOS SYNDROME (*see* CUTANEOUS ASTHENIA).

EHRLICHIA canis, 'or a closely related species', was identified in 14 human patients (13 of whom had recently been bitten by ticks) suffering from fever, rigors, myalgia, and gastro-enteritis. Tests showed leukopenia and thrombocytopenia. (Fishbein, D. B. & others. *JAVMA* (1987) **190,** 1608.)

EHRLICHIOSIS. Infection with species of Ehrlichia, a rickettsia.

Canine ehrlichiosis has as its vector the brown dog tick. (*See* TICK-BORNE FEVER of cattle, and CANINE TROPICAL PANCYTOPENIA.)

EICOSANOIDS. Arachidonic acid, a polyunsaturated fatty acid present in most body cells of domestic animals, can be oxidised to the prostaglandins, prostacyclin, thromboxanes and leukotrienes. These compounds, collectively known as the eicosanoids, are involved in inflammatory and allergic conditions, in reproductive and perinatal processes, with platelet aggregation and vascular homeostasis, kidney function, fever, certain tumours and many other normal and disease conditions.

EIMERIA (*see* COCCIDIOSIS).

ELASTIC BANDS (*see* RUBBER BANDS).

ELASTICITY, EXCESSIVE, OF SKIN, in dogs. (*See* CUTANEOUS ASTHENIA.)

'ELASTRATOR'. An instrument used to stretch a strong rubber ring so that it may be placed over the neck of the scrotum for the purpose of castration.

ELBOW is the joint formed between the lower end of the humerus and the upper ends of the radius and ulna.

ELECTRIC FENCES (*see under* PASTURE MANAGEMENT).

ELECTRIC SHOCK, 'STRAY VOLTAGE', and ELECTROCUTION. Faulty electrical wiring and earthing have led to to drinking-bowls, water pipes, mangers, etc, becoming 'live'. In some instances this has led to the death of **cows** from electrocution following a short circuit.

'Stray voltage'. In one incident these led to cows refusing concentrates in the parlour – not because they were unpalatable, as at first thought, but because cows wanting to eat were deterred by a mild electric shock.

This 'stray voltage' has been associated with intermittent or unexplained periods of poor performance, increased milking time, and 'an increased prevalence of mastitis.' 'Stray voltage' was detected in 32 out of 59 dairy farms in Michigan, following investigations requested by dairymen or veterinarians. (Kirk, J. H. & others. (1984) *JAVMA* **185,** 426.)

Electrocution. Deaths from electrocution may occur outside buildings. In one case 30 cows and heifers were found dead beneath an electric pylon. It seems that the cattle had used a metal stay as a rubbing 'post', and that it had become loose and then come in contact with the high-voltage lines that the pylon was carrying.

Pigs. Metal troughs becoming electrically 'live' led to 20 pigs becoming paralysed after a severe thunderstorm in England, the VI Service reported. Injuries apparently resulted from panic and crushing. In another case 22 out of 32 pigs in one pen were found piled up around the trough, close to which was a burnt-out live wire. The carcases were bloated and the skin bluish. Additional post-mortem findings may include external burns, numerous haemorrhages affecting many internal organs, black unclotted blood, and congestion/oedema of the nervous system, fractur of lumbar vertebrae or of the pelvis. In pigs at any rate rupture of the urinary bladder may occur. (*See* Giles, N. and Simmons, J. R., *Vet. Rec.* (1975), **97**, 305.)

Horses. A New York insurance agency stated that in 1981 0·96 per cent of its claims in respect of the death of horses were for lightning strike, and 0·27 per cent for electrocution. The previous year the figures were 0·86 per cent for lightning, and 2·1 per cent for electrocution, respectively.

In Canada a veterinarian was asked to call to see a horse which appeared to be suffering from colic. On arrival at the farm he was told that the animal had died minutes after she had telephoned. Earlier the same day, she explained, a mare in foal had died instantly in the same spot in front of a small barn; and another had died there too. Suspecting electrocution, she had switched off the barn's power supply.

Subsequently an inspector found that the builder of the barn had made a serious mistake when carrying out the electrical work, so that what was supposed to be the earth line was anything but safe. The situation had become more dangerous after recent excavation in front of the barn, where the earthing plate had been accidentally dug up and replaced horizontally across the path to the barn. The horses had died on the first wet day after the work was completed; but their owner recalled that previous to that they had shied or tended to bolt when passing the spot. (Brackett, J. (1983) *Canadian Veterinary Journal* **24**, 66.)

Dogs and cats. Electrocution is not uncommon, and almost invariably results from puppies or kittens chewing through the insulation of electric wiring (e.g. of vacuum-cleaner, table-lamp, etc). Burns to the mouth and lips are seen; a tan to grey discoloration being noticeable. Oedema of the lungs may be caused, with dyspnoea. Sixteen of 26 dogs that were treated survived, and were discharged from hospital within two or three days. Mortality rate for all the dogs in the survey was 38 per cent. None of seven cats died. (R. J. Kolata and C. F. Burrows. *Journal of the American Animal Hospital Association* (1981) **17** 219).

Electrocution is used for purposes of euthanasia in the case of dogs and cats, but recent research has shown that if the apparatus in use is to be humane in its effects – not causing paralysis initially without loss of consciousness – certain safeguards must be fulfilled. (*See* EUTHANASIA.)

Lightning stroke. Cattle, sheep, and horses are most often affected. Usually death occurs instantly, and the animal is often found with a bunch of grass between its teeth. Usually, but not invariably, there are external scorch marks, with subcutaneous lesions beneath. The other signs are as those given above under electrocution.

ELECTRIC WIRING in farm livestock buildings (*see* ELECTRIC SHOCK).

ELECTRO-CARDIOGRAM (ECG) is a record of the variations in electric potential which occur in the heart as it contracts and relaxes. This record is obtained by placing electrodes on either side of the chest wall or on the two forelegs, the skin being first wetted with salt solution; these are then connected with one another through an instrument known as the electro-cardiograph, which records on to a moving photographic film. The normal electro-cardiogram of each heart-beat shows one wave corresponding to the activity of the auricle, and four waves corresponding to the phases of each ventricular beat. Various readily recognisable changes are seen in cases in which the heart is acting in an abnormal manner, or in which one or other side of the heart is hypertrophied. This record, therefore, forms a useful aid in many cases of cardiac disease.

Electro-cardiography has been described as a useful aid to pregnancy diagnosis in the mare – useful 'where thoroughbred mares more than 5 months pregnant are presented for sale' (*see under* TWINS); and also for monitoring heart rate during anaesthesia.

ELECTRO-CAUTERY is useful for operations where space is restricted, such as removing small tumours, etc., in mouth, nose, or throat, and to check haemorrhage in the deeper parts of wounds, and sometimes for disbudding. (*See also* CRYOSURGERY.)

ELECTRO-IMMOBILISATION of animals is a technique developed in Australia, but not yet approved for use in the UK, since there is some doubt as to whether it is humane or not.

The technique has been used for castration, dehorning, and spaying. It depends, states the BVA, on 'the passage of short duration current pulses between electrodes inserted under the skin and positioned across nerve pathways. The effect is to immobilise the muscles in tetany and, it is claimed, block pain sensation, thus providing restraint and anaesthesia sufficient to facilitate stock handling and surgery.'

The BVA deprecates the use of electro-immobilisation until such time as there is scientific evidence that cruelty is not caused. The Farm Animal Welfare Council takes a similar view.

ELECTRO-THERAPY

High-frequency currents. This form of electrotherapy has had probably most application to treatment of animals. It has advantages in that it is painless in application; no control measures are necessary other than means to hold the animal reasonably quiet. The duration of treatment is usually about 5 to 20 minutes daily or for shorter periods twice daily.

Good results are claimed in the treatment of various forms of paralysis in dogs and horses, muscular atrophy, chronic skin diseases of a non-parasitic nature, enlargements of joints and painful conditions in the limbs due to ligamentous or tendinous adhesions following injury, arthritis, rheumatism, and various inflammatory changes in peripheral nerves.

A modification of high-frequency treatment is known as diathermy. In this, electric currents pass into the deeper tissues and can be made to produce internal warmth. (*See* DIATHERMY.)

Faradic currents are used to produce rhythmic muscular contractions in the treatment of muscle, tendon and joint injuries in the horse, etc. (*See also* LIGHT TREATMENT, X-RAYS, IONIC MEDICATION, IONTOPHORESIS, CANCER, STUNNING.)

ELECTROCUTION (*see under* ELECTRIC SHOCK).

ELECTROLYTE. Any compound which, in solution, conducts an electric current and is decomposed by it. (*See under* IONIC MEDICATION, NORMAL SALINE, DEHYDRATION.)

ELECTRON MICROSCOPE. These costly and complex instruments have made it possible to study and photograph viruses, bacteriophages, and the structure of bacteria. The instrument makes use of a high-voltage 'electron gun', with electro-magnets taking the place of lenses. The 'specimen' is prepared in the form of a finely divided suspension on a cellulose supporting film, mounted on metal gauze, and the electron microscope subjects it to a high degree of vacuum. The electron image is focused on a fluorescent screen, which is then replaced by a photographic plate. Magnification may be up to ×300,000, and by means of photographic enlargement and the use of projection slides, a total magnification approaching ×1,000,000 can be achieved.

ELECTROPHORESIS. Starch gel electrophoresis is a method of separating certain constituents of blood serum in such a way that they form visible and identifiable patterns which can then be 'read' and recorded.

It has been used in the investigation of infertility in cattle. The mating of animals presenting certain serum patterns resulted in a higher rate of fetal mortality than the mating of other animals. This technique, therefore, may become valuable in planned breeding of the future in order to avoid incompatibility and wastage.

ELECTUARY is a soft paste made by compounding drugs with treacle, sugar, or honey. It is used as a convenient method of applying drugs to the throat and pharynx of animals, and has much the same effect as lozenges in human beings. In pigs, where dosing is very difficult and often dangerous, purgative or other medicines are often given as electuaries, and antiseptic mouth applications are sometimes made up in the same way for all animals. To relieve sore throat in the horse an electuary of extract of belladonna, potassium chlorate, and aniseed, made up into a paste with treacle, is much used and serves to soothe the inflamed surface. The electuary is applied by means of a flat stick, and is smeared upon the back of the tongue, upon the teeth.

ELEPHANTS, DISEASES OF. These include anthrax, multiple abscesses, blackleg, botulism, elephant pox, enzootic pneumonia, influenza, myasis, parasitic gastro-enteritis, pasteurellosis, rabies, salmonellosis, stephanofilarial dermatitis, schistosomiasis, surra, tetanus, trypanosomiasis, tuberculosis.

ELISA is the abbreviation for the system of enzyme-linked immunosorbent assay, developed by the Swedish scientists Engvall and Perlmann. It is likely to supersede radioimmuno-assay (RIA); enzymes linked to antibodies or antigens replacing the isotypes used in RIA. ELISA tests are now widely used in laboratories. (*See, for example,* AUJESZKY'S DISEASE.) ☞

ELIXIR is a diluted tincture made pleasant to the taste by the addition of aromatic substances – sugar or glycerine.

ELIZABETHAN COLLAR. Usually made of cardboard, the shape of a lampshade, and designed to fit over the dog's head and to be attached to its collar, with the object of preventing the animal interfering with wounds, skin lesions, or dressings.

EMBOLISM. The plugging of a small blood-vessel by blood-clot fragments originating from elsewhere in the body, and carried along in the bloodstream. Bacteria, worm larvae, air-bubbles, and fat, are other causes of embolism. The importance of the embolism depends upon the situation. In the brain it may cause apoplexy. In other organs the area that was supplied by the little vessel before it became blocked by the embolism ceases to function, and if the blood-supply is totally cut off it dies, or degenerates, becoming an 'infarct'. (*See also* GLASS EMBOLISM, THROMBOSIS CATHETER EMBOLISM.)

EMBROCATIONS (*see* LINIMENTS).

EMBRYO (*see* FETUS, and next two entries.)

EMBRYO TRANSFER. The development and application of current techniques followed research into methods of freezing and thawing mammalian embryos.

Frozen embryos. Research at the Agricultural Research Council's Unit of Reproductive Physiology and Biochemistry, Cambridge, by Mr L. E. A. Rowson, FRS, FRCVS and colleagues, led in 1973 to the birth of a healthy Hereford bull calf, 'Frosty' – the first large mammal to be born after being frozen as an embryo.

Fertilised eggs (blastocysts recovered on days 10 to 13 of pregnancy) had been removed from a cow and, after treatment with the cryoprotective (anti-freeze) agent dimethylsulphoxide, were cooled slowly (0·2°C per minute) to a final temperature of −196°C. Six days later, thawing was carried out and 2 eggs transferred to the uterus of a Hereford × Friesian cow (the host mother). Only one of these eggs developed; but this one resulted in the calf illustrated.

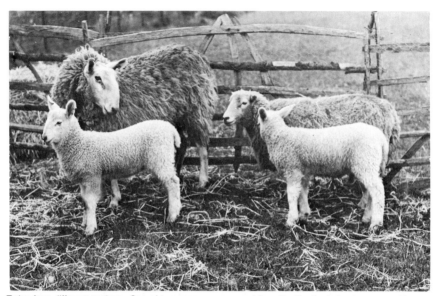

Twins from different mothers. One of two eggs was removed from the Border Leicester ewe and transplanted into the Welsh ewe.

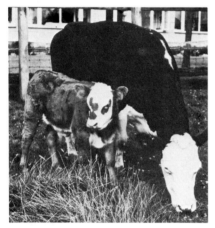

The calf 'Frosty' and his 'host mother'.

In 1974 the first frozen-embryo lambs were born. In 1978 the ARC announced the birth of a calf which, as an embryo, had been deep-frozen for a month.

Transference. This technique was in commercial use in cattle in 1974. Briefly, it consists in stimulating super-ovulation – the production of a number of eggs at one time – by the female; removing these eggs from the female; keeping them alive for the necessary length of time; and in introducing one such egg into another female. The technique, developed at Cambridge, had already in the 1950s been successfully carried out in sheep – ewes having produced young of which they were not, in the full sense the mothers; and it was extended to cattle later, again by L. E. Rowson and colleagues.

Sheep eggs have been exported from England to South Africa in a rabbit, and used to produce lambs whose true parents had never left England.

Fertilised pig eggs, obtained in Canada, have produced a litter of three in a sow at Weybridge.

Limiting factors had been the high costs of the necessary surgery, the cost of buying and feeding the recipient cows, and the very high standard of management required for both donor and recipient animals.

Its advantages were summarised (1974) by J. M. Bowen, Colorado State University, as follows: (1) increased number of offspring from valuable females; (2) rapid progeny testing of females; (3) induction of twinning; (4) the investigation of causes of infertility; (5) transport of cattle ova from one state or country to another; and (6) an increased rate of genetic improvement.

The technique. Five days before oestrus is due the donor animal is treated with pregnant mare's serum (PMSG) to produce superovulation. When oestrus occurs insemination is carried out two or three times, using fresh rather than frozen semen.

On day six, when the eggs are at the morula stage, consisting of 8 to 32 cells each, and looking under the microscope like blackberries, they are flushed out of the Fallopian tube after surgical exposure of this and the uterus, the cow being under fluothane general anaesthesia.

It may be possible to recover 8 to 12 ova, and an attempt is made to select the normal ones. (For example, by culturing them in TCM 199 for 1 or 2 days after recovery. In that time further development will have occurred; eggs which do not show this are discarded.)

The recipient animals must be at exact oestrus synchronisation with the donor. The transplant is made by puncturing one horn of the anaesthetised recipient's uterus with a small glass pipette containing one ovum in a synthetic medium, TCM199. This liquid is forced out of the pipette, carrying the ovum with it.

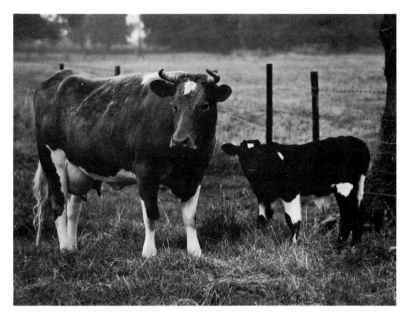

Transplantation. As a seven-day embryo this calf was stored for a month at a temperature of −196°C before being transferred, non-surgically, to the recipient cow seen in the Agricultural Research Council picture.

NON-SURGICAL TRANSFER. Four out of eight heifers at the Agricultural Institute, Belclare, Co. Galway, became pregnant following a non-surgical technique for the transfer of fertilised cow eggs. Reporting (*Vet. Rect.* (1975), **96**, 490–1) this success, Dr J. M. Sreenan commented: 'To be of value, egg transfer techniques must be capable of operation at farm level.' In fact, the actual egg transfer was carried out by a technician from a commercial A I centre using 'normal artificial insemination procedures'.

The fertilised eggs were drawn singly into 0·25 cc insemination straws, which were slightly shortened and then 'loaded into the insemination gun and the outer sheath put in place in the normal fashion. The gun was then introduced through the cervix and forward into each uterine horn. The fertilised eggs were expelled by use of the plunger.'

In each of the four animals mentioned above, it was a single pregnancy. However, the technique should prove valuable in obtaining artificial twinning. (Twinning rates of 73 and even 75 per cent have followed bilateral *surgical* egg transfer.)

Non-surgical transfer of a mare's egg has also been successful. The mare was one of three which became pregnant in Poland following transport of mares' eggs in rabbits from Britain. Transplantation (surgical in the other two cases) was effected by an Agricultural Research Council team in 1975 – the first successful transfer in the mare ever recorded.

A technique for the non-surgical *recovery* of eggs from the donor cow has been developed at the A R C's Institute of Animal Physiology, and involves use of a 2- or 3-way catheter having an inflatable cuff. The catheter is passed through the cervix and on into one of the horns of the uterus,

which is then sealed with the cuff. Fluid is flushed into the horn. It is possible by this method to recover 50 per cent of the eggs available – as good a result as that obtained by surgery. In 1978 a calf was born following this procedure and transplantation.

Sows. A day 7 hatched blastocyst of a Chinese Meishan, frozen at −196°C and then thawed, survived to farrowing. (Kashiwazaki & others. *Veterinary Record* (1991) **128**, 256.)

Pregnancy in sows has been achieved with blastocysts frozen at −35°C. (Hayashi & others. *Veterinary Record* (1989) **125**, 43.)

In 1979 the first **inter-species transfer** of embryos was carried out at the Thoroughbred Breeders' Association's equine fertility unit at Cambridge. This resulted in one pony mare foaling a donkey (gestation period about 346 days or about 15 days longer than for a foal) and two donkeys gave birth to pony foals (born after 346 and 361 days' gestation period, respectively). (*See* PLACENTA for the objects of this research by Dr W. R. Allen).

USE OF A LAPAROSCOPE. Bringing the reproductive tract to exterior at laparotomy, for the purpose of embryo transfer, inevitably involves some degree of surgical trauma, and often leads to the formation of post-operative adhesions involving the uterus and ovaries. In 1985 McKelvey, W. A. C. & others (*Veterinary Record* **117**, 492) transferred embryos from ewes by a laparascopic technique, which resulted in a pregnancy rate of 75 per cent.

'The reduced surgical trauma and operating time have benefits in terms of animal welfare, as well as for the economics of the embryo transfer industry.'

EMBRYOLOGY is the study of the development of the embryo within the body of the female.

EMESIS means VOMITING (which see).

EMETINE is one of the alkaloids or active principles of the drug ipecacuanha.

EMPHYSEMA. An abnormal presence of air in some part of the body. The term is applied to the presence of air in the subcutaneous tissues following a wound but, more commonly, to two abnormal conditions of the lungs: destructive (vesicular) emphysema and interstitial emphysema.

Destructive (vesicular) emphysema is a condition of the lung characterised by an abnormal enlargement of the air spaces, accompanied by destructive changes in the alveolar wall. This condition occurs in dogs with chronic bronchitis and in horses with chronic obstructive pulmonary disease (see 'BROKEN WIND'). The cause of this form of emphysema is not known, but has been variously attributed to obstructive inflammatory lesions of the bronchioles, ischaemic atrophy of alveolar septa, exposure to poisonous gases and fumes, and damage to the lungs by enzymes. Destructive emphysema is irreversible and may progress to respiratory failure and death. The main symptom is respiratory distress on exertion, with a marked expiratory effort.

Interstitial emphysema. Air is present in the connective tissue of the lung – a state of inflation of the interstitial (interlobular) tissue. The air is found in the lymphatics, under the pleura in the interlobular septa, and around blood vessels, sometimes in the form of large bullae 10 cm or more in diameter. Air may track as far as the hilum of the lung and gain access to the mediastinum from where, in exceptional circumstances, it may even spread to subcutaneous connective tissue – usually in the shoulder region or over the upper part of the chest.

Interstitial emphysema is a common condition in cattle, especially in association with parasitic bronchitis (HUSK) or with 'FOG FEVER'. Increased effort, in response to obstructed airways, overexertion and violent struggling, causes a marked increase in pressure within the alveoli. Rupture then occurs, allowing air to escape into the interstitial tissue on inspiration, but impeding its leaving on expiration. When the lung lobules become surrounded by interstitial emphysema their ability to inflate during inspiration is restricted, and this may lead to respiratory distress. If the cause of the emphysema is removed, however, the air is gradually absorbed and the animal slowly returns to normal.

EMPYEMA. A collection of purulent fluid within a cavity. (See PYOTHORAX, PLEURISY.)

'EMTRYL' is the proprietary name of a drug, containing dimetridazole, used in the prevention and treatment of swine dysentery, and had clearance under the Medicines Act for use as a growth promoter for pigs.

ENAMEL (see TEETH).

ENARTHRODIAL JOINTS are those of the ball-and-socket type which allow movement in nearly any direction. Examples include the shoulder joint between the *scapula* and the *humerus*; and the hip joint in which the nearly spherical head of the *femur* fits into the cup-shaped cavity called the *acetabulum* on the pelvis.

Enarthrodial joints are, in joint classification, one type of Diarthrodial joints – synovial or true joints.

ENCEPHALITIS. Inflammation of the brain may be brought about through the activity of bacteria such as those of strangles, listeriosis, but especially during infection with viruses, such as those of rabies, canine distemper, etc. (*See under* BOVINE, EQUINE, CANINE, FELINE, etc., and TOXOPLASMOSIS.)

The symptoms of encephalitis include fever, excitement, delirium, convulsions, paralysis, and loss of consciousness. Several symptoms are common to MENINGITIS. (*See also* SLEEPER SYNDROME.)

FIRST-AID. Keep the animal quiet – in a darkened room if showing excitement, and avoid noise or handling the patient.

ENCEPHALITOZOON *cuniculi.* An intracellular protozoal parasite. It develops in macrophages, brain, kidney and other tissues of rabbits, dogs, rodents, primates.

In carnivores severe nephritis, encephalitis and a high mortality are associated with transplacental infection.

In a Norwegian outbreak 1500 blue fox cubs died (33 per cent of the litters), although the parents showed no signs of infection.

In the UK foxhound puppies have died, and in Tanzania two spaniel puppies which had shown rabies-like signs.

DIAGNOSIS. An ELISA test. W. S. Hollister and colleagues found by its means 51 positive samples out of 248 sera from stray dogs.

ENCEPHALOMALACIA. A group name for the degenerative diseases of the brain. Causes include the copper deficiency of swayback, horse-tail and bracken poisoning, metallic poisoning, and mulberry heart disease of pigs. Another example of encephalomalacia is 'Crazy chick' disease.

ENCEPHALOMYELITIS means inflammation of both the brain and the spinal cord.

ENCEPHALOMYELITIS, VIRAL, OF PIGS. This term covers the group of diseases known as Teschen disease, Talfan disease, and *Poliomyelitis suum*, which may possibly be all caused by the same virus, though this remains uncertain.

Believed to have originated in Czechoslovakia, Viral Encephalomyelitis of pigs is now encountered throughout most of Europe. In Britain and Denmark, only a small percentage of pigs become infected, and illness is far milder than in some other countries.

Symptoms include fever, stiffness, staggering gait, paralysis, and those of encephalitis generally.

ENCEPHALOMYOCARDITIS VIRUS. Antibodies to this have been found in the serum of more than 28 per cent of normal pigs in the UK. It is a picorna virus, a pathogen also of rodents and human beings, and has caused outbreaks of illness in pigs in Australia, USA, Panama. (D. V. Sangar *et al. Vet. Rec.* (1977), **100**, 240.)

ENCHONDROMA means a tumour formed of cartilage. (*See* TUMOURS.)

ENCYSTED. Enclosed in a cyst.

ENDARTERITIS. Inflammation of the inner coat of an artery. (*See* ARTERIES, DISEASES OF.)

ENDO- is a prefix meaning situated inside.

ENDOCARDITIS means inflammation of the smooth membrane that lines the inside of the heart. It occurs especially over the heart valves. (*See* HEART DISEASES.)

ENDOCRINE GLANDS. These secrete hormones – chemical substances which are carried by the blood and influence the action of tissues or organs other than those in which they were produced. (*See* HORMONES; also under the name of individual endocrine glands, *e.g.* ADRENAL, THYROID, PARATHYROID, PITUITARY, THYMUS, PANCREAS.)

ENDOMETRITIS means an inflammation of the mucous membrane that lines the uterus. (*See* UTERUS, DISEASES OF.)

ENDORPHINS. Morphine-like, natural analgesics produced in the body. Acupuncture is said to stimulate their release into the bloodstream. (*See also* TWITCH.)

ENDOSCOPE. An instrument used for viewing the interior of an organ, and for facilitating the extraction of a foreign body, e.g. from the oesophagus; and for assistance with other surgery, including embryo transfer. (*See also* LAPAROSCOPY.)

ENDOTHELIUM is the membrane lining various vessels and cavities of the body, such as the pleura, pericardium, peritoneum, lymphatic vessels, blood-vessels, and joints. It consists of a fibrous layer covered with thin flat cells, which render the surface perfectly smooth and secrete the fluid for its lubrication.

ENDOTOXINS are those toxins which are retained within the bodies of bacteria until the latter die and disintegrate.

ENDOTRACHEAL ANAESTHESIA (*see* ANAESTHESIA).

ENDRIN. A highly toxic insecticide of the chlorinated hydrocarbon group. It has caused fatal poisoning in cattle, dogs, fish, and birds.

ENERGY (*see* CALORIE, CARBOHYDRATES, META-BOLISABLE ENERGY, JOULES).

ENROFLOXACIN. An animal test certificate (ATC) was issued by the Veterinary Medicines Directorate permitting the use of enrofloxacin under 'controlled conditions' in turkeys, chickens, pigeons and parrots; but not in laying birds, as residues in eggs could be 'a potential threat to the food chain.' (Dr J. M. Rutter, Veterinary Medicines Directorate.)

ENSILAGE (*see* SILAGE).

ENTEQUE SECO. A wasting disease of cattle, sheep and horses. It occurs mainly in Argentina, but also in Uruguay and possibly Brazil. It may be identical with Manchester wasting disease (Jamaica) and Naalehu disease (Hawaii).
CAUSE. A plant, common on wet land, known as duraznillo blanco (*Solanum melacoxylon* or *glaucum*). Poisoning may arise from the deliberate eating of the leaves or the accidental consumption of dead, fallen leaves during grazing of the underlying pasture plants. It is particularly dangerous when growing in association with white clover.
It produces an arteriosclerosis, with calcification in heart, aorta, lungs, etc.
SIGNS. Emaciation occurring over weeks or months, and an abnormal gait.

ENTERALGIA is another name for colic.

ENTERITIS (*see* DIARRHOEA *and* INTESTINES, DISEASES OF).

ENTEROCELE (*see* HERNIA).

ENTEROLITHS are stones that develop in the intestines, being formed by deposition of salts round a hard metallic or other nucleus. (*See* CALCULI.)

ENTEROSTOMY means an operation by which an artifical opening is formed into the intestine.

ENTEROTOXAEMIA. An acute disease of calves, lambs, goats; and occasionally of piglets and foals.
CAUSE: Toxins emanating from the intestines and present in the bloodstream. The toxins involved are from four strains of *Clostridium welchii* and from some strains of *E. coli.*
SIGNS: Severe enteritis, with dysentery in some cases, and sudden death in others.
PREVENTION. A vaccine is available.

Calves seldom survive for more than a few hours.

Goats show a sudden drop in milk yield, dysentery, and death within 36 hours. There is also a sub-acute type of the disease lasting 7 to ten days, and followed by recovery.

Sheep. The disease affects both unweaned lambs and sheep one to two years old.

ENTEROVIRUSES. A group of smaller viruses pathogenic to animals and causing disease in cattle, pigs and ducks (duck hepatitis).

ENTROPION (*see* EYE, DISEASES OF).

ENURESIS (*see* INCONTINENCE).

ENVIRONMENT (*see* HOUSING OF ANIMALS, PASTURE MANAGEMENT, EXPOSURE, RAINFALL, ALTITUDE, HEAT-STROKE, ANHIDROSIS, TROPICAL DISEASES, VENTILATION, CALF HOUSING.)

ENZOOTIC refers to a disease present (endemic) among animals in a particular region, country, or locality. For example, braxy and louping-ill are enzootic in the south and west of Scotland and the north of England. Compare **epizootic** (epidemic), in which a disease spreads rapidly through large numbers of animals over a wide area.

For Enzootic Abortion of Sheep, *see under* ABORTION, ENZOOTIC.

ENZOOTIC BOVINE LEUKOSIS (*see* BOVINE LEUKOSIS).

ENZOOTIC OVINE ABORTION is caused by *Chlamydia psittaci*. (*See under* ABORTION, ENZOOTIC.)

ENZOOTIC PNEUMONIA OF PIGS. This was formerly described as Virus Pneumonia of Pigs (VPP), but the cause is now generally regarded as being *Mycoplasma hyopneumoniae*. However, 'Kasza *et al.* (1969) described an apparent synergism between *M. hyopneumoniae* and porcine adenovirus. *Haemophilus* species are frequently present in enzootic pneumonia-like lesions but may be replaced by *Pasteurella multocida* at some stage to produce a more severe type of lesion.' From the above it will be appreciated that while a mycoplasma may be the primary cause, other organisms may be involved to a varying degree. (*See* RESPIRATORY INFECTIONS OF THE PIG, SYNERGISM.)

Many pigs reaching the bacon factories are affected with some degree of pneumonia, so that the matter is of the very greatest economic importance.

SIGNS. When the disease is first introduced into a herd, pigs of all ages (from 10 days upwards) go down with it, and many die. Where the disease is already present, deaths are few. Symptoms, which may easily be overlooked or ignored, then consist merely of a cough. There is, in addition, a certain degree of unthriftiness which in extreme cases may amount to stunted growth. In all cases one may expect the liveweight gain to be reduced. Sometimes pigs which contract the disease earlier in life quite suddenly develop acute pneumonia at 19 to 26 weeks of age, known as 'secondary breakdown'. Affected animals lose their appetite and often become prostrate; breathing rapidly with a temperature over 105°F. A number die if left untreated, but the majority have a fluctuating fever for a few days and then recover.

PREVENTION. An attack of this pneumonia is not followed by immunity, and there is no means of preventive inoculation. All that can be done is to try to avoid buying in infected stock. Litters are best kept in arks on pasture, and any sows showing a cough eliminated. Weaned pigs should not be brought into a fattening house where pigs with pneumonia are present. (*See* DUSTY ATMOSPHERE, SWINE INFLUENZA.)

A health-control scheme for pig herds claiming freedom from enzootic pneumonia was introduced in 1959.

DIAGNOSIS. A complement fixation test has been devised.

ENZOOTIC PNEUMONIA OF SHEEP (*see* PASTEURELLOSIS, PNEUMONIA OF SHEEP.)

ENZYMES are formed by living cells, and are complex organic chemical compounds which facilitate or speed biochemical processes in the animal body, including those of digestion. Some enzymes are also produced by the normal bacterial inhabitants of the intestinal canal. Each has a specific use in splitting up either proteins, carbohydrates, fats, or crude fibre. The best known are the ptyalin of saliva and diastase of the pancreatic juice, which break down starches into soluble sugars, pepsin from the gastric juice and trypsin from the pancreas, which break complex proteins into simple amino acids, and lipase in the intestines which attacks fats. (*See* DIGESTION.) Enzymes are used in the cleaning of badly infected wounds. (*See* STREPTODORNASE.)

Some enzymes detoxify poisons, breaking them down into relatively harmless compounds. The differing susceptibility of cat and dog, for example, to phenol is due to the former animal lacking a particular enzyme which the dog has. (*See* TAURINE.)

Some enzymes are injurious (*see* thiaminase *under* THIAMIN).

(*See also* BLOOD ENZYMES, and CREATINE KINASE for enzymes used in diagnosis.)

EOSINOPHIL is the name given to white cells in the blood-stream containing granules which readily stain with eosin, a histological dye. The nucleus of this leukocyte is lobular. Eosinophils, basophils, and neutrophils are collectively known as polymorphonuclear leukocytes. As well as these circulating cells, eosinophils are found in the pituitary and pineal glands.

In a normal horse, one cubic inch of blood contains between 5 and 8 million eosinophil white cells – compared with about 160 million other white cells, and 128,000 million red cells.

Eosinophils increase in numbers during certain chronic infections and infestations with parasites. They contain hydrolytic enzymes. 'Unlike neutrophils, eosinophils have low phagocytic capacity and are not good at killing micro-organisms.' (*Lancet*) (*See* BLOOD.)

EOSINOPHILIA means that an abnormally large number of eosinophils are present in the blood-stream. This may occur during severe parasitic infestation in horses and dogs, in certain wasting conditions, and in disease of the lymph system.

EOSINOPHILIC GRANULOMA. A complex in cats. The name covers at least three different lesions, of a chronic nature.

Eosinophilic ulcers usually occur on the upper lip, or commissure of the lips, gums, palate, pharynx and tongue. Reddish-brown in colour, they have raised edges. They are not malignant (compare 'rodent ulcer' in man which is a basal cell carcinoma.)

Eosinophilic plaques may occur anywhere on the body but are most common on the abdomen and inside of the thigh. The plaques are red, with raised edges, and ulcerate. They are extremely itchy.

Linear granulomas are seen mainly on the hind legs and in the mouth, and are yellowish-pink in colour. Itching is not usually present. As with the ulcers mentioned above, females seem more prone to this granuloma than are males. In the mouth lesions are 'more nodular' and have to be differentiated from bacterial or mycotic infections and also carcinoma. (Lloyd M. Reedy, *Carnation Research Digest*, 1982).

EOSINOPHILIC MYOSITIS (*see under* MUSCLES, DISEASES OF).

EPERYTHROZOON FELIS. A blood parasite found in cats in Britain, and first reported in 1959. (*See* FELINE INFECTIOUS ANAEMIA.)

EPERYTHROZOON PARVUM. A blood parasite of the pig, which gives rise to fever, anaemia, and sometimes jaundice. It can be transmitted from pig to pig by lice. It occurs in Britain and USA. Other species of this parasite affect sheep, and cattle in Africa. In the UK *E. wenyoni* has been isolated from anaemic cattle. (*See also* HAEMOBARTONELLA.)

EPHEDRINE is an alkaloid derived from the Chinese plant *Ma Huang*, or prepared synthetically. It stimulates the heart and central nervous system and relaxes the bronchioles. It is used for asthma in dogs.

EPHEMERAL FEVER (THREE-DAY SICKNESS). An acute, infectious, and transient fever accompanied by muscular pains, and lameness which has a tendency to shift from limb to limb. The disease was first described in South Africa in 1867 and has been seen in Africa, Asia and Australia. In 1967–8 considerable economic loss was caused by an outbreak among beef and dairy cattle in northern and eastern Australia.

CAUSE is a rhabdovirus. The disease is sudden in onset and attacks a large percentage of the cattle in affected districts, taking the form of an acute epizootic; then, in a few weeks, it dies down again as quickly as it arose. The disease is transmitted by insects, including Culicoides midges. The incubation period is 2–10 days.

SIGNS. The disease is ushered in by a suddenly occurring rise of temperature which may reach 107°F. This is accompanied by loss of appetite, cessation of rumination, rapid respirations, a quick and full pulse (which, however, may become very weak later), and a staring coat. The affected subject stands with head down. The attitude of the patient is rather characteristic, the four legs being placed far under the body and the back

arched, suggestive of the position of a horse suffering from laminitis. There may be a discharge from eyes and nose.

In milking cows, the milk yield is much diminished, but abortion is not a common complication. Many animals prefer to lie down rather than remain on their feet, and once down are most reluctant to get up again. The symptoms along with the elevated temperature continue like this for about three days – hence the name. There is usually a considerable loss of condition.

In Australia the mortality is seldom more than 0·5 per cent.

PREVENTION. Vaccines are used in Japan.

EPI- is a prefix meaning situated on or outside of.

'EPIDEMIC DIARRHOEA'. The provisional name for a disease, probably caused by a virus, resembling Transmissible Gastro-Enteritis (TGE) of pigs, except that unweaned pigs are not affected. It is therefore less serious than TGE.

'EPIDEMIC TREMORS' is the colloquial name for a virus disease of poultry characterised by an unsteady gait. (*See* AVIAN ENCEPHALOMYELITIS.)

EPIDEMIOLOGY. This has been defined as the systematic characterisation and explanation of patterns of disease, and the use of this information in the resolution of health problems. International reporting services, as carried out by WHO and OIE, play their part; and the use of computers has helped; e.g. during the outbreak of foot-and-mouth disease on the Isle of Wight in 1981.

EPIDERMIS (*see* SKIN).

EPIDIDYMIS is a structure situated within the scrotum and in which the sperms mature after leaving the testicle. The epididymis has as its outlet the *Vas deferens*. (*See* TESTIS.)

EPIDIDYMITIS means inflammation of the epididymis. (*See also under* RAM.)

EPIDIDYMITIS and VAGINITIS, CONTAGIOUS ('Epivag'). A venereal disease of cattle in Kenya and Southern Africa, and an important cause there of infertility and sterility.

CAUSE. Possibly a double infection with a virus and a mycoplasma; possibly a campylobacter.

SIGNS. There may be a yellowish discharge from the vagina, or merely a redness of the mucous membrane. In the bull, enlargement of the epididymis occurs over a period of months.

CONTROL. Slaughter of infected bulls, and use of AI.

EPIDURAL ANAESTHESIA is a form of spinal anaesthesia induced by the injection of a local anaesthetic solution into the epidural space of the spinal canal.

The technique is used in bovine obstetrics; the injection being made between the first and second coccygeal vertebrae. (*See also* ANAESTHETICS, ANALGESICS.)

EPIGASTRIUM is the region lying in the middle of the abdomen, immediately over the stomach. (*See* ABDOMEN.)

EPIGLOTTIS is a leaf-like piece of elastic cartilage covered with mucous membrane, which stands upright between the back of the tongue and the entrance to the glottis, or larynx. It plays an important part in the act of swallowing, preventing solids and fluids from passing directly off the back of the tongue into the larynx.

Epiglottic entrapment in the horse is diagnosed more and more frequently due probably to the wider use of endoscopy and greater expertise in its use. Affected horses have a history of decreased exercise tolerance and they make abnormal inspiratory and expiratory noises. For diagnosis and surgical correction *see* R. M. Ordidge, *Vet. Rec.* (1977), **100**, 365.

EPILEPSY is a chronic nervous disorder characterised by a sudden complete loss of consciousness, associated with muscular convulsions. This is particularly a disease of the dog, although other domesticated animals may be affected upon rare occasions. The *cause* of primary or idiopathic epilepsy is a genetic one, whereas secondary epilepsy may be caused by trauma, neoplasia, infections, cardiovascular disease, or metabolic conditions.

The disease 'can be controlled completely in about one-third of affected dogs, and considerably improved in another third. Phenobarbitone or primidone are recommended for treatment. (Frey, H-H. *Veterinary Record* (1986) **118**, 484.)

In a series of 260 cases of suspected central nervous system lesions, studied by Dr Phyllis Croft, 167 were shown by electro-encephalogram to be examples of epilepsy.

Secondary epilepsy may be the result of a head injury, and can occur whenever scar tissue is formed in the brain.

'Fits', practically indistinguishable from true epileptic seizures, frequently occur when puppies are cutting their permanent teeth about the ages of 2 to 6 months, and also when there are large numbers of round or tape worms present in the intestines. (*See also* FITS, HYSTERIA, ENCEPHALITIS, POISONS, HEART DISEASE.)

SIGNS. Attacks usually commence without any warning. The limbs are sometimes held out rigidly, and sometimes moved as if the animal were running or galloping. The animal champs its jaws; the eyes are fixed and staring, or the eyeballs may roll, and the pupils are dilated. There is usually a good deal of salivation from the mouth. The rectum and the bladder are usually evacuated involuntarily. The dog regains consciousness in 1 to 2 minutes; in a few cases consciousness may not be completely lost. The first fit often occurs between the age of 1 and 3.

TREATMENT. After consciousness returns the dog should be placed in a quiet room away from other dogs or human beings. Treatment should be left to a veterinary surgeon. (*See* LARGACTIL, MYSOLINE.)

EPINEPHRIN (*see* ADRENALIN).

EPIPHORA is a condition in which the tears, instead of passing down the tear-duct to the inside of the nose, run over on to the cheek. It may be due to a blocking of the tear-duct, generally from inflammation of its lining membrane following conjunctivitis etc., or by a grass seed. (*See* EYE.)

It is a symptom of naphthalene poisoning in cattle. In the smaller animals, a grass seed may be the cause of blockage.

EPIPHYSEAL FRACTURE is one which occurs along the line of the epiphyseal cartilage, and results in the epiphysis of a bone becoming separated from the shaft or diaphysis. These fractures may occur in any young animals before complete ossification has occurred. (*See* FRACTURES and BONE, DISEASES OF.)

EPIPHYSIS means the spongy extremity of a bone which is attached to the shaft for the purpose of forming a joint with the similar process of the adjacent bone. An epiphysis is covered on its surface by the cartilage, is developed from a separate centre of ossification, and in a young animal is connected with the shaft of the bone by a plate of cartilage that disappears in the adult, being replaced by bone. (*See* BONE – growth of.)

EPIPHYSITIS may occur in young calves affected with 'joint-ill'; and has been reported in adult cattle housed on slatted floors. The cattle were lame, and inflammation and necrosis were found involving the distal epiphysis of the large metatarsal bones. It also occurs in horses.

EPISOMES (*see* PLASMIDS).

EPISPASTICS are substances which produce blistering on the skin.

EPISTAXIS means bleeding from the nose. (*See* GUTTURAL POUCH DIPHTHERIA, HAEMORRHAGE.)

EPITHELIOGENESIS IMPERFECTA. An inherited condition in which there is a gap in the epithelium which readily bleeds and then heals by scar tissue. It has been seen in foals, calves, piglets, lambs, and kittens.

EPITHELIOMA is a type of malignant tumour. (*See* CANCER.)

EPITHELIUM is the layer or layers of cells of which skin and mucous membranes are formed. The epithelial tissues take many forms. (*See* SKIN *and* MUCOUS MEMBRANE.)

'EPIVAG'. A venereal disease of cattle in Kenya and Southern Africa; Contagious Epididymitis and Vaginitis. (*See* EPIDIDYMITIS.)

EPIZOOTIC is a term applied to a disease which affects a large number of animals in a large area of land at the same time and spreads with great rapidity. For example, foot-and-mouth disease and cattle plague. (*See* O.I.E.)

EPIZOOTIC CEREBROSPINAL NEMATO-DIASIS. A disease of horses in Asia, caused by the migrating larvae of the roundworm *Setaria equina*. (*See* ROUNDWORMS.)

EPIZOOTIC LYMPHANGITIS. Synonyms: Lymphangitis epizootica, 'African glanders', 'Japanese farcy', and 'Neapolitan farcy'.

This is a chronic contagious disease of the horse family (*Equidae*). Rare cases have been recorded in cattle, and also in man.
DISTRIBUTION. It occurs widely in Asia, in Africa, and has also been described in America. It was unknown in Great Britain until 1902, when it was brought into the country by army horses returning from the South African war. The disease was made a notifiable one by the Epizootic Lymphangitis Orders of 1904 and 1905, after which it was rapidly eradicated. Apart from very occasional reports following the 1914–18 War, it has not occurred in Britain since.
CAUSE. A fungus *Histoplasma* (Cryptococcus) *farciminosa*, which gains entry into the body through a wound, either on the skin or of a mucous surface. The disease is spread by flies, grooming tools, or by any materials which have come into contact with diseased animals or their infective discharges, such as cloths, sponges, and even pails of antiseptic solution!
INCUBATION PERIOD. Under natural conditions at least one month, but more commonly three or more, may elapse from the time of contamination of a wound till the onset of the symptoms. Even by means of experimental inoculation, incubation takes one month.
SIGNS. The first signs of the disease are often thickenings or 'cording' of a lymphatic vessel and the enlargement of the adjacent lymph nodes. A fore-limb is usually the site of the lesions, which include granulomas, nodules which discharge a creamy pus and ulcerate. Ulcers may form on the mucous membrane of the nose; occasionally on vulva or scrotum.

The disease, which runs a slow course lasting weeks or months, has to be differentiated from glanders. A few horses recover.
TREATMENT. In the UK this is not allowed. The disease is NOTIFIABLE.

EPIZOOTIC PULMONARY ADENOMATOSIS (*see under* JAAGSIEKTE).

EPSOM SALTS is the popular name for sulphate of magnesium, a saline LAXATIVE. (*See* LAXATIVES.) Epsom Salts are also useful as a first-aid treatment of lead and carbolic acid poisoning.

EPULIS is a tumour of the gum (or involving the jaw bones).

EQUID (*see under* EQUINE).

EQUINE BACK LESIONS (*see* HORSES, BACK TROUBLE).

EQUINE BILIARY FEVER. This disease is caused by two distinct parasites: *Babesia caballi* and *B. equi*. The former species resembles *Babesia bigemina* in size and morphology, and causes a

disease similar to Texas fever but which is milder and more amenable to treatment than that caused by *B. equi*. This is a smaller species than *B. caballi* and causes a disease which is highly virulent for adult horses and other species of the horse family, but is mild in young animals. Recovered animals are in a state of premunition, and inoculation of colts as a means of protection later in life is commonly practised.
DISTRIBUTION. The disease is found in Russia and various parts of Europe, India, Africa, South America, and South Africa.
SIGNS. At the beginning of the disease there is a sharp rise in temperature to about 107°F. During this period the parasites are multiplying in the blood. In a few days the temperature falls and anaemia sets in. In the horse this is usually masked by an intense icterus, though not in the donkey and mule. Haemoglobinuria, and constipation followed by diarrhoea, are frequent symptoms, and are succeeded by rapid emaciation. The animal may die during the initial fever (2 to 5 days) or from anaemia and emaciation about the eleventh day or later. Complications are frequent.
TREATMENT. Complete rest, an injection of Pirevan or Piroparv or of a broad-spectrum antibiotic.
TRANSMISSION. In Southern Europe *B. caballi* is transmitted by *Dermacentor reticulatus* and *D. silvarum*; in South Africa *B. equi* is transmitted by *Rhipicephalus evertsi* and *R. bursa*. Other species and genera of ticks probably act as vectors of *B. equi* in other countries.

EQUINE BLOOD TYPES. 'Transferrin is an ideal protein for blood-typing because it can exist in 7 different forms or alleles in the horse. They are called D, F^1, F^2, H, M, O, and R. All horses have two transferrin alleles; these may be the same, e.g. DD, OO, etc, or they can be any combination of two different ones, e.g. DR, F^2O, HM, etc. There are therefore in all 28 possible transferrin types. Whatever an animal's transferrin type may be, it always receives one half from the sire and one half from the dam, e.g. F^2 from the sire and R from the dam would give a transferrin type F^2R, or D from each would give DD.' – (A. M. Scott, Animal Health Trust Equine Research Station, reprinted from *The British Racehorse*, 1968.)

EQUINE COITAL EXANTHEMA. A venereal disease of horses caused by a herpes virus. (*See table under* HERPESVIRUS.)

EQUINE CONTAGIOUS METRITIS. A venereal disease which appeared in Britain in 1977, and is of a type previously unknown. This highly contagious disease reduced the conception rate among mares visiting the National Stud at Newmarket from 91 per cent (1976) to 42 per cent in 1977.
CAUSE. A Gram-negative cocco-bacillus, known as the CEM organism. This has been isolated from the cervix, urethra and clitoris. The organism is apt to persist in the clitoral fossa after clearance from other parts of the mare's urogenital tract, and routine sampling at this site is therefore necessary or diagnosis may fail to be confirmed.

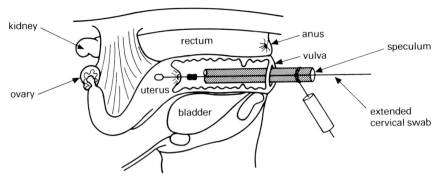

Diagram showing the technique of collecting a cervical swab via a tubular speculum. The swab is passed as far into the open oestrous cervix, and beyond, as possible.

CONTROL. A code of practice for control of the infection was formulated by the Horserace Betting Levy Board in 1977, and supported by the Ministry of Agriculture and the Thoroughbred Breeders' Association.

CERVICAL SWAB TESTS are a routine diagnostic and preventive measure on stud farms. Among techniques described by S. W. Ricketts (*Veterinary Record* (1981) **108,** 46) is that shown in the diagram.

CARRIERS. Testing the blood for CEM antibodies, and inoculating smegma from mares and stallions under test into other mares should be of help, stated Dr T. W. Swerczeck, University of Kentucky.

Measures to control the spread of contagious equine metritis (CEM) in *non-thoroughbred* mares were announced at a meeting organised by the British Equestrian Federation in 1978. They were:

1. Stallions should be swabbed for CEM before the start of the covering season according to the recommendations set down by the various horse and pony breed societies.

2. Stallion owners should insist on being informed of the 1977 breeding history of all mares before they are brought to the stud.

3. Mares should be swabbed in heat at least once. The swabs should be cultured for the organism of CEM as well as other causes of infertility. The mare should not be covered until the result of the culture is known.

4. Mares infected with CEM or in contact with a confirmed case in 1977 should have three sets of swabs taken at a minimum interval of seven days, one set being taken during heat.

5. Clinical examinations and diagnostic tests should be carried out early in the stud season to give time for treatment and further examinations for freedom from infection.

6. Stallion owners should reserve the right to call in their own veterinary surgeon for further examination of a visiting mare at the expense of the owner.

7. Owners of native ponies on their native heath should avoid introducing into the herd stallions or mares which have had contact with thoroughbred breeding stock during the 1977 season, until proved to be free of infection.

8. The risk of contracting infection is greatest when cross breeding involving thoroughbred animals is taking place and breeders using their horses for this purpose should be particularly vigilant, especially in the case of a discharge from a mare or where a mare returns to service too soon. A high standard of stud hygiene is vital in all establishments. (*See also* clitoral sinusectomy *under* CLITORIS.)

EQUINE DYSAUTONOMIA (*see* GRASS SICKNESS).

EQUINE EHRLICHIOSIS. (*See* POTOMAC HORSE FEVER.) The tentative name given to a transmissible disease of horses first recognised in California. The causal agent resembles that of tickborne fever of cattle. Oedema of the extremities is a symptom.

EQUINE ENCEPHALITIS. A virus disease occurring in North America, South America, Russia, Far and Middle East. It affects horses, but chickens, pheasants, etc., act as a reservoir of infection. Man can be infected. Four or five viruses are known to exist. Paralysis of the head and neck muscles is a feature. Treatment consists in the use of antiserum in large doses. Mosquitoes transmit this disease, or group of diseases; the horse is an 'accidental' host. (*See also* NEAR EAST ENCEPHALITIS, VENEZUELAN.)

The deaths of thousands of horses in Mexico and the USA in 1971 led to further restrictions on the import of horses into the UK.

Equine encephalitis was prevalent throughout the USA in 1975. The viruses are St Louis Encephalitis (SLE), Western Equine Encephalitis (WEE), and Eastern Equine Encephalitis (EEE). 'Generally speaking', commented an official report, these viruses 'follow a bird–mosquito cycle, with an occasional spill-over to mammalian hosts. SLE appears in humans, and WEE/EEE appear in both humans and horses.' Rodents may be affected, too. The three virus infections cannot be differentiated on clinical grounds; laboratory tests are essential.

(For symptoms, *see under* ENCEPHALITIS.)

CONTROL. There is a very effective chick embryo vaccine.

Public health. In Canada a disastrous outbreak occurred in Manitoba in 1941, when 509 human cases were reported, with 78 deaths; 12 of them among children. Of 27 infants, many became mentally retarded, and suffered convulsions, spasticity, and hemiplegia. In 1975 the disease re-appeared in Manitoba, but human cases numbered only 14, and there were no deaths. (Equine cases totalled 277.)

In man the disease takes the form of an aseptic meningitis, with some deaths among the very young and the very old.

EQUINE FILARIASIS. Infestation of horses with the filarid worm, *Seturia equina*, the larvae being carried by mosquitoes and biting flies. It occurs in South and Central Europe, and Asia.
SIGNS. Malaise and anaemia, or fever, conjunctivitis, and dropsical swellings.

EQUINE GAIT ANALYSIS. The Animal Health introduced the Kaegi computerised gait analysis system to help in the diagnosis of equine lameness. The idea was that of a Swiss inventor, Bruno Kaegi, and was developed to assess the paces of a trotting horse. The system was expected to provide an objective measurement of the degree of lameness affecting a horse, and also a comparison between the limbs, and was described as 'of great potential for purchase and pre-insurance examinations'.

EQUINE GENITAL INFECTIONS in the mare.
A survey carried out in 1964 by Lord Porchester's Veterinary Committee, for the Thoroughbred Breeders' Association, showed the following infections:

	Per cent	Approx. percentages of all mares swabbed
Beta-haemolytic Streptococcal infections	49	9·3
Klebsiella pneumoniae	8	1·6
Escherichia coli and coliforms	16	3·3
Pathogenic staphylococci	11	2·0
Corynebacterum sp.	3	0·6
Mixed infections	10	1·9
Fungal infections (all types)	3	0·6

In taking swabs 'it is quite possible to find mares with negative cervical swabs carrying *Klebsiella aerogenes* in the vestibule, urethra or clitoris,' so swabs must be taken not only from the cervix. (R. E. S. Greenwood and D. R. Ellis, *Vet Rec.* (1976), **99**, 439.)

Abortion caused by the virus of Equine Rhinopneumonitis has also occurred in the UK for several years; most outbreaks being associated with imported or visiting mares. Contagious equine metritis (CEM) is an important uterine infection described under EQUINE CONTAGIOUS METRITIS and due to the C.E.M. organism.

Other infections include: *Klebsiella aerogenes, Pseudomonas* species; and see also LISTERIOSIS, LEPTOSIROSIS, and BRUCELLOSIS. Fungal infections have rarely been reported, and include *Aspergillus fumigatus* and *Candida albicans.*

EQUINE HERPESVIRUSES. These include EHV1, the Equine Rhinopneumonitis or 'equine abortion' virus. Primarily affecting the respiratory system, this virus is the cause of much illness in young horses. EHV 3 causes Equine Coital Exanthema. (EHV 2 is probably non-pathogenic.) (*Vet. Rec.* (1976) **98**, 153.) EHV 1 has caused ataxia and paresis.

EQUINE HYDATID DISEASE (*see* HYDATID DISEASE).

EQUINE INFECTIOUS ANAEMIA. Synonyms: pernicious equine anaemia, swamp fever, horse malaria, etc.

A contagious disease of horses and mules during the course of which changes occur in the blood, and rapid emaciation with debility and prostration are evident. It occurs chiefly in the Western States of America and the North-Western Provinces of Canada, as well as in most countries of Europe, and in Asia, and Africa. The first case in the UK was reported from Newmarket in 1975.
CAUSE. A virus. The horse is commonly infected by biting insects, *e.g.* horse flies, stable flies, mosquitoes. Infected grooming tools – if they cause an abrasion – or syringes, hypodermic needles (or even contaminated vaccines) are other means of transmission. Virus may be present in urine, faeces, saliva, nasal secretions, semen, and milk.

The disease is prevalent in low-lying, swampy areas, especially during spring and summer months.

The virus may cause illness in man (who may infect a horse); also in pigs.
SIGNS. After an incubation period of two to four weeks, equine infectious anaemia gives rise to intermittent fever (with a temperature of up to 106°), depression and weakness. Often there are tiny haemorrhages on the lining of the eyelids and under the tongue. Jaundice, swelling of the legs and lower part of the abdomen, and anaemia may follow. In acute cases, death is common. In chronic cases there may be a recurrence of fever, loss of appetite, and emaciation.

The Newmarket case was dealt with under the Infectious Diseases of Horses Order 1975, which enables restrictions to be placed on suspected animals, infected places, and contact horses.

About 50 per cent of horses in a stud or stable may become ill with this disease, and the mortality rate can very between 30 and 70 per cent or so.

It should be added that some horses do not show symptoms but become latent carriers of the infection, passing it on to others.

No treatment has so far been proved to be efficacious, and recovered animals become carriers. Vaccines are ineffective.
DIAGNOSIS may be confirmed by means of the agar gel immunodiffusion precipitation (Coggins') test. Horses imported into the UK from the USA must have passed this test with a negative result. (*See* NOTIFIABLE DISEASES.) Equine infectious anaemia 'may be confused with other infections including trypanosomiasis, anthrax, equine rhinopneumonitis abortion, African horse sickness, the equine encephalitides, leptospirosis

and piroplasmosis' (D. G. Powell, *Vet. Rec.* 1976, **99**, 7).

CONTROL: where possible, test and slaughter reactors in order to eradicate the disease. (*See* Issel & Coggins (1979) *JAVMA* **74**, 7 for further information.)

EQUINE INFLUENZA. A common and highly infectious disease of horses. Provided that they have not been worked while ill, mortality from influenza is usually nil, except in foals infected during the first few days of life. There is surely a danger in referring to equine influenza as 'The Cough' or 'Newmarket Cough' if those collo-quialisms give rise to the idea that it is only a cough and not an illness. Owners should appreci-ate that influenza viruses need to be treated with respect; also that there are many other causes of coughing in horses. (*See* COUGH.)

CAUSE. A virus was first isolated in Prague in 1957. One of a similar type was isolated in the 1963 outbreak in Britain, and is now known as A/Equi/1. Also referred to as the Cambridge strain, it was also found in the USA. In the 1963 outbreak in the USA another virus, believed to have come from South America, was isolated. This is called A/Equi/2 or the 'Miami strain'. This virus appeared in Britain for the first time in the 1965 outbreak. (*See* EQUINE RESPIRATORY VIRUSES.)

SIGNS. The temperature rises to a degree or two above normal, or even as high as 106°F. Often the first symptom observed by the owner is the cough, at first of a dry type but later becoming moist. Coughing may last for 1 week, or persist for 3 weeks. In mild cases there may be virtually no other symptoms and – if rested – the horse makes an uneventful recovery.

In less mild cases the animal has a dejected appearance and very little appetite. Sometimes there is probably pain in the muscles, for the horse may show difficulty or clumsiness in lying down and getting up, or may appear stiff.

A foal born to a mare during the course of an attack of influenza, or as the first symptoms are beginning to appear, will appear normal for 4 or 5 days; but then the temperature rises to 105° or more, the foal ceases to feed, and within a couple of days its breathing becomes very laboured. Death can be expected when the foal is about 9 or 10 days old.

TREATMENT. First-aid measures call for rest, warmth and, if appetite fails, several small feeds a day. Professional advice should always be ob-tained. Antibiotics may be used in order to pre-vent any complications caused by bacteria.

In the foal, hyperimmune serum has proved effective in saving life **when given between 60 and 80 days after birth.** Antibiotics may also be used liberally during the first 3 to 4 days of life in order to try to avoid complications arising from second-ary infection.

When the disease has already appeared in a stable, it is wise to rely upon the thermometer rather than the cough as the first sign of infection in a horse. The temperature may be up 12 hours before coughing starts, and if the fever is detected early the animal can be rested with all the greater chances of the influenza remaining mild.

PREVENTION. A reliable vaccine, containing both A/Equi/1 and A/Equi/2 viruses, is avail-able. It is recommended that foals are vaccinated when between 3 and 6 months old. In-foal mares should be vaccinated at least 3 weeks before they foal. Horses should be vaccinated 3 weeks before they go to sales, etc., where they are likely to be exposed to infection. Newcomers to a stable, especially 2- or 3-year-olds, should also be vac-cinated. Immunity is developed in 98 per cent of vaccinated animals within 2 to 3 weeks, and should last for about a year.

Some apparent 'breakdowns' in horses vac-cinated against equine influenza may be due to the fact that some outbreaks of coughing are due to other infections, *e.g.* Rhinopneumonitis.

EQUINE LYMPHOSARCOMA. Eleven cases in-volving the thoracic cavity were described. The clinical changes included inappetence (dysphagia was present in three cases) weight loss, pectoral oedema, dyspnoea, pleural effusion and dis-tension of the jugular veins. In two cases there were signs of abdominal disease. Post mortem examination revealed lesions in the abdomen as well as the chest in eight cases. (Mair, T. S., Lane, J. G. & Lucke, V. M. (1985) *Equine Veterinary Journal* **17**, 428.)

EQUINE MYOGLOBINURIA (Azoturia) is seldom seen in horses under four years old, and practically never in those that are out at pasture.

CAUSE. The direct cause of the disease is as yet unknown, but when horses that have been in con-tinuous work are suddenly rested for a few days, fed very well meanwhile, and then returned to work or exercise, there is a risk of azoturia.

It has been suggested that the cause is an accumulation of glycogen in muscle, liberating excessive amounts of lactic acid during exercise.

SIGNS. The hind-limbs suddenly become stiff and weak or staggering, and there is a tendency to 'knuckle-over' at the fetlocks. The muscles of the hindquarters become tense, hard, and often pain-ful. They feel like wood to the hand. Colicky symptoms are observed in some cases, but they pass off after a short time. The urine is a wine-red or coffee colour. In some cases the urine is re-tained, and it is necessary to relieve the bladder by the passage of a catheter. The temperature is gen-erally elevated in severe cases, but seldom reaches more than 104°F.

The horse should be taken from work at once when the stiffness is noticed. It should be placed in a loose-box for preference with plenty of bedding, and if the weather is at all cold one or two rugs should be applied.

If the horse has to be taken home, this should be done by horse box. **If the horse is walked for any distance, a fatal outcome is likely.**

TREATMENT. An antihistamine or cortisone may be used in treatment; and the application of hot packs, etc., to the loins and over the hard muscles, gives relief.

PREVENTION. When horses are out of work they should be given some amount of exercise, and have their concentrated diet restricted.

Equine respiratory viruses

Virus classification	Virus	Disease produced
Myxovirus	*Myxovirus influenzae A/equi 1 *Myxovirus influenzae A/equi 2	Equine influenza
Picornavirus	*Rhinovirus 1 Rhinovirus 2	Rhinitis; Pharyngitis
Herpesvirus	*Equine herpesvirus 1 (EHV 1)	Rhinopneumonitis
	*Equine herpesviruses 2, 3, 4 etc. ('Slow growing herpesviruses'; 'Cytomegaloviruses'.)	Pathogenicity uncertain; often present in the respiratory tract
Adenovirus	Adenovirus	Pneumonia and acute respiratory illness. Suspected infection reported from USA, Australia and Germany
Paramyxovirus	Parainfluenza 3 virus	Acute upper respiratory infection. Unconfirmed reports of occurrence in N. America
Coronavirus	Infectious bronchitis-like agent	Acute upper respiratory infection. Unconfirmed reports of occurrence in N. America
Orbivirus	African Horse Sickness virus	African Horse Sickness
Pestivirus	Equine arteritis virus	Equine viral arteritis

*Infections recognised as occurring in Britain.
(This table is reproduced, by courtesy of Dr H. Platt, from a paper he gave at the 1971 BVA Congress, amended in 1986.)

Atypical equine myoglobinuria. This syndrome affects mostly horses at grass. (Compare EQUINE MYOGLOBINURIA.) There is a sudden onset of stiffness unrelated to exercise. Affected horses or ponies are reluctant to move, and many become recumbent; some dying. Appetite is not lost and water is drunk. Pulse and respiration rates also remain normal as a rule. Dark chocolate-coloured or red urine is passed. (Patricia Harris, Animal Health Trust, 1985.)

EQUINE PAPULAR DERMATITIS. Possibly caused by a virus, this has been seen in thoroughbreds in Australia. Firm, multiple papular swellings appear which recede after 2 to 3 weeks.

EQUINE PIROPLASMOSIS is another name for biliary fever of the horse, which is due to one of two protozoön parasites, *Piroplasma* (or *Babesia*) *caballi*, or *Nuttallia equi*. (*See* EQUINE BILIARY FEVER.)

EQUINE RESPIRATORY VIRUSES. The table shows the viruses known to cause disease of the horse's respiratory system. (*See table above.*)

EQUINE SARCOID. (*See* SARCOID.)

EQUINE VERMINOUS ARTERITIS. This is a swelling of the cranial mesenteric artery, commonly encountered in horses, and resulting from thickening and fibrosis of the arterial wall due to the effects of migrating Strongyle worm larvae. Thrombosis and embolism may follow the stenosis, or reduced lumen, of the artery. Infarction and ischaemia of the bowel may result. Rupture of the artery at this site is very rare indeed. (The term 'verminous aneurysm', which persisted in the veterinary literature until the late 1970s, or beyond, is a misnomer).
 (L. B. Jeffcott. *Equine Vet. J.* (1980) **12**, 34.
SIGNS often occur during or shortly after work

and include the sudden onset of abdominal pain, fever, flaring of the nostrils, a pulse rate of 70–80, and turning the head towards the right flank.
 Following recovery from one attack, abdominal pain may return at frequent intervals over weeks or months. The horse may become bad-tempered, be unwilling to back or turn in a small circle, may remain recumbent for long periods, and may hesitate before jumping.
TREATMENT. Dr Greatorex, at the Royal Veterinary College, used intravenous injections of 6 per cent dextran 70 in 5 per cent dextrose solution as an anti-clotting agent. Of 57 horses, 49 recovered completely; the other 8 failing to respond. (*See table overleaf.*)

EQUINE VIRAL ARTERITIS. This is a highly contagious disease in which damage is caused to the arteries, especially the smaller ones.
SIGNS include fever, conjunctivitis, oedema of the lungs and also affecting the legs and other parts of the body. Haemorrhagic enteritis, with abdominal pain and diarrhoea, may occur. Over 50 per cent of pregnant mares abort. Horses which recover are likely to become carriers. A vaccine is available. (*See* HORSES, IMPORT CONTROLS.)

EQUINE VIRAL RHINOPNEUMONITIS. A disease recognised in America and Europe and caused by the equine herpesvirus–1 (*see* EQUINE RESPIRATORY VIRUSES).
SIGNS include slight fever, cough, and nasal discharge. These are seen in weaned foals and yearlings; though some infections are subclinical. In the mare, some strains of EHV–1 cause abortion, often after the gestation period has passed the eighth month. What gives the disease its alternative name of 'Equine Virus Abortion', is the fact that pregnant mares exposed for the first time to the infection may abort.
 Indeed the term 'abortion storms' has been used, since 40 to 60 per cent (or even more) of the mares in a stud may abort. Usually such an

Breed, age and sex of 57 cases of equine verminous arteritis

Breed	No. of Cases	0–1	1–2	2–3	3–6	6–9	9–12	12+	Male	Female
Arabs	7	1	2	—	3	—	1	—	4	3
Hackneys	1	—	—	—	—	—	1	—	1	—
Hunters	9	—	—	—	6	2	—	1	7	2
Palominos	4	—	—	1	2	1	—	—	2	2
Ponies	13	1	1	—	7	3	1	—	11	2
Thoroughbreds	22	2	—	2	4	10	3	1	16	6
Trotters	1	—	—	—	—	1	—	—	1	—
Totals	57	4	3	3	22	17	6	2	42	15

(J. C. Greatorex, *Vet. Rec.* (1977), **101**, 184.)

occurrence is a sequel to an outbreak of severe and extensive nasal catarrh when the in-foal mares were between 4½ and 7 months pregnant.

It must be emphasised, however, that these 'abortion storms' are exceptional, and have become more so, both on the Continent and in the USA, in recent years.

Abortions may occur at any time from 4½ months of pregnancy right up to the normal foaling date, but 8½ to 10 months is the most common period. Mares show no other symptoms at this time. Subsequent foaling is nearly always normal.

The virus is present in the aborted fetus, fluids, and membranes. It cannot survive more than a fortnight in the absence of horse tissue. On straw, concrete floors, etc., it dies within a week. But when dried on to horse hairs, it has been shown to be infective for up to 6 weeks. The stallion is not, it is believed, involved in the spread of the disease – first reported in the UK in 1961.

A 1974 report attributed cases of acute paresis and paralysis in horses in Canada to this virus.

EQUISETUM POISONING (*see* HORSE-TAILS, POISONING BY).

EQUIVALENTS, TABLES OF. In Great Britain the metric system of weights and measures has been adopted as the more accurate and convenient manner by which drugs and medicines can be dispensed, and other measurements recorded.

Measures of length
Abbreviations: inch = in, foot = ft, yard = yd, millimetre = mm, centimetre = cm, metre = m
$$1 \text{ in} = 2\cdot5399 \text{ cm}$$
$$(= 2\cdot54 \text{ approx.})$$
$$1 \text{ ft} = 30\cdot4794 \text{ cm}$$
$$(= 30\cdot48 \text{ approx.})$$
$$1 \text{ yd} = 91\cdot4383 \text{ cm}$$
$$\text{or } 0\cdot914 \text{ m}$$
To convert:
in to cm, multiply by 2·54
yd to m, multiply by 0·914
$$10 \text{ mm} = 1 \text{ cm}$$
$$1 \text{ cm} = 0\cdot3937 \text{ in}$$
$$1 \text{ m} = 1 \text{ yd } 0 \text{ ft } 3\cdot37 \text{ in}$$
To convert:
cm to in, multiply by 0·39
m to yd, multiply by 1·09

Measures of weight
Abbreviations: grain = gr., dram = dr., ounce = oz, pound = lb, milligram = mg, gram = g, kilogram = kg

(Apothec.) 1 gr. = 0·0648 g
$$= 64\cdot8 \text{ mg}$$
$$1 \text{ dr.} = 3\cdot888 \text{ g}$$
$$= 3888 \text{ mg}$$
(Avoir.) 1 oz = 28·35 g
$$1 \text{ lb} = 453\cdot592 \text{ g}$$
$$= \text{approx. } \tfrac{1}{2} \text{ kg}$$
To convert:
oz (Avoir.) to g, multiply by 28·35
lb (Avoir.) to g, multiply by 453·6
lb (Avoir.) to kg, multiply by 0·454
oz (Troy) to g, multiply by 31·104
$$1 \text{ mg} = 0\cdot0154 \text{ gr.}$$
$$1 \text{ g} = 15\cdot4323 \text{ gr.}$$
$$= 0\cdot0321 \text{ oz (Avoir.)}$$
$$1 \text{ kg} = 2\cdot2046 \text{ lb (Avoir.)}$$
To convert:
g to oz (Avoir.), multiply by 0·0352
g to gr., multiply by 15·432
kg to lb (Avoir.), multiply by 2·2046

Measures of capacity
Abbreviations: fluid dram = fl.dr., fluid ounce = fl.oz, ounce = oz, pint = pt, gallon = gall., cubic centimetre = cc (scientifically cm³), gram = g, millilitre = ml, litre = l
$$1 \text{ fl.dr.} = 3\cdot544 \text{ cc or ml}$$
$$1 \text{ fl.oz} = 28\cdot412 \text{ cc or ml}$$
$$1 \text{ oz (Troy)} = 31\cdot1034 \text{ g}$$
$$1 \text{ pt} = 567\cdot933 \text{ cc or ml}$$
$$\text{or } 0\cdot568 \text{ l}$$
To convert:
fl. oz to cc or ml, multiply by 28·412
pt to cc or ml, multiply by 568·0
gall. to l, multiply by 4·54
$$1 \text{ cc or ml} = 1 \text{ gram of distilled water}$$
$$\text{at } 4°\text{C.}$$
$$= 0\cdot061 \text{ cubic inches}$$
$$= 0\cdot352 \text{ fl.oz}$$
$$= 16\cdot896 \text{ minims (imperial)}$$
$$1 \text{ l} = 61\cdot0 \text{ cubic inches}$$
$$= 1\cdot7607 \text{ pt}$$
$$= 35\cdot196 \text{ fl.oz}$$
To convert:
cc (or ml) to oz, multiply by 0·352
l to pt, multiply by 1·76
l to fl.oz, multiply by 35·196

Other equivalents:
1 gall. of water weighs 10 lb and occupies 277·274 cubic inches (4·54 l or 4540·0 ml or cc)

Measures of area
A hectare (10,000 square metres) is a little less than 2½ acres.
A square kilometre (1000 metres × 1000 metres) is about ⅜ of a square mile.

(*See also* SI UNITS, MICRON, NANOMETRE.)

ERGOMETRINE is the most powerful of the active constituents of ergot in producing muscular contractions of the uterus. It is used to stimulate a sluggish uterus during parturition and to control uterine haemorrhage following parturition.

ERGOT is the small mass of horn which is found amongst the tuft of hair which grows from the back of the fetlocks of horses. It is produced by cells which are similar to those which form the horn of the hoof, and it is considered by some authorities to be the remains of what once was the hoof of another digit which the horse has now lost.

ERGOT, FUNGAL. There are several species of ergot, including *Claviceps fusiformis*, which infests the bullrush millet, and *C. purpurea* – a parasite of rye and other cereals, such as maize. (Please note: there is no effective treatment in advanced cases.)

ERGOT OF MUNGA, the bulrush millet, is in southern Zimbabwe an important cause of loss to the pig industry. The sow's udder fails to enlarge and become functional, and piglet mortality is heavy as a result of the absence of milk or *agalactia*. Sows show no other signs of ill health. The alkaloidal composition of this ergot is believed to differ from that of *Claviceps purpurea*.

ERGOT OF RYE is a fungus which attacks the seed of rye or other cereal, subsists upon it, and finally replaces it. The fungus is called *Claviceps purpurea*, and is artificially cultivated on account of its medicinal properties. Its medicinal preparations are used to stimulate the wall of the uterus during parturition when there is inertia, and are also useful for checking haemorrhage by causing constriction of the arterioles. The crude ergot is unsafe to use. In parturition the active principle ergometrine is employed both in human and animal work to increase the force and efficiency of labour pains.

ERGOT POISONING occurs through eating cereals upon which the fungus is parasitic, such as rye and various kinds of maize, etc., and through taking foods made from affected plants (*e.g.* maize meals). Extensive outbreaks have occurred in various parts of the United States of America, in Germany, Austria, and other parts of Europe. Abortion and gangrene of the extremities in cattle have been seen in Britain.
SIGNS. The characteristic feature of poisoning due to *Claviceps purpurea* is that there is irritation and pain in the extremities of the body, and later, areas of the skin of these parts become gangrenous, and may slough off.

Two forms are recognised: in the first, convulsive symptoms due to stimulation of the nervous system are seen; and in the second, gangrene occurs.

Horses that have eaten large amounts of ergotised hay develop symptoms during the first 24 hours after feeding. The animal becomes dull and listless, a cold sweat breaks out on the neck and flanks, the breathing is slow and deep, the temperature is below normal, the pulse is weak and finally imperceptible, and death occurs during deep coma. When lesser amounts have been taken over a longer period there may be diarrhoea, colic, vomiting, and signs of abdominal pain. Pregnant animals may abort, and lose condition.

Trembling, general muscular spasms, loss of sensation of the extremities, convulsions and delirium, may be seen.

In the gangrenous form there is coldness of the feet, ears, lips, tail, combs and wattles of birds, and other extremities, a loss of sensation in these parts, and eventually dry gangrene sets in. After a day or two the hair falls out, teeth drop out, the tips of the ears and tail may slough off, and the skin of the limbs, or even the whole of the feet, may be cast off. Death occurs from exhaustion, or from septicaemia.

Ergot-contaminated feed may result in reduced fertility and agalactia in the sow. (*See also under* ERGOT OF MUNGA.)

ERYSIPELAS, SWINE (*see* SWINE ERYSIPELAS).

ERYSIPELOID. Human infection with *Erysipelothrix rhusiopathiae*, the cause of swine erysipelas.

ERYTHEMA is a redness of the skin, the surface blood-vessels of which become gorged with blood.

ERYTHROCYTE is another name for a red blood cell.

ERYTHROCYTE MOSAICISM. The mixture of two blood types in each of non-identical twins.

ERYTHROLEUCOSIS. This is a transmissible virus-associated type of cancer occurring in poultry. It is associated with the fowl paralysis group of diseases. It was described and named in 1908, three years before the Rous sarcoma made history. (*See under* LEUCOSIS COMPLEX.)

ERYTHROMYCIN. An antibiotic which has a bacteriostatic action against Gram-positive organisms. It is used when penicillin-susceptible strains have developed resistance. This drug is usually considered too irritant to be given parenterally, but is used in intramammary injections.

ERYTHROPOIESIS. The formation of red blood cells in the bone marrow, stimulated by the hormone **Erythropoietin** secreted by the kidneys.

ESCHAR is an area of body tissue that has been killed by heat or by caustics.

ESCHERICHIA COLI. This is the modern name for *Bacillus coli*. For further information *see* E. COLI.

ESCUTCHEON. The anal region of an ox, with special reference to the direction of growth of hair.

ESERINE (*see* PHYSOSTIGMINE).

ESTER. A compound formed from an alcohol and an acid by elimination of water, *e.g.,* ethyl acetate.

ESTRADIOL and ESTRONE are hormones secreted by the ovary (interstitial cells and Graäfian follicles) which bring about oestrus and, in late pregnancy, stimulate development of the mammary gland.

ESTRUMATE. A proprietary name for the prostaglandin analogue Cloprostenol. (*See* CLOPROSTENOL and CONTROLLED BREEDING.)

ESTRUS (*see* OESTRUS).

ETHANOL POISONING was suspected as the cause of severe depression in five puppies which had been shampooed with a dishwashing detergent liquid. A sixth puppy had died. A blood concentration of 0·075 ethanol was found. The five survivors responded immediately to treatment with 1·5 mg/kg doxapram hydrogen chloride given intravenously. It was suggested that enough of the normal skin lipid was removed by the detergent to allow substantial absorption of ethanol. (Del Mar, E. (1984) *Veterinary Medicine/SAC* **79**, 318.)

ETHIDIUM BROMIDE. A trypanocide given by intra-muscular injection. This drug is also used in the treatment of 'Heather Blindness' (Contagious Ophthalmia) in sheep and Bovine Keratitis.

ETHIONINE. This inhibits protein synthesis in the liver and, when given to fasted calves, appeared to cause changes in the blood similar to those seen in naturally occurring 'Fatty liver syndrome' of cattle. (Buermans, H. J. & Black, W. D. (1983), *American Journal of Veterinary Research* **44**, 2208.)

ETHMOID is a bone which separates the nasal cavity from that of the brain. It is spongy in nature and contains numerous cavities, some of which communicate with the nose and serve to carry the nerves of the sense of smell.

ETHOLOGY. The study of the behaviour of animals in their normal environment. Applied ethology is an important aspect of animal welfare, and includes experiments to determine animals' preferences and also their reactions to farming practices.

ETHYL CHLORIDE is a clear, colourless liquid, produced by the action of hydrochloric acid upon alcohol. Extremely volatile, it rapidly produces freezing of the surface of the skin when sprayed upon it. It is used to produce insensibility for short surface operations, such as the removal of warts or small tumours, the lancing of painful abscesses, the removal of thorns or foreign bodies, etc. It is put up in glass or metal tube provided with a fine nozzle. Ethyl chloride is sometimes used as a general anaesthetic for the extraction of teeth. Insensibility is easily induced, but is of only short duration, and rapidly passes off when the administration ceases.

ETHYLENE is a colourless inflammable gas which is sometimes used as an anaesthetic in small animals. Ethylene glycol, the 'antifreeze' used for cars, is highly poisonous for dogs and cats. (*See* 'ANTIFREEZE'.)

ETIOLOGY is the study of the cause(s) of disease.

ETORPHINE (*See* 'IMMOBILON').

EUROPEAN BROWN HARE SYNDROME. This has been reported from several EC countries, including the UK.
CAUSE. Picorna-like virus particles have been isolated in the UK.
SIGNS. Dullness, loss of fear of people, and nervous disorders such as ataxia. The death rate has been high. (Chasey, D. & Duff, P. *Veterinary Record* (1990) **126**, 623.)

EUROPEAN COMMUNITY (EC). This was formerly known as the European Economic Community (EEC), created by the Treaty of Rome in 1957, with six member states. The UK became a member in 1973. In 1991 the membership had grown to twelve countries.

The EC has been defined as a group of nations which have abandoned a significant part of their national sovereignty in return for a share in a much larger trading block.

More than 60 directives concerning animal health have been issued over the past six years.

Additionally, veterinary professional directives, covering training, freedom of movement, and what are called rights of establishment, have been issued.

In June 1991 the EC directives were extended to cover meat inspection food hygiene, and slaughterhouses.

The EC has over-ridden some UK legislation, postponed legislation relating to the use of stilbenes in small-animal practice, and intervened over size/design of battery cages for hens.

Fears have been expressed that the UK's freedom from rabies will be threatened by the EC's attitude towards rabies – endemic on the Continent.

However, the European Parliament (as distinct from the EC) has supported the idea of a system of dog registration.

EURYTREMA. A fluke. (*See* PANCREAS, DISEASES OF).

EUSTACHIAN TUBES are the passages, one on each side, which lead from the throat to the middle ear, and serve to maintain an even atmospheric pressure upon the inner surface of the 'eardrum' or tympanum. They open widely in the act of swallowing, and during a yawn. Each has a sac or diverticulum connected with it in the horse, and in certain conditions these become filled with pus from a strangles abscess or from some other suppurating source near, when operation becomes necessary to evacuate the pus and prevent it doing damage by burrowing into the middle ear or surrounding parts. (*See* EAR.)

EUTHANASIA as applied to animals, is a means of producing death free from ante-mortem fear or suffering. The term mainly applies to dogs and cats and other pets, although, strictly speaking, the humane slaughtering of animals for food purposes, and the humane destruction of horses or other animals kept for working purposes, should also fall within the meaning of the word.

Methods of achieving euthanasia were discussed and reviewed at a 1975 symposium organised by the Universities' Federation for Animal Welfare (UFAW).

Injection of drugs (small animals). This is the method preferred by most veterinarians, and barbiturates are widely used; *e.g.,* sodium pentobarbitone solution (200 mg per ml) given intravenously at a dosage of 1 ml per kg bodyweight. 'Equally satisfactory', said Dr J. Sandford, is a saturated solution of magnesium sulphate at a dosage of 2·5 to 4 mg per kg. If an intravenous injection is not practicable, anaesthetics such as ketamine* or the mixture of steroids known as Saffan† were recommended by Dr Sandford. 'They have the advantage of acting very rapidly following intramuscular administration.' They must, however, be followed by a lethal injection of another agent. (Arnolds introduced Termineze for the euthanasia of dogs and cats. It contains 400 mg/ml quinalbarbitone sodium and 25 mg/ml cinchocaine hydrochloride, for use at a dose rate of 0·25 ml/kg bodyweight.) (Arnolds Ltd.)

Injection of drugs (large animals). If an intravenous injection is practicable, an over dose of chloral hydrate may be given. Or if barbiturates are preferred, 'while sodium pentobarbitone solution is quite satisfactory in sheep and young cattle, for adult cattle and horses the rapid injection of a small volume of sodium thiapentone solution to cause collapse and loss of consciousness within a few seconds may be easier if restraint is difficult, to be followed by injection of a

*Ketalar, Parke Davis.
†Glaxo Laboratories.

secondary agent to cause cardiac arrest', commented Dr Sandford, who stressed the need for careful restraint.

For **animals which cannot be handled,** tranquilliser/anaesthetic mixtures may be administered intramuscularly by means of a projectile syringe. Etorphine is an example.

Carbon dioxide. Miss J. MacArthur described a new apparatus consisting of two open-topped, glass-fronted chambers separated by a central division. In the first section a mixture of 70 per cent CO_2 and 30 per cent O_2 is passed through a bottle containing warm water before it enters the first chamber through a copper pipe along its base in which there are drilled a series of small holes. After allowing the gas mixture to fill the chamber for 3 minutes, the animal in a cage, to which it has become adapted by being left in it for a short time, is lowered into the gas mixture. Within 20 seconds unconsciousness supervenes mostly without struggling. The cage is then lifted from the first chamber and placed gently into the second chamber in which a mixture of pure CO_2 has flowed for 3 minutes beforehand, filling the chamber. Death occurs within 3 minutes. This apparatus is also very well suited to the euthanasia of other small animals such as puppies, mice, rats, gerbils, guinea pigs and hamsters. Carbon dioxide, used in this way, would appear to be far preferable to chloroform, which many animal welfare societies use in their lethal chambers for disposing of unwanted cats.

Car exhaust fumes have also been used, for cats, and death occurred within about a minute. This was quicker than a 70 per cent CO_2 30 per cent O_2 mixture, and appeared to cause the cats less 'discomfort'. (Simonsen, H. B. and others. *British Veterinary Journal* (1981) **137**, 274).

Electrocution can be humane for canine euthanasia, provided that the dog is 'stunned by passing an adequate electric current through the brain before allowing the current to go through the body to cause stoppage of the heart', said Dr Phyllis G. Croft at the 1975 symposium. She emphasised that lethal cabinets for electrocution should be made strictly in accordance with British Standards specification, and not modified – as had been done in the recent past. Such modifications or differences in design could lead to apprehension and pain before death, which defeats the whole purpose – namely euthanasia as opposed to mere destruction of the dog.

Captive-bolt pistol. This was also discussed at the UFAW symposium. Correctly used, this type of 'humane killer' can be a valuable means of euthanasia for the larger animals, and also for the dog – though the method has obvious disadvantages from the point of view of a dog-owner wishing to be present.

The following advice may be useful for animal-owners or others in remote places where no veterinarian is available and who have to shoot an animal.

For horses and cattle the point aimed at is *not* in the middle of the forehead, between the eyes; a shot so placed passes into the nasal chambers or air sinuses, down into the mouth and throat, and misses the important vital centres. The correct spot is higher up than this. Two imaginary lines should be drawn, each running from one eye to the opposite ear across the front of the forehead, and the point of their intersection is the most vital spot. A shot aimed about parallel with the ground and directed at this spot enters the brain cavity, destroys the brain and the beginning of the spinal cord, and passes on into the neck, where its energy is expended. Otherwise, if for some reason this part is not accessible, the next best place to aim at is the base of one ear, the direction being again parallel with the ground. In the case of horned cattle, the presence of the horn may deflect the shot, and in them it is better to shoot into the base of the brain from behind, directing the charge downwards and forwards. When pigs have to be shot the middle line of the head is not altogether the best place, because there is a strong crest of bone running downwards in this position; the shot should be placed a little above and a little nearer the centre of the skull than the eye. For dogs and cats the centre of the forehead should be aimed at, for in these animals the brain is of relatively larger size, and more easily accessible.

Minimising stress. Mr E. H. Shillabeer, writing in the *Veterinary Record*, had some excellent advice to offer on this. 'Since 1970 it has been my custom to show a surviving companion animal its euthanased former companion whenever possible.'

'Acceptance of the situation by the surviving dog (or cat) certainly appears to shorten their period of "grief" or unsettled behaviour.'

'I also press strongly for the owner's presence at euthanasia because I believe that the animal's stress is thus minimised. If a house call is feasible, that is preferable too as I am always helped by a veterinary nurse to make the procedure as stress-free as possible for all concern.'

EXANTHEMATA is an old name indicating diseases that are characterised by a rash or eruption. (*See under* VESICULAR, and EQUINE COITAL EXANTHEMA.)

EXCHANGE TRANSFUSION (*see* BLOOD TRANSFUSION).

EXCIPIENT means any more or less inert substance added to a prescription in order to make the remedy more suitable in bulk, consistency, or form for administration.

EXCORIATION. Destruction of small areas of skin or mucous membrane.

EXERCISE is a matter of great importance in the preservation of health. It is obvious that the methods of domestication, which have made such enormous modifications in the characteristics of horses, cattle, sheep, pigs, and dogs, have also so altered their modes of life that exercise is a matter

over which they themselves often have no control. Lack of sufficient exercise is most serious in young animals, especially calves, pigs, and puppies. They do not grow and develop as they should.

Females of all species must have regular exercise during pregnancy, for otherwise the tone of the uterine wall and other muscles of the body is lost, and there is a risk of trouble occurring at parturition.

Over-exercise, especially if an animal is not in a fit condition, is, on the other hand, equally bad. Efforts beyond the animal's strength are apt to bring about dilatation of the heart, or lead to exhaustion; even, rarely, to death if a horse is taken out hunting when unfit.

Heavy draught horses should get a short walk for 10 to 15 minutes twice daily when standing idle, or they may be turned out into a paddock or yard for the greater part of the day. Cattle tied up in stalls should receive a minimum of 10 to 20 minutes' exercise out of doors twice daily. When shut in loose-boxes they do not require to be let out every day, for they can move about to a certain extent in the box, and get some exercise in that way. Breeding sows and boars kept in pig-houses where space is limited always thrive better when allowed into a yard for some part of the day, or when allowed into a paddock to graze. House-dogs need different amounts of exercise according to their breeds and ages. Young dogs of the sporting breeds never do well unless they receive at least 1 hour's sharp walk morning and night when on the leash, or about half this period when allowed to range at liberty. Older dogs and those of pet breeds need less, but generally speaking, the more exercise the dog gets the better health it will enjoy. (*See also* SHEEP-DOGS, MUSCLE, subheading 'Condition'.)

EXERCISING HORSES. Horses must be gradually introduced to exercise or work, because over-exertion of an unfit or of a partly fit horse may have serious and permanent consequences. To get a riding horse fit it is usual to begin with daily walking exercise, with only an occasional trot for the first month or so. As the horse becomes fitter the duration of the exercise is lengthened, and the animal is made to walk, then given a sharp trot or a short gallop, and finally another walk home each day for a further 2 to 4 weeks. From this stage it proceeds to one when the gallop is of longer duration on alternate days, and then, later, the horse gets a stiff gallop every day for perhaps half an hour or so. In some stables there is a system of morning and afternoon exercise for each horse, but much must be left to the individual requirement of each animal, and to the judgment of the trainer. After a time, varying up to four months or more in some cases, the horse arrives at its maximum pitch of perfection, and then begins to 'go stale'. The art of the race-horse trainer enables him to judge the length of time it takes for each individual horse to arrive at his best at such a time as will allow him to enter for the race for which he is being trained. Every horse-trainer has his own individual methods, and as these are by no means hard-and-fast rules, nothing more than the merest outline can be given here.

The 'condition' of a horse, by which is meant its capacity for doing work, cannot be retained indefinitely; there comes a time when it begins to perform less and less well, and is said to have 'gone stale'. This is an indication that a rest is required.

Overtraining in the racehorse. This, and stress, should be regarded as a common cause of poor performance, Dr S. Perrson said at the 1981 BEVA congress; and could be regarded as a clinical entity. Affected horses appeared to 'fade' at the end of a race. They also showed signs of stress before racing. It was possible to identify the overtrained horse by studying its blood oxygen uptake levels, pulse/work relationship, total red cell volume changes, and blood cortisol levels. Once identified, such a horse should be exercised more slowly and gradually worked up to previous levels. (*See also* RACEHORSES.)

EXFOLIATION. The separation in layers or scales of dead bone or of skin.

EXOCRINE (*see* GLANDS).

EXOPHTHALMOS. Bulging of the eyeballs. In America it has been observed as a hereditary defect in certain Jersey cattle in the USA; and in Britain in certain Shorthorn herds – the condition being preceded by a squint. (*See* EYE, DISEASES OF.)

EXOSTOSIS. An outgrowth from a bone, usually the result of some form of inflammation. (*See* BONE, DISEASES OF.)

EXOTOXINS. Toxins which diffuse readily from the bodies of bacteria during their lifetime.

EXPLOSIVE, PLASTIC (PE4) POISONING. (*See* CYCLONITE). (*See also* DYNAMITE).

EXPORTING ANIMALS (*see* IMPORTING /EX-PORTING, *and also under* HORSES).

EXPOSURE to intense cold can usually be well tolerated by the animal which is well fed. More food is required during very cold weather in order to maintain the body temperature. Windbreaks are important, but the tendency is for their number to decline in the interests of larger fields and units more suited to mechanisation. Animals denied shelter from very cold winds, and at the same time inadequately fed, are most liable to disease of one kind or another. (*See also* SHEARING, FROSTBITE, FEED BLOCKS, SHEEP.)

EXTRAVASATION. An escape of blood or lymph from the vessels which ought to contain it.

EXTRINSIC ALLERGIC ALVEOLITIS (*see* FARMER'S LUNG, 'BROKEN WIND', ALLERGY).

EXUDATE. A fluid which seeps into a body cavity or the tissues, often as a result of disease.

EYE

Eye. The eyes are set in deep cavities known as 'bony orbits', whose edges are prominent and form a protection to the eyeball. In the pig, dog, and cat the edge of the bony orbit is not complete posteriorly, but in the other domesticated animals it forms a complete circle. The two orbits are separated from each other in the middle line of the skull by only a very small space, and posteriorly the nerves leaving each eye (optic nerves) converge and meet each other on the floor of the brain cavity, so that each eye is intimately associated with its fellow behind, though they are set on opposite sides of the skull when viewed from the front. Lying inside the orbit but around the eyeball proper there is a large quantity of 'periorbital fat' upon which the eye rests as though upon an elastic cushion, and by virtue of which it is endowed with great mobility. The eye is protected by two main eyelids and in many cases by a small rudimentary 'third eyelid', 'haw', or *nictitating membrane*, which is found at the inner corner. The eyelids meet at the outer and inner 'canthi'. The external canthus is rounded, but the internal canthus is narrowed to form a U-shaped bay or recess, called the 'lacrimal lake'. Just within the inner canthus and attached to the nictitating membrane of which it forms a part, is a small rounded pigmented prominence known as the 'lacrimal caruncle', which is formed of modified skin, and which often bears one or two tiny hairs. (*See also* HARDERIAN GLAND.)

Eyelids. Each of the two main eyelids consists of four layers: on the surface there is skin similar to that which covers the adjacent part of the face, but thin, loose, pliant, and bearing extremely fine hairs; below this is a layer of thin subcutaneous tissue, and then comes the second or muscular layer which is instrumental in opening and shutting the eyelids; the third layer is fibrous, and along the free edge of the lid this layer is denser and forms the 'tarsus' of the eyelid, in the substance of which is embedded a row of glands, called the 'tarsal glands', numbering 45 to 50 in the upper and 30 to 35 in the lower lid of the horse (small cysts are occasionally formed in connection with these glands which appear as rounded, painful swellings upon the surface of the lid); the fourth layer consists of the delicate mucous membrane called the 'conjunctiva', which rubs over the surface of the eyeball (also covered by conjunctiva) and tends to remove any dust, particles of debris, etc., that may collect on the moist surface. The two layers of conjunctiva are continuous with each other, being reflected off the eyelid on to the anterior surface of the eyeball, and forming little pockets (upper and lower) in which oat-chaffs sometimes lodge and are difficult to

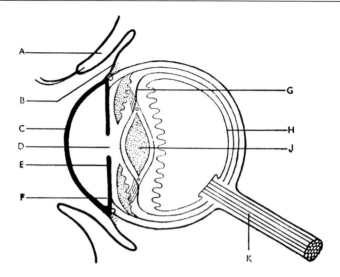

The Eye: a sectional view. A, indicates the eyelid; B, conjunctiva; C, cornea; D, pupil; E, iris; F, ligament of the iris; G, ligament of the lens; H, retina; J, lens; K, optic nerve. Next to the retina (H) comes the hyaloid membrane, then the choroid coat and (the outermost) the sclerotic coat.

remove; normally these pockets should contain small amounts of fluid, forming tears. Any excess secretion of tears reaches the nasal cavity by the 'lacrimal duct', the two openings of which can be seen towards the inner canthus along the free margins of each of the lids. The third eyelid is situated at the inner angle of the eye, consisting of a semilunar fold of the conjunctiva, which is supported and strengthened by a small roughly crescentic plate of cartilage. Ordinarily this eyelid covers only a very small part of the surface of the eye, but in certain diseases, such as tetanus, the pressure by the muscles of the eyeball upon the orbital fat displaces the third eyelid, and it may reach across the eye to the extent of almost one inch.

In the cat, the appearance of the third eyelid (nictitating membrane), like a curtain partly drawn across a window, is a common sign of general ill health and is due to absorption of fat in the vicinity and is not usually a disease of the eye. (*See also* 'DRY-EYE' under EYE, DISEASES OF.)

Front of the eye. If the lids of a horse's eye be separated widely the 'white' of the eye comes into view. The white appearance is due to the sclerotic coat, composed of dense white fibrous tissue, shining through the translucent conjunctival covering. In the centre of the white is set the transparent oval 'cornea', through which the rays of light pass on their way to the inner parts of the eye. (In the pig, dog, and cat the cornea is practically circular in outline.) Behind the cornea lies the beautifully coloured 'iris', with a hole in its centre, the 'pupil', which looks black against the dark interior of the eye. The edge of the pupil is often irregular in outline, owing to the presence of 'nigroid bodies'. The shape of the pupil and the colour of the iris vary in each of the domesticated animals, and in individuals of the same or different breeds. In the horse and ox the pupil is

roughly oval, or even egg-shaped, with the larger end inwards, and the colour of the iris is either a warm chocolate brown, greyish-blue, very dark or almost black, or else appears variegated with patches of white. In some horses, though rarely in cattle, there may be an absence of pigment matter in the iris, and the horse is then said to be 'wall-eyed' or 'ring-eyed'. In the pig, dog, and cat the pupil is rounded when fully dilated, but in the cat the contracted pupil (*e.g.* during the day or in a strong light) resolves itself into a vertical slit; the contracted pupil of the dog and pig is round. Lying between the anterior surface of the eye, the cornea, and the iris, in a space known as the 'anterior chamber' of the eye, which is filled with a clear lymph-like fluid known as the 'aqueous humour'.

Coats of the eyeball. The eyeball, as already mentioned, rests upon a pad of fat within the cavity of the orbit, where it is held in position through the agency of seven ocular muscles and the optic nerve around which they are arranged. There are three layers forming the ball of the eye: (*a*) THE SCLEROTIC COAT, which is outermost, is composed of dense white fibrous tissue, which gives its appearance to the white of the eye in front. This coat completely encloses the ball, except for a small area through which emerges the optic nerve, while in front it is modified so as to form the transparent cornea. It maintains the shape of, and gives strength to, the ball of the eye. The cornea, which has a greater curvature than the rest of the ball, bulges out in front. The whole cornea is somewhat like a window let into the front of the sclerotic coat.

(*b*) THE CHOROID, or vascular coat, lies within the sclerotic, and consists of three parts. The choroid membrane, which forms more than two-thirds of a lining to the sclerotic, consists mainly of a network of vessels which nourish the sclerotic coat and the interior of the eyeball. Its general colour is bluish-black, but an area a little above the level of the end of the optic nerve has a remarkable metallic lustre and is known as the 'tapetum'. The colour of the tapetum is variable, but generally it has a brilliant iridescent bluish-green colour shading imperceptibly into yellow. The choroid membrane is prolonged forwards into the 'ciliary body', a very complex structure which forms a thickened ring opposite the line where the sclera merges into the cornea. To this line of junction the ciliary body is firmly attached by the ciliary muscle, which by its contraction and relaxation moves the ciliary body to and fro over the sclerotic, so as to allow the lens of the eye which is suspended from, or rather, 'set into', the ciliary body, to alter its shape in such a way that it is able accurately to focus rays of light, coming from an object before the eye, on to the retina. The farthest forward part of the choroid coat is 'iris', lying in front of the lens and behind the cornea.

The iris consists partly of fibrous tissue and partly of muscle fibres, arranged radially and circularly, with pigment cells interspaced throughout. These fibres by their contraction serve to narrow or dilate the pupil, according to whether the light entering the eye is strong or weak, and according as the animal looks at a near or distant object.

(c) THE RETINA, or nervous coat, is the innermost of the three coats of eyeball. After the optic nerve has pierced the sclerotic and choroid coats, it ends by a sudden spreading out of its fibres in all directions to form the retina, which also contains some blood-vessels and pigment cells. The retina, in microscopic sections, is seen to consist of no less than ten layers.

The rods and cones convert light waves into nerve impulses. The rods are very sensitive under night vision and near darkness. The cones achieve (under good light) detailed vision and differentiate between colours.

The 'visual purple' is a pigment called rhodopsin, synthesised from retinene (a pigment related to carotone) and a protein. Under bright light the fading of the 'visual purple' involves a conversion of rhodopsin into vitamin A plus protein by means of an enzyme.

Contents of the eyeball, viz. aqueous humour, vitreous humour, and crystalline lens. Occupying the space between the iris and the cornea, *i.e.* the anterior chamber of the eye, there is a clear watery, lymph-like fluid which serves to maintain the contours of the cornea. It is being constantly secreted and drained away, and eventually reaches the veins of the eye. Behind the iris lies the 'crystalline lens', which acts as does the lens of a camera, with the exception that it can alter the curves of its surfaces and therefore is able to change its refractive powers. It is composed of layers arranged like the leaves of an onion to some extent. The lens is held suspended by its capsule, which is attached to the ciliary body already mentioned. Behind the lens the cavity of the ball of the eye is filled with a viscid, jelly-like, tenacious fluid called the 'vitreous humour'. It maintains the intra-ocular pressure by which the eyeball retains its shape.

The lacrimal system provides a means whereby the eye surface is maintained free from dust and other foreign material. It consists of the lacrimal gland which secretes the clear fluid popularly known as 'tears'; excretory ducts, from 12 to 16 in number; and the two lacrimal ducts which open into a lacrimal sac from which begins the nasolacrimal duct which carries the secretion down into the nose. The gland lies towards the upper outer aspect of the orbit; secretes the clear salty, watery fluid which flows out through the excretory ducts to reach the conjunctival sac and bathe the surface of the eye. The secretion is finally received by the two lacrimal ducts, the openings of which lie one in each eyelid about a third of an inch from the inner canthus. These open into the lacrimal sac, from which takes origin the long nasolacrimal duct which conveys the secretion down into the lower part of the corresponding nasal passage, just within the nostril.

Accommodation. All the rays of light proceeding from a distant object may be looked upon as being practically parallel, while those coming from a near object are divergent. The difference between *distant* and *near* in this connection can be taken as about 20 feet from the animal. A 'near' object can be seen anywhere between 20 feet and 4 to 5 inches from the eye, but nearer than this it loses its distinction. Parallel rays of light do not require any focusing on the retina other than is provided by the surface of the cornea, and when an animal looks at a distant object the lens capsule which is attached to the ciliary process retains the lens in a temporarily flattened condition and the ciliary muscle is relaxed, so that no great strain is put upon the eye. Rays of light from an object near at hand, however, which are divergent, require to be brought to a point of focus upon the retina, and as they pass through the lens their direction is changed on account of the convexity of the lens. The amount of this convexity is determined by the divergency of the rays, and is automatically provided for through the pull of the ciliary muscle upon the ciliary body. As the function of the muscle is to pull the ciliary body forwards, the tension upon the ligament of the lens is lessened and the capsule of the lens slackens, so that the lens, by its inherent elasticity, is allowed to bulge with a greater convexity upon its anterior surface. The greater the convexity, the more are the rays of light refracted, and the more convergent do rays which pass through it become. (*See also* VISION.)

Lens (*see* illustration of EYE).

EYE, INJURIES AND DISEASES OF. All such injuries and diseases can be of economic importance to farmers, since the productive efficiency of affected animals is likely to be reduced, owing to stress, pain, or infection – or all three. Milk yield may decline in the dairy cow. If the animal's sight is seriously impaired, feeding may become difficult, with consequent loss of bodily condition.

Blepharitis. Inflammation of the edges of the eye-lids, and usually accompanies conjunctivitis. Its causes, symptoms, and treatment are similar to those of that disease.

Blindness. There are many causes of this, including disease of the retina, of the optic nerve, and of the brain. Blindness may be congenital or acquired, temporary or permanent. Vitamin A deficiency may be responsible, and also poisoning by rape and other plants, and by substances such as lead. Blindness in the dog and cat may result from carbon monoxide poisoning, and persist for some time; it may also result from metaldehyde poisoning. (*See also under* QUININE, MALE FERN, BRIGHT BLINDNESS of sheep.)

'Day blindness' (Hemeralopia). Stated to be due to an autosomal recessive gene, this eye disease is common in the Alaskan malamute dog, and has been reported also in miniature poodles. The blindness occurs during bright light, although in dim light the animal can see.

Horses. The sudden onset of blindness in one or both eyes has been reported as a result of optic nerve atrophy, following trauma. Signs are: dilated, fixed pupils, and a lack of the menace reflex. Within three to four weeks the optic disc becomes paler, and the retina's blood vessels markedly decreased. There is a rupture of the nerve axons. (Martin, L. & others. (1986) *Equine Veterinary Journal* **18**, 133.)

'Night blindness' (nyctalopia) is a condition that sometimes affects horses and mules in countries where the glare of the sunlight is very intense during the day. At night such animals are quite unable to see, and will stumble into objects that are easily discernible to human beings. **Camels** are seldom affected, owing to the effective protection afforded to the retina by the overhanging eyelids and deeply placed eyeballs. (For the condition in the **dog** *see under* 'NIGHT BLINDNESS'.)

Opacity of the cornea will, of course, prevent light rays reaching the retina, as happens in keratitis, so that partial or complete blindness results. Similarly, partial or complete blindness may result from a cataract. Other causes have been mentioned on the preceding pages, *e.g.* dislocation of the lens, glaucoma, etc. **In cattle and sheep**, cerebrocortical necrosis. **In sheep**, other causes of blindness include: infectious keratitis or con-

tagious ophthalmia ('Heather Blindness'); pregnancy toxaemia; and the effects of eating bracken, as described under BRIGHT BLINDNESS of sheep. (For an African disease *see* BLOUWILDEBEESOOG.)

Poultry. Blindness may be the result of excessive ammonia fumes from deep litter, or it may be associated with fowl paralysis, salmonellosis, aspergillosis, etc. Cataract, followed in some cases by liquefaction of the lens, occurs during outbreaks of avian infectious encephalomyelitis. (*See also under* LIGHTING OF ANIMAL BUILDINGS.)

'Blue eye' (*see* CANINE VIRAL HEPATITIS).

Cancer, either of sarcomatous or carcinomatous nature, is sometimes found in connection with the conjunctiva. Tumours appear as red hard swellings, painless when small, but not when large. These neoplasms often grow at a rapid rate, and may infiltrate the surrounding tissues, sometimes affecting the bones of the orbit. Cancer of the eye is a common condition in Hereford cattle. In Australia, Dr D. J. Richards, B V Sc has commented: 'It has been suggested that several factors may contribute to the development of cancer eye in cattle. These include age, irritation of the eyes by dust, sand, insects or chemicals, sunlight, lack of eye-lid pigmentation and virus infection. Some authorities believe that cattle may be genetically prone to the condition, while others feel that poor nutrition is another factor as the condition appears to occur more frequently following a drought.' (*See* TUMOURS.)

The beginning of 'Cancer Eye', as it is sometimes colloquially known, may be a raised area of skin or a wart. Either may become malignant, developing into a typical carcinoma – the type of cancer occurring in this eye disease of Herefords. However, in the USA a survey was carried out; the eyes of 48 Hereford cows being examined at 6-monthly intervals for two years. Over half the cows showed preliminary signs of 'cancer eye', but – without any treatment – one third of the growths had disappeared by the time of the last examination.

It may be of interest to mention that in the USA a form of cryosurgery has been developed to treat cancer of the eye. The technique is a highly skilled one and requires special thermo-couples to monitor the very low temperatures.

H. E. Farris treated 718 cases of eye cancer by this means. In 609 of the cases, a single freeze caused total regression of 66 per cent of the growths. In 109, treated by a rapid freeze to −25°C, a natural thaw,. and then a re-freeze, the 'cure rate was 97 per cent'.

Cataract. The condition is by far the most common in the horse and dog in old age, although it is also met with in other animals, and it may occur at almost any time of life. It consists of a coagulation of the plasma of the cells in the lens with loss of transparency. A bluish, cloudy appearance of the eye results and vision becomes blurred.

CAUSES include over-exposure to X-rays, nuclear radiation, and, more commonly, diabetes or naphthalene and other forms of poisoning. Cataract must also be looked upon as a change characteristic of old age.

TREATMENT. Cataracts were removed by phacofragmentation and aspiration from one or both eyes of 56 dogs. Vision improved immediately in 53 of the dogs: after two years 25 of 29 dogs still had vision, and after four years five of seven dogs. The surgery was unsuccessful in dogs with severe anterior uveitis with secondary glaucoma, retinal detachments, and fibropupillary membrane formation. (Miller, T. R. & others *Journal of the American Veterinary Medical Association* (1987) **100**, 157.)

Coloboma is a congenital and hereditary defect – a notch, gap, hole, or fissure in any of the structures of the eye. In other words, at birth a part of the eye is missing. Bilateral coloboma is common in Charolais cattle, often involving the optic disc. The condition can be recognised only with an ophthalmoscope, and does not deteriorate with the passage of time. Effect on vision varies from very slight to (rarely) blindness.

Conjunctivitis, or inflammation of the conjunctival membranes, is an extremely common condition among animals, and probably constitutes the commonest trouble to which the eyes are subject. In cattle, conjunctivitis is often the first symptom of Cattle Plague, Ephemeral Fever, and Ondiri disease (Bovine Infectious Petechial Fever).

Conjunctivitis is one symptom associated with many specific infections, such as distemper in the dog (*and see* EYEWORMS).

CAUSES.   The presence of dust, sand, pollen, seeds, lime, pieces of chaff, in the atmosphere of a stable or field, is probably one of the commonest causes in the larger farm animals, but such agents as flies, worms, and ticks, must also be noted in addition to the above. In the cat two infections which cause conjunctivitis – *Haemophilus parainfluenzae* and *Moraxella lacunata* – are transmissible to man, in which illness may also be caused. (*See* FELINE EYE INFECTIONS.)

Chlamydia psittaci was isolated from 30 per cent of swabs from 753 cats suffering from conjunctivitis.

SIGNS. The first signs of conjunctivitis are redness and swelling of the lining membranes of the eye-lids, excessive discharge of tears, and a tendency for the animal to keep its eyelids shut.

FIRST-AID. Clean away the discharges by bathing with a warmed eye lotion. (If only one eye is affected, the cause may be a foreign body that has lodged in the eye.) The best way to apply lotions, whether to the horse, dog, or other animal, is to use a perfectly clean piece of cotton-wool soaked in the solution and squeezed above the eye so that the drops trickle into it. Cases of conjunctivitis should never be neglected, for the inflammation may spread to the cornea, resulting in KERATITIS.

Dislocation of the lens is a condition in which the crystalline lens becomes displaced forwards into the anterior chamber. It occurs in dogs, especially Sealyhams and rough-haired terriers, and at first is very hard to recognise. The dog runs into stationary objects without any obvious reason. Casual examination of the eyes reveals no change and the condition may not be suspected for many months. Later, the owner becomes aware that sight is failing in the dog and careful examination reveals a 'wobbly lens' in the eye. Operation may do much to restore some degree of vision and save the eye, but neglect almost invariably results in the development of glaucoma (*see* GLAUCOMA) and the affected eye may have to be surgically removed.

Technically, lens dislocation may be classified as congenital, primary, secondary, or traumatic. Secondary cases not uncommonly follow cataract or glaucoma; but most cases occur spontaneously in adult life. (Animal Health Trust).

'Dry eye' (Keratoconjunctivitis sicca) is a condition in the dog arising from a partial failure of tear production and leading to roughening of the corneal surface with a consequent lack of lustre. 'Artificial tears' may have to be provided, or a surgical operation performed involving parotid duct transplantation. (Professor D. D. Lawson, 1978 BVA Congress.) The condition has been linked to the use of SULPHASALAZINE (which see) for the treatment of idiopathic colitis in dogs.

Ectropion means a turning-out of one or both eye-lids, so that the conjunctiva is exposed. It is a common condition in bloodhounds and St Bernards, and is in them regarded as practically normal. It is also treated by operation, but a part of the conjunctiva from within the edge of the lid is removed instead of part of the skin from the outside, as in entropion.

Entropion. Turning in of the eyelid, often the lower one, so that it rubs upon the cornea, causing inflammation. The condition is common in dogs – often an inherited defect occurring in many breeds.

In newborn lambs entropion is occasionally seen and, if bilateral, can lead to eventual blindness and starvation. It can be corrected by Michel clips. (F. A. Earles, *Vet. Record* (1984) **114**, 193.) It is treated by a plastic operation such as is performed for trichiasis.

Epiphora is another name for what is commonly called 'watery eye' or 'overflow of tears'. It is generally due to some obstruction to the drainage of tears through the lacrimal duct to the nose, but it is also an accompanying symptom of most forms of mild inflammation of the conjunctiva or cornea, and of naphthalene poisoning in cattle; and of atopic disease in the dog.

Foreign bodies in the eye have already been referred to under CONJUNCTIVITIS. Severe irritation may be caused by a piece of grit or a grass seed or husk. Pain and irritation may be shown by the dog pawing his face.

TREATMENT. If a hair, bristle or tip of an awn, for instance, can be seen on folding back the eyelid, or if a white spot (sometimes indicating the site of a thorn's penetration) or what appears to be 'a white film' is visible on the surface of the eye, the best **first-aid** treatment is a drop of olive-oil. (Cod-liver oil will do, but not any oil!) Boracic acid lotion is worse than useless (except for the mechanical washing out of grit); what is needed is a lubricant to reduce the harmful friction, and this is where the oil helps. Removal of a foreign body is best accomplished with the aid of a local anaesthetic, and professional help should be obtained.

Occasionally the object may be removed by taking the corner of a clean handkerchief, winding it into a point, and lifting the offending body out with it. It is always best to seek professional assistance and have the foreign body removed under a local anaesthetic. The use of a suitable eye lotion will be helpful afterwards.

Glaucoma is a condition in which the tension of the fluid contents of the eyeball is greatly in excess of the normal. It is associated with obstruction to the drainage system of the eye, in which fluid continues to be secreted but the excess is not removed. It may follow cases of progressive retinal atrophy. It eventually results in swelling and bulging of one or both of the eyes, and blindness results. Secondary glaucoma is more common and caused by an eye disease, of which the most frequent is lens dislocation. (*See also under* EXOPHTHALMOS.)

Harderian gland, displaced. In the dog this gland sometimes becomes enlarged and displaced, owing to blockage of its ducts or to a nearby swelling, when it becomes visible at the corner of the eye as a reddish lump. It may then require surgical removal.

'Heather blindness' is a colloquial name for the equivalent of IBK in sheep. *Rickettsia conjunctivae* is a common cause.

TREATMENT. Shade and fly-control aid recovery, but veterinary treatment of IBK is necessary.

Boracic and similar eye lotions are useless in treating IBK or 'Heather Blindness'. Ethidium bromide, used twice daily for 5 days, can save the sight, and is as effective as chloramphenicol in the disease of cattle.

Horner's syndrome. The pupil of one eye appears smaller than normal, the upper eyelid may droop, the lower lid may be raised, and the nictitating membrane ('third eyelid') protruded across part of the eye.

The cause is some lesion affecting the sympathetic nerves of the eye; for example, a tumour of the spinal cord, chronic otitis, bite wounds, bee stings. Some cases are transient, as with wounds and bee stings.

Infectious bovine keratoconjunctivitis (IBK) is a convenient name for a group of eye diseases with a world-wide distribution, and includes 'New Forest' disease. What they have in common is conjunctivitis and keratitis.

CAUSES: Bacteria, viruses, mycoplasmas, rickettsiae, fungi, and *Thelazia* worms – any of these alone or in combination may produce IBK. In addition, the sun's rays, dust particles, and chemical irritants may all predispose to, or exacerbate, the condition. IBK is commonly transmitted by flies and, in Africa, by two species of moth which feed on secretions and exudate from the eye. Some infective agents are present on the healthy eye, and become active only when the eye is damaged or irritated in some way.

Moraxella (*Haemophilus*) *bovis* is a common bacterial cause of IBK. Some American research has suggested that *Moraxella* may not cause keratitis unless the virus of bovine rhinotracheitis is present also.

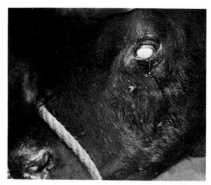

Complete opacity of the cornea due to IBK. The animal was blind.

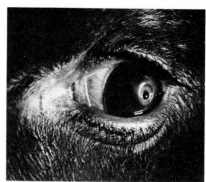

A keratocoele in a three month old calf with IBK. (With acknowledgements to Professor Clifford Formston, and the Royal Veterinary College.)

Iritis means inflammation of the iris, a condition which is very often associated with inflammation of the ciliary body, when the term *iridocyclitis* is used. The chief symptoms are dullness of the iris, congestion of the blood-vessels around its margin, a lessened response to varying intensities of light, and usually a firmly contracted pupil. Occasionally, especially during inflammation of the cornea, the iris adheres to this structure – a condition known as *anterior synechia*; while more frequently the iris adheres to the lens, which lies behind it, and the condition is spoken of as *posterior synechia*. The aqueous humour is often cloudy and may appear purulent, little flocculi of lymph being seen floating in the anterior chamber or sticking to the posterior surface of the cornea. There is always great pain, fear of light (*photophobia*), and the animal hangs its head and is dull and listless.

Keratitis. Inflammation of the cornea may follow conjunctivitis, or it may arise from an injury to, or infection of, the cornea itself. A thorn, for example, may pierce the surface layers of the cornea and remain invisible until a faint whitish ring appears around its protruding part. Should a larger area of the cornea be involved, **opacity** becomes obvious. (Animal-owners often refer to it as 'a film over the eye'; but in fact the opacity stems from inflammation *below* the surface.) Keratitis may be caused by trauma of various kinds, e.g. a whip lash, a kick or blow; or by irritant skin dressings which are not prevented from running into the eyes, or by lime, sparks, or by continuous irritation by a foreign body such as a grass awn, piece of glass or grit. It may arise during the course of certain diseases, such as distemper in dogs and influenza in horses; it can be produced by the presence of *Thelazia* worms, or by fly-borne infections; frost-bite is said to be the cause of it in ewes on hills during severe weather, when it is called 'snow blindness'; turning-in of the eye-lids (*entropion*) may give rise to it in the dog.

Keratomycosis is keratitis due to a fungus, and is uncommon. If, however, tissue resistance is reduced by treatment with corticosteroids (which are immunosuppressive), any fungi present on the cornea may become pathogenic. It may be only when corneal ulcers fail to respond to conventional treatment that keratomycosis is suspected. Natamycin may prove helpful. *Fusarium solani* is implicated in most equine cases, sometimes Candida species; but several other fungi may be involved. (*See also* HYPERKERATOSIS.)

In the early stages, inflammation of the cornea results in symptoms very similar to those seen in conjunctivitis; the production of tears, closing of the eyelids, pain and swelling, being noticed. When the eye is examined, however, the surface of the cornea is found to have lost its lustre. There may be a bluish haze, and an opacity, varying from pin-head size to the whole of the cornea – when the animal becomes completely blind in that eye, for the time being, anyway. The appearance of blood vessels where none are normally seen is another feature of keratitis and occurs before opacity becomes complete. There may be ulceration of the cornea, and even penetration. If the latter should occur, a **keratocoele** (hernia) may form endangering the whole eye, since infection, or escape of the aqueous humour, may sometimes occur.

Myiasis (*see* UITPEULOOG, a disease occurring in South Africa).

New Forest disease. (Infections Bovine Keratitis). Success has been claimed for treatment involving 'the injection of 2 to 5 ml of an antibiotic preparation into the subconjunctival tissues of the upper eyelid. Cortisone (1 ml) may also be injected if corneal ulceration has not occurred. In this practice, penicillin, oxytetracycline and chloramphenicol have given equally beneficial results. . . . In more than 1,000 cases treated in this way . . . 90 per cent recovered following a single injection.' (Giles, M. B. de, *Vet. Rec.* (1976), **98**, 31.)

Opacity of the cornea may result from oedema of the cornea following infection with CANINE VIRAL HEPATITIS; and see KERATITIS below.

Ovine infectious keratoconjunctivitis. This occurs worldwide. In a field survey carried out by the University of Liverpool's veterinary staff, the microflora of 240 clinically unaffected eyes from sheep in ten flocks were compared with those of 240 clinically affected eyes from twelve natural outbreaks. Totals of 16 and 17 genera of bacteria were recovered, including *Branhamella ovis, E. coli*, and *Staphylococcus aureus*. Mycoplasma and Acholeplasma were isolated from both groups. (Dr G. O. Egwu & others. *Veterinary Record* (1989) **125**, 253.)

Pannus is a complication of keratitis in which blood-vessels bud out from the margins of the cornea and run in towards the centre of the eye, stopping at the edges of an ulcer if such exists. Pannus is a condition which always takes a long time to clear up, and even months after there may be seen a dullness of the cornea, due to the tiny vessels that still exist but are invisible to the naked eye.

Partial displacement. Pekingese and other dogs with prominent eyes sometimes suffer a traumatic partial displacement of the eye from the orbit, as a result of being struck by a car or of some other accident. The globe may become trapped by the eyelids which become located behind it.

FIRST-AID. The owner should bandage the eye with bandage moistened in saline solution (a teaspoonful of ordinary salt to a pint of water). Professional aid is urgently required.

TREATMENT. This requires a general anaesthetic and re-positioning of the eye where possible. If the cornea, etc, has been badly damaged, the only course is enucleation of the eye. After suturing of the eyelids over the vacant socket, the result will not appear unsightly to the owner.

Periodic ophthalmia (*see under this heading*). (*See also* OPHTHALMIA.)

Progressive retinal atrophy, or so-called 'Night Blindness', is a hereditary condition which was common in some strains of Irish Red Setter. The blood vessels of the retina undergo progressive atrophy and the animal suffers from impaired vision in consequence. To endeavour to correct this the pupil dilates widely, even in daylight, and the dog's expression become staring. At night or at dusk, the dog is unable to avoid objects and blunders into them, but during full daylight it appears to see quite well.

No treatment can arrest the progressive degeneration and the dog gradually becomes blind. In severe cases puppies may show first symptoms soon after weaning.

Neither dogs nor bitches which show the condition should be used for breeding. Breeds affected include Collies, Griffons, Poodles, Retrievers, Sealyhams, Cocker and English Springer Spaniels.

The disease also occurs in cats, *e.g.* Abyssinian and Siamese. A few years ago, 25 per cent of Abyssinian cats were found to be affected. Dr K. Narfstrom stated that the earliest signs are not recognised until the cat is 18 months old or more; and the advanced form takes another 18 months to develop. (*See also* TAURINE.)

Ptosis is an inability to raise the upper eyelid, usually associated with some general disease, such as distemper in dogs or 'grass sickness' in horses. It may also arise after injuries when the nerve supplying the muscles of the upper lid (3rd cranial nerve) is paralysed. (*See* GLUTTERAL POUCH DIPHTHERIA.)

Retention cysts are produced in the thickness of the eye-lid owing to blockage of a tarsal gland.

Sclerotitis (Scleritis), or 'blood-shot eye', is inflammation of the sclerotic coat of the eyeball. It often accompanies conjunctivitis when the latter is at all severe. It is treated as for conjunctivitis.

Stye, or hordeolum, is a condition in which a small amount of pus collects in the follicle around the root of one of the eyelashes. One after another may form in succession, owing to the spread of infective material from follicle to follicle.

Trachoma. A term used in human medicine for a granular conjunctivitis, often followed by keratitis and pannus.

Trichiasis. Turning in of the eyelashes so that they irritate and inflame the conditions. The condition is common in dogs and sometimes a hereditary defect. It is treated surgically, by means of an operation in which an elliptical piece of skin is removed from the outer surface of the eyelid, and the edges sutured together. This causes the lashes to turn outwards, where they will not irritate or inflame the cornea.

Warts occur in connection with the eye-lids comparatively frequently in horses, cattle, and dogs, and sometimes become malignant, spreading at a rapid rate and causing interference with sight or the movement of the eye-lids. Owing to the malformation which they may cause when numerous, warts should always be removed before they attain a large size or before they have time to spread.

EYELIDS (*see under* EYE).

EYEWORMS. In cattle *Thelazia* worms are one cause of I B K. Species include *T. skrjabini* and *T. gulosa*, found behind the third eyelid and in the ducts of associated glands. From 1 to 67 worms were found in eyes examined at a U K abattoir in 36·9 per cent of 287 cattle heads examined. Other species of *Thelazia* infest dogs, cats, and man. (J. B. R. Arbuckle & L. F. Khalil, (1976) *Vet. Rec.* **99,** 376.) The same authors reported (1978) finding *T. Lacrymalis* in 28 per cent of horses whose eyes were examined at an abattoir.

F

FACE FLIES (*see under* FLIES).

FACIAL DEFORMITY (*see under* HOLOPROSEN-CEPHALY (of lambs and pigs)).

'FACIAL ECZEMA' is a synonym used overseas for light sensitisation in cattle and sheep. (*See* LIGHT SENSITISATION.)

FACIAL NERVE is the seventh of the cranial nerves, and supplies the muscles of expression of the face. It is totally a motor nerve.

FACIAL PARALYSIS. In the case of unilateral 'facial paralysis', which very often follows accidents in which the side of the face has been badly bruised, the muscles on one side become paralysed but those on the opposite side are unaffected. This absence of antagonism between the two sides results in the upper and lower lips, and the muscles around the nostrils, becoming drawn over towards the unaffected side, and the animal presents an altered facial expression. The ear on the injured side of the head very often hangs loosely and flaps back and forward with every movement of the head, and the eyelids on the same side are held half shut. (*See also under* GUTTURAL POUCH DIPHTHERIA and LISTERIOSIS.)

FACTOR 1. *See under* CLOTTING of blood, where other factors are mentioned.

FACTORY CHIMNEYS. Smoke from these may contaminate pastures and cause disease in grazing animals. (*See* FLUOROSIS, MOLYBDENUM.)

'FADING' is the colloquial name for an illness of puppies, leading usually to their death within a few days of birth. Symptoms include: progressive weakness which soon makes suckling impossible; a falling body temperature; and 'paddling' movements. Infected puppies may be killed by their dams. One cause is canine virus hepatitis; another is a canine herpes virus; a third may be a blood incompatibility; a fourth Bordetella; a fifth is hypothermia or 'chilling' in which the puppy's body temperature falls. A possible sixth cause may be *Clostridium perfringens* infection. (*See also under* PUPPIES, HERPES.)

Kittens. A similar syndrome may be caused by the feline leukaemia virus.

FAECES, EATING OF (*see* COPROPHAGY).

FAECES, FEEDING OF. Poultry manure is now used as cattle feed on a large scale in many parts of the world. (*See* POULTRY WASTE, DRIED.)

FAINTING FITS, or SYNCOPE are generally due to cerebral anaemia occurring through weakened pulsation of the heart, sudden shock, or severe injury. It is most commonly seen in dogs

and cats, especially when old, but cases have been seen in all animals. (*See* HEART STIMULANTS.)

FALCONS, DISEASES OF. Avian pox has been found in imported peregrine falcons, giving rise to scab formation on feet and face and leading sometimes to blindness. Tuberculosis is not uncommon, and may be suspected when the bird loses weight. (A tuberculin test is practicable and worth carrying out, owing to the risk of infection being transmitted to other falcons and to people handling them.) Frounce and inflammation of the crop are two old names for a condition, caused by infestation with *Capillaria* worms, which can be successfully treated. Frounce causes a bird to refuse food, or to pick up pieces of meat and flick them away again, swallowing apparently being too painful; there is also a sticky, white discharge at the corners of the beak and in the mouth.

Abnormal gait and spontaneous bone fractures may arise as a result of calcium deficiency through birds being fed an all-meat diet not containing bone. This deficiency may be prevented by sprinkling sterilised bone meal or oyster shell on the meat, or feeding laboratory-bred mice, J. E. Cooper has suggested (*Vet. Rec.* (1975), **97**, 307).

FALLOPIAN TUBES. These, one on each side, run from the extremity of the horns of the uterus to the region of the ovary.

FALSE PREGNANCY (*see under* PSEUDO-PREGNANCY).

FAM. A useful disinfectant approved for use in outbreaks of fowl pest, foot-and-mouth disease, and tuberculosis.

FAN FAILURE leading to heat stroke. (*See* CONTROLLED ENVIRONMENT HOUSING.)

FARCY (*see* GLANDERS).

FARM, OPERATIONS ON THE. In the U K it is illegal for castration of horse, donkey, mule, dog or cat to be carried out without an anaesthetic. (*See* ANAESTHESIA, LEGAL REQUIREMENTS; CASTRATION.) Only a veterinary surgeon is permitted to castrate any farm animal more than 2 months old; with the exception of rams, for which the maximum age is 3 months.

Only veterinary surgeons are permitted to carry out a vasectomy or electro-ejaculation of any farm animal; likewise the desnooding of turkeys over 21 days old, decombing of domestic fowls over 72 hours old, to detoe fowls and turkeys over 72 hours old, remove supernumary teats of calves over 3 months old, or disbud or dishorn sheep or goats.

Certain overseas procedures are prohibited in the U K, namely – freeze dagging of sheep, penis amputation and other operations on the penis, tongue amputation in calves, hot branding of cattle, and the devoicing of cockerels. Very short docking of sheep is also prohibited (*see* DOCKING).

FARM ANIMAL WELFARE COUNCIL. This was established by the government of the United Kingdom in 1979, under the chairmanship of Professor R. J. Harrison MD, DSc, FRS, to keep under review the welfare of farm animals on agricultural land, at markets, in transit and at the place of slaughter, and to advise on any legislation or other changes that may be necessary. (*See also* WELFARE CODES.)

FARM CHEMICALS (*see* SPRAYS USED ON CROPS, FERTILISERS, METALDEHYDE).

FARM TREATMENT AGAINST WORMS (*see* WORMS).

FARMS, VETERINARY FACILITIES ON (*see* VETERINARY).

'FARMER'S LUNG'. A disease due to the inhalation of dust, from mouldy hay, etc., containing spores of e.g. *Micropolyspora faeni*. Giving rise to faulty gas exchange, 'farmer's lung' has been recognised in man, cow and horse. Technically, it is one of the illnesses classified as *extrinsic allergic alveolitis*. Precipitating antibodies to *M. faeni* develop in the serum. Repeated exposure results in an immunological reaction on the walls of the alveoli, giving rise to respiratory distress.

FARROWING. The act of parturition in the sow.

FARROWING CRATES. The use of these is helpful in preventing overlying of piglets by the sow, and so in obviating one cause of piglet mortality; but they are far from ideal. Farrowing rails serve the same purpose but perhaps the best arrangement is the circular one which originated in New Zealand. (*See* ROUND HOUSE.)

Work at the University of Nebraska suggests that a round stall is better, because the conventional rectangular one does not allow the sow to obey her natural nesting instincts, and may give rise to stress, more stillbirths and agalactia.

FARROWING RATES. In the sow, the farrowing rate after one natural service appears to be in the region of 86 per cent. Following a first artificial insemination, the farrowing rate appears to be appreciably lower, but at the Lyndhurst, Hants AI Centre, a farrowing rate of about 83 per cent was obtained when only females which stood firmly to be mounted at insemination time were used. In 1966 the national (British) average farrowing rate was 65 per cent to a first insemination.

FASCIA is the name applied to sheets or bands of fibrous tissue which enclose and connect the muscles.

FASCIOLIASIS. Infestation with liver flukes.

FAT. Normal body fat is, chemically, an ester of three molecules of one, two, or three fatty acids, with one molecule of glycerol. Such fats are known as glycerides, to distinguish them from other fats and waxes in which an alcohol other than glycerol has formed the ester. *See also* LIPIDS (which include fat) and FATTY ACIDS. For fat as a tissue, see ADIPOSE TISSUE. A LIPOMA is a benign fatty tumour. For other diseases associated with fat, *see* STEATITIS, 'FATTY LIVER' SYNDROME; *also* OBESITY, DIET.

FAT SUPPLEMENTS in poultry rations can lead to TOXIC FAT DISEASE (which see). (*See* LIPIDS for cattle supplement; *also* ECZEMA in cats.)

FATIGUE (*see* EXERCISE, MUSCLE, NERVES).

FATTY ACIDS. These, with an alcohol, form FAT (which see). *Saturated* fatty acids have twice as many hydrogen atoms as carbon atoms, and each molecule of fatty acid contains two atoms of oxygen. *Unsaturated* fatty acids contain less than twice as many hydrogen atoms as carbon items, and one or more pairs of adjacent atoms are connected by double bonds. *Polyunsaturated* fatty acids are those in which several pairs of adjacent carbon atoms contain double bonds.

FATTY ACIDS, ESSENTIAL. Evening primrose oil, Dr D. H. Lloyd BVetMed has stated, can ameliorate allergic skin disease and improve coat condition in dogs and cats.

FATTY DEGENERATION A condition in which there is an excess of fat in the parenchyma cells of organs such as the liver, heart, and kidneys.

'FATTY LIVER SYNDROME' OF CATTLE. This may occur in high-yielding dairy cows immediately after calving. It is then that they are subjected to 'energy deficit' and mobilise body reserves for milk production. This mobilisation results in the accumulation of fat in the liver, and also in muscle and kidney. In some cases the liver cells become so engorged with fat that they actually rupture.

An important consequence of this syndrome may be an adverse effect on fertility. A study at the I R A D, Compton, showed that cows with a severe fatty liver syndrome had a calving interval of 443 days, as compared with 376 days for those with a mild fatty liver syndrome.

Complications such as chronic ketosis, parturient paresis (recumbency after calving), and a greater susceptibility to infection have been reported overseas, but Dr I. H. Reid's view, as expressed at the 1980 B.V.A Congress, was that more research would be needed to confirm or refute a connection between fatty liver and increased susceptibility to infection.

Dr C. J. Roberts, also of Compton, described this as a true 'production disease'.

'FATTY LIVER HAEMORRHAGIC SYNDROME'. This is a condition in laying hens which has to be differentiated from F L K S (below) of broiler-chicks. This condition in hens is improved by diets based on wheat as compared with maize; whereas FLKS is aggravated by diets based on wheat. Heat stress may be a partial cause. Death is due to haemorrhage from the enlarged liver.

FATTY LIVER/KIDNEY SYNDROME OF CHICKENS. A condition in which excessive amounts of fat are present in the liver, kidneys, and myocardium. The liver is pale and swollen, with haemorrhages sometimes present, and the kidneys vary from being slightly swollen and pale pink to being excessively enlarged and white.
CAUSE. FLKS was shown in 1974 to respond to biotin (*see* VITAMINS), and accordingly can be prevented by suitable modification of the diet.
SIGNS. A number of the more forward birds (usually 2 to 3 weeks old) suddenly show symptoms of paralysis. They lie down on their breasts with their heads stretched forward; others lie on their sides with their heads bent over their backs. Death may occur within a few hours. Mortality seldom exceeds 1 per cent. The best birds appear to be affected.

FAUCES is the narrow opening which connects the mouth with the throat. It is bounded above by the soft palate, below by the base of the tongue, and the openings of the tonsils lie at either side.

FAULTY NUTRITION (*see* NUTRITION, FEED BLOCKS, DIET, LAMENESS in cattle, BLINDNESS).

FAULTY WIRING of farm equipment has led to cows refusing concentrates in the parlour, not because they were unpalatable as at first thought, but because the container was 'live' so that cows wanting to feed were deterred by a mild electric shock. (*See also* EARTHING and ELECTRIC SHOCK.)

FAVUS is another name for 'honeycomb ringworm'. (*See* RINGWORM.)

FEATHER PICKING, or FEATHER PULLING in poultry and in cage birds, particularly parrots, is in many cases due to the irritation caused by lice or to the ravages of the depluming mite. In such cases the necessary anti-parasitic measures must be taken. It occurs in birds penned up, due to a lack of exercise and facilities for scratching, to keep them occupied. Errors in nutrition also play a part, a monotonous diet predisposing to it. Lack of adequate animal protein in the diet of young growing chicks, especially when kept under intensive conditions, may cause the vice. Once the birds start pulling the feather they sooner or later draw blood, and an outbreak of cannibalism results. Treatment consists of isolating the culprit if it can be found at the beginning and feeding the birds a balanced diet containing green food. The addition of blood meal in the mash in many cases acts as a specific. The use of blue-glass in intensive houses has stopped the habit in some cases, but it is not always effective. In dealing with cage birds, variation of the diet, salines in the drinking water, and keeping the birds in the dark for a time sometimes has the desired effect, but once the habit is confirmed it is very difficult to control.

FEATHERS, PROCESSED. At packing stations it has become the practice to collect and process *together* feathers and poultry offal. In order to obtain feather protein in a form useful as food, such a high temperature has to be employed that the feeding value of the offal is destroyed. Accordingly, this material should not be sold as 'meat meal' or bought as an ingredient for rations on account of its alleged protein value.

FEDESA. The European Federation of Animal Health.

FEED ADDITIVES (*see* ADDITIVES).

FEED BLOCKS. These 'self-help' lick blocks, placed out on pasture, are useful especially on hill farms for preventing loss of condition and even semi-starvation in the ewe.
Most feed blocks contain cereals as a source of carbohydrate, protein from natural sources supplemented by urea, minerals, trace elements, and vitamins. In some blocks glucose or molasses is substituted for the cereals as the chief source of carbohydrate. A third type contains no protein or urea but provides glucose, minerals, trace elements, and vitamins; being especially useful in the context of hypomagnesaemia (and other metabolic ills) in ewes shortly before and after lambing.
One manufacturer commented that there was a danger of farmers thinking too rigidly in terms of feed blocks and roughage only. This could result in bare maintenance; and for cattle on winter grazing he would normally recommend 2–3 lb cereals if some daily liveweight gain were to be achieved. A sudden cold spell could call for additional carbohydrate.
The need for adequate feeding of cereals to lowland ewes a few weeks before and after lambing – in addition to the cereal content of the block – is stressed by most feed block manufacturers.

FEEDING (*see* DIET, *and* FAULTY NUTRITION).

FEEDING-STUFFS. These must be stored separately from fertilisers, or contamination and subsequent poisoning may occur.
The safe storage period on the farm of certain feeds is given under DIET.
Poultry and rats and mice must not be allowed to contaminate feeding-stuffs, or SALMONELLOSIS may result in stock eating the food. If warfarin has been used, this may be contained in rodents' urine and lead to poisoning of stock through contamination of feeding-stuffs. (*See also* TOXOPLASMOSIS.)
Unsterilised bone-meal is a potential source of salmonellosis and anthrax infections.
(*See also* ADDITIVES, CONCENTRATES, DIET, MOULDY FOOD, MYCOTOXICOSIS, CUBES, SACKS, *and* LUBRICANTS, MEDICINES ACT.)

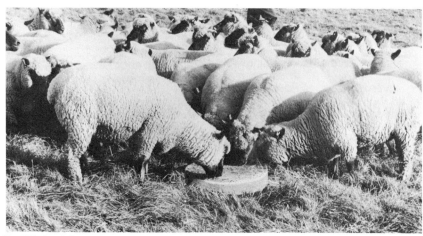

Feed Blocks: A Coopablok in use.

FEEDLOTS involve the zero-grazing of beef cattle on a very large scale. By 1973 in the USA there were already feedlots of 100,000 head each, and many more containing tens of thousands of cattle. Veterinary problems arise when these cattle are brought to the feedlot from range or pasture, and fed on grain. Shipping fever is a common ailment; likewise liver abscesses.

FELINE BABESIOSIS Young cats may develop immunity to *Babesia felis*, older cats often have recurrent illness. Subclinical infections occur. When symptoms are present they include lethargy, loss of appetite, and anaemia; and occasionally jaundice. The disease can prove fatal. (R. C. Weiss & F. W. Scott. *American Journal of Veterinary Research* (1981) 382.) (*See* BABESIOSIS.)

FELINE ANAEMIA (*see* ANAEMIA, TOXOPLASMOSIS, HAEMOBARTONELLA, FELINE LEUKAEMIA, FELINE BABESIOSIS).

FELINE CALICIVIRUS DISEASE. This is virtually indistinguishable from FELINE VIRAL RHINOTRACHEITIS. However, tongue ulceration is more common in FCD than in FVR, while the converse is true of coughing. Paw lesions may occur in FCD, not in FVR. (Povey, C., *Vet. Rec.* (1976), **98**, 293.)

FELINE CANCER. Cancer is an important disease of cats, and an American estimate suggests a rate of 264 per 100,000 cats per year. In 31 per cent of cases of cancer the site is the lymph nodes, followed by 16 per cent involving the bone marrow. Skin cancer accounts for 7 per cent, mammary gland cancer for 5 per cent. (Elizabeth M. Hodgkins, University of California). (*See also under* CANCER for figures relating to mammary gland tumours, benign and malignant.)

Feline skin cancer. Mast cell tumours have previously been reported to be malignant and ultimately fatal. However, in 14 cases none of the tumours metastasised to lymph nodes or viscera, none recurred at a previous excision site and none

contributed to the death of a cat. (Buerger, R. G. & Scott, D. W. (1987) *Journal of the American Veterinary Medical Association* **190**, 1440.)

FELINE DIABETES (*see* DIABETES).

FELINE DYSAUTONOMIA (Key–Gaskell syndrome). A condition in cats first recognised at Bristol University's department of veterinary medicine in 1981–82.
SIGNS include depression, loss of appetite, prominent nictitating membranes, nostrils dry and encrusted – suggesting a respiratory disease. Constipation and a transient diarrhoea have both been reported; also incontinence in some cases. The pupils are dilated and unresponsive to light. There may be difficulty in swallowing and regurgitation of food; and a key finding is enlargement of the oesophagus. According to Glasgow University's research workers, the prognosis seems to depend on the degree of this 'megalo-oesophagus'. Lesions include loss of nerve cells, and their replacement by fibrous tissue, in certain ganglia.
CAUSE, in early 1985 unknown; but Professor Gaskell and A.T.B. Edney have pointed out that the syndrome has some striking similarities with GRASS SICKNESS in horses and, like the latter, appears to be prevalent only in the UK; with a few cases reported from Scandinavia.
TREATMENT involves countering dehydration by means of glucose-saline, offering tempting food or feeding liquid foods by syringe, use of eyedrops containing pilocarpine to obtain pupil constriction.
PROGNOSIS. The recovery rate is stated to be about 25 per cent, but may take weeks or months. Cats with a greatly enlarged oesophagus, persistent loss of appetite, or bladder paralysis are the least likely to survive.

FELINE ENCEPHALOMYELITIS. This has been reported in Sydney, Australia, and is characterised by non-fatal cases of hind-leg ataxia, and sometimes by side-to-side movements of head and neck. On *post-mortem* examination, demyelinating lesions and perivascular cuffing involving the brain and spinal cord were found. The cause is thought to be a virus, but efforts to transmit the disease failed.

FELINE EYE INFECTIONS. Conjunctival swabs obtained from 39 cats with conjunctivitis and from 50 clinically normal cats were examined microbiologically. Non-haemolytic streptococci and *Staphylococcus epidermis* were isolated from both groups while beta-haemolytic streptococci, rhinotracheitis (feline herpes 1) virus, *Mycoplasma felis* and *Chlamydia psittaci* were isolated from cases with conjunctivitis. Organisms were isolated from 14 of the diseased cats and from two of the normal animals. (Shewen, P. E and others *Canadian Veterinary Journal* (1980) **21**, 231.)

FELINE GINGIVITIS. This can be mild and transient. Sometimes the term is applied not to an inflammation of the gums but merely to a hyperaemia – an increased blood flow – which, Dr Rosalind Gaskell has said, may alarm the owner but does not hurt the (young) cat.

Gingivitis can also be acute or chronic; easily treatable, or highly intractable.

One of the commonest causes of gingivitis in middle-aged or elderly cats is the accumulation of tartar on the surface of the teeth. If neglected, the tartar will gradually encroach on to the gums, causing these to become inflamed. Unless the tartar is removed, a shrinkage of the gums is likely to follow. As the gum recedes from the teeth it leaves pockets or spaces into which food particles and bacteria can lodge, exacerbating the inflammation, causing halitosis and leading to the roots of some teeth becoming infected.

The yellowish tartar deposits can become so thick and extensive that eventually they completely mask the teeth. A cat in this condition undoubtedly suffers much discomfort, finds eating a little difficult, and may have toothache. Health is further impaired by the persistent infection. The cat becomes dejected.

Even in such advanced cases, removal of the tartar (and of any loose teeth) can bring about almost a rejuvenation of the animal.

This form of chronic gingivigts, then, can be successfully overcome by treatment and, indeed, prevented if an annual check of the teeth is carried out by a veterinary surgeon.

Intractable gingivitis. Some cases of this are associated with a generalised illness rather than merely disease of the mouth. For example, chronic kidney disease, and possibly diabetes, may cause ulcers on the gums (as well as elsewhere in the mouth).

Some strains of the feline calicivirus may also cause gum and tongue ulceration. Bacterial secondary invaders are likely to worsen this, especially if the cat's bodily defence systems have been impaired by, say, the feline leukaemia virus, some other infection, or even stress.

Antibiotics or suphonamides are used to control the bacteria; vitamins prescribed to assist the repair of damaged tissue and to help restore appetite, and other supportive measures taken. However, some cases of feline gingivitis do not respond.

It is likely that *all* the causes of feline gingivitis have not yet been established. Further research will no doubt bridge the gaps in existing knowledge, and bring new methods of treatment and a better prognosis. (*See also* FELINE STOMATITIS.)

FELINE HERPESVIRUS (*see* FELINE VIRAL RHINO TRACHEITIS *and* FELINE INFLUENZA).

FELINE IMMUNODEFICIENCY VIRUS (FIV). (Formerly known as the Feline T-lymphotropic Lentivirus (FTLV).) It was discovered in California by N. C. Pedersen & colleagues, and it has been detected in the UK, Switzerland, and the Netherlands.

The virus is said to establish a permanent infection, and may eventually produce clinical signs. The prognosis is poor.

As the virus causes immunodeficiency, secondary infections account for many of the clinical signs.
SIGNS. Anorexia, weight loss, lethargy, nervous signs such as twitching and persistent licking of the lips.
DIAGNOSIS. An ELISA test. The feline leukaemia virus can produce chronic illness with similar signs, so testing for FeLV antibodies is needed for a differential diagnosis.

FELINE INFECTIOUS ANAEMIA. This disease, caused by parasites of the genus Perythrozoon, has been reported in the UK, USA and S. Africa. It is treated with antibiotics. Organic iron preparations and vitamin B_{12} are also used.

Infection with *Haemobartonella felis* has been described in the USA in cats 1 to 3 years old, and successfully reproduced experimentally. It is believed that many adult cats carry the parasite and that the disease lies dormant until some debilitating condition lowers the cat's resistance. In Britain, the causal agent has been named *Eperythrozoon felis*.

The symptoms may include: fever, anaemia, loss of appetite, depression, weakness, and loss of weight. Anaemia may be severe enough to cause panting.

For diagnosis and staining techniques, see *Veterinary Record*, Sept. 12, 1970. Blood smears are essential, and must be repeated. The parasites are in blood only 10–15 days after infection.

FELINE INFECTIOUS ENTERITIS or PANLEUKOPENIA. Formerly often known as Feline Distemper. Cats of all ages are susceptible. Survivors appear to acquire lifelong immunity.
CAUSE. A parvovirus, indistinguishable from mink enteritis virus. Resistant to heat and disinfectants, the virus can survive outside its host for a year.
SIGNS. Loss of appetite, vomiting, intense depression, and prostration; the animal prefers to lie in cold places, cries out, and rapidly loses weight. The temperature, at first 105°F or more, becomes subnormal in 12 to 18 hours, and death commonly occurs within 24 hours. The cat may pass no motions throughout its illness, but usually there is diarrhoea in the later stages. Dehydration is rapid. In newborn kittens, the brain

may be affected giving rise to a staggering gait. In a few cases (which often recover) the tongue becomes ulcerated.

It seems that a mild form is common as many older cats have immunity without previous severe illness.

DIAGNOSIS may be confirmed by laboratory means – examination of bone marrow and blood smears. Poisoning, toxoplasmosis, intestinal foreign bodies, septicaemia have to be differentiated.

PREVENTION. A vaccine is available.

TREATMENT. Whole blood given intravenously at 20 ml per kg or hyperimmune serum at 6–10 ml per kg, and lactated Ringer's solution, with anti-emetics every few hours, plus broad-spectrum antibiotics, vitamins, and baby foods are recommended by Dr Charles Povey MRCVS, Ontario Veterinary College, University of Guelph. In a cattery, isolation of in-contact animals and rigid disinfection must be practised. (*See also* NURSING.)

FELINE INFECTIOUS PERITONITIS. This disease was first described in the USA in 1966, and has been encountered also in the UK. It is a slowly progressive and fatal disease of young cats, and sometimes of older ones also, caused by a coronavirus.

SIGNS. Fever, depression, loss of appetite, gradual loss of weight leading to emaciation, distension of the abdomen due to exudate. Occasionally, diarrhoea and vomiting occur. There may be distressed breathing and, towards the end, jaundice.

There is also a 'dry' form – much harder to diagnose, which may involve liver, kidneys, eyes, and brain. A granuloma in a kidney is found in some of these cases.

POST-MORTEM FINDINGS. The abdominal cavity contains fluid and its lining membrane is inflamed. Whitish flakes of fibrin may be present in the fluid, and the liver may show white spots. The chest may also contain fluid. In some cases there are granulomatous changes in several organs or tissues.

DIAGNOSIS. Differentiation from leukaemia/lymphosarcoma and toxoplasmosis has to be made.

FELINE 'INFLUENZA'. The name is loosely applied at present to respiratory infections involving more than one virus. It commonly occurs in cat-breeding and boarding establishments, and in cats which have been taken to a show; the infection(s) being highly contagious. Secondary bacterial invaders account for many of the symptoms. It was suggested by R. C. Povey, (*Veterinary Record*, 1969, **84**, 335), that

'Cat flu' =

FELINE VIRAL RHINOTRACHEITIS and/or

FELINE CALICIVIRUS

+ Secondary bacteria

SIGNS. Sneezing and coughing. The temperature is usually high at first; the appetite is in abeyance; the animal is dull; the eyes are kept half-shut, or the eyelids may be closed together; from the nose there is a certain amount of discharge, thin at first and thicker and creamy later on; condition is rapidly lost. If pneumonia supervenes the breathing becomes very rapid and great distress is apparent; exhaustion and prostration follow, and death usually takes place in from 3 to 6 or 7 days.

TREATMENT. Isolation under the best possible hygienic conditions is immediately necessary in every case. There should be plenty of light and fresh air, and domesticated cats need to be kept fairly warm. A woollen or flannel coat or body bandage may be necessary in highly bred and delicate cats. Medicinal treatment is not to be advocated unless the symptoms warrant it. Cats are difficult animals to dose, except by skilled persons, and very often the struggles occasioned by attempts at administration of medicines do more harm than the medicines do good.

Often one of the sulpha drugs given twice daily in butter or small amounts of fish or meat, gives satisfactory results. Food should be light and easily digested. (*See* NURSING, HYDROLISED PROTEIN.)

Owing to the very highly contagious nature of feline 'flu, disinfection after recovery must be very thorough before other cats are admitted to the premises; and where death has occurred, at least 6 weeks should be allowed to elapse before a new cat is purchased.

FELINE JUVENILE OSTEODYSTROPHY is a disease, of nutritional origin, in the growing kitten. (It may occur, too, in young wild feline animals reared in captivity.)

CAUSE. The disease has been reproduced by feeding a diet deficient in calcium and rich in phosphorus; *e.g.* kittens fed exclusively on a diet of minced beef or sheep heart have developed the disease within 8 weeks.

SIGNS. The kitten becomes less playful and reluctant to jump down even from modest heights; it may become stranded when climbing curtains owing to being unable to disengage its claws; lameness, sometimes due to a green-stick fracture; pain in the back, making the kitten bad-tempered and sometimes unable to stand. In kittens which survive, deformity of the skeleton may be shown in later life, with bowing of long bones, fractures, prominence of the spine of the shoulder blade, and abnormalities which together suggest a shortening of the back.

FELINE LEUKAEMIA. This is caused by a virus discovered by Professor W. F. H. Jarrett in 1964. The virus gives rise to cancer, especially lymphosarcoma involving the alimentary canal and thymus, and lymphatic leukaemia. Anaemia, glomerulonephritis, and an immuno-suppressive syndrome may also result from this infection, which can be readily transmitted from cat to cat. Many cats are able to overcome the infection. The virus may infect not only the bone marrow, lymph nodes, etc., but also epithelial cells of mouth, nose, salivary glands, intestine, urinary bladder. Cats inoculated experimentally with Fe L V may not develop leukaemia until 4 years later. There is at present no evidence that Fe L V can infect man, though it will grow in cultures of human cells.

Kittens of up to 4 months of age are more likely to become permanently infected with FeLV than older cats, but many cases do occur in cats over 5 years old.

Many cats which have apparently recovered from natural exposure to the virus remain latently infected, but keep free from FeLV-associated diseases. Such cats may infect their kittens via the milk.

Most deaths of FeLV-positive cats are not directly attributable to this virus, but to other viral or bacterial infections which, in the ordinary way would not prove fatal to the cat; but which are rendered far more serious owing to the immunosuppression caused by the virus.

SIGNIFICANCE OF FLV. This was diagnosed in tissues taken post mortem from 1095 cats. As expected, there were significant associations between FeLV infection and anaemia, tumours of the leukaemia/lymphoma complex, feline infectious peritonitis, bacterial infections, emaciation, FeLV-associated enteritis, lymphatic hyperplasia and haemorrhage. However, there were unexpected associations with icterus, several types of hepatitis, and liver degeneration. (Reinacher, M. & Theilen, G. (1987) *American Journal of Veterinary Research* **48**, 939.)

SIGNS. These include a gradual loss of condition, poor appetite, depression, anaemia. Breathing may become laboured due to the accumulation of fluid within the chest. A persistent cough, and vomiting, are other symptoms.

DIAGNOSIS. FeLV infection can be detected by a fluorescent antibody test, an ELISA test, electron microscopic examination of tissues, and by isolation of virus. A saliva test kit is available from Norden Laboratories. An under-tongue saliva sample is taken, and placed in the test reagent, when a colour change takes place.

CONTROL. It is possible to prevent the spread of the disease to susceptible cats by a 'test-and-removal' system. By means of the fluorescent antibody test, it is possible to identify an infected cat. This is removed from the household for euthanasia, and other cats in the same household are then tested. If FeLV-positive, they too are removed, even if clinically healthy. Retesting of the FeLV-negative cats is necessary after 3 and 6 months. If still FeLV-negative, they can be considered clear, and new cats introduced on to the premises, if desired. (Hardy, W. D. *et al.*, *Nature* (1973), **263**, 326).

The virus may persist in the bone marrow of cats which have obstensibly recovered. Such a latent infection can be reactivated by large doses of corticosteroid; and the virus can be recovered by cultivation of bone marrow cells. FeLV is not transmitted from cats with a latent infection.

Professor W. F. Jarrett FRS and colleagues developed an experimental vaccine, and in 1983 a commercial vaccine was in process of development by several companies.

In the USA a vaccine has been available for some years. A course of three injections is required. The vaccine is stated to protect about 80 per cent of cats against challenge by the FeLV; which compares with 13 per cent unvaccinated cats being naturally resistant to the virus in a control group.

At the end of 1988 the French company Virbac introduced a genetically engineered vaccine under the brand name Leucogen. Two injections at a fifteen-day interval are stipulated.

FELINE MILIARY DERMATITIS (*see* ECZEMA).

FELINE PANLEUKOPENIA (*see* FELINE INFECTIOUS ENTERITIS).

FELINE PNEUMONITIS A name given to *Chlamydia psittaci* infection in cats. It causes sneezing and other symptoms occurring in the human cold, and is common in boarding and other catteries, where spread is by aerosol infection. Immunity develops, but some recovered cats may become 'carriers'.

FELINE PYOTHORAX (*see* PYOTHORAX).

FELINE SPONGIFORM ENCEPHALOPATHY (FSE). This has been defined as a degeneration of the grey matter of the brain stem, with the formation of microscopic cavities known as *vacuoles.*

The first known victim of this disease was a Siamese seen at Bristol University in 1990.

By September 2, 1991 MAFF had reported one case in Scotland, and nineteen others in the UK. (*See* SPONGIFORM ENCEPHALOPATHIES.)

SIGNS. An unsteady gait, with a tendency to fall; then being unable to get to its feet without help. Four other cats in the same household remained well.

CAUSE. A *Lancet* editorial article commented: 'All the spongiform encephalopathies have a feature in common – the involvement of an aberrant form of a normal cell protein called *prion protein.*'

A prion has been defined as a self-replicating infectious protein. (Dr S. P. Prusiner, writing in *Science* in 1982.)

FELINE STOMATITIS. Inflammation of the cat's mouth.

CAUSES. There is a variety of causes – not all of them yet known. Dr R. M. Gaskell stated at the 1983 BVA Congress that there may be a background of kidney disease or, some suggest, diabetes.

Viruses associated with stomatitis in the cat include the feline calicivirus and the rhinotracheitis virus; and a chronic ulcerative stomatitis might be due to immunosuppression by the feline leukaemia virus, for example.

SIGNS. These include difficulty in swallowing, halitosis, excessive salivation, loss of appetite, and sometimes bleeding.

TREATMENT. The aim is to limit secondary bacterial infection by means of ampicillin, for example, or sulphonamide, or tylosin. A supplement of vitamins A, B, and C may help. If the cat will not eat, subcutaneous fluid therapy will be required.

Chronic stomatitis in elderly cats may be due to EOSINOPHILIC GRANULOMA, or malignant growths such as squamous-cell CARCINOMA or FIBROSAR-COMA. (*See also* FELINE GINGIVITIS.)

FELINE UROLOGICAL SYNDROME (FUS).

A case control study was made of 345 cases of FUS seen at the Danish Veterinary School between 1965 and 1970. Of these 190 had urethral obstruction and 155 had cystitis. Both conditions were more common in castrated males and in cats aged between 4 and 6 years of age. (Willeberg, P., *Nord. Vet.-Med.* (1975), **27**, 1.)

Both cystitis and obstruction of the urethra may have one feature in common: the formation of sand-like material, composed of varying proportions of crystalline and organic matter. The crystals are usually struvite (ammonium magnesium phosphate hexahydrate). Calculi or 'stones' also sometimes occur in the cat, but less commonly than the sand-like deposits.

CAUSE. Various theories have been advanced to account for FUS. It has been suggested that a virus or viruses may be involved; that a high level of magnesium in the diet could cause FUS. The effects of heredity and castration have also been mentioned.

Dr Mark L. Morris and Dr Lon D. Lewis, consultants on veterinary diets in the USA, stated that the reason why FUS is more likely to occur when a cat is fed an ordinary commercial dry, rather than canned, food is that these dry foods are lower in calories and digestibility than many canned foods. 'This increases the amount of dry food that the cat must eat to meet calorie requirements and, therefore, increases the amount of magnesium consumed and excreted in the urine.'

In the USA 60 per cent of cats are fed on dry commercial cat foods, and the magnesium content of most of these is several times the quantity which the cat actually needs. It is this excess which leads to magnesium being excreted and the sand-like struvite crystals being formed in the urinary bladder.

Drs Morris and Lewis do not regard viruses or bacteria as a cause of FUS, though both may be present in the urine. The crystals may form around them or cell debris.

Low-magnesium 'Prescription Diets' are now available. (Hills Pet Products Ltd.', London.)

Dr M. F. Tarttelin, of Massey University, New Zealand, urged that greater emphasis should be placed on the fact that cats are obligate carnivores, and should therefore receive a diet with a high meat content. Such a diet maintains urine pH in the acid range (pH 5 to 6), at which struvite crystals are uncommon.

However, he stated, many commercial dry diets produce an alkaline urine. 'It is probable that the alkalinity is related to the cereal content of dry foods, which contain an excess of potassium salts.' It is the metabolism of these, he stated, which produces an alkaline urine; and he concluded that urine pH is even more important than the magnesium content of the diet.

(Urine acidifiers are now being used in some dry cat foods.)

Smaller and more frequent meals are advocated, as he found that fasting raises urine pH.

(Tarttelin, M. F. *Veterinary Record* 1987, **121**, 227 and 245).

SIGNS. The owners may notice the cat straining to pass urine, with only very little to be seen in the litter tray. The urine may be blood-stained. Cat-owners sometimes mistake FUS for constipation.

Other signs include loss of appetite, dejection, restlessness. Signs of pain will be shown if the abdomen is touched, owing to distension of the bladder.

Urethral blockage is an emergency requiring immediate veterinary attention; in default of which there is the great risk of collapse, leading to unconsciousness. The bladder may rupture, causing additional shock, and leading to peritonitis.

TREATMENT. Skilled manipulation can sometimes free a plug (often a mixture of organic material and the struvite crystals) blocking the end of the penis. If this fails, or the obstruction is further back, a catheter will have to be passed. If catherisation fails, it will be necessary to empty the bladder by means of aspiration or incision.

PROGNOSIS. There are cases in which, after removal of the urethral obstruction, the latter does not recur. Unfortunately, in between 20 and 50 per cent of cases, recurrence does take place. After two or three such recurrences, the owner has to decide whether euthanasia would be best for the cat, rather than have it subjected to even more catherisations; or whether to opt for a URETHROSTOMY operation. (The potential benefits and risks are referred to under that heading.)

POST-OPERATIVE TREATMENT includes giving not only an antibiotic but also a urine-acidifier, in pill form, in an attempt to dissolve the remaining crystals.

A low-magnesium diet is also recommended and, in the USA and the UK, proprietary preparations are on sale to meet this requirement. (*See* PRESCRIPTION DIETS).

FELINE T-LYMPHOTROPIC LENTIVIRUS (*see* FELINE IMMUNODEFICIENCY VIRUS).

FELINE VESTIBULAR SYNDROME, IDIOPATHIC.

Seventy-five cases were seen between 1975–84 at the New York State College of Veterinary Medicine.

SIGNS. Head tilt, ataxia, nystagmus, and occasionally vomiting. Duration of signs was only up to 24 hours; only one hour in two cats. (Burke, Elizabeth E. (1985) *JAVMA* **941**, 187.)

FELINE VIRAL RHINOTRACHEITIS.

This disease was discovered in the USA and first recorded in Britain in 1966. Severe symptoms are usually confined to kittens of up to 6 months old. Sneezing, conjunctivitis with discharge, coughing and ulcerated tongue may be seen. Bronchopneumonia and chronic sinusitis are possible complications. Cause: a herpes virus.

Infection may occur in a latent form, and there may be a link between this virus and feline syncytia-forming virus. (Ellis, T. M. (1982) *Research in Veterinary Science* **33**, 270.)

Treatment may include the use of a steam vaporiser, lactated Ringer's solution to overcome de-hydration, and antibiotics. Vitamins and baby foods may help.

FEMINISATION in the male dog may occur as the result of a sertoli-cell tumour of a testicle. (See SERTOLI-CELL TUMOUR.)

FEMUR is the bone of the thigh, reaching from the hip-joint above to the stifle-joint below. It is the largest, strongest, and longest individual bone of the body. The bone lies at a slope of about 45 degrees to the horizontal in most animals when they are at rest, articulating at its upper end with the acetabulum of the pelvis, and at its lower end with the tibia. Just above the joint surface for the tibia is the patellar surface, upon which slides the patella, or 'knee cap'. Fractures of the head of the femur are common.☛

FENBENDAZOLE. An effective anthelmintic used in cattle, horses, pigs, dogs and cats. (See WORMS, FARM TREATMENT.)

FERNS other than bracken occasionally cause poisoning in cattle. For example, *Dryopteris filixmas* (male fern) and *D. borreri* (rusty male fern) give rise to blindness, drowsiness and a desire to stand or lie in water. Poisoning is occasionally fatal. (See also BRACKEN.)

FERRET (*Mustela putorius furo*). In the UK the breeding season begins in March and continues until the end of August. As 'persistently high oestrogen levels associated with prolonged oestrus can cause a fatal pancytopenia, there would seem to be a special need to control oestrus in the jill when not kept for breeding,' and this can be achieved either by spaying or by a single injection of 0·5 ml of proligestone (Delvosteron; Mycofarm) subcutaneously over the shoulder/ base of the neck to cover the whole season. (Oxenham, M. & Evans, J. M. (1985) *Vet. Record* **116**, 300).

Other diseases of ferrets include: CANINE DISTEMPER, BOTULISM, ABSCESS formation.

FERRITIN concentrations in serum are closely related to total body iron stores, and ferritin immunoassays can be used to assess the clinical iron status of human beings, horses, cattle, dogs, and pigs. (Weeks, B. R., Smith, J. E. & Phillips, R. M. (1988) *American Journal of Veterinary Research* **49**, 1193.)

FERTILISATION (see REPRODUCTION).

FERTILISERS should not be stored near feeding-stuffs, as contamination of the latter, leading to poisoning, may occur. In Australia, 17 out of 50 Herefords died after gaining access to the remains of a fertiliser dump. A crust of superphosphate and ammonium sulphate had remained on the ground.

For the risk associated with unsterilised bonemeal, see under ANTHRAX and SALMONELLOSIS.

Hypomagnesaemia is frequently encountered in animals grazing pasture which has received a recent dressing with potash. (See also BASIC SLAG, FOG FEVER.)

FERTILITY (see CONCEPTION RATES, FARROWING RATES, INFERTILITY, CALVING INTERVAL).

FESCUE. In New Zealand and the USA a severe hind-foot lameness of cattle has been attributed to the grazing of *Festuca arunincea*, a coarse and unpalatable grass which grows on poorly drained land or on the banks of ditches, and being tall stands out above the snow. In typical cases, the left hind-foot is affected first, and becomes cold, the skin being dry and necrotic. Symptoms appear 10 to 14 days after the cattle go on to the Tall-Fescue-dominated pasture. Ergot may be present, but is not invariably so.

It was suggested in 1971 in Australia that 'fescue foot' may be associated with a potent toxin produced by the fungus *Fusarium tricinctum*. This toxin is now known as Butenolide.

FETAL INFECTIONS. Examples of these are TOXOCARIASIS in bitches; and TOXOPLASMOSIS *in utero* of cows, ewes, sows, bitches and cats.

FETAL MEMBRANES. (See CHORION, AMNION, ALLANTOIS; *also* UTERUS, DISEASES OF *and* EMBRYOLOGY.)

FETAL RESORPTION (see MUMMIFICATION).

FETLOCK-JOINT is the joint in the horse's limb between the metacarpus or metatarsus (cannon bones) and the first phalanx (long pastern bone). At the back of this joint are situated the sesamoids of the first phalanx. (See BONES.)

FETUS. For an outline description of the development of the fetus, see under EMBRYOLOGY. For fetal circulation, see the diagram under CIRCULATION OF THE BLOOD. (See also FREEMARTIN.)

FEVER is one of the commonest symptoms of infectious disease, and serves to make the distinction between *febrile* and *non-febrile* ailments.

Examples of *specific fevers*: equine influenza, distemper, braxy, blackquarter, or swine fever.

When fever reaches an excessively high stage, *e.g.* 107°F, in the horse or dog, the term *hyperpyrexia* (excessive fever) is applied, and it is regarded as indicating a condition of danger; while if it exceeds 108° or 109°F for any length of time, death almost always results. Occasionally, in certain fevers or febrile conditions, such as severe heat-stroke, the temperature may reach 112°. (See also under TEMPERATURE.)

There is usually a certain amount of shivering, to which the term 'rigor' is applied, but this is very often not noticed by the owner. The stage of rigors is followed by dullness, the animal standing about with a distressed expression or moving sluggishly. Later, perspiration, rapid breathing, a fast, full, bounding pulse, and a greater elevation of temperature are exhibited. Thirst is usually marked; the appetite disappears; the urine is scanty and of a high specific gravity; the bowels are generally constipated, although diarrhoea may follow later; intense injection of all the visible mucous membranes, *i.e.* those of the eyes, nostrils, mouth, occurs. (*See also* HYPERTHERMIA.)

Fever may perhaps have a beneficial effect. It was noticed in the last century that patients in a Russian mental hospital, suffering from neurosyphilis, improved as regards their paresis during a fever outbreak; and 'malaria therapy' was introduced at a later date. Experiments with newborn mice show that fatal infection with Coxsackie B1 virus can be modified to a subclinical infection if the animals are kept in an incubator at 34°C and thus attain the same body temperature as 8–9-day-old-mice. (Teisner, B., Haahr, *see Nature*, 1974, **247,** 568.) Similarly, *puppies infected with canine herpes virus survive longer and have diminished replication of virus in their organs if their body temperature is artificially raised to that of adult dogs.* (Carmichael, L. E., Barnes, F. D., Percy, D. H., *J. infect. Dis.*, 1969, **120,** 669.)

FIBRE, IMPORTANCE OF (*see under* DIET).

FIBRILLATION means contraction of individual bundles of muscle fibres without relation to the whole.

FIBRIN is a substance upon which depends the formation of blood-clots. (*See* CLOTTING OF BLOOD, PLASMA.)

Fibrin is found not only in coagulated blood, but in many inflammatory conditions. Later it is either dissolved again by, and taken up into, the blood, or is 'organised' into fibrous tissue.

FIBRINOGEN, PLASMA. Concentration of this is increased in inflammatory conditions, especially lesions of serous surfaces and in endocarditis. (*See also* CLOTTING OF BLOOD.)

FIBROBLAST. A flat, irregularly-shaped connective-tissue cell.

FIBROMA is a tumour consisting of fibrous tissue. (*See* TUMOURS.)

FIBROSIS. The formation of fibrous tissue, which may replace other tissue. (*See also* CIRRHOSIS.)

FIBROUS TISSUE is one of the most abundant tissues of the body, being found in quantity below the skin, around muscles and to a less extent between them, and forming tendons to a great extent; quantities are associated with bone when it is being calcified and afterwards, and fibrous tissue is always laid down where healing or inflammatory processes are at work. There are two varieties: white fibrous tissue and yellow elastic fibrous tissue.

White fibrous tissue consists of a substance called 'collagen' which yields gelatin on boiling, and is arranged in bundles of fibres between which lie flattened star-shaped cells. It is very unyielding and forms tendons and ligaments; it binds the bundles of muscle fibres together, is laid down during the repair of wounds, and forms the scars which result; it may form the basis of cartilage, and it has the property of contracting as time goes on and may cause puckering of the tissues around. *Yellow fibrous tissue* is not so plentiful as the former. It consists of bundles of long yellow fibres, formed from a substance called 'elastin', and is very elastic. It is found in the walls of arteries, in certain ligaments which are elastic, and the bundles are present in some varieties of elastic cartilage. (*See* ADHESIONS, SCARS, WOUNDS.)

FIBULA is one of the bones of the hind-limb, running from the stifle to the hock. It appears to become less and less important in direct proportion as the number of the digits of the limb decreases. In the horse and ox it is a very small and slim bone which does not take any part in the bearing of weight, while in the dog it is quite large, and with the tibia, takes its share in supporting the weight of the body.

FILARIAL WORMS (*see* FILARIASIS).

FILARIASIS is a group of diseases caused by the presence in the body of certain small thread-like Nematode worms, called filariae, which are often found in the blood-stream. Biting insects act as vectors. (*See* HEARTWORM and TRACHEAL WORMS for canine filariasis; also EQUINE FILARIASIS; and BRAIN, DISEASES OF.).

Parafilaria bovicola causes bovine filariasis in Africa, the Far East, and part of Europe. The female worm penetrates the skin, causing subcutaneous haemorrhagic lesions that resemble bruising. Eggs are laid in the blood there. Downgrading of carcases at meat inspection is a cause of significant loss. Ivermectin is useful as a control measure.

FILOVIRUS (*see* MONKEYS, DISEASES OF.)

FIMBRIAE. Specific surface antigens. They can be used in vaccines against *E. coli*, for example. (*See under* GENETIC ENGINEERING.)

FINNISH LANDRACE SHEEP have been imported into the U K for experimental and commercial breeding. They are remarkable for high prolificacy, triplets being common, and 4 or 5 lambs not rare. (*Illustration opposite.*)

FIRE-EXTINGUISHERS. These are required under the terms of the Animal Boarding Establishment Act, 1963.

FISH, DISEASES OF. There are now nine diseases covered by the Diseases of Fish Act, and all are notifiable in Britain: furunculosis and columnaris (bacterial); infectious pancreatic necrosis, viral haemorrhagic septicaemia, infectious haematopoietic necrosis and spring viraemia (viral); whirling disease (protozoan); ulcerative dermal necrosis and erythrodermatitis, of unknown cause.

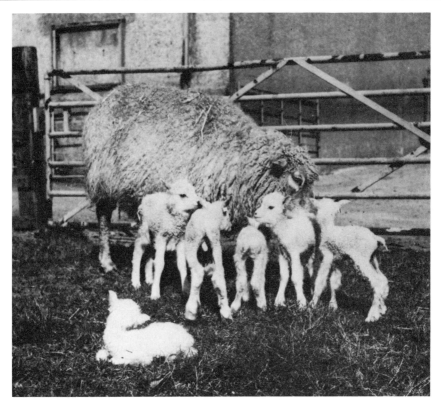

A Finnish Landrace ewe and her litter. (With acknowledgements to the AFRC's Animal Breeding Research Organisation.)

On a fish-farm in England 4,900 rainbow trout died from CEROIDOSIS (which see) over a 4-month period. Affected fish swam on their sides or upside down, and often rapidly in circles. A few were seen with their heads out of water, swimming like porpoises. (Holliman, A. & Southgate, P. *Veterinary Record* (1986) **119**, 179.)

Aquarium fish may be affected with fish tuberculosis, caused by *Mycobacterium piscium, M. platpoecilus,* or *M. fortuitum.* These cause a granulomatous condition which can prove fatal. Skin infection may develop in people handling diseased fish. (L. Leibovitz. *J A V M A* (1980) **176**, 415). (*See also* PETS, WHIRLING DISEASE, *and* SPRING VIRAEMIA OF CARP.)

FISH MEAL is largely used for feeding to pigs and poultry, although it is also added to the rations for dairy cows, calves and other farm livestock. It is composed of the dried and ground residue from fish, the edible portions of which are used for human consumption. The best variety is that made from 'white' fish – known in the trade as white fish meal. When prepared with a large admixture of herring or mackerel offal it is liable to have a strong odour, which may taint the flesh of pigs and the eggs of hens receiving it.

Fish meal is rich in protein, calcium, phosphorus, and contains smaller amounts of iodine and other elements useful to animals. It contains a variable amount of oil. It forms a useful means of maintaining the amount of protein in the ration

for all breeding females and for young animals during their period of active growth. From 3 to 10 per cent of the weight of food may consist of white fish meal. When pigs are being fattened for bacon and 'fattening-off' rations are fed, the amount of fish meal is reduced, and during the last 4 to 6 weeks it is customary to discontinue it entirely. Pigs may, however, continue to receive an amount of white fish meal up to one four-hundredth of their live weight without producing any recognisable taint in the flesh.

Many investigations have emphasised the very great economic value of fish meal for animals fed largely upon cereal by-products. It serves to correct the protein and mineral deficiencies of these and enable a balanced ration to be fed. It serves a very useful purpose by enabling more home-grown cereals to be fed and largely replaces protein-rich imported vegetable products. (*See also* AMINO ACIDS, DIET.)

FISH OILS. Live-stock owners should beware of feeding inferior fish oils, which often cause illness owing to their quickly becoming rancid, in place of good quality cod-liver oil. (*See* RANCIDITY.)

FISH, POISONING OF. This may occur through liquor from silage clamps seeping into streams, etc. The following, in very small concentrations, are lethal to fish: DDT, Derris, BHC (Gammexane), Aldrin. Many agricultural sprays may, therefore, kill fish; and likewise snail-killers used in fluke control. Virtually all the 450,000 trout in one pond died. The owner of the trout farm reported that they had been leaping out of the water on to the banks. The Devon V.I. Centre's findings suggested that the inadvertent contamination by excessively chlorinated water, into the stream supplying the trout farm, was to blame. In Hampshire the flushing of drains with a chlorine preparation led to similar trouble in river trout. The autopsy findings were 'scalding of the flanks, fins, and gills'. (*See also under* RO-TENONE for deliberate poisoning of fish.) (*See also* AFLATOXINS.)

FISH SOLUBLES. Concentrated and purified stickwater, the liquid which is pressed out of fish during oil-extraction and meal-making processes.

FISTULA is an unnatural narrow channel leading from some natural cavity, such as a duct of the mammary gland, or the interior of the rectum or anal gland, to the surface. In cows, treads by neighbours, tears by barbed wire, bites or other injury to the teats, sometimes result in milk escaping from the side of the teat. In dental fistula, which occurs in cats and dogs most commonly, but is also seen in the horse, an abscess develops at the root of a molar tooth, and the pus burrows upwards and bursts through the skin on to the surface of the face.

Occasionally a fistula heals, but often it is extremely hard to close, especially if it has persisted for some time. Surgery may be necessary.

FISTULOUS WITHERS is a condition in which a sinus develops in connection with the withers of the horse. It may follow an external injury and infection with bacteria, when, on account of the poor blood-supply, local necrosis (death) of the ligaments above the vertebrae, or of the summits of the spinous processes, with suppuration, sets in. Organisms identical with those causing abortion in cows – *Brucella abortus*–are often found, and numerous pus-forming organisms can generally be identified. In other cases, filarial worms have been found embedded in the ligament, and are responsible for those cases which arise without any previous history of injury to this part of the body.
SIGNS. At first there is noticed pain and swelling over the withers, perhaps more obvious on one side than the other, and working horses resent the application of the collar, or show a lessened inclination for work. Later on the swelling usually bursts, but it may appear to subside in a few cases. The openings which are left when the purulent material is discharged may heal over in time, but other swellings form and burst as before. In many cases one or two openings remain permanently and a thin stream of pus is constantly discharged. This runs down over the shoulders and scalds the skin, causing the hair to fall off. As a rule there is not a great deal of pain so long as the sinus remains open, and the horse is not usually affected to any great extent in his general health. In very severe forms the pus may burrow downwards.

TREATMENT. Fistulous withers is always a serious condition which should be treated before great and perhaps irreparable damage has been done to the tissues involved. Old-standing cases are notoriously difficult to treat, and many have to be destroyed.

The application of poultices and blisters to the outside is absolutely useless. Penicillin has not proved very efficacious; better results may follow the use of other antibiotics or the sulpha drugs. 'S19' vaccine is useful. Otherwise, extensive surgery may be necessary.

The treatment generally takes from 2 weeks (in very slight cases) to as long as 3 months or more, where the sinuses are deep and bone is involved, and cases are always better if they can be sent to a veterinary hospital for treatment.

FITS is another name for convulsive seizures accompanied usually by at least a few seconds of unconsciousness. Dr Phyllis Croft has commented on epilepsy: 'Typically, the dog is relaxed or even asleep at the time when the fit occurs, and the first phase consists of a tonic spasm of voluntary muscle with arrest of respiration; this lasts 30 to 40 seconds and is succeeded by clonic contractions of limb muscles ('galloping'). After this the dog usually appears to be exhausted for a period varying from a few seconds to a few minutes, with a gasping form of respiration. Some dogs then get up and appear normal almost immediately, while others wander restlessly for half an hour or more, bump into furniture and eat greedily if they find any food. The pattern of the fit is reasonably consistent in any one dog, but varies considerably from one dog to another. In between these fits, the dog appears to be entirely normal.'

Fits may be associated with epilepsy – the most common cause in adult dogs. They may occur during the course of a generalised illness such as canine distemper or rabies; may follow a head injury; be associated with a brain tumour; or follow some types of poisoning. In puppies, hydrocephalus is a cause of fits, but more commonly cutting of the teeth or infestation with parasitic worms.

Deprivation of drinking-water may cause convulsions in dogs as in pigs. (*See* SALT POISONING.)
TREATMENT. Anti-convulsant drugs, such as primidone or phenytoin, may be successful; the dose being the lowest found to control fits over a period. In dogs in which these drugs produce side-effects, phenobarbitone may be tried, though it may cause whining in some dogs. Diazepam is useful, given intra-muscularly alone, as with barbiturates. (*See* CONVULSIONS, EPILEPSY, HYSTERIA.)

FLAGELLA. Whip-like processes possessed by certain bacteria and protozoan parasites and used for purposes of movement.

'FLAIL CHEST'. A condition which may result when one or more ribs are fractured in two places; the damaged area moving slightly inwards on inspiration, and outwards on expiration.

'FLAT PUP' SYNDROME is a condition in which puppies can, at 2 to 3 weeks, use their front legs normally, but the hind-legs are splayed out sideways.

FLAVINE COMPOUNDS, among which are acriflavine, euflavine, and proflavine, are derivatives of aniline. Acriflavine, the hydrochloride of diamino-methyl-acridinium, is an orange-red crystalline powder, soluble in water and forming a powerful antiseptic solution in strengths of 1 in 1000. It stains horn and skin tissues bright yellow. It has been used to control bacterial infection, and stimulate healing, in open wounds.

FLAVOMYCIN. A feed antibiotic. (*See* ADDITIVES.)

'FLEA COLLARS' for dogs and cats are impregnated with a parasiticide, which varies with the manufacturer. Sendran (propexur) is reportedly effective against fleas, lice, and ticks, and capable of ridding a dog of all three within 48 hours. Dichlorvos, used in resin strips attached to the dog's collar is claimed to be effective against fleas for up to 3 months. Animal-owners should select a reliable make, for sometimes ineffective collars appear on the market, and should check their effectiveness; and should also watch for any signs of skin inflammation as a few animals are allergic to some of the chemicals used.

FLEAS are members of the Order *Siphonaptera*, and are degenerate forms of two-winged insects.

The eggs are mostly laid on the floor or bedding; but a few may be laid on the body of the host, from which they fall. They appear as white specks, and pop when burst. Hatching takes from two days (in summer) to 12 days or so.

When fully grown, the legless larva spins a cocoon, in which the pupa develops. The adult flea emerges when conditions of temperature and moisture are favourable. It can remain alive in the cocoon for up to a year.

If infestation is suspected, but not a single flea can be seen, combing may gather some black or dark brown flea faeces. These will form a reddish halo if placed on moistened cotton wool.

Pulex irritans is the human flea, but is frequently found on dogs and cats, and occasionally pigs and horses.

Ctenocephalis canis is the dog flea, but is often found on man and cat. It can transmit *Dipylidium caninum*, as also may the cat flea, *C. felis*, and the human flea, *Pulex irritans*. All these fleas cause severe irritation, and in young or debilitated animals may cause anaemia if numerous. Sensitisation to flea-bites is an important cause of ECZEMA.

In a survey of flea-infested dogs in Dublin, of 128 dogs 86 had dog fleas only; 24 were infested entirely by the human flea; 12 by both dog and human fleas; 4 by cat fleas; and 2 by both dog and cat fleas. (K. P. Baker & C. Hatch. *Vet. Record* (1972), **91**, 151.)

In another survey, carried out at the Royal Veterinary College, London, fleas were recovered from 20 per cent of 193 dogs examined *post mortem*. Three species were found: *Ctenocephalides felis felis*, *C. canis*, and *Orchopeas howardi*. (W. P. Beresford-Jones. *Journal of Small Animal Practice* (1981), **22**, 27.)

Spilopsyllus cuniculi, the European rabbit flea, infests also cats and occasionally dogs.

It was introduced in 1966 into Australia, as a vector of myxomatosis, in order to reduce the rabbit population.

Reproduction of the flea is partly dependent on the reproductive hormones of the rabbit, and so the greatest numbers are present during the rabbit's pregnancy.

In cats *S. cuniculi* attach to the ear pinna causing an itchy dermatitis, but do not breed even on pregnant cats. (Studdert, V. P. & Arundel, J. H. *Veterinary Record* (1988) **123**, 624.)

Archaoppsylla erinacei, the hedgehog flea, only occasionally and temporarily infests dogs, but may cause an allergic dermatitis in them. Cats might become infested too.

Echidnophaga gallinacea, the 'stick-tight' or chicken flea, is usually found attached in dense masses to the head of a fowl or the ear of a dog or cat. Man, horses, and cattle are occasionally infected. It is a common parasite throughout the

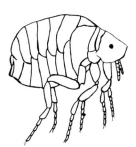

Echidnophaga gallinacea. × 30.

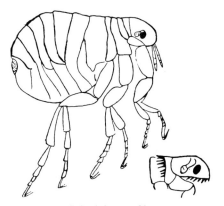

Pulex irritans. × 20.
Inset: head of dog flea.

tropics and is frequently the cause of death in poultry. The female flea, after fertilisation, inserts its mouth parts into the cuticle of the host, and remains there. Ulcers may form; and in any case the flea is difficult to move.

Tunga penetrans, the true jigger flea, differs only in slight details from the last species. The female, however, penetrates the skin, and lying in an inflammatory pocket with an opening to the exterior, becomes as large as a pea. It is found in Africa and America in man and all the domestic mammals, especially the pig. In the Republic of Zaire, for example, localisation of jiggers in the teats of sows has led to death of piglets from lack of milk, to painful enlargement of the udder – with sometimes mastitis.

The presence of the flea may, in addition to being very painful, give rise to ulceration and even gangrene.

The eggs are laid in the ulcers; and the larvae crawl out and pupate on the ground.

Destruction of fleas (*see* INSECTICIDES). Bedding must be destroyed or disinfected and the surrounding floor boards and cracks cleaned thoroughly or the animal will shortly be reinfested. This is even more important than ridding the host of fleas. (*See also* 'FLEA-COLLARS'.) Precautions must be taken with cats, and especially kittens. Owners should follow closely manufacturers' instructions if using an aerosol spray, etc., and should look for the words 'Safe for cats' on proprietory packages. B H C has caused poisoning, and is banned in the UK. Selenium sulphide shampoos offer an alternative.

Flea spray. A new aerosol for the control of fleas in the house introduced by Ceva Ltd. 'Acclaim' contains methoprene and is claimed to prevent the emergence of adult fleas from pupae, thus breaking the life cycle. It is also claimed to be completely safe to mammals. It should be applied as a fine spray to bedding, carpets, curtains and upholstery.

FLIES are mostly, but not exclusively, members of the Order *Diptera* – the two-winged flies.

Even the common housefly can transmit infection such as anthrax and tuberculosis, and also various species of parasitic worms. The stablefly's role in the production of summer mastitis is well known, and other flies, such as the sheep headfly, may be responsible for cases of this disease too. The autumnfly (and almost certainly others) can transmit an eye worm of cattle, and also the infective agent *Moraxella bovis* which causes the more commonly recognised contagious keratitis or 'New Forest disease'.

The approach of a cloud of flies, such as the headfly, will cause cattle to cease grazing and huddle together. The movement or presence of a mass of even non-biting flies over the animal's body represents a further cause of 'worry' or restlessness; and both the headfly and the autumnfly feed on secretions from eyes, nose, etc., and on the serum exuding from small wounds.

Biting flies cause not merely irritation but, as we all know from personal experience, pain. Biting especially on the lower parts of the limbs, and on the flanks, stableflies may make several punctures before taking their blood meal. The size of this may be such as to cause anaemia if there are many stableflies present. Additionally, biting flies may transmit various infections which further reduce the animal's condition; and cattle may be sensitised to the secretions poured

into the bite wound, so that an allergy arises with sometimes the production of serious skin lesions which, in turn, may attract other flies.

Saw fly poisoning. Within four days of being moved to new pasture, a flock of 250 sheep on the Danish island of Sjaelland had sustained 50 deaths. The pasture had many birch trees, which were heavily infested with larvae of the blue-back sawfly (*Arge pullata*). Veterinary investigation confirmed that a toxin present in these was the cause of death, following internal haemorrhage and acute hepatitis.

The sawfly was first reported in Denmark in 1974, stated Dr S. M. Thamsborg and colleagues; but sawfly poisoning of cattle and sheep has been recognised since 1955 in Australia, where heavy losses have occurred. Goats are susceptible also.

The sawfly larva is bright yellow with black dashed lines on the back. It defoliates birch trees, and then drops to the ground to pupate or search for more food. (*Vet. Rec.* (1987) **121**, 253.)

Order diptera. Insects which have one pair of wings.

SIMULIUM (BUFFALO GNATS). The flies of this genus are small thick-set hump-back flies – hence their name. They are often black or reddish-brown in colour. The female mouth parts are short and stout, and are formed for cutting and stabbing. The females at certain times appear in swarms and attack cattle, horses and other animals.

The eggs are laid in water. The larvae, which are aquatic and creep about like leeches, can only live in running well-aerated water. In still water they are asphyxiated. The larva when mature spins a silky cocoon which is attached to water weeds. In this the pupa lies loosely, breathing by means of extruded gill-tufts. The larval stage lasts for 3 to 4 weeks and the pupal stage for 1 to 3 weeks; but the larvae can live over winter and do not pupate until the following spring or summer. The fly is very active in Central Europe, where cattle may die in 2 hours after attack. They show laboured breathing, stumbling gait, rapid pulse, and swellings in pendulous places. In less severe cases loss of appetite, abortion, depression, and temporary or permanent blindness may result.

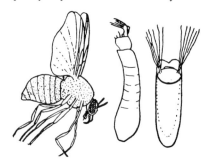

Simulium. Adult larva, and pupa. The adult fly is magnified × about 10.

SANDFLIES. Two-winged flies, of which the blood-sucking females transmit infections, including that of LEISHMANIASIS (which see, and illustration).

MOSQUITO. The mosquito, the carrier of malaria and yellow fever to man, is also of importance in tropical veterinary medicine, transmitting diseases such as 'AVIAN MALARIA', HEARTWORM of dogs, BLUETONGUE, EQUINE ENCEPHALOMYELITIS, AFRICAN HORSE SICKNESS, RIFT VALLEY FEVER (*see under these headings*). In temperate climates, too, mosquitoes are important disease vectors.

Four genera of mosquitoes are of veterinary importance; AEDES, ANOPHELES, CULEX, and MANSONIA.

Eggs are laid on the surface of water or floating vegetation, either singly (*Aedes* and *Anopheles*) or as 'rafts' of eggs.

Larvae undergo three moults, and develop only in water, in which they are highly mobile.

Larvae-eating fish, such as *Alphanus dispar*, are being used in the Nile Delta and elsewhere for mosquito control. (*See also* DDT and DIELDRIN).

MIDGES, BITING (CULICOID). *See* separate entry in alphabetical sections.

GADFLIES. THE TABANIDAE. The family of the gadflies is a large and important one, as the females are blood-suckers.

The eggs are laid in masses on leaves and plants near water. The larvae are more or less aquatic, but towards maturity they live in damp earth or decaying vegetation. The larva is cylindrical, pointed at both ends, and with most of the segments carrying pseudo-pods or false feet. The pupa resembles that of a moth. In temperate climates development takes nearly a year. The males feed on plant juices, but the females are blood-suckers, and in addition carriers of various diseases, as for example, trypanosomiasis, swamp fever in horses, and filariasis in man.

The bite is painful, and causes much irritation to horses and cattle, causing gadding, decrease in milk yield, and so on. No remedies are really satisfactory, although nets have been used with some success on horses.

If the pools most commonly frequented by these flies are covered with a thick layer of paraffin oil, the flies are killed. If this plan is adopted early in the season the numbers can be kept under control.

TABANUS can mechanically transmit surra and other blood diseases such as anthrax. Another species transmits swamp fever in horses.

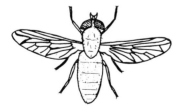

Tabanus. × 2.

HAEMATOPOTA. This is also a world-wide genus. The species have smoky wings, and include the British clegg or horse-fly which, in addition to being a veritable pest to horses, inflicts a very painful bite to man.

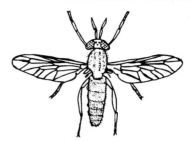

Haematopota. × 3.

CHRYSOPS is distinguished by its long slender antennae, and its green or golden eyes spotted with purple. It is found all over the world, including Britain. This genus is the carrier of the parasite of Calabar swelling in man. It also can inflict a very painful bite.

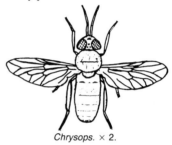

Chrysops. × 2.

The non-biting two-winged flies have an even greater significance to man and his animals than the biting flies.

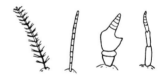

Culex Simulium Tabanus Chrysops.

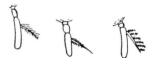

Musca Sarcophaga Glossina.

Antennae of various flies. The small hair seen in the lower row is the 'Arista'.

MUSCIDAE. The flies belonging to this family are smallish to medium-sized flies. The type of this family is *Musca domestica*.

MUSCA DOMESTICA. The great majority of flies found in houses belong to this species. It is a medium-sized fly with four black stripes on its back, and a sharp elbow in the fourth wing vein. The eggs are laid, about 120 in a batch, preferably in horse manure, but occasionally in human or other excreta. They hatch in 24 hours, and the issuing larva (or maggots) feeds and moults and finally becomes full grown in 4 to 5 days. It leaves the manure at this stage, and crawls to a dry spot where it pupates. The puparia are more or less barrel-shaped and dark brown in colour.

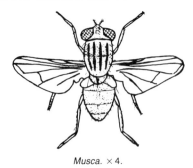

Musca. × 4.

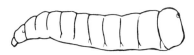

Larva

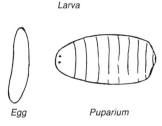

Egg   Puparium

Diagram to illustrate the life-history of *Musca domestica*.

In 4 or 5 days in summer the adult fly emerges. The shortest time on record between the laying of the egg and the appearance of the adult is 8 days; but 10 to 12 days is more normal. In 3 to 4 days the female is ready to lay eggs. The fly lives over the winter in the pupal stage, although in kitchens and warm places adults may be seen at every season of the year.

The house-fly can transmit disease by swallowing bacterial spores, and either bringing them up in their vomit or passing them out in their faeces; or by carrying them about on its hairs and legs. Two species of stomach worm are carried by this fly, in which they pass part of their life-cycle. Among other organisms known to be carried by this fly are anthrax, tuberculosis, and many species of worm eggs. (*See* FLY CONTROL.)

HEADFLY. This is a non-biting fly which, as its name *Hydrotaea irritans* suggests, is a cause of great irritation to cattle, sheep, etc., especially since so many head flies often settle on the same animal. The fly will take advantage of any abrasion on the sheep's skin. Both fly repellents and headcaps have been used and compared at the Redesdale Experimental Husbandry Farm. 'Headcaps gave good and sometimes complete protection,' but are inconvenient in use. Pine-tar oil is a useful repellent.

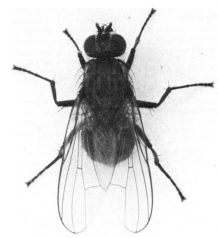

The Headfly. (Crown copyright photograph.)

The headfly is responsible for carrying bacteria to cows' teats (especially when already damaged by biting flies or other causes), and appears to have an important role in producing 'Summer Mastitis'. (*See* MASTITIS.)

FACE FLIES. These 'autumn flies' (*Musca autumnalis*) plague beef and dairy cattle, and horses, at pasture, feeding on watery secretions from nostrils and eyes.

DIPTEROUS LARVAE or MAGGOTS– MYIASIS. Of very great importance to the veterinary surgeon and the agriculturist are those non-biting muscid flies which have taken on a parasitic existence in their larval stages.

Myiasis means the presence of dipterous larvae (or other stages) in organs and tissues of the living animal and the disorders and destruction of tissue caused thereby. (*See* 'STRIKE'.)

The myiasis-producing flies are now usually divided into three groups – specific, semi-specific, and accidental.

Specific: This group consists of flies which *must* breed in living tissue. It includes:

Chrysomyia bezziana,
Cordylobia anthropophaga,
Wohlfahrtia magnifica,
Booponus intonsus, and all the
Oestridae.

Semi-specific: This group consists of flies which, normally breeding in carcases, *may* live in the living animal. It includes the blow-flies, the sheep-maggot flies, and some of the flesh-flies.

Accidental: This group includes all flies the larvae of which, accidentally swallowed with the food, *may* live in the intestine.

The more important of the above flies are considered below.

'BLOW-FLIES' – *Calliphorinae* – are largish muscids of a metallic green or yellow colour.

'COMMON BLOW-FLY' or '*blue-bottle*' – *Calliphora* sp. – has reddish palps, black legs, and a bristly thorax. Their general colour is dark blue with lighter patches on the abdomen. The colour, however, is not lustrous. The ova are usually deposited in decaying animal matter, but occasionally in living tissue.

'GREEN-BOTTLE FLY' – *Lucilia sericata* – is the British sheep-maggot fly. It is also found in Australia and America.

Lucilia caesar, a common species in Europe, does not 'blow' sheep in this country, but does so in countries such as Russia, where other species are absent. Other species of *Lucilia* in India and Australia occasionally are also implicated.

'COPPER-BOTTLE FLY'. *Lucilia cuprina*, the strike fly attacks sheep in Australia and South Africa.

These are of a bright metallic or bluish-green colour, with many strong bristles on the thorax arranged in two parallel rows. There are no stripes on the thorax or abdomen. The cheeks are not hairy as in *Calliphora*.

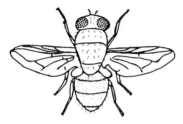

Lucilia. This fly is larger than the house-fly and smaller than the blow-fly.

This genus blows wool, but occasionally infects wounds.

Chrysomyia bezziana, found in India, Africa, and the Philippines, is a metallic greenish-blue blow-fly, closely related to *Lucilia*, but with dark transverse abdominal bands and with fewer and less-developed thoracic bristles. The metallic sheen is more brassy than in *Lucilia*. This fly breeds only in living tissue – in discharges from natural orifices, or in sores and cuts. Up to 500 eggs may be laid at one time. They hatch in about 30 hours, and the larvae rapidly reach maturity, crawl out and pupate on the ground. Several other species of this genus are semi-specific myiasis flies, normally breeding in decaying matter. These include *C. albiceps*, a notorious sheep-maggot fly in Australia.

'SCREW-WORM FLY' – *Callitroga americana* – in America, can be distinguished from the old-world species by the three well-marked blue dorsal stripes on the thorax and dark hairs on the abdomen. It is of a dark bluish-green colour, with a well-marked yellowish-red face. (*See also* FLY CONTROL.)

This species will lay eggs in decaying animal or vegetable matter, but will also oviposit in any diseased tissue, in wounds in the vulvae of freshly calved cows, the umbilical cord of calves, and so on. The ova hatch in 24 hours, and the maggot matures in 4 to 6 days. The pupal stage on the ground lasts 3 to 10 days. The maggot resembles a blue-bottle maggot, but the deeply cut constrictions between segments and the prominent rings of spines give it its popular name.

As soon as the egg hatches, the larva starts burrowing into the flesh. It can penetrate the sound tissue of living animals, and may even lay bare the bones.

'TUMBU FLY', *Cordylobia anthropophaga*: a specific myiasis fly in Africa, attacking many hosts. It is a dirty brownish-yellow blow-fly with blackish markings. Eggs are laid in dust and rubbish on which the host, usually a dog, is accustomed to lie. The small larva may live apart from the host for 10 days, but it may eventually burrow into the epidermis or die. It moults in this position, and forms a **'tumbu'** below the skin with an opening to the exterior through which it breathes. The 'tumbu' does not suppurate unless the larva dies. The larva emerges in about 7 or 8 days, and 2 or 3 days later it pupates. The adults emerge in about 20 days. This fly does not burrow into the deeper tissues. The scrotum is a common site of the maggot. Putting a drop of oil or Vaseline over the breathing hole will force the larva to protrude, when it can be removed.

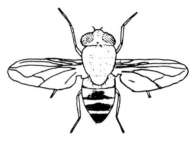

Cordylobia. × 2½.

Booponus intonsus is a light yellow specific myiasis fly found in the Philippines, which is somewhat allied to *Cordylobia*. It infects bovines and goats.

The eggs are laid on the hairs on the lower parts of the legs; and the larvae make their way to the coronet and bury themselves in the flesh. The larvae resemble the screw-worm. The larval period seems to last 2 or 3 weeks, when it leaves the host and pupates in the ground. The pupal life is 10 days.

The larvae cause a considerable lameness with numerous superficial wounds and distortion of the horn. The larva is called the 'foot maggot'.

'FLESH FLIES' – *Sarcophidae* – are closely related to the *Muscidae*. The body is more elongated than the blow-flies, and they are usually grey in colour, with a mottled abdomen and a striped thorax. They generally bring forth living larvae instead of laying eggs. Two genera are important.

Sarcophaga spp. These are large grey flies with red eyes and square chequered markings on the abdomen. The third segment of the antenna is long. All the species normally breed in decaying animal matter, but may be found in old festering wounds. They are found throughout the world.

Wohlfahrtia magnifica resembles the preceding genus, but has well-defined round spots on the abdomen. The third segment of the antenna is short and the arista is without bristles. It is widely distributed in Russia, Asia Minor, and Egypt. The larvae never attack carcases, but are *always* found in wounds and natural cavities of living animals. The fly deposits living larvae on sores and discharges.

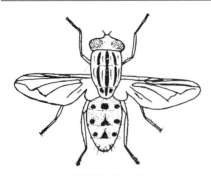

Wohlfahrtia. × 3.

In Australia the most important sheep-maggot flies are *Calliphora augur*, a large orange-coloured fly; *Calliphora stygia*, the common sheep-maggot fly, often called the 'golden-haired blow-fly'; and *Chrysomyia albiceps* var. *putoni*, the larva of which is known as the 'hairy maggot'.

Injuries due to maggots. The injuries due to maggots may be roughly divided into two classes – larvae attacking wounds and discharges, and larvae attacking the wool of sheep. The first class of injuries are found on any animal, including man. The flies usually, but not always select old sores. Some, such as *Chrysomyia americana*, the 'screw-worm', will penetrate into the sound tissue, and prefer fresh wounds or carcases. The infected wound usually has a watery discharge.

Prevention is obviously most important. (*See also under* MYIASIS.)

BLOOD-SUCKING MUSCID FLIES. These flies, which resemble the house-fly in general appearance, are responsible for an enormous amount of damage to farm animals. When one considers that they include such flies as the tsetse fly, the stable-fly, and the horn-fly, this is easily understood.

STOMOXYS. This genus is mainly confined to Africa and Asia, but one species, *S. calcitrans*, the **stable-fly**, is world-wide in its distribution.

Stomoxys breeds in stable manure and in other places where moisture and organic material is found. The eggs hatch in 2 to 3 days, and the larva, which is similar to but smaller than *Musca*, becomes full-grown in 2 to 3 weeks. The pupal stage lasts 9 to 13 days. Development is more rapid in the tropics, where the time between egg and adult may be reduced to 12 days.

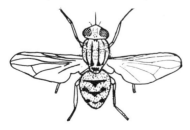

Stomoxys. × 3.

This fly is a serious pest to horses and other animals. It will also bite man. Apart from the extreme irritation of its bite, it can transmit anthrax, surra, and other diseases. It is also the intermediate host of *Habronema microstomum*, a worm parasite of horses.

HAEMATOBIA. *H. stimulans* is a common blood-sucking parasite of cattle, and occasionally horses and man, in Europe. It resembles *Stomoxys*, but has spatulate palps as long as the proboscis, and has hairs on both sides of the arista. It breeds in fresh cattle dung. The larva becomes full-grown in 6 to 9 days, while the pupal stage lasts 5 to 8 days.

LYPEROSIA. *L. irritans* is very closely related to *Haematobia*, but can be distinguished from it by the absence of bristles from the under side of the arista. It is found in Europe (including the U K) and America. It is a very serious pest to cattle, clustering round the base of the horns, a habit which gives the fly its popular name of **horn-fly**. The irritation caused by their bites is estimated to cause a drop in milk yield amounting in some cases to 50 per cent. The flies breed in fresh cow dung. Flies emerge in about 15 days after the egg is deposited. The maggots must have moisture, and can be destroyed by any means which will dry the manure quickly. The horn-fly seldom goes far from its host, and may be destroyed by attaching splash-boards to ordinary dippers. The fly leaves the cattle at the moment of entering the bath, but the dip, caught and flung back by the splash-board, drenches and destroys the flies. The hotter and more excited the cattle the closer the flies stick and the greater number killed. Any oily dip is suitable. (*See also* FLY CONTROL.)

TSETSE FLIES (GLOSSINA). The flies of this genus, are, with one exception (found in Arabia), confined to Africa. They are the notorious carriers of trypanosomiasis in man and animals. *Glossina* resembles a large stable-fly; but has a feathered arista, long slender palps, a slender shaft to the proboscis, and a peculiar wing venation. The life-history is unusual. The female produces one living larva at a time and deposits it when full-grown. It immediately pupates. One female produces only about a dozen larvae in her life.

Over a dozen species of glossina are known. The most important are: *G. palpalis*; *G. morsitans*; *G. brevipalpis*; *G. longipalpis*; *G. pallidipes*; *G. tachinoides.*

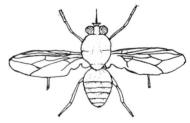

Glossina. × 2½.

BOT AND WARBLE FLIES. *Oestridae.* The bot family consists of hairy, heavy flies with rudimentary mouth parts. The female attaches the egg, or, in the case of the nostril flies, places the larva on a suitable host, and the remainder of the larval life is parasitic. When mature the larvae leave the host and pupate on the ground.

These flies may be placed in three groups according to the habitat of the larva:

(1) In the alimentary canal –
   Gastrophilus, the horse bot.
   Cobboldia, the elephant bot.
(2) In the head sinuses –
   Oestrus, the sheep nostril fly;
   Rhinaestrus, the horse nostril fly;
   Cephalomyia, the camel nostril fly; and others.
(3) In the subcutaneous tissue –
   Hypoderma, the warble-fly;
   Dermatobia, the macaw worm fly; and others.

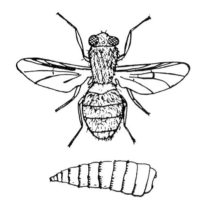

Gastrophilus. (Adult fly × 2½, and 'Bot' × 2.)

BOT FLIES (GASTROPHILUS). The flies of this genus are large and hairy, with large compound eyes and three ocelli. The females have an elongated ovipositor which is bent under the body when at rest. Four species are of importance.

G. intestinalis (*G. equi*), the common horse bot, has cloudy wings; it deposits its eggs on any part of the horse, but especially on the distal ends of the hairs. The eggs require moisture and friction (supplied by licking) before they will hatch.

G. nasalis (*G. veterinus*) is smaller, more hairy, and has a rusty coloured thorax. It oviposits usually at the proximal ends of hairs under the jaw. It lays one egg and flies to a distance, returning later to lay another.

G. haemorrhoidalis has a bright orange-red tip to the abdomen. It deposits its eggs only at the base of the small hairs on the lips of the horse. The eggs may hatch without moisture or friction.

G. pecorum resembles *G. intestinalis*. In colour it is yellowish-brown to nearly black with brownish-clouded wings. Its habits are similar to that species.

The distribution of the first three is universal, but the last seems to be restricted to Europe and South Africa.

The life-history of the species of this genus is not fully understood yet. Some of the newly hatched larvae *may* pierce the skin or buccal mucous membrane. In any case the larvae are found in various parts of the alimentary tract. Each species has its own special preference. *G. intestinalis* is usually found in the stomach,

occasionally the duodenum; *G. nasalis* prefers the duodenum, but has been found in the pharynx and stomach; *G. haemorrhoidalis* is found in the stomach, duodenum, rectum, and even in the anus; while *G. pecorum* usually occurs in the pharynx or stomach, but may be recovered from any part.

Bots when present in large numbers in the stomach or intestine, or even in small numbers about the pharynx and anus, may cause a considerable suffering to their host by mere mechanical obstruction. The adult fly worries the horse considerably especially the species *G. nasalis* and *G. haemorrhoidalis*, and may cause loss of condition.

Treatment. Formerly, carbon disulphide, administered in autumn and early winter by stomach tube and followed by warm saline. Recently, a dichlorvos formulation* has proved effective (also against round worms). Withholding water 4 hours before and after dosing is recommended when treating against bots. In 1983 an ivermectin paste was introduced (*See* AVERMECTINS, IVERMECTIN.)

Some control is possible by regular removal of the 'nits' from the lower limbs of grazing horses during summer.

OESTRUS. *Oestrus ovis*, the sheep nostril fly, is somewhat larger than the house-fly and is greyish yellow to brown in colour. It is found practically all over the world. It deposits eggs, or larvae. The hovering female 'strikes' at the nostrils, and the

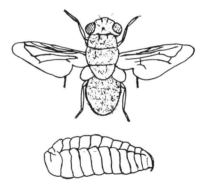

Oestrus. (Fly × 2; maggot × 1.)

young larvae crawl up the nose, and may lodge in one of the sinuses of the skull. It remains there until fully grown, when it is sneezed out and pupates in the ground.

Prevention is carried out by means of an application of tar to the nostrils. This may be applied by means of a salt lick, access to which may only be obtained by smallish holes (2 inches) smeared with tar. Ploughing a single furrow across a sheep pasture, allows the sheep to protect their nostrils from the flies 'strike', and gives some measure of protection. Some anthelmintics are effective.

RHINOESTRUS. *Rhinoestrus purpureus* (*R. nasalis*), the horse nostril fly, is common in Central Europe and North Africa. It is a smallish fly with the body covered with small tubercles, and is

* 'Equigard' pellets given in the feed.

closely related to *Oestrus*. The female deposits a number of living larvae at one time in the eyes or the nose of the horse (and occasionally man). The larvae may be found about the cranial cavities or even in the pharynx or larynx. Russian Gadfly is a synonym.

HYPODERMA. Two species of warble-flies, *Hypoderma bovis* and *H. lineatum*, are found in cattle (and occasionally in the horse). Both are very extensively found in Europe and America.

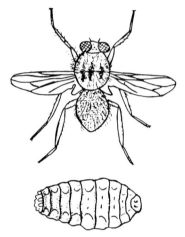

Hypoderma. (Fly × 2; and 'Warble' × 1½.)

Hypoderma bovis is a largish fly with yellow hair just behind the head. The under part of the abdomen is nearly black, while the tail end is orange yellow. The legs have few hairs.

Hypoderma lineatum is rather smaller with a reddish-orange tail and rough hairy legs.

H. bovis lays its eggs one on the base of each hair at a time. The fly has a most terrifying effect on cattle, and causes them to gallop madly in all directions. *H. lineatum* irritates animals less than does *H. bovis*. The ova are generally deposited while the animal is lying in the shade. A number of eggs – up to fourteen – are laid on the same hair, and are often in full view.

In both cases larvae emerge in several days and pierce the skin. They travel up through the connective tissue and finally reach the back. Under the skin the larvae form a small swelling (about the middle of winter), which moves about at first, but gradually becomes still and enlarges. A small opening appears in the centre through which the larva breathes. In spring the larva falls to the ground and pupates. Several weeks later the adult fly emerges.

The presence of the larvae may decrease the milk yield by 10 per cent to 20 per cent, cause a considerable depreciation in flesh near the points where the larvae are, and enormously reduce the value of the hide. The adult fly also causes loss through the mad chasing about of cattle. (*See also under* WARBLES.)

Hypoderma diana is a warble-fly affecting deer.

DERMATOBIA. *Dermatobia hominis*, the macaw worm-fly, is a parasite of cattle and other domesticated animals (and occasionally man) in tropical America. It is a medium-sized fly, grey or steel-blue in colour, with pale brown wings. The female lays its eggs on the body of some blood-sucking arthropod, usually a mosquito. This carrier attacks an animal 5 or 6 days later, and the larvae, rapidly escaping from their shells, pierce the skin of the host, and form a local tumour near where they were deposited. In a month or so they emerge and pupate.

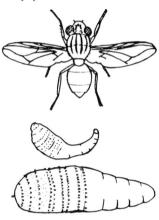

Dermatobia. (Fly and maggots × 1½.)

PUPIPARA. This family, which includes the sheep ked and the New Forest fly, was so called because live larvae are produced which pupate at once. The adults in this case are blood-sucking parasites with a hard integument with a broad neckless head and very stout legs ending in grasping claws. Wings are present or absent. Two genera are important.

Hippobosca equina, the New Forest fly or horse ked, has wings which, however, are seldom used, the fly preferring to run swiftly between the hairs of the host. It is a typical member of the group.

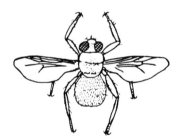

Hippobosca. × 2.

PARAGLE FLY. *Paragle redicum*, an anthomyiid fly, lays its eggs in canine faeces, and the white specks have been mistaken for tapeworm segments. Larvae may also be passed alive through the canine (and also the human) gut. (Urquhart, H. R. and others, 1984, *Veterinary Record* **114,** 68.)

Hymenoptera. Insects which have two pairs of wings.

SAWFLIES. These have four wings and a saw-like ovipositor. The larvae are said to be poisonous if swallowed.

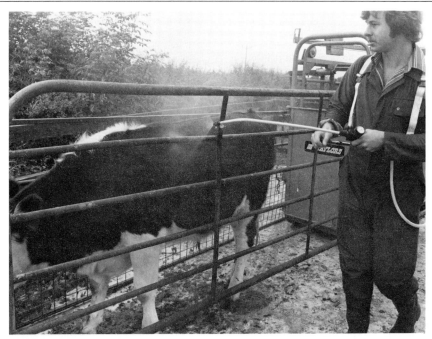

Fly control by means of a knapsack sprayer, using a Shell insecticide, Barricade, based on a synthetic pyrethroid.

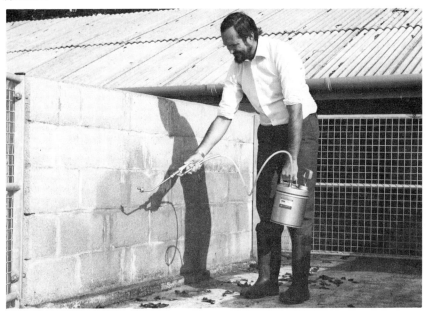

For housed stock, spraying walls may suffice. The preparation being used is Stomoxin P, a Wellcome Foundation product based on a synthetic pyrethroid and stated to be 10 times more lethal to house flies than DDT.

Fly control measures. Perceptive farmers have for many years realised the harmful effects of fly infestation on livestock, but only now is the full importance of these effects becoming widely recognised. Controlled field trials, comparing the productivity of treated and untreated cattle, have convincingly demonstrated the advantages that can be gained by modern fly-control methods. Moreover, recent developments in in-

secticides and application methods have made fly control a far more practicable and cost-effective undertaking.

Flies interfere with normal rest and feeding. The approach of a cloud of flies often causes cattle to cease grazing and huddle together. All countrymen are familiar with the sight of cattle 'gadding'; and swarms of black fly (*Simulium ornatum*) may not merely cause store cattle to break out of fields, or rush round them, but can actually kill cattle.

The horse fly (*Tabanus*), like the stable fly (*Stomoxys*), has a painful bite, and the wounds inflicted attract other flies, which exacerbate the 'worry' situation and often transmit even more infection. Some animals become sensitised to the secretions of biting flies, so that an allergy results. One example of this is the 'sweet itch' of horses caused by biting (*Culicoid*) midges.

Flies are notorious for spreading livestock diseases. Even the common house fly (*Musca domestica*) can transmit anthrax, tuberculosis, and the larvae of some parasitic worms. The headfly (*Hydrotaea irritans*) is among several species that may transmit the bacteria that cause 'summer mastitis'. All too often this leads to gangrene of part of the udder, usually with the permanent loss of use of one quarter – and to great pain and occasionally death of the cow.

Besides interfering with grazing, the headfly causes infested sheep to scratch, rub and knock their heads, often breaking the skin. Open wounds then attract other flies, increasing the tendency to self-mutilation. Sometimes the whole poll region becomes raw. Pine-tar oil has been used as a repellent; and headcaps for protection, but they are inconvenient to use.

Plastic tags impregnated with synthetic pyrethroids have been used to great effect in the reduction of 'fly-worry' in cattle. For sheep too, it was found at the Moredun Institute that tags containing cypermethrin and permethrin were effective in controlling the severity of damage caused by headflies.

The activities of the autumn fly (*Musca autumnalis*) are very similar to those of the headfly. Both flies feed on secretions from nose, mouth, eyes and wounds, and are among several species that transmit the various pathogens causing 'New Forest disease'. This involves an acute and painful conjunctivitis, with inflammation also of the cornea, which becomes opaque, so that cattle are often rendered temporarily blind. Complications may result in permanent eye defects and impaired sight; but even without them the disease causes stress and, since it interferes with feeding, loss of condition can be appreciable.

Other bacterial diseases spread by flies include salmonellosis and brucellosis; while viral diseases such as swine fever and foot-and-mouth have in the past been similarly transmitted in the UK. The larvae of some flies also parasatise animals; for example the 'green-bottle' fly causing strike in sheep, and the sheep nostril fly, and the horse bot flies. The mere approach of warble flies cause cattle to stampede, and the larvae undoubtedly cause pain during their migration through the cow's body, and probably irritation while present in the skin swellings, or warbles. In a few instances, cows die following the accidental crushing of larvae in the warbles, and larvae occasionally seriously damage the spinal cord.

Deterring and killing flies. The number of flies entering a milking parlour can be reduced by a spray-boom erected over the doorways, and a plain water mist, produced by ordinary sprinklers or misters, has been recommended by MAFF for use in collecting yards where a spray-boom over the parlour entrance is impracticable. Such measures, however, do not reduce the total fly population of the farm – they do not kill. Electric fly traps do, and a few farmers have installed them in piggeries and dairy cattle buildings. Which flies are electrocuted will obviously depend on the feeding and resting habits of the various species.

Of far wider application, and the most effective weapon against farm flies, is the insecticidal spray. This can be used to convert a livestock building into one big fly trap. Many long-established insecticides are suitable for this purpose, but the newer ones obviously have an initial advantage, in that flies will not have had time to develop resistance to them.

For housed stock, spraying walls may suffice; but beef and dairy cattle at grass will be the target of flies coming from their resting places among trees. Fly control, if it is to benefit grazing animals, therefore requires application of an officially approved insecticide direct to their backs. For this purpose, the synthetic pyrethroids have a promising future.

Developed at the Rothamsted Experimental Station in Hertfordshire, under the auspices of the National Development Corporation, these new insecticides are chemically allied to the active ingredients of pyrethrum, but are more potent as fly-killers and are also light-stable so that they stay effective longer in the sun.

In 1978 Shell Chemicals UK introduced Outflank, a formulation of the synthetic pyrethroid permethrin for use as a spray on the walls of buildings. In 1979 the Wellcome Foundation introduced another permethrin-based formulation, Stomoxin, for spraying – after dilution – direct on to the animal. Stomoxin is stated to be 10 times more lethal to house flies than DDT, and up to five times more so than organo-phosphorus insecticides; and to present no threat to food.

UK field trials with Stomoxin involved over 10,000 cattle. A spray arch was used on seven of the 48 farms, on many of which a hand lance connected to a tractor-driven sprayer was a popular method; three farmers simply used watering cans to apply the insecticide to the cows' backs.

Fly control for horses and ponies. Barricade (Shell) was officially approved as the first synthetic pyrethroid formulation for spraying on to these animals. It is based on cypermethrin.

In 1985 Beecham Animal Health introduced a PVC fly band, impregnated with cypermethrin, for threading on to either the browband or the crownpiece of a headcollar.

Success has been claimed for a special ear tag impregnated with 8 per cent cypermethrin, and developed by Shell, for cattle at pasture.

Whether measured in terms of reduced animal suffering, or farmers' incomes, or a lowered incidence of diseases – some of which are of public health as well as economic importance – fly control is very worthwhile. If further evidence of its effectiveness were needed, any doubter should note the encouraging progress of MAFF's five-year plan to eradicate warble flies from the UK. A Meat and Livestock Commission survey has shown that the average level of infestation fell from 34·3% in May 1978 to 8·6% by May 1979. Not only were fewer cattle infested, but the average level of warbles in each was greatly reduced. Since, though to a much lesser extent, horses, as well as cattle, suffer from warble-fly larvae, the campaign – if it succeeds – will benefit them and their owners.

Overseas, an automatic sprayer, operated by a photo-electric cell, has been successfully used at Pennsylvania State University, both on range and in cowshed doorways.

The release of sterile male flies from aircraft has been used on a large scale in Puerto Rico to control the screw-worm fly.

In tropical regions simple fly traps are used; but also the spraying of ground with DDT and dieldrin (stated WHO in 1980) for the control of tsetse flies and human trypanosomiasis; but *see also under* TROPICS.

In 1985 over 60 million genetically engineered blowfly maggots were due to be dropped on a small island off the south Australian coast, in an attempt to eradicate sheep blowflies, 'currently costing farmers A$150 million annually, *New Scientist* reported. The maggots were altered so that females which mate will produce blind or sterile offspring – hereditary characteristic which will 'confer genetic death on future generations.' (*See also* DIPS and DIPPING.)

FLOODS (*see* PASTURE CONTAMINATION, SALMONELLOSIS, WATER-DROPWORT).

FLOOR (*see under* BEDDING (for pigs), HOUSING OF ANIMALS).

FLOOR FEEDING OF PIGS. This practice is attractive to the pig farmer since it saves the cost of troughs and also saves space; the normal feeding passage becoming a catwalk over the pigs' sleeping quarters.

From a health point of view, the precise composition of the concrete floor may prove important. In an outbreak of illness among pigs in Eire, with anaemia, gastric ulceration, and haemorrhage, the cause was thought to be the 'pit sand' (with a high iron content) with which the concrete was made, giving rise to iron poisoning once the surface layer had been licked off.

More important is the fact that loss of appetite in pigs – a common symptom of many diseases – may not be noticed. With trough-feeding, it is easy to see which pigs are uninterested in food.

Feeding pellets instead of meal may also cause trouble – digestive upsets. The method may involve more stress than conventional systems.

FLOOR SPACE. As a rough guide, the following *minimum* figures may be given: bacon pig, 6 square feet; veal calf, 12 square feet; laying hen on deep litter, 2½ square feet.

FLOOR SWEEPINGS in mill or barn have been added to feed and caused fatal poisoning. For example, pigs have died in this way from nitrate poisoning, and cattle from mustard seed poisoning.

'FLOPPY' LABRADORS. The colloquial name for an inherited muscle disease of both black and yellow Labrador retrievers. The condition has been seen both in the UK and the USA. Inheritance is associated with an autosomal recessive gene, and leads to 'a deficiency of type II muscle fibres.' (Ruth McKerrell. 1986 BVA Congress paper).
SIGNS. Poor exercise tolerance, especially in cold weather, a stiff hopping gait, with sometimes collapse. Signs have been shown as early as 8 weeks of age, but in other cases after several months.

FLOUR (*see* AGENE PROCESS).

FLOUR MITE INFESTATION (*Acarus farinae*). Infestation of animal feeds by these mites can cause a significant loss of nutrient value, as explained under DIET. Like forage mites of various species, flour mites can also cause an irritating parasitic skin disease of animals. In one incident 36 police horses were stabled in a building which was cleaned and whitewashed before their arrival. Unfortunately a feed barrow was overlooked and still contained oats left over from the previous year. New oats of high quality were delivered in sacks, and the delivery man opened one sack and topped up the barrow. After he had gone, new oats continued to be put on top of what was left in the large feed barrow, which was never completely emptied. A fortnight after the horses' arrival, the last four in the line showed signs of head and neck irritation. One horse had rubbed one side of its neck bare; two others had dermatitis on the poll and alongside the mane.

Examination of the bottom layer of the barrow's contents revealed an enormous number of flour mites, and these were also isolated from the skin lesions. (Norval, J. & McPherson, E. A. (1983) *Veterinary Record* **112**, 385.)

An unsuspected cause of diarrhoea in dogs may be dog biscuits or meal, stored in large bins, and heavily infested with forage mites. As flies may carry nymphal forage mites, fly control is important in reducing such infestations.

The finding of forage mites and/or their eggs in dog faeces was made in the parasitology department of the Royal Veterinary College, England, by Dr M. T. Fox and colleagues. They pointed out that on several occasions the forage mite eggs had been mistaken elsewhere for the eggs of Strongyle worms from dogs reported as unresponsive to anthelmintics. However, the mite's egg is nearly double the size of the worm's egg.

Flour mites (*Acarus siro* and *A. farinae*), the house/furniture mite (*Glycyphagus domesticus*), and the mould mites (*Tyrophagus putrescentiae* and *T. longior* may also be involved. (Fox, M. T. & others. *Veterinary Record* (1986) **118**, 459).

FLUID REPLACEMENT THERAPY (*see under* DEHYDRATION).

FLUKES and FLUKE DISEASE (*see* LIVER FLUKES, LUNG FLUKES, SCHISTOSOMIASIS for Blood Flukes, PANCREAS, DISEASES OF; and RUMEN FLUKES.)

FLUORESCENT (*see under* TETRACYCLINES which make bone fluoresce, and *under* WOOD'S LAMP which shows ringworm-affected hairs fluorescing). For the fluorescent antibody test, *see under* RABIES *and* IMMUNOFLUORESCENT MICROSCOPY.

FLUORESCIN (FLUORESCEIN) is a useful diagnostic agent in injuries and ulcers on the cornea of the eye. A weak solution is dropped into the eye and the injured area can be seen clearly demarcated from the surrounding healthy cornea.

FLUORINE. This element occurs in body tissues and in some natural water supplies. Excess of fluorine causes mottling of the teeth. (For fluorine poisoning, *see* FLUOROSIS.)

FLUOROACETATE POISONING. Sodium mono-fluoroacetate ('1080') is used to kill rats and mice, and it is in this connection that poisoning in domestic animals and man may arise. The drug causes distress, yelping, sometimes vomiting, and convulsions in the dog. Treatment consists in the administration of nembutal. The dose of '1080' which was found to kill one dog in two was 0·66 mg per kg. '1080' is banned in the UK.

In 1963, two outbreaks of fatal poisoning involving numerous dogs, cats, cattle and a pony were attributed to the agricultural insecticide fluoroacetamide.

FLUOROSIS or chronic fluorine poisoning is of economic importance in cattle, sheep, etc., grazing pastures contaminated by fluorine compounds emanating from iron and steel works and other industrial plant. It has also been reported in dairy cattle receiving mineral supplements with a high fluorine content, the result of incorporation of rock phosphate. This is something which animal feed manufacturers should guard against, and they should offer guarantees concerning maximum fluorine content in their products.
SIGNS. There is severe lameness, and a resulting loss of condition; milk yield is greatly reduced. The teeth may become mottled, and the bones become particularly liable to fracture. Cows may stand with their legs crossed in cases of fracture of the pedal bones. Hip lameness is probably more common.
ANTIDOTE. Calcium aluminate is of some *limited* value as an antidote to fluorine poisoning.

FLUOTHANE is a trade name for HALOTHANE.

FLURBIPROFEN. Fluriprofen, Flurbiprofen and Ibuprofen are non-steroidal anti-inflammatory drugs (Froben and Brufen; Boots Medical) used in human medicine, and sometimes given to dogs by their owners, or eaten by dogs with access to the tablets, with resultant poisoning – sometimes fatal. Stomach ulceration and kidney failure have been caused.

FLUSHING OF EWES aims for rising metabolism in breeding ewes some 6 to 3 weeks before service, by putting them on to protein-rich feed. The purpose is to intensify subsequent oestrus and thereby ensure that each ewe is in fit condition to breed.

In some recent experiments, doubt has been cast on the efficacy of flushing.

FOALING (*see* PARTURITION).

FOALS are young horses of either sex until the time they are one year old. Male foals are known as 'colt foals', and female foals are called 'filly foals'. Most foals are born between March and June in Britain, although quite a number (especially thoroughbreds) are dropped earlier than this. Thoroughbreds are conventionally aged as from 1st January of the year in which they are born, and all other horses from the 1st May, irrespective of whether they were actually foaled before or after these dates.

Generally speaking, foals run with their dams at grass during the summer, and are weaned at from 4 to 6 months of age. With weakly foals, however, and in the case of highly bred pedigree animals, it is not uncommon to allow them to run with their dams until nearly Christmas-time, so that they may get an exceptionally good start in life.

As a rule, foals will begin to eat grass when they are between 3 weeks and a month old, although some start earlier and some later than this. At about 6 weeks to 2½ months they will begin to eat dry corn from mangers along with their mothers.

FOALS, DISEASES OF.

Diarrhoea may occur as a result of changes in the mare's milk, due to metritis or laminitis, for example; or as a result of the dam grazing avidly upon rich spring grass, etc.

So-called 'foal heat' diarrhoea is common and occurs 7 to 10 days after birth, and accordingly often coincides with the mare's first *post-partum* oestrus; but the precise cause has not been established.
Salmonella typhimurium may cause a subclinical infection; or acute and severe diarrhoea or septicaemia, the latter often following the former. (*See* SALMONELLOSIS.)
Escherichia coli is another cause of acute diarrhoea in the foal. (*See* E. COLI.)
Corynebacterium equi is probably a more common cause of pneumonia than of diarrhoea; nevertheless the latter can be severe. Clostridial

enterotoxaemia occurs; likewise campylobacter infections.

Viruses causing diarrhoea in foals include a CORONAVIRUS and a ROTAVIRUS. The latter may be associated with a profuse, watery diarrhoea and lymph node enlargement, sometimes followed by death. (*See also* GLOBIDIOSIS.)

Navel-ill and Joint-ill. These are colloquial terms for dangerous infections which may attack the foal within the first fortnight of its life. Pain and swelling at the navel, with sometimes abscesses along the umbilical vein, may occur; but Joint-Ill (Polyarthritis) symptoms may be noticed first. Often the hock and stifle joints are painful and swollen, there is fever, and the foal is obviously ill.

Treatment includes the use of appropriate antibiotics (but *not* corticosteroids, which have an immunosuppressive effect).

Organisms causing Septicaemia and Joint-Ill
Escherichia coli
Actinobacillus equuli
Streptococcus zooepidemicus
Klebsiella pneumonia, etc.

(with acknowledgements to Dr Hugh Platt).

Septicaemia is always a danger likely to arise with or after the last two conditions. Septicaemia due to *Actinobacillus equuli* infection (**'Sleepy foal disease'**) may occur within the first three days of life. The foal becomes dull, disinclined to suck, has stupor, diarrhoea, and prostration and death quickly follow. Polyarthritis may occur in foals which survive a little longer.

Haemolytic disease. This results from an incompatibility between the blood of sire and dam, and the consequent production of antibodies which reach the foal in the colostrum and break down the foal's red blood cells. These become so reduced in number that not only is there jaundice but often also a fatal anaemia. If trouble from this cause were anticipated, the use of a foster-mother might save the situation but, obviously, this is seldom practicable. Moreover, unless the mare has previously had a 'jaundiced foal', there will be no inkling of what is in store. If she has, however, it is possible to test her blood against the sire's during pregnancy and obtain a fairly good idea as to their incompatibility or otherwise. Treatment must be undertaken quickly and consists in exchange transfusion – the removal of up to 5 pints of the foal's blood and the simultaneous injection of up to 6 pints of a compatible donor's blood, previously bottled. The transfusion requires special apparatus and takes about 3 hours to complete. Recoveries following this treatment have been spectacular.

Worms. Both strongyles (red worms) and ascarids may cause trouble in foals. The former give rise to malaise, cough, unthriftiness, tiredness, and sometimes abdominal pain; the latter to diarrhoea and intermittent colic, among other symptoms. The Animal Health Trust recommends that foals be dosed every 4 weeks, alternately for ascarids and strongyles, until the age of 1 year.

Bone diseases in foals include VALGUS (described under BONE, DISEASES OF); and RICKETS which can render the growth-plate more vulnerable to injury.

Skin diseases. Congenital or inherited conditions include *Epitheliogenesis imperfecta* and ICTHIOSIS. ALOPECIA is sometimes a complication of STRANGLES; to which URTICARIA is an occasional sequel.

Tyzzer's disease (which see) may also have jaundice as one symptom; others being dullness, disinclination to suck, a 'sleepiness' common also to 'Sleepy foal disease', possibly convulsions, diarrhoea. Death may occur suddenly before symptoms have shown. It is thought that mice may transmit the infection.

Pneumonia, due to *Corynebacterium equi,* occurs sporadically in the UK. A suppurative broncho-pneumonia, with abscesses in the lungs and pulmonary lymph nodes, it may be associated with 'Joint-ill' and osteomyelitis.

Combined antibacterial drug treatment is recommended for foals suffering from pneumonia caused by *Corynebacterium equi.* The response to treatment should be monitored clinically and radiographically and it is recommended that treatment should be continued for two weeks after the foal is both clinically and radiographically normal. The preferred combination of antibiotics is the oral administration of erythromycin estolate (25 mg/kg four times daily) plus rifampin (10 mg/kg twice daily). Erythromycin can also be combined for synergistic effect with sodium benzylpenicillin (100,000 iu/kg, intravenously, four times daily) or with ampicillin (11 to 15 mg/kg, intravenously, four times daily). (Prescott, J. F. & Sweeney, C. R. (1985) *Journal of the American Veterinary Medical Association* **187,** 725.)

Rhinopneumonitis. A congenital infection with EHV 1 virus is a case of early death in foals. (*See* EQUINE RHINOPNEUMONITIS.)

Muscular dystrophy (*see under* MUSCLES, DISEASES OF).

Pervious urachus, or 'leaking at the navel', is a condition in which the communication between the urinary bladder and the umbilicus or navel outside, which should close at the time of birth, remains patent and allows urine to dribble from it. The urine blisters the skin around, becomes decomposed and gives rise to a foul odour, and ultimately results in considerable swelling and suppuration around the navel. It should be treated by operation as soon as it is noticed, and kept clear by the application of antiseptics.

Combined immunodeficiency (CID) occurs in some Arab foals. (*See* IMMUNODEFICIENCY). (*See also under* HERNIA, VALGUS, *and* TYZZER'S DISEASE.)

FODDER BEET (*see* POISONING).

FODDER MITES (*see* FLOUR MITES).

FOETAL, FOETUS (*see* FETAL, FETUS).

FOG (*see under* SMOG *and below*).

'FOG FEVER'. The colloquial name derived from the word 'fog', meaning the second crop of grass taken from pasture already cut once that season for hay or silage, has caused much confusion, since it has been applied to several different syndromes in cattle.

Dr R. G. Breeze and his veterinary research colleagues at the University of Glasgow defined (1976) fog fever as acute pulmonary emphysema occurring in adult cattle which had been moved from poor to lush grazing in the autumn.

They regard fog fever as similar to, if not identical with, the acute bovine pulmonary emphysema encountered in North American adult cattle (of beef type) moved from range to lush pasture: and they differentiate fog fever from the effects of parasitic bronchitis, and also from extrinsic allergic alveolitis caused by micro-organisms in mouldy hay (what had previously been sometimes referred to as 'the farmer's lung type of fog fever'). They agree that the lesions of fog fever may be virtually indistinguishable from those of one stage of parasitic bronchitis (husk). **CAUSE.** Unknown; possibly the result of production of toxic indoles after ruminal fermentation of the ingested amino acid L-tryptophan in grass. (Breeze, R. G. *et al, The Veterinary Bulletin* (1976), **46**, 243.)

Veterinary research workers at the University of Glasgow reported on their investigation of 30 cases of fog fever. The disease was seen during August–November, and typically affected mature single suckler beef cows. In every instance the disease followed a change of pasture, and about 90 per cent of cases occurred within a fortnight of such a change. Except for two cases which arose on *Brassica* crops, all followed movement from a poor to a better grass field. 'Commonly,' commented Dr I. E. Selman, Dr H. M. Pirie and colleagues, 'hungry cattle had been moved from rough or poor permanent grazing to good lush fields, in most cases hay or silage aftermath. The fields on which fog fever arose had usually received at least one application of an artificial fertiliser during the year. On the relatively few occasions when the disease arose on non-fertilised grass, the mean interval between the introduction of cattle to the field and the onset of respiratory signs was significantly longer than when the disease was encountered on fertilised grass.'

Two clinical forms of fog fever were observed, and in neither was coughing an important symptom. The mild form affected up to 50 or 60 per cent within affected groups of cattle, and was often missed by farmers, as the animal remained bright though breathing rather rapidly. In the severe form of fog fever, the degree of respiratory distress varied greatly, was often severe, and resulted in a 30 per cent mortality, with death commonly occurring within the first 2 days of the illness. (*Vet. Rec.* (1974), **95**, 139.)

POST-MORTEM. Lesions include pulmonary congestion, oedema, and hyaline membranes, interstitial emphysema and diffuse alveolar epithelial hyperplasia.

A fog-fever-like condition in sheep, 6 months old, was seen in Sweden. All became ill within 3 days of being moved from poor to lush pasture.

FOGGAGE. Aftermath, 'fog'. Grass grown for winter grazing.

FOLIC ACID. One of the vitamins of the B-complex. (*See* VITAMINS.) The importance of folates in fetal development has been recognised only since the 1960s. They are essential in the metabolism of several amino-acids and in the formation of nucleic acids.

FOLLICLE is the term applied to a very small sac or gland, *e.g.* small collections of lymphoid tissue in the throat and the small digestive glands on the mucous membrane of the intestine. The hair follicle is the depression in the skin in the lowest part of which is situated the hair papilla from which it grows. The Graäfian follicle is the little sac in the ovary which encloses an ovum. (*See* SKIN; OVARY.)

FOLLICLE STIMULATING HORMONE (FSH). This is secreted by the anterior lobe of the pituitary gland, and stimulates the development of the Graäfian follicles in the ovary, and controls the secretion of oestrogens from the ovary. In the male animal FSH stimulates sperm production in the testicle.

FOLLICULAR MANGE is another name for demodectic mange due to the parasite *Demodex canis*, which lives in the hair follicles of the skin, and causes mange in dogs particularly. (*See* MITES.)

FOMENTATION (*see* POULTICES).

FOMITES is a term used to include all articles that have been in actual contact with a sick animal, so as to retain some of the infective material and be capable of spreading the disease. Bedding material, fodder, mangers, stable or byre utensils, clothing, grooming tools, the clothes of an attendant, or even the attendant himself, may all be fomites.

FOOD ALLERGIES (*see* ALLERGIES, FATTY ACIDS).

FOOD CONVERSION RATIOS. These express the number of pounds of food required to obtain a liveweight gain of 1 lb. For bacon pigs, the period taken is usually that from weaning to slaughter.

If FCRs are to be used as a basis of comparison as between one litter and another, or one farm's pigs and another's it is essential that the same meal or other foods be used; otherwise the figures become meaningless.

FOOD INSPECTION in countries such as Denmark and the USA has long been carried out entirely by members of the veterinary profession. In the UK this has been only partly so. However, EC requirements are likely to speed the change in 1992. Meat inspection duties include pre-slaughter inspection of food animals, and the examination of organs and tissues as well as inspection of the dressed carcase. Laboratory facilities are essential. For conditions which render meat dangerous as food, *see* TUBERCULOSIS, SALMONELLOSIS, ANTHRAX, TRICHINOSIS, HYDATID DISEASE, etc.

FOOD-POISONING IN MAN (*see* SAL-MONELLOSIS; CAMPYLOBACTER; ROTAVIRUS; *also* BOTULISM).

In England and Wales during 1981 there were 568 confirmed outbreaks of salmonellosis, 50 of *Clostridium perfringens* infection, 13 of *Staphylococcus aureus* and 9 of *Bacillus cereus* and other species. There were also 16 outbreaks of Campylobacter infection arising from milk, and 16 of salmonellosis from milk. (*See also* YERSINIOSIS, LISTERIOSIS). The latter has been increasingly reported among the very young, the elderly, and those immuno-suppressed. A number of outbreaks in North America have been linked to dairy produce and raw vegetables. (*See also* MILK-BORNE DISEASE.)

An analysis was based on 1044 outbreaks of food poisoning that were reported in England and Wales between 1970 and 1979. The aetiological agents included *Salmonella* species (38 per cent), *Clostridium perfringens* (37 per cent), *Staphylococcus aureus* (12·7 per cent) and *Bacillus* species (5·1 per cent). The place of consumption included family houses (19·7 per cent); restaurants, hotels, clubs, holiday camps (17·1 per cent); banquets, dinners, receptions (12·2 per cent); hospitals (11 per cent); institutions (9·3 per cent); schools (8·8 per cent); canteens, meals-on-wheels (8·5 per cent) and shops, bakeries and take-aways (7·7 per cent). Preparation of food in advance of consumption, combined with improper storage and inadequate cooking, cooling and reheating were the most common factors in these outbreaks. Infected food handlers did not play a significant role except in instances of *Staph aureus* food poisoning. (Roberts, D. *Journal of Hygiene*, 1982, **89,** 491.)

FOODS AND FEEDING (*see* DIET AND DIETETICS, NURSING OF SICK ANIMALS; RATIONS; *also* CAT FOODS).

FOOL'S PARSLEY POISONING.

Although a member of the Natural Order *Umbellifera* – very many of the members of which are poisonous (*e.g.* Water Hemlock, Water Dropwort, and Hemlock) – the extremely common Fool's Parsley (*Aethusa cynapium*) is not a frequent cause of poisoning of animals. It is dangerous when fed to rabbits, if it is pulled in the early green succulent stage before the flowering tops are formed.

Under ordinary circumstances herbivorous animals do not readily eat fool's parsley, for at the time when its growth is most luxuriant (*i.e.* in spring) there is generally an abundance of grass, which they prefer.

SIGNS. In cows, there have been seen a loss of appetite, salivation, fever, uncertain gait, and paralysis of the hindquarters. In horses, an instance has been recorded in which a number of animals ate the plant in quantity; those which had white muzzles and feet became attacked with diarrhoea and all white areas of the body became severely inflamed, but other horses of a whole-colour remained unaffected. (*See* LIGHT SENSITISATION.) In other cases stupor, paralysis, and convulsions have been noticed.

FIRST-AID. Drenches of strong black tea or coffee should be given so that the tannic acid in them may combine with the alkaloids of the plant and form inert substances.

FOOT-AND-MOUTH DISEASE (EPIZOOTIC APHTHA, MALIGNANT APHTHA, and APHTHOUS FEVER)

is an acute febrile disease of cattle, sheep, goats, and pigs, which is characterised by the formation of vesicles in the mouth and feet, and sometimes on the skin of the udder or teats of females.

Very rarely lesions of foot-and-mouth disease occur in man (and have to be differentiated from HAND, FOOT-AND-MOUTH DISEASE). Except in children, foot-and-mouth disease is usually mild in the human subject.

Hedgehogs are susceptible to infection, which they may spread to farm live-stock. Birds and rats may also be concerned in the spread of infection; also coypu. Rats, hamsters, chickens, rabbits and suckling mice can be infected experimentally.

Wild herbivores, including deer, and many animals kept in zoological gardens, are susceptible to infection; and grey squirrels.

Foot-and-mouth disease has occurred in almost every country in the world where cattle are kept. It has been endemic in countries of South America, the continent of Europe, Asia, and Africa.

The disease is not characterised by high mortality. Usually less than 5 per cent of adult animals die from foot-and-mouth disease. In young animals mortality may, however, be as high as 50 per cent.

From the farmer's point of view, most of the economic loss comes through failure of beef animals to put on weight, loss of milk in dairy cows, etc. From a national point of view, where control measures are rigorously applied, the disease involves heavy expenditure on diagnostic services, vaccination, compensation to owners, quarantine, disposal of carcases, etc.

CAUSE. Foot-and-mouth disease is caused by an Aphthovirus of which seven types are recognised – including the three known as O, A and C, which cause outbreaks of the disease in Britain, and four more which so far have been confined to Asia and Africa – Asia and Sat 1, Sat 2, and Sat 3. In 1960 the type Asia 1 virus caused serious outbreaks in Israel, the Lebanon and Syria, and fear was expressed that it might invade Europe. Sat 1 virus appeared in Israel, Syria, Jordan, and Turkey during 1962. In 1966 the A22 strain, which had been causing disease in Turkey and Iraq, appeared in Sussex. The sub-type O_1 was responsible for the great epidemic in Britain during 1967–68. The Asia 1 type reached Turkey in 1973, posing a threat to Europe.

No cross-immunity is exhibited between *types*, and only partial cross-immunity between *sub-types* within a type.

In 1973 the Wellcome Laboratory, Pirbright (England), had in culture over 140 different *strains* of foot-and-mouth disease virus, of which 33 had been classified as official subtypes. Of these strains, nearly 120 had been adapted for growth in BHK21 (baby hamster kidney cells).

The virus is present in the vesicles and in the discharges which come from them when they burst; and since there is nearly always an excessive secretion of saliva from an animal affected with lesions in the mouth, it is through the medium of contamination with saliva that the disease is perhaps most readily spread. As well as this, however, the urine, faeces, and small amounts of serum from lesions in the feet, are factors in the spread to other animals.

The virus can survive for very considerable lengths of time, and may be spread by a host of intermediate objects which have been in contact with affected animals: Hides, hair, wool, hay, straw, sacks and packing fabrics generally, milk, manure, animals (especially cats and dogs, hares, rabbits, rats, mice, and birds). Migratory birds in their flights from one country to another may act as carriers. Spread by wind, watercourses, tourists and their vehicles, are all possible means of spread. Much of the spread of the disease during the 1967–8 epidemic has been attributed to wind. Airborne transmission of the virus over wide areas of sea is considered feasible, given favourable conditions. Rain and snow are also considered important too.

Bulk collection of milk was also implicated. The virus may be excreted in milk before symptoms in the cow have appeared or become obvious.

People who handle infected cattle and do not take the precautions to disinfect their hands and change their clothing afterwards, will distribute the virus.

Experiments at Pirbright, have shown that when examining infected pigs some of the foot-and-mouth virus reaches the human nose, and may remain there for 24 hours, or even 48 hours. During this period the virus may be transferred to any other (uninfected) pigs which the person is handling or examining. In other words, the nose of man can be a hazard in the spread of the disease.

The virus can survive in frozen liver or kidney for 4 months or more. The use of swill containing scraps of meat, bones, or other animal tissue for feeding to pigs is a very important factor in the spread of foot-and-mouth disease, and because of the number of outbreaks traced to swill, the Ministry of Agriculture imposes a requirement upon those who use swill that it shall have been boiled for at least 1 hour before being fed.

The virus can survive in bull semen stored at low temperatures.

The period for which the disease lies latent after infection (*i.e.* the incubation period) varies from 1 to 15 days, but the majority of cases show symptoms between the 2nd and the 6th day after having been exposed to infection. Infection usually takes place through the alimentary canal.

An important feature of the disease in relation to its spread is the excretion of virus before symptoms become evident to the owner of the animal.

This is characteristic of the O_1 virus. With pigs, experimental work at Pirbright has shown that 10 days may elapse between excretion of virus and the development of lesions. With cattle and sheep, the figure may be 5 days; or an average of 2½ days.

SIGNS. At first, animals are noticed to become dull, refuse their food, lie about in a sluggish manner, and milk cows suddenly give a lessened flow of milk. Their temperatures rapidly rise to 104° or 105°F in the case of cattle, and fever is maintained until the crop of vesicles form, after which it subsides. A few hours after the initial dullness has been noticed affected animals usually commence to salivate profusely – long ropes of stringy saliva hanging from the mouth.

The animal frequently smacks its lips in a characteristic manner, yawns, and protrudes its tongue. As a rule the combination of these symptoms leads an owner to examine his cattle, particularly their mouths, and the blisters are found in all stages of development. Some are just forming, some are well formed, some have recently burst, but the mucous membrane that formed their covering is still adherent, and in the oldest the mucous membrane has been cast off from their surfaces and shallow ulcer-like areas are left. The commonest situations are on the dental pad and in the upper incisor region, on the tongue, especially around its tip, and on the insides of the cheeks and gums. The blisters each run a similar course; for a few hours they gradually rise, then they burst, liberating a small amount of yellowish, straw-coloured serum (which should be regarded as highly infective and as containing the virus), and there remains behind a shallow, eroded, red, raw, ulcer-like area, to the edges of which little pieces of mucous membrane remain adherent for a short time until they are removed by the movements of the mouth. In from 6 days to a fortnight or so these areas heal, and the lesions disappear. As a rule adjacent areas become confluent, and in bad cases large irregular, ragged, red patches form, from the surfaces of which the mucous membrane has disappeared. The lesions are always extremely painful, and on this account the animal is prevented from feeding. Generally, it can still drink, and it will often take liquid or very soft food, but it refuses dry food entirely.

LAMENESS may be the first sign of the disease. Foot lesions generally appear 4 or 5 days after the vesicles form in the mouth. In these, blisters form around the coronets, between the claws.

Sheep and Pigs. Foot lesions usually begin either at the coronet or at the heels instead of between the claws as in cattle. In the pig the muzzle and end of the snout may show lesions.

Animals in milk – cows, ewes, and sows – may develop characteristic lesions upon their teats or upon the skin of the udder. The lesions are similar to those forming in the mouth, but they take

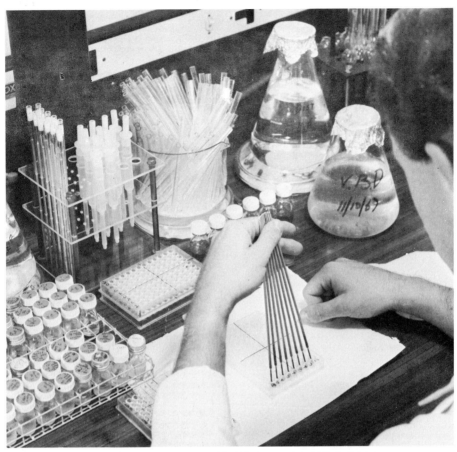

A complement fixation test for type determination. (World Reference Lab. (AVRI), Pirbright.)

longer to mature. In some cases the whole of the tip of the teat shows a single large blister, which is soon burst by milking or sucking. Subsequently an eroded appearance remains, until healing is established. Milk secretion rapidly diminishes. Permanent udder damage may result from the disease. The pain is usually acute, and the milk – contaminated with the exudate and with discharges from the lesions – is highly infective to young animals.

The illness may cause animals to lose much weight, or to cease to grow. Abortion, infertility, and diabetes are occasional complications.

Foot-and-mouth disease may be the cause of **sudden death** in pigs, cattle and sheep.

DIFFERENTIAL DIAGNOSIS. It is necessary by laboratory tests to distinguish between foot-and-mouth disease and Swine Vesicular Disease and Vesicular Stomatitis.

CONTROL. Vaccination is practised in countries where a slaughter policy is unworkable; not *vice versa*, as might be thought by those who condemn the slaughter policy without having studied the reasons for it.

A vaccination policy, without slaughter, is adopted in countries where the disease is endemic and its incidence high. 'Overall' vaccination is seldom practicable for reasons of cost, so 'frontier' vaccination or 'ring' vaccination (of all susceptible animals within a given radius of an outbreak) are usually practised.

A slaughter policy obtains in Great Britain, Canada, USA, Norway, Eire, and Northern Ireland – countries where the disease is not endemic. Such a policy, involving compensation to owners of compulsorily slaughtered animals, is normally far less costly than vaccination.

VACCINE BANK. The United Kingdom, Australia, New Zealand, Finland, Ireland, Norway and Sweden in 1985 formally established a foot-and-mouth disease vaccine bank. The participating countries are all free from the disease and do not normally vaccinate against it, but should an outbreak occur a supply of vaccine could be obtained immediately from the Animal Virus Research Institute at Pirbright. What is actually 'banked' is not vaccine but a concentrated f-&-m antigen which can quickly be reconstituted into vaccine. There are half a million cattle doses of each of five virus types.

The bank will contain the equivalent of 0·5 million cattle doses each of type A (A24) (Cruzeiro), type A (A22) (Iraq), type C (C1) (Oberbayern 1973) and O (O1) (Lausanne).

CONTROL MEASURES IN BRITAIN. In Great Britain this disease is scheduled under the Diseases of Animals Acts, and all outbreaks must be promptly reported to the Local Authorities and to the Ministry of Agriculture. Strict isolation is at first ensured, and the affected animals are slaughtered and burned or buried. In-contact animals are slaughtered. The premises are carefully cleansed and disinfected under supervision, and re-stocking is not allowed for at least 28 days after the last animal was slaughtered; the time actually varies with local conditions. During the time the cattle are being slaughtered and while disinfection is proceeding, no unauthorised person is allowed upon the premises, and every one leaving the farm (Infected Place) is required to disinfect himself as thoroughly as possible.

Meanwhile, in a radius of about 10 miles around an infected farm an Infected Area is declared. No susceptible animals are allowed to leave the area, and no movement is permitted except under licence for slaughter within 96 hours; no animals are allowed to be driven across the public highway within the radius; no markets, fairs, shows, sales, etc., are allowed to take place within the area; fox-hunting and other field-sports are forbidden, and owners of animals are advised to confine themselves upon their own premises as much as possible and to prevent the entrance of unauthorised persons.

Normally, the Infected Area remains as such for 21 days, being contracted to a radius of 5 miles after 14 days.

When the disease has spread, or threatens to spread over a wide area, the Ministry may declare a Controlled Area. In this, animals may be moved only under licence, and only into an Infected Area. Markets are banned (except for animals to be slaughtered immediately).

It is also advisable that hides, wool, hair, horns, hoofs, bone-meal, and animal manures from foreign parts, should be effectively sterilised either before leaving the country of origin, or else upon arrival at the ports of those countries free from the disease.

NORTHUMBERLAND COMMITTEE REPORT. Following the disastrous epidemic of 1967–8, which involved 2397 outbreaks and payments in compensation, to owners of compulsorily slaughtered animals, of about £27m, a committee was appointed under the chairmanship of the Duke of Northumberland to review the policy and arrangements for dealing with the disease (which, in this epidemic, had resulted in the slaughter of over 211,000 head of cattle; 108,000 sheep; and 113,000 pigs; and 50 goats).

The Northumberland Committee recommended continuation of the slaughter policy; but that this should be reinforced by a ring vaccination scheme if a meat import policy, calculated to reduce substantially the risks of primary outbreaks, were not implemented. (*See under* RING VACCINATION.)

DISINFECTANTS. For the current list *see Diseases of Animals* (*Approved Disinfectants*) *Orders.* HMSO.

FOOT-BATHS FOR CATTLE. A foot-bath with 1¼-inch pipes laid horizontally 2 inches apart,

even if filled with plain water, will help to detach mud; the pipes forcing the claws apart.

Caution: A 5 per cent formalin foot-bath is often recommended for the control or prevention of foul-in-the-foot, but it is important not to exceed that strength or to put the cows through it too often. One of MAFF's VI centres recently reported that on one farm 90 out of 100 cows developed severe inflammation at their heels because they were walked through a 4–7 per cent formalin foot-bath twice daily for two weeks. Fifty of those cows developed further lesions, a few of which had not healed a month later.

Use of a footbath – especially in winter but beneficial in summer too – was advocated as the best and easiest contribution which a dairy farmer could make towards reducing herd LAMENESS (which see), by Kelly & Whitaker. They emphasised its proper use, admitting that improper use of a footbath could do more harm than good. Apart from too frequent use of a Formalin footbath, contamination with dung and slurry can render it harmful.

Provision must be made in the planning stage for ease of filling, cleaning, and disposal of the Formalin solution. It is convenient to have the footbath installed at the parlour exit, so that cows become completely familiar with it and readily walk through it, whether filled or empty. (It would not be desirable to have the footbath at the *entry* to the parlour, owing to fumes from the Formalin.)

Kelly & Whitaker suggest dimensions for the footbath as follows: length, about 10 ft; width 3 ft 6 inches; depth 9 inches. They consider the ideal is to have two successive footbaths, the first containing plain water, and the second a solution of 5 per cent Formalin.

A more recent recommendation is a 1 per cent solution for routine use as an aid to reducing herd lameness.

FOOT-BATHS FOR SHEEP are used for the purpose of treating or preventing foot-rot and the foot lesions of orf.

The bath consists of a shallow trough made of concrete or wood, measuring about 6 to 9 inches wide, 4 to 6 inches deep in the middle and tapering at each end to about 1 inch depth, and about 10 to 15 feet long (or more). It is built in connection with a sheep-pen or fold, in which the sheep may be first collected, and from which they may be driven one at a time through the bath. Hurdles or a fence along each side of the trough prevent the sheep from leaving it while being driven through. No drying pen is necessary, as the small amount of poison carried out on the feet is not sufficient to impregnate the pastures to any serious extent.

The solutions most often used for foot-baths are 3 per cent formalin solution; or copper sulphate, 4 to 8 per cent. As a preventative of contagious foot-rot a three-weekly run through a foot-bath gives excellent results. (*See* FOOT-ROT.)

Caution: A striking example of overdoing foot-bath use was the disastrous use of formalin in a foot-bath to treat lameness in a flock of 150 ewes. 'As the lameness increased', MAFF stated, 'so did the frequency and strength of the formalin liquid until the entire flock was crippled and had to be slaughtered'.

FOOT OF THE HORSE. There is truth in the old saying, 'No foot, no horse,' although at first sight this may seem picturesque exaggeration. From the horse, man demands a capacity for movement, and this of necessity entails sound organs on which movement depends, and of these the feet are not the least important.

It will be the aim here to give some account of the anatomy and physiology of the normal foot; an account of the commoner diseases will be found under their respective headings, such as CORNS, QUITTOR, LAMINITIS, SANDCRACK, SEEDY TOE, BRUISED SOLE, INJURIES FROM SHOEING, etc.

Skeleton of the foot consists of the lower part of the second phalanx, the whole of the third phalanx, and the sesamoid of the third phalanx or 'navicular bone'. (*See under* BONES.) From the posterior angles of the third phalanx (coffin-bone) project two roughly quadrilateral plates of cartilage, one on either side, which are known as the 'lateral cartilages'. These are important structures in the absorption of shock and in preserving the elasticity of the foot as a whole. Under certain conditions they become ossified, when the name 'side-bones' is applied. The three bones above mentioned are bound together by a series of ligaments which, while they allow free mobility in normal directions, prevent unnatural movements which might rupture the capsules of the coffin-joint. Lying between the two lateral cartilages and behind the third phalanx there is a fibro-elastic structure known as the 'plantar cushion' or *digital torus*, which, although, strictly speaking, it is not part of the skeleton of the foot, will be considered here for convenience. This plantar cushion is composed of extremely elastic, dense, fibrous tissue, poorly supplied with blood-vessels and not greatly sensitive, and is one of the chief shock-absorbing structures of the foot. From above it is pressed upon by the descending deep flexor tendon, when the foot comes to the ground; from below it is pressed upwards by the horny frog; it cannot expand forwards to any great extent, because of the presence of the coffin-bone; and since it is practically a rubber-like buffer, it expands backwards and sideways. On either side of it, however, are the lateral cartilages, and these are pressed outwards in the process and carry with them the horny wall at the heels. These structures collectively can be likened to the bare foot of man.

Sensitive structures. Covering the parts above described and accurately moulded to them (just as the sock of a man is moulded to the foot) are the sensitive parts which nourish the horny hoof. These are, around the hoof-head above the coronary band, a *periopic matrix*, from fine projects on the surface of which is nourished the *periople*, a layer of hard varnish-like horn which prevents undue evaporation from the wall; around the coronet, from one heel to the other, a bolster-like structure about four-fifths of an inch wide known as the *coronary band*, or *coronary cushion*, which nourishes and from which grows the horn

of the wall; running down the inside of the wall all the way round and turning inwards and forwards at the heels, a *laminar matrix*, which is provided with laminae or 'leaves' which interdigitate with corresponding laminae on the inside of the wall; covering the lower surface of the coffin-bone, and nourishing the sole of the hoof, a *solar matrix*, or *sensitive sole*, and covering the lower surface of the plantar cushion and nourishing the frog, a *furcal matrix*, or *sensitive frog*. The term *pododerm* is applied collectively to these sensitive structures. The pododermic tissues are in reality modified skin, but instead of growing hairs as does the skin in other parts of the body, they produce numerous minute tubular horn fibres which are firmly united to each other.

Horny structures. Considered collectively the horny parts of the foot form what is known as the 'hoof' – composed of practically the same material as the horns or claws of other animals, and being in reality modified skin – is a protective, slightly elastic casing which protects the softer parts of the foot from concussion, friction and injury. It is composed of the wall, the sole, and the frog.

The wall is all that portion which can be seen when the foot rests upon the ground. It gives the foot its form. Its horn is hard, solid, only slightly elastic, and affords protection to the sensitive laminar matrix below it.

The inner surface of the wall has about 600 horny leaves or *laminae*, which dovetail with the sensitive laminae forming a firm union between wall and matrix. The upper edge of the wall is thin, flexible, and grooved for the lodgment of the coronary cushion. The lower edge is called the 'bearing surface', and is the part to which the shoe is fitted.

The sole is that part of the hoof which is nourished by the sensitive tissue covering the solar surface of the coffin-bone. It is divided into a body and two branches, and is roughly crescent-shaped. The sole is markedly vaulted in normal feet, especially in hind-feet, but in very many old horses it becomes flat or even convex; when excessively convex it is called a 'dropped sole'. The outer border is bevelled to correspond to the slope of the wall, but is separated from it by the *white line* of soft horn which acts as a kind of cementing substance between the wall and the sole. This line is of great importance in shoeing, as it indicates the thickness of the wall, and is used as a guiding line through which the nails can be driven with safety. In the posterior part of the sole there is a V-shaped notch, between the branches of which lie the bars and the frog.

The frog is an exact mould of the lower surface of the plantar cushion which it protects. It is a roughly triangular wedge-shaped mass filling up the space between the bars and the V-shaped notch of the sole. It projects downwards more than the sole, and receives the greatest amount of the concussion in the normal foot; it is only seldom injured, however, for its horn is of very elastic consistency. The ground surface presents a very well-marked *median cleft*, which corresponds to an elevation in its upper (inner) surface

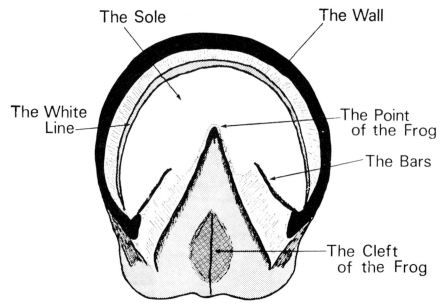

The Sole

The Wall

The White Line

The Point of the Frog

The Bars

The Cleft of the Frog

Diagram of the underside of a hoof. (With acknowledgements to *The UFAW Handbook on the Care and Management of Farm Animals* Churchill Livingstone (Longman Group).)

which is commonly known as the 'frog stay', and which aids in the attachment of the frog to the overlying parts.

FOOT-ROT OF CATTLE. This name is used in the USA for what in Britain is called FOUL-IN-THE-FOOT. *Bacteroides nodosus* has been isolated from some foot lesions of cattle in Britain.

FOOT-ROT OF PIGS. Thirty per cent of casualty pigs at one UK slaughter-house had abscesses (a common reason for condemnation of meat) and twelve per cent of these abscesses were on the feet.

In a survey covering over 6000 pigs 30 per cent of the lesions were erosion of the heel, 24 per cent of the toe, and 21 per cent of the sole. Fine cracks to deep fissures constituted another 2·7 of the lesions. (See diagram under BIOTIN.)

CAUSES. These include excessively rough concrete, some of which can be abrasive. Softening of the horn under damp, dirty conditions is another factor; and nutrition may be involved in some instances.

FOOT-ROT OF SHEEP is a disease of the horny parts and of the adjacent soft structures of the feet. The organism primarily responsible is *Bacteroides nodosus*. The disease is commonly prevalent on wet, marshy, badly-drained pastures, in old folds or sheep pens. Wet soil, however, does not cause foot-rot but merely facilitates infection. This is a mixed one, with *B. necrophorus* causing sufficient damage to permit the entry of *B. nodosus*.

In Australia two forms of foot-rot are recognised, in both of which *B. nodosus* is always present. The type of foot-rot which develops depends upon the proteolyptic capacity of the infecting strain of *B. nodosus*. In **benign** foot-rot the

infecting strain is of low proteolytic activity and the resultant disease is limited and does not spread under the hard horn, although it might cause lifting of the sole of the foot. In **virulent** foot-rot the infecting strain is of high proteolytic activity and results in extensive separation of the hard horn, with the clinical appearance of classical foot-rot. (Dr D. F. Stewart.)

It appears that transmission of foot-rot infection from cattle to sheep is possible.

B. nodosus cannot survive in the soil or on pasture for more than a fortnight.

SIGNS. Lameness is the first noticeable feature. At first the sheep manages to put the foot to the ground, but after a time it goes on three legs only, the pain having greatly increased.

When the foot is examined there will either be found a swelling over the coronet or an area of the horn of the hoof is found to be soft, painful on pressure, 'rotten-looking', and a variable amount of foul-smelling discharge is present.

If neglected the horn will begin to separate from the underlying sensitive tissues, and will eventually be shed. Sometimes the disease penetrates into the foot, affecting the ligaments or even the bone. One, two, three, or all four feet may be affected. If the two fore-feet are attacked the sheep very often assumes the kneeling position for feeding. If the two hind feet, any three feet, or all four are affected, standing becomes an impossibility, and the sheep, still retaining its appetite, will feed from the sitting position, crawling forward a few inches at a time to a new piece of grazing.

PREVENTION. Foot-rot can be eradicated. Leave contaminated pasture free of sheep for 3 weeks. Isolate and treat all infected or suspected sheep. The feet of heavy sheep should not be allowed to get overgrown during wet weather; turning on to a bare fallow or stubble field, or

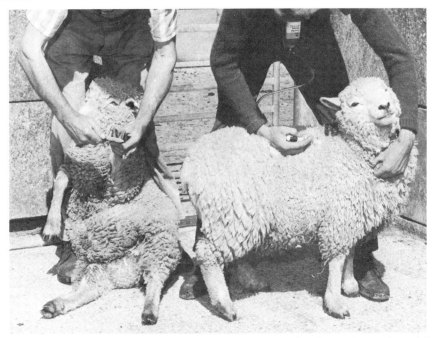

The old and the new in foot-rot treatment. Two injections with Wellcome Foot Rot vaccine at an interval of six weeks replace the laborious paring and cutting of feet necessary with existing methods of control.

walking along a hard road, is advocated by some to wear away the feet, but is not a very practicable proposition. The better way is to round up the sheep and pare each foot individually once every 6 weeks or 2 months.

Research initiated in Australia led to the development of a vaccine, which is now commercially available, and is prepared from cultures of *B. nodosus.*

Tasman's 'Footwax' vaccine contains 10 strains of inactivated *Bacteroides nodosus* with an oil adjuvant.

TREATMENT. It is advisable to separate the infected from the healthy, passing the latter through a foot-bath and changing the pasture to as high ground as possible. If the lame sheep can be shut up in a strawed yard, in pig-courts, or in pens, given hand-feeding and individual attention daily, they recover much better than if they are left out in the open and only attended to occasionally. The feet should be carefully trimmed, all necrotic horny material removed. When all the 'rotten' substance has been removed the foot should be cleansed in a solution of an antiseptic, and an astringent antiseptic dressing applied. **The use of foot-rot vaccine may obviate much time-consuming work on treating diseased feet,** however.

Where vaccine is not available, one may apply an antibiotic preparation – either a tincture or other liquid preparation of chloramphenicol, or an ointment containing Terramycin. (*See also* FOOT-BATHS.)

The shepherd should take care to ensure that he does not spread the disease to other sheep through the medium of his hands or knife; he should wash both after dealing with each case, and all parings,

diseased tissue, and infected swabs should be collected in a pail and burned. Neglect of these precautions often results in a continuance of new cases in a flock.

FORAGE MITES (*see* MITES).

FORAMEN is a hole or opening. The word is applied particularly to holes in bones through which pass nerves or blood-vessels. The *foramen magnum* is the large opening in the posterior aspect of the skull through which passes the spinal cord to enter the *foramina* in each of the vertebrae of the spine. The *nutrient foramina* are the holes in the shafts, etc., of the bones which penetrate to the marrow cavity, by which blood and lymph vessels and nerves pass to and from the marrow cavity.

FOREIGN BODIES. This term includes a grass seed in the ear, nose, beneath the skin between the toes or beneath the eye-lid, in the prepuce or penis of the cat; a needle embedded in the tongue; a chop bone wedged in a dog's mouth; a piece of bone lodged in the gullet; a piece of wire in the reticulum; pebbles in a dog's stomach; lead shot and airgun pellets. (*See* AWNS; *under* CHOKING, STOMACH, DISEASE OF, etc.)

Foreign bodies also include a broken-off portion of an intravenous needle within a vein, or of a catheter. Miniature 'button batteries', swallowed by small children, have caused an obstruction of the oesophagus, and also mercury poisoning; and a similar risk could be expected in dogs and cats.

FORMALIN is a gaseous body prepared by the oxidation of methyl alcohol. For commercial purposes it is prepared as a solution of 40 per cent strength in water. Formalin is a powerful antiseptic, and has the quality of hardening or fixing the tissues. The solution in water gives off gas slowly, and this has an irritant action on the eyes and nose.

Formalin is used for preserving pathological specimens, occasionally as a disinfectant, and for the production of formaldehyde gas for fumigation of buildings. A 3 per cent solution of formalin has been used in a foot-bath in the treatment of foot-rot in sheep. Its application, however, may cause considerable pain if it reaches sensitive tissues. (*See also under* FOOT-BATHS, DISINFECTION.)

FOSSA is an anatomical term applied to a depression in a bone which lodges some other structure, such as part of the brain in the skull. It is also used to describe grooves or pockets in soft tissues, such as the renal fossa of the liver in which is lodged the right kidney.

FOUL-IN-THE-FOOT (called FOOT-ROT in the USA). Technically known as interdigital necrobacillosis, the lesion takes the form of a swelling which tends to force the claws apart. The whole length of the space between the claws may be involved, with one or two fissures in the skin evident, and a slough of dead tissue.

CAUSE. *Corynebacterium pyogenes*, or *Bacteroides* organisms – only as a mixed infection – are the cause, entering tissues through a wound or through devitalisation of the skin from frost, mud, decomposing urine or faeces, or other irritants.

SIGNS. There is nearly always well-marked lameness. Hind-feet are more often affected than fore-feet, probably owing to their greater liability to soiling from urine and faeces, in which the necrosis bacillus can generally be easily found. In many cases a cow will suddenly stop walking, and shake the affected foot as though she desired to dislodge a stone or other hard object which has become wedged between the claws.

TREATMENT. This calls for professional aid. The intravenous injection of sulphamezathine. (*See* FOOT-ROT, FOOT-BATHS.)

FOWL CHOLERA. Synonyms: Cholera gallinarium, Avian pasteurellosis, Pasteurellosis of the fowl. Haemorrhagic septicaemia of the fowl. This is a contagious disease of fowls, usually epizootic in type and characterised by sudden onset, high fever, extensive blood extravasations into the different organs, and severe diarrhoea. The disease occurs all over Europe, in North and South America, in most parts of Africa, and in Asia. All common fowls, including domestic poultry (chickens, ducks, geese, guinea-fowl, turkeys, pigeons, pheasants, and fancy birds), are susceptible. Most common wild birds are also liable to infection and serve to spread the disease. Rabbits and mice may also contract it under special circumstances.

CAUSE. *Pasteurella multocida*.

SIGNS. After a brief incubation period (usually 2 to 4 days) the birds may be seen to stagger and

fall down, or more commonly are just found dead. In the less acute type, which perhaps is the more common, the birds are seen to look ill, to stand apart from the rest, droop their wings, refuse both food and water; the combs, wattles, and ear lobes become discoloured, and there is great nervous prostration. A discharge comes away from the eyes and nose, a frothy saliva from the mouth, and there is usually severe diarrhoea. The respirations become rapid; the temperature may reach 110°F or 111°F. The feathers are ruffled and draggled, and those of the hinder parts of the body are soiled with faecal discharges. Vomiting may take place, and in from 1 to 3 days the affected birds usually die. In other cases the symptoms are more sub-acute, and the disease may run on for from 7 to 9 or 10 days, but as a rule ends fatally. In the more chronic type it may take several weeks before death ensues. In acute outbreaks from 90 to 95 per cent may die, although in others the death-rate may be only 20 per cent.

FOWL-PARALYSIS (*Neuro-lymphomatosis*). (*See* MAREK'S DISEASE.)

FOWL PEST. This term usually refers to NEWCASTLE DISEASE (which see), but also includes FOWL PLAGUE.

FOWL PLAGUE (*see* AVIAN INFLUENZA).

FOWL-POX (AVIAN CONTAGIOUS EPITHELIOMA and AVIAN DIPHTHERIA) is a virus disease in which wart-like nodules appear on the comb, wattles, eyelids, and openings of the nostrils.

The disease attacks the fowl most often, but other domesticated birds are all susceptible, likewise wild and domesticated pigeons. It occurs in almost all parts of the world. (*See* POX.)

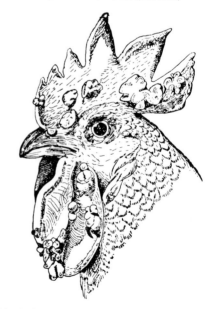

Head of cock affected with avian contagious epithelioma. Wattles and comb are mainly affected.

The virus infects the skin through abrasions, and may be transmitted by insect vectors (especially mosquitoes). Various secondary organisms are usually responsible for deaths.

The period of incubation is usually between 3 and 12 days, and bad housing conditions, severe weather, and poor feeding serve to lower vitality and render an outbreak much more serious.

SIGNS. There are three types of lesions: (i) nodular eruptive lesions on comb and wattles; (ii) a cheesy, yellowish membrane in the mouth and throat; (iii) oculo-nasal form (possibly due to a different virus).

The mouth lesions consist of patches of a greyish, fairly firm, cheesy-looking material, which is of considerable thickness, and not easy to detach. This is the 'false membrane'. In many cases the entrance to the trachea is partially blocked with these deposits, and the breathing is consequently obstructed. The smell from the mouth is always foul.

TREATMENT is economically unsound. The best measures consist of the slaughter of all affected birds and the inoculation of the healthy ones with 'pigeon-pox vaccine'.

PREVENTION. Newly purchased birds should be isolated for 3 weeks before being added to the flock, and after returning from shows, laying trials, etc., the same procedure should be adopted.

Vaccination can be done at 6 weeks of age; or, more usually, between 3 and 5 months of age.

FOWL TYPHOID. This is an acute infectious disease of fowls (also of ducks, geese, turkeys, game and wild birds) caused by the *Salmonella gallinarium*. The disease has a world-wide distribution, but has been virtually eradicated from the U K.

Most outbreaks occur in pullets near point of lay, but birds of all ages are susceptible – even chicks. The disease is usually introduced into a flock by the purchase of 'carrier' fowls, and thereafter spreads by contamination of food and water with the droppings of such birds. The incubation period is from 4 to 6 days.

SIGNS are not always characteristic. There is generally marked drowsiness, loss of appetite, and great weakness. The fowls prefer to sit about in dark corners. The comb and wattles are sometimes pale and anaemic; but they may in other cases be markedly congested. Diarrhoea is usually present. Death, following progressive weakness, results in from 4 to 14 days after the onset of the symptoms. The percentage mortality varies from about 20 to 30 per cent, and many or most of the recovered birds become 'carriers', which serve to spread the disease to other birds.

DIAGNOSIS. A dead fowl should be sent to a poultry research laboratory.

If fowl typhoid is diagnosed, samples of blood from the surviving and apparently healthy birds should be submitted to the agglutination test, and all reactors should be isolated and destroyed; the carcases being burned or buried in quicklime. The remaining birds should be treated with furazolidone for 10 days, moved to fresh premises, and re-treated.

PREVENTION. '9R' vaccine.

After removal of the reacting birds, the houses, utensils, etc., should be disinfected.

FOX, DISEASES OF. In Europe, N. America and other parts of the world, wild foxes often become victims of rabies, and spread this disease to farm live-stock which they may attack. A history of aggressiveness and the frequenting of populated areas does not, however, point conclusively to rabies; distemper may be the reason. (*See also* FOX ENCEPHALITIS *below, and* CHASTEK PARALYSIS.)

The fox acts as host of the roundworm *Toxocara canis* and of the *Toxascaris leonina*, and if silver fox cubs are reared by a cat, they may become infected with *Toxocara mystax* of the cat. The fox harbours the dog tapeworms *Taenia serialis*, and *T. multiceps*, and *Echinococcus granulosus*. Leptospirosis occurs in foxes in the U K and may be spread to farm livestock. (Five strains have been isolated.) Flukes may infest foxes.

FOX ENCEPHALITIS is of veterinary interest and commercial importance on the fox ranches of North America, where these animals are bred for their fur. The disease is considered identical with Rubarth's disease of dogs.

SIGNS. Young foxes in good condition are most frequently affected. A violent convulsion is followed by a lethargic or 'sleep-walking' state. This may be followed by excitability and more convulsions – during which the slamming of a door or any loud noise may prove fatal. The illness runs a very rapid course, from 1 hour to 3 days, 24 hours being the average duration.

CONTROL. By means of serum and preventive inoculation.

This disease, or one caused by a similar virus, may have accounted for the deaths of (wild) foxes in Britain in 1959 and 1960; but during this period, many young foxes are believed to have died as the result of eating birds poisoned by Dieldrin. Symptoms are similar.

FOXGLOVE POISONING (*see* DIGITALIS POISONING).

FRACTURES. *Simple fractures* are the commonest variety, and consist of those in which the bone is broken clean across, with or without tearing and laceration of the soft parts surrounding it, but without any wound leading from the fracture through to the skin. They are spoken of as being transverse, longitudinal, or oblique, according to the direction of the break.

Compound fractures are those in which the skin is injured, so that a direct or indirect communication between the fracture and the outside air exists. The broken end of the bone very often penetrates through the skin and is found exposed. Bleeding is apt to be severe; infection of the ends of the bones with pathogenic organisms may occur.

Incomplete fractures are those in which the bone is broken only partly across, or in which the tough periosteum (the tissue covering the bone) is not torn. This variety occurs in the shin-bones (tibiae)

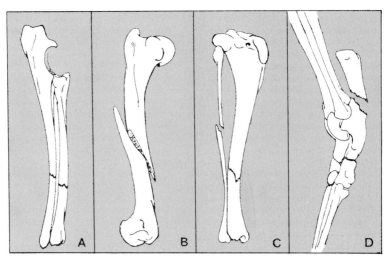

Classification of fractures. A. Transverse fracture with excellent stability after reduction. B. Oblique fracture with no stability after reduction. C. Slightly oblique fracture which, by virtue of the irregularity of the fracture line, provides a useable degree of stability after reduction. D. A typical distracted fracture. (*With acknowledgements to the British Veterinary Association.*)

of horses which have been kicked, and in the bones of young animals. In these the bone cracks like a twig half-way across, and then splits for some distance along its length, just as does a branch which has been cut half-way through and then bent; these fractures are known as 'greenstick fractures'.

Fissured fractures are mere cracks in the bone which are found in the skull and face bones after blows or falls. They are usually not serious unless haemorrhage accompanies them and the blood-clot presses upon a nerve or on the brain itself.

Deferred fractures occur when the bone has actually been fractured, but the fractions do not separate until or unless some extra severe strain is put upon the part.

Distracted fractures are those in which muscular contraction causes the detached fragment to be drawn away from the main body of the bone.

Depressed fractures also occur in the skull bones as a rule, and consist of fractures in which a fragment of bone is forced in below the level of the surrounding surface. They may give rise to very serious symptoms when the depressed portion presses upon the brain substance.

Complicated fractures are those in which there is some other serious injury produced in addition to the fracture, *e.g.* dislocation of the dog's hip along with fracture of the shaft of the femur, tearing of a large nerve, etc.

Comminuted fractures are those in which there is much splintering, the term *sequestra* being applied to those splinters of bone which are separated and eventually die.

Impacted fractures are those in which, after the break has occurred, one fragment is jammed inside another, usually at an angle.

Ununited fractures are those in which, after the usual time has elapsed for the fracture to heal, it is found that union has not taken place. The failure to unite may be simply due to 'delayed union', on account of debility or illness or due to the fact that the limb or other member is not kept at rest sufficiently for the process of healing to occur. In other cases of ununited fracture a piece of muscle or other tissue becomes placed between the broken ends of the bones and effectively prevents their union.

CAUSES. Disease, such as osteomalacia, in which there is a reduction in the density of bone and of its tensile strength, is one cause. However, the common cause is external violence. (*See also* ELECTRIC SHOCK.)

Horses. Kicks, falls, blows, errors in judgment during jumping, putting their feet into rabbit-holes when galloping, accidents when the animal collides with some stationary object, or is struck by a vehicle.

Fractures incurred by 53 racehorses at a New York track were found to be due to three lesions; namely, osteochondrosis, chondro-osteo necrosis, and degeneration of tendons and ligaments. (Krook, L. & Maylin, G. *Cornell Veterinarian* (1988) **78**.)

Cattle. Fractures result from injuries during fighting, slipping, and falling when struggling, running, or during service, from jumping fences, hedges, ditches, from crowding accidents at markets, etc., and from crushes in cattle-trucks.

Fracture of the third phalanx in a medial front claw is commonly associated with fluorine poisoning, and causes cattle to stand with their legs crossed. (*See also* SHOEING.)

Pigs and Sheep. The causes are usually similar, but legs are broken more easily. Careless use of the shepherd's crook, are responsible for many. Falling over precipices and getting a limb fast in a gate, fence, or hurdle, may also result in a broken bone.

Dogs and Cats. Of 298 cats brought, on account of fractures, to a small-animal hospital in London over a two-year period, over 90 per cent of them had been injured in road accidents. The bones most frequently broken were the femur (28 per cent of the cats), pelvis (25 per cent), and jaw (11 per cent). 'Treatment proved satisfactory in the great majority of cases.' (Philips, I. R. *J. Small Anim. Practice*, (1979), **20**, 661.)

In a survey of 26 feline fractures diagnosed at the Universiti Pertanian Malaysia, the femur, jaw, tibia, pelvis, and spine were the most common sites of fracture, in that order.

Of 61 dogs covered by the same survey, the femur, tibia, pelvis, radius and ulna were the bones most often involved. Nearly half the cases were the result of road traffic accidents; with six being ascribed to nutritional causes, four to falls, and one to a bullet wound. (Wong, W. T. *Veterinary Record*, 1984, **115**, 273.)

SIGNS. The chief signs of a fracture are *uselessness of the part, crepitus of the fragments*, and sometimes *unnatural mobility* and *deformity*. If a limb is affected there is usually an unnatural mobility, inability to sustain weight, distortion or deformity, shortening of the length, a thickness or swelling at the seat of the fracture (due to overlapping of the fragments), and a variable amount of pain. (*See also* FRACTURES OF SPECIAL PARTS.)

HEALING OF FRACTURES. When the bone breaks, many vessels, both in its substance and in the periosteum, are torn, and accordingly a large clot of blood forms around the ends, between them, and for some distance up the inside of the bone. Later, great numbers of white blood cells find their way into this clot, which becomes 'organised', blood-vessels and, later, fibrous tissue being formed in it (*soft callus*). Next, lime salts are gradually deposited in this fibrous tissue, which thus develops into bone (*hard callus*). In this process a thick ring of new bone forms round the broken ends, filling up all crevices; and when union is complete, this thickening is again gradually absorbed, leaving the bone as it was before the injury.

In racing greyhounds badly fractured scaphoids have been removed and replaced by acrylic implants. In the USA Dr R. D. Bloebaum reported the use of a **titanium-alloy implant** which enabled a greyhound to race again 43 times before retirement from the track.

TREATMENT. Reduction and apposition are brought about by manipulation of the fractured bones under anaesthesia. Immobilisation is then effected by means of plaster of Paris, and various proprietary mixtures impregnated into bandages. Splints of metal, leather, wood, or cardboard, padded with cotton-wool, are useful, especially with dogs and cats. (*See* SPLINTING MATERIALS.)

Special types of extension splints, having transverse pins which transfix the bone, have been used with success in appropriate cases. Medullary pins, driven down the marrow cavity of long bones; wiring; and plating, have all been used with success. (*See* BONEPINNING.)

Whenever splints, plaster, or other bandages are being applied to fractured limbs it is essential to ensure that the surface of the skin is well padded with cotton-wool, and that the pressure is

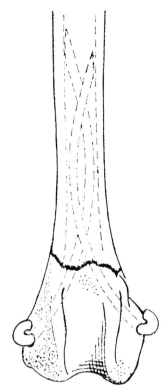

Two Rush-type intramedullary pins used to repair a supracondyloid fracture of the femur.

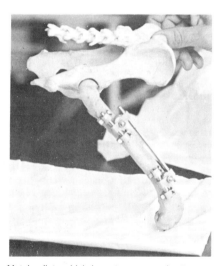

Metal splints which have transverse pins to penetrate and fix the bone are used in treating fractures in small animals, and have succeeded in cases where the older methods would have been of no avail.

evenly distributed. Failure in this respect may result in parts of the skin becoming gangrenous through obstruction to the blood-flow.

BONE GRAFTS. These are being used to a limited extent in veterinary surgery to repair fractures of the femur, humerus, tibia, radius and ulna; and in one case to replace bone lost to sequestrum formation in an infected fracture. Dr K. R. Sinibaldi described his technique in 26 cases, and used it to replace comminuted fragments, to lengthen bones, correct delayed or faulty union.

The allografts were harvested aseptically from healthy dogs, autoclaved the same day, and stored at between − 10 and − 20°C in a domestic freezer for use up to one year later. Ordinary bone-plating techniques were used. Clinically normal function was achieved in 24 of the dogs. (Sinibaldi, K. R. (1989) *Journal of the American Veterinary Medical Association* (1989) **194**, 1570.)

Fractures of special parts.
1. THE CRANIUM. Little and others reviewed the clinical features of fractures of the head of 21 horses; 14 had a history of a severe traumatic incident while seven were found with an injury when stabled or at pasture. Surgical treatment was successful in most cases in which fractures involved bones of the jaws and face. Fractures involving the cranial cavity or the cranial nerves were difficult to treat and usually carried a poor prognosis. (Little, C. B. & others, *Australian Veterinary Journal*, (1985), **62**, 89.) (*See also* CONCUSSION.)
2. THE FACE BONES. May be simple or serious according to bones involved. Nasal bones, often fractured from accidents, and accompanied by swelling, pain, haemorrhage, difficulty in breathing, much watering of the eyes. Jaw-bones broken from falls, kicks, etc., and usually interfere with feeding. Lower jaw fractures usually result in an open hanging mouth, escape of saliva, altered expression, and frequently loose teeth, torn lips, and haemorrhage are in evidence. Bones of orbit fractured by falls on to side of head, collisions, etc.; interference with vision and with movements of lower jaw, in most cases serious. Treatment necessitates operation usually; removal of broken pieces, elevation of depressed portions, removal of loose teeth, wiring or plating broken parts together; removal of eye, etc. Feeding must be carefully undertaken when jaws are injured; sloppy food, mashes, etc., for horse, hand-feeding for dog.
3. THE VERTEBRAE. Commonest in horse and dog through accidents, *e.g.* getting cast in stall, casting for operation (muscular action), run-over accidents in dogs, falls from heights, blows from sticks. They result in paralysis, if a vertebra is fractured, or in local disturbance if only a process is affected. There is often a fatal termination, or a need for euthanasia. Tail-bones often broken in dogs and cattle through getting caught in doors, gates, fences, etc.
4. THE RIBS. Due to external violence usually, but first rib sometimes broken through muscular action in a side-slip and violent recovery, when it often results in radial paralysis. (*See* RADIAL PARALYSIS.) Otherwise broken ribs show little or nothing characteristic except local pain and deformity, unless many involved, when breathing may be short and difficult. (*See* 'FLAIL-CHEST', PNEUMOTHORAX.)

5. THE PELVIS. In 123 cases of fracture of the pelvis in dogs in one practice, all were the result of road accidents. Twenty-eight of the dogs were treated surgically, and 66 conservatively. The conclusion drawn was that, although the majority of patients would recover without surgery, the latter could reduce the time taken for recovery especially with multiple fractures on both sides of the pelvis. (Denny, H. R. *Journal of Small Animal Practice*, 1978, **19**, 151). Occurs sometimes during service in bull and stallion when their hind-feet slip from under them and they fall backwards on to buttocks. Least serious when only external angle of ilium ('point of hip') involved.
6. THE SCAPULA. Fractures uncommon. Mostly occur through neck of bone, or on the projecting spine. Clothing of muscles impedes diagnosis but assists recovery, acting as natural bandage.
7. THE HUMERUS. Lameness intense in all animals; usually limb quite useless. Horses and cattle do not make good recoveries except when young, but other animals more satisfactory. (*See* BONE-PINNING.) Absolute rest essential; horses may be slung.

In a series of 130 cases in dogs and cats, most animals with proximal, shaft and supracondylar fractures had excellent results. The poor prognosis associated with distal articular fractures was most often because of failure of the fixation device in the supracondylar area. The best results were achieved with a plate on the caudal and medial surface of the distal humerus. (Bardet, J. F., Hohn and others, *Veterinary Surgery*, 1983, **12**, 73.)
8. THE RADIUS AND ULNA. One or both bones may be broken; fracture of ulna less serious unless elbow-joint involved. In dogs, if one broken the other acts as a natural splint. Lameness always marked, and pain on pressure. Local swelling usually noticed, and deformity. Bandaging useful and advisable. Young horses placed in slings. Bone-pinning has been carried out successfully in the dog and the horse.
9. CORONOID PROCESS (lower jaw). One hundred and thirty cases of fragmented coronoid process in 109 dogs were studied. Sixty-eight cases were treated surgically by medial elbow arthrotomy and 62 were treated with rest and anti-inflammatory drugs. Surgical treatment did not decrease the incidence of lameness after treatment, but the dogs treated surgically were more active and less lame than those treated without surgery. Young dogs with mild lameness due to fragmented medial coronoid processes probably do not benefit from surgery, but dogs with chronic, moderate or severe lameness have a better prognosis if they are treated surgically. (Read, R. A., Armstrong, S. J., O'Keefe, J. D. & Eger, C. E. (1990) *Journal of Small Animal Practice* **31**, 330.)
10. BONES OF KNEE. Seldom fractured except from shrapnel, bullets, etc., Impossible to bring about recovery without stiffening of joint (ankylosis). Occurs rarely in dogs, from very severe crushes; in such cases recovery very problematical.

11. THE METACARPALS. Generally not very serious in dog. In horse good recoveries made when fracture is clean across without complications or splinters. Those occurring in middle of cannon most satisfactory. Limb bandaged; horse slung; plaster left in position for at least 6 weeks. Usually little or no resulting callus or blemish when well set.

12. THE PASTERN BONE. May be transverse, oblique, or longitudinal ('split pastern'), often comminuted. Severe lameness always. Simple transverse fractures satisfactory if temperament of horse will allow rest and slinging; oblique, longitudinal, and all comminuted cases unsatisfactory, and if recovery occurs usually some deformity or blemish left.

13. THE SECOND PHALANX, COFFIN- AND NAVICULAR BONES. Fractures in these bones are rare; caused by direct violence, and sometimes follow operation of neurectomy (unnerving), and seen in cattle as a result of weakening of bone through FLUOROSIS. Fracture of coffin-bone if simple and joint surfaces not involved makes good recovery as a rule, since hoof acts as splint and bandage. Fracture of second phalanx (short pastern bone) usually very unsatisfactory.

Seventy-three phalangeal fractures were diagnosed in 71 cattle. Twenty-four cattle had injured themselves on slatted floors. Closed fractures were treated conservatively by orthopaedic shoeing of the adjacent claw. Digital amputation was necessary in 27 cases. (Köstlin, R. & Petzoldt, F.-J., *Tierärztliche Umschau*, (1985), **40**, 864.)

Most fractures of the navicular bone are sagittal and minimally displaced but the prognosis is poor because the fibrous callus causes permanent lameness. Such fractures in five horses were repaired by inserting a 50 mm screw which exerted compression between the two fragments. The pilot hole was drilled and the screw implanted precisely along the transverse axis of the navicular bone by means of a mechanical guide; the process was monitored by image intensifying fluoroscopy. After 11 weeks the fractures had healed without superfluous callus formation. (Nemth, F. & Dik, K. J., *Equine Veterinary Journal*, (1985), **17,** 137.)

14. THE FEMUR. Very common in dogs after street accidents. Shaft, neck, or one of the trochanters may be involved. Frequently in dogs dislocation of the hip-joint accompanies fracture. Extreme lameness, shortening of the limb, local swelling, and great pain on movement usually seen. There may or may not be crepitus. In horse, fracture of pelvis very often accompanies fractured femur and makes diagnosis difficult. Usually necessitates euthanasia in large animals, but in small animals recovery may be either partial or complete. (*See* BONE-PINNING.)

15. THE PATELLA. Is a very serious condition. Results in a lowering of the affected stifle and inability to advance the limb. There is great pain and much swelling over the stifle. Only treatment is union of the fragments by wire sutures; difficult to perform, and seldom does complete recovery follow.

16. THE TIBIA. Many fractures of tibia become compound from sharp points of broken bones penetrating through the skin. (*See* BONE-PINNING which has been used successfully in dog, cat, and horse.)

17. BONES OF HOCK. Fracture of os calcis (point of hock) – the epiphyseal summit becomes torn away from the rest of the bone by an undue pull of the Achilles' tendon (hamstring). Fractures of other bones of hock are less common (with the exception of the SCAPHOID in the racing greyhound). (*See* SCAPHOID; BONES, ARTIFICIAL; WIRING.)

18. THE LOWER BONES OF THE LEG. What has been said as applied to the fore cannons, pasterns, and coffin-bones, etc., is almost equally applicable to the hind-limbs, but in a hind-limb a similar fracture is more serious than in a fore-limb. (*See* SPLINTING.)

FRANCISELLA (*see* TULARAEMIA).

FREE RADICALS. Highly reactive molecules, formed in the presence of oxygen and capable of damaging living tissue. They have been implicated in human heart disease and arthritis. They may also be a cause of sudden death of pigs: those being transported for long distances or subject to other forms of stress. However, protection can be given by feeding vitamin E, which 'scavenges' radicals, Drs Garry Duthie and John Arthur Free of the A F R C stated.

FREEMARTIN. Until 1977 it was reasonable to define a freemartin as a sterile heifer born twin to a normal bull calf; the most widely accepted explanation being that sex hormones from the earlier developing male twin pass across to the female twin, with the result that sexual differentiation of both male and female proceeds under control of male hormones.

However, as long ago as 1917 it had been suggested that hermaphrodites might occur in female *single* births, as a consequence of early fetal death and resorption of the male twin in the uterus. During the 1970s chromosome analysis had revealed the presence of both male and female cells in single-born bull calves. Dr Wijeratne and colleagues were the first to demonstrate this condition – technically known as *secondary chimerism* – in single-born freemartins. (*Primary chimerism* can occur where two sperms fertilise the same ovum.)

Not every female fetus having a male twin sharing the uterus will become a freemartin, because in some instances death of the male twin fetus occurs before about day 39 of pregnancy – when a common blood supply may become established. Moreover, in between 5 and 10 per cent of heterosexual twin pregnancies a common blood supply is not established.

Blood samples were taken from 36 heifers not in calf after three or more inseminations or natural service, and chromosome analysis of these animals' white cells showed that 12 of the heifers had both male and female chromosomes. Five of these heifers were single-born. In three which were slaughtered, abnormalities of the reproductive tract were formed.

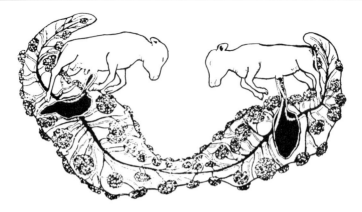

The bovine freemartin.

Two of the slaughtered heifers had shown normal oestrous cycles, and had reproductive organs apparently normal on clinical examination; but one of them, with 5 per cent male cells, had her cervix closed by a fibrous band or hymen; the other which had 12 per cent male cells was sterile on account of fibrous bands blocking the horns of the uterus. Both heifers possessed functional ovaries. The third heifer, with 45 per cent male cells, had a normal vagina, enlarged clitoris, seminal vesicles and sex organs having both ovaries and testes in primitive form.

'Presuming that 5 per cent of all heifers reared for breeding are infertile, the probable prevalence of single-born freemartins in this heifer population is about 0·9 per cent.' (W. V. S. Wijeratne, I. B. Munro, and P. R. Wilkes. *Vet. Record* (1977), **100**, 333.)

About 90 per cent of heifer calves born twin to a bull calf are freemartins. Many freemartins can be detected on clinical examination, since the vagina is often only a third of the normal length and, in addition, there is often an enlarged clitoris and a vulval tuft of hair.

The condition is associated with anastomosis of the placental blood-vessels (*see* diagram).

Pig freemartins may also occur. (*See also* H-Y ANTIGEN.)

FREEZE-BRANDING (*see* BRANDING).

FREMITUS is a sensation which is communicated to the hand of an observer when it is laid across the chest in certain diseases of the lungs and heart. Friction fremitus is a grating feeling communicated to the hand by the pleura or pericardium when it is roughened as in pleurisy or pericarditis.

FRESCON (N-Tritylmorpholine) has been developed for control of the amphibious snails which transmit liver fluke (*Fasciola hepatica*), a parasite of sheep and cattle.

FROG (*see* FOOT OF HORSE).

FRONTAL BONE of the skull. A roughly quadrilateral plate-like bone which forms part of the roof of the cranium and passes forward between the eyes to meet the nasal bones. In the horned breeds of cattle and sheep it is extended laterally to form the horn cores. (*See* BONES, *also* SINUSES OF SKULL.)

FRONTAL SINUS (*see* SINUSES OF SKULL).

FROST-BITE may affect any animal exposed for long periods to severe cold. As a result of this cold the body reacts by a constriction of surface blood-vessels, in order to minimise heat loss and maintain body temperature. This leaves exposed parts of the skin susceptible to freezing. The part, such as the tips of ears, or the tail, becomes numb, and may be completely frozen. Pain is not felt at this stage (but occurs during the thawing process). In some instances natural recovery takes place, but in others gangrene follows and ear-tips, tails, and the wattles and combs of poultry may slough off.

An animal-owner may have no reason to suspect frostbite until the appearance of gangrene and sloughing. (*See* GANGRENE.) Nowadays massage, rubbing the part with snow have been abandoned as likely to do more harm than good in human medicine; and immersing the part in warm or hot water is equally to be avoided. (*See* CHILBLAIN.)

FRUSEMIDE. A diuretic suitable for the treatment of some cases of OEDEMA.

'FRYING PAN' DEATHS. Overheated fat gives off acrolein, which can be highly poisonous and was, indeed, used in chemical warfare in 1914–18. A dog died after being shut up in a kitchen for half an hour with a smoking chip pan. *Ante-mortem* symptoms were distressed breathing and cyanosis.

Five cockatiels died within half an hour following exposure to fumes from a 'non-stick' frying pan coated with plastic polytetrafluoroethylene. Within an hour the birds' owner became ill with 'polymer fume fever', but recovered. In this case the pan contained water only – no fat. (Blandford, T. B., *Vet. Rec.* (1975), **96**.)

FUCOSIDOSIS. A lysosomal storage disease caused by the absence of an enzyme – alpha-L-fucosidase.

It is an inherited disease in the English Springer Spaniel, affecting mainly those between 18 months and 4 years old. The signs of this ultimately fatal disease include ataxia, change in temperament, depression, apparent deafness and impaired sight. Swallowing may be difficult. Loss of weight occurs. (Herrtage, M. E., BVA Congress, 1986.)

FUMES (*see* CARBON MONOXIDE, 'FRYING-PAN' DEATHS, SLURRY, ANAESTHETICS, AEROSOLS).

FUMIGATION (*see* DISINFECTION).

FUNDUS is the base or innermost part of a hollow organ distant from its opening.

FUNGAL DISEASES. Broadly speaking, these include both the invasion of tissues by fungi, and also the effects on organs of fungal poisons (*see* MYCOTOXICOSIS).

Ringworm offers a good example of the invasion of tissues by pathogenic fungi; one should, perhaps, say *potentially* pathogenic fungi, for many are present in the alimentary canal of healthy animals, and cause lesions only when circumstances favour invasion or multiplication. (*See* MASTITIS – Mycotic, for an example of the latter.)

(*See also* ASPERGILLOSIS, BLASTOMYCOSIS, HISTOPLASMOSIS, MUCORMYCOSIS, MONILIASIS, STREPTOTHRICOSIS, CRYPTOCOCCOSIS, FUSARIUM, MORTIERELLA, COCCIDIOMYCOSIS, RHINOSPORIDIOSIS, SPOROTRICHOSIS.)

FUNGAL TOXINS (*see* MYCOTOXICOSIS).

FUR MITES (*see* MITES).

FUR, SWALLOWED (*see* HAIR BALLS).

FURAZOLIDONE. A drug used in the treatment of Blackhead and Hexamitiasis.

FURFURACEOUS is a term applied to skin diseases which produce a bran-like scaliness.

FURUNCULOSIS. The presence of boils (abscesses). In the dog, the term is applied sometimes to abscesses/cysts between the toes. (*See* INTERDIGITAL CYSTS.) Perianal furuncolosis also occurs in dogs.

FURZE, or GORSE (*Ulex europaeus*), which is a very common and plentiful shrub in waste lands in Great Britain, was formerly often cut and used as fodder after chaffing or bruising. The plant contains a very small proportion of a poisonous alkaloid which is called *ulexine*, and is practically identical with *cystine* from broom. It is a nerve and muscle poison, but it is seldom present in dangerous amounts. (*See* BROOM POISONING for signs.)

FUS (*see* FELINE UROLOGICAL SYNDROME).

FUSARIUM. Mouldy shelled maize containing *F. moniliforme* has caused diarrhoea and ataxia in cattle; and in broilers the same species, contaminating maize and wheat, has with *F. culmorum*, *F. Tricinctum*, and *F. nivale*, been implicated in poor growth rate, poor feathering, and abnormal behaviour. Fusarium species may also cause kerato-conjunctivitis (*See under* EYE, DISEASES; *also* MYCOTOXICOSIS, and ZEARALENONE.)

FUSIFORMIS (Bacteroides.) (*See* BACTERIA – table, *and* FOOT-ROT).

G

GAD-FLY, 'GADDING' (*see* FLIES, WARBLES). In Britain, warble flies are on the wing from late May onwards.

GAIT, ABNORMAL (*see* ATAXIA, DYSMETRIA, 'GOOSE-STEPPING', LAMENESS).

GALACTAGOGUE A preparation, usually a herbal one, given in the hope of increasing milk production in cows.

GALACTOCELE is a cyst-like swelling in the mammary gland caused by the obstruction of the milk-duct which normally carries the milk from the area to the milk sinus at the base of the teat. The condition is seen in sows and bitches, but is rare in cows.

GALL-BLADDER is the little pouch-like sac in which bile produced by the liver is stored until it is required during the process of digestion. It is a hollow pear-shaped organ lying in a depression on the posterior surface of the liver. The gall-bladder is not present in the horse and in animals of the horse tribe, but is found in the other domesticated animals.

Blockages of the bile-duct by liver flukes or by gall-stones may result in jaundice as well as severe local inflammation. Acute inflammation of the gall-bladder is painful, and there is danger of rupture or gangrene.

A case of spontaneous perforation of the gall-bladder was reported by Lipowitz. Vomiting, abdominal tenderness, and loss of appetite were present for several days before jaundice appeared. Paracentesis and radiography revealed ascites. Treatment consisted of cholecystectomy, abdominal lavage and drainage, and antibiotics. An uneventful recovery followed.

'GALL SICKNESS' (*see* ANAPLASMOSIS.)

GALL-STONES, which are also known as BILIARY CALCULI, are concretions which are formed in the gall-bladder or in the bile-ducts of the liver. As a rule they are hard, brownish in colour, coated with mucus, and of a more or less rounded shape. They may be composed of cholestrol, cholestrol and bile pigments, or of pigment and lime salts. One or several may be present, causing pain and jaundice.

Gallstones are more prevalent in sheep than in cows, cats, and horses, and more than twice as prevalent as the 5 per cent found in a systematic study of gallstones in dogs. (Petruzzi, J. & others. *Journal of Comparative Pathology* (1988) **98** 367.)

In human medicine ursodeoxycholic acid has been used to dissolve gallstones.

GALVANISED BINS, used to store swill, have led to zinc poisoning in pigs. (*See* ZINC POISONING.)

GALVAYNE'S GROOVE (*see* DENTITION, horse's).

GAME BIRDS, MORTALITY. This may be considered under two headings:

From farm chemicals. The most important of these are dieldrin, aldrin, and heptachlor, used as seed dressings; some of the organo-phosphorus insecticides such as schradan; dimethoate; the 'nitro-type' of weedkillers such as DNC, which stains the carcase yellow. (*See* DDT.)

DDT and even the relatively safe insecticide BHC can, if used in too high a concentration, prove lethal. Pheasant poults have died as a result of being treated for lice with a 5 per cent gamma benzene hexachloride dusting powder.

The organo-phosphorus insecticides, mentioned above, do not necessarily act quickly. Death may occur eight weeks after eating the poisoned food. The symptoms shown by poisoned birds include: ruffled feathers, saliva around the beak, high-stepping gait or unsteadiness on the legs, distressed breathing, and paralysis.

Spraying an orchard with either DDD or DDT has caused heavy game bird losses. A partridge was found dead in a field where blackcurrants had been sprayed with the insecticide Endrin. It was reported from the farm that eight or nine partridges died within a few hours of eating earthworms which came to the surface of the soil soon after spraying. Rat poisons may perhaps be included in the term 'farm chemicals'. Owls die after eating poisoned rodents.

From natural causes. Impacted gizzard, roup, tuberculosis, aspergillosis, swine erysipelas, fowl-pox, fowl cholera, fowl typhoid, infectious sinusitis. 'Gapes' is another cause of death; in the USA, Equine Encephalomyelitis. Deaths from Fowl Pest (Newcastle disease) have been reported in the UK; Blackhead in pheasants and partridges.

'GROUSE DISEASE' is the colloquial name for infestation with *Trichostrongylus tenuis*, which can cause disease when food supplies fail.

LOUPING ILL, transmitted by sheep ticks, is generally fatal to red grouse, and can reduce stocks to very low densities. Red grouse (*Lagopus lagopus scoticus*) are 'the commonest game birds on British heather moorland. In maximising stocks of wild grouse, management techniques include burning heather in narrow strips to provide a patchwork of long heather for cover, and short heather – the preferred food. Draining of wet moors improves heather growth, but many boggy patches should be left to ensure enough insects for the chicks.' Cotton grass can be grown for the sake of the flower-heads as a dietary supplement for laying hens. (Moss, R. & Watson, A. Institute of Terrestial Ecology, Kincardineshire.)

A nine-day outbreak of **INCLUSION-BODY HEPATITIS** resulted in an 18 per cent mortality among 1000 intensively reared pheasant poults (19 days old when the outbreak began). This virus disease had been recorded in chickens in the UK previously, but not in pheasants.

An outbreak of **SALMONELLOSIS** killed 50 per cent of 2800 pheasant poults, deaths beginning in 3-day-olds. The infection was one of *S. typhimurium*, An antibiotic achieved control later.

COCCIDIOSIS is an important disease of pheasants and other game birds, and causes a high mortality in chicks 2 to 4 weeks old.

YERSINIOSIS is another important disease of pheasants.

MONILIASIS causes lethargy, stunted growth and a heavy mortality in partridges. Treatment with formic acid, sprayed on food, has proved successful in treatment. (*See also* BOTULISM.)

GAMETES. These are the ova and spermatozoa, and contain half the number (haploid) of chromosomes present in all other body cells (diploid).
Gametocide for bird control. (*See* TEM.)

GAMMA CAMERA, PROBE (*see* RADIO-ISOTOPES).

GAMMA GLOBULIN is a protein fraction of the blood serum which contains the antibodies against certain bacteria or viruses. (*See* COLOSTRUM, IMMUNOGLOBULINS.) It can be prepared in a concentrated form and can be used to give protection against infection.

GAMMEXANE products contain the gamma isomer of benzene hexachloride, a highly effective, persistent insecticide. (*See* BENZENE HEXACHLORIDE; *also* BHC POISONING.)

GANGLION is a group of nerve cell bodies.

GANGRENE means the death (necrosis) of a part of the body accompanied by putrefaction. In *primary gangrene* the organisms which cause the necrosis also bring about the putrefactive changes. In *secondary gangrene* the putrefaction is caused by organisms which have invaded dead tissue (*e.g.* following a burn). There are two varieties of gangrene, *dry* and *moist*; dry gangrene is a condition of mummification in which the circulation stops and the part withers up, while in moist gangrene there is inflammation accompanied by putrefactive changes.

Infection following necrosis may lead to gangrene after burns, scalds, frostbite, crush wounds, puncture wounds, etc.

Poisoning by ergot results in the same condition in the most distant parts of the body, *e.g.* the feet, tip of tail, ears, and the combs and wattles of poultry.

SIGNS. There is at first a degree of pain when the affected part is handled, and in a short time it becomes reddened and swollen. Later it turns blue or black, the hair falls from it, and there is a distinct line of demarcation between the gangrenous and the healthy surface. Around the dividing line there is usually some degree of inflammation, and pus production.

Moist gangrene is considerably more serious, since it is accompanied by putrefaction and the absorption of toxins. The whole area turns black or greenish, the hair falls out, an offensive smell is evident, and much fluid exudes from the decomposing tissues. A high temperature, disturbed heart's action, and rapid breathing, are shown. (*See also* GAS GANGRENE.)

TREATMENT is mainly surgical, backed up by the use of appropriate antibiotics or sulphonamides. In advanced cases humane destruction becomes necessary. (*See also* FROST-BITE.)

GANGRENOUS DERMATITIS. A disease of poultry, often associated with Infectious Bursal Disease and Inclusion-Body Hepatitis, which usually affects birds between 25–50 days of age.

GANJAM ULRUS. The Indian name for a Bunyavirus infection transmitted by ticks.

GAPES is a disease of young chickens and turkeys particularly, although all the domesticated and many wild birds may also be affected, which is due to *Syngamus trachea*.

The presence of worms in the bronchial tubes and trachea of the bird causes it to gasp for breath or 'gape', from which the name of the disease originated. Part of the life-history of the worm is passed in the body of the earthworm, and young chickens eating earthworms may become affected. (*See also under* CAPILLARIASIS.)

Thiabendazole, given in the feed, is an effective method of treatment.

GARDEN CHEMICALS. Birds, dogs, and cats may be poisoned as a result of the use of pesticides. For the poisoning of birds, *see preparations listed under* GAME-BIRDS. Dieldrin is highly toxic for cats, and like DDT, should not be used on them or in their vicinity. In fact, all the CHLORINATED HYDROCARBONS are best avoided in places where small domestic animals or their food may become contaminated.

For the dangers of slug-baits, *see* METALDEHYDE POISONING. (*See* ORCHARDS for the dangers of fruit-tree sprays. For seed dressings, *see under* SEED CORN.) (*See also* PARAQUAT, HERBICIDES.)

GARDEN NIGHTSHADE POISONING results from animals eating *Solanum nigrum*, which is found in many parts of the world. Its toxicity appears to vary in different localities. The berries contain an active alkaloidal glycoside called *solanine*, which is readily converted into sugar and the poisonous *solanidine* by the action of the gastric juices in the stomach.

SIGNS. Staggering, loss of sensation and consciousness, and sometimes convulsions. First-aid: strong black tea or coffee.

GARRON. A useful type of horse for hill-farm work and carrying deer. Garrons do not constitute a separate breed, but were a cross between Western Island ponies and the Percheron. Nowadays, the Garron is regarded as a larger version of the Highland pony.

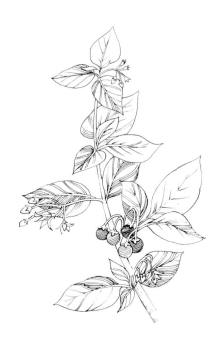

Garden Nightshade (*Solanum nigrum*), also known as
Black Nightshade, has small purple flowers, and large
black shiny berries, several of which are attached to a
single stalk. Height: 4 to 6 ft.

GAS (*see* AIR, BLOAT, CARBON MONOXIDE, OZONE,
ANAESTHETICS, SLURRY, NITROGEN DIOXIDE, etc.)

GAS GANGRENE is an acute bacterial disease
due to the inoculation of wounds with organisms
belonging to the 'gas gangrene' group. This group
comprises anaerobic organisms, most of which
produce a gas when living in the animal body, and
all of which are associated with decomposition of
the tissues invaded.

Gas gangrene may attack any of the domestic
animals and man. The horse is least resistant and
the cow least susceptible.

CAUSES. Gas gangrene is produced by the *Clostridium oedematiens, Cl. welchii, Cl. septicum, Cl.
Chauvei* gaining access to the tissues of an animal
through a small wound; after castration or docking, etc.

SIGNS. A few hours after the organisms gain entrance the area of invasion is found swollen, hot,
painful on pressure, and may crackle when
handled. This latter effect is due to gas formation
below the skin. The skin and underlying tissues
rapidly become discoloured.

In a series of nine cases in horses, the signs were
fever, depression, painful muscular swellings,
and toxaemia. All were dehydrated. Colic had
been evident in 6 of the horses; laminitis in 2.
Infection had followed intra-muscular injections
in 8 of the horses, and a puncture wound in 1. The
Clostridia isolated were: *chauvoei*, 1; *septicum*, 2;
and *perfringens* (6). (Rebhun, William C.
JAVMA, (1985), **187**, 732.)

PREVENTION. Immunisation can be effected.
(*See also* BRAXY, BLACKQUARTER.)

GASTRALGIA. Pain in the stomach.

GASTRECTASIS. Dilatation of the stomach.

GASTRECTOMY is an operation for the
removal of the whole or part of the stomach.

GASTRIC means anything connected with the
stomach, *e.g.* gastric ulcer, gastric juice.

GASTRIC ULCERS. These are seen in pigs in
some cases (but not all) of SWINE FEVER. They
have also been found in piglets under a fortnight
old, due to *Rhizopus microsporus*, isolated both
from stomachs and bedding. (*See* MUCORMYCOSIS.)
Associated with this infection may be another
fungal one – MONILIASIS – caused by the yeast-
like organism *Candida albicans*.

Gastric ulcers may also be produced by the
toxin of *Aspergillus flavus* (see AFLATOXIN.), and
by COPPER POISONING.

For gastric ulcers in cattle, *see under* STOMACH,
DISEASES OF – Abomasum – *and* RUMEN, DISEASES
OF.)

GASTRITIS. Inflammation of the stomach.

GASTROCNEMIUS is the large muscle which
lies behind the stifle-joint and the tibia and fibula,
and ends in the tendon Achilles or 'hamstring'
which is attached to the 'point of the hock'.

GASTRODISCUS. Amphistome flukes, *e.g. G.
aegyptiacus*, are common parasites of horses and
pigs in the tropics and subtropics. A heavy infestation has caused collapse in the horse.

GASTRO-ENTERITIS is inflammation of the
stomach and intestines. It is an acute condition
commonest in young animals. It may be specific
or due to irritant organic or inorganic poisons.
(*See also* HAEMORRHAGIC, PARASITIC, and
TRANSMISSIBLE GASTROENTERITIS; also DIAR-
RHOEA.)

GASTROPEXY. A surgical operation to prevent
a recurrence of torsion of the stomach. In dogs it
has been carried out after spot coagulation of the
surface of the fundus by diathermy. The stomach
is fixed in its normal position against the diaphragm by 7 to 10 rows of silk sutures (7 or 10 to a
row).

The incision into the abdominal wall is closed
by absorbable synthetic sutures.

This operation is also known as Fundupexy.

(Frendin, J. & Funkquist, B. *Journal of Small
Animal Practice* (1990) **3**, 78.)

GEL is a colloid substance which is firm in consistency, although it contains much water; *e.g.* ordinary gelatin.

GELATIN SPONGE is prepared as a haemostatic, and can be left in a wound; complete
absorption taking place in 4 to 6 weeks. The
sponge may be sterilised in dry heat, and applied
either dry or moistened with normal saline, an

antibiotic solution, or a solution of thrombin. Absorbable Gelatin Sponge complies with the requirements of the British Pharmacopoeia.

GELBVIEHS. This German Yellow breed, as it is also known, was evolved by crossing Swiss breeds with German breeds, and is dual-purpose, averaging nearly 800 gallons of milk at 4 per cent butterfat. Fattening stock give a daily liveweight gain of 2·5 lb and are ready for the butcher at 405 days in Germany.

GELDING is a castrated horse.

Occasionally a horse which has had both testicles completely removed shows stallion-like behaviour, when it is known as a 'false rig'. Such an animal may mount mares and achieve both erection and intromission. The chasing, or rounding up, of mares, and nipping them, may also occur. This behaviour is not hormonally induced or hormone dependent; and the old idea that it is due to being 'cut proud' can no longer be accepted. 'The thesis put forward is that the behaviour shown is part of the normal social interaction between horses.' (Cox, J. E. *Veterinary Record*, (1986), **118,** 353.) 'False rigs' and cryptorchids may show similar behaviour.

Blood samples were taken before, and 30 to 100 minutes after an intravenous injection of human chorionic gonadotrophin from 104 horses with either sexual and/or aggressive male behaviour but which had no palpable or visible testes. The concentration of testosterone in the second sample classified all but eight horses as either geldings (<40 pg/ml) or cryptorchids (>100 pg/ml). Surgical investigation confirmed the diagnosis in 23 geldings and 47 cryptorchids while the remaining horses were not operated on. (Cox, J. E. (1975), *Equine Veterinary Journal*, **7,** 179.) (*See also* CASTRATION – Immuno-castration, for treatment of an aggressive cryptorchid stallion.)

GENERIC PRODUCTS. Those sold under their pharmacopoeic names rather than brand names.

GENES. The biological units of heredity, arranged along the length of the CHROMOSOMES (which see). (*See also* CELLS.)

GENETICS, HEREDITY, and BREEDING

GENETICS, HEREDITY, and BREEDING.

Introduction. The science of genetics deals with the physiology of heredity, the mechanism by which resemblance between parent and offspring is conserved and transmitted, and with the origin and significance of variation, the mechanism by which such resemblance is modified and transformed. It seeks to define the manner in which the hereditary characters of the individual are represented in the fertilised egg in which the individual has its beginning.

Stock-breeding is a craft concerned with the maintenance of the desirable qualities of a stock, the improvement of these qualities generation by generation, and the elimination through breeding of qualities which are held to be undesirable. The problems of the geneticist and of the stock-breeder are identical though their interests are dissimilar.

The geneticist has made much progress by studying the inexpensive, quickly maturing, very highly fertile animals such as the mouse, rat, guinea-pig, rabbit, and above all the fruit fly *Drosophila*.

A better understanding of heredity was rendered possible by the concept that the individual as a whole was not the unit in inheritance, but could be regarded as a definite orderly combination of independently heritable units.

Breed was now interpreted as signifying different combinations of independently heritable characters all drawn from the common source of the stock in which modern domesticated cattle had their origin, just as different arrangements and combinations of letters make different words, though all words are made up of letters derived from a common source – the alphabet.

The breeder has employed the methods of hybridisation and in-breeding associated with selection in the creation of the modern breeds. He has practised inbreeding with selection in order that the desired type of his stock may be fixed, and he has sought hybrid vigour in outcrossing. The geneticist has employed these very same methods in his studies. The method of genetics is character-analysis. The object of the breeder is character-synthesis.

Instead of the hereditary mechanism being a simple affair as was first thought, it is one of the most complex.

Phenotype and **Genotype.** Allan Fraser MD, DSc, when senior lecturer in animal husbandry at Aberdeen University, once drew a helpful analogy between heredity and a game of cards, with each card representing a gene, and Honours cards representing genes most desirable to a breeder.

A game of cards is preceded by the shuffling of packs, and so also is the conception of an animal preceded by a shuffling of genes. Each pack is then halved – just as before sperm and ovum meet, and the number of genes in both is halved by what is called the reduction division. Fertilisation then reunites the two half packs to form one new pack. The cards in this represent the genes in the new individual animal.

'The cards in any one hand or the gene sample in any individual animal are the result of pure chance – no one can predict how the run of the cards or of the genes will go.'

Of two animals, sharing the same sire and dam, one may have a much better genotype, be a more valuable breeding animal than its full brother or sister. (This is shown in the diagram below, under the heading 'Inheritance and High milk yields'.

If the cards dealt at conception be called the unalterable genotype of the animal, the playing of that hand may be called the environment, which includes climate, nutrition, exposure to infections, stocking rates, and every aspect of husbandry and animal management.

Some stockmen can make a surprisingly good job with poor genetic material; others a sorry job with the best stock; but of course the most skilful stockman cannot improve upon the hand of genes once dealt.

Genotype can be defined as the entire array of genes carried by an individual (or, in another sense, the genetic constitution of an individual with respect to any limited number of genes under examination).

Phenotype means the appearance and/or the performance of an individual. Phenotypic variation of a population results from the combined effects of inheritance and environment. Genetic variation is that part of the phenotypic variation which is due to genes.

Homozygous and **Heterozygous**. In order to illustrate one of the simpler aspects of heredity in relation to stock-breeding, *the appearance of red calf in a herd in which the fashionable coat colour is black, and in which all red animals are eliminated,* will serve as an example.

Black-and-red coat colours in cattle constitute a typical pair of Mendelian characters, black being the dominant and red being the recessive member of the pair. A red calf can only be produced by black parents when both of these are heterozygous in respect of their coat-colour character. For the character black-coat colour there is a determiner or factor. This factor may be present in the zygote in the duplex state, having been conveyed thereinto by both egg and sperm. When the factor for black is present in the duplex state the individual that arises for that fertilised egg or zygote is spoken of as being homozygous for the character black-coat colour. On the other hand, into the zygote there may have been brought a factor for black from one parent and a factor for red, the alternative character, from the other parent. Under these circumstances, of these two factors, that for black and that for red, it is the former alone that determines what the coat colour shall be. Black is said to be dominant in its relation to red. Homozygous and heterozygous blacks will be indistinguishable on inspection. If two heterozygous blacks are mated there will occur on the average in every four, 3 black calves to 1 red. To explain this 3:1 ratio it is assumed that *half of both male and female gametes* of such

heterozygous individuals (*i.e.* sperm and ovum) carry the factor for the dominant character *black*, and the other half the factor for the alternative recessive *red*, and the two sorts of egg and of sperm occur in equal numbers. If it is assumed that for every pair of factors that correspond to a pair of characters only one can pass into the ripe gamete, it follows that a 3:1 ratio in the next generation will be obtained, and of the individuals exhibiting the dominant character one will be homozygous for that character and two heterozygous, whilst the individual exhibiting the recessive character must of necessity carry the factor for that character in the duplex state, since if in its hereditary constitution it carries a factor for the dominant, it will exhibit the dominant character. It is possible by examining the records of the coat colours of the offspring to define the hereditary constitution of the parent in respect of the coat colours black and red. The following matings are possible:

Homozygous black to homozygous black will give none but blacks, all homozygous.

Homozygous black to heterozygous black will give all blacks, of which 50 per cent will be homozygous and 50 per cent heterozygous.

Homozygous black to homozygous red will give all heterozygous blacks.

Heterozygous black to heterozygous black will give 25 per cent homozygous blacks, 50 per cent heterozygous blacks, and 25 per cent reds.

Heterozygous black to red will give 50 per cent heterozygous blacks and 50 per cent red.

Red to red will give all reds, of necessity homozygous. The only mating of blacks that can yield a red calf is that of two individuals heterozygous in respect of this coat-colour character.

The coat-colour character has to be considered quite apart from all the rest of the characters that in their association make the animal what it is. An individual is a pure black when it is in respect of this character homozygous, when in its hereditary constitution the determiner or factor for this character has been received from both its parents.

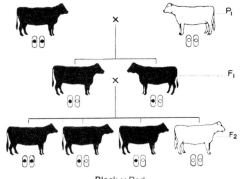

Black × Red
(Red is necessarily white in the diagram.)

Inheritance through multiple genes. The above example shows how a character, coat colour, may be inherited through single genes. This is the mechanism of heredity at its simplest. Most characters, however, including many of economic importance to the farmer, are inherited in a far more complex manner through multiple genes.

Multiple genes may have an additive effect as regards the expression of some character; or they may interact, one with another, in the production of a character, inheritance of which is even more complex.

Inheritance and **High milk yields**. It seems that it is easier to increase the butter-fat content and solids-not-fat content than it is to increase the milk yield through breeding. The heritability of milk yield is not as high as that of some other characters.

There is a correlation between high yields and body size, but conformation is by no means always associated with high yields. A few of the highest yielding cows have had, to put it mildly, an unfashionable conformation.

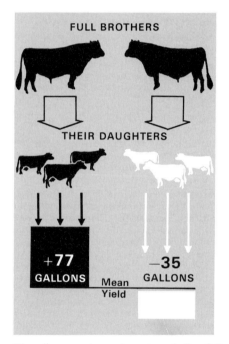

The diagram shows how two bulls, full brothers, may influence milk production in their daughters in opposite ways. It also shows how the 'gene lottery' can make nonsense out of the expectations of a breeder.

For this reason, progeny testing has proved of the greatest importance in the selection of bulls, each of which – through A I – may have not 100 offspring but tens of thousands.

It is possible for a farmer to use (by means of A I) a bull with the proved ability to produce daughters with a high milk yield, as compared with the yield resulting from use of an improved or average bull. Proven bulls are listed in terms of 'a bonus of 50 or of anything up to 100 gallons' and also in terms of a butterfat 'bonus'). (*See also* PROGENY TESTING.)

There have been many scientific papers reporting association between blood groups and production characters in cattle and other animals. The work on transferrin and milk yield is one

example; that of blood groups and milk yield another. 'None of the effects found was large enough to be of practical value in selecting to milk yield,' stated Dr R. L. Spooner and colleagues (*Anim. Prod.* 1973, **16**, 209–14), in their paper 'Apparent Heterozygote Excess at the Amylase I locus in cattle.' They described a technique of detecting Amylase I genotypes in sera by electrophoresis in starch gel as a promising method of future selection for milk yield. (*See also* BLOOD TYPING, ELECTROPHORESIS.)

Selection is the systematic choice of animals in a population (defined in the genetic sense as a group of interbreeding animals sharing a common gene pool, *e.g.* a closed herd, an A I district, a breed) as parents for the next generation.

Family selection means the selection of individuals on the performance of their relatives (sibs, half-sibs, or progeny); *i.e.* selection between families instead of between individuals.

Genotypic selection is that based on progeny testing with a very large number of progeny, so that the breeding value of the parent is exactly known.

Inbreeding may be defined as the mating of individuals more closely related than the average relationship of the population.

Both crossbreeding and inbreeding are methods of bringing about genetic change.

Inbreeding was practised by the early developers and improvers of livestock breeds in order to fix the type of their animals. 'Perhaps it is as well that they were unable also to fix performance,' commented, in the A B R O report for January 1974, Dr Gerald Winer and Dr Susan Hayter.

Inbreeding can be expected to increase the proportion of animals homozygous for a given desired character. As the process proceeds, however, individuals with undesirable characters are likely to appear – animals which are abnormal in some respect, sterile, or weak. Inbreeding could prove disastrously expensive if the proportion of such animals were high. (Test mating of a bull to related or carrier females may be carried out in order to detect specific genes such as lethal factors; the carriers then being culled from the herd.)

Prolonged inbreeding will lead to disappointing regression, diminution of vigour, decreased fertility, and a reduction in body size.

The fusion of two inbred lines. By inbreeding for a specific character, and by practising rigid selection for two, three, or more generations, a strain of relatively homozygous individuals for the selected character can be created. If two such strains are developed separately but simultaneously for two different but highly desirable characters, and if these two strains are then crossed, the resulting progeny can be expected to possess both desirable characters to a useful degree. The mechanism has been notably successful in producing strains of poultry with large egg size and high annual yields, and has been exploited commercially.

When the generation in which the two desirable characters are expressed is bred from again, an

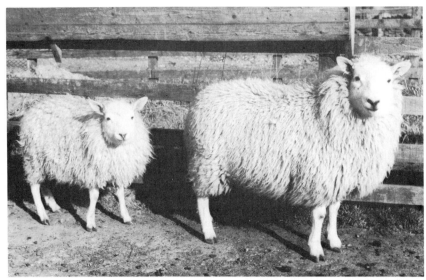

The effect of inbreeding and crossing. These two sheep were sired by the same ram, but the smaller one was highly inbred (59 per cent) and when 10 months old had attained little more than 40 per cent of the weight of its half-sib (right), which was a 3-way cross of inbred lines, its dam being a 2-way line cross. These hoggs are of Cheviot × Welsh extraction. (Animal Breeding Research Organisation photograph, with acknowledgements to Dr Gerald Wiener and Dr Susan Hayter.)

immediate reassortment of characters occurs, and only in a small percentage of the individuals will the desirable characters be expressed. The others are most likely to be useless.

Hybrid vigour (Heterosis), usually demonstrated by increase in size, better live-weight gains and greater resistance to disease and in the earlier attainment of sexual maturity, occurs in the first cross-bred generation out of the mating of two widely dissimilar pure-bred parental stocks. Hybrid vigour is an indication of heterozygosis. The two parental breeds must be within reason as dissimilar in their characterisation as possible; then in the pooling of those hereditary constitutions there will be a very considerable degree of heterozygosis in the first cross-bred offspring; the desirable characters are pooled, and in respect of those characters exhibited by the two parents the offspring will be heterozygous.

If the first crosses which exhibit this hybrid vigour so markedly are interbred, their offspring will not exhibit this vigour to the same extent.

'Nicking'. Two individuals not remarkable in themselves may produce superior offspring. This fact can be explained on the assumption that the mating brings together the chance association of factors which are complementary or supplementary, and that these in conjunction determine characters that are greatly esteemed.

'Pedigree and purity'. Pedigrees and registration in the appropriate herd book have been an essential part of breeders' work in all but 'commercial' herds. The system has been of service, though not free from abuse. Pedigrees have from time to time been falsified or genuine mistakes made (including use of the wrong semen in 'AI work'), and until the advent of blood typing there was no means of checking such errors.

It is easy to exaggerate the importance of

'family name' or of remote ancestors; and in terms of production traits or characters 'the concept of "purity" of pure breeds is not only something of a myth, but might actually be detrimental to the possibilities for improvement.' (ABRO report, January 1974.)

Chromosomes. A male can be distinguished from a female not only by external appearances and by differences in the architecture of the reproductive system, but also by differences in the organisation of the cells of which their bodies are composed.

The nucleus of the resting cell appears in stained microscopic preparations as a vesicle containing a network of delicate threads upon which are borne, like beads upon a tangled skein, minute masses of a deeply staining material known as **chromatin**. As the cell proceeds to divide into two, this tangled mass of fine threads resolves itself into a constant number of filaments of definite shape and these become progressively shorter to assume the form of stout rods known as **chromosomes**. The number of chromosomes is usually some multiple of two, and is constant and characteristic of the species to which the individual belongs, e.g. Dog 78; Horse 64; Cow 60; Sheep 54; Pig 38; Cat 38.

(The study of chromosomes is known as CYTO-GENETICS, which see.)

The **gametes,** egg and sperm respectively, differ remarkably in size and form, but they are alike in that each contains half the number of chromosomes that is characteristic of the somatic cells of that species.

At fertilisation, the characteristic number is restored, and in the case of each pair one member is derived from one parent, the other from the other. In this distribution of the chromosomes one finds a mechanism by which offspring may inherit from both parents by means of the constituent genes.

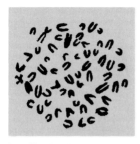

A bull's lymphocyte in metaphase of mitosis. (With acknowledgements to Dr C. R. E. Halnan
and to the *Veterinary Record*.)

It is possible to distinguish male from female
by differences in the chromosome content. While
all other pairs of chromosomes consist of two
chromosomes exactly alike in size and shape, one
pair differs in the two sexes. As they influence sex
determination, these chromosomes are referred to
as the sex-chromosomes.

The ovum (or egg) contains the X chromosome.
The sperm may contain either the Y chromosome,
which will produce male offspring (XY), or the X
chromosome, which will produce female offspring (XX).

In most female mammals the paired sex-
chromosomes are identical, and called the X
chromosomes on account of their shape.

In the male, the sex-chromosomes are dissimilar, one being the X chromosome and the
other the Y.

The autosomes are all the other chromosomes
except the sex-chromosomes.

Genetic aspects of infertility. A brief mention
of these will be found under the succeeding paragraphs. Chromosome screening (*see* CYTOGEN-
ETICS) and, to a lesser extent, blood-typing are
likely to be of increasing value in eliminating a
proportion of bovine infertility due to hereditary
causes. (*See also* INFERTILITY.)

Inheritance of twinning. It is mainly cows over
three years old which have twins, and although
twinning may be a desirable character for the
farmer it is not one which is easy to obtain through
breeding. It seems that there is a rather low level
of genetic variation in frequency of twinning, and
that prospects for rapidly increasing litter size in
dairy cattle do not at present seem good.
(ABRO, 1974). In some breeds of sheep, and perhaps also in cattle, it may not be the ovulation
rate which is the limiting factor but, as indicated
above, the survival rate of fertilised eggs.

Heritability of certain traits. The following
table, compiled at the Animal Breeding Research

Trait	Heritability
	%
Litter size at weaning	7
Average weaning weight	8
Daily gain, after weaning	0
Food conversion	5
Average backfat	50
Percentage of lean meat	45

Organisation, shows the degree of heritability of
certain traits sought by the pig breeder.

It will be seen that litter performance has a low
heritability, and must be achieved by suitable
crossbreeding. The crossbred sow has a marked
superiority in this respect.

Lethal and semi-lethal factors. Lethal factors
have been defined as genes, which when present in
the homozygous condition cause the death of the
embryo, and when present in the heterozygous
conditions cause a serious impairment in the individual often leading to non-survival.

Lethals may be dominant or incompletely
dominant, but many are certainly recessive. They
are not always recognised since they may cause
death of the embryo early in development, and
the mating may be regarded as having been infertile – another illustration of the difficulty of de-
fining the genetics of infertility.

Several lethals are met with in cattle, such as
parrot-mouthed, in which calves die at a few
hours of age; amputated, in which calves are born
dead with legs and lower jaws absent.

Semi-lethals include over-shot jaws in calves.

Heredity and disease. 'DISEASES exhibit a spectrum according to the genetic influence. Canine
haemophilia is entirely genetic. Swedish gonad
hypoplasia is mainly genetic, mastitis is mainly
environmental and injuries are entirely environmental. Simply dividing diseases into genetic and
non-genetic is, therefore, inaccurate.

Recessive inheritance. Many diseases are inherited
as autosomal recessives. Neither parent is usually
affected, but the disease comes from both; the
sexes are affected equally, inbreeding is often
being practised, the incidence is generally low
and exact genetic ratios are obtainable. Few diseases, however, fulfil all the criteria of simple
recessives.

Diseases due to sex-linked recessives, *e.g.*
canine haemophilia, are uncommon in domestic
mammals and, not being transmitted by unaffected males – the carrier female transmits the disease to half her male offspring – are unlikely to
be a major problem. In poultry, however, sex-
linked abnormalities such as familiar cerebellar
degeneration are transmitted by the male to half
his female progeny and are relatively common.

Diseases such as cryptochidism and inter-sexes
are sex-limited and sometimes regarded as due to
recessives, the homozygote only expressing itself
in one sex. While both parents are probably involved their exact inheritance is unknown and
cryptochidism is certainly subject to environmental modification.

Irregular inheritance. Many defects have a complex inheritance. Sporadic abnormalities, which
increase on inbreeding, such as chicken 'crooked
toes' or pig 'kinky tails', are called pheno-devi-
ants, and are probably caused by recessives exhibiting a threshold of manifestation.

Dominant inheritance. The disease usually comes
from one affected parent, and half its offspring
are affected. Few dominant diseases are known in
live-stock, except in poultry. Irregular domin-
ants, exemplified by 'curved limbs', where an unaffected male transmits defective offspring out of

unrelated females and less than half are affected, do, however, occur. Environment or modifying genes may effect the genes' penetrance.

Semi-dominant inheritance. Several diseases are due to semi-dominants, the heterozygote being distinguishable from both homozygotes. A single dose of a semi-dominant gene produces a Dexter, a double dose a bulldog calf, and the homozygous normal allele produces a long-legged Dexter. Some American dwarfs are due to semi-dominants.' (Dr G. B. Young, Animal Breeding Research Organisation, 1967.)

Genetic defects. In the 1976 annual report for ABRO, Dr Young commented: 'All breeds of livestock harbour some genetic defects, but their incidence is usually low. From time to time, however, specific defects become more frequent in certain breeds, and give cause for concern.'

Cattle. Dr Young gave the following examples with reference to British breeds.

Arthrogryposis in Charolais cattle. This defect is characterised by twisted limbs, cleft palate, and twisted spine. In France about 1 per cent of Charolais cattle are affected. AI records show that while many bulls transmit an occasional defect of this nature, a few sire about 5 per cent of offspring having this abnormality.

Another defect encountered in some Charolais cattle involves the eyes. (*See* Coloboma under EYE, DISEASES OF.)

Decapitated sperms. This defect causes the rejection for AI in Britain of many Hereford bulls 'with superior test performance' because their semen contains a high percentage of sperms with the head separated from the tail.

Tibial hemimelia. A dog-sitting position in the newborn Galloway calf is suggestive of this defect, which involves bones missing from the hind legs (but has to be differentiated from another defect involving the pelvis, which also prevents the calf from standing on its hind legs). It is estimated that about 16 per cent of Galloways now carry the gene which transmits this defect. (The Galloway Breed Society has an excellent scheme, requiring compulsory insurance and compulsory slaughter of any bulls leaving offspring with this defect.) (*See also* MANNOSIDOSIS.)

Sheep. Genetic defects include *Achondroplasia* in some South Country Cheviot flocks. A 'squashed-in' face, shortened forelimbs and defective hooves are characteristic of these 'dwarf lambs'.

Cerebellar ataxia is seen in some Border Leicester flocks, and these 'daft lambs' have a staggering gait and incoordination of the head. This is due to a recessive gene.

'GENETIC ENGINEERING'. 'This usually means the recombination of genes from different organisms into one organism in a way that would never occur naturally; e.g. from a plant into an animal. However, in practice, the terminology also includes genetic deletions, although these may occur quite naturally.' (*AFRC News* 1989.)

J. M. Rutter commented: 'Recent advances in our knowledge of nucleic acids have led to the creation in the laboratory of new combinations of genetic material. This has been achieved by splicing together DNA from entirely different sources to form hybrid molecules that are less likely to occur during evolutionary processes.'

Micro-organisms virulent for cattle (for example) will, if they can be adapted to grow in laboratory animals, become less virulent for the original host, and may have usefulness for later vaccine purposes. One method of adapting the micro-organisms to grow in laboratory animals is to fuse, artificially, cells to form a HETERO-KARYON (which see).

The AFRC's Institute for Research on Animal Diseases, Compton, in work on East Coast Fever, have artificially fused bovine lymphoid cells, infected with *Theileria parva*, to mouse and hamster cells growing *in vitro*. The resultant heterokaryons contained normal macroschizonts of the parasite. Parasitised mouse and hamster cells have also been formed in this way. It is hoped that such cells can be cloned to develop a small-animal line infected with *T. parva*.

Uses. Genetic engineering has provided information on the molecular basis of gene action, on bacterial virulence and bacterial resistance. In agriculture it offers the hope of being able to transfer from bacteria to plants the genes which confer the ability to fix nitrogen – and so reduce farmers' dependence on scarce and costly nitrogen fertilisers.

In the UK, at the AFRC's Unit of Nitrogen Fixation, genes for nitrogen fixation were transferred with the aid of a PLASMID (which see) from a naturally occurring nitrogen-fixer *Klebsiella pneumoniae* to *E. coli*, 'which had never fixed nitrogen before. The plasmid, of the exchangeable class, was able, when transferring, to take along fragments of its host's chromosomes, including pieces bearing the nitrogen-fixation genes.'

In the UK, at the AFRC's Unit of Nitrogen Fixation

'Some of the new nitrogen-fixing *E. coli* strains converted these fragments of *Klebsiella* chromosome into new, separate plasmids. Geneticists in the Unit therefore constructed, by ordinary genetic manipulations, plasmids carrying nitrogen-fixation genes which would transfer themselves alone, without the aid of another plasmid.' (*AFRC Research Review.*)

In 1974–5 they obtained an F-prime plasmid which transfers itself among the coliform bacteria, but this work led to a nitrogen-fixing salmonella. A P-prime plasmid transfers itself among a very much wider range of bacteria, including *Rhizobium* and *Pseudomonas*.

'In veterinary medicine the greatest potential lies in the preparation of completely safe viral vaccines. An initial degree of success has already been achieved with foot-and-mouth virus. The specific viral protein, free of infectivity, has been produced by a genetically manipulated *E. coli*.' (Sir William Henderson, DSc, FRCVS, FRS). It has been demonstrated that this protein from a bacterial culture is capable of stimulating antibody production in animals. The method offers the possibility not only of safer, cheaper and more effective vaccines than are currently

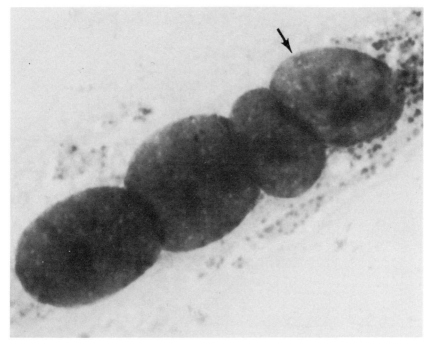

A bovine/hamster heterokaryon formed by the fusion of *T. parva*-infected bovine lymphoid cells and baby hamster kidney cells. The cell contains three hamster nuclei and one bovine nucleus (arrowed) with a prominent nucleolus. The intracytoplasmic masses are macroschizonts of *T. parva*. (×1600). (With acknowledgements to the AFRC's Institute for Research on Animal Diseases.) Monoclonal antibodies from mouse hybridomas have been produced by the AFRC for use in blood typing in cattle.

available, but also of vaccines against infections for which no such protection exists at present.

RECOMBINANT DNA TECHNIQUES. This involved three lines of research: (1) recognition and isolation of extrachromosomal DNA, or plasmids; (2) the manipulation of DNA with 'restriction' enzymes which selectively split DNA into fragments which could then be rejoined; (3) reinserting the fragmented DNA into living cells so that it became part of the genetic material of the cells.

In this way, genetic instructions for producing mammalian enzymes could be transferred into *Escherichia coli*, the cell most used for propagating such plasmid vectors, to produce insulin, for example.

The next step was to develop synthetic nucleotides, actually to construct genes. This has been done successfully and nucleotides of up to 500 characters have been constructed.

'In the future,' Dr Tim Harris stated (1983), work will be done towards using yeast and mammalian cells, with less emphasis on *E. coli*.'

Another technique in genetic engineering involves **monoclonal antibodies.** These are produced by fusing antibody-producing cells from an immunised donor with another type of white blood cell, thereby producing hybrid cells which in tissue culture could provide the desired antibodies. Among potential uses are, again, vaccines, but also diagnostic reagents; for blood-typing, in race-horses, for example.

Potential dangers. Professor Paul Berg's committee of scientists (*see Nature* (1974), **250**, 175)

urged that two types of experiment should be deferred for the present: (1) the introduction of genes for antibiotic resistance or bacterial toxin production into bacterial strains not already carrying them, and the construction of new combinations of antibiotic resistance to clinically useful antibiotics; (2) linkage of DNA from tumour-producing or other animal viruses to autonomously replicating DNA elements such as bacterial plasmids or other virus DNA.

GENITAL ORGANS (*see* diagrams for PENIS and UTERUS).

GENOME. A complete set of chromosomes derived from one parent; or the total gene complement of a set of chromosomes.

GENOTYPE. This can mean the entire array of genes carried by an individual; or the genetic constitution of an individual with respect to any limited number of genes under examination; or (more loosely) the individual within a given genotype. (*See also under* GENUS.)

GENOTYPIC SELECTION is that based on progeny testing with a very large number of progeny so that the breeding value of the parent is exactly known. The expression is also loosely used as a synonym for progeny testing without this proviso.

GENTIAN, which is mainly used as the dried and powdered root of the Yellow Gentian plant (*Gentiana lutea*), is a bitter tonic, for horses and cattle as an appetiser.

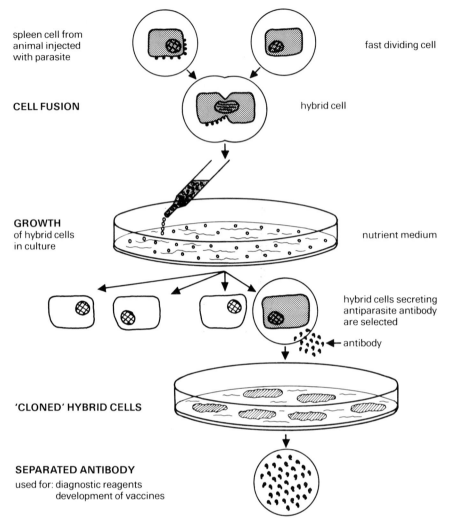

spleen cell from animal injected with parasite

fast dividing cell

CELL FUSION

hybrid cell

GROWTH of hybrid cells in culture

nutrient medium

hybrid cells secreting antiparasite antibody are selected

antibody

'CLONED' HYBRID CELLS

SEPARATED ANTIBODY
used for: diagnostic reagents
              development of vaccines

'Hybridoma' technique for producing antibodies to parasite antigens (diagrammatic). Spleen cells from mice previously injected with parasite, and secreting antibody to the parasite, can be fused with other cells to form hybrid cells that live and multiply. From these a cell line is selected by 'cloning' (i.e. a colony that represents the progeny of a single cell is isolated) which secretes appropriate antiparasite antibody. (With acknowledgements to *WHO Chronicle* (1982), **36**.)

GENTIAN VIOLET. A stain used in microscopical work and a valuable antiseptic, of use against fungal and bacterial skin infections. (*See also* CRYSTAL VIOLET *under* ANTISEPTICS.)

GENUS is a group of species. One of the species is chosen as being typical, and referred to as the genotype.

GERBILS (*see* PETS).

GERM CELLS. The gametes, *i.e.* ovum or sperm.

GESTATION (*see* PREGNANCY).

GETAH VIRUS. A mild infectious disease of racehorses, characterised by fever, dermatitis, and oedema of the limbs, appeared in Japan in 1978, and was found to be due to Getah virus. Anti-

bodies to it had previously been detected in man, horses, pigs, and birds; none of which showed symptoms.

GIANT CELLS. Seen in various infections, *e.g.* the poxes, these multinucleate cells are formed by cell fusion, stimulated by viruses. Giant cells can be obtained *in vitro* in cell cultures, as well as being found in the body.

GIANT HOGWEED (*Heracleum mantegazzianum*). This plant grows to a height of up to 12 feet, and has white flowers. The stem is hollow, and has reddish/purple blotches. Human contact with the plant, and subsequent exposure to sunlight, leads to dermatitis; and the poisoning is a result of LIGHT SENSITISATION (which see). A suspected case of this was seen in a goat, which was subdued, refusing food or water, and salivating profusely. Severe ulceration was found in its mouth. Two sheep were sensitive to the cut stems of the plant and developed mouth ulcers. (Andrews, A., Giles and Thomsett, *Veterinary Record*, (1985), **116, 205.**)

Circumstantial evidence suggested involvement of this plant in week-old ducklings which had foot and beak lesions. Two ducklings with white beaks could manage only 'open-beak' breathing; whereas the beaks which were pigmented, in the other five ducklings, were not affected. The foot lesions consisted of large blisters. (Harwood, D. G., *Veterinary Record*, (1985), **116, 300.**)

GIARDIA. A genus of flagellate protozoa.

GIARDIASIS. In dogs a low-grade infection with *Giardia canis* may interfere with the absorption of fat and vitamin A; while if large numbers of *G. canis* are present there is likely to be chronic diarrhoea (sometimes dysentery), with resulting dehydration.

The flagellate parasite occurs in two forms: the trophozoite, which divides by binary fission, and is seldom seen in the faeces; and the cyst form which is found in the faeces but is not easy to identify.

Metronizadole is used in treatment.

In the USA *G. lamblia* is a common cause of human gastro-enteritis. The infection is usually via drinking-water, but can also be child-to-child.

GID, or STURDY, is a condition in sheep, and occasionally in cattle, due to the presence in the brain of tapeworm cysts. The sheep become infected through swallowing unhatched eggs of the dog tapeworm *Taenia multiceps*. The eggs are passed out in the dog's faeces. As the cysts (coenuri) develop, they press upon brain cells and give rise to nervous signs, such as staggering, circling, blindness. The name Sturdy derives from the 'sturdy' manner in which an affected sheep may struggle when caught. (*See* COENURIASIS.)

GILCHRIST'S DISEASE. Infection in man with *Blastomyces dermatitidis*. (*See* BLASTOMYCOSIS.)

GILT. A female pig intended for breeding purposes and up to the time she has her first litter.

GIMMER (*see under* SHEEP).

GINGIVITIS. Inflammation of the gums (*see* MOUTH, DISEASES OF; *and also* FELINE GINGIVITIS).

GIZZARD (*Ventriculus*). The thick-walled, muscular stomach, which has a tough keratin lining. The gizzard's main function is to grind food, and in this it is assisted by swallowed grit and small stones. (*See under* GRIT.)

GLANDERS is a specific, contagious, and inoculable disease of the horse family (equidae), but also liable to be contracted by other mammals, including man, and characterised by the formation of nodules in the lungs, liver, spleen, or other organs; ulcerations of the mucous membranes, especially those of the upper air passages, accompanied by changes in the lymphatics and also by skin lesions. It is due to the entrance and growth in the body of the glanders bacillus *Pseudomonas mallei* (formerly known as *Pfeifferella mallei*).

History. Glanders has been known as a serious disease since about 450 BC, when it was mentioned by Hippocrates, and its contagious nature was pointed out by Vegetius (a veterinary writer) in the fourth century.

Distribution. Glanders has been distributed to practically every country in the world at some time or other, and was once a usual concomitant of wars. It became prevalent, both in the United Kingdom and in South Africa, after the South African war. In the year 1892 there were more than 3000 cases of glanders recorded in Great Britain, in 1904 between 2000 and 3000, while only nine outbreaks were recorded in the year 1923, and none since 1926.

Glanders is still endemic in Mongolia, other parts of Asia, East Africa and South America.

The donkey is the most susceptible to the disease and nearly always suffers from the acute form, from which it dies in from 2 to 3 weeks.

In the horse, glanders occurs in an acute or a chronic form, the latter existing for months or even years before it finally kills its victim; however, under modern conditions it is rare to allow the disease to run its natural course. The mule is intermediate in susceptibility between the donkey and the horse, but usually shows the acute type. Dogs and cats may become infected if fed upon meat from a horse which had glanders. The camel is susceptible, though natural cases are very rare. Of experimental animals the guinea-pig is the most susceptible.

Horses can be infected naturally by three different channels:

1. By the digestive tract, through the medium of infected food and water. This is by far the commonest method of spread.

2. By inhalation (rarely) when some abrasion of the respiratory passage is present.

3. By skin infection.

Glanders in man is a distressing and nearly always fatal disease, and may be contracted by stable-men. Laboratory workers handling infected material or pure cultures of the organism are especially liable to infection, so that every precaution against this contingency has to be taken; in fact, the glanders bacillus is amongst the most dangerous of all disease-producing bacteria cultivated.

The causal organism is present in all the lesions, though it does not – except the rare cases – circulate in the blood-stream.

INCUBATION PERIOD. This may last several months in the horse.

SIGNS. The signs of glanders in the horse are very varied. The disease may run an acute course of only 2 to 3 weeks, but by far the greatest number of cases met with are of a sub-acute or chronic nature. A horse may be affected and show no outward sign of disease, and yet perhaps it may have nodules in one or both lungs.

Glanders may be of the nasal, pulmonary, or glandular form, of the type producing skin lesions (farcy), or an admixture of these, and it may also become generalised. One of the dangers of the disease is that a horse may work for weeks or even months with 'open' lesions – not losing a great deal of flesh nor appearing very ill – and so spread the disease to healthy horses with which it comes into contact.

Glandular enlargements. When farcy is present the glands inside the axilla or inside the groin may be somewhat enlarged and even painful to the touch. In entire horses the testicles often become enlarged and painful, or even the seat of glanderous abscesses.

Nasal Symptoms. There may be a nasal discharge, thin and watery in the early stages, but later becoming thick, greyish, or yellow and oily.

Examination of the nose in these cases is dangerous, as man may easily contract the disease by this means.

Farcy. In this form of the disease the skin is involved. It is usually chronic in nature, but farcy buds and subcutaneous swellings may complicate the most acute form of the disease shortly before death. This complication is especially common in the mule, which often succumbs to the disease before the farcy buds have time to burst. In chronic farcy there is usually swelling of one or more limbs, more frequently a hind one. The lymphatic glands of the affected limb become enlarged, the lymph vessels corded, and usually a chain of farcy buds develops along their course.

In acute glanders there may be all the signs of an acute broncho-pneumonia, a high temperature, a rapid loss of flesh, rapid and sometimes noisy breathing, followed by death in a few weeks; in fact, this is the common form seen in the donkey and often in the mule, with or without the complication of farcy.

DIAGNOSIS. This is confirmed by means of the mallein test.

TREATMENT. In Yugoslavia, success has been reported with Sulphathiazole, but in most western countries treatment is not permitted; the policy being one of slaughter and eradication.

GLANDS. A term loosely applied to a number of different organs. In each there are epithelial cells which have a secretory function (e.g. tear production). Glands are often classified as either *endocrine* (ductless) or *exocrine* glands – which usually have ducts to carry their secretion to an epithelial surface. (*See* ENDOCRINE GLANDS, HORMONES.)

A description of the various glands will be found under headings such as THYROID, LIVER, MAMMARY GLANDS, OVARIES, PANCREAS, SALIVARY GLANDS, TESTIS, etc. Sweat and sebaceous glands are referred to under SKIN.

Lymphatic glands are nowadays more often referred to as Lymph Nodes.

GLASS EMBOLISM. Fluids for injection may contain glass particles. Glass gets in not during manufacture of the vial, but when the latter is broken. In human medicine the risk of glass embolism has been stressed, and it has been suggested that, as a wise precaution, time should be allowed for glass particles to settle before filling the syringe.

GLASS, SOLUBLE. Soluble glasses containing copper and selenium have been used in BOLUSES (which see).

GLASSER'S DISEASE. An infection and swelling of the hock or knee joints, or both, in the pig. There is fever, lameness and a disinclination to move. Death is usually a sequel, unless early treatment with *e.g.* penicillin is undertaken. Glasser's disease is differentiated from 'Joint-Ill'. Pigs of 5 to 14 weeks old are chiefly affected. The cause is *Haemophilus suis*, or a mycoplasma, or both.

GLAUBER'S SALTS is the popular name for sodium sulphate, a saline purgative.

A dose of 4 ounces is said to be dangerous in the pig, and fatal poisoning has occurred with Glauber's salt given in three daily doses.

GLAUCOMA (*see under* EYE, DISEASES OF).

GLENOID CAVITY is the shallow socket on the shoulder-blade into which the humerus fits, forming the shoulder joint.

GLIOMA is a tumour which forms in the brain or spinal cord. It is composed of neuroglia, which is the special connective tissue found supporting the nerve cells and the nerve fibres. (*See* TUMOURS.)

GLIOSIS. A proliferation of ASTROCYTES (which see). It may follow a brain injury.

GLOBIDIOSIS. A disease characterised by enteritis and closely resembling coccidiosis. It occurs in Africa, SW Europe, the USA, and Australia. The cause is (species of) *Globidium*. Cysts may be formed in the skin or underlying tissue. Horses, cattle, and sheep are affected. In horses severe diarrhoea may be caused. Fatal cases of *Globidium* (*Eimeria*) *leuckarti* have occasionally been recorded in horses in the UK and Ireland since 1973.

GLOBULIN is a protein fraction of the blood plasma, associated with immunity. (*See also* GAMMA GLOBULIN.)

GLOMERULUS is a small knot of blood-vessels, and from which the excretion of fluid out of the blood into the tubules of the kidney takes place. (*See* KIDNEY.) Glomerulo-nephritis is referred to under KIDNEYS, DISEASES OF.

GLOSSECTOMY, PARTIAL. A surgical operation to remove part of the tongue following severe laceration by a sharp bit. Before the operation the horse had been unable to eat or drink for several days. (Mohammed, A. & others, University of Maiduguri, Nigeria. (*Vet. Rec* (1991) **128** 355.)

GLOSSITIS. Inflammation of the tongue.

GLOSSOPHARYNGEAL NERVE is the 9th cranial nerve, which in the main is sensory. It is the nerve of taste for the back of the tongue, of sensation in a general way for the upper part of the throat, as well as for the middle ear, and it supplies the parotid gland.

GLOTTIS is the narrow opening at the upper end of the larynx. (*See* AIR PASSAGES, CHOKING, LARYNX.)

GLOVES, SURGICAL. Surgical glove powder (sterilised maize starch) can cause an iatrogenic starch peritonitis. In a comparative study of various methods of washing, brushing and rinsing, a routine involving a one minute povidine-iodine surgical scrub followed by a rinse under sterile running water (500 ml) for 30 seconds removed 99·8 to 100 per cent of the original starch grain count and also provided the surgeon with a reassuring autotactile stick signal (separation of opposing forefinger and thumb as total removal of starch is about to be achieved). Glove stickiness disappears when tissue fluid of patient coats gloves. Rinsing gloves in water alone leaves about 10 per cent of the original starch on the gloves. (Fraser, I. (1982), *British Medical Journal*, **284**, 1835.)

GLUCAGON. This is a polypeptide hormone secreted by alpha-cells in the islets of Langerhans of the pancreas, and increases the amount of glucose in the blood.

GLUCOCORTICOIDS. Hormones, from the cortex of the adrenal gland, concerned with the formation of glucose. Cortisol (hydrocortisone) is one of the most important of these. Excessive secretion of glucocorticoids is a feature of Cushing's disease.

GLUCOSE is the form of sugar found in honey, grapes, fruits, etc., and in diabetes mellitus it is passed in the urine. It is the form in which sugar circulates in the blood-stream, and is very useful as an injection or drench when there is a deficiency of circulating sugar in the blood or an excess of ketones. (*See* ACETONAEMIA.) Glucose is a most valuable food to give during the course of acute illnesses, since it puts no strain upon the digestive system yet provides fuel for the muscles, etc. Glucose saline is given as a drink or administered *per rectum* or by subcutaneous injection during the course of jaundice, gastro-enteritis, etc. (*See* SUGARS.)

GLUTEAL is the scientific name applied to the region of the buttocks, and to structures associated, such as gluteal arteries, muscles, nerves.

GLYCERIDES (*see* FAT).

GLYCERIN, or GLYCEROL, is a clear, colourless, odourless, thick liquid of a sweet taste, obtained by decomposition and distillation of fats. It dissolves many substances and has a great power of absorbing water.

USES. Given by the mouth, diluted, it has been used with success in the treatment of pregnancy toxaemia in ewes and of acetonaemia in cattle. Internally, glycerin acts as a laxative to the dog in moderate doses. It is soothing and antiseptic to inflamed mucous membranes in the mouth and throat. In amounts of ½ to 1 ounce it is useful as a rectal injection to induce passage of impacted faeces in obstinate constipation in the dog, and it may be used for the same purpose in foals and calves. For these purposes it may be given diluted with a little water, or it may be used in the pure state. It is also used as a basis for the compounding of various electuaries for the horse and dog, and it is sometimes incorporated into cough mixtures for the smaller animals. It forms a basis for certain skin dressings when it is desired to soften the skin surface and encourage the absorption of other drugs.

It is also used as a diluent for semen. (*See under* ARTIFICIAL INSEMINATION.)

GLYCOGEN is an animal starch found specially in the liver as well as in other tissues. It is the form in which carbohydrates taken in the food are stored in the liver and muscles before they are converted into glucose as the needs of the system require.

GLYCOL, ETHYLENE (*see under* 'ANTIFREEZE' for poisoning in dog and cat).

GLYCOSIDES. These are the cause of poisoning by some plants, and include: (1) *cyanogenetic glycosides*, which can release hydrocyanic acid and are present in laurel, linseed, etc.; (2) other glycosides such as are present in foxgloves and mustard; and (3) *saponins* in 'Lords and Ladies' (*Arum maculatum*).

GLYCOSURIA means the presence of glucose in the urine. It is seen in diabetes mellitus (*see* DIABETES), and in some other conditions, and in all animals after severe shocks. (*See also under* URINE, ABNORMAL CONDITIONS OF.)

GLYCYRRHETINIC ACID. Obtained from liquorice, it has been used for reducing inflammation and is cheaper than cortisone preparations.

GNATHOSTOMA SPINIGERUM. A roundworm infecting dogs, cats, wild carnivores, and man. It forms a nodule about 1½ cm in diameter in the gastric mucosa, and in a cat (suspected of having rabies) it caused anorexia, nausea, and convulsions, coma and death.

GNOTOBIOTICS, the name given to germfree laboratory animals reared according to techniques developed by Professor J. A. Reyniers of Notre Dame University, Chicago. Such animals have been used in the investigation of certain diseases. (*See also* SPF, DISEASE-FREE.)

GOADS, ELECTRIC. These are preferable to the use of carelessly or sadistically wielded sticks, and are a help. The points should be spring-loaded, as otherwise they can be jabbed into the animal – when the purpose and object of an electric goad are defeated.

GOAT WARBLE FLY, *Przhevalskiana silenus*, parasitises goats and horses in many European and eastern countries. *Hypoderma aeratum* and *H. crossi* are other species which cause warble lesions.

GOATLING. A female between one and two years old.

GOATS: Disbudding of kids. This is carried out under general anaesthesia. (*See* ANAESTHESIA for goats); and the iron used for disbudding is heated by gas (or electricity) to a 'cherry-red' heat.

GOATS, DISEASES OF. (*See under the following headings:* ACETONAEMIA, AGALACTIA, BRUCELLOSIS, CAPRINE ARTHRITIS-ENCEPHALITIS, CONTAGIOUS CAPRINE PLEURO-PNEUMONA, CASEOUS LYMPHADENITIS, CHLAMYDIA (for abortion), 'CLOUDBURST', COCCIDIOSIS, CRYPTOSPORIDIOSIS, CYSTICERCOSIS, ENTEROTOXAEMIA, JOHNE'S DISEASE, MASTITIS, ORF, PARASITIC BRONCHITIS, PARASITIC GASTRO-ENTERITIS, PREGNANCY TOXAEMIA, Q FEVER, RICKETS, RINDERPEST, SALMONELLOSIS, SWAYBACK, TUBERCULOSIS, YERSINIOSIS, LOUPING ILL, SCRAPIE, OSTEODYSTROPHIA FIBROSA, MANNOSIDOSIS, LISTERIOSIS, MYCOPLASMOSIS, RINDERPEST, LIVER FLUKES, GOITRE.)

GOATS' MILK, CHEESE. Goat's milk is often substituted for cow's milk for children suffering from a suspected allergy to cow's milk. However, unless the milk is pasteurised, there is a risk of human illness arising; especially from infection with *Brucella melitensis*, but also from *Yersinia pseudotuberculosis* – one cause of mastitis in goats. Goat's milk may contain louping-ill virus, *staphylococci, E. coli*; and, since goats are not immune to tuberculosis, even tubercle bacilli. In the UK the statutory tests applied to cow's milk are not applied (1986) to goat's milk. Goat's milk cheese is also a source of *B. melitensis* infection.

GOATS AS GRAZERS with sheep (*see* PASTURE MANAGEMENT).

GOITRE is a condition, associated with an iodine deficiency, in which the thyroid gland enlarges in size. It is seen in puppies, foals, and lambs, and also in calves, and it appears to be commoner in some districts than in others. Swellings may appear below the larynx, usually one on either side, and beyond the local enlargements there may be no definite symptoms shown. Some cases respond to the administration of thyroid extracts, and iodine internally, while some clear up spontaneously without treatment.
(*See* IODINE, CALCIUM SUPPLEMENTS, THYROID GLAND.)

Lethargy is a notable symptom of goitre in the dog, in which the disease often occurs in the 3 to 5 year age group, especially in the bigger breeds.

Some pastures and foodstuffs may give rise to goitre. (*See* GOITROGEN.) Goitre seems particularly common in Dorset Horn sheep.

A number of cases of supposed 'goitre' prove upon careful examination to be tumour growth in some part of the throat, not necessarily in connection with the thyroid gland though cancer of the thyroid is not uncommon in the dog.

Goitre also occurs when, instead of a deficiency of thyroxin, there is a state of *hyperthyroidism*, or too much thyroxin. (*See* THYROID GLAND, DISEASE.)

In goat kids some supposed cases of goitre prove to be hyperplasia of the THYMUS gland.

In other animals 'goitre' may be a misdiagnosis for neoplasms in the throat region.

GOITROGEN, GOITROGENIC FACTOR is one which gives rise to goitre. Both kale and cabbage contain goitrogens and must therefore not constitute too large a proportion of an animal's ration over a period. The same applies to turnips. Iodine licks may be advisable. (*See* IODINE DEFICIENCY.)

GONAD is a gland which produces a gamete, *i.e.* the ovary or testis.

GONADOTROPHIC indicates something which stimulates the gonads – testes and ovaries. (*See below and* HORMONES.)

GONADOTROPHINS are hormones which have a gonadotrophic effect in the body. (*See* HORMONES.)

Chorionic gonadotrophin effects luteinisation and is used in the treatment of functional uterine haemorrhage, cases of habitual abortion, and to induce descent of the testes in cases of cryptorchidism.

Serum gonadotrophin contains a follicle-stimulating hormone which affects the gonads of both sexes. It is used in the treatment of sterility, anoestrus, and hypoplasia of the gonads.

GOOSE INFLUENZA. A disease common in Hungary, and first recorded in Britain in 1970; when it caused a mortality of up to 70 per cent among birds under a month old. Symptoms: dullness, loss of appetite, thirst, and a nasal discharge.

'GOOSE-STEPPING'. In the pig this can be a symptom of a deficiency of pantothenic acid, one of the B group of vitamins. In cattle it may be a symptom of familial ataxia. (*See* GENETICS, DEFECTS.)

GOSSYPOL is a toxic substance present in cotton-seed cake or meal unless removed efficiently before manufacture.

Gossypol poisoning gives rise to loss of appetite, gastro-enteritis, ascites, pulmonary oedema, convulsions and death.

Birth control. Already in the 1950s it was known that gossypol could impair spermatogenesis, but not ovulation, in rats. In the 1980s research workers in China, in a search for possible male human contraceptives, included gossypol in their list, and sought to enhance the depressive effect on spermatogenesis while at the same time reducing gossypol's toxicity. The World Health Organisation was encouraging this research, which led to a highly purified acetic acid preparation of gossypol being offered to scientists in other countries.

Previously, gossypol had been considered as a contraceptive for possible use in dogs and cats; and the idea might be revived if results with the new preparation are successful.

GOUT, the metabolic disorder *Hyperuricaemia*, of man, is associated with an excess of urates in blood and tissue fluids which in some, but by no means all cases, leads to the deposition of crystals of sodium urate in joints. Subsequently an acute gouty arthritis may follow. A genetic factor, associated with an enzyme deficiency, may be involved. Gout has to be distinguished from lead poisoning (Scott, J. T., *British Medical Journal*, (1983), **287**, 78.) Gout may occur in the dog. (*See also* 'VISCERAL GOUT' in poultry.)

Calcium gout. (*Calcinosis circumscripta.*) This has been recorded in dogs and monkeys as well as in man, and involves the deposition of calcium salts and the appearance of fibrous tissue around the deposits. Firm, painless nodules occur under the skin of the limbs and feet and at the elbow. Ulceration, with a gritty discharge, may occur. The cause is unknown. Diagnosis may be assisted by radiography. Calcium-gout occurs mainly in large breeds of dog, *e.g.* Alsatians. It also occurred in 32 piglets of 17 herds in Switzerland at the age of several days to 4 weeks. Signs were cough and dyspnoea in all cases; some showed weight loss and hunched backs. The respiratory and circulatory system evinced severe changes, with calcinosis in elastic fibres of lungs, atrial walls, and arterioles. Older piglets also showed inflammatory changes. Milder changes were seen in stomach, kidneys, and muscles. (*Schw. Arch. Tierhlk.* (1975), **117**, 9.)

GRAÄFIAN FOLLICLE. The mature ovarian follicle. (*See* OVARIES.)

GRAFTS (*see* SKIN GRAFTING, IMMUNITY, H-Y ANTIGEN, MAJOR HISTOCOMPATIBILITY SYSTEM).

GRAINS, BREWERS'. Brewers' grains are a by-product of brewing, consisting of the exhausted malt, and are used wet in some cases, where they can be easily obtained from a nearby brewery, or as dried grains. They are useful as a feeding-stuff for cattle, pigs, and sheep, but must be introduced gradually into the ration. Wet grains are almost entirely used for feeding milk cows. They must be used fresh as they deteriorate on keeping. Dried grains keep well, and are suitable for horses, about 5 to 10 lb daily, and to sheep, up to ½ lb.

GRAINS, DISTILLERS'. Distillery grains are produced as a by-product during the manufacture of whisky in a manner somewhat similar to brewers' grains in the manufacture of beer. They are sold either wet or dry, but are much to be preferred dry, since the wet grains are liable to contain considerable amounts of raw alcohol, which may lead to intoxication of animals eating them. The amounts and uses are similar to brewers' grains.

GRAM-NEGATIVE bacteria are those which do not retain the violet of Gram's stain (haematoxylin, eosin, and aniline methylene violet). Bacteria which do retain the violet are called Gram-positive. This staining differentiation provides an important means of classifying bacteria into two groups. (Nuclei are stained blue, cytoplasm red, and Gram + bacteria violet by this staining method, devised by a Danish physician.)

'GRAMOXONE'. The proprietary name of a herbicide containing PARAQUAT (which see).

GRANULAR VULVOVAGINITIS (*see under* VULVOVAGINITIS).

GRANULATIONS are small masses of cells of a constructive nature containing loops of newly formed blood-vessels which spring up over the surfaces of healing wounds. What is commonly called 'proud flesh'. Granulation tissue also occurs internally, forming GRANULOMAS at the site of lesions. (*See also* WOUND TREATMENT.)

GRANULOMA. A tumour composed of granulation tissue. (*See* EOSINOPHILIC GRANULOMA, and 'LICK GRANULOMA' for important conditions in cats and dogs, and 'SWAMP CANCER').

Occasionally a granuloma is seen as the result of a *Staphylococcus aureus* infection involving the skin of cats and dogs, or the mammary glands of cattle and goats, or the equine spermatic cord. One case involved a gastric ulcer in a cat.

GRASS (*see under* PASTURE MANAGEMENT, LEYS, DRIED GRASS, HAY, 'HAYFLAKES', HAYLAGE, SILAGE). **Grass seeds as foreign bodies** (*see* AWNS).

GRASS SICKNESS is a provisional name for a disease of horses which has been recognised in the central and eastern areas of Scotland since 1907, and has spread to Wales and to many parts of England; also in Sweden. It occurs in horses after they are put on to the grass between the months of April and September. Of recent years practically all breeds of horses have been affected, including ponies.

CAUSE. Various theories advanced include: (1) degeneration of certain ganglia of the sympathetic nervous system due to a virus; (2) a fungal toxin; (3) a drastic reduction in peptide-containing autonomic nerves, though what produces this is not known.

Pathognomic lesions in the autonomic nervous system can be experimentally produced by intra-peritoneal injection of 500 ml serum from acute cases of grass sickness into normal horses. The serum injections do not, however, cause the **stasis of the gastrointestinal tract which is typical of the disease.** Examination of sera from acute cases of grass sickness revealed a compound of small molecular weight which does not occur in the serum of normal horses or in cases of colic. This substance may be a neurotoxin but the experimental methods used did not confirm this. Johnson, P., *Research in a Veterinary Science*, (1985), **38**, 329.

N. T. Hodson and colleagues suggested a fourth cause, namely: overactivity of the sympatho-adrenal system and stress, *e.g.*, sweating, muscle fasciculation, tachycardia and increased plasma catecholamines. It is known that many types of stimuli caused by environmental, emotional or physical (trauma, disease) factors act as stressors and that general arousal will cause a common response in both parts of the sympatho-adrenal system.

Two sets of circumstances are thought by clinicians to be involved in its aetiology. First, stress caused by travel to new surroundings, particularly in excitable young thoroughbred mares about to foal; and secondly changes in the external environment such as cold and wet weather following warm and sunny weather. Similar changes are known to cause stress and increases in both plasma catecholamines and corticosteroids in laboratory animals. (Hodson, N. P & others, *Veterinary Record*, (1986), **118**, 148.)

SIGNS. The disease may be (1) *peracute*, with death occurring in 8 to 16 hours, and periods of great violence being shown when the animal may be a danger to people looking after it; (2) *sub-acute*. The horse becomes dull and listless and off its food. It may have an anxious expression, and roll from pain. Later there may be a discharge from the nostrils, and an excessive amount of salivation. Swallowing is difficult. There may be localised twitching and sweating. No faeces are passed. Attempts at vomiting are made. Food material becomes impacted in the large intestine.

The illness lasts for from 2 to 5 days, when death or the chronic stage supervenes. The mortality is high; (3) *chronic*. The signs are similar, except that constipation is not complete, and also some food may be eaten. The horse becomes progressively thinner, until in the later stages it has a tucked-up 'greyhound' appearance. The horse may live for a variable period in this state; some last only a few weeks, but others linger on for six months or more.

DIAGNOSIS. Administration of a barium preparation, followed by radiography, demonstrated serious malfunction of the oesophagus. 'Taken in conjunction with other clinical findings, this evidence was specific enough to confirm the diagnosis, without the need for an exploratory laparotomy, enabling euthanasia to be effected without delay.' (Animal Health Trust.)

TREATMENT. Recovery is uncommon, and seldom complete. Euthanasia is usually indicated. No medicinal treatment is of any avail so far as is known at present. The only measures that can be recommended are those that concern the animal's comfort.

'GRASS STAGGERS, TETANY' (*see under* HYPOMAGNESAEMIA).

GRASS, TURNING OUT TO (*see under* YARDED CATTLE).

GRASSLAND MANAGEMENT (*see under* PASTURE MANAGEMENT).

GRAVE'S DISEASE is another name for exophthalmic goitre.

GRAZING BEHAVIOUR. A study, made at Cornell University, of Aberdeen-Angus and Hereford cows at pasture (receiving no supplementary feed) showed that:

1. The average grazing time was 7 hours and 32 minutes, of which 4 hours and 52 minutes were spent in actual eating, and the balance in walking and selecting herbage during the process of grazing. During the hours of darkness the cattle grazed for 2 hours and 28 minutes.

2. In a pasture of 6 acres the cow travelled 2·45 miles, of which 1·96 were during daylight hours and 0·49 during darkness.

3. The cows lay down for 11 hours and 39 minutes, but this was divided into nine periods ranging from less than 1 hour to more than 6 hours. The time spent in chewing the cud averaged 6 hours and 51 minutes.

4. The calves, which were about 3 months old, were suckled three times a day at intervals of 8 hours, and for 15 minutes at a time.

5. Droppings were deposited on an average twelve times a day and urine nine times.

6. Under the conditions prevailing, the cows drank water once a day only. This may be accounted for by the luxuriant pasture herbage consisting of Kentucky bluegrass and wild white clover with an average water content of 72 per cent.

7. The cows showed no inclination to extend the grazing period beyond 8 hours even when the amount of herbage consumed fell to 45 pounds a day. 'It is evident that a mechanical factor is involved in grazing management and that one of the basic principles of good pasture management is to provide the live-stock with pastures in a condition which will permit them to gather the optimum amount of food within a normal period of 8 hours' grazing.

'We may speculate upon the potential productivity of British pastures if we ever achieve a degree of efficiency in grazing management which will permit mature cattle to consume daily the normal maximum of about 150 lb of green herbage. This should be sufficient for maintenance and the production of about 50 lb of milk or possibly for the production of 5 lb liveweight increase daily.' (Professor D. R. Johnstone-Wallace.)

Recent work, however, and especially that in New Zealand, has proved that the time dairy cattle graze and ruminate is very flexible, and that the feed intake varies much less from day to day than the time spent in grazing. The cow has, in fact, a capacity to change her grazing habits to suit both her environment and her own bodily needs.

The quartering of a field by horses into parts for grazing and parts for defaecation has been described by E. L. Taylor, who adds that cattle avoid the grass in the proximity of faecal pats. 'The fineness of this perception of contamination is shown by a helminthologist's observation that cattle were able to detect minute traces of faeces such as he was not able to see.'

GRAZING MANAGEMENT (*see* PASTURE MANAGEMENT).

GREASY HEEL. This is a chronic fungal skin infection seen in horses mainly during the winter; with lesions occurring below the fetlock.
CAUSE. *Dermatophilus congolensis*, which 'invades the epidermis but does not destroy the germinating layer,' so that regeneration occurs, to be followed by renewed invasion and desquamation. Lesions extend and there is pus formation; the hair becoming matted and tufted.

Greasy heel occurs in horses with marked feather, such as Shires, stabled in unhygienic, damp stables, or grazing pasture liable to flooding. In ungroomed horses at grass, the tufting may be mistaken for normal coat condition. (Professor K. P. Baker).
FIRST-AID, pending veterinary advice: Clip all the hair away from the affected areas, and thoroughly wash the leg with soap and water containing washing soda. Burn the hair. Wash the hands, as the infection is transmissible to man. Isolate horse under dry conditions. (*See also* POX, DERMATOPHILUS.)

'GREASY PIG DISEASE' is a form of seborrhoea, sometimes labelled 'eczema', occurring in piglets. It was thought to be associated with a vitamin B deficiency, and many cases were claimed to respond dramatically when treated accordingly. It is now regarded as a staphylococcal infection. Bites, abrasions, tattooing, and lice infestation may facilitate entry of the organism through the skin.

Often only some piglets in a single litter on the farm are affected. Symptoms include dullness, loss of bloom, and soft, greasy spots on the reddened skin of the snout, ears, around the eyes, and sometimes on the abdomen. The spots join up and spread, and after a few days the piglet may have a largely greasy and brown body, with thickened and cracking skin. Severely affected cases die within a few days; survivors are seldom an economic proposition as recovery takes several weeks and may be incomplete.
PREVENTION. Clipping the teeth of piglets, boiling tattooing instruments, and providing concrete which is smooth (and preferably not bare). To be successful, veterinary treatment with a suitable antibiotic has to be undertaken very promptly if it is to succeed. Long-standing cases are best slaughtered. There is no vaccine available.

'GREEN-BOTTLE' FLY (*see* FLIES).

GREENSTICK FRACTURE is one in which the bone fractures incompletely somewhat similar to the break of a green stick. They mostly occur in young animals. (*See* FRACTURES.)

GREYFACE. The term often applied to a Border Leicester × Scottish Blackface cross.

GRISEOFULVIN. An antibiotic, which can be given by mouth, effective against ringworm and other fungal diseases. Dosing over a 3-week period may be necessary in the treatment of ringworm in calves. It is advisable not to use griseofulvin in pregnant animals, as there is some risk of malformed offspring resulting.

GRIT FOR POULTRY. Insoluble grit – sand, flint grit, tiny pebbles – is necessary for the grinding of the food in the gizzard; poultry possessing no teeth. Flint grit should be provided at the rate of 1 lb per 100 birds, and is best broadcast with the grain every 2 or 3 months; except for battery birds, which require a monthly ration. Where gravel is available, no special flint grit need be provided.

Soluble limestone grit is given in order to supply calcium for bone formation and eggshell production, and it dissolves in the gizzard within 48 hours. It is not necessary for chicks, growers or birds in early lay if they are receiving commercial mash or pellets without corn. Too much limestone grit can be harmful.

GROOMING. The objects of grooming horses, cattle, and dogs, especially when kept shut up in buildings, are fourfold: it is undertaken for the purpose of cleanliness, for the prevention of disease of the skin, to stimulate the skin circulation, and to remove waste products of metabolism.

Horses
Quartering. This consists of going over the horse's body with a dandy-brush and removing the coarse adherent particles of bedding, dried dung, etc., as a preliminary before the horse leaves the stable for morning exercise. At the same time a cloth and a pail of water are used to wipe away discharges from the eyes, nose, and dock, in this order, and to remove any urine stains from other parts of the body. Quartering is usually only carried out in highclass stables, where the horses go out for a short walk before the men have had their breakfasts, or when a horse is not going to work but is to be turned out to grass for the day. (*See* SPONGES.)

Dandy-brushing. The dandy-brush is made of stiff, coarse, whisk fibre, generally of the yellow variety, with the bristles not close together. It removes the coarser particles of matter from the coat, and stirs up the finer debris, as well as disentangling matted hairs. Owing to its stiffness it is not used over the head, but each side of the neck, the whole of the body, and the four quarters are well brushed. It should be used in the left hand for the near side of the animal, and in the right hand for the off-side. It is advisable to make short, vigorous sweeps, turning the wrist at the end of each sweep, so that the material collected in the bristles is thrown out of the coat. Care is necessary when the under-sides of the body and the insides of the legs of thin-skinned or ticklish horses are being groomed with the dandy, for they may kick if this rough brush is used carelessly.

Body-brushing and curry-combing. The body-brush is made from finer whisk fibre than the dandy, the bristles are set much closer together, and they are softer and more flexible. There is usually a strap across the back of the brush into which the hand is thrust, so that a better grip can be obtained. The curry-comb is made of metal, either in the form of a square plate with a series of alternately toothed and smooth ridges set across it, or it may be oval with crenated ridges running round it. The former variety is provided with a handle, and the latter has a strap across its back like the body-brush. The body-brush is used all over the horse's body, head, and neck. It picks up the finer particles of matter left behind by the dandy-brush and holds them between the fine bristles. To clean the brush it is necessary every three or four sweeps to draw it across the face of the curry-comb and transfer the dirt to the latter. The body-brush should be used in long firm sweeps, without any turn of the wrist. While grooming the near side, the body-brush is held in the left hand and the curry-comb in the right, and for the off-side the positions are reversed.

Wisping. A wisp is a small mat of plaited straw or hay, which is used to beat out fine dust from the coat, scour and polish the surface hair, and to promote a better skin and superficial circulation. When properly applied it acts as massage to the surface of the body, and gives the coat a fine shine.

Combing the mane and tail. For this purpose a bone or metal comb is used, fashioned after the familiar manner of a toilet comb, with stouter teeth. The mane is combed a few strands at a time, both from the outside and also from the inside (with the teeth through the whole thickness of the mane), so that the hair may be laid straight and all tangles removed. Afterwards the tail is treated similarly. When a few unruly strands will not lie in position it is usual to damp the fibres of the water-brush (which is not unlike a small, fine dandy-brush pointed at each end) and lay the strands with the damp brush. Neither the mane nor the tail, however, should be soaked with water.

Rubbing or shining is carried out either with a stable-rubber, which is a piece of towelling about 18 inches square, or with a chamois leather. During this process the hairs of the coat are laid straight all over the body, any loose pieces of hay or straw from the wisp are removed, and the final gloss is put on to the coat.

Cleaning out of the feet. The last operation of grooming consists of picking up each of the feet and removing any adherent dung, etc., by means of a hoof-pick and brushing out the sole of each foot with the water-brush. If desired, the walls of the hoofs may also be blackened or oiled at this time. This operation should be left till last, just before the horse leaves the stable, for otherwise he may collect fresh dung in his feet. It is an important matter not to neglect this cleaning out of the feet, for if there is a cake of dung in the soles of each foot, not only is it extremely untidy, but small stones are liable to be picked up and may cause injury to the soles.

Parts often neglected. When examining a horse to discover the thoroughness or otherwise of the grooming it is usual to take a white handkerchief and to rub it along the coat; the size of the particles of grey debris which adhere to its surface are in inverse ratio to the efficiency of the grooming – *i.e.* the larger the particles the less efficiently has the horse been groomed. The following parts should be carefully examined: under the forelock, the poll, jowl, under the mane, between the fore-legs, behind the elbows, along the belly, inside the thighs, in the hollows of the heels, and around the dock and between the buttocks.

To dry a wet horse. When a horse returns to a stable soaked with rain, snow, or sweat, it is very advisable that it be dried to avoid the risk of chill through too rapid evaporation of the moisture in the coat. First of all it should be given a warm drink.

The harness is next removed and the surface of the body scraped down with a sweat-scraper. This is a flexible ribbon of copper provided with a handle at either end. The scraper removes the excess water from the coat, and may be used to scrape away adherent mud from the legs and belly, but it should not be used over bony prominences, owing to the danger of abrading the skin. Two or three hay wisps are made ready, and the horse is vigorously wisped down all over. As one wisp becomes wet it is discarded and another taken. Sometimes a coarse, rough towel is used instead of a wisp. In about ten minutes all the moisture that can be removed by this means will have been removed, and the rest must be allowed to evaporate. An armful of straw is arranged across the horse's back, and a rug is thrown over all, and girthed up. The straw allows a certain amount of ventilation under the rug, and prevents too rapid cooling and chilling. In about two hours' time the rug should be removed, a second wisping should be given, and a new dry rug should be applied. If the feet and legs are very wet, especially if there is much feather, they should be bandaged with woollen stable bandages, and a little bran or sawdust may be sprinkled on to the wet hair below the bandage. Sometimes a horse's feet are washed immediately after coming in from work, especially if they are coated with mud; when this is carried out, care should be taken to see that they are well dried again afterwards, for frequent washing predisposes to grease, eczema, and other skin conditions, through maceration of the surface epithelium.

Milk cows. The general principles as given for the horse apply almost equally to cattle, and especially to milk cows kept in byres, where they are unable to lick and clean themselves as they do in nature. As a rule the process is not so thorough as for horses, only a dandy-brush and a curry-comb being used.

Dogs. When grooming it is always advisable to begin by combing and brushing the coat in the wrong direction (against the lie of the hair), so as to remove pieces of dirt, débris, etc., which have become lodged under a lock of the coat and to finish by brushing and combing in the direction in which it is desired that the hair shall eventually lie.

In the spring, and again in the autumn, when the coat is changing, both dogs and cats require more careful grooming than they do at other times of the year, for at these times when they are casting their coats there is always a good deal of dead and loose hair to be removed to make way for the new young coat.

Cats benefit from regular grooming. With long-haired breeds, it is essential.

GROOTLAMSIEKTE. A disease of sheep in SW Africa, associated with a prolonged gestation period, and caused by a poisonous shrub (*Salsola tuberculata.*)

GROUNDNUT MEAL. During 1960 many turkeys fed in Britain on proprietary feeding-stuffs died, and the cause was traced to Brazilian groundnut meal – not all samples of which, however, proved harmful. Calves and pigs also died. In calves, groundnut poisoning resembles that of ragwort.

The toxic factor has been identified as the toxin (called Aflatoxin) produced by the common mould *Aspergillus flavus*, and may contaminate groundnuts from other countries also.

'The mould can grow on decorticated groundnuts when their moisture content exceeds about 9 per cent, or on meal at about 16 per cent. It usually develops on the nuts after they are harvested, particularly if drying is delayed and the shells damaged. However, if harvesting is delayed the nuts may become toxic in the ground, and if the nuts are stored at a moisture content in excess of 9 per cent they can also become toxic.' (*World Crops.*)

Pigs of from 3 to 12 weeks are particularly susceptible, and pregnant sows to a lesser extent.

It was found that cows fed on hay and a concentrate ration containing 20 per cent toxic groundnut meal excreted a toxin in the milk which produced the same biological effect in ducklings as aflatoxin. There is evidence strongly suggesting that aflatoxin may be a carcinogen, giving rise to cancer of the liver. A 100 per cent incidence of carcinoma of the liver was found in pigs in Morocco in 1945 which survived illness following the feeding of a mixture of oil-cakes. The same effect has been observed in rats.

Groundnut meal contains an alkaloid Arachine, which can cause a fatal hepatitis in dogs, and temporary paralysis in frogs and rabbits. (*See also* AFLATOXINS.)

GROWTH HORMONE (*see* SOMATOTROPHIN).

GROWTH PLATES. These are described under BONE – growth of. (For growth-plate defects, *see* BONE, DISEASES OF, and VALGUS.)

'GROWTH PROMOTERS'. Substances which, given in animal feeds, increase feed conversion efficiency or result in better daily liveweight gains, or both. A growth-promoter product (Elanco) in the form of a BOLUS containing MONENSIN (which see) was introduced in 1986 for cattle. (For types and examples, *see under* ADDITIVES; *also see* SOMATOSTATIN, STILBENES, SURFACTANTS, HORMONES IN MEAT PRODUCTION; WORMS, FARM TREATMENT AGAINST.)

GROWTHS (*see* TUMOURS, CANCER, GRANULOMA).

GUARNIERI BODIES (*see* INCLUSION BODIES).

GUINEA-PIG. Also known as a Cavy, the guinea-pig is technically a rodent, *Cavia porcella*, originating from South America; but is better known as a children's pet, a laboratory animal, and as one bred for show purposes.

Breeds include: English, Abyssinian and Peruvian.

Diseases include tuberculosis, pseudotuberculosis (yersiniosis), salmonellosis, leptospirosis, streptococcal pneumonia, toxoplasmosis, a viral infection of the salivary glands, and fascioliasis. Mange due to Trixacarus and lice infestations also occur. (*See* PETS.)

Guinea-pigs cannot synthesise vitamin C and so, like people, are liable to have scurvy.

The teeth of guinea-pigs grow continuously, and sometimes deviations from the normal cause loss of appetite; as may an accumulation of hair in the sulci of the gums.

GUINEA WORM. (*Dracunculus medinensis*) a nematode parasite which infects man, subhuman primates, dogs, cattle and horses. This parasite is found in Africa, the Middle East, India, Pakistan and Iran. The intermediate hosts are several species of the crustacea *Cyclops*, which live in ponds and wells, etc.

D. insignis infects carnivores in the USA and southern Canada.

The pads of a dog's feet may be severely affected by female guinea worms.

GULLET (*see* OESOPHAGUS).

GUMBORO DISEASE. This takes its name from a town in Delaware, USA. It affects broiler chickens of 1 to 5 weeks of age. The disease has been recorded in Britain. (*See* INFECTIOUS BURSAL DISEASE.)

GUMS, THE. The colour of these is dependent on the blood circulating within them, and provides useful clues to the veterinarian engaged on the detective work which goes into each diagnosis. Very pale gums suggest anaemia or internal haemorrhage. Gum pallor may be seen too in cases of leukaemia, shock after an accident, in warfarin poisoning, or failure of the left side of the heart. A yellowish tinge suggests jaundice. A blue or purple discoloration (*cyanosis*) indicates a shortage of oxygen in the circulating blood. (*See* CYANOSIS; and, for inflammation of the gums, Gingivitis under MOUTH, DISEASES OF.) For a common tumour of the gum, *see* EPULIS.

GUNSHOT INJURIES. In the small-animal practice teaching unit of the University of Edinburgh, records showed that over the previous five years there were 23 cases in which the animal had been shot, as detected by surgical and radiological means. Of 11 canine cases, seven involved shotgun pellets and four airgun pellets. One poodle died following lacerations to abdominal organs, and a lurcher developed a fatal fungal disease of the chest after shotgun injuries.

Of 10 feline cases, seven were injured by airguns. One cat had a femur fractured by a single pellet; and the periodic collapse of another cat was suspected to be due to an injury somewhere in the chest. Of three cats wounded by shotguns, one was put down because of spinal injury; another had a urethral obstruction.

A cat found lying in the street was thought to have been hit by a car. However, a veterinary examination revealed only a slight puncture wound on the right side of the chest. The cat was in pain, and there was no femoral pulse. A metallic object was suggested on radiography, and found to be a BB shot inside the aorta, which was incised and sutured. The cat was able to walk with difficulty after two weeks, and appeared completely recovered after five months. (Horton, C. R. & others, *Veterinary Medicine/SAC*, (1978), **73**, 321.)

Many animals are wounded without their owners knowing, and the pellets are often detected only when X-rayed for some entirely different reason.

In Canada the owner of a Labrador took it to a veterinary clinic on account of a swollen leg with skin wounds; explaining that the dog had been struck by a car two or three days previously. However, radiographs showed that, while there were multiple fractures, their cause was not a car but a shotgun.

Accidental or malicious shooting of dogs and cats often leads to serious **eye injury**, usually with some permanent impairment of vision. To give some examples, an 11-month old dog, shot with a 12-bore, suffered injury to the iris of one eye; the iris becoming partly adherent to the lens (*posterior synechia*). Six weeks after the accident the rest of the iris was mobile, and the pupil able to respond to light. An opaque pigmented spot remained on the cornea where it had been penetrated.

Another dog received one lead shot in the lens and another in the vitreous body of one eye. Seven months later a cataract had developed.

A third dog needed amputation of a part of the iris protruding through the shot wound in the cornea, which needed sutures.

'GUT-TIE' is the colloquial name for a type of hernia in which a piece of bowel becomes entangled in the spermatic cord following castration of cattle.

GUTTURAL POUCH. A diverticulum of the Eustachian tube developed from the pharynx.

Diseases of the guttural pouch include fungal infections, which may be followed by paralysis of the cranial nerves; and also a haemangioma, which may have a similar result. With both, the signs include difficulty in swallowing and the return of food and water through the nostrils. (*See also below.*) (*See* EAR, MIDDLE.)

GUTTURAL POUCH DIPHTHERIA was described as a disease entity by W. H. Cook in the UK in 1966. He stated that it is characterised by diphtheritic membrane formation in the guttural pouch. GPD has been encountered in horses from 2 months to 18 years old – in ponies, cobs, hunters, and thoroughbreds. It may prove fatal within a week, or may be chronic, with symptoms shown over a period of 7 months or more, he stated.

SIGNS. Epistaxis (nose bleeding) was present in 17 out of the 22 horses examined by Cook. 'Haemorrhage in every case occurred spontaneously while the horse was at rest in the stable. It is generally recurrent and may be mild, severe, or fatal.'

Pharyngeal paralysis. 'Ten of the 22 horses have shown difficulty in swallowing. Attempts to eat solid food result in coughing and the discharge of food material from mouth and nostrils. Drinking may be difficult. Water is conveyed back into the bucket via the nostrils.'

Laryngeal hemiplegia. 'Evidence of this was present in 10 out of the 22 horses. Five of the survivors made an abnormal inspiratory noise when exercised.'

Soft palate paresis. 'In racehorses this is shown by the sudden onset of respiratory obstruction during a race.'

DIAGNOSIS. This involves an examination of the guttural pouches by endoscope.

TREATMENT. Irrigation may be tried, and antibiotics used systemically.

GUTTURAL POUCH MYCOSIS can usually be successfully treated with benzimidazole drugs given by mouth. A specially designed catheter has been used for local treatment with antifungal agents. (Church, S. & others, *Equine Veterinary Journal*, (1986), **18**, 362.)

GYRUS. A convolution of the brain.

H

HABRONEMIASIS. Infection of horses with worms of the genus *Habronema*, the cause of 'summer sores' and a usually mild chronic gastritis. (*See* ROUNDWORMS in Horses.)

HAEMANGIOMA is a tumour composed of blood-vessels. In the liver of adult **cattle** small haemangiomata are not uncommonly found, but they are seldom of any practical importance. (*See also under* GUTTURAL POUCH for haemangioma in **horses**.)

HAEMANGIOSARCOMA. Cardiac haemangiosarcoma. A malignant tumour which may give rise to fatal internal haemorrhage, and has been found in the lung, spleen, liver, kidney, brain, etc., of dogs. Thirty-eight cases of this were seen at one veterinary hospital. In 16 **dogs** it was found on exploratory thoracotomy; in 22 the diagnosis was made only at autopsy. In 9 dogs in which the tumour could be resected, survival time averaged four months. Metastases were found in 16 of the dogs. (Aronsohn, M. H., *JAVMA*, (1985), **187**, 922.)

HAEMATEMESIS. Vomiting blood. When the latter is from a lesion of the stomach or oesophagus it is bright red; but when it has lain in the stomach for some time, and been partly digested it resembles coffee-grounds.

HAEMATIDROSIS. The presence of blood in the sweat.

HAEMATOCELE. This usually refers to the testicle following an injury which has ruptured the smaller blood-vessels. Blood from them then collects in the cavity of the scrotum, in the loose cellular tissue, or in the outer coat of the testicle itself.

HAEMATOCRIT VALUE. This means the percentage by volume of whole blood that is composed of erythrocytes. It is determined by filling a graduated haematocrit tube with blood – treated so that it will not clot – and then centrifuging the tube until the red cells are packed in the lower end. As a rough guide, values range as follows: sheep, 32; cow, 40; horse and pig, 42; dog, 45.

HAEMATOMA. A swelling containing clotted blood under the skin, or deeper in the musculature, following serious bruising; for example, after an animal has been struck by a car. Haematomas also occur in cases of warfarin poisoning and canine haemophilia. (*See also under* EAR, DISEASES OF for haematomas in cats and dogs resulting from scratching of the ear.)

HAEMATOPEDESIS (*see* HAEMATIDROSIS).

HAEMATOPHAGOUS. This adjective applies to parasites which feed on blood, such as ticks, fleas, and vampire bats.

HAEMATOTHORAX means an effusion of blood into the pleural cavity.

HAEMATOZOA is a general name applied to the various parasites of the blood.

HAEMATOZOON CANIS, a coccidia-like parasite found in countries where the tick *Rhipicephalus sanguineus* is present.
SIGNS: anaemia, fever, hindleg weakness, dyspnoea; sometimes epistaxis.

HAEMATURIA is any condition in which blood is found in the urine. (*See* URINE, ABNORMAL CONDITIONS OF.)

HAEMOBARTONELLA. Also known as Eperythrozoon. A single-celled parasite of the blood. *H. felis* is the cause of feline infectious anaemia; *H. canis* of the corresponding disease of dogs, in which the parasite complicates many cases of canine parvovirus infections. (*See also* EPERYTHROZOON for the infections in farm animals.) Diagnosis is not easy as the parasites may not be present in the first blood samples examined. Antibiotic treatment is usually successful; a vitamin B_{12} preparation often being given simultaneously.
The infection was demonstrated in 38 cats which could be divided into four groups. Group A were feline leukaemia virus-free and healthy carriers of Haemobartonella, with no anaemia.
Group B were also FeLV-free but had other disease.
Group C were FeLV-positive but had no other disease; Group D were FeLV-positive and did have other disease. (Bobade, P. A. & others. *Veterinary Record* (1988) **122**, 32.)

HAEMOGLOBIN is a complex organic compound containing iron, and gives the red colour to the red blood cells. (*See* METHAEMOGLOBIN.) Haemoglobin has the function of absorbing oxygen from the air in the lungs and of transporting oxygen to the tissues.
It exists in two forms, *carboxyhaemoglobin*, found in venous blood, and *oxyhaemoglobin*, found in arterial blood that has been in contact with oxygen. This oxyhaemoglobin, a weak compound of haemoglobin and oxygen, is broken down in the tissues, yielding to the cells its oxygen, and becoming once more haemoglobin.
In some forms of anaemia there is a great deficiency in haemoglobin. (*See* BLOOD, ANAEMIA, RESPIRATION.)

HAEMOGLOBIN REACTIVE PROTEIN. This appears in the blood serum when an abscess is present in the body, and disappears when the abscess disappears. It forms the basis of a diagnostic test for internal abscesses (*e.g.* of the liver), as explained under BLOOD TYPING.

HAEMOGLOBINURIA. The presence of haemoglobin in the urine, such as occurs in azoturia, red-water fever, leptospirosis of calves, poisoning by an excess of kale or cabbage.

HAEMOLYSIS means the destruction of red blood cells and the consequent escape from them of Haemoglobin. It occurs gradually in some forms of anaemia and rapidly in poisoning by snake venom. Some chemical and bacterial toxins cause haemolysis.

HAEMOLYTIC. Relating to haemolysis. For Haemolytic Disease of foals, *see* FOALS, DISEASES OF. Haemolytic Disease in pigs and dogs is similar in its effects. In cattle, it may account for some cases of abortion.

HAEMOPHILIA (*see* CANINE HAEMOPHILIA).

HAEMOPHILUS INFECTIONS include *Haemophilus somnus* causing the 'sleeper' syndrome in feedlot cattle in the USA. (*See* 'SLEEPER'.) The organism has also been isolated from cases of pneumonia, metritis, and abortion in cattle; and in Canada it is commonly found in the genital tract of bulls. *H. somnus* has been found in semen samples from Danish bulls also. In pigs in the UK *Haemophilus parasuis, H. parainfluenzae* and *H. parahaemolyticus* are often associated with chronic respiratory disease, including a painful pleurisy. *H. parahaemolyticus* may also cause an acute illness and sudden death.

Infection with *H. pleuropneumoniae* has been increasingly detected in Britain, as have the reported number of outbreaks of acute pleuropneumonia due to this organism.

HAEMOPOIESIS,-ETIC. Relating to the formation of red blood cells.

HAEMOPTYSIS means the expulsion of blood from the lower air passages, generally by coughing. The blood so expelled is bright red in colour and is frothy, thus differing from that which has been expelled from the stomach. It is seen in tuberculosis. (*See also* 'BLEEDER' HORSES.)

HAEMORRHAGE (*see* BLEEDING; PROTHROMBIN; INTERNAL HAEMORRHAGE; *and* HAEMORRHAGIC DISEASE).

HAEMORRHAGIC DIATHESIS. An inherited tendency, transmissible to either sex, to bleeding from the nasal and other mucosa. It has been reported in the dog (as well as in man). Thrombocytopenia is not involved.

'HAEMORRHAGIC DISEASE' OF DOGS (*see* CANINE TROPICAL PANCYTOPAENIA, DIARRHOEA, HAEMANGIOSARCOMA, CANINE HAEMOPHILIA and HAEMORRHAGE).

HAEMORRHAGIC ENTERITIS OF TURKEYS. This disease or syndrome has appeared in the UK, USA, Australia, Rhodesia, and South Africa. There is an increased incidence during hot weather. An adenovirus accounts for many cases.

HAEMORRHAGIC FEVER with renal syndrome (HFRS). An important human disease caused by Hantaan or related viruses, and occurring in Europe, the USA, and the Far East. Human mortality varies from 0.5 to 18 per cent. In Belgium staff at a research institute were infected by laboratory rats; but voles are the main source. In the USA urban rats have been implicated. (WHO).

SYMPTOMS. They can be like the effects of a mild influenza attack; but in many cases they are those of a serious illness characterised by dizziness, vomiting, back pain, haematuria, acute kidney failure, and shock.

HAEMORRHAGIC GASTRO-ENTERITIS OF PIGS. One syndrome involves the sudden death of growing pigs, with autopsy findings of haemorrhage into the small intestine, and sometimes volvulus.

Whey-feeding is especially associated with this syndrome, but it can occur also in meal-fed pigs.

J. N. Todd and colleagues of MAFF's veterinary investigation centre, Bristol, described their findings in 50 cases of intestinal haemorrhage in pigs between two and six months old from whey-feeding units. In 47 of the pigs a *post mortem* finding was a twisting of the intestinal mesentery – the membrane which supports the intestines.

The hypothesis of Mr Todd and his colleagues is that in whey-fed pigs 'rapid gas production occurs in the colon after feeding and the consequent distension of this organ results in its displacement, which in some cases leads to volvulus, and, to the death of the animal'. The haemorrhage is, they consider, a consequence of the twisting and occlusion of the mesenteric veins. Pig breeders both in this country and in New Zealand have noticed that affected pigs (including some which recovered) showed distension of the abdomen. This suggests that gas formation is the first stage, and *not* the result of the twisting.

Preliminary experiments in the Bristol VI laboratory indicate not only that whey is highly fermentable but that it may contain substantial quantities of 'dissolved' gas which may be rapidly released.

Haemorrhage from the intestine is an important feature of another syndrome described by Dr R. J. Love and other veterinary research workers at the universities of Sydney, New South Wales. An outbreak involved 372 adult pigs in the breeding units of a minimal-disease piggery in Australia; 186 pigs died. Some had been seen to be passing blood; others died without any symptoms being observed.

This syndrome has the somewhat cumbersome name **Proliferative Haemorrhagic Enteropathy** (PHE), and has been described also by several research workers in the UK. PHE is associated with adenoma-like changes in the small intestine similar to those seen in necrotic enteritis and inflammation of the ileum, the last part of the small intestine. (*See also* PORCINE ADENOMATOSIS.)

HAEMORRHAGIC SEPTICAEMIA (PASTEUR-ELLOSIS). This is present in most tropical countries, and is especially important in Asia. Outbreaks tend to occur at the beginning of the monsoon rains. Buffaloes and cattle are the animals mainly affected, but the disease occurs also in camels, goats, sheep, pigs and horses.
CAUSE. *Pasteurella multocida* Type 1, and possibly other serotypes. Stress due to exhaustion, under-feeding, and transport may predispose animals to infection.
SIGNS. After a very short incubation period (two days or less), buffaloes and cattle become dull, lose their appetite, salivate profusely, and have a high fever. Visible mucous membranes become dark red. The tongue may swell and protrude from the mouth. Oedema results in hot, painful swellings in the regions of the throat, brisket, and dewlap. Death, in this most acute form, usually follows dyspnoea, and occurs in from a few hours to three or four days. Mortality is very high. In less acute cases there may be dysentery or broncho-pneumonia.
TREATMENT can seldom be carried out in time to save life, but sulphonamide drugs and antibiotics may help if given early.
CONTROL. Oil-adjuvant vaccines are useful. (*See also* PASTEURELLOSIS, SHIPPING FEVER.)

HAEMOSIDERIN. An iron-protein compound. It appears to be the form in which iron is stored until needed for haemoglobin.

HAEMOSTATICS are means taken to check bleeding, and may be either drugs applied to the area, or mechanical devices, etc. As regards human medicine, 20 agents were scrutinised 'but only three, ethamsylate, εe-aminocaproic acid, and tranexamic acid – emerged with any clinical credibility'. (*Lancet* Aug. 20 1977 416.) (*See* HAEMORRHAGE, GELATIN SPONGE.)

HAIR (*see* SKIN).

HAIR-BALLS sometimes cause indigestion in **calves,** especially those aged about 6 weeks to 4 months. The hair may be in the form of a ball or in loose masses, sometimes mixed with milk curds, sand, binder twine, etc. Bad management encourages calves to lick their own or other animal's hair. The condition rarely proves fatal both in calves and pigs. (However, the owner of an animal, on finding a hairball, may erroneously decide that that is the cause of death, which may in fact have been caused by some infection.)
SIGNS. Are usually vague, but may include grinding of the teeth, an unnatural gait, and in chronic cases a general loss of condition, although the appetite remains fairly good. Convulsions may also occur.
PREVENTION. Ensure a well-balanced diet, adequate minerals and roughage, and attend to any skin disease. (*See* SALT LICKS.)

TREATMENT is surgical and often successful if carried out early.
  Cats. Hair/fur balls sometimes result in impaction of the intestine. Less commonly this occurs also in the dog. (*See also* TRICHOBEZOAR).

HAIR, CLIPPING OF THE (*see* CLIPPING OF ANIMALS).

HAIR, DISEASES OF (*see* ALOPECIA, RINGWORM, DERMATOPHILUS, SKIN DISEASES).

HAIR DRYERS. Hot air from these has been used for removal of maggots from wounds following the desired debridement.

'HAIRY SHAKER' DISEASE is transmissible disease of lambs in New Zealand, resembling Border Disease (which see).

HALF-BRED. This term usually means the cross of a Cheviot ewe × Border Leicester.

HALOTHANE. A volatile anaesthetic used for horses, dogs, cats, laboratory animals and, to a lesser extent, in cattle. 'It is a potent respiratory depressant. One of the more important properties is its effect on the vasomotor centre, which is markedly depressed, causing a degree of hypotension. This fact is of considerable importance in that the lowered blood pressure may help to prevent shock. Fluothane should therefore not be used in conjunction with other hypotensive drugs (*e.g.* chlorpromazine).' (J. R. Campbell and D. D. Lawson.) (*See* ANAESTHETICS.)

HALOTHANE TEST. 'The anaesthetic halothane can detect a single gene affecting stress susceptibility and production traits,' Dr A. J. Webb of the AFRC's Animal Breeding Research Organisation, Edinburgh, commented with reference to the porcine stress syndrome. (*see* PALE SOFT EXUDATIVE MUSCLE).
  'The halothane test is relatively easy to carry out under farm conditions. Pigs of around 8 weeks of age are made to breathe the anaesthetic through a face mask for a total of three minutes. If they remain relaxed throughout this period, they are scored as negative, or "stress resistant". If the muscles of the hind leg become rigid during the three minutes, the pigs are scored as positive, or "stress susceptible". In this case the halothane must be turned off immediately, or the reaction may reach an irreversible stage which can kill the pig. Positive and negative reactors normally recover fully within five minutes of the test.' (*Pig Breeders' Gazette.*)

HAM (*see* GLUTEAL, MUSCLES and, for abscesses, INJECTIONS).

HAMARTOMA. A tumour-like malformation composed of an abnormal mixture of the normal tissue components of the organ from which the Hamartoma arises. Pulmonary hamartomas have been found in animals, with either vascular or cartilaginous tissue predominating. It is a rare congential defect.

HAMMONDIA HAMMONDI. A coccidian parasite, antigenically related to *Toxoplasma gondii*, of cats. The parasite has a 2-host life-cycle. Hosts also include rodents, dogs.

HAMPSHIRE. A black pig with a white belt, from Kentucky, USA. The origins of the breed were probably nineteenth century Old English.

HAMSTERS. Two species have become popular domestic pets; namely the dwarf Russian (*Phodopus sungorus*), and *Mesocricetus auratus.*

The former, also known as the striped, hairy-footed hamster, comes from Siberia, central Asia, and northern China.

Diseases include tumour formation affecting mouth, skin, and mammary glands, and leading to rapid loss of weight; indeed, to emaciation in many cases.

Weight loss as a result of broncho-pneumonia or of tooth-trimming also occurs.

Cystic ovaries, in hamsters prevented from breeding, result in an enlarged abdomen and a haemorrhagic discharge from the vulva.

Synthetic-fibre bedding material sold for hamsters has caused severe injury, sometimes necessitating euthanasia.

In the *Mesocricetus auratus* species, the main health problem is 'Wet Tail', a fairly common and often fatal disease; so named because of diarrhoea and consequent staining of the tail.
ANAESTHESIA: Halothane appears to be well tolerated, with rapid recovery, when used for spaying, etc. (Lawrie, A. M. & Megahy, I. W. *Veterinary Record* (1991) **27**, 128).

Hamsters and human health. They occasionally carry the virus of Lymphocytic Choriomeningitis (LCM).

Sixty people, aged from 3 to 70, became ill following the despatch by an Alabama breeder of LCM-infected hamsters (via wholesalers) to shops in seven states of the USA. Of 60 patients, 55 kept hamsters as pets, and 4 worked for wholesalers or retail shops. An outbreak, involving 48 people, was also reported from Germany, the cause being medical laboratory hamsters. (*See also under* LYMPHOCYTIC CHORIOMENINGITIS, and PETS.)

HAND. A unit of measurement for the height of a horse, as measured at the withers. A hand is four inches. Under 1981 UK legislation, metrication was introduced, resulting in rounded equivalents; *e.g.* 12 hands = 122 cm; 10½ hands = 107 cm. (*See* HORSES, MEASUREMENT OF.)

HAND, FOOT, AND MOUTH DISEASE. A disease of man, first described in 1957, which has to be differentiated from rare human infection with foot and mouth disease. The cause is Coxsackie A9 virus (or A5, A10 or A16). (See *Lancet* for October 7, 1972).

HANTAVIRUS. A genus containing the Hantaan and related viruses. (*See* HAEMORRHAGIC FEVER with renal syndrome, HFRS.)

Hantavirus infection in animals. A single feline case in the UK was recorded in 1983, but since then the veterinary faculty of Liverpool University carried out a survey of serum samples taken from 41 pet cats brought for treatment, and from 12 young cats for neutering. Six were shown to have antibody to the virus in their bloodstream.

One of 7 stray cats from Leeds, and 7 of 85 feral cats in various parts of England and Wales were likewise Hantavirus antibody-positive.

The virus can cause chronic illness in cats, especially in those infected also with the feline leukaemia virus or the feline immunodeficiency virus.
SOURCES OF INFECTION: voles and rats.

Human Hantavirus infection. In many parts of Europe a mild form, *Nephropathia epidemica*, has been recorded; but a severe form appeared in Greece and Bulgaria. There may be internal haemorrhage and kidney disease in some cases.
SOURCES 'probably include' aerosols of the virus from saliva, urine, faeces, and lung secretions; also bites by rodents.

Laboratory infections from rats kept there, and from Hantaan tissue culture, are a recognised hazard. (*Lancet* **336**, 407.)

Farm workers, water sports enthusiasts, sewage farm workers, and laboratory personnel have seropositivity rates of up to 21 per cent.
SYMPTOMS, appearing two or three weeks after exposure, comprise conjunctivitis, with erythema of face, neck and upper chest. In the severe form, fever, headache, nausea and vomiting are typical; with moderate or severe kidney disease.

It was suggested by Kudesiu, G. and others (*Lancet* (1988) June 18th 1397) that people with suspected leptospirosis should have their blood tested also for Hantavirus.

HAPLOID refers to the reduced number of chromosomes in the ovum and sperm – half the (diploid) number in the somatic cells. (*see* MEIOSIS.)

HAPTEN. A small molecule that cannot by itself initiate an immune response, but which can do so when linked to a 'carrier', *e.g.* a protein such as albumin. (*See* IMMUNE RESPONSE, B CELLS.)

HARD PALATE (*see* PALATE).

HARDERIAN GLAND. A sebaceous gland which, in some animals, acts as an accessory to the lacrimal gland. Normally the Harderian gland is completely covered by the third eyelid, but in dogs obstruction to the flow of material from the gland not uncommonly causes its enlargement and projection beyond the third eyelid, when it appears as a red, roundish mass. In some cases it may be necessary for the gland to be removed under local or general anaesthesia. (*See also* EYE, DISEASES OF.)

'HARDWARE DISEASE'. The colloquial American name for traumatic pericarditis of cattle caused by metal objects, such as pieces of baling wire, nails. (*See under* HEART, DISEASES OF.)

HARE-LIP. This deformity is seen in puppies of the toy breeds and in sheep. When the cleft in the lip is wide, sucking is impossible and the young puppies often die from starvation. In less severe cases they obtain some nourishment, but never thrive as well as the others in a litter. The malformation is generally associated with 'cleft palate'. (*See* CLEFT PALATE.)

HARES may harbour the liver fluke of sheep, *Fasciola hepatica*, and the cystic stage of the tapeworm *Taenia multiceps packi* of the dog, and of *Taenia pisiformis*. In some countries (*e.g.* Denmark), hares are a source of *Brucella abortus suis* infection to pigs. Some European hares also harbour *Br. melitensis*.

In the UK, Orf-like lesions have been seen (and confused with myxomatosis). Other diseases include aspergillosis, streptococcal endocarditis, toxoplasmosis, and coccidiosis. Louping-ill virus and/or antibody has been found in English hares, and also Q fever antibody. Avian tuberculosis is another occasional finding.

In order to prevent the introduction of *Brucella suis* and also of *Pasteurella tularensis* infections, the Hares (Control of Importation) Order 1965 was enacted in the UK. (*See* TULARAEMIA.)

For a virus which killed many hares in 1991 both in the UK and the European mainland.

HARVEST MITES (*see under* MITES).

HASSALL'S CORPUSCLES (*see* THYMUS GLAND).

HAVERHILL FEVER. The name given in human medicine to sporadic cases of rat-bite fever resulting from contamination of food. The causal bacteria are *Streptobacillus moniliformis* and *Spirillum minus*. Rats are usually sub-clinical carriers.

HAW (*see end of section headed* EYE).

HAWKS (*see* FALCONS).

HAY. There are two general classes of hay: that from grasses only, and that containing leguminous plants such as clover, lucerne. (*See* LEYS, PASTURE MANAGEMENT.) Hay is a very important, but nowadays perhaps a somewhat under-rated, article of diet for cattle. (*See part in heavy type under* DIET/**Fibre.**) Hay is sometimes put down on very lush pasture where bloat is anticipated. As well as assisting in bloat prevention, it will help to obviate hypomagnesaemia and acetonaemia also. The feeding of hay together with green fodder crops is said to reduce the risk of scouring, especially when large quantities of the fodder are being eaten and during wet weather. When kale or rape are being fed in quantity hay is most necessary in the diet. Hay made from leys is evidently not very palatable, for it is refused by the sick cow which will often relish even not very good hay made from old pasture.

'Tripoded hay has four or five times as much carotene as good hay made in the swathe, and barn-dried hay is even better. On the other hand, swathe hay has more vitamin D than other types if made in good weather. Badly-damaged swathe hay is deficient in both carotene and vitamin D, and there may well be a case for adding vitamins A and D as well as minerals to any cereals used to make good the losses in poor hay.' – T. H. Davies.

There would certainly seem to be more scope now for barn hay-drying though the relatively high costs of this and also of hay-towers are likely to limit wide application of these two methods. The first essential, in any event, is of course high-quality grass to make into hay.

In 1972 an ADAS regional nutrition chemist, G. Alderman, commented that three-quarters of the 2,800,000 acres of hay made in England was of sub-maintenance quality. 'Average quality is inadequate for the bare maintenance of an average Friesian cow, which will require 2 lb of cereal supplement.' At the other extreme is, as Professor Ian Moor pointed out, the hay with a crude protein content of 19·98 per cent which obtained for the Hillsborough Research Station, Northern Ireland, a daily liveweight gain of 2·14lb daily in bullocks fed *hay only.*

Mouldy hay can be dangerous (*see* ASPERGILLOSIS and FARMER'S LUNG.) Hay which contains sweet clovers, or vernal, and has become overheated or mouldy, may have a dangerously high DICOUMAROL content and give rise to HAEMORRHAGIC SYNDROME OF CATTLE (which see). Fatal poisoning has also occurred in stock fed hay containing RAGWORT or FOXGLOVES.

'HAY FEVER' (*see* ATOPIC DISEASE).

'HAYFLAKES'. In appearance, hayflakes resemble chopped hay but retain the quality of dried grass. They are not chopped so short that the fibrous quality of grass is destroyed, nor so long that storage space becomes difficult. They can be stored loose in the barn for self- or easy feeding; or they can be baled.

HAYLAGE is a registered trade name for material which has been wilted down to 40–50 per cent dry matter, precision chopped to ½-inch nominal length, and processed through a Harvestore tower silo.

HCH. Hexachlorocyclohexane. (*See* BHC which consists of five isomers of HCH.)

In Britain HCH-containing sheep dips have been withdrawn from the approved list.

HEADFLY (*see* FLIES).

HEAD-TILTING. In cats this sign occurs in cases of a foreign body present in an ear. (*See* EAR, DISEASES OF, under *Shaking the head.*) (*See also* FELINE VESTIBULAR SYNDROME.)

'HEAD GRIT' (*see* 'YELLOWSES').

HEAD INJURIES. These may result in concussion (*see under* BRAIN, DISEASES OF) or secondary EPILEPSY (which see) in the dog. Lesions may include an intracranial haematoma, a depressed fracture of the skull, scar tissue, etc.

HEALING OF WOUNDS (*see* WOUNDS).

HEALTH SCHEMES FOR FARM ANIMALS.
These can lead to increased profitability, especially in the large units which are commonplace today.

As Professor C. S. G. Grunsell, of the University of Bristol Veterinary School, once wrote: 'At the outset it is necessary to consider the definition of health. In the case of farm livestock it can no longer be accepted as simply a state in which disease is absent, and is now more accurately regarded as a state of maximum economic production.' Similarly, in the same context, infertility could be defined as a failure to breed as often or as regularly as the farmer would wish. In financial terms, such failure has been costed by the Milk Marketing Board; for example, missing a single heat period can mean a loss of over £5.

Reference is made elsewhere to the PIG HEALTH SCHEME, confined to MLC's nucleus and reserve herds, and to the Enzootic Pneumonia Scheme introduced in 1959.

In Iowa, USA, a pig health scheme, operated by veterinary surgeons in private practice, has found favour among producers and costs the equivalent of 72½p per pig weaned. This can include worming sows; spraying against external parasites; vaccination against swine fever, erysipelas, and leptospirosis; and boar fertility.

A study in Canada had shown that the farmer received between 150 and 500 per cent return on invested funds from an effective health programme (the major variable being the degree of co-operation by the farmer). In an Australian health scheme there was an improved reproductive performance estimated to be worth £4 per cow after the first two years.

Currently on farms in the UK health schemes are in operation. For example, many large dairy units receive weekly or fortnightly visits, when cows are presented to the veterinary surgeon for pregnancy diagnosis and treatment. He will also advise on preventive measures.

This is further exemplified at BOCM Silcock's Knaptoft Farm where it has been the custom for the veterinary surgeon to examine: (1) all cows not seen on heat 40 days after calving; (2) cows with erratic heat periods; (3) all cows 8 weeks after the last service for pregnancy diagnosis. (*See also* POULTRY HEALTH SCHEME.)

HEARING (*see* EAR, last paragraph; *also* ULTRASOUND *and* TELEVISION SETS).

HEARTBEAT (*see* PULSE RATE).

HEART DISEASES. As in man, heart troubles are very much more common in old age. However, even young animals may suffer from faulty heart action due to congenital defects.
SIGNS. Irregularity in the heart-beat, some difficulty in breathing without obvious changes in the lungs or pleura, breathlessness when compelled to exert themselves, a tendency to swelling of the dependent parts of the body (*e.g.* along the lower line of the chest and abdomen and 'filling' of the limbs), are among the signs. A cough is sometimes a symptom of valvular disease.

Congestive heart failure. Disease of the right side of the heart often gives rise to ascites, sometimes to swelling of one or more limbs due to oedema. Engorgement of the veins often occurs, with enlargement of the liver. The animal becomes easily tired and may lose weight. Ultimately congestive heart failure is likely to occur. This may also result from left-sided failure due to myocarditis or mitral valve incompetence.

In small animals treatment consists in reducing exercise, and giving diuretics.

A common cause of heart failure in dogs is degeneration of a MITRAL VALVE (which see).

Pericarditis is an inflammation of the membrane covering the exterior of the heart. It may be 'idiopathic', when its cause is not known; or it may be 'traumatic', when it is due to a wound; or it may follow a general infection (*e.g.* 'Heart-water') or a local infection (*e.g.* pleurisy) or an abscess in a remote part of the body. Pericarditis may be 'dry', in which case the two opposing surfaces of the membrane are covered by a layer of fibrin; or oedema may accompany this condition, in which case fluid fills up the pericardial sac and, when no more distension of the sac can occur, presses upon the outside of the heart itself.

Pericarditis has been reported in very young pigs at grass. 'The piglet, often in good condition and not anaemic, dies suddenly about 2 to 3 weeks of age.' (*See also* 'MULBERRY HEART'.)

Tamponade. A rapid accumulation of blood in the pericardium, suddenly arresting heart function.

Either acute or chronic tamponade was the presenting sign in 42 cases of pericardial effusion reviewed by Berg and Wingfield. Their patients were large dogs with an average age of nine years.

Twenty-four of the cases were associated with neoplasia, eight with benign idiopathic effusions. six with primary heart disease, and two with trauma.

Echocardiography was found to be the best way of detecting pericardial effusion; and the idiopathic effusions responded well to pericardiectomy. (Berg, R. J. & Wingfield, W., *J. American Hospital Assoc.*, 1984.)

Congenital heart disease in dogs and cats is usually indicated by a cardiac murmur; the site and nature of which shows whether a valve or a shunt is involved.

Shunts include 'holes' in the heart, and patent *ductus arteriosus.*

Radiography and Doppler ultrasound are helpful in diagnosis.

Surveys of a total of 580 dogs with congenital heart disease showed that 28 per cent had patent *ductus arteriosus*; 16 per cent had pulmonary stenosis; 9 per cent had persistent right aortic arch; over 7 per cent had a ventricular septal defect; and over 7 per cent had stenosis of the aorta. (Patterson, D. F. *Journal of Small Animal Practice* (1989) **30**, 153.) (*See* HEARTWORMS also.)

Deficiency of vitamin E is one cause of sudden cardiac arrest in cattle.

SIGNS. These are not always characteristic, but they include breathlessness, pain on pressure of the left side of the chest, a jugular pulse (seen along the jugular furrow with each heart-beat), and oedema. On listening to the heart a variation in the normal sounds may be heard, or they may be altogether masked by the presence of the fluid. A tinkle is sometimes audible over the region of the heart; friction sounds indicate the presence of dry pericarditis; and irregularity or even palpitation may be noticed.

Traumatic pericarditis of cattle. Sometimes when the animal is thought to be suffering from simple digestive disturbance, it is found that a nail or piece of wire has been swallowed and arrives in the reticulum.

A distance of about only two inches separates the heart from the reticulum, so that the foreign body is liable to penetrate the pericardium.

Attacks of pain may occur, the appetite is irregular, but after a time the animal regains its normal health, since an adhesion has occurred around the hole in the reticulum wall, and the inflammation subsides. A cow may die suddenly before symptoms of pericarditis appear, or soon afterwards.

TREATMENT is sometimes feasible by surgically opening the rumen and removing the piece of metal.

PREVENTION: In Switzerland the percentage of cows slaughtered on account of traumatic pericarditis was greatly reduced following use by Dr E. Schneider of magnets for the treatment of traumatic reticulitis. He used magnets weighing 114 g, 90 mm long and 15 mm in diameter. He introduced the magnets *per os* 10 minutes after a subcutaneous injection of atropine sulphate. Without this he found that only 53 per cent of the magnets dropped at once into the reticulum. The correct siting of the magnets was checked with a compass.

Myocarditis is inflammation of the heart muscle. In the pig it is seen in HERZTOD disease, for example; in cattle, in MUSCULAR DYSTROPHY. (*see also* CANINE PARVOVIRUS and MYOCARDIUM.)

Endocarditis is an inflammation of the membrane lining the heart. It frequently leads to the development of nodules on the valves.

The nodules result in an incomplete closing of the valves, and since the fibrin deposited upon them tends to become converted into fibrous tissue (*organised*), the growths slowly increase in size. They are seen in chronic erysipelas of pigs (*see* SWINE ERYSIPELAS.)

The valvular insufficiency can be diagnosed by auscultation. Congestive heart failure may be the outcome (sometimes embolism); but compensation takes place, and the animal may live a long time with faulty valves.

Bacterial endocarditis is a cause of death in cattle, especially in South Wales. (*See* HEART WORM for another cause of endocarditis in the dog.)

Valvular diseases form a most important and common group of heart disorders, and although the power of compensation already referred to may so neutralise the ill-effects of a narrowed valve, or one which leaks, severe strains or exertion, or even trying conditions such as parturition may precipitate ill effects. Very often when an animal 'drops dead', perhaps after running a race, or while undergoing some departure from its normal mode of life, the actual cause is afterwards found to be a diseased heart valve. Fainting fits are not by any means rare in incompetence of the tricuspid valves, in which condition may occur. Congestion of the lungs may be brought about by incompetence of the auriculo-ventricular valve on the left side of the heart (mitral insufficiency). This same condition may lead to a chronic asthmatical cough in old dogs, which is occasionally mistaken for bronchitis.

Canine heart repair. Skeletal muscle transplants were used to replace or repair defects in the left ventricle of dogs; some of which were kept alive for over a year. At autopsy the transplants were found to be in good condition, according to a report in *Circulation.*

Hypertrophy, or enlargement of the heart takes place as the result of some constant simple strain, such as occurs in race-horses, hunters, and sporting dogs; or as the result of backward pressure from a diseased valve, and which entails the 'compensation' of valvular disease; or it may be due to resistance to the flow of blood in some diseased organ or tissue, which results in high blood-pressure. (*See* COMPENSATION.)

Hypertrophy of the left ventricle, leading to heart failure, may in the dog follow *Leptospira canicola* infection.

Dilatation of the heart may precede hypertrophy, *i.e.* when it occurs before the heart muscle has had an opportunity to increase to meet the extra demands upon it, and it very frequently follows hypertrophy, especially when there is some devitalising process at work which hinders the proper nutrition of the organ.

Hypertrophy may be a beneficial condition in any animal, and, except when it is due to valvular trouble, need not cause any worry to the owner. It is sometimes excessive in horses; in some instances the heart may weigh as much as 25 lb instead of the 7 or 8 lb of the normal. Degenerative changes may follow hypertrophy when the animal becomes less active during later life.

Congenital defects. These include a patent *Ductus arteriosus* (*see* diagram of fetal circulation *under* CIRCULATION, *and also* LIGAMENTUM ARTERIOSUM.) (*See too* ECTOPIA CORDIS.) Tetralogy of Fallot consists of (1) stenosis of the pulmonary valve; (2) a defect in the septum which separates the two ventricles; (3) the aorta over-riding both ventricles; (4) marked hypertrophy of the right ventricle.

The signs are often vague: in kittens, for example, a failure to thrive, inability to cope with exercise. More serious defects result in the death of newborn kittens.

Functional disorders: Palpitation is a condition in which the heart beats fast and strongly, due to fright, for example.

Bradycardia is a condition of unusually slow action of the heart. **Intermittency** or **irregularity** is an exceedingly common condition among animals, and as a rule appears to cause them no inconvenience whatever. In some horses at rest in the stable the heart constantly misses every third, fourth, or fifth beat, a long pause taking the place of the pulsation, but when at exercise or work the normal rhythm is restored.

Heart-block is a condition in which the conducting mechanism between atrium and ventricle (atrio-ventricular bundle of His) is damaged in whole or part, so that the two beat independently of each other.

Rapid heart action may be due to some temporary irritability in the heart muscle; it is distinguished from the rapid pulsation of a fever, by the absence of high temperature and by the normal strength of the pulse. The condition is known as **Tachycardia**.

Cardiac flutter and fibrillation are conditions of great irregularity in the pulse, due to the atria emptying themselves, not by a series of regular waves, but by an irregular series of flutters or twitches instead, which fail to stimulate the ventricles properly.

Five cases of atrial fibrillation are described in horses after racing. In four of them, which had performed poorly during their races, the arrhythmias disappeared spontaneously within 24 hours; these cases were regarded as paroxysmal. In the fifth horse, which won its race, the arrhythmia persisted for at least 45 hours after the race and it was regarded as an example of persistent atrial fibrillation. Treatment with quinidine sulphate restored the sinus rhythm. Paroxysmal atrial fibrillation may cause a sudden decrease in racing performance. (Holmes, J. R., *Equine Veterinary Journal*, (1986), **18,** 37.)

Diagnosis of heart disease is based largely on the character of the pulse and heart sounds. Murmurs, for example, indicate valvular incompetence, cardiac dilatation, or congenital lesions. Muffled sounds may indicate fluid in the pericardium (or pleurisy).

Additionally radiography and cardiography are used in diagnosis. (*See* PACEMAKERS as a possibility of treating some canine patients.)

HEART STIMULANTS. These include nikethamide (Coramine), pholedrine sulphate, adrenalin, caffeine, digitalis.

HEARTWATER, also known as BUSH SICKNESS (Boschziekte), VELD SICKNESS, and INAPUNGA, is a specific disease of cattle, sheep, and goats transmitted by the 'bont-tick' (*Amblyomma hebraeum*), in South Africa, and *A. variegatum* in Kenya. The disease is characterised by the accumulation of a large amount of fluid in the pericardial sac and nervous symptoms.

In 1980 the existence of Heartwater in many islands of the Carribbean was discovered; previously the disease had been known only in Africa. The tick involved is *Amblyomma variegatum*, introduced into Guadeloupe with cattle from Senegal in the 1980s.

CAUSE. Infection with *Rickettsia ruminantium* (*Cowdria ruminantium*) which possesses an ultra-visible stage which is taken into the body of a feeding bont-tick, and is transmitted to other animals upon which the tick feeds at a later state of its life-history.

INCUBATION. After sheep and goats have been bitten by infected ticks, a period of between 11 and 18 days elapses before any symptoms are shown; in cattle the disease appears between 20 and 25 days after infestation with ticks. These periods are influenced by the stage of the disease in the animal supplying the infected blood to the ticks, and also by individual susceptibility, which is less in native-bred cattle than in those imported from other countries, and especially those brought from Great Britain.

SIGNS.

(1) Sheep and goats.

Sheep and goats at first show nothing more than a rise in temperature (which gradually increases to 107°F, falling each evening 2 or 3 degrees lower), a general dullness, prostration, and lack of appetite, and as these conditions are common to many other diseases the difficulty of diagnosis is great. The affected animals isolate themselves from the rest of the flock, lie about in secluded spots, cease to ruminate, and when handled or driven are very easily tired and lie down.

Many animals show peculiar nervous symptoms, which vary in different individuals; some may bleat almost continuously; others champ the jaws as if feeding, moving the tongue backward and forward between the lips; others lick the ground; some turn in circles until they finally fall to the ground and lie prostrate or perform galloping movements with their limbs; while others, show profuse salivation. Convulsions are not uncommon, especially when the animals are handled. Death usually follows soon after convulsions make their appearance.

(2) Cattle.

The symptoms in cattle are very similar to those seen in sheep. The nervous form in which peculiar masticatory movements are made by the mouth is common. Animals show a tendency to bite at their feet or legs, especially when lying on the ground, and biting the ground is also seen. A number of animals in the early stages may show a dangerous tendency to charge any human being approaching them. In cattle the disease is usually at its height about the fourth day after the first rise in temperature, and death usually occurs about the sixth day. Hyper-acute cases occur in cattle, and the animal is found dead on the veld.

AUTOPSY. Fluid in the pericardial sac surrounding the heart (hence the name – heartwater); but while this is usually found in sheep and goats, it may be absent in the case of cattle. In typical instances there is also a collection of similar fluid in the thoracic and abdominal cavities. Both the pericardium, and the endocardium which lines the heart, may show several small or a few large 'petechiae', *i.e.* areas where a slight amount of haemorrhage has taken place.

PREVENTION. Entirely successful results have followed measures taken against the ticks which transmit the disease. These consist in '*five-day dippings*'.

Antibiotics and sulphadimidine are used in treatment.

HEARTWORMS. *Dirofilaria immitis* is a common parasite of dogs in Central Europe, Russia, Australia, America, and Asia, and the worm larvae are transmitted by various mosquitoes and gnats. The adult worms reach a length of up to 12 inches (females) and inhabit the right side of the heart, causing some degree of endocarditis and a variety of symptoms, *e.g.* cough, hind leg weakness, collapse on exercise, laboured breathing, anaemia, emaciation.

This infestation is known as canine filariasis or Dirofilariasis. The kidneys and urinary tract may be affected. (*See also* EYE, DISEASES OF.)

In Canada, 560 dogs (1·79 per cent of those tested) were found to have heartworms in 1981.

'About 20 per cent of dogs are infected with adult worms without having microfilariae,' Robert Lewis, of the University of Georgia, stated.

The point that heartworms can cause devastating cardio-pulmonary effects in **cats** was made at a meeting of the American Heartworm Society. It was also recognised that the disease could be present without microfilariae, not only during the prepatent period; for adult worms may be males, 'geriatric females', or of one sex only.

There have been reports of Dirofilaria worms being recovered from the brains of cats. One such report referred to a cat with ataxia which died 48 hours later. At autopsy 3 heartworms were found in the heart, 3 in the brain, and 4 in a kidney.

DIAGNOSIS. An ELISA test has been developed at the University of Pennsylvania, based on the detection of antibodies to heartworms, and is claimed to be extremely accurate, and obviously helpful when no microfilariae are present. Radiography has also been recommended for diagnosis of occult cases by Dr Robert Lewis, of the University of Georgia, who commented that about 20 per cent of dogs are infected with adult worms, without having microfilariae.

TREATMENT AND CONTROL. Of five dogs dosed with ivermectin one day after artificial infection with 50 infective larvae of *Dirofilaria immitis*, none harboured any heartworms when killed 201 days later. The five control dogs had an average of 11 worms each at post mortem examination. The authors conclude that treatment with ivermectin at monthly intervals would prevent heartworm disease. (Blair, L. S. Williams, E. & Ewanciw, D. V., *Research in Veterinary Science* (1982) **33**, 386.)

In the UK ivermectin is not licensed for use in dogs, and thiacetarsamide (Caparsolate; Abbot) is used on a limited scale for imported dogs; also Nanocide (Cooper).

Another canine heartworm is *Angiostrongylus vasorum* which inhabits the pulmonary artery and the right ventricle of the heart. Symptoms include malaise and large subcutaneous swellings. Slugs and snails may act as intermediate hosts.

A 3-year-old dog, which died suddenly after an acute attack of dyspnoea, was found to have an *Angiostrongylus vasorum*. (Dr A. J. Trees, Liverpool School of Tropical Medicine. *Veterinary Record* (1987) April 25th).

'HEAT' (*see* OESTRUS. For the suppression of 'heat' in the bitch, *see* OESTRUS, SUPPRESSION OF.)

'HEAT' DETECTION IN COWS (*see under* OESTRUS, DETECTION OF).

HEAT EXHAUSTION. A syndrome in which there is an electrolyte and water depletion in the body. (*See* HEAT-STROKE.)

HEAT LOSS from the body occurs by radiation, by conduction and by convection from the skin, and by evaporation from the skin and lungs. The normal body temperature is controlled partly by alteration of the rate of metabolism, and partly by constriction of the surface blood vessels when the animal is exposed to cold, and also by shivering which generates heat. There comes a point, however, as body temperature falls still further, at which shivering ceases. Then the danger of hypothermia may not be recognised. (*See* BEDDING for pigs; HYPOTHERMIA.)

Sensible loss of heat. This is the heat which animals lose by convection, conduction, and radiation. It does not include heat lost by vaporising water from the skin and respiratory passages.

HEAT-STROKE is a condition associated with excessively hot weather, and, especially under conditions of stress. It occurs in domestic animals when taken to tropical countries from temperate countries, especially when recently unloaded from transport ships and subjected to great excitement in unfamiliar surroundings; it is seen in cattle, sheep, and swine travelling by road or rail, and it frequently occurs at agricultural shows; dogs may be affected when they have been left in a car parked in the sun, and with windows closed or almost closed. There is a failure to lower body temperature. (*See* CAR, PARKED; also HYPERTHERMIA, TROPICS.)

SIGNS. The animal is usually suddenly attacked with a great lethargy and inability for work or movement. The gait is staggering, and if the animal is made to move it falls to the ground. Convulsions may occur, and if the temperature is taken it is found to be very high, perhaps as much as 108°F in the horse. Death often takes place in a few hours, but some cases last as long as 3 days. If recovery occurs great dullness for a number of weeks is very liable to follow.

TREATMENT. Removal to a cool place, douching the head and neck with cold water from a hosepipe. Ice cubes may be used for the smaller animals. Internally, a dose of pholedrine sulphate.

An animal may die as a result of combined heat-stroke and heat-exhaustion, or either separately. (*See* HEAT-EXHAUSTION.)

HEBDOMADIS serogroup (*see* LEPTOSPIROSIS).

HEDGEHOGS are of veterinary interest in that they are susceptible to natural infection with foot-and-mouth disease, which they transmit to other animals.

Hedgehogs, like horses, are the natural hosts for *Leptospira bratislava*. A possible case of this infection in a dog, previously vaccinated against leptospirosis, but known to have access to hedgehogs, occurred.

SIGNS included thirst, variable appetite, weakness of the hindquarters, followed by vomiting, dysentery and jaundice. Complete recovery took six weeks. Leptospirosis was confirmed following blood tests, which also suggested *bratislava*, though this was not isolated; antibiotics have been used in the initial treatment. (Thomas, S., *Veterinary Record* (1980), **106**, 233.)

A UK survey of mortality in hedgehogs (*Erinaceus europaeus*) showed that 47 per cent were road casualties. Thirty-nine had salmonellosis. Other zoonoses were ringworm (*Trichophyton erinacei*) and *Yersinia pseudotuberculosis* in a very small proportion of the hedgehogs. Lungworms, flukes (*Brachylaemus erinacei*), tapeworms (*Rodentolepsis erinacei*), ticks, fleas, and mange mites (Caparinia tripilis) were other parasites found.

Three hedgehogs had died of metaldehyde poisoning. (Keymer, I. F. & others. *Veterinary Record* (1991) **128**, 245.)

A safe, simple method of dealing with 'rolled-up' hedgehogs, for the purpose of examination or treatment against external parasites, was described by Dr Nancy Kock, International Wildlife Veterinary Services, California. Her method is to place the animal in an aquarium tank (containing a parasiticide dip solution if needed), when it will immediately unroll and begin swimming. Using protective gloves, the hedgehog can then be grasped by the scruff of its neck like a kitten. Once held firmly like that, it was unable to roll up again, making examination easy. (Kock, N., *Veterinary Record* (1985), **117**, 136.)

ANAESTHESIA. Fenatyl citrate + fluanisone (Hypnorm; Crown) by subcutaneous injection is suitable for anaesthetising hedgehogs.

HEIFER. A year-old female up to her first calving.

HEINZ BODIES in red cells are seen in cases of haemolytic anaemia caused by, *e.g.* an excess of kale in dairy cattle. **Heinz-body anaemia** has also been seen in cats as a result of poisoning by methylene blue, formerly used in America as a urinary antiseptic. This form of anaemia has also been linked with onions, and a case was reported in a puppy which preferred raw onions and other vegetables to conventional dog foods. After a change of diet the puppy became well, and no longer tended to collapse after exercise. Heinz bodies are present in cats poisoned by paracetamol.

HELLEBORES. There are four hellebores of importance to the owners of animals, and the three are liable to some confusion. **Black hellebore** is the dried rhizome and rootlets of the Christmas rose, or bear's-foot, *Helleborus niger*. It may be eaten by live-stock when garden trimmings are thrown out on to fields to which livestock have access. It contains two very irritant glycosides – *helleborin* and *helleborein*. **Stinking hellebore** (*Helleborus fetidus*) and **Green hellebore** (*H. virids* or *Veratrum viride*), are sometimes the cause of live-stock poisoning. The latter, along with **White hellebore** (*Veratrum album*), plants of the United States of America, contain several alkaloids. They are depressants of the motor nervous centres.

Poisoning by hellebores. Symptoms are stupor, convulsions, and death when large amounts have been taken, and purgation, salivation, excessive urination, attempts to vomit, great straining and the evacuation of a frothy mucus, when smaller amounts have been eaten. Cows give milk which has a bitter taste and which is liable to induce diarrhoea or purgation in animals and man drinking it. Rumenotomy in cattle and sheep may be indicated, in order to remove parts of the swallowed plant. Affected cow's milk is likely to have a purgative effect in people drinking it.

In Idaho, USA, ewes eating *Veratrum californicum* give birth to lambs with harelip and hydrocephalus.

This 'Western false hellebore' is teratogenic, due to the presence of cyclopamine in its roots and leaves. It causes the deformity known to ranchers as 'monkey face lamb disease', which can be avoided by preventing pregnant ewes foraging on the plant a fortnight after conception. The fetus is also at risk on days 19 to 21 from early embryonic death, and between days 28 to 33 when stenosis of the trachea may result, together with shortening of metacarpal and metatarsal bones. So 'ranchers should prevent sheep feeding on the plant until 33 days after the rams have been removed from the flock.' (Keeler, R. F. & others, *Veterinary Medicine*, (1986), May 449.

HELMINTHS (*see* ROUNDWORMS, TAPEWORMS, FLUKES).

HEMERALOPIA (*see* EYE, DISEASES OF).

HEMIPLEGIA means paralysis limited to one side of the body only. (*See under* GUTTURAL POUCH DISEASE for facial and laryngeal hemiplegia in horses.)

In the cat (and dog) paralysis limited to one side of the body may be the result of cerebral thrombosis, haemorrhage, or embolism – plugging of an artery in the brain. The affected cat may fall over (always to the same side), or move in a circle. A tilting of the head and nystagmus (a jerky involuntary movement of the eyeball) have also been recorded. Fortunately, extremely few cat owners will ever encounter these conditions.

HEMIVERTEBRA ('wedge-shaped' vertebra) has been recorded in dogs. (*See* SPINE, DISEASES OF.)

HEMLOCK POISONING. As a rule animals will not eat Hemlock on account of the mousy odour and disagreeable taste, but in the spring, when green herbage is scarce and when the fresh shoots of the plant are plentiful, young cattle are sometimes affected.

The toxic principles of hemlock are a group of volatile alkaloids; the most important being *coniine*. Others include N-methyloconiine, coniceine, and conhydrine. They are present in the flowers, fruits, and leaves.

Hay containing hemlock is not likely to cause poisoning, owing to the volatility of the alkaloids.

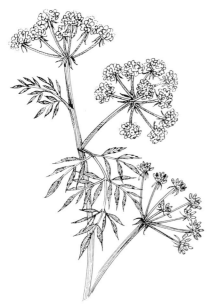

Hemlock (*Conium maculatum*). The flowers are creamy white, and the stem is distinguished by purplish spots. Height: 4 to 6 ft.

SIGNS. They cause initial stimulation and then depression of the central nervous system. Dilation of the pupils, weakness and a staggering gait are seen first; later breathing becomes slow and laboured. Before death the animal may be paralysed and unable to rise from the ground, though consciousness usually remains.

The mousy odour, detectable in the breath and urine of poisoned animals, assists diagnosis.

FIRST-AID. *See* ALKALOIDS.

Hemlock poisoning in the pregnant cow can result in deformity in the calf, and the same cause was suspected by MAFF in piglet deformities where the sow had access to rough grazing.

HEN YARDS (*see under* POULTRY).

HEPARIN. A naturally occurring anticoagulant.

HEPATISATION means the solidified state of the lung that is seen in pneumonia, which gives it the appearance and consistence of the liver.

HEPATITIS. Inflammation of the liver. (*See* LIVER.)

Hepatitis in the horse occurs after Infectious Equine Encephalomyelitis, especially where vaccines or sera have been used.

Hepatitis in dogs. (*See* CANINE VIRUS HEPATITIS.) (*See also under* DUCK HEPATITIS.)

HEPATOZOON. A single-celled parasite transmitted by the tick *Rhipicephalus sanguineus. H. canis* infects both dogs and cats, often causing anaemia, fever, and occasionally paraplegia. Other species infect rodents.

HEPTACHLOR. A constituent of chlordane, a chlorinated hydrocarbon, and used also as an insecticide on its own. It is stored in the body fat, and in the tissues is converted into heptachlorepoxide, 4 times as toxic to birds as Heptachlor itself.

HERBICIDES (*see* PARAQUAT, DIQUAT, MONO-CHLOROACETATE, WEEDKILLERS, POISONING).

HEREDITY (*see* GENETICS).

HERMAPHRODITE. An animal in which reproductive tissue of both sexes is present. A lateral hermaphrodite has an ovary on one side, and a testicle on the other; whereas a bilateral hermaphrodite has an ovary and testicle (or a combined ovary-testis) on each side. (*See also* INTER-SEX.)

A hermaphrodite rabbit served several females and sired more than 250 young of both sexes. In the next breeding season the rabbit (housed in isolation) became pregnant and produced seven healthy young of both sexes. (Frankenhuis, M. T. & others. *Veterinary Record* (1990) **126** 598.)

HERNIA. In a typical abdominal hernia there are always the following parts: a 'ring', or opening in the muscular wall of the abdomen, which may have been brought about as the result of an accident or may have been present at birth; and secondly, a swelling appearing below the skin, composed of the 'hernial sac' and its contents.

The contents vary according to the situation, size, and nature of the hernia, but the following organs or parts of them are most commonly herniated: a loop of bowel with its attached mesentery; omentum, either the whole or a part (very common in dogs); the stomach; the urinary bladder; the spleen or liver (through the diaphragm); the uterus, either when non-pregnant or with its contained fetus or fetuses; and sometimes a kidney in the cat.

(For strangulated hernia, see under the heading 'Signs' below.)

Umbilical hernia. The opening in the abdominal wall is a natural one which should, however, have closed at birth. If given time, it may still do so. In the puppy, for example, only a persistent or irreducible umbilical hernia will need surgical intervention – owing to the risk of a piece of omentum having its blood circulation interfered with, or bowel becoming obstructed or strangulated – both serious conditions requiring immediate surgery.

Inguinal hernia, which is practically the same as scrotal hernia, but at a less advanced stage, is almost wholly confined to the male sex in all animals, except the bitch, where a horn of the uterus may, upon occasion, come down through the inguinal canal. Inguinal and scrotal forms of hernia may be either congenital or acquired; congenital forms (most common in young animals) result through some failure of the inguinal canal, through which the testicle descends, to close properly; while acquired forms (commoner in adults) result from such accidents as slipping sideways with the hind-feet, injuries to the abdomen from falls, blows, and kicks.

Femoral hernia is very rare, but sometimes occurs in performing dogs which have been trained to walk upon their hind legs for considerable periods of time. The vertical position of the body imposes an unusual strain upon the muscles at the fold of the thigh, and they give way. It is always acquired.

Perineal hernia is almost exclusively confined to the dog. It may occur in either sex, usually as the result of much straining occasioned by constipation or diarrhoea, chronic coughing or asthma, bronchitis, etc., and in old male dogs suffering from enlarged prostate glands.

Ventral hernia is almost invariably the result of a serious injury to the muscular portion of the abdominal wall. It is commonest in mares, especially those used for breeding purposes. Very often there is little or nothing to be noticed if the mare is injured when non-pregnant, but when pregnancy follows and the tension upon the abdominal wall increases, the muscular part gives way and a large mass appears along the lower line of the abdomen. In cows it very often results from horngores from neighbours; in such, the skin remains intact but the muscle is torn and a swelling appears at the seat of the injury. Hernia due to a gore is probably commonest in the region of the flank, where the muscle is naturally thin.

Mesenteric hernia. This is rare in cattle ('probably because of the thickness of the mesentery') but not in horses. In a case involving a cow, intestine was herniated through a tear or defect in the mesentery; resulting in incarceration. A laparotomy was performed, and the defect enlarged to permit extrication of the intestine. The cow recovered. (van der Velden, M. A., *Veterinary Record*, (1984), **115**, 414.)

Diaphragmatic hernia may occur in any animal, but is commonest in the dog and the cat. It usually results from jumping downwards from a great height – an act which throws the full weight of the abdominal contents forward against the diaphragm when the animal lands on its feet; but it may also occur in road accidents.

The rent may be in the muscular or tendinous portion of the diaphragm, but it very frequently involves one or other of the natural openings (*hiati*), giving passage to the oesophagus, the vena cava, or the aorta, although a hernia through an enlarged aortic hiatus is very rare on account of the powerful nature of the diaphragm in its upper parts.

SIGNS. The symptoms vary much, depending upon the particular organ which is protruded, upon the size of the opening, which may or may not compress the hernia, and upon the condition of the latter. In very many cases among animals herniae contain either omentum or a loop of bowel, or both. The swelling may be present at birth, or it may appear suddenly or gradually at almost any time during life. To the touch it may present one of several sensations: (1) in the simple form it feels soft, fluctuating (as if it contained fluid), painless, neither hot nor cold, and causes no discomfort to the animal when being handled; if it be pressed upon it can usually be returned to the abdominal cavity, though it will reappear as soon as the pressure is released; in small animals it will disappear when they are laid upon their backs, and remain out of sight until they regain their feet; (2) when the structures are adherent to the skin which covers them, return to the abdomen is impossible, no diminution in size can be appreciated with manipulation, no definite ring can be determined as a rule, and there is no increase in size with exertion, but otherwise an *adherent hernia* presents the same appearances as a simple one; (3) in the strangulated form, which may supervene upon a hitherto simple hernia, there are very definite and serious symptoms of general disturbance: breathing fast and distressed, an anxious expression is visible on the face, and the swelling shows a marked tenseness and pain when being handled. It may be red and inflamed-looking at first, but later it very frequently becomes bluish. After about 12 to 24 hours gangrene sets in; the swelling becomes cold and painless to the touch; the temperature falls sub-normal, and the animal becomes alarmingly weak. Death usually follows shortly after, unless the strangulation is relieved by operation and perhaps amputation of the strangulated portion of bowel. An obstructed hernia is usually merely the preliminary of strangulation.

TREATMENT. Palliative treatment, such as is so very common in human beings consisting in the application of trusses, bandages, etc., is of no use whatever where animals are concerned. With young animals of any species it is usual to leave herniae alone provided they are not acute, for it very often happens that during the growth and development of the young creature the hernia disappears of its own accord, and the hole in the abdominal wall heals over. There is, however, always a danger that, as the result of some extra exertion, heavy feeding, boisterous playfulness, fighting, etc., strangulation may occur, and the condition may demand immediate attention.

The most rational method is one in which the animal is anaesthetised, skin incised, the contents returned to the abdomen, the peritoneal sac obliterated if it is present, the edges of the ring carefully sutured so that they will form a strong union, and finally the skin wound closed.

The operation for a strangulated hernia differs from that for a simple one in that it is necessary to enlarge the tight ring, to allow restoration of the circulation. If the bowel is obviously gangrenous the dead portions may be removed and the ends united to each other, but the chances of recovery are small, for peritonitis will most probably have started within the abdomen.

Some of the herpesviruses of man, domestic animals and poultry*

Recommended label	Traditional name	Associated disease
Human herpesvirus 1	Herpes simplex type 1	Herpetic sores etc.
Human herpesvirus 2	Herpes simplex type 2	Genital herpes and cervical cancer
Human herpesvirus 3	Varicella-zoster	Chicken pox and shingles
Human herpesvirus 4	Epstein-Barr virus	Burkitt's lymphoma and infectious mono-nucleosis (glandular fever)
Canine herpesvirus 1	Canine herpesvirus	Herpes of dogs (neo-natal deaths, respiratory infection, genital lesions)
Feline herpesvirus 1	Feline rhinotracheitis virus	Respiratory disease
Equid herpesvirus 1	Equine abortion virus	Abortion
Equid herpesvirus 2	Cytomegalovirus	Nothing or respiratory disease
Equid herpesvirus 3	Coital exanthema virus	Coital exanthema
Equid herpesvirus 4		Respiratory disease
Bovid herpesvirus 1	Infectious bovine rhino-tracheitis/infectious pustular vulvo-vaginitis	Upper respiratory tract infection; vaginitis, abortion etc.
Bovid herpesvirus 2	Bovine mammillitis virus	Mammillitis and pseudo-lumpy skin disease
Bovid herpesvirus 3	Malignant catarrhal fever virus (wildebeeste herpes virus)	Malignant catarrhal fever in cattle (Africa)
Bovid herpesvirus 4	Jaagsiekte virus pulmonary adenomatosis	Metritis, abortion, respiratory disease
Pig herpesvirus 1	Pseudorabies virus	Aujeszky's disease
Pig herpesvirus 2	Inclusion body rhinitis (cytomegalo) virus	Rhinitis
Phasianid herpesvirus 1	Infectious laryngo-tracheitis virus	Laryngotracheitis in poultry
Phasianid herpesvirus 2	Marek's disease virus	Marek's disease (fowl paralysis)

*Based on the recommendations of the Herpesvirus Study Group, International Committee for the Nomenclature of Viruses. (Dr W. B. Martin, *Vet Rec.* (1976) **99** 352.) and updated 1991 by G. P. W.

When a mare has developed a large ventral hernia during pregnancy nothing should be done until she has foaled, but after that, if the hernia is not too large, it should be operated upon before she is allowed to breed again.

HERPESVIRUSES cause, for example, Aujeszky's disease, jaagsiekte, feline rhino-tracheitis. (*See the table above and also under* MONKEYS *and* FADING.)

HERZTOD DISEASE. A heart condition in pigs, which has similarities to Mulberry Heart.

HETEROKARYON. A cell containing nuclei of two different species (an example of 'genetic engineering'). (*See* GENETICS.)

HETEROPLASTIC tissue is that which is abnormal, different in structure, or from another individual in the case of a graft (**heteroplastid**). Heteroplastic bones are those which are not parts of the skeleton, *e.g.* the *Os penis* in the dog, and the *Os cordis* (one of two small bones in the cow's heart). **Heteroplasm** is normal tissue found in an abnormal situation.

HETEROSIS. Hybrid vigour.

HETEROZYGOUS Relating to a heterozygote, which is produced from unlike GAMETES and has one gene (*see* ALLELES) dominant and the other recessive for a particular characteristic.

HETP. An organo-phosphorus insecticide used in agriculture and horticulture. Similar to TEPP (which see).

HEXACHLOROBENZENE. Used as a seed-dressing, it has given rise to a form of PORPHYRIA (which see) in children in Turkey, and might similarly affect livestock.

HEXACHLOROCYCLOHEXANE. The group name for several isomers each having the formula $C_6H_6Cl_6$. The most important of them is BENZENE HEXACHLORIDE. (*See* HCH, BHC.)

HEXACHLOROPHANE. An antiseptic used as an ingredient of medicated soap to kill bacteria on the skin.

HEXAMINE is a substance made by the action of ammonia upon formalin. It is excreted by the kidneys, and as it sets free formalin in an acid medium it has some antiseptic qualities when the urine is acid.

HEXAMITIASIS. An intestinal disease of turkeys occurring in the USA and in Britain.
CAUSE. *Hexamita meleagridis.*
SIGNS. Day-old poults may be affected, but more commonly the disease attacks turkeys a few weeks old. The feathers become ruffled, the birds listless with drooping wings. The droppings become liquid and frothy. Birds stand silent and motionless with eyes closed. Loss of condition is rapid, with marked dehydration. In young birds mortality may reach 100 per cent. Recovered birds may act as carriers.
TREATMENT. Tinostat has given some success. Antibiotics, furazolidone.

HEXOESTROL. The trade name for a synthetic oestrogen said to be more active than stilboestrol. (*See* STILBOESTROL, HORMONES IN MEAT PRODUCTION, STILBENES, CAPONISING, etc.)

HEXOSES are monosaccharide carbohydrates and include GLUCOSE, fructose, galactose, and mannose. Monosaccharides also include the pentoses, *e.g.* arabinose, ribose. (*See* SUGAR.)

HEXYLRESORCINOL. A urinary antiseptic, effective for alkaline as well as acid urine. It is not suitable for cats.

HIATUS HERNIA (*see under* HERNIA).

HIBITANE. Chlorhexidine, a valuable disinfectant effective against some bacteria which cause mastitis in cattle.

HIDROSIS. Sweat secretion, either normal or abnormally profuse.

HIGH-RISE SYNDROME (*see* CATS FALLING.)

HILUM, or (incorrectly) **HILUS,** is a term applied to the depression on organs such as the lung, kidney, and spleen, at which the vessels and nerves enter or leave, and round which the lymph nodes cluster.

HINNY. The offspring of a stallion and a female ass.

HIP-JOINT is the joint formed between the head of the femur, or thigh-bone, and the depression on the side of the pelvis called the acetabulum.

'HIP DYSPLASIA' IN DOGS. This term, current among dog breeders, covers a number of abnormal conditions of the acetabulum and head of the femur.
Some of these conditions are hereditary.
They include: (1) *Subluxation*, in which the head of the femur is no longer firmly seated within the acetabulum. Deformity of the head of the femur gradually develops. The symptoms include: a reluctance to rise from the sitting position, and a sawing gait, observed when the puppy (most often an Alsatian, sometimes a Golden Retriever or Boxer) is 4 or 5 months old.
(2) *Oestochondritis dissecans* is seen in terriers with short legs, poodles, and Pekingese. It is possibly identical with Perthe's Disease. Muscular wasting and lameness is observed, usually in one limb.
(3) *Slipped Epiphysis.* This also causes pain and lameness at 4 to 6 months, but is difficult to distinguish from (2).
(4) *Congenital dislocation*, in which the acetabula are too shallow to retain the heads of the femurs in position. Reported in the Black Labrador. A false joint forms in time. (*See also* PERTHE'S.)

HISTAMINASE. An enzyme obtained from extracts of kidney and intestinal mucosa, capable of inactivating histamine and other diamines. It has been used in treating anaphylactic shock and other allergic conditions due to, or accompanied by, the liberation of histamine in the body.

HISTAMINE. An amine occurring as a decomposition product of histidine (*see* AMINO-ACIDS) and prepared synthetically from it. Histamine is widely distributed in an inactive compound form in the body, particularly in the lungs, liver, and to a lesser extent in blood and muscle. As a result of trauma, burns, or infection, it may be liberated from the skin, lungs, and other tissues. Histamine dilates capillaries, reduces blood pressure, increases any tendency to oedema, stimulates visceral muscles and gastric and pancreatic secretions. Histamine toxicity is shown by engorgement of the liver, shock, and a tendency to urticaria-like skin lesions. (*See also* ANTIHISTAMINES, ALLERGY, MAST CELLS.)

HISTIDINE. An amino-acid from which histamine is derived by bacterial decomposition.

HISTIOCYTES. Another name for macrophages. (*See under* BLOOD, leukocytes.)

Histiocytosis. In New Zealand two types have been described: (I) an infectious one, diagnosed histologically; and (II) a skin disease characterised by many itchy plaques, affecting dogs.
Treatment with PREDNISOLONE was successful in most cases. (Thornton, R. N. & Tinsdale, C. J. *New Zealand Veterinary Journal* (1988) **36,** 192.)

HISTOCOMPATIBILITY (*see* MAJOR HISTOCOMPATIBILITY SYSTEM).

HISTOPLASMOSIS. A fungal disease, caused by *Histoplasma capsulata*, which gives rise to loss of appetite, diarrhoea, emaciation, and liver enlargement. It occurs in dogs and man chiefly. In man, often infected by venturing into bat-infested caves in Central and South America, and in Africa, lesions first occur in the lungs, but – in serious cases – other organs may be affected.

The mycelial phase, found in soil, produces two kinds of spores: *microconidia* and *macronidia*. The latter enter the body by inhalation.

HISTOSTAB. An antihistamine.

HOCK is the tarsus, a joint composed of 6 or 7 bones, between the tibia and the cannon bone of the hind-limb. (*See under* BONE.)

HODGKIN'S DISEASE is a form of cancer involving the lymph nodes, bone marrow and sometimes other tissues.

HOG. A male pig after being castrated.

HOG CHOLERA (*see* SWINE FEVER).

HOGWEED (*see under* GIANT).

HOGG. An uncastrated male pig. (*See also under* SHEEP.)

HOGGET (*see under* SHEEP).

HOLLY. The Veterinary Investigation Service, Truro, found that a holly leaf was causing an obstruction in both pharynx and larynx of a lamb. The farmer had lost five five good lambs in three weeks while they had been grazing under holly trees.

HOLOPROSENCEPHALY. A rare congenital brain malformation, accompanied by various facial deformities. The condition appears to be inherited in an autosomal recessive manner. (Roth, I. J. & others. *Australian Veterinary Journal* (1987) **64**, 271.)

HOLSTEIN-FRIESIAN. This breed of cattle in the USA and Canada has its origin in animals imported from the Netherlands most between 1857–87. They are also known as American or Canadian Holsteins or Holsteins.

HOMATROPINE is an artificial alkaloid prepared from atropine. Its sole use is to dilate the pupil of the eye for careful examination of the deeper parts of that structure. It is more suitable than atropine, as it does not interfere with vision for such a length of time as does atropine.

HOMEOSTASIS. Maintenance of the body fluids (as opposed to fluid *within* cells) at the correct pH and chemical composition.

HOMOGRAFT REACTION. The process by which an animal rejects grafts of another's tissue. (*See* IMMUNE RESPONSE *and* KIDNEYS, function.) The term Allograft is now regarded as preferable to Homograft.)

HOMOZYGOUS (*see* GENETICS).

HONEY. This appears to have an antibiotic effect and to be a successful dressing for bedsores in human patients.

Some honeys contain PYRROLIZIDINE ALKALOIDS (which see).

HOOF (*see* FOOT OF THE HORSE).

HOOF-PRINTS, and other places where the soil is exposed below the turf, are on wet pastures a common habitat of the snails which act as intermediate hosts of the liver-fluke. Dressing with 28 lb of finely-powdered bluestone, mixed with 1 cwt of dry sand, to the acre, will reduce the snail population if done each year in June and repeated in August.

HOOF REPAIR WITH PLASTICS. A technique used in the USA enables a plastic material to be bonded with the horn, so that this can be built up. Cracks, deformities, and cavities can be repaired, using an acrylic substance in the form of a white powder, together with one of two types of fluid.* With one, the acrylic assumes in about 5 minutes the hardness of wall horn; with the other, that of the frog tissue. The former can be rasped and nailed; the latter rasped or trimmed with a knife. Large defects should be repaired with a series of layers in order to avoid damage from heat generated by the process. The latter is described in the *Journal of the American Veterinary Medical Association*, **147**, 1, 340.

HOOKWORMS. These include *Uncinaria stenocephala*, present in temperate regions (including the UK), and the more pathogenic *Ancylostoma caninum* in warmer climates. Infestation occurs either through skin penetration or by ingestion of larvae in bitch's milk, etc. (Jacobs, D. E. & others *Veterinary Record* (1989) **124**, 347) (*See also* ROUNDWORMS.)

HOOSE (*see* PARASITIC BRONCHITIS).

HORDEOLUM. A stye. (*see* EYE, DISEASES OF).

HORMONES are substances which upon absorption into the blood-stream influence the action of tissues or organs other than those in which they were produced. The internal secretions of the ovary, testicles, thyroid, parathyroid, adrenal, pituitary body, and the pancreas are examples of hormones. (*See* ENDOCRINE GLANDS.) The placenta is also a source of one or more hormones.

Most animal hormones are either polypeptides (small proteins) or steroids, and the two groups have different modes of action.

The inter-action of the hormones is far-reaching and complex. In health, a delicate balance – the 'endocrine balance' – is maintained. In ill health this balance may be disturbed by an insufficiency of one particular hormone or by excess of another. Some hormones are antagonistic to each other, so that an excess of one amounts to much the same thing as too little of another. In some conditions, such as 'milk fever' in the cow, a number of endocrine glands are believed to be involved; the imbalance being far from a simple one. The thyroid might be regarded as the 'master gland'; its secretion profoundly

---

*Hoof Repairing Material: H. D. Justi Division, Williams Gold Refining Co., Inc., Philadelphia, USA.

influencing growth, sexual development, immunity, and the rate of metabolism. Yet the thyroid is itself stimulated by a hormone secreted by the anterior pituitary gland – an example which illustrates the interdependence of the whole endocrine system.

An animal's disposition and its hormone secretions are closely linked. Fear or anger, for example, will cause an outpouring of adrenaline – the 'fight or flee' hormone. And, probably, the animal's 'endocrine make-up' determines to some extent its capacity for, or tendency to, anger, fear, etc., as it does for sexual appetite.

Insulin (*see* PANCREAS, DIABETES, HORMONE THERAPY). *Glucagon* (*see* PANCREAS).

Thyroxine (*see under this heading and* THYROID GLAND).

Adrenalin (*see under this heading and* ADRENAL GLANDS). *Aldosterone* (*see* ditto). (*See also* GLUCO-CORTICOIDS.)

Hormones of the anterior pituitary lobe stimulate the gonads (gonadotrophin), thyroid, adrenals, the skeleton, and milk secretion, etc.

Pituitary Gonadotrophin influences both the ovary and testis. In the latter it stimulates development of the sperm-secreting tissue and of actual sperm production, and of the interstitial tissue and the secretion of male sex hormones. In the ovary it stimulates growth of the ovarian follicles and development of corpora lutea. Pituitary Gonadotrophin is thus considered as having two parts or principles: FSH (Follicle Stimulating Hormone) and LH (Luteinising Hormone).

Chorionic Gonadotrophin. This is a hormone resembling that of the anterior pituitary but formed in the placenta and excreted in the urine of pregnant women. The action of this hormone is predominantly luteinising.

Serum Gonadotrophin (PMS) is a hormone similar to the above but predominantly follicle-stimulating, obtained from the serum of pregnant mares.

Pituitrin is the hormone from the posterior lobe of the pituitary, and comprises a pressor principles (*vasopressin*), which acts upon the heart and circulation, causing a rise in blood-pressure, and an oxytocic principle (*oxytocin*) which stimulates involuntary muscles such as those of the intestines and of the uterus (when pregnant). (*See also under* ANTI-DIURETIC HORMONE.)

Natural oestrogens are hormones obtained from the follicles of the ovary and include *oestrin* and its chemical variants *oestrone, oestriol, oestradiol*, etc. At puberty oestrin brings about development of the teats, udder, vagina, etc. Oestrin is, to some extent, antagonistic to luteal hormone and the parathyroid secretion.

Synthetic oestrogens have a similar effect to the above. They include stilboestrol, hexoestrol, and dienoestrol.

Progestin, progesterone, or the *luteal hormone* is produced by the corpus luteum. This hormone stimulates preparation of the lining of the uterus for pregnancy, and by counteracting other hormones ensures the undisturbed maintenance of the gravid uterus; meanwhile suppressing oestrus, and – with the oestrogens – stimulates development of the udder and onset of lactation.

Androgens are sex hormones, *e.g. testosterone* secreted by the testes, and hormone(s) secreted by the adrenal supplementing, it seems, the action of testosterone. The latter is responsible for the development of secondary sexual characters, is capable of counteracting the female sex hormones, and apparently inhibits the deposition of fat.

HORMONE THERAPY is of value in cases where a true endocrine failure or imbalance is at fault, but it is obviously not a panacea. Moreover, the indiscriminate use of hormones is fraught with danger, and if persisted with may give rise to the production of ANTIHORMONES (which see). Therapy, as opposed to 'chemical caponisation', should be carried out by a veterinary surgeon only.

The uses of *insulin, thyroxine, adrenalin*, and *pituitrin* are described under these headings, and extracts of *thyroid* and *parathyroid* gland are similarly dealt with. Apart from these, considerable use is made in veterinary practice of the sex hormones. (*See* HORMONES *above.*)

Chorionic Gonadotrophin is used in the treatment of nymphomania due to cystic ovaries, of cryptorchidism, and also of pyometra and of some cases of infertility due to a deficiency of luteinising hormone. In the mare and cow a single dose given intra-muscularly will usually correct nymphomania.

Serum Gonadotrophin (PMS) is used in cases of anoestrus and infertility, and to obtain an extra crop of lambs. (PMS = pregnant mare's serum.)

Progesterone is used to prevent abortion or resorption of the fetus occurring as a result of luteal deficiency. It is also used to treat cases of cystic ovaries, and may be tried to relieve uterine haemorrhage. Luteal hormone preparations are given either intramuscularly (if in oil) or by implantation (if in tablet or pellet form).

Synthetic oestrogens were formerly used in cases of retention of the afterbirth, in some cases of pyometra, uterine inertia and dystokia, and in order to cut short lactation. Some synthetic oestrogens can be given by the mouth. In the dog stilboestrol was used in treating enlarged prostate; in the bitch stilboestrol diproprionate may be used by intra-muscular injection after mating to prevent conception.

Testosterone propionate is of use in sexually under-developed young males, and in adult males it may be given to improve fertility or to overcome impotence. In castrated or androgen-deficient males it may be of service in obesity, alopecia, and possibly eczema. In the female it may be used to cut short oestrus in racing bitches and mares, to suppress lactation, and in the treatment of pyometra. It has been used with success in the treatment of alopecia (baldness) in spayed cats and also in the bitch (non-spayed). (*See* CORTICOSTEROIDS, SYNCHRONISATION OF OESTRUS.)

HORMONES IN MEAT PRODUCTION. In America 2000 out of 9000 lambs died as a result of urethral obstruction after receiving 12 mg stilboestrol by injection.

In a Welsh experiment the implanted group was approximately 40 per cent heavier than that of the non-implanted control animals, and fetched an extra 45p per head at December prices. In other experiments fattening hoggs have shown an added increase of 33 per cent over 30 days on turnips, and of 42 per cent over 150 days on turnips and concentrates. Lamb carcases are generally leaner. (*See also* TWINNING.)

In 1973, under the name Finaplix, a formulation of trenbolone acetate was introduced on the UK market. This product is an anabolic and one of a number of natural and synthetic *male* hormones, claimed to give very slight side-effects as compared with female sex hormones, and to be safer from the point of view of the meat consumer. The implant is made into the loose skin at the base of the ear 60–70 days before slaughter.

The question is often asked: why castrate an animal and then implant a sex hormone? The manufacturers of Finaplix comment: 'Not everyone wishes to fatten bulls, with the attendant risks to life and limb; and the bull tends to have heavy front-end development. The implant results in a good back-end where the more expensive meat is.' (*See also* ANABOLIC STEROIDS, SOMATOSTATIN.)

In 1984 Syntex Pharmaceuticals introduced Synovex-S for use in steers. The implant contains progesterone and oestradiol benzoate.

Human health hazard. Following reports of cases in USA of adenocarcinoma of the vagina in adolescent girls whose mothers had been treated with stilboestrol during pregnancy, the Veterinary Products Committee in the UK began consideration of the risks to human health which might arise from residues of stilboestrol and other oestrogens in meat.

'A practice has arisen,' says the Committee in its report for 1971, 'of injecting 200–300 mg or more of stilboestrol into veal calves some 4 weeks before slaughter. This is a significant departure from previous practices, and we were advised by the Medical Research Council that it might well give rise to an appreciable hazard to the health of consumers, particularly women taking contraceptive pills.' A proposal was accordingly made to prohibit the sale, supply and import of oestrogens for injection into cattle under 6 months old; but this prohibition proved difficult to effect.

In the USA in 1972 a ban (already applied in 21 other countries) was imposed on the use of stilboestrol in animal feeds, owing to the dangers of carcinogenic residues in the livers of implanted animals.

HORN FLY. *Lyperosia irritans* is a parasite of cattle in America, Hawaii, and Europe. Heavy infestations of cattle have been reported in the UK. (*See* FLIES.)

HORNER'S SYNDROME (*see* EYE, DISEASES OF).

HORNS, INJURIES TO. In the horned breeds of cattle, sheep, and goats, injuries to the horns are not uncommon. In spite of the great strength of the horns of cattle, fracture of the horn cores, from fighting, collision, etc., may arise with comparative ease when the force has been applied in a lateral or transverse manner. Very frequently the horn itself remains apparently intact, but the bony core is fractured, and the injury is not suspected until the animal is noticed bleeding profusely from one nostril, *i.e.* that on the same side as the injured horn. Sometimes the tip of a horn may be broken clean off, and the external haemorrhage is liable to be alarming.

HORSE BOTS. A survey carried out in Ireland showed that during the months October–May (inclusive), 90 per cent of horses slaughtered at an abattoir near Dublin, and just under 67 per cent of those at an abattoir near Belfast, were infected with *Gastrophilus intestinalis*. Over 28 per cent of horses at the former abattoir harboured *G. nasalis*; but none of those in the Ulster abattoir. (C. Hatch *et al. Vet. Rec.* (1976) **98** 274.)

Horse bots have been known to infect the liver, causing hepatitis and jaundice.

As bot flies have only one generation per year, Dr Hatch and colleagues suggest that a single annual treatment of horses, preferably during early winter, would remove most if not all the bots. (*See under* FLIES.)

A paste preparation of IVERMECTIN (which see) was introduced in 1983 for the control of bots.

HORSE-MEAT. Uncooked liver, lungs, etc., may be a source of the hydatid cysts of the tapeworm *Echinococcus granulosus* of the dog. (*See also under* MEAT STAINED GREEN.)

Dogs and cats have occasionally been poisoned, some fatally, after being fed horse-meat containing barbiturates or chloral hydrate (administered to the horse for purposes of euthanasia). Signs include drowsiness and muscular incoordination.

Human cases of TRICHINOSIS (which see) have followed the eating of horse-meat served rare.

HORSE-POX (*see* POX).

HORSES, BACK TROUBLES IN. A deterioration in a horse's performance or ability to jump may be the result of chronic back pain or discomfort. This may alter the animal's behaviour or temperament. Some may become fractious when handled or worked. Some may resent any weight on their backs at all. (Dr Leo Jeffcott has stressed the need for a complete history of the animal, since problems in schooling and equitation may be the real trouble, and to rule these out details of management, tack, performance, and previous temperament need study).

Dr Jeffcott, of the Animal Health Trust's Equine Research Station, Newmarket, has stated (*In Practice* (1979) 1 5 4) that seven of the most common causes of equine back trouble involve the thoracic and lumbar regions of the spine. Lesions may be grouped as in the table overleaf.

Three types of ACUPUNCTURE (which see) were found to be equally useful in the treatment of horses with chronic back pain. Three groups of fifteen horses suffering from this condition for between two and 108 months were treated by (1) needle acupuncture (once a week for 8 weeks); or

DEFORMITY OF VERTEBRAL COLUMN	Scoliosis, lordosis, kyphosis, synostosis (congenital vertebral fusion).
SOFT TISSUE INJURIES	Strain/damage to supraspinous ligament of the back; myositis; or cramp; sacroiliac strain.
FRACTURES	Dorsal spinous processes – single or multiple; bodies of vertebrae and neural arch.
OTHER BONE DAMAGE	Ossifying spondylosis; crowding or overriding of the dorsal spinous processes; osteoarthritis and fusing of the dorsal spines, transverse and articular processes.
MISCELLANEOUS	Skin lesions – sitfasts; warbles beneath saddle area.

Major causes of back troubles in horses. (With acknowledgements to Dr L. Jeffcott.)

(2) laser acupuncture (once a week for eleven weeks); or (3) injection acupuncture (once per week for 9 weeks).

Pain was reduced in thirteen horses in group 1; in eleven in group 2; and in thirteen in group 3; and they were able to resume training and competition work (Klide, A. M. & Martin, B. B. *JAVMA* (1989) **195**, 1375.)

HORSES, COMMON CAUSES OF DEATH IN.
Records of consecutive post-mortem examinations, carried out at the University of Liverpool Veterinary Field Station between 1958 and 1980, showed that in 480 horses the following conditions accounted for 10 or more deaths:
Alimentary system. Perforations 21, specific and nonspecific enteritis 21, volvuli 18, strangulated hernias 15, malabsorption due to atrophic enteropathy 14, intestinal obstructions 13, parasitic enteritis 12.
Locomotor system. Fractures 25, septic arthritis 12.

Nervous system. Grass sickness 51.
Cardiovascular system. Verminous arteritis 14, haemorrhage 13.
Haemopoetic system. Lymphosarcoma 12.
Miscellaneous. Pyaemia or septicaemia 14.

The following conditions were *not* considered to have caused death in the 480 horses, but were found 30 times or more:
Alimentary system. Parasitic peritonitis 93, gastrophilus larval infestation 82, parasitic enteritis 54, hepatic hydatidosis 44, and gastric ulceration with no gastrophilus present 37.
Cardiovascular system. Verminous arteritis 146.
Respiratory system. Pneumonia 31. (Baker, J. R. and Ellis, C. E. (1981) *Equine Veterinary Journal*, **13**, 43 and 47.)

HORSES, DISEASES OF.
These include: Acne, contagious; aneurysm; anhidrosis; anthrax; asthma; azoturia; blouwildebeesoog; blue nose disease; borna disease; 'broken wind'; brucellosis; chronic catarrhal enteritis; colic; Comeny's

---

infectious paralysis; coronary thrombosis; dourine, entéqué seco; epizootic lymphangitis; equine biliary fever; equine contagious metritis; equine contagious pleuropneumonia; equine Ehrlichiosis; equine encephalomyelitis; equine filariasis; equine genital infections; equine infectious anaemia; equine piroplasmosis; equine rhinopneumonitis; equine verminous arteritis; equine viral arteritis; fistulous withers; foals, diseases of; glanders; grass sickness; grease; guttural pouch diphtheria; horses, back diseases in; horses, loss of condition in; horses, spinal cord disease in; horses, worms in; horse sickness, African; hyperlipaemia; Japanese B. encephalitis; Kimberley horse disease; laminitis; louping-ill; mal de caderas; mal du coit; periodic ophthalmia; 'poll evil'; potomac horse fever; pox; purpura; rabies; rhinosporidiosis; senkobo; strangles; stringhalt; summer sores; tetanus; tuberculosis; Tyzzer's disease; ulcerative lymphangitis; urticaria. (*See under these headings and also under* RACEHORSES. *See also* 'ROARING', *and under* EPIGLOTTIS; *and* TRANSIT TETANY.)

There have been cases of Q FEVER in Iran.

Diseases of the equine liver (*see* RAGWORT POISONING, LIVER-FLUKES, AFLATOXINS, HYDATID DISEASE).

HORSES, FEEDING OF. Horses at grass are likely to be contented horses, for they can feed at intervals during both day and night (as they do in the wild state), with exercise as an appetiser. A stabled horse is denied these opportunities. (However, horses do need shelter in winter; or at least to be rugged.)

'Horses are fussy feeders, and can be affected by the age, composition and type of pasture – all of which influence dry matter intake.' (*See* end of PASTURE MANAGEMENT for grasses most suitable for horses.)

With concentrate feed 'the aroma, freshness, and physical characteristics influence both initial acceptance and continued consumption.' (David Frape, *In Practice*, May 1980.)

(*See* DIET for preparation of feeds, palatability, and deterioration in storage, etc.; *also* LUCERNE, LINSEED, HAY, HYDROPONIC 'GRASS'.)

The horse can only eat relatively small quantities of feed at a time. The number of feeding times per day should therefore be increased with increasing work load because otherwise the horse cannot get enough feed to cover requirements. In addition, the horse chews its feed thoroughly and therefore requires relatively long feeding times (about 1 hour). A horse under an average work load requires per day about 2 kg feed (air-dry weight) per 100 kg body weight.

Horses in all phases of life can largely cover their nutrient requirements by sufficiently long daily *grazing* on a good pasture. If the pasture is of poor quality the nutrition of horses will be deficient unless supplemented.

Oats are the most widely used cereal for feeding horses, and do not need processing for adults, but should be crimped or rolled for foals. Barley, wheat and maize are used to a lesser extent. Barley should be crimped or rolled, wheat

should be rolled, and maize cracked. If included in horse feeds, beans should be split or kibbled.

Cereals are rich in starch, comparatively poor in protein, and mostly provide too little calcium but too much phosphorus. This mineral imbalance is also found in bran, which should not form a significant proportion of the ration.

Hay and oats feed rations are sufficient to cover the requirements of adult horses both for maintenance and for work, gestation and lactation, only if the feed rations are of good quality. If of poor quality, mares in the late phase of gestation may suffer from a deficiency in minerals, whereas lactating mares and young horses may suffer from a deficiency not only in minerals but also in energy and in high-grade digestible crude protein.

For safety reasons (as a safeguard against undetected poor quality of feed rations) it is therefore advisable to supplement both grazing and hay and oats feeding of horses in all phases of life with minerals and trace elements (mineral supplement feed).

Mares at the peak of lactation and young horses up to 6 months after weaning, if they are fed on hay and oats, require feed supplementation with high-energy low-fibre concentrate feed containing high-grade protein, *e.g.,* dried skimmed milk.

Regardless of the stage of life and of performance requirements, all horses should be given all necessary vitamins as a supplement to the feed. This is the only way to avoid uncertainties or actual deficiencies in vitamin supply which may arise owing to the variability of vitamin contents of feedstuffs. In addition, over and above a sufficient supply of minerals, all horses should have free access to common salt in the form of mineral licks.

A way 'to avoid deficiency situations when feeding horses on hay and oats rations is to replace the oats partly or entirely by a compound feed for horses. With such *hay/oats /compound feed* rations or *hay/compound feed* rations, no further supplementation is required provided the compound feed contains the necessary ingredients.' (Roche Information Service.)

David Frape has commented as follows:

Maintenance rations. *Crude protein* requirements are relatively low, and can be met by cereal grains. More than half the diet can be hay. (Horse hays in the UK average between 4 and 7 per cent crude protein.) When the latter is low, however, 'protein digestibility tends to be low, so that the minimum requirements may not be met even for maintenance'. *Energy* requirements can be met by good-quality hay.

'Growth, lactation and work each have different nutrient requirements.' For work, or lactation, gut capacity is insufficient for energy requirements to be met from bulky, but good-quality, hay.'

For growth. The *protein* requirements of a young, growing horse are much greater than those referred to under Maintenance above. Both digestibility and amino-acid content are important. 'Diets containing only poor-quality protein should be supplemented with LYSINE (which see), or some soya could be substituted for linseed.'

Pregnant/lactating mares. 'In America, under poor range conditions, where grazing provides inadequate protein, feed blocks supplying 50 g urea daily improve a pregnant mare's condition.'

'During the last third of pregnancy, *energy* requirements increase above those of maintenance. The mare should still be able to consume daily 1 kg of hay and ¼ to ½ kg cubes per 100 kg of body weight. (Levels of feed for thoroughbreds need to be 30 per cent higher than those for pleasure horses.)'

During peak lactation a 500-kg mare may produce over 3 gallons of milk daily and, if she is also undertaking some work, her *energy* demands are considerable. Requirements for concentrate cubes during the third month of lactation may reach 1½ to 1¾ kg per 100 kg body weight.'

In a BVA Congress paper J. H. Lees, of the University College of Wales, commented on the acceptance, even by traditional horse owners of proprietary concentrates for their horses. For novices these concentrates are a boon, since they are likely to be well balanced. Some concentrates contain soya-bean meal, which is a good source of lysine in which home-mixed rations are often deficient.

Horses do need some long hay in addition to concentrates to provide bulk, assist peristalsis, and mitigate the boredom which can lead to habits such as crib-biting.

In recent years silage has, to a very limited extent, become an item of horses' diet. Care must be taken to avoid any mouldy samples, and it may take a week for a horse to accept silage.

J. H. Lees also mentioned the use of hydroponics by a few horse-owners, who lay down eight trays to grow mats of barley seedlings. 'These are harvested at the eight-day stage, when the flag is 8 or 9 inches high, and growing from a 2-inch accumulation of roots and barley husks.' This food is relished, and parasite-free.

Food preferences of ponies. Studies of the feed preferences of ponies should help to predict the acceptability and intake of rations containing sucrose, grains or by-product feedstuffs. Given a choice between oats, maize, barley, rye and wheat six mature pony mares preferred oats, with maize ranking second and barley third. Wheat and barley were liked least but when the choice was restricted to these two grains the ponies feed intake was not greatly depressed. Given oats or oats plus 2 per cent or 10 per cent sucrose, four of six pony geldings selected the sweetened oats but one disliked sucrose and the other selected from one feed bucket regardless of its content. The six pony mares preferred a basal diet containing 54 per cent maize, 20 per cent whole oats, 10 per cent wheat bran, 8 per cent soyabean meal, 7 per cent molasses and 1 per cent limestone when it was supplemented with 20 per cent of distillers' grain, but not when it was supplemented with 20 per cent beetpulp, 20 per cent blood meal or 20 per cent meat and bone meal. They did not prefer the same basal diet containing 20 per cent alfalfa meal, although horses are reported to prefer alfalfa pasture to other legumes. (Hawkes, J. & others, *Equine Veterinary Journal*, (1985), **17**, 20.)

The following rules should be adhered to as far as the feeding of horses in Great Britain is concerned:

(1) Water before feeding (*see* WATERING).

(2) Feed in small amounts and as often as the nature of the work or other circumstances will allow.

(3) Do not work immediately after the horse finishes feeding. An hour should be given for a full feed.

(4) Give the first feed of the day early, and give the majority of the bulky food at the last feed of the day, so that the horse can eat it at its leisure.

(5) Always buy the best quality of food obtainable; it is false economy to use inferior foodstuffs.

(6) Inspect the teeth periodically, and have any errors corrected at once.

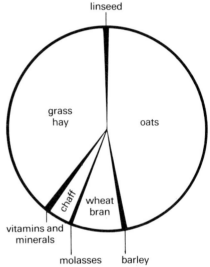

Average weekly composition of traditional feed given to thoroughbreds in training – percentage by weight. (With acknowledgements to David Frape and *In Practice*.)

HORSES, IDENTIFICATION OF. In the USA thoroughbreds are identified by blood typing, coat colour markings, and chestnuts (not fraud-proof). Whorls (trichoglyphs) are also a valuable means of identification. (*See* WHORLS.)

HORSES, IMPORT CONTROLS. In 1975 the UK introduced import controls designed to prevent the introduction of four diseases which were, at the same time, made notifiable: namely, equine infectious anaemia, equine encephalomyelitis, African horse sickness, and dourine.

The Equine Animals (Importation) Order was amended in 1974 to prohibit import from the USA of horses unless negative to blood tests (before leaving the USA) for *Babesia caballi* and *B. equi*.

In 1974 general licences were issued for any horses imported into Great Britain from France, Northern Ireland and the Republic of Ireland. In 1983 the general licensing system was extended to the following countries: Austria, Belgium, Denmark, Federal Republic of Germany, Finland,

Italy, Luxembourg, Netherlands, Norway, Portugal, Spain, Sweden and Switzerland. (Each horse must be accompanied by the correct Health Certificate stipulated in the general licence.)

The Importation of Equine Animals Order 1979 defines equine animal as horse, ass, zebra or any cross-breed thereof, and prohibits imports except under licence.

New regulations made in March 1985 require that horses imported from the USA must be isolated before export for at least 30 days on premises situated outside Kentucky which satisfy prescribed criteria. Blood samples for testing for equine infectious anaemia, vesicular stomatitis, and equine viral arteritis must be taken not less than 21 days after the beginning of isolation but within 15 days of export.

New health regulations which must be satisfied when horses are permanently imported into Great Britain from 13 European countries came into force in 1985.

Under the terms of a new general licence controlling imports from all 13 countries, *i.e.*, Austria, Belgium, Denmark, Federal Republic of Germany, Finland, Italy, Luxembourg, Netherlands, Norway, Portugal, Spain, Sweden and Switzerland, an importer will be required to ensure that the horse is kept on the same premises during the 30 days preceding import. This will help to reinforce existing safeguards against the introduction of equine viral arteritis and will bring the regulations for horse imports from these countries into line with those applying to imports from the USA and Canada. To assist importers a model health certificate will be included as part of the licence.

The new licence will not cover species other than horses. Other equine animals such as asses, mules, donkeys and zebras may only be imported under specific licence from the appropriate agriculture department.

The illegal importation of zebras from Africa into Spain in 1987 has resulted in HORSE-SICKNESS, AFRICAN occurring there every autumn.

HORSES, INFECTIOUS DISEASES OF, ORDER 1975 (*see* HORSES, IMPORT CONTROLS).

HORSES, INFERTILITY IN (*see* EQUINE CONTAGIOUS METRITIS, UTERINE INFECTIONS).

HORSES, LOSS OF CONDITION IN. When ponies and other riding horses lose condition, a veterinary surgeon should be consulted, for the possible causes are many and a professional diagnosis is important. Some pony owners, inexperienced or otherwise, may be underfeeding their animals, not supplying enough drinking water, or overworking them. Appetite may be depressed because of pain – perhaps in the joints or feet, perhaps associated with brucellosis. The teeth may need attention. Chronic grass disease will result in loss of condition. Migrating red worm larvae may be causing circulatory disturbance, or the animal may have a severe infestation of worms in the intestine. Bots may be present in the stomach. Chronic disease of liver or kidneys may be present; or cancer or tuberculosis. These and many other conditions may be causing the pony to be unthrifty.

A scheme of *regular* visits by a veterinary surgeon (often on a contract basis) can help to keep horses and ponies in good condition. (*See* HORSES, DISEASES OF.)

HORSES, LUNG HAEMORRHAGE. A study carried out at the Animal Health Trust's equine research station confirmed the high incidence of blood pigment present in tracheal washes from 'normal' racehorses, and indicated that exercise-induced subclinical bleeding from the lungs occurs in British as in other racehorses. (*See* RACEHORSES, EXERCISE.)

HORSES, MEASUREMENT OF. (*See* HAND). As Mr D. F. Oliver pointed out at the 1980 BVA Congress, the precise height of a horse may determine whether it is worth thousands of pounds or only hundreds. 'The value of a horse which "measures in" may well be in the order of £35,000; if "measured out" only £500,' he said. The use of a spirit level, to check the level of the ground, is now required in the UK. The horse must be measured from both sides, and the mean taken. Some horses resent the slightest pressure on their withers; others are taught to crouch at such pressure – both making accurate measurement extremely difficult. Horses should be familiarised with the measuring standard. (*See* HANDS.)

Horses should be examined for 'over-preparation of the foot' and measuring postponed if they are found in this condition.

The heights of 89 horses were measured at the withers before and after half a furlong of trotting exercise. The average height increase after the exercise was 1·75 cm; the horses returning to their 'resting height' within seven minutes. (Hodges, A. A. & others, *Veterinary Record*, (1986), **118**, 121.)

The British Veterinary Association withdrew its support for the scheme in November 1988.

HORSES, SPINAL CORD DISEASES IN. A survey based on 81 horses examined at the New York State College of Veterinary Medicine, Cornell University between January 1974 and July 1976 revealed 20 (25 per cent) cases of injury including cervical vertebral stenotic myelopathy (CSM) (11 cases), compressive myelopathy (four), occipitoatlantoaxial malformation (two), cervical vertebral osteomyelitis (two) and cervical injury (one). Of the 37 (45 per cent) inflammatory lesions equine protozoal myeloencephalitis (EPM) was the most common. Organisms were seen in 16 of the 32 cases. There were also 23 (28 per cent) cases of equine degenerative myeloencephalopathy (EDM).

CSM occurred particulary in young male thoroughbreds and horses that were large for their age and breed. They were identified accurately by measuring (on radiographs) the minimum saggittal diameter at the level of each vertebra (it should exceed 16 mm) and also between adjacent vertebra in the flexed position (it should exceed 13 mm).

EDM was characterised by the onset of progressive symmetric ataxia, spasticity and paresis in animals, particularly Arabs, under two years of age. EDM was distinguished from CSM and other conditions with focal lesions because of differences in the patterns of pelvic and thoracic limb gait deficits.

EPM was most frequent in young mature standard-bred and thoroughbred horses in the spring and summer. In addition to ataxia and paresis there is frequently acute to chronic progressive asymmetrical defects in the gait and evidence of sensory deficits, loss of reflexes and muscle atrophy. Tetraplegia was associated with severe lesions in the spinal cord or brain stem. The protozoon parasite involved is probably a coccidian; morphological and serological evidence mitigates against the suggestion that EPM is a form of toxoplasmosis. (Mayhew, I. G., Delahunta, A., Whitlock, R. H., Krook, L. & Tasker, J. B. (1978). *Cornell Veterinarian.* **68.** Supplement 6.)

HORSES, WORMS IN. The following list shows those adult worms regarded as of most importance. (The list of small strongyles totals 11 and their names are omitted here.)

Adult Worms in the Intestines
Of considerable importance.
1. Large strongyles
    Strongylus edentatus
    Strongylus equinus
    Strongylus vulgaris
2. Small strongyles
    Adults mainly in Other Tissues
Echinococcus granulosus (larval stage)
Dracunculus medinensis
*Draschia megastoma** (larval stages in the skin)
Dictyocaulus arnfieldi
Fasciola spp.
Habronema spp. (larval stages in the skin)
    (With acknowledgements to M. C. Round, and the Animal Health Trust.) (*See* ROUNDWORMS, IVERMECTIN, FLUKES, TAPEWORMS.)

HORSE-SICKNESS, AFRICAN. This disease was first recorded in Europe in 1982. (AFRC).
CAUSE. A virus, transmitted by the biting midge *Culicoides imicola*, which is common in Africa, Asia, and the Middle East.
SIGNS. There are four types of the disease that can be recognised clinically: (1) Horse-sickness fever. With this the temperature rises about one degree per day, until it reaches its maximum – up to 106°F – over a period of 12 to 14 days; (2) The pulmonary form ('dunkop') in which the breathing becomes laboured, with nostrils fully distended, and death occurring in three days or so; (4) The oedematous or cardiac form, locally known as 'dikkop' or thickhead; and (5) the mixed form which is comparatively rare.

Complications include blindness and/or paralysis of the oesophagus.
PREVENTION. A vaccine is available.

*Frequently, but incorrectly, called *Habronema megastoma.*

Certain complications are comparatively common in cases of horse-sickness, and of these paralysis of the oesophagus, which leads to an inability to feed and swallow properly, and blindness are common.
TREATMENT. All that can be done is to treat the symptoms.
PREVENTION. *Protection against night-flying insects* is of the greatest importance. A vaccine is used.

HORSE-TAILS, POISONING BY. In different localities and under different conditions there may be considerable variation in the chemical composition of species of *Equisetum*, with results accordingly. It would appear that on the continent of Europe and in Great Britain *Equisetum palustre* and *E. sylvaticum* are the most dangerous, and that in America *E. arvense* is most to be feared, particularly when they are fed among hay.
(For pathology, symptoms, and treatment, *see* BRACKEN POISONING, THIAMINASE.)

HOSPITAL-ACQUIRED DISEASE (*see* NOSOCOMIAL, IATROGENIC, ANTS (Pharoah's), SALMONELLOSIS).

HOUND ATAXIA. In 1981 this condition was reported in England, and affected hounds kept in hunt kennels, where their diet was mainly paunch. When this became difficult to obtain, and ceased to be the main item of diet, the ataxia ceased also. (Drs Palmer, A. C. & Medd, R. K. *Veterinary Record* (1981) **109** 43.)

HOUNDS (*see* MEAT, KNACKER'S; HOOKWORMS, ORF, BOTULISM; HORSE-MEAT; SALMONELLOSIS, AUJESZKY'S DISEASE).

HOUSE DECORATING, POISONING. In one case, old lead primer was stripped by means of an electric sander, which dispersed particles of the primer so that the air soon contained a toxic amount of lead. One infant and one cat suffered lead poisoning as a result.

In another case, the purchaser of a house had the downstairs floors professionally treated against woodworm. Six pedigree cats were accordingly kept upstairs for six weeks. Even so, four weeks after being admitted to the downstairs rooms, five of the cats died from dieldrin poisoning.

HOUSE PLANTS, poisoning in cats and dogs may be caused by the needles from Christmas trees, holly, mistletoe, laurel, oleander, azalea, lily-of-the-valley, rhododendron, honeysuckle and hydrangea.

HOUSING OF ANIMALS. This is, obviously, a vast subject, and for detailed information reference should be made to the bibliographies given in the special feature 'Farm Animal Housing' in the *Veterinary Record* (1983) **113**, 554–596. (*See also* TROPICS.)

Two things must be said at the outset. The first is that, generally speaking – given windbreaks, the possibility of shelter in inclement weather

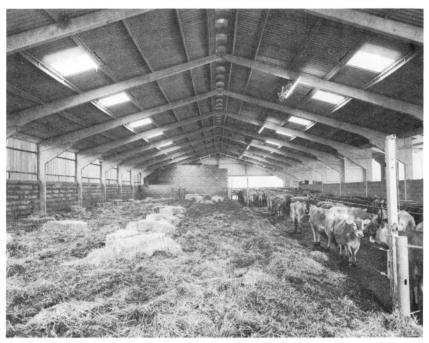

A modern dairy unit, with lying area, parlour and dairy under one roof. Note the Yorkshire boarding to the left of the picture – a means of ensuring good ventilation and an absence of condensation.

and of shade in summer, the avoidance of muddy conditions and of overstocking – animals kept out-of-doors are likely to be healthier than those which are housed for long periods. In the past, housing of animals so often meant overcrowding in dark, damp, draughty or ill-ventilated buildings. Under such conditions disease is almost inevitable – rickets, pneumonia or scours in calves; infertility in the bull; agalactia in the sow; tuberculosis in the dairy cow. Some modern and costly buildings still have ventilation defects, leading to condensation inside and resulting in ill-health of the housed stock. The use of Yorkshire boarding can obviate both the condensation problem and much of the pneumonia.

The second thing is that, from a health point of view, not every 'development' is an advance. Commercial competition may dictate the overcrowding of chickens to the point where feather-picking has to be counteracted by red lighting or debeaking; this may lead to short-term economic gains, but it is the antithesis of good animal husbandry, and the solving of the veterinary problems raised must be viewed accordingly. Intensivism can surely be pushed to a stage where not research, but only a return to good husbandry, will succeed in reducing the incidence of disease – and also, incidentally, the size of the drug bill.

On the other hand, the dairy cow has undoubtedly benefited from another dictate of economy – the change from cowshed to the yard-and-parlour system – for instead of being yoked or closely chained for long periods, she is free to move around; and such exercise is in itself important. (*See* CUBICLES FOR COWS.)

Cattle were housed on slatted floors in

England in 1860 – with straw; the current revival of the practice, without straw, may lead to hygromata, damaged teats or injured legs to an extent not readily admitted in the first flush of enthusiasm; and it is, of course, important that there should not be a draught blowing through the slats, or the money saved on straw will be lost in other ways.

Intensivism has led to development in forced-draught ventilation, and to the efficient insulation of walls and roof of animal houses by means of Polystyrene, Fibreglass, and other substances. (*See under* CONTROLLED ENVIRONMENT.)

It costs over four times as much to keep an animal warm by feeding concentrates – 'an internal fuel' – as by warming the live-stock house. Minimum economic temperatures are given below.

Housing has an important bearing upon the feeding of animals. Pigs, for instance, confined on concrete have no opportunity for the normal scavenging which can obviate mineral or vitamin deficiencies, and special rations accordingly become necessary for such housed animals. Vitamin A and B deficiencies are particularly likely to occur. In store cattle, lack of a vitamin A supplement causes blindness on many farms.

Residual infection is obviously important, and advice is given on this under SALMONELLOSIS and DISINFECTION. In a building used for calves and pigs, or pigs and turkeys, for example, a cross-infection between the species may arise with a particular strain of *E. coli*. On land surrounding buildings it is worth remembering that the worm *Trichostrongylus axei* is common to cattle, sheep, horses, and goats.

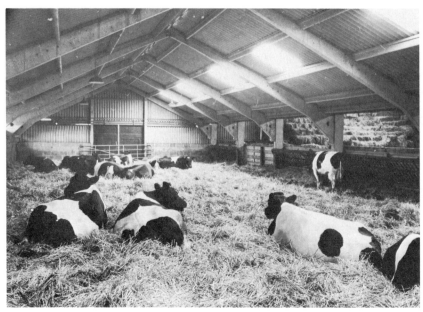

Cattle on deep litter in a covered yard.

Cattle. An adjustable open-ridge method of ventilation is still recommended as the best for cowsheds. In winter, the optimum temperature inside appears to be within 44–55°F. Milk yields are said to be depressed when the temperature falls below freezing point. In summer, there is an upper limit of about 77°, at which point cattle begin showing distress. High humidity, at a temperature above 60°, appears to diminish milk yield.

For young calves, the temperature should not be allowed to fall below 60°F. (*See* CALF HOUSING.)

For covered yards, ventilators should be provided at the highest point, with a gap of 2 feet between the top of the walls and the eaves. Open-fronted covered yards should not have a gap.

Pigs. Given adequate straw, the most primitive arks on range will yield better results than a cold, damp house. A warm environment will reduce the risk of overlying by the sow. While different optimum temperatures have been given by different research workers, it seems that 70° is about the figure to aim at in the farrowing house. For artificial rearing, a temperature of 86° has been recommended for the first 4 days. Cold, damp floors result in liver disorders which do not appear in buildings where the pigs have a warm, dry bed. Pregnant sows are better not housed. (*See* CONCRETE, HYPOTHERMIA.)

For fattening pigs, an optimum temperature would appear to be about 65°; and 60° should be the minimum. Humidity does not appear to have an adverse effect, though few authorities recommend it. Good ventilation is advocated.

Sheep. In general, the disease problems associated with the housing of sheep have been less serious than might have been expected, and there is a credit side as well as a debit side. For example, if lambs are born and reared to market weight indoors, there is far less risk of worm infestation causing trouble. It is recommended that pens should not contain more than 15–25 ewes, grouped according to lambing dates.

Ewes and hoggs housed for the winter after grazing should be wormed during the first week. If it is a liver-fluke area, dosing against flukes is advisable 6 weeks after housing.

Lambs *must* be protected against lamb dysentery, and any from unvaccinated ewes should be given antiserum.

Infestation with lice may be aggravated by housing and spread more rapidly. Since it can cause serious loss of condition, dipping or spraying before housing is recommended.

E. coli infections are as much a threat to the housed lamb as to the housed calf. Overcrowding and dirty conditions at lambing predispose to coli septicaemia, which is usually a sequel to navel infection. In early weaned lambs, the quality of the milk substitute is important if scouring is to be avoided; and measures should be taken to minimise contact between housed sheep and their dung. Slatted floors, regular cleaning, copious use of bedding material, periodical disinfection – all help in this direction.

Good ventilation can go a long way towards reducing the risk of acute pneumonia. In lambs and older sheep this is often associated with Pasteurella infection, sometimes aggravated by lungworm infestation. Pasteurella pneumonia vaccine *may* be effective in prevention, but is useless against other forms of pneumonia – which can be caused by other bacteria, moulds, and viruses. With reference to the latter, para-influenza 3 vaccine may well have a place.

Infections which give rise to abortion may prove more troublesome indoors than out, and vaccination against enzootic (*Chlamydial*) abortion seems worthwhile. (*See also* COPPER

POISONING *and under* SHEEP BREEDING *and* INTENSIVE.)

Poultry. Chickens probably do best at temperatures between 55° and 65°F. Egg-production declines at temperatures below 40° or above 75°F. A relative humidity of 50 per cent is considered the optimum for grown birds. A cold, dry house is better than a warm, wet one. Ventilation requirements vary; for example, a bird may need as much as 1 cubic foot per minute per lb bodyweight in the hottest weather, but only one-sixth of this in the coldest weather. (*See also under* CHICKS, NIGHT LIGHTING.)

For other aspects of housing, *see under* CONCRETE, LEAD POISONING, WOOD PRESERVATIVES, CUBICLES, BULL HOUSING, LOOSE BOXES, DEEP LITTER, INTENSIVE LIVE-STOCK PRODUCTION, YORKSHIRE BOARDING, WATER.

HUCKLEBERRY POISONING (*see* GARDEN NIGHTSHADE POISONING).

HUMANE DESTRUCTION OF ANIMALS (*see* EUTHANASIA).

HUMERUS is the bone of the foreleg between the shoulder-joint and the elbow-joint. It has a rounded head which, with the corresponding depression of the scapula, forms the 'ball-and-socket' shoulder-joint. At the opposite extremity it forms with the radius and ulna the hinged elbow-joint.

HUMORAL IMMUNITY is that conferred by the immunoglobulins derived from the B cells of the reticulo-endothelial system, and is differentiated from Cell-mediated Immunity associated with T-CELLS. (*See also* IMMUNE RESPONSE, COLOSTRUM, IMMUNOGLOBULINS.)

HUMOUR is a term applied to any fluid or semi-fluid tissue of the body, *e.g.* the aqueous and vitreous humours in the eye.

HUSK is a disease of cattle, sheep, and goats characterised by bronchitis, which is caused by lungworms. (*See* PARASITIC BRONCHITIS.)

H-Y ANTIGEN. This is present in the gonads of the bovine freemartin – a discovery made at the Sloan Kettering Institute for Cancer Research – and possibly, acting as a hormone, 'induces XX cells in the female gonad to assume testicular organisation'. (*Lancet* Nov. 6, 1976). The antigen was discovered on the acrosome of mouse sperm. It apparently accounts for the rejection of male grafts by females of the same species.

HYALINE MEMBRANES. A fibrinous exudate from the epithelium of the bronchioles, found in stillborn animals and those dying soon after birth.

HYALURONIDASE. An enzyme which breaks down the hyaluronic acid forming part of the material in the interstices of tissue, and so facilitates the absorption of injected fluids. It assists the

rapid distribution of drugs injected either subcutaneously or intramuscularly. It has been used in the treatment of urinary calculi.

HYBRID. At one time this word meant a cross between two inbred lines; recently it has been used to describe a simple cross between two different breeds.

For a comparison between a hybrid and a chimera (with reference to fertile mules) *see* CHIMERA.

HYBRIDOMA (*see* GENETICS – 'Genetic Engineering'; *also under* RABIES, diagnosis).

HYBRID VIGOUR (*see* GENETICS; BLOOD-TYPING and T-CELLS.)

HYDATID DISEASE is caused by the cystic larval stage of the tapeworm *Echinococcus granulosus*, of which the dog and fox are the usual hosts. Eggs released from tapeworm segments passed in the faeces by these animals are later swallowed by grazing cattle, sheep and horses, which may become infested also through drinking water contaminated by wind-blown eggs.

In Australia an anti-hydatid disease campaign has proved successful; though in New South Wales there is a sylvatic strain which circulates predominantly between wild dogs and wallabies. Eighteen wild dogs were trapped, of which eleven were found to be infected. By contrast, only one of 76 domestic dogs examined during the same period was found to be infected. (Morrison, P. & others. *Australian Veterinary Journal* (1988) **65**, 97.)

People become infested through swallowing eggs attached to inadequately washed vegetables, and possibly eggs may be inhaled in dust or carried by flies to uncovered food. The handling of infested dogs is an important source. In Beirut the risk is put at 21 times greater for dog-owners than others, by the World Health Organisation, who state also that in California nomadic sheep rearers are 1000 times more likely to have hydatid disease than other inhabitants of the state. (WHO Technical Report 637, 1970).

There have been successful campaigns to control human hydatid disease in both Cyprus and Iceland; by compulsory treatment and/or banning of dogs.

Swallowed eggs hatch in the intestines and are carried via the portal vein to the liver. Some remain there, developing into hydatid cysts; others may form cysts in the lungs or occasionally elsewhere, *e.g.* spleen, kidney, bone marrow cavity, or brain. Inside the cysts brood capsules, containing the infective stage of the tapeworm develop, and after 5 or 6 months can infest dog or fox.

In Wales, where the incidence of hydatid disease is relatively high, farm dogs and foxhounds are important in its spread.

Only some seven people are known to die from this disease in England and Wales each year – a figure which would probably be higher were diagnosis less difficult. Condemnation of sheep and cattle offal from this cause runs into hundreds of thousands of pounds annually. Routine worming of dogs is essential for control. *E. granulosus* is far from being a typical tapeworm, as it has only three or four segments and a total length of a mere 3–9 mm, so that the dog-owner will not notice the voided segments.

(*See* WALLABIES.)

A problem of diagnosis also arises, in that this worm's eggs are indistinguishable from those of *Taenia* tapeworms. Previously, Professor M. J. Clarkson has pointed out, one could dose dogs with arecoline hydrochloride and examine the faeces for the presence of the intact tapeworm, but in Britain this anthelmintic is no longer obtainable, having been replaced by more modern drugs which destroy the tapeworm but leave it unrecognisable. (M. J. Clarkson. *In Practice*.) (For effective anthelmintic treatment of dogs, *see* DRONCIT.)

Equine hydatidosis in Britain is caused by a strain of *E. granulosus* which has become specifically adapted to the horse as its intermediate host, and is often referred to now as *E. granulosus equinus*. This apparently is of low pathenogenicity for man.

In a survey covering 1388 horses and ponies examined at two abattoirs in the north of England, 8·7 per cent were infected. Prevalence of infection was closely related to age; rising from zero in animals up to two years old to over 20 per cent of those over eight years old.

Sixty-six per cent of the infected animals had viable cysts. Prevalence appears to be greatest in central and north-west England. (G. T. Edwards, *Vet. Record* (1982), **110**, 511.)

Treatment of human patients. 'Hydatid disease is one of the rare parasitic conditions that can be treated only by surgery . . . However, the result is often incomplete, with frequent local recurrences or accidents of secondary dissemination. Repeated interventions are often mutilating and do not guarantee a definite cure.' (A. Bekhti and others. *British Medical Journal* (1977) **2**, 1047). They used mebendazole successfully in four patients, but WHO points out that while success has been obtained in some, others have died despite it.

HYDRALAZINE. An arterial dilator, useful in treating dogs with failing heart due to mitral regurgitation (usually caused by fibrosis of the valve). (Kittleson, M. D., *JAVMA*, (1985), **187**, 258.)

HYDRARGYRUM (*see* MERCURY).

HYDROCELE means a collection of fluid present within the outer proper coat of the testicle (tunica vaginalis) or within the spermatic cord.

HYDROCEPHALUS is a condition in which a large amount of fluid collects within the brain cavity of the skull. It may be present before birth (*congenital hydrocephalus*), in which case the large size of the head may present an obstruction to parturition. In the congenital form which is met with in foals, calves, and puppies, there is a large prominent swelling over the forehead, and a rounded dome-like cranium. Animals born in this condition are usually dead, or if they are living they die soon after birth. It may become necessary to puncture the swollen skull and evacuate the fluid before delivery can be effected.

In the *acquired form*, which is chiefly met within the horse and dog, the fluid collects in the ventricles of the brain, or under the meninges, as the result of meningitis, or the presence of a tumour, which has interfered with the free circulation of the cerebro-spinal fluid, or has produced an exudate from the engorged blood-vessels.

When due to meningitis it is usually an acute condition, and its symptoms are masked by those of the meningitis; when due to other causes in which there is obstruction to the flow of cerebro-spinal fluid it is usually chronic, and the symptoms are those of pressure on the brain. The animal becomes gradually dull, sleepy, insensitive to its surroundings. Convulsions may occur, and during one of these death is liable to take place. (*See under* HELLEBORES.)

HYDROCHLORIC ACID is normally present in the gastric juice, to the extent of about 2 parts per 1000 (*see* DIGESTION). In the concentrated form it is like all other mineral acids, a corrosive and irritant poison.

HYDROCYANIC ACID (HCN), and its salts – sodium and potassium cyanide – are among the most deadly poisons, and very rapid in their effects.

SIGNS. If taken by mouth, or given by injection, there is a rapid acceleration of the breathing (and occasionally coughing). A poisoned dog or cat will utter a cry and collapse, the limbs extended fully. There is an odour of bitter almonds. There may be convulsions. Respiratory failure ensues, and death may occur within seconds.

Hydrocyanic poisoning may occur from the ingestion by grazing animals of plants containing a cyanogetic glycoside. (*See* GLYCOSIDES). Poisoning is then less acute, and signs are not always indicative of the cause.

TREATMENT. In acute cases, death occurs in dogs and cats before treatment can begin. If a smaller quantity of the poison has entered the body, or if poisoning is the result of the cyanogetic glycosides, (and this is known in time), an intravenous injection of a 1 per cent solution of sodium nitrite, followed by 25 per cent sodium thiosulphate has been recommended for the dog and large animals. Repeat doses at half that rate. (Garners', Toxicology.)

HYDROGEN PEROXIDE. An antiseptic, with some effect against viruses, due to the release of oxygen. It is unsuitable for the irrigation of cavities or deep wounds. (*See* OXYGEN EMBOLISM.)

HYDROMETRA. The accumulation of a watery fluid within the uterus, sometimes sufficient to push other organs aside and to cause swelling of the abdomen of rabbits. This idiopathic condition has also been seen in cats.

HYDRONEPHROSIS is a condition in which the capsule of the kidney, or even the kidney itself, becomes greatly distended with urine which is unable to pass along the ureter into the urinary bladder owing to some obstruction in that channel, such as calculus, a twist, or owing to the pressure of some organ near by. The kidney swells in size, and causes pressure upon the surrounding organs with pain over the lumbar region, and in severe cases a bulging of the muscles just behind the last rib. It is treated by either the removal of the whole kidney, provided the other one is healthy, or else by the removal of the obstruction.

HYDROPERICARDIUM syndrome (Angara disease) has had a devastating effect on the broiler poultry industry of Pakistan for the past few years. The disease has typically been seen in three- to six-week-old growing broiler chicks and results in up to 60 per cent mortality. The syndrome is characterised by the accumulation of clear, straw-coloured fluid in the pericardial sac, a swollen and discoloured liver and enlarged kidneys with distended tubules.
Cause. An unidentified infectious agent which appears to require the presence of an adenovirus to produce the lesions. (M. Afzal, R. Muneer, G. Stein *Veterinary Record* (1991) **128,** 591)

HYDROPONIC 'GRASS', consisting of a mat of barley seedlings harvested at the eight-day stage, has been used for horse feeding, and is usually eaten with relish. It is highly nutritious, very digestible and parasite-free. (J. L. Lees, University College of Wales.) (*See under* HORSES, FEEDING OF.)

HYDROPS AMNII and HYDROPS UTERI (*see* UTERUS, DISEASES OF).

HYDROSALPINX. An accumulation of serous fluid in the Fallopian tube. It is stated to be a common cause of permanent sterility in gilts in America.

HYDROTHORAX means a collection of exudate in the chest, *i.e.* in the pleural cavity. This is one of the results of certain forms of pleurisy.

'HYENA DISEASE'. A disorder in cattle of the development of the skeleton, mainly localised in the hind limbs, as a result of which calves have a back resembling that of a hyena. It was first reported in France in 1975. Two theories as to its cause are current: (1) that it is a metabolic disease; (2) that a virus (possibly that of bovine virus diarrhoea/mucosal disease) is involved. (Espinasse, J. & others, *Veterinary Record*, (1986), **118,** 328.)

HYGIENE. (*See* INFECTION, VENTILATION, HOUSING, WATER-SUPPLY, DIET AND DIETETICS, DISINFECTION, SLURRY, etc.)

HYGROMA is a swelling occurring in connection with a joint, usually the knee or hock, and the result of repeated bruising against a hard surface (*see* CAPPED HOCK, etc.).

Hygroma in cattle may arise through an insufficiency of bedding, or through faulty building design. (*See also* CALLOSITIES.)

Hygroma of the elbow in large dogs was successfully treated by means of the following technique. A 6-mm diameter Penrose drain was passed through incisions made dorsally and ventrally into the hygroma, and secured firmly to the skin. Dressings were changed every 4 to 5 days, and the drain taken after 2 or 3 weeks. The wounds healed satisfactorily, and the hygroma was obliterated in 18 cases out of 18. Dr D. E. Johnston cautioned against use of corticosteroids, aspiration, and excision. (*JAVMA* (1975) **167** 213.)

HYGROMYCIN B. An antibiotic used in the USA as an anthelmintic, and claimed to be effective against large roundworms and whipworms.

HYMEN, IMPERFORATE. Imperforate hymen in thoroughbred fillies, with consequent accumulation of fluid in the uterus, has led to symptoms varying from acute abdominal pain, sweating, and attempts to lie down and roll, to discomfort when urinating. Immediate relief followed necessary surgery in the more serious case; pulse and respiration rates returning to normal within 10 minutes, with feeding resumed. (*See also* 'WHITE HEIFER DISEASE'.)

HYOID is the name of the bone which gives support to the root of the tongue and to the larynx. It has some similarity to the letter **U.**

HYOSCYAMUS (*see* HENBANE).

HYOSTRONGYLUS RUBIDUS. A parasitic worm of pigs.

HYPER- is a prefix indicating excess.

HYPERAEMIA. Congestion. An excessive amount of blood in a part of the body.

HYPERAESTHESIA. Over-sensitiveness to bright light, sudden noise or touch. It occurs in diseases such as rabies, tetanus, hypomagnesaemia.
Feline hyperaesthesia may result also from poisoning by, for example, benzoic acid.
SIGNS: Aggressiveness, excitement.

HYPERBARIC (*see* OXYGEN).

HYPERCALCAEMIA. An excess of calcium in the blood.
CAUSES. In dogs these include cancer, an excess of vitamin D, osteolytic lesions, kidney failure, excess parathroid hormone, Addison's disease, severe hypothermia, and blastomycosis.
In man, additional causes of hypercalcaemia include acromegaly, increased thyroid gland activity, long-term immobilisation, too much vitamin A, treatment with thiazide diuretics, tuberculosis, sarcoidosis, histoplasmosis, coccidiomycosis, and silicone-induced granuloma.

The above causes were given by Dr Steven Dow and others, who described four cases in dogs associated with blastomycosis, a hitherto unknown cause. In all four the lungs were extensively affected, and kidney function impaired.

SIGNS. Emaciation, anorexia, and dehydration were seen in one of their cases, a 3-year-old dog. Body temperature was 103·8, heart rate 108 beats per minute, and a respiratory rate of 48. No bone lesions were detected by radiography. Blastomyces organisms were found both in a lymph node and in the urine.

TREATMENT. Amphotericin-B was given over a 4-month period, during which the serum calcium concentration fell from 12·5 mg/dl to 11·5 mg/dl on day 98. A year and a half later the dog remained free from blastomycosis. (Dow, S. W. & others, *JAVMA* (1986), **188**, 706.)

HYPERCAPNIA. The presence in the blood of a raised level of carbon dioxide.

HYPERCHLORHYDRIA is a form of indigestion associated with excessive secretion of hydrochloric acid.

HYPERGLYCAEMIA. An excess of sugar in the blood. (*See* DIABETES MELLITUS.)

HYPER-IMMUNE SERUM. The serum of an animal which has been hyper-immunised by repeated injections of a toxin or vaccine. It is rich in antibodies, and is used for curative treatment of *e.g.* tetanus.

HYPERKERATOSIS means an excess of horn or KERATIN (which see). The specific disease is also characterised by hardening of the skin.

CAUSE. The disease is due to poisoning by minute quantities of chlorinated naphthalene compounds (and possibly other chemical substances also). These are found in many wood-preserving compounds, in insecticides, lubricants, and electrical insulation material. These substances bring about a secondary vitamin A deficiency. In America the disease has followed the feeding of pellets prepared by machinery lubricated with grease or oil containing naphthalene compounds – an indication of the minute quantities sufficient to cause trouble. Usually, however, the disease is a sequel to housing stock in recently creosoted buildings. (For the disease in pigs, *see also* ZINC and CALCIUM SUPPLEMENTS.)

SIGNS. A thickening of the skin, sometimes with loss of hair, on neck and shoulders. In calves, stunted growth, a discharge from the eye (often with a corneal opacity), frothing at the mouth, weakness and emaciation occur, and death may precede any obvious skin changes.

TREATMENT. Vitamin A will assist recovery.

HYPERLIPAEMIA. A fatal disease of ponies. It was first reported in Europe, then in Australia. Mares affected in late pregnancy or early lactation.

SIGNS. Depression, weakness, loss of appetite, diarrhoea, and terminal convulsions.

AUTOPSY findings: Liver much enlarged, yellow and friable. (Thilsted, J. P., *Modern Veterinary Practice* (1982) **63**, 467.)

HYPERMETRIA. A high-stepping gait. (*See* COENURIASIS.)

HYPEROXALURIA. An excess of oxalates in the urine. This accompanies L-glyceric aciduria in a recently recognised kidney disease of kittens 5 to 9 months old.

Acute kidney failure develops together with atrophy of nerves supplying muscles.

SIGNS: extreme weakness, affecting standing and walking.

CAUSE: a recessive gene.

HYPERPARATHYROIDISM (*see* PARATHYROID GLANDS.)

Of 21 dogs suffering from this, 20 had an adenoma, and one a carcinoma.

SIGNS. Thirst, listlessness, weakness, loss of appetite. (Berger, B. & Feldman, E. C., *Journal of the American JAVMA* (1987) **191**, 350.)

HYPERPLASIA is the term applied to abnormally great development of some organ or tissue.

HYPERPOTASSAEMIA. Too high a level of potassium in the blood-stream. This may be brought about artificially, with fatal results, by the mistaken use of potassium iodide intravenously instead of sodium iodide.

HYPERPYREXIA means a high degree of fever. (*See* FEVER, TEMPERATURE.)

HYPERSENSITIVITY. Once an animal has been 'primed' or sensitised by an antigen, further contact with this will boost the immune response – but may also provoke tissue-damaging reactions. (*See* IMMUNE RESPONSE, ALLERGY, PENICILLIN, SENSITIVITY TO, ANAPHYLAXIS, SERUM SICKNESS).

HYPERTENSION. High arterial blood pressure. In dogs kidney disease is the most common cause of hypertension.

SIGNS. Detachment of the retina, or bleeding from it, may be the first indication. The dog may suddenly go blind

Long-term effects may include enlargement of the left ventricle of the heart and kidney failure. (Dimski, D. S. & Hawkins, E.C. *Compendium of Continuing Education* (1989) **10** 1152.)

HYPERTHERMIA. A body temperature greatly in excess of the normal, as occurs in fevers.

HYPERTHERMIA, MALIGNANT. When some dogs of the Great Dane breed, some pigs of the Piétrain breed, and some human beings (about 1 in every 10,000 people) are anaesthetised with Halothane, their body temperature rises to a point at which – unless the anaesthesia is discontinued – the hyperthermia is likely to prove fatal.

Hyperthermia may occur in animals poisoned by chlorinated hydrocarbon insecticides. (*See also* HEAT-STROKE, TROPICS, FEVER.)

Malignant hyperthermia may also develop as a result of stress. 'This change is consistent with a fault in the regulation of muscle cell calcium ions.' (Nelson, T. E. *JAVMA* (1991) **198** 989.)

HYPERTHYROIDISM. Excessive activity of the thyroid gland. (*See* THYROID GLAND.)

HYPERTONIC (*see under* ISOTONIC).

HYPERTROPHIC PULMONARY OSTEO-PATHY (Marie's disease). This was first described in man in 1890. It has been reported in the dog (*see also* ACROPACHIA) and in the horse. In the latter it has occurred in the absence of either tuberculosis or tumours. In Africa, the roundworm *Spirocera lupi* has been reported as associated with the condition in the dog.

In the dog the disease takes the form of a non-oedematous swelling of all four legs. It is associated with tumours of the lung. Severing of the vagus nerve has been recommended in cases (the majority) where surgical removal of the lung lesions is not possible, and has led to a reduction of the bone enlargement in the limbs, and of the swelling, pain, and lameness. Euthanasia may, of course, be preferable.

HYPERTROPHY means extra size or development of an organ or tissue.

In certain valvular diseases of the heart when obstruction to the free flow of blood occurs, the muscle wall of the heart becomes increased in thickness and strength, and a compensation results. In the training of horses the trainer aims at getting the maximum efficiency from the skeletal muscles, which under the influence of judicious training and feeding become hypertrophied.

After one organ of a pair has been removed, as, for instance, the kidney or the ovary, the remaining organ becomes increased in size so as to be able to perform practically the same amount of work as was previously done by the pair.

HYPERVITAMINOSIS. Disease associated with an excess of a particular vitamin. For example, chronic hypervitaminosis A occurs in cats fed exclusively or virtually so, on an all-liver diet. (*See under* CAT FOODS.)

HYPHAEMIA. An infusion of blood into the anterior chamber of the eye.

HYPO- is a prefix indicating a deficiency.

HYPOADRENOCORTICISM (*see* ADDISON'S DISEASE.)

HYPOCALCAEMIA (*see* MILK FEVER; TRANSIT TETANY; LAMBING SICKNESS IN EWES, ECLAMPSIA, METABOLIC PROFILES). ☞

HYPOCHLORITES are widely used as disinfectants, being relatively non-toxic and non-irritant to the skin. Their efficacy depends upon the amount of available chlorine, which is more active against viruses than most disinfectants.

Hypochlorites are unable to penetrate grease and are often combined with detergents. Sodium hypochlorite is useful for disinfecting premises after an outbreak of a virus disease. (*See also* TEAT-DIPPING ANTISEPTICS.)

HYPOCUPRAEMIA. A condition in which there is too little copper in the blood-stream. This occurs in SWAYBACK in lambs, and is also associated with serious ill health in cattle. On the Shropshire–Cheshire border, for example, hypocupraemia is accompanied by scouring and stunted growth. Two-year-old heifers have been mistaken for 8-month-old calves. In Caithness hypocupraemia is liable to occur on 75 per cent of the farms unless precautions are taken. Scouring is not a common symptom there but calves of the beef breeds show a stilted gait and progressive unthriftiness. (For further information, *see* COPPER.)

HYPOCUPROSIS. A disease caused by a copper deficiency. (*See above* and COPPER.)

HYPODERMIC (*see* INJECTIONS.)

HYPOGLOSSAL NERVE is the 12th cranial nerve and supplies the muscles of the tongue, together with others nearby.

HYPOGLYCAEMIA is a deficiency of sugar in the blood. It may occur in states of starvation, but is of special importance in connection with the administration of insulin, which is injected to lower the blood sugar from an abnormal amount, and which, if given in too large doses, may produce too great reduction with symptoms of nervousness, breathlessness, and excitement. In human medicine hypoglycaemia may be a sequel to the use of sulphonamides, *e.g.* sulphadiazine. These symptoms are relieved by taking some food containing sugar and by an injection of adrenalin, which checks the action of insulin. (*See* BABY PIG DISEASE.)

HYPOKALAEMIA. A deficiency of potassium in the blood. (*See* 'DOWNER COW' SYNDROME.)

HYPOMAGNESAEMIA. A condition in which there is too little magnesium in the bloodstream.

Hypomagnesaemia is of particular importance in cattle, and occurs when a herd is turned on to lush spring grass after being stall fed during the winter, but an interval of a few days elapses before symptoms appear. Hypomagnesaemia occurs in bulls as well as in cows, and also in beef calves and sheep. It is encountered during the late autumn or winter in yarded animals receiving fodder crops in large amounts with little or no good hay, sometimes – but not invariably – after a snowfall or cold, wet spell. (*See also under* BEDDING FOR CATTLE.)

Hypomagnesaemia has apparently been more common in the Ayrshire than in other British breeds of cattle. Cows which have had several calves are more prone to it than heifers.

It is not uncommon in ewes within a month of lambing.

Hypomagnesaemia is commonly seen in animals grazing pastures which have recently received a heavy dressing of nitrogenous or potash fertiliser.

It appears to be associated with a high protein diet and too little fibre. Whole milk is not by itself an adequate source of magnesium for a rapidly growing young animal, and the condition may accordingly occur in calves. (*See* OMASUM.)

SIGNS. Shivering, a staggering gait, excitement, convulsions, and paralysis may precede death. In a less acute form of Hypomagnesaemia the animals appear 'nervy' – responding violently to sensations of touch or sound – and there may be muscular tremors.

TREATMENT. This must be prompt and consists in the intravenous injection of magnesium salts. Successful in perhaps 75 per cent of cases. Great care is necessary, however, in giving the injection and even approaching the animal – which may otherwise die at the prick of the needle.

An enema of up to five tablespoonfuls of magnesium chloride in a ¼-litre of arm water is recommended by the Tennessee State University.

Magnesium can also be given in the drinking water, using a proprietary product 'Aquatrace'.

PREVENTION. The feeding of magnesium-rich supplements 3 weeks before early spring grazing and for 1 week or so afterwards; or, in sheep, the use of a magnesium lick, from a month after service till a month after lambing. (For adult cattle a daily dose of 2 oz per head of calcined magnesite, mixed with damp sugarbeet pulp, is recommended.) A mixture of magnesium acetate solution and molasses may be offered *ad lib.* from ball feeders on pasture, as an alternative. Magnesium 'bullets' are also used. Top-dressing pasture with calcined magnesite (about 10 cwt per acre) is helpful. (*See* MAGNESIUM, MILK FEVER.) Magnesium can also be given in the drinking water, using 'Aquatrace'.

HYPOMYELINOGENESIS CONGENITA IN SHEEP. A congenital disease of lambs, characterised by trembling or twitching, staggering, and sometimes shaking of the head.

HYPONATRAEMIA. A deficiency of sodium in the blood.

HYPOPARATHYROIDISM, nutritional secondary. (*See* CANINE and FELINE JUVENILE OSTEODYSTROPHY.)

HYPOPHOSPHATAEMIA. A condition in which the level of blood phosphorus is too low. (*See* MILK FEVER, 'DOWNER COW' SYNDROME.)

HYPOPHYSIS. The pituitary gland. Hypophysectomy is removal of the pituitary.

HYPOPLASIA. Under-development. Hypoplasia of the genital organs is one cause of sterility.

HYPOTENSION. Low arterial blood-pressure.

HYPOTENSIVE DRUGS are used to reduce high blood pressure.

HYPOTHALAMUS. A part of the brain below the thalamus which acts as a thermostat, maintaining body temperature. It also influences blood circulation, urinary secretion, and appetite. (*See* BRAIN.)

HYPOTHERMIA. An abnormally low body temperature. In human surgery this is deliberately induced, by various means, for operations on heart or brain. A technique used in human surgery for operations within the dry heart. The venous blood is cooled in a circuit outside the body (a method now preferred to the use of ice packs or refrigerated blankets) until a body temperature of $68° – 77°F$ is obtained, when the flow of blood to the heart can be stopped for several minutes to allow the operation to proceed.

HYPOTHERMIA, ACCIDENTAL. The chilling of newborn animals, or of those under a general anaesthetic, is a life-threatening condition. Warmth is essential. (*See also under* SHEEP BREEDING – Lamb survival; and HOUSING OF ANIMALS.)

HYPOTHYROIDISM. A condition associated in cattle with a high incidence of aborted, still-born, or weakly calves. (*See also* GOITRE.)

HYPOVOLAEMIA. A diminished volume of blood. (*See* SHOCK.)

HYSTERECTOMY. A surgical operation for removal of the uterus. Usually the ovaries are removed at the same time. (*See* OVARIO-HYSTERECTOMY.)

HYSTERIA (CANINE). The disappearance of this disease from the UK has been attributed to the abandonment of the use of agenised flour in the manufacture of dog biscuits. (The agene process involved the bleaching of flour with nitrogen chloride.)

It has been suggested that some cases may have been due to the use of flour, containing the spores of *Tilletia tritici*, in dog-biscuit manufacture.

SIGNS: The dog would suddenly 'appear to go mad', racing round with a fixed stare, barking or howling.

(For distemper-like signs, *see* MENINGITIS.)

I

IATROGENIC DISEASE is that caused by treatment; for example, the side-effects of some drugs. Adverse drug reactions were suspected in 130 of 39,541 cases treated at the Veterinary Hospital, University of California, Davis. In 66 cases there was reasonable evidence to link the reaction observed to the drug. Antibiotics and antiparasiticides were incriminated 21 times with anaphylaxis being most commonly observed reaction. There were three deaths following the administration of procaine penicillin (inadvertently i/v) to a lamb, potassium penicillin (10,000 units/Kg) to a cat and oxytetracycline (25 mg/kg) to a cow. Anaesthetic and related agents were involved 20 times. Severe clonic convulsions developed in five cats receiving more than 80 mg ketamine hydrochloride; cardiac arrest, hypotension, dyspnoea and muscular rigidity in two horses given xylazine (1 mg/kg i/v) and severe bradycardia and respiratory arrest in two dogs given fentanyl-droperidol. Anti-cancer drugs were implicated in 10 cases with the most dramatic reactions being observed in five dogs treated with 5-fluorouracil. One of these died as a result of neural toxicosis. (Ndiritu, C. G. and Enos, L. R. (1977), *Journal of the American Veterinary Medical Association,* **171,** 335.) (*See also* SIDE-EFFECTS, DRUG INTER-ACTIONS.)

IBK. Infectious Bovine Keratitis (Infectious Ophthalmia of cattle). (*See under* EYE, DISEASES OF.)

IBR. Infectious Bovine Rhinotracheitis. (*See* RHINOTRACHEITIS.)

IBUFROFEN. A non-steroidal anti-inflammatory drug, much used in human medicine, but which can cause a sometimes fatal gastric ulceration in dogs. The same is true of flurbiprofen.

ICE, ICE CUBES. Of use in cases of haemorrhage from the stomach, as an aid to control bleeding from wounds, and as an application in cases of meningitis, paraphimosis.

ICELANDIC PNEUMONIA (*see* PULMONARY ADENOMATOSIS, *also* MAEDI/VISNA).

ICHTHYOSIS is a condition of the skin in the dog, especially over the elbow and hocks in which large and irregular cracks appear. These become filled with dirt, and suppuration results.

ICTERUS (*see* JAUNDICE).

IDAZOXAN. A drug used to reverse the effect of XYLAZINE (which see), and very quick in its action.

IDENTICHIP. An electronically coded microchip, the size of a grain of rice, encased in implant-grade glass. It is inserted in the loose skin of the neck of the animal (under local anaesthesia).

The microchip is encoded with the animal-owner's address, etc., kept on a central computer register.

Electronic scanning devices, called 'readers', will enable veterinary surgeons and animal welfare registered staff to have direct access to the register.

This Pet Registration Scheme is conducted by Animalcare Ltd., of Common Road, Dunnington, York YO1 5RU.

IDENTIFICATION OF CATTLE. Nose prints, taken in the same manner as finger-prints, have been used in New Zealand. This may have value in black-skinned animals for which tattooing is of little value. (*See also* BRANDING.)

IDIOPATHIC is a term applied to diseases to indicate that their cause is unknown.

Idiopathic feline vestibular syndrome (IFVS). (*See under* FELINE VESTIBULAR.)

IDIOSYNCRASY. An untypical reaction to a drug or to a food; in a behavioural sense, a quirk.

IgA is an antibody/immunoglobulin found in the blood serum and also in secretions from mucous membranes. (*See* SECRETORY IGA.) IgG and IgM are other immunoglobulins. (*See* IMMUNO-GLOBULINS.)

ILE DE FRANCE. A French breed of sheep.

ILEITIS. Inflammation of the ileum.

ILEOCAECAL refers to the junction between ileum and caecum, that is, between the end of the small intestine and the commencement of the large. The so-called ileocaecal valve is formed by the caecum in such manner that while food material may readily travel from ileum into caecum, it is difficult for it to pass in the opposite direction.

ILEUM is the last arbitrary division of the small intestine. (*See* INTESTINES.)

Inflammation of the ileum – which becomes thickened and stiff, almost like a piece of rubber hose – is a cause of death in piglets 2 to 4 months old. It has been suggested that there is a hereditary predisposition to this condition, which often affects the whole litter. In many instances, the trouble is recognised only at the bacon factory, having caused no *apparent* illness in the pigs. Those that die, on the other hand, do so from perforating ulcers and peritonitis, after showing evidence of thirst, a bluish colour of the skin, and collapse. (*See* PORCINE INTESTINAL ADENO-MATOSIS.)

ILEUS. The intestinal obstruction which can follow failure of PERISTALSIS.

ILIAC. Relating to the flank. (*See* ARTERIES.)

ILIUM is another name for the haunch-bone, the outer angle of which forms the 'point of the hip'. The ilium is the largest and most anteriorly situated bone of the pelvis. (*See* BONE.)

IMBALANCE. A term used to describe, for example, a faulty calcium–phosphorus ratio in the food of an animal; or an excess of one hormone in the blood-stream, or a deficiency of another – with resulting disease. (*See* RICKETS, OSTEOFIBROSIS, INFERTILITY, METABOLIC PROFILES, CALCIUM SUPPLEMENTS, DOGS' DIET.)

'IMMOBILON' (Reckitt & Colman) is a combination of two drugs to provide anaesthesia. There are two formulations:
(1) 'Small Animal Immobilon' combines etorphine hydrochloride with methotrimeprazine and, given by intramuscular injection, provides analgesia and immobilisation useful for a wide variety of diagnostic and therapeutic procedures, such as the suturing of wounds, setting of fractures, dentistry, and minor surgery.

Dogs. Immobilon does not, like morphine, cause excitement, vomiting, or defaecation. It does, however, act as a respiratory depressant, and slows heart action.
(2) 'Large Animal Immobilon' is a combination of etorphine with acepromazine. It is convenient to administer, provides useful anaesthesia and recumbency, but not complete muscular relaxation.

Horses. Immobilon is a respiratory depressant to an extent which may lead to a shortage of oxygen in the tissues. Heart action is accelerated, and blood pressure raised.
Side-effects in horses. The animal sometimes becomes recumbent again after four hours or so. Prolapse of the penis is another side-effect. (*See under* PENIS.)
Immobilon is reversible in its effects by means of 'Revivon' (diprenorphine hydrochloride).

PRECAUTIONS. 'Immobilon' is highly toxic for people. A veterinary surgeon died within fifteen minutes after accidental self-inoculation when a colt made a sudden violent movement. (Unfortunately the victim was not carrying 'Revivon'.)
Recommended precautions include the wearing of gloves to avoid skin contamination (which has required hospital treatment), protection of the eyes, and the presence of someone to administer naxalone and diphrenorphine.

IMMUNE-MEDIATED DISEASE include: PEMPHIGUS, FELINE INFECTIOUS PERITONITIS, MYASTHENIA GRAVIS. THROMBOCYTOPENIA and POLYARTHRITIS may also, in some instances, be immune-mediated diseases. (*See* AUTO-IMMUNE DISEASE.)

IMMUNE RESPONSE, THE. This is a term used in Immunology, which is the study of the body's reaction to the presence of foreign substances.

Such substances (usually polysaccharide or protein) are present in bacteria, viruses and other parasites, but are dissimilar to any substances occurring naturally in the host's body. The foreign substances act as *antigens* and give rise to *antibodies*. This is the immune response.
When antigen enters the body, the immune response may take two forms: (1) **Humoral** immunity, which involves the synthesis and release of antibody into the blood and other body fluids; and (2) **Cell-mediated** immunity, involving the production of 'sensitised' lymphocytes which have the antibody on their cell surfaces. (*See* IMMUNOGLOBULINS, INTERFERON, INFECTION.)
Antibodies combine with (and for all practical purposes neutralise) the antigens. In this way an animal may overcome infection.
Lymphocytes play an important part in the immune response, attacking cells containing the antigens. This happens in graft rejection and organ transplants, in reaction to malignant tumours, and in infections where bacteria, viruses or other parasites are present inside host cells.
B lymphocytes are the precursors of the plasma cells which secrete antibodies. B cells have antibody-like receptors on their surfaces which aid in the recognition of specific antigens. (*See under* BLOOD, B-CELLS, T-CELLS, RETICULO-ENDOTHELIAL, ANTIBODIES, IMMUNOGLOBULINS *and* SECRETORY IgA.)

IMMUNISATION is the process of artificially producing resistance to a given infection; generally by means of a vaccine, sometimes by means of an antiserum or antitoxin. (*See* IMMUNITY, VACCINES, ANTISERUM.)
Side-effects. Immunisation is not always attained without side-effects. (*See* SERUM SICKNESS, ANAPHYLACTIC SHOCK.) In human medicine both serum shock and serum neuritis may occasionally follow the use of equine antitetanus serum or of antitoxin made from this. (*See Lancet,* Nov. 27, 1965.)

IMMUNITY is the power to resist infection or the action of certain poisons. This immunity is either (1) inherited; (2) acquired naturally; or (3) acquired artificially.

Natural immunity. There are some species of animals that are not affected by diseases or by poisons that are dangerous to others. The snake-killing mongoose of India possesses an immunity against cobra venom; the pigeon can withstand large doses of morphine without harm; fowls are resistant to tetanus; the horse does not become affected with foot-and-mouth disease; rats are not attacked by tuberculosis; the ox is immune from glanders; man is not affected by swine fever and many other diseases that are fatal to the lower animals, while, with the exception of the monkey, animals are not susceptible to syphilis. It is probable that species immunity cannot be broken down even by massive inoculation of the causal agent.
A degree of immunity to locally occurring infections is transmitted to it by the medium of the colostrum in its mother's milk. (*See* COLOSTRUM, IMMUNOGLOBULINS.)

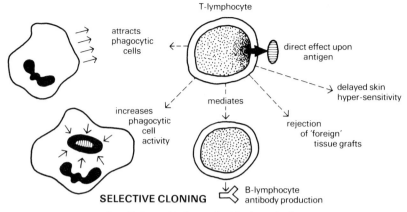

Specific immunity: humoral antibody production

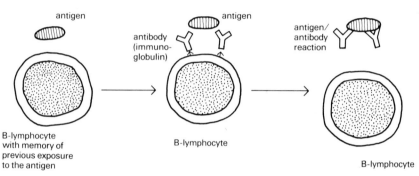

Specific immunity: cell-mediated immune response.

Acquired immunity results from an attack of some disease from which the animal has recovered. It is probable that most diseases confer a certain amount of immunity, but this varies greatly. It may be lifelong, or virtually so, as in sheep pox, swine fever or erysipelas. In most instances, however, its duration is less, and in some only temporary. *E.g.* cattle may be attacked by foot-and-mouth disease several times during their lives, and horses after recovery from one attack of tetanus may have a second natural attack. The immunity conferred by recovery is liable in many of the virus diseases (*e.g.* Bluetongue), and in some protozoal diseases to break down in the presence of massive infection subsequently. Recovery from a disease involves a process of natural immunisation against that disease, the toxins or other antigens present in the body being destroyed by antibodies elaborated by the body tissues.

Artificially acquired immunity is of two varieties, either active or passive.

(*a*) *Active immunity* may be artificially produced by inoculating an animal with a vaccine (*i.e.* dead or attenuated bacteria or virus) or with a toxoid.

(*b*) *Passive immunity* is that form of artificial immunity obtained by injecting into the body of one animal blood-serum drawn from the body of another animal which has previously been rendered actively immune by injecting particular antigens. The serum contains antibodies or 'anti-toxins', which enable an in-contact animal to resist an infection, or enable an already infected animal to overcome the infection, so that an attack of illness – if it occurs at all – is milder than it would otherwise have been. (*See* ANTI-SERUM.) A young animal may acquire passive immunity through the colostrum of its dam which had been immunised with this purpose in mind. (For an example, *see* LAMB DYSENTERY.)

The immune system normally 'learns' to discriminate between self and non-self antigens early in development, leading to the normal state known as self-tolerance. A newborn mouse or rat injected with large numbers of cells from a genetically foreign individual will grow up tolerant of the foreign alloantigens of the donor, so that, for example, it will accept a skin graft from the donor which would normally be rejected. It has been shown that this induced state of 'neonatal tolerance' is maintained by suppressor T cells. (AFRC.)

There are many complexities involved in immunity, which is far from being the simple subject it may here appear. (*See* IMMUNE RESPONSE, ORIFICES.)

IMMUNODEFICIENCY. This may involve a specific factor, such as antibody or lymphocytes; or a non-specific factor such as a complement component. In either case the deficiency results in

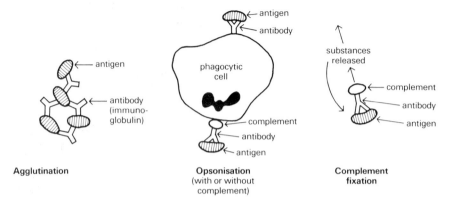

Agglutination

Opsonisation
(with or without
complement)

Complement
fixation

Specific immunity immunoglobulin activity.

some failure of the IMMUNE RESPONSE (which see), so that viral, bacterial or fungal disease may ensue.

Deficiencies of immunity can be either primary, due to congenital dysfunction of the immune mechanism; or secondary.

Primary immuno-deficiency has been studied more fully in humans than in animals, although a condition of foals called 'Inherited combined immuno-deficiency in foals of Arabian breeding' has been documented in America.

Theoretically, if the deficiency is mainly of *B-lymphocytes*, the animal is likely to have measurably low levels of immuno-globulins and a deficiency of lymphoid follicles in lymph nodes. Such an animal would be susceptible to pyogenic bacterial infection, but would be able to cope with most viral infections.

Conversely, if the deficiency is mainly of *T-lymphocytes*, the animal will have reduced 'delayed skin hypersensitivity' and will be more susceptible to viruses.

Foals affected by the inherited *combined* immuno-deficiency frequently suffer from adenoviral pneumonia due to their inability to resist infection.

Secondary partial immuno-deficiency is much more common, and is being increasingly recognised as an important cause of failure to recover completely from certain diseases.

Severe malnutrition, certain viral infections, exposure to X-rays, and cortico-steroid therapy can all lead to a reduction in the immune response. (Source: ICI's *Spectrum* (1982) **1**, issue 8). (*See also* IMMUNOSUPPRESSION.)

IMMUNOFLUORESCENT MICROSCOPY. This is a useful laboratory method of diagnosis, described as specific and very sensitive. It enables a virus to be identified during the course of an unknown infection. It can demonstrate the presence of swine fever virus, for example, even before the appearance of symptoms. Results can be obtained within a matter of hours.

The principle involved is that antigens in tissues are identified by using their ability to respond to, and fix, the homologous antibody previously labelled with a fluorescent tracer which does not affect its properties.

The method has demonstrated swine fever virus using impressions from lymph nodes taken from pigs killed during the first 60 hours after experimental infection. The virus is revealed first in the cytoplasm as a diffuse granular fluorescence; later bright, fluorescent particles become visible within the nucleus.

The term fluorescent antibody test is applied to this technique. (*See also under* RABIES.)

IMMUNOGLOBULINS – found in blood, colostrum, and most secretions – are proteins produced by PLASMA cells (which see) in response to stimulation by antigens, and play an important part in the IMMUNE RESPONSE (which see). Immunoglobulins inactivate or destroy antigens. In cattle four classes of immunoglobulin had (by 1978) been recognised: IgG, IgM, IgA, and IgE. 'This immunoglobulin is found in very low concentrations in serum but binds to basophils and mast cells, and possibly protects against parasitic infections. Specific antigen stimulates IgE-coated cells to release histamine resulting in local or sometimes systemic inflammation.' (*See* ALLERGY, REAGINIC ANTIBODIES.) (Dr M. R. Williams.) 'Parasite antigens are a potent stimulus for induction of anti-parasite antibodies of the IgE class, and parasite infection can potentiate a pre-existing antibody response to an unrelated antigen.' (Williams, M. R., (1976), *Lancet*.) (*See also under* IGA *and* SECRETORY IGA; *and* COLOSTRUM.)

IMMUNO-STIMULATION (*see* LEVAMISOLE, BCG).

IMMUNOSUPPRESSION. Suppression of the immune response, leading to greater susceptibility of an animal to pathogens, such as may occur in trypanosomiasis, influenza, distemper, and brucellosis, and *see under* CORTISONE, ANERGY, LEVAMISOLE, SPLEEN.)

The occurrence of *anergy* following certain viral infections is worth emphasising; affected animals showing a reduced cell-mediated response, especially following infections by viruses having a cytotoxic effect on lymphoid cells; e.g. Newcastle disease virus'. (Source: I C I.)

Immuno-suppressants include CORTICO-STEROIDS; cytotoxic drugs such as CYCLOPHOS-PHAMIDE; PURINE-based drugs; and GOLD compounds.

IMPACTION is a condition in which two things are firmly lodged together. For example, when after a fracture one piece of bone is driven within the other, this is known as an impacted fracture; when a temporary tooth is so firmly lodged in its socket that the eruption of the permanent one below is prevented, this is known as dental impaction. Impaction of rumen or of colon means that food materials have become tightly packed into these organs. (*See* STOMACH, DISEASES; INTESTINES, DISEASES; and COLIC in horses.)

IMPETIGO is a skin disease of dogs and cattle particularly, characterised by the formation of painless pustules, shallow, thin-walled, and usually projecting upwards above the level of the surface of the skin. It is seen in puppies affected with worms, distemper, and teething troubles, in bitches and cows after parturition, when the mammary glands are usually affected, and in other animals. (*See also* ACNE.)

IMPLANTATION. This term is used in connection with the application beneath the skin of pellets composed of, or containing, synthetic hormones. (*See* HORMONES IN MEAT PRODUCTION, CAPONISATION.) (*See also* IDENTICHIP.)

IMPLANTS. An acrylic implant has been used to treat a facial deformity in a horse.

An acrylic implant, using material intended for the repair of human dentures, was cast *in situ* to repair a split hard palate, following a dog-bite. (This technique obviated the conventional method of taking a plaster cast first and then moulding the implant.) (Coles, B. H. EVSc., & Underwood, Lisbeth C. BVSc.)

IMPLANTS, BIODEGRADABLE, rod-shaped and made of polyglycolic acid were used for fixing a comminuted fracture of the calcaneus in a dog, and a comminuted fracture of the distal shaft of the tibia in a cat. The fractures healed in six weeks without complications and the animals used their injured legs earlier and seemed to feel less pain than patients operated with metallic implants. Metallic implants often cause decalcification of the bone around an implant, and the implant may loosen before the fracture has healed; in contrast bone tissue grows into the biodegradable implants and they dissolve, main-

taining a rigid contact between the bone and the implant. Axelson, P. & others. *Journal of Small Animal Practice* (1988) **29**, 249.)

IMPORTING/EXPORTING ANIMALS. Many animal-owners – including sophisticated travellers completely familiar with passports, visas, and vaccination certificates – overlook the fact that they cannot legally take their pet animals with them across any and every national frontier. Some governments exercise a total ban on the import of certain species of animal; others require prior vaccination and production of a certificate; others insist upon an animal going straight into quarantine on arrival.

Australia and New Zealand, for example, will admit dogs only from each other's territories or from the UK.

Pet animals. An import licence must be obtained *in advance* for any dog, cat, or other pet animal which it is proposed to take **into the UK.** (The address for licence application is: Import Licence Section, MAFF, Government Buildings, Toby Jug Site, Hook Rise South, Tolworth, Surrey, England.) It is worthwhile taking a dog, etc., into the UK only if the traveller expects to stay more than 6 months, for that is the length of the compulsory quarantine period. One can sum up the position as 'UK holidays for people, yes (and welcome); for pets, no', the reason being the risk of introducing rabies. Expatriates returning to the UK must similarly obtain a licence and be prepared to pay for 6 months' quarantine – necessary also where a UK resident takes his pet animal on holiday abroad with him and then brings it back. Smuggled or unlicensed animals can be destroyed or re-exported or put in quarantine at the owner's expense. The Export of Animals (Protection) Order 1981 laid down certain welfare requirements for the export of cattle, sheep, goats, and pigs from Great Britain.

There are restrictions on the import of cattle and semen on account of BLUE-TONGUE and other diseases.

Sheep. Regulations about importing sheep into the UK, made in 1984, require a period of one-month on-farm isolation following release from the reception/quarantine station. During the isolation period testing for Maedi/Visna, *Brucella ovis*, and *Mycoplasma agalactiae* is carried out; with slaughter or re-export required for positive reactors.

(*See also* HORSES, IMPORT CONTROLS; BIRDS, IMPORT OF; RABIES; QUARANTINE.)

IMPOTENCE. Causes include malformation of the genital organs, weakness, starvation, constrictions resulting from injuries or operations, or it may be only a temporary phase in the life of the animal from which it recovers with rest and good food. (*See also* PENIS, INFERTILITY.)

IMPRINTING. This is a mental process in which an inborn tendency in the animal causes it to attach itself to a set group of objects or a single object within a few hours after birth. It is a very important process if the young lamb or calf is to be properly suckled and cared for.

IN VITRO. In the test-tube.

IN VIVO. In the living body.

INCISOR. There are no upper incisor teeth in domesticated ruminants. (*See* TEETH.)

INCLUSION BODIES. Round, oval, or irregular-shaped structures of a homogeneous or granular nature, found in cells during the course of virus infections. *E.g.*, Negri bodies in nerve cells in rabies, Bollinger bodies in epithelial cells in fowl pox.

INCLUSION BODY HEPATITIS. A virus disease of chickens, and also of intensively reared pheasant poults. In broilers the disease may appear at about 5–7 weeks of age, giving rise to an increased mortality but with some birds remaining healthy.

INCOMPETENCE is a term applied to the valves of the heart when, as a result of disease in the valves or alterations in the size of the chambers of the heart, the valves are unable to close the orifices which they should protect. (*See* HEART DISEASES.)

INCONTINENCE. Faecal and urinary incontinence may both follow injury to the spinal cord (*see* PARALYSIS). Faecal incontinence alone in the dog and cat may result from DIARRHOEA, STRESS, or possibly weakness of the *sphincter ani* in old animals.

Urinary incontinence may be associated with a dog with an enlarged prostate gland relieving bladder pressure indoors. (*See also under* DIABETES INSIPIDUS.) Old dogs may be unable to avoid incontinence at night, owing to kidney lesions. A rare cause is an ectopic ureter. (*See* URETER.)

Occasionally urinary incontinence is a sequel to spaying of the bitch, and is attributed either to a hormonal effect or to adhesion between the vaginal stump and the bladder or urethra. (*J. Small Anim. Pract.* (1980) **21** 287.)

In the cat, chronic nephritis in the elderly animal is a common cause, as in the dog. The animal is obliged to drink more, and to pass urine during the night-time. Stress may be a factor too; for example the appearance of an aggressive entire tom cat in the neighbourhood, being left alone for long periods, or the addition of a baby or another cat to the household. (*See also* POLYDIPSIA.)

INCO-ORDINATION is a term meaning irregularity in movement. Various muscles or, in some instances, portion of one muscle contract or fail to contract without relation to each other or to the whole. Deliberate purposive movements are no longer possible or are carried out imperfectly.

INCUBATION PERIOD. The time that elapses between infection and appearance of symptoms of a disease.

The average incubation periods for the commoner infectious diseases are:

Anthrax	12 to 24 hours or more
Black-quarter	1 to 5 days
Braxy	12 to 48 hours
Distemper	3 days to 3 weeks
Dourine	15 to 40 days
East Coast fever	10 to 20 days
Erysipelas (swine)	2 to 3 days
Foot-and-mouth disease	2 to 12 days
Heart-water	11 to 18 days
Influenza	3 to 10 days
Lymphangitis, epizootic	8 days to 9 months
Piroplasmosis, British bovine	14 days at earliest
Piroplasmosis, other forms	Up to 3 weeks
Pleuro-pneumonia, contagious bovine	3 weeks to 3 months
Pleuro-pneumonia, contagious equine	3 to 10 days
Rabies	10 days to 5* months
Rinderpest	4 to 5 days
African horse-sickness	6 to 8 days
Strangles	3 to 8 days
Surra	5 to 30 days
Swine fever	5 to 15 days
Tetanus, horse	4 days to 3 weeks
Tetanus, ox	5 to 8 days
Texas fever	6 weeks
Tuberculosis	2 weeks to 6 months

(* but *see under* RABIES)

Caution. It is always wise to allow at least a week more than the longest incubation period given before an animal that has been in contact with an infection and has not developed the disease is allowed to resume its place with other healthy animals. (*See also* INFECTION, ISOLATION, QUARANTINE.)

INDICATOR. A substance used in chemistry, etc., to show by a colour change that a reaction has taken place. (*See also* COMPLEMENT FIXATION TEST.)

INDUCTOTHERM an electrical apparatus used in the treatment of sprained tendons, etc. (*See* DIATHERMY.)

INFARCTION means the changes which take place in an organ when an artery becomes suddenly plugged, leading to the formation of a dense wedge-shaped mass in the part of the organ that was originally supplied by that artery. (*See* EMBOLISM.)

INFECTION. Exposure to infection may or may not be followed by disease, depending upon whether the potential host animal has or has not a useful degree of immunity against that particular infective agent, whether the animal is well nourished, not under stress, and has not any other major infection, disease, or defect which might lower its power to resist the new infection. (*See* IMMUNOSUPPRESSION, IMMUNODEFICIENCY.)

The virulence or otherwise of the infective agent, and the quantity of it, will also have a bearing upon whether disease will follow. For example, a heifer vaccinated against *Brucella abortus* will normally be able to resist exposure to these organisms; but her immunity might break down if challenged by a massive dose of *Br. abortus*.

With rabies, for example, there is a 'threshold' dose of virus, and below this the infected animal will not become rabid (at any rate in the absence of stress).

Susceptibility to infection is also influenced by genetics. For example, *see* K_{88} and MAREK'S DISEASE.

Concurrent infections. The average farm animal is host to several different parasites at one and the same time – including viruses, mycoplasmas, bacteria, fungi, and worms. Accordingly, when one speaks of a calf having pneumonia, it is unrealistic to imagine that, say, the parainfluenza 3 virus (causing the inflammation of the lungs) is the calf's sole resident parasite.

Some parasites may be present in relatively small numbers and not be causing active disease. Some, owing to the host's powers of resistance – the immune response – may be on the decline. Others may have a sudden opportunity for multiplication and increased activity as the host's resistance becomes lowered by some additional infection or by stress arising from cold, insufficiency of good food, poor ventilation, or the rigours of transport, etc.

Again, infections should be thought of as not merely mixed but changing all the time, developing, and with complex interactions between a number of factors, including management ones. (*See under* RESPIRATORY DISEASE IN PIGS.)

In respiratory diseases there is often a synergism between viruses and certain bacteria. In canine distemper, for instance, *Bordetella bronchiseptica* is quick to invade in the wake of the canine distemper virus and produce bronchitis. Foot-rot in sheep is often a mixed bacterial infection, with *Fusiformis necrophorus* causing sufficient damage to permit the entry of *B. nodosus*. A worm (liver fluke) and bacteria may both be involved in production of 'Black Disease'.

Experimental work at the Institute for Research on Animal Diseases, Compton, has shown that fluke-free cattle can withstand an intravenous dose of 10^8 *Salmonella dublin*, whereas those infested with liver fluke are killed by this same dose.

Clinical and sub-clinical infections. Exposure to infection may lead to overt or *clinical* disease in which symptoms are in evidence; or there may be a *sub-clinical* infection in which few if any symptoms – detectable without laboratory aids – are shown. A good example is sub-clinical mastitis. (*See* MASTITIS IN THE COW.)

Infection may persist in an animal which has recovered from a disease and is no longer showing symptoms but is excreting the infective agent. Such an animal is known as a *carrier*. For example, a bull may be a carrier of brucellosis; a dog of leptospirosis; a horse of equine infectious anaemia; a cat of feline leukaemia.

Routes/modes of infection. An animal may breathe in air containing droplets in which the infective agent is present; *e.g.* influenza virus or tubercle bacillus. This is sometimes called an aerosol infection.

The oral route provides a common mode of infection. Infective material may be licked, an infected carcase eaten, or a cow may eat feed contaminated with salmonella organisms or anthrax spores. (In some instances, an infective agent, such as salmonella, is already in the intestine but becomes pathogenic when its bacterial competitors are mostly destroyed by an antibiotic. *See* DIARRHOEA – Horse.)

Spirochaetes and hookworm larvae are examples of parasites which can enter the host through unbroken skin. Small, even insignificant, wounds can be followed by tetanus. Biting flies can transmit diseases (*see under* FLIES), and ticks are notorious vectors. Dog bites and cat scratches can lead to rabies, the virus of which can penetrate intact mucous membrane.

Infection may be transmitted at mating, *e.g.* brucellosis by the carrier bull. Dourine in the horse, and venereal tumours in the dog, are two other examples of infections transmitted at coitus. Congenital infections also occur.

Inter-species infections. Many microorganisms have a wide range of possible hosts, *e.g.* the rabies virus, the influenza viruses, the anthrax bacillus. Infections from man *to* farm animals are ANTHROPONOSES (which see). Farmers may also be interested in diseases which arise in one species following their use of buildings which previously housed another species. For example, turkeys have become infected in this way with swine erysipelas, which also affects game birds. (*See also under* HOUSING OF ANIMALS.) With cattle kept in association with pigs (as in North America), acute interstitial pneumonia may occur in cattle due to the pig worm *Ascaris suum*. (*See also* DOG KENNELS.)

Infections transmissible from animals to man are listed under ZOONOSES. In Britain, those of importance to farmers and stockmen include: Brucellosis, Q-fever, canicola fever, Weil's disease (leptospiral jaundice), louping ill, anthrax, erysipelas, tuberculosis, salmonellosis.

Blood-cells which counter infection. When bacteria gain entrance through a wound in the skin, for example, they are attacked by white blood-cells (leucocytes). The first to attack are *neutrophils*, which have their origin in the bone marrow. They pass through the walls of the capillaries and engulf the bacteria. *Monocytes* perform a similar task when they have turned into *macrophages*, but in addition to engulfing bacteria they also dispose of disintegrating neutrophils. *Lymphocytes* (T-cells or B-cells) also reach the site of infection; see LYMPHOCYTES. (*See also* INTERFERON, IRON-BINDING.)

Other aspects of infection are dealt with under separate headings such as ANTIBODY, COLOSTRUM,

FOMITES, IMMUNE RESPONSE, IMMUNITY, ISOLATION, NOTIFIABLE DISEASES, NURSING, DISINFECTION.

INFECTIOUS BOVINE KERATO-CONJUNCTIVITIS (see EYE, DISEASES OF).

INFECTIOUS BOVINE RHINOTRACHEITIS
(see under RHINOTRACHEITIS).

INFECTIOUS BRONCHITIS OF POULTRY.
CAUSE: A coronavirus, *Haemophilus gallinarum*.
SIGNS: Breathing difficulties which may be evident only at night. A reduced egg yield. Misshapen eggs may be laid following recovery. Mortality is usually low and due to secondary infections such as *E. coli*.
PREVENTION: Combined vaccines against this disease and INFECTIOUS BURSAL DISEASE, and against INFECTIOUS BRONCHITIS and NEWCASTLE DISEASE, are available. (Glaxo).

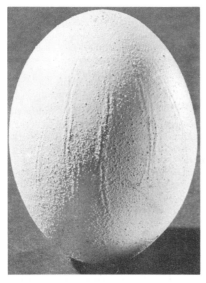

Infectious bronchitis can result in a marked deterioration in egg quality with consequent heavy economic loss. The illustration shows some of the effects, which include roughening and scoring of the shell. Shells may also be distorted and thin, or soft shelled eggs may be laid by infected birds. (With acknowledgement to Glaxo Laboratories Ltd.)

INFECTIOUS BURSAL DISEASE (IBD) of
chicks, a subclinical infection can have an immuno-suppressive effect which may interfere with vaccination against Newcastle disease. IBD has a world-wide distribution, and is also known as GUMBORO DISEASE. It affects broilers 1–5 weeks old, with symptoms of listlessness and diarrhoea. Mortality may be fairly high at the beginning of an outbreak.

The disease has been endemic in the UK for over 17 years, but until 1988 it had not caused significant losses. However, in that year a highly virulent strain of IBD virus appeared.

In 1990 it was causing heavy losses in both egg and broiler production.

INFECTIOUS LARYNGOTRACHEITIS (see under AVIAN).

INFECTIOUS NASAL GRANULOMATA IN CATTLE.
In certain parts of India cattle in restricted areas (sometimes in single herds only) may become affected with this condition. Large tumour-like masses develop in connection with the frontal sinus and the turbinated bones in the nasal passages.

The cause is a Schistosome, *S. nasalis*, which is present in the veins of the nasal mucous membrane.
TREATMENT. Intravenous injection of tartar emetic repeated 5 or 6 times at weekly intervals. Lithium antimony thiomalate intra-muscularly has now replaced tartar emetic to some extent.

INFECTIOUS NECROTIC HEPATITIS (see BLACK DISEASE).

INFECTIOUS PUSTULAR VULVOVAGINITIS
(see under VULVOVAGINITIS).

INFECTIOUS STUNTING SYNDROME (see STUNTING).

INFECTIVE DRUG RESISTANCE.
Resistant strains of bacteria may arise as a result of chromosomal mutation. In 1959 Japanese workers demonstrated another type of resistance transmissible from a resistant bacterial cell to a sensitive one merely by contact. (See ANTIBIOTIC RESISTANCE.)

INFERTILITY.
Insidious but great losses are directly due to failure to breed on the part of otherwise promising animals. The immediate loss to the individual owner of live-stock is not so apparent as with certain specific diseases, but it is infinitely greater than the loss accruing from any other single specific or non-specific disease. This loss is made up by the keep of the barren animals, the absence of offspring, reduction of the milk supply, and interference with breeding programmes. (See also CALVING INTERVAL.)

Causes. The most common and important causes of infertility can be grouped for convenience under the following headings.
1. FEEDING AND CONDITION. Under-feeding is a common cause of infertility in heifers. There must be adequate protein of good quality in the diet, and adequate vitamin A (and perhaps C), plus adequate copper, iodine, and other trace elements. These include manganese. A diet rich in calcium but poor in phosphorus may, in the in-calf cow, lead to resorption of the fetus. (See also CALCIUM SUPPLEMENTS.)

Excessive fat, on the other hand, may also lead to infertility or to inability on the part of the male to accomplish coitus. (See also 'FATTY LIVER SYNDROME'.)

In cows, temporary infertility may apparently be closely associated with the feeding at about the time of service. Cows losing weight are likely to be affected, especially if fed on poor-quality hay or silage. With *ad lib.* feeding systems, heifers and more timid cows may not be receiving enough roughage. Kale is sometimes responsible.

In ewes, infertility and fetal death are always serious in many hill areas, the result – to quote Dr John Stamp – 'of keeping pregnant sheep under conditions of near-starvation during the winter months when weather conditions are atrocious'. (*See* DIET, FLUSHING OF EWES, STILL-BORN, REPRODUCTION, VITAMINS, KALE, SELENIUM.)

II. ENVIRONMENT AND MANAGEMENT. A sudden change of environment, close confinement in dark quarters (formerly the lot of many a bull), lack of exercise may all predispose to, or produce, infertility. Abnormal segregation of the sexes and the use of vasectomised males (for purposes of detecting oestrus) are other factors. A low level of nutrition may cause a quiescent or dormant state on the part of the ovaries. At the same time there are seasonal cycles of sexual activity, and a 'failure to breed' during the winter months may be natural enough, even if the farmer regards it as infertility. This 'winter infertility', as it is often called, may be influenced by temperature, length of daylight, lack of pasture oestrogens, underfeeding, etc. At this season, heifers often have inactive ovaries, while in cows irregular and 'silent' heats give low conception rates.

Infertility may result from the oestrogenic effects of red clover in the UK, as well as from subterranean clovers in Australia.

III. DISEASES OF THE GENITAL ORGANS IN FEMALE. This is a very long list, and includes some of the commonest and most important conditions which bring about infertility.

Inflammation or other disease of the ovaries. Ovaritis; the non-maturation of Graäfian follicles, from any cause, and the presence in the ovary of cysts (which often form from a corpus luteum), are causes of infertility; another is blocked Fallopian tubes.

Persistent corpora lutea. Not only do they apparently predispose to uterine infection, but they inhibit the ripening of the next Graäfian follicles, and therefore ovulation cannot occur. Spurious oestrus may be shown, but service is always unsuccessful. (*See under* OVARIES, DISEASES OF; HORMONES *and* HORMONE THERAPY.)

Inflammation of the uterine mucous membrane. A large number of cases of infertility can be ascribed to infection of the uterus (metritis) or the oviduct by organisms. **(For a list of the infections which cause infertility,** *see under* ABORTION. **For infections causing infertility in the mare,** *see under* EQUINE GENITAL INFECTIONS.)

When the condition is mild, following a previous calving, it may disappear spontaneously, but in many instances it persists and becomes chronic. Associated with inflammation of the mucous membrane of the uterus or oviduct is often a persistent corpus luteum in the ovary. Carelessness during parturition, the use of unclean instruments or appliances, decomposition of retained membranes, and other similar factors, also bring about infection of the uterus. *Brucellosis* though not necessarily itself a cause of sterility, by lowering the vital resistance of the uterus, favours infection by a multitude of other organisms which normally may be non-pathogenic. The details of uterine infection, including salpingitis (inflammation of the oviduct), in the causation of sterility, are highly technical, but, generally speaking, it may be said that the presence of organisms in the uterus, or the presence of the products of their activity, either kills the spermatozoa, or renders the locality unsuitable for anchorage of the fertilised ovum (or ova), with the result that it perishes.

Abnormalities of the cervix may prevent conception – mechanically when the lumen is occluded or plugged by mucus of a thick tenacious nature, and pathologically when there is acute inflammation of the mucous membrane of the cervix, or even of the whole uterus. Scirrhous cervix – where much fibrous tissue is laid down in the cervix – when very advanced may cause sterility, but by itself is not usually of great importance. It is much more serious as a hindrance to parturition. (*See, for example*, RING-WOMB of the ewe.) Cysts and fibrous bands in the os are seldom sufficiently extensive to occlude the passage through the cervical canal. Occlusion may, however, occur as the result of swelling and congestion of the mucous membrane, due to infection and inflammation. In such cases the sperms are unable to penetrate into the uterus, and fertilisation does not occur. This may also be the result of acidity (and thickened mucus) following a mild infection, and sometimes syringing the vagina a short time before service with a weak alkaline solution (*e.g.* 5 per cent bicarbonate of potassium) proves successful. (*See* 'WHITES', 'EPIVAG'.)

Tumours, either malignant or benign.

Specific disease, such as tuberculosis in cattle, or in mares. Contagious equine uretritis. (*See* VULVO-VAGINITIS.)

IV. HEREDITARY ABNORMALITIES IN THE FEMALE. *Freemartin* (*see under* this heading).

Hypoplasia of the ovaries of cows may occur as an inherited condition in the female. It may involve one or both ovaries, causing either infertility or complete sterility. The uterus, also, may be hypoplastic. (*See also under* GENETICS.)

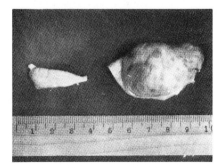

Hypoplasia of the left ovary of a cow of the Swedish Highland breed. Compare its size with that of the normal right ovary from the same animal. (The ruler is graduated in centimetres.)

Endocrine failure. Heredity may be involved.

Hermaphroditism.

'*White heifer disease*' (*see under this heading and diagram below*).

It was stated in 1967 that 10 per cent of female pigs are sterile. Group studies have shown that 25

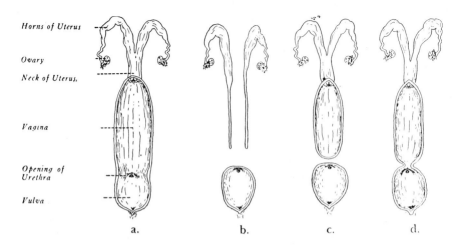

Malformation of the genital organs leading to sterility are shown in the diagram and compared with the normal. a, normal organs; b, the ducts fail to unite to form a vagina; c, vagina formed but does not open into the vulva; d, narrow passage between vagina and vulva. (This diagram is reproduced with acknowledgement to Dr G. F. Finlay, University of Sydney.)

to 50 per cent of infertile gilts had abnormalities of the genital tract sufficient to cause sterility, and two-thirds of these were regarded as hereditary.

V. DISEASE OF THE GENITAL ORGANS IN MALE.

Orchitis, or inflammation of the testicle, and *Epididymitis*, inflammation of the epididymis, due to injury from kicks, or to infection from external wounds, or from specific infection, such as *brucellosis* or *trichomoniasis* in the bull. (*See* TESTICLE, DISEASES OF; VENEREAL INFECTIONS.)

Tumours of the testicles may destroy the tubules or prevent spermatogenesis, and on the penis, or in connection with the prepuce, may act as purely mechanical agents, which prevent coitus by the male.

Adhesions between penis and prepuce, the result of acute or chronic balanitis, though rare, may cause mechanical inability to protrude the penis and fertilise the female. (*See also under* PENIS.)

Inflammation in the secondary sexual glands – i.e. in prostate, seminal vesicles, or other glands – may occlude the vasa deferentia or ejaculatory ducts, and cause inability to pass semen, while in other cases the semen may be so altered as to cause death of the sperms in the female passages.

Affection of the prepuce, such as balanitis, and injuries accompanied by laceration or severe bruising, may cause temporary sterility, but when recovery occurs fertility returns. (*See also under* PENIS.)

VI. HEREDITARY ABNORMALITIES IN THE MALE.

Cryptorchidism, in which one or both testes do not descend into the scrotum, is a well-known cause of infertility in the male. When one testis properly descends, and is fully developed, conception may follow service, and a sire suffering from this disability has upon some occasions been regularly used in a flock or herd; but when the rig animal has both organs retained, although sexual desire may be emphatic, service is usually unsuccessful. The condition unfits a male animal for use as a breeding sire, since there is evidence that it is a hereditary unsoundness. (*See* HORMONE THERAPY.)

HYPOPLASIA or under-development of the male sex organs, particularly of the testis, is an important cause of sterility. It may involve both testicles or only one.

ENDOCRINE FAILURE may arise as a result of an inherited predisposition. In bulls this may occur in later life, rendering them sterile *after* they have produced a number of progeny which, in their turn, may perpetuate this form of infertility.

Hermaphrodism, or *Hermaphroditism*, in which an animal possesses both male and female organs, but is without a full complement of either, is usually, but not always, associated with sterility. (*See also* GENETICS, INTERSEX.)

VII. PHYSICAL OR PSYCHICAL INABILITY OR DISTURBANCE.

Under this heading are grouped a number of conditions which are difficult to classify elsewhere. Some occur in the male, some in the female, and some are common to both sexes.

Incompatibility between the blood of sire and dam may be responsible for some cases of abortion in cattle, etc. (*See* HAEMOLYTIC DISEASE.)

Old age. When an animal reaches a certain age reproduction becomes impossible. The periods of oestrus cease. Breeding ceases earlier in the females than in the male.

Discrepancies in size between male and female may result in failure to breed. The penis may be too short, or too large; the vagina may be too long or too small; the female may not have the strength to carry a heavy male; or the male may not be tall enough to reach the female.

Injuries to the back, hips, hind legs, or feet of the male, and sometimes to the same regions of the female, may be severe enough to prevent successful coitus. Progressive spinal arthritis is a common condition in bulls. (*See also* BREEDING OF ANIMALS; REPRODUCTION; EMBRYOLOGY; UTERUS, DISEASES OF; HORMONE THERAPY; GENETICS;

VENEREAL DISEASES; ANOESTRUS; ABORTION; MUM-
MIFICATION.)

INFLAMMATION may be briefly defined as the
reaction of the tissues to any injury, short of one
sufficiently severe to cause death. There are four
cardinal symptoms of inflammation, viz. heat,
pain, redness, and swelling, to which may be
added interference with function. (*See* ABSCESS,
WOUNDS, ALLERGY.)

For the inflammations of special organs *see
under* PNEUMONIA, PLEURISY, PERITONITIS, MAM-
MARY GLAND, etc.

For anti-inflammatory drugs, *see* CORTICO-
STEROIDS, CORTICOTROPHIN, CORTISONE, IBU-
FROFEN, FLURBIPROFEN, GLYCYRRETINIC ACID,
ANTIHISTAMINES, CALAMINE.

INFLUENZA. Scientifically, this term is now
applied only to diseases caused by a myxovirus.
The World Health Organisation was much
exercised as to what happens to the virus of
human influenza between epidemics. It has long
been known that there is a relationship between
this disease and swine influenza. The human influenza virus (Type A) was isolated from the
parasitic pig lung-worm. Larvae of these lungworms are harboured by earthworms – the only
known intermediate hosts – which live for as long
as ten years.

In 1957 WHO stated: 'In the inter-epidemic
periods, the virus is not found in the tissues of the
pigs. However, earthworms taken from infected
pig farms seem to carry inapparent viruses, and
these can develop, in pigs eating the worms, into
normal viruses capable of being isolated from the
respiratory system. The question, therefore, arises
whether the pigs are, in fact, the virus reservoirs,
rather than being secondarily infected by the
human virus, as some have maintained.' (*See also*
SWINE INFLUENZA.)

In 1972–3 WHO drew attention to the accumulating evidence that influenza viruses of mammals
and birds play an important part in the emergence
of new viruses which cause outbreaks of illness in
man in several continents.

The recovery from pigs in Taiwan in 1970 of
influenza virus indistinguishable from that
causing Type A Hong Kong influenza epidemics
in man in 1968 provided the first direct evidence of
the inter-species transfer of influenza viruses. Pigs
experimentally inoculated with that virus transmitted it to pen mates. Moreover the Taiwan virus
taken from pigs readily infected human volunteers, who developed antibodies effective against
virus from both pigs and people.

It is now suggested that the Hong Kong human
influenza virus did not arise by mutation from a
pre-existing human strain, but that it probably
arose from the mixed infection in a mammal or
bird with an animal influenza virus and a human
Type A Asian strain. The animal virus may have
provided certain subunits or components; the
other sub-units having come from a human strain.

'Sera collected in 1967 and 1972 from people in
the 0–100 age-group showed haemagglutination-
inhibition (HI) antibody to swine virus
A/Iowa/15/39 (Hsw1N1) in greatest number and

with highest titre in people born before 1918. The
recently isolated A/New Jersey/10/76 (Hsw1N1)
virus showed a result comparable to that of the
Swine/1930 virus in sera of 1972. On the analogy
of the findings in 1968, when the Hong Kong virus
became epidemic in human populations and antibody to this virus was found in sera of people over
70 years, the suggestion is made that the recurrence of swine virus as an epidemic agent of
human influenza may be expected around 1986.'
(Dr N. Masurel, *Lancet* (1976, July 31.)

1986. Recommended vaccines should contain
the following antigens, WHO stated:
A/Philippines/2/82(H3N2)-like strain; A/Chile/
1/83(H1N1)-like strain; B/USSR/100/83-like
strain.

Influenza in the horse – (*see under* EQUINE IN-
FLUENZA). Pneumonia in calves may be caused by
a virus of influenza-type.

In the dog parainfluenza virus SV5 has been
isolated in the USA, UK from dogs with upper
respiratory disease. (*See* 'KENNEL COUGH'.)

Avian strains of type A influenza virus cause a
number of diseases in hens, ducks, turkeys, etc.
During 1980 and 1981 nine subtypes of influenza
A virus were isolated from birds in Britain,
usually as a result of investigations of disease or
death. However these viruses were shown to be of
low virulence for chickens. Highly pathogenic
avian influenza virus had been isolated from
turkeys, mainly in Norfolk, in 1979; and was the
cause of economically devastating outbreaks
among turkeys in the USA between 1977 and
1979. (D. J. Alexander. *Vet. Record* (1982) **111,**
319.) (*See* AVIAN INFLUENZA.)

'INFLUENZA', CAT (*see* FELINE INFLUENZA).

INFRA-RED lamps are used in the creeps of piggeries and in poultry brooders. Either 'bright' or
'dull' emitters are available; the latter being preferred for chick-rearing. They have many advantages, but a power-cut can cause severe losses.
(*See also under* LIGHT TREATMENT; TOES, TWISTED.)

INGUINAL CANAL is the passage from the abdominal cavity to the outside down which pass
the spermatic cords and their associated structures in the male, while in the female the vessels
of the mammary gland pass through the canal to
the udder. It is a slit-like opening, about 5 inches
long in the horse, and is directed downwards, inwards, and forwards. It is bounded behind by a
strong band called the inguinal or *Poupart's* ligament. The canal is important, because if it is
dilated from any cause some part of the small
intestines may pass through it, resulting in
inguinal hernia. (*See* HERNIAS.) It serves as the
opening through which retained testicles are
removed in the 'rig' or cryptorchid animal.

INGUINAL REGION is the region of the inguinal
canal, that is, that part of the posterior and
uppermost division of the abdominal wall which
lies in below the brim of the pelvis. The scrotum,
penis, and their vessels, etc., are situated in the
inguinal region in the male horse, and in the
female the mammary glands with the vessels that

supply them. In some animals, such as the dog and boar, the scrotum is farther back, *i.e.* in the perineal region, while in the bull and ram the penis is farther forwards.

INHERITED DEFECTS/DISEASES are referred to under GENETICS. *See also* DEFORMITIES, and HORSES, CONFORMATION DEFECTS.

INJECTIONS may be hypodermic or subcutaneous, intradermal, intra-muscular, intravenous (into a vein), intraperitoneal (into the abdominal cavity), epidural. Precautions must be taken against the introduction of bacteria, dirt, etc. The hair should be clipped away at the site of injection, and the skin cleaned with spirit or an antiseptic. Needles and syringes should be sterilised before use, unless of the disposal type intended for once-only use and already sterilised and in a sealed wrapper.

Where the material to be injected is already fluid, this is generally guaranteed sterile by the manufacturers, and is put up in sealed vials. In cases where the drug has to be dissolved in water first, only water that has been recently boiled and allowed to cool should be used, and solution of the drug should take place in a perfectly clean vessel. Neglect of these precautions is likely to be followed by the formation of an abscess at the point of injection or even by septicaemia.

The syringe having been filled with the drug in solution, a fold of the skin is picked up between the thumb and forefinger of the left hand, and the needle is inserted into the middle of this fold. The nozzle of the syringe is slipped into the head of the needle and the piston is slowly but firmly pressed home so as to expel the contents into the loose tissues under the skin. Care should be taken that all air-bubbles are excluded from the barrel of the syringe, as it is unwise to introduce them.

With herd inoculations on the farm in mind, a device was introduced in 1982 under the proprietary name Sterimatic, to reduce the risk from contaminated needles on syringes or multi-dose injection 'guns'. A retractible sleeve with a sterilising cap fits over the needle to protect the operator. Both the site of the injection and the needle are, it is claimed, sterilised automatically after every injection; the needle needing replacement only after some 50 injections.

PRECAUTIONS. Restless animals should always be secured so that they will not make a sudden plunge when the needle is introduced, and break the stem of the needle. Abscesses in hams are common in pigs, and doubtless result from anti-anaemia intra-muscular injections made without due precautions as to cleanliness and to broken-off needles.

The sciatic nerve may be damaged as the result of an intra-muscular injection into a pig's ham. This site should be avoided, and it has been recommended that the injection be given into the muscles of the neck, just behind the ear, and not into fatty tissue. (Van Alstine, W. G. & Dietrich, J.A. *Compendium of Continuing Education* (1988) **10** 1329.) They reported that within one to eight weeks of an injection of an antibiotic into the ham of 180 4-week-old pigs, 180 had paralysis of that leg.

Care must be taken not to make what should be a subcutaneous injection into the chest. This danger was illustrated when a farmer injected 500 lambs, using a multidose syringe intended for cattle, and with a ¼-inch needle. Within a week 17 of the lambs had died; autopsy showing pyothorax and a pure growth of *Corynebacterium pyogenes*. The Perth VI Centre demonstrated on a dead lamb, that it was possible to reach the pleural cavity with the above cattle syringe, especially in thin lambs; and suggested that probably many other 'vaccine failures' had been due to inadvertent injections into the chest. 'Alternative sites, such as the side of the neck, would appear to offer a much reduced chance of complications.' (Appleyard, W. T. & others, *Veterinary Record* (1986), **119**, 283.)

With intravenous injections of chloral hydrate, for example, severe tissue damage can follow if some of the drug enters the vein wall or surrounding tissue.

Inoculations should not be carried out in a dusty shed. (*See* ANTHRAX.)

With stable compounds the route of administration has little influence on the end result; not so, however, with unstable ones. 1000 mg per kg of thalidomide produces no central depression in mice when given subcutaneously. The same dose given intraperitoneally gives rapid and profound sedation. Clearly, if one pharmacological action can depend on the route of administration, another may. (K. Hellman, *Lancet*, February 19, 1966.) (*See also* AMPOULE, DETERGENT RESIDUE, PANJET, *and* ENEMA.)

Accidental self-inoculation may occur owing to the sudden violent movement of a large animal. People have been infected with BRUCELLOSIS in this way; and a veterinary surgeon died from IMMOBILON. Additionally, adjuvanted oil-based vaccines may cause ill-effects in farmers and others accidentally self-inoculated.

INJURIES (*see* ACCIDENTS, WOUNDS, FRACTURES, BLEEDING, SHOCK).

INJURIES FROM SHOEING. These are not always the fault of the smith. There are some horses with such bad feet that it may be quite impossible to shoe them without running the risk of injuring the sensitive structures in the process. The nails, toe-clips, or even the shoe, may inflict damage.

(1) **THE NAILS** may produce lameness either by actually penetrating the sensitive laminae – a condition called 'pricking'; or, by being driven too close to the laminae, they may press upon the sensitive structures – a condition known as 'binding'.

Pricking may be only slight when the farrier knows that the nail has stabbed the quick and immediately withdraws it. All nail injuries should receive prompt attention, for they are usually amenable to treatment in the early stages; but if neglected they rapidly suppurate, causing the horse great pain and often permanent damage.

Binding is not so serious. Generally it suffices to remove the shoe, allow the horse to remain barefooted for a day or so, and then to replace the shoe, taking special care that the nails are not driven too coarsely upon the second occasion. The lameness in this case very often only appears two or three days after the horse has been shod, and is attributed to some other cause.

(2) THE CLIP may produce lameness by being driven too coarsely, and either burning the sensitive structures when being fitted, or pressing upon them unduly when hammered into position afterwards. When side-clips are used, *i.e.* one on each side of the foot, if they are forced home too far the foot is jammed in between two rigid structures which will not allow it to expand and contract with each movement of the foot, and lameness results. The shoe should be removed, the horse given a day or two's rest, the clips altered, and the shoe reapplied, when he will usually go sound. If burning is suspected, the same procedure may be adopted. If the shoe loosens till it is only holding by one nail, or if the shoe is partially torn off, the horse may tread on the clip which penetrates the sole of the foot and inflict a very severe wound. This is treated as for pricking, the area being pared out.

(3) THE SHOE may cause injury if it has an uneven surface and presses upon one part too much. This is particularly liable to happen when the horn of the foot is weak and thin. Horses with flat feet, or those with dropped sole, may develop bruises of the sole if the web of the shoe presses upon the outer circumference of the sole, where it joins the white line. In such cases the shoe should be removed and the unevenness corrected, or the bearing surface of the foot should be eased. Some horses may require to be shod with a barshoe, so that the frog may take some of the weight off the affected part, and others need a run at grass.

Burning of the sensitive parts of the foot may occur through the carelessness of the smith, not by making the shoe too hot, but by holding it in position on the foot for too long a time, so that it may 'bed itself in'. This is a most reprehensible practice and should not be tolerated. The injury usually results in a separation of the horn from the sensitive tissues below, and some weeks pass before the horse can resume his work again. (*See* CORNS, BRUISED SOLE.)

INNOMINATE is the bone of the pelvis and the structures associated with it. The pelvis is composed of six separate bones, three on either side, viz. ilium, pubis, and ischium.

INOCULATION (*see* INJECTIONS, VACCINATION, INFECTION, *and* IMMUNITY).

INSECTICIDES. The late 1970s saw the introduction of the synthetic pyrethroids (e.g. cypermethrin and permethrin) – a notable advance in the field of insecticides.

Large animals. These insecticides for the protection of large animals are discussed under FLIES and FLY CONTROL.

The introduction of IVERMECTIN was another major advance; being not only a valuable anthelmintic but also a systemic insecticide, which can be given by mouth or by injection, and is effective against lice, fleas, and parasitic mites.

Small animals. Insecticides are available in formulations for application as wet shampoos, aerosol sprays, dry dusting powders, and 'flea collars'. Active ingredients include: permethrin, pybuthrin, derris, gamma BHC, iodofenphos, bromocyclen, carbaryl. Most of these ingredients are found in both wet shampoos and dry dusting powders. Aerosol spray ingredients include permethrin, bromocyclen, dichlorvos, propoxur. Dichlorvos and diazinon (both organophosphorus compounds) are used in 'flea collars'.

Manufacturers' instructions should be strictly followed, and **only preparations stated to be safe for cats** should be used on those animals.

Over-exposure of animals to insecticides, either through too frequent use or use of excessive quantities, can lead to poisoning. (*See* CHLORINATED HYDROCARBONS, ORGANO-PHOSPHORUS POISONING; *also* PERMETHRIN.)

Accidental poisoning. DDT fell into disrepute in the UK, USA, Australia and New Zealand, but is still used for ground spraying in Africa (*see* DDT). The use of unsuitable insecticides can lead to fatal poisoning in cattle, etc. (*See* TEPP.) Poisoning may occur following absorption of an unsuitable insecticide spray through the skin. This, or inhalation of spray droplets, may lead to dangerously contaminated milk. In the USA the following insecticides are *not* recommended for dairy and cowshed use on account of this risk: DDT, aldrin, dieldrin, chlordane, lindane, methoxychlor, toxaphene, and heptachlor. (*See* CHLORINATED HYDROCARBONS.)

Some insecticides may be safe for one species of animal but fatal to another. For example, on a farm in New York State an insecticide spray containing thiophosphate had no effect on 50 chickens, but killed over 7000 ducklings.

Dieldrin, used as a seed dressing, has caused fatal poisoning in wood-pigeons and other wild birds. Lambs have been killed by ALDRIN (which see). (*See* BHC, DDT, DIELDRIN, DERRIS, TEPP, PARATHION, PYRETHRUM, SYSTEMIC, NANKOR, FLY CONTROL, CARBAMATES, CHLORINATED HYDROCARBONS, GAME-BIRDS, etc.)

Insecticide resistance. In about the year 1946 house flies showed resistance to DDT, and by 1970 some 250 species of fly affecting man, his animals or crops, had developed resistance to one or more of the organochlorines, *e.g.* dieldrin, organo-phosphates; or carbamates.

Most cases of resistance apparently depend on a single gene, and are developed mostly following large-scale use of insecticides in control programmes. (*See also under* FLY CONTROL.)

INSECTS. For a general description of these, *see* FLIES.

INSULATION OF BUILDINGS, FLOORS (*see under* HOUSING OF ANIMALS).

INSULIN is a hormone secreted by part of the pancreas, where it is produced by the Islets of Langerhans. It is used in the treatment of diabetes in dogs and cats. (*See* DIABETES.)

INSULINOMA. A tumour affecting cells of the Islets of Langerhans in the pancreas, which may lead to collapse, convulsions, coma and death in the dog as a result of hypoglycaemia. (A. C. Palmer, *Vet. Rec.* (1972), **90**, 167.)

INSURANCE. In the UK there is now a wide choice of comprehensive insurance policies available to animal-owners. Farmers can insure against the risks of foot-and-mouth disease or brucellosis, for example, through policies underwritten by Lloyds or by Pet Plan Insurance (also in London). There is insurance for horses. Dog- and cat-owners can avail themselves of policies covering veterinary fees, third-party liability, theft or death of an animal from illness or accident. Policies can be issued through veterinary surgeons. With the possibility of having to pay for a major operation or prolonged treatment, such policies can minimise the owner's financial outlay, and are a safeguard against unexpected and sometimes large expenses.

INTENSIVE LIVE-STOCK PRODUCTION. This means, generally speaking, having farm animals indoors to a greater extent, and also having them within a smaller space inside a building.

The economic *advantages* claimed for intensive live-stock production are the economies of scale through reducing costs of labour and equipment per animal housed; lower feed costs through bulk buying and home mixing; the ability to afford skilled management and labour; also a saving in acres of valuable land.

The *disadvantages* are the effect on stock of large concentration, disease, cannibalism and all the problems of stress, and intensive feeding methods.

Intensive live-stock production was the subject of a government enquiry. (*See under* BRAMBELL.)

The following describes potential hazards and health problems, and should not be regarded as condemnation of all current farming methods!

Poultry. De-beaking, badly done, can reduce resistance to infection. Birds de-beaked and unable to take a dust bath are prone to severe infestation with lice and mites, both now commonly resistant to the commonly used parasiticides; and infestation is a problem in battery houses. Lack of exercise is conducive to fatty degeneration of the liver in battery birds. Among birds crowded together on deep litter coccidiosis and worm infestations are apt to be serious. Faulty ventilation often gives rise to a harmful concentration of ammonia in houses where there is litter, and also predisposes to infectious bronchitis, and other respiratory infections. The greater the concentration of birds, the greater the stress, it seems; and the more chance of an increasing proportion both of susceptible birds and of 'carriers' of various infections.

Beef cattle. In calf-rearing units, salmonella infections cause a high proportion of the deaths of bought-in calves. Bronchitis is also an important cause of losses, which often amount to 7 per cent.

In units taking in 12-week-old calves, respiratory disease, principally virus infections, are important. Other conditions encountered include: foul-in-the-foot, infectious bovine keratitis, and bloat.

If trough space is too limited, inflammation of the eyes may be caused by cattle flicking their ears into their neighbours' eyes – simulating the effects of infectious bovine keratitis.

Among veal calves, pneumonia and a peracute coliform septicaemia are major causes of losses. Anaemia, parasites, and a form of anaphylactic shock are also among the hazards of rearing.

Pigs. These animals are particularly prone to the effects of stress (discussed under that heading), and of confinement in poorly ventilated buildings which favours respiratory infections such as enzootic pneumonia.

Dr D. W. B. Sainsbury has strongly advocated the use of farrow-to-finish pens which accommodate pigs from birth to slaughter day and obviate four or five moves to strange surroundings with its accompanying stress.

Sheep. Respiratory troubles, including various forms of pneumonia, are a danger in buildings where ventilation is poor. There are some very successful flock houses, with one end virtually open, where disease problems have been minimal; foot-rot being controlled by regular use of a foot-bath. In such buildings, the ewes lamb indoors, to the great advantage of the shepherd. Straw is used for bedding. Yorkshire boarding assists ventilation.

Lameness. Intensive systems of farming tend to ignore the social behaviour of animals to the detriment of their health. Two good examples involving lameness in cattle were described by Mr G. P. David of Shrewsbury veterinary investigation centre. In the first case 12 heifers which had been used to being in a small social group outside in a straw yard were abruptly transferred at calving and put in with cows in modern concrete based cow cubicles. Five became acutely lame with septic and aseptic laminitis and solar ulceration. In two the condition was so severe that they had to be slaughtered, but the other heifers improved when they were transferred to straw yards.

Mr David explained that the outbreak was thought to be related to the sudden introduction to concrete surfaces and uncomfortable cubicles which reduced the time that the animals lay down. Increased activity caused by behavioural interactions with the established cows was probably also a factor.

The second case involved an outbreak of solar ulcerations in 90 per cent of a small herd of dairy cows. It coincided with the occupation of a new cubicle house with concrete based lipless cubicles. When given an opportunity the cows 'voted with their feet' and returned to their old earth-floored cubicles.

(*See also* HOUSING OF ANIMALS.)

INTERCOSTAL. Between the ribs.

INTERCURRENT is a term applied to one disease which occurs during the course of another disease already present, and modifies its course or increases its severity.

INTERDIGITAL CYST, or INTERDIGITAL ABSCESS, is a condition commonly affecting the feet of dogs, in which abscesses about the size of a pea or larger appear in the spaces between the digits of the paws. It most often affects Spaniels, Airedales, Scots terriers, Sealyhams, Dandie Dinmonts.
CAUSES are generally held to be an infection of the hair follicles between the toes, or to grit penetrating the skin there. In some instances the lesion may be a true cyst.
SIGNS. The dog licks his foot, and upon examination a swelling (which is painful) is noticed in the inter-digital space. Within a couple of days or so, the swelling may discharge a little blood-stained pus. If the lesions have been repeatedly forming, they may suddenly cease, and the dog remains free from them for perhaps months at a time. Unfortunately, recurrences are likely at varying intervals.
TREATMENT. The foot is bandaged to keep the wound clean, dressed daily until there is no more discharge and the wound has healed. Some encouraging results have been obtained by the professional use of CRYOSURGERY.)

INTERDIGITAL NECROBACILLOSIS (see 'FOUL-IN-THE-FOOT').

INTERFERON. A substance which inhibits the multiplication of viruses within living cells. The first chicken interferon was discovered in 1957, but hopes that interferons could be immediately used in medicine were not fulfilled.
Many cells produce interferon as a defence mechanism against further spread of viral infection. 'The stimulus seems to be double-stranded R NA, released during replication of most R NA and DNA viruses.' (Lancet, Nov. 20, 1976). Interferon does not prevent the virus from entering a cell, but 'specifically inhibits translation of viral messenger R NA.'
While interferons have, in limited trials, afforded protection against some virus infections, their use is still not practicable on anything but a limited scale; and research turned more to discovering non-toxic interferon inducers – which would stimulate production by the body of interferons – rather than on using interferons obtained by artificial means.
In 1982 WHO commented: 'In malignant disease, complete regression of tumours has rarely been achieved by interferon treatment, and no response has been observed in the majority of (human) patients.
'Interferons are not a panacea for the cure of human virus infections or cancer.'

Until recently, interferon has been a very scarce and expensive commodity. However, recombinant DNA techniques have made possible the production of interferons in larger quantities and at a much reduced cost; and their use in veterinary medicine is likely in the near future.
Interferon is being used in several countries as an adjunct to post-exposure prophylaxis of human rabies; but WHO's 1982 words remain valid.

INTERNAL HAEMORRHAGE may result from rupture of some large blood-vessel; or it may be the result of an injury to some organ that is richly supplied with blood, such as the liver or spleen. In either case the bleeding occurs into one of the body cavities and the blood is lost to the tissues of the animal. (See also HAEMANGIOSARCOMA, and diseases with names beginning with the word HAEMORRHAGIC, WARFARIN POISONING.)
SIGNS of severe internal haemorrhage include extreme pallor of mouth and mucous membrane lining the eyelids, coldness of the skin, rapid breathing, or a series of gasps, collapse, and a pulse becoming weak, slow, and then imperceptible. (See SHOCK.)
TREATMENT of severe internal haemorrhage can seldom be undertaken in time to save life. When the internal bleeding is less profuse, success may be achieved with ADRENALIN, BLOOD TRANSFUSION or DEXTRAN, VITAMIN K.

INTERSEX. An individual with characteristics intermediate between those of a male and a female. In cattle, examples include the FREEMARTIN (which see); XY gonadal dysgenesis (in which there are no gonads); and testicular feminisation. A case of the latter, described by Dr S. E. Long, was a single born cow showing signs of virilism and found to have abdominal testes, some undeveloped Mullerian duct derivatives, a normal vagina, and a 60XY genotype in all tissues examined.
In a canine example of intersex, the os penis was absent, the penis could not be extruded from the prepuce, and no testicles were present in the scrotum. A laparotomy revealed a uterus and ovaries.
(See under TRISOMY for the case of an intersex Spanish-bred horse, 'considered to be a mare,' which had the characteristics of a pseudo-hermaphrodite male.)

INTERSTITIAL is a term applied to cells of different tissue set amongst the active tissue cells of an organ. It is generally of a supporting character and formed of fibrous tissue. The term is also applied to diseases which specially affect this tissue, as interstitial nephritis. (See under KIDNEYS, DISEASES OF – Chronic nephritis.)

INTERVERTEBRAL DISC PROTRUSION (see under SPINE and NANDROLONE).

INTESTINAL ADENOMATOSIS (*see under* PORCINE).

INTESTINES.

Horse. (1) Small Intestine. This measures about 70 feet, and is divided into a fixed portion – *duodenum*, and a more or less free portion – *jejunum* and *ileum*. Its diameter varies from 1½ to 3 inches when moderately distended, and its capacity is about 12 gallons.

(2) Large Intestine. This extends from the end of the ileum to the anus, and measures about 25 feet in length. Its diameter varies in different parts from about 3 inches in the small colon to nearly 20 inches across the widest part of the caecum. It is divided into *caecum, large colon, small colon,* and *rectum*. The caecum is a large blind sac lying on the right side of the abdomen and extending downwards and forwards to within a hand's-breadth from the sternum. It is shaped somewhat like a reversed comma, having both its entrance and exit near the base, and has a capacity of about 8 gallons. Foodstuff enters it by the ileo-caecal valve, and leaves by the *caeco-colic valve*, whence commences the large colon.

Cows. The intestines lie entirely to the right of the middle line of the abdomen. (1) Small intestine, measuring 130 feet in length, lies in the lower part of the right side of the abdomen, filling in the spaces left between more fixed organs. (2) Large intestine is much smaller than in the horse, and not so complicated. The caecum lies in the upper posterior part of the abdomen, with its blind sac posteriorly in or near the pelvic inlet. The caecum is about 2½ feet long and is followed by the colon (there is no small colon in the ox), which has a length of about 35 feet. The colon is arranged like the coils of a watch-spring, with each coil double, consisting of one part running towards the centre – *centripetal*, and a corresponding part running from the centre – *centrifugal*.

Sheep. The intestines of the sheep are similar to those of the cow.

Pigs. (1) Small Intestine. This varies from 50 to 65 feet in length, and mainly lies on the left side and floor of the abdomen, with some coils pushed across on to the right side of the body. (2) Large intestine is about 15 feet long and considerably wider than the small bowel.

Dogs. The intestines are short in this animal, only reaching a length of about 15 or 16 feet, of which the small intestine measures 12 to 14 feet. The small intestine occupies the right side of the abdomen and part of the floor. From here the colon has a short course upwards towards the head, turns across to the left side of the body, and then runs backwards to end in the rectum.

Structure. In all animals the intestines, both small and large, are constructed of four main coats. They all consist of an inner mucous membrane lining, a submucous coat, a middle muscular coat, and an outer peritoneal one.

Mucous membrane coat. This is the soft, moist, velvety lining which is found in all parts of the intestine. (*See* BRUSH BORDER, PEYER'S PATCHES, VILLUS.)

Muscular coat. There are two definite layers of muscle fibres in the wall of the bowel. The innermost of these has its fibres all running in a circular manner round the submucous coat, and the outer layer has fibres running lengthwise. In the large intestine some of these longitudinal fibres are collected into distinct bands called 'taenia', which being somewhat shorter than the other fibres cause a certain amount of puckering of the bowels. The muscular arrangement of the intestines is very important, as it is owing to it that all the movement of the bowels occurs. In health it is continually contracting and expanding, shortening and lengthening, and moving the food either onwards or backwards. During the process the food is squeezed and churned and most thoroughly mixed with the digestive juices. The movement is called 'peristalsis' when it tends to move the food towards the anus, and 'antiperistalsis' when it is in the opposite direction.

Peritoneal coat forms the outermost covering of the bowel. It is continuous for the whole length of the canal from the pylorus to the anus, except for certain comparatively small regions where, for example, the duodenum and the caecum are bound directly to the roof of the abdomen or to other organs by fibrous tissue. It is a tough membrane with a layer of smooth glistening cells on its outer surface which rub against similar cells on the surfaces of adjacent organs and reduce friction to a minimum. (*See* PERITONEUM.)

Attachments. The intestines are hung or held in position by folds of peritoneum which bind them, directly or indirectly, to some part of the abdominal wall. The fold in which the free part of the small intestine hangs is called the 'mesentery of the small intestine', and it is through this that the blood and lymph vessels and the nerves enter and leave the bowel. It is composed of two layers, in the middle of which pass the vessels.

FUNCTIONS (*see* DIGESTION).

INTESTINES, DISEASES OF. Intestinal inflammation, or ENTERITIS, is a common disease in all animals, and may take an acute or chronic form. In either case the chief symptom is diarrhoea. In acute enteritis, diarrhoea leads to DEHYDRATION; while in the chronic form, the animal ceases to thrive and the abdomen becomes permanently 'tucked up'. The causes and treatment of enteritis are given under DIARRHOEA.

PERFORATION of part of the intestine may follow ulceration, itself a complication of some cases of enteritis. Perforation may also follow stabbing injuries such as goring by bulls, war injuries to horses, farm and road accidents, or the swallowing of sharp-pointed objects. (*See* FOREIGN BODIES.) Perforation of the wall of the intestine is obviously a very serious condition and an immediate threat to the animal's life, since bacteria which accompany partly digested food escaping from the intestine will cause PERITONITIS (which see).

Necrosis and infarction may be detected by assessing the serum levels of CREATINE kinase (which see). (*See also* VOLVULUS, INTUSSUSCEPTION, COLIC.)

INTESTINE, OBSTRUCTION. This may result from an impacted mass of food material. (*See* IMPACTION.) In the dog, for example, a hard mass containing spicules of bone may render defaecation impossible, and an enema will be necessary if a dose of medicinal liquid paraffin does not achieve the desired result. In the cat a mass of fur may similarly cause obstruction. FOREIGN BODIES of many kinds, including string, are another cause.

Wood chewing. A bad habit of some horses, whether stabled or at grass, which can lead to obstruction of the small intestine.
SIGNS. Colic, passage of stomach contents down both nostrils.
TREATMENT. Enterotomy under a general anaesthetic. This, in one of two cases, produced an enterolith 'as hard as coal, and black.' (Green, P. & Tong, J. M. J. *Veterinary Record* (1988) page 186.)

Duodenal obstruction in cattle, though not common, has been described by Van der Velden. In most cases the obstruction is due to decreased motility of the duodenum, caused by inflammation of the duodenal wall and preperforative peritonitis, resulting from duodenal ulcers or penetrating foreign bodies respectively.

Other causes. A strangulated HERNIA is a serious cause of obstruction; compression of blood vessels and nerves making matters worse. INTUSSUSCEPTION, in which a part of the intestine becomes turned in on itself (like the finger of a rubber glove may do) is fraught with similar dangers. VOLVULUS, or the twisting of a loop of intestine, is another cause. All these conditions may be followed by GANGRENE and PERITONITIS. Prompt surgical treatment is necessary to save life.

A growth affecting either the lumen of the intestine so blocking it, or the exterior and so constricting it, is another possibility. (*See* TUMOURS, CANCER.)

Signs. intestinal obstruction can be expected to cause depression, loss of appetite, dehydration, fever, some degree of toxaemia, vomiting, and pain.

TYMPANY (distension of the intestine with gas) may occur in some cases of intestinal obstruction. In brood mares tympany of the large intestine may predispose to rupture of the caecum (or other part) from pressure exerted by the fetal hind feet at the onset of parturition, an AHT report suggested in 1983. (*See also* COLIC for diseases in horses.)

INTRACRANIAL is the term applied to structures, diseases, or operations associated with the contents of the cranium.

INTRADERMAL. Into the thickness of the skin as in intradermal injections.

INTRAMEDULLARY. Within the marrow cavity of long bones. Thus, intramedullary pins – used in the treatment of fractures.

INTRAMUSCULAR. Within a muscle; *e.g.* Intramuscular injection.

INTRA-PERITONEAL INJECTIONS are those made direct into the abdominal cavity.

INTRATHECAL. Into a sheath; intraspinal.

INTRATRACHEAL. Into the 'windpipe'. (*See also* ENDOTRACHEAL ANAESTHESIA.)

INTRAVENOUS INJECTION. An injection direct into a vein, a technique employed in anaesthesia and where much fluid has to be injected. (*See also* INJECTIONS.)

INTUSSUSCEPTION is a form of obstruction of the bowels in which a part of the intestine turns in on itself in the way which may happen with the finger of a rubber glove. It occurs mostly in horses, puppies and kittens, causes obstruction of the intestine and great pain.

If the condition is not relieved it leads to stopping of the blood-supply in that part of the bowel which is enclosed, and death. Symptoms include loss of appetite, uneasiness due to abdominal pain, straining, and blood in the faeces. In the dog a sausage-like swelling may be palpated in the abdomen, or there may be protrusion from the anus of a turgid, cylindrical mass having four thicknesses of bowel wall. Treatment involves manipulation under anaesthesia (after laparatomy in most cases), and sometimes the surgical removal of the innermost portion of the bowel and an end-to-end anastomosis.

Caecal intussusception. Two cases of this in ponies led, respectively, to pain followed by sudden death; and to pain lasting three weeks from the time of a veterinary examination. The first case was found at autopsy to have intussusception of the base of the caecum; the second had the entire caecum invaginated into the colon. In both animals the lesions had been present for a long time. (Milne, E. M. & others. *Veterinary Record* (1989) **125** 148.)

INVOLUTION. A change back to its normal condition which an organ undergoes after fulfilling its normal function, *e.g.* involution of the uterus following pregnancy.

IODIDES are salts of iodine. Sodium iodide is used in the treatment of actinobacillosis, and formerly it was used with other drugs in the treatment of oedema, and of ringworm. Taken in excess, iodides cause a condition known as 'iodism' or iodine poisoning. The symptoms of this are diarrhoea, loss of appetite, emaciation, total refusal of water, a dry, scurfy condition of the skin with a loss of hair, and in some cases catarrh of the nasal mucous membranes.

IODINE is a non-metallic element which is found largely in seaweed. It is prepared in the form of a dark violet-brown scales, which are soluble in alcohol and ether.
USES. Pure iodine in the form of scales is never used. The ordinary tincture of iodine that is a common household remedy contains 2½ per cent of iodine.

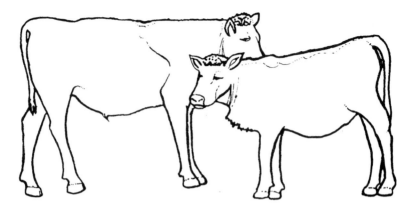

Iodine deficiency – comparison of body size between the normal and deficient animal.

A mild IODOPHOR, *e.g.* Iosan CCT, is used for teat-dipping in modern dairy hygiene for the prevention of mastitis.

Internally it is a violent irritant poison. (*See also under* RADIOACTIVE IODINE.)

IODINE DEFICIENCY ON THE FARM. Iodine is required by the body for the formation of thyroxine, the hormone produced by the thyroid gland, and the common sign of iodine deficiency is goitre. Acute iodine deficiency occurs in fourteen of the United States. In Britain, typical iodine deficiency is not common in farm stock, although in some areas the question of iodine intake below the optimum for health and fertility is of economic importance. The remedy is to provide salt licks or mineral mixtures containing traces of iodine. This is particularly important when large quantities of kale, cabbage, or turnips are fed. (*See* TRACE ELEMENTS.)

IODO-CASEIN. An artificially prepared thyroid active protein sometimes used instead of thyroxine.

IODOPHOR. An 'iodine-bearer'. (*See under* IODINE and MASTITIS – teat-dipping.)

IONIC MEDICATION, IONTOPHORESIS involves the use of an electric current to cause substances to pass through the skin and subcutaneous tissues for curative purposes. The substance used must be soluble in water. A continuous current is necessary. Electrolytes which have been used include sodium chloride, magnesium sulphate, copper sulphate, methylene blue, quinine sulphate, and adrenalin. These are made into solutions in which pads of felt or lint are soaked, and the pads are applied to the area to be treated. One electrode is laid over the pad, and another applied to some suitable part of the body, and the current is applied. This causes a disintegration of the electrolyte into its constituent ions, which are driven through the skin and exert their curative action on the tissues of the area.

USES. Ionisation has been used to stimulate sluggish ulcers to heal, in the treatment of demodectic mange, to soften scars, to exert local antiseptic or germicidal actions, to allay pain, and to induce local construction of vessels in treating inflammatory changes.

IONISING RADIATION REGULATIONS 1985. These were introduced in the UK and cover the inspection of X-ray equipment in veterinary practices, from a safety point of view.

IONOPHORES. These include monensin, narasin, salinomycin, and lasalocid. 'The ionophores are so-called because of their capability to combine with particular ions and to transport these ions through biological membranes.
Ionophore poisoning (*see* MONENSIN).

IRIS is the muscular and fibrous curtain which hangs behind the cornea of the eye and serves to regulate the amount of light that is allowed to reach the inner parts of the eye. It possesses radiating and circular fibres which, when they contract under the influence of light, enlarge and decrease the size of the pupil respectively. (*See* EYE.)
Iridectomy. An operation by which a part or the whole of the iris is removed.

IRITIS. Inflammation of the iris. (*See* EYE.)

IRON is a TRACE ELEMENT (which see) – essential for life. Over half the body's iron is contained in the haemoglobin of the red blood-cells. Iron is additionally present as beta-globulin transferrin in the blood plasma, in the myoglobin of muscles, and in enzymes.

Iron also has a role in bodily resistance to infection. Iron-binding proteins (*see below*) can be shown to inhibit the growth of bacteria *in vitro*. 'Probably,' stated *The Lancet* (Aug. 10, 1974), 'the ability of micro-organisms to compete successfully with the host for iron is a feature of pathogenicity, and ability of the host to limit availability to the pathogen is associated with resistance to infection.'

Bacteria (*e.g.* salmonellas and tubercle bacilli) and some fungi also produce iron-binding substances.

IRON-BINDING PROTEINS include conalbumin, a constituent of egg-white; transferrin, in blood plasma; lactoferrin, in milk, tears, saliva, bile, seminal secretions, cervical mucus, and in the granules of neutrophils. All these proteins inhibit the growth of bacteria.

IRON POISONING. This may occur from over-dosage, or from the eating by a pet animal of an iron preparation left within reach. (*See also under* FLOOR FEEDINGS OF PIGS, for the danger of concrete made with sand rich in iron.)

Horses have died very soon after receiving an intra-muscular injection of an organic iron preparation.

Piglets have been poisoned by iron-dextran preparations given to prevent anaemia and ASYMMETRIC HINDQUARTER SYNDROME may develop following organic iron injections.

In the dog, ferrous sulphate or ferrous gluconate in doses as low as 0·3 or 0·75 gramme respectively of ferrous iron per kg bodyweight, have caused severe illness with diarrhoea, vomiting and ulceration of stomach and intestine.

IRRADIATION. Exposure to X-rays, radio-active material, ultra-violet, or infra-red rays. Husk (lungworm) larvae have been irradiated for vaccine purposes. (*See* PARASITIC BRONCHITIS; *also* 'RADIATION SICKNESS', IONISING RADIATION.)

IRRIGATION is the washing out of wounds or cavities of the body by means of large amounts of warm water containing some antiseptic in solution.

ISCHAEMIA. Local anaemia.

ISCHAEMIC CONTRACTURE (*see under* MUSCLES, DISEASES OF).

ISCHIUM is the bone which forms the most posterior part of the pelvis, and forms the point of the buttock.

ISCHURIA means insufficiency in the amount of urine passed, due either to suppression of excretion in the kidneys or retention in the bladder.

ISLETS OF LANGERHANS (*see* PANCREAS).

ISOFLURANE. A colourless liquid with an ether-like smell, non-explosive and non-inflammable in clinical concentrations, used as an anaesthetic by inhalation for dogs and horses. It gave satisfactory anaesthesia in all 22 dogs and 21 horses undergoing various types of surgery, and recovery from the anaesthetic was rapid. In horses 'it was particularly smooth, with the patients spending a greater part of their recumbency in the sternal position, as opposed to lateral recumbency, before standing in a well coordinated manner.' (Jones, R. S., *Veterinary Record* (1986), **119**, 8.)

ISOLATION is an important procedure in the control of the spread of infectious disease. On a farm it is advisable, where practicable, to keep newly bought stock separate from previously existing stock for two or three weeks, so that if

infectious/contagious disease occurs it may be possible to prevent its spread to the old stock. (*See* INCUBATION, INFECTION, QUARANTINE, NOTIFIABLE DISEASES.)

ISOQUINOLINIUM chloride lotion has been used in the treatment of ringworm in cattle.

ISOTONIC is a term applied to solutions which have the same power of diffusion as one another. An isotonic solution used in medicine is one which can be mixed with body fluids without causing any disturbance. An isotonic saline solution for injection into the blood, so that it may possess the same osmotic pressure as the blood serum, is one of 0·9 per cent strength or containing 80 grains of chloride of sodium to the pint of water. This is also known as normal or physiological salt solution. An isotonic solution of glucose for injection into the blood is one of 5 per cent strength in water. Solutions, which are weaker than or stronger than the fluids of the body with which they are intended to be mixed, are known as hypotonic and hypertonic respectively.

ITCHINESS (*see* PRURITUS).

-ITIS. A suffix added to the name of an organ to signify inflammation of that organ.

IVERMECTIN, the most active of the AVERMECTINS (which see), is a potent anthelmintic, effective at very low dosage, which can be given orally or by subcutaneous injection. Ivermectin also gives control of lungworms in addition to external parasites such as warbles, lice, and sarcoptic mange mites on pigs, for example. Effective against mature and immature roundworms of cattle, including *Ostertagia* larvae; against ticks, mange mites, warbles, etc. Horses can be dosed orally with a paste formulation of ivermectin for the control of roundworms and horse bots. (*See* WORMS, FARM TREATMENT AGAINST; HORSE BOTS.)

Formulations of ivermectin (Ivomec from MSD Agvet) are available in the UK for sheep, pigs, cattle and horses; but not for dogs or cats. A new pour-on formulation of Ivomec was introduced in 1991 for the control of internal and external parasites of cattle.

Warning. MSD Agvet has warned that animals must not be slaughtered for human consumption within 28 days of the last treatment; nor should it be used in cows producing milk or in the 28 days before calving.

The product contains isopropyl alcohol which is highly inflammable. Protective clothing (including gloves) must be worn when liquid Ivermectin products are applied.

Ivermectin poisoning in dogs has occurred as a result of ignoring manufacturers' recommendations.

Stuart M. Easby reported a case in a collie, which had been injected with Ivomec by a friend of the owner. The bitch was in a coma for seven weeks. On veterinary examination, the next day the signs were dilated pupils, ataxia, and depression; with no response to sound, and apparent blindness. Four days after the injection, complete coma had developed. Only the swallowing reflex was present. The bitch was maintained, after preliminary treatment, on oral glucose and hydrolised protein solution given by the owner.

Twitching of an ear when spoken to was the first response on day 26. By five weeks she was eating, able to stand if lifted, but still blind. At seven weeks, her sight had returned and she appeared normal again.

IXODES is the generic name of one of the varieties of ticks that infest animals. (*See* TICKS.)

J

JAAGSIEKTE. A disease of adult sheep, first recognised in South Africa. (*See* PULMONARY ADENOMATOSIS.)

JACK BEANS may cause poisoning if fed raw. (*See* LEGUME POISONING.)

JACOBSON'S ORGAN. Also known as the vomeronasal organ, this is thought to determine the flavour of food in the mouth by smell rather than taste. The organ has two small tubes which extend from the floor of the nasal cavity to the level of the 2nd/4th cheek tooth. It is present in cat, dog, horse, etc.

JANET. A female mule.

JAPANESE B ENCEPHALITIS. This disease is present in Nepal and other regions of Asia.
CAUSE: a Flavivirus.
SIGNS: the eyesight of horses is affected first. Later they become drowsy. Many die, and the recovery of others is seldom complete.

Experimentally, the disease has been transmitted to cattle, sheep, goats, and pigs. In the latter it may result in abortion or stillbirths.

The disease is a zoonosis, and for its prevention in people a vaccine has been used. In a 1984 issue of the *Journal of the Royal Army Medical Corps*, Dr. A. Henderson reported that only minimal side-effects followed the use of vaccine in 1,152 British subjects.

Dr J. L. Sanchez and colleagues at the Walter Reed Army Institute of Research, Washington, suggested that two doses give reasonable protection for short visits to areas where the disease is endemic, but advised a booster dose after three months.

JAUNDICE is a yellowish discoloration of the visible mucous membranes of the body (eye, nose, mouth, and genital organs).

The symptom of jaundice (icterus) may indicate the destruction of red-blood cells due to parasites, such as may occur in cases of Biliary Fever and Surra in the horse; Red-water in cattle; Malignant Jaundice (canine babesiosis); also in leptospiral jaundice (*See* LEPTOSPIROSIS), and canine viral hepatitis.

In cats jaundice is seen in the dry form of feline infectious peritonitis, toxoplasmosis.

Jaundice may indicate an incompatibility between the blood of sire and dam causing haemolytic jaundice of the new-born foal or piglet.

When bile cannot enter into the small intestine by the bile-duct from the liver in the usual way, it becomes dammed back, is absorbed by the lymphatics and the blood vessels, carried into the general circulation, and some of its constituents are deposited in the tissues. (*See* GALL-STONES, *also*

under GALL-BLADDER, DISEASES OF, CIRRHOSIS; LIVER, DISEASES OF, EQUINE BILIARY FEVER).

It may be seen during poisoning with copper, mercury, phosphorus, chloroform, or lead, and after some snakebites. Aflatoxins may cause jaundice.
(*See also* JAUNDICE, LEPTOSPIROSIS; JAUNDICE OF THE NEW-BORN *under* FOAL DISEASES; *and* BILIARY FEVER.)

JAUNDICE, LEPTOSPIRAL, OF DOGS (*see* LEPTOSPIROSIS IN DOGS).

JAUNDICE, LEPTOSPIRAL, OF OTHER ANIMALS (*see under* LEPTOSPIROSIS).

JAVA BEAN POISONING. The 'Java' beans, *Phaseolus lunatus*, were once imported in large amounts. The beans are of varying origin, and differ in colour, thus: *Java* beans are as a rule reddish-brown, but they may be almost black; *Rangoon* or *Burmah* beans are smaller, plumper, and lighter in colour (so-called 'red-Rangoons' are pinkish with small purple splashes).

The active poisonous agent in the beans is a substance called *Phaseolunatin*, which is a member of a group of *cyanogenetic glucosides*.
SIGNS. These are exactly the same as those given under HYDROCYANIC ACID, which see.

JAW. The upper jawbones are two in number and are firmly united to the other bones of the face. The lower jaw – or mandible or coronoid process – is composed of a single bone in horse, pig, dog, and cat, but in the ruminants the fusion between the right and left sides does not occur until old age. Each of the jaws presents a number of deep sockets or 'alveoli' which contain the teeth. (*See* DISLOCATIONS, FRACTURES, MOUTH, TEETH; *also* ATROPHIC MYOSITIS *and* EOSINOPHILIC MYOSITIS – both given in the Section headed MUSCLES, DISEASES OF.)

JAW, diseases of. For overshot and undershot jaws, see under TEETH, Diseases.

'Lion jaw' (Craniomandibular osteopathy). A disease seen mostly in West Highland terriers. Eating becomes difficult, mouth-opening painful.
(*See* 'BOTTLE-JAW'.)

JEJUNUM is the central portion of the small intestine. (*See* INTESTINE.)

JENNY. A female ass.

JEQUIRITY POISONING. This is caused by the red and black seeds of the climbing plant *Abrus precatorius*, which grows in Australia, Asia, and South America. It gives rise to cyanosis and pin-point-size haemorrhages from the skin, and diarrhoea.

In sheep diarrhoea is *not* a major symptom.
TREATMENT. When once well established,

Johne's disease is invariably fatal, and no treatment is effective or worthwhile.

PREVENTION. Attention should be paid to the prevention of infection to other animals, especially calves. Pastures that are suspected of being heavily infected should be left without stock for 4 or 5 months. All infected litter should be stored in a dung-pit which is not accessible to other animals, and should be used for cultivated land. Loose-boxes, sheds, etc., that have housed a case should be carefully disinfected and diseased animals should be fed after healthy ones. Ponds and water-courses should be fenced to prevent fouling by faeces, water for drinking being pumped out.

A vaccine became available to UK veterinary surgeons in May 1964. It is intended for use in calves up to a month old in problem herds. Care has to be taken to minimise its interference with interpretation of the tuberculin test. Vaccination is being practised in Iceland, Holland, Belgium, and France.

In Norway a vaccination campaign to control the disease in **goats** was begun in 1967. Between then and 1982 some 130,000 goats had been vaccinated, and the infection rate reduced from 53 to 1 per cent. Kids are vaccinated at the age of two to four weeks. (Saxegaard, F. & Fodstat, F. H., *Veterinary Record* (1985), **116**, 439.)

DIAGNOSIS. The disease can usually be diagnosed on clinical evidence, with some confirmation afforded by microscopic examination of the faeces. 'In 30 to 50 per cent of clinically affected cows, typical clumps of acid-fast bacilli can be found,' Dr Gilmour stated, and 'the complement fixation test is positive in about 90 per cent of cattle with advanced disease.' The fluorescent antibody test is equally useful.

Unfortunately, diagnosis of the carrier state is not possible with any certainty. 'There is no single test which can conclusively detect the presence or absence of *M. johnei* – therefore the limited value of the available tests for import and export certification must be recognised.'

'The complement fixation test is positive in only a small proportion of carriers and, more important, it gives rise to false positive results.' The fluorescent antibody test would need to be repeated – a single test is of no value.

The difficulty in identifying 'carriers' makes Johne's disease a difficult one to control.

JERSIAN. Also known as a F-J hybrid, this is a beef cross obtained from a Jersey bull on a Friesian cow. (In New Zealand, the reverse cross is used.)

JETTING is a technique developed in Australia, involving the application of insecticide under pressure by means of a jetting gun – a handpiece with four needle jets for combing through the wool. The pressure used is 60 to 80 lb per square inch, which can be achieved by an ordinary medium/high-volume agricultural sprayer.

In Britain, jetting was demonstrated at the 1965 Royal Show, and many advantages were claimed for it.

Jetting has, however, not displaced dipping to any extent in the UK, where spraying has been found inefficient in the control of sheep scab.

JIGGER flea. (*See under* FLEAS – *Tunga penetrans.*)

JOHNE'S DISEASE is a chronic infection, involving the small and large intestines, affecting cattle particularly, but sometimes sheep, goats, and deer, characterised by the appearance of a persistent diarrhoea, gradual emaciation, and great weakness. The infection has been set up experimentally in the rabbit. It may occur naturally in the pig, and *post-mortem* findings may at first suggest tuberculosis.

CAUSE. The acid-fast *Mycobacterium johnei*.

Experimentally, sheep can be infected with as few as 1000 *M. johnei* bacilli. These then multiply in the intestinal mucosa for the first two or three months after infection. Some animals are then able to overcome the infection completely, others becoming carriers, with the bacilli remaining in the intestinal mucosa and lymph nodes. Some of the carriers eventually become clinically ill with Johne's disease. (Gilmour, N. L. J., *Vet. Rec.* (1976), **99**, 433.)

SIGNS. The disease is very slow in onset. Cattle that have become infected may not show symptoms for as long as two years after the last case occurred on that farm.

Pointers to the disease are an unexplained drop in milk yield (often months before other symptoms appear); and diarrhoea in an individual adult animal.

Loss of condition, general unthriftiness, a harsh, staring coat are then seen, with diarrhoea. The temperature fluctuates a degree or two above normal. Appetite is variable. In the last stages emaciation becomes very marked, and the animal becomes progressively weaker.

JOHNIN. A diagnostic agent used for JOHNE'S DISEASE.

JOINT-ILL. NAVEL-ILL or POLYARTHRITIS is a disease of foals, lambs, and calves, in which abscesses form at the umbilicus and in some of the joints of the limbs, due, in the majority of cases, to the entrance of organisms into the body by way of the unclosed navel. There are numerous organisms associated with the disease, the commonest of which are streptococci, staphylococci, Pasteurella, *E. coli*, the necrosis bacillus, and *see under* FOALS, DISEASES OF.

SIGNS. Usually the young animal becomes dull, takes no interest in its dam, refuses to suckle; the breathing is hurried; the temperature rises from 2° to 4°F above normal; the foal prefers to lie stretched out on its side, and may have attacks of either diarrhoea or constipation. If the navel is examined it is found to be wet and oozing with blood-stained serous material, or it may be dry, swollen, painful to the touch, and hard, owing to abscess formation within. In cases that appear later in life there may be no umbilical symptoms. In the course of a day or so, one or more of the joints swells up. The joints most commonly attacked are the stifle, hip, knee, hock, shoulder and elbow, but it may be seen in any of the others. The swelling is tense, painful, hot, and oedematous. There is the danger of a fatal septicaemia.

Ten calves with internal umbilical abscesses were seen in one practice over a period of eight years. The primary infection had obviously occurred at, or soon after, birth; but once the umbilicus had sealed over, external signs were not evident, and the umbilical remnant appeared normal.

The calves were usually presented as unthrifty, depressed and slow in their movements. Their temperature was invariably normal. (Shearer, A. G., *Veterinary Record* (1986), **118,** 480.)

PREVENTION. Attention must always be paid to the cleanliness of the foaling-box, the calving-box, and the lambing-pen. Where climatic and other conditions are favourable the pregnant females should be allowed to give birth to their young out of doors. Lambing-pens should without fail be changed to a fresh site every year.

Investigations undertaken by the Animal Health Trust suggests that thoroughbred foals in the UK suffer severe illness as a result of being deprived of a not inconsiderable volume of blood when the navel cord is ruptured by human agency prematurely. Severance of the cord, it seems, is always best left to the mare. The use of strong disinfectants applied to the stump of the navel cord is likewise deprecated.

An application of a sulphanilamide dry dressing may be safer than iodine solution.

When cutting the cord, it is necessary to maintain the strictest cleanliness. Scissors should be sterilised, and tape scrupulously clean.

TREATMENT. Antibiotics and antiserum, Tiamulin. The umbilicus is opened up, and evacuated, disinfected. Isolation and other hygiene measures are needed.

All pails, and other feeding utensils that are liable to get infected, should be washed out with boiling water or steamed before future use, and the pen or box that houses a case should be occasionally washed out with disinfectant. (*See also* FOALS, DISEASES OF.)

JOINTS fall into two great divisions, namely, (*a*) movable joints, and (*b*) fixed joints. In a *movable joint* there are four main structures. Firstly, there are the two bones whose junction forms the joint; secondly, there is a layer of smooth cartilage covering the ends of these bones where they meet, which is called 'articular' cartilage; thirdly, there is a sheath of fibrous tissue known as the 'joint capsule', which is thickened into bands of 'ligaments' which hold the bones together at various points; and finally, there is a closed bladder of membrane, known as the 'synovial membrane', which lines the capsule and produces a synovial fluid to lubricate the movements of the joint. Further, the bones are kept in position at the joints by the various muscles passing over them. This type is known as a *diarthrodial joint*.

Some joints possess subsidiary structures such as discs of fibro-cartilage, which adapt the bones more perfectly to one another where they do not quite correspond, and allow of slightly freer

movement, *e.g.* the stifle-joint. In others, movable pads of fat under the synovial membrane fill up larger cavities and afford additional protection to the joint, *e.g.* the hock-joint. In some the edge of one bone is amplified by a margin of cartilage which makes dislocation less of a risk than otherwise, *e.g.* the hip and the shoulder-joints.

In the *fixed joints* a layer of cartilage or of fibrous tissue intervenes between the bones and binds them firmly together (*synarthrodial joint*). This type of joint is exemplified by the 'sutures' between the bones that make up the skull. Classified among these fixed joints are the *amphiarthrodial joints*, in which there is a thick disc of fibro-cartilage between the bones, so that, although the individual joint is really capable of but limited movement, a series of these, like the joints between the bodies of the vertebrae, gives the column, as a whole, a very flexible character. In this connection it is noticeable that the movement in the region of the neck may be much more free than in some of the true movable joints, such as between the small bones of the hock or carpus.

Varieties. Apart from the division into fixed and movable joints, those that are movable are further classified. *Gliding joints* are those in which the bones have flat surfaces capable only of a limited amount of movement, such as the bones of the carpus and tarsus. In *hinge-joints* like the elbow, fetlock, and pastern, movement can take place around one axis only, and is called flexion and extension. In the *ball-and-socket joints*, such as the shoulder and hip-joints, free movement can occur in any direction. There are other subsidiary varieties, named according to the shape of the bones which enter into the joint.

JOINTS, DISEASES OF.

Arthritis means inflammation which involves all the structures of the joint, *viz.* synovial membrane, capsular ligaments, cartilages, and the ends of the bones that take part in the formation of the joint. Arthritis is a general term which includes osteoarthritis and rheumatoid arthritis. Arthritis often begins as a synovitis (*see* SYNOVITIS, under this section), but the degree of inflammation is severe enough to extend to the structures around the synovial membrane. Its causes, symptoms, and treatment are similar to those given for synovitis, but it sometimes leads to ankylosis and fixation of the joint. (*See* CORTISONE.) The joints that are most often affected are the stifle, hock, knee, and fetlocks, but the shoulder, hip, elbow, and the lower joints of the digit are not infrequently the seat of disease as well. Among diseases that are associated with joints, and which are treated in separate sections, are: NAVICULAR DISEASE, SLIPPED SHOULDER, SLIPPED STIFLE, HYGROMA OF THE KNEE, CAPPED ELBOW, CAPPED HOCK, KNUCKLING OF THE FETLOCK, and JOINT-ILL; *see also below and* BURSITIS, ANKYLOSIS, FRACTURES, DISLOCATIONS, GLASSER'S DISEASE, 'HIP DYSPLASIA', SWINE ERYSIPELAS, etc.

Rheumatoid arthritis. This can be important in the dog, and may occur at any age from two years. Symptoms may be vague at first; the animal appearing depressed, with a poor appetite, and often some degree of fever, but with no lameness. Eventually the latter symptom appears, sometimes involving several joints, sometimes affecting only one limb and then shifting to another. There may be crepitus – a grating sound – when the limb is moved.

Diagnosis depends upon radiography and – as in human medicine – there are certain laboratory tests, the results of which provide additional criteria for deciding whether the condition really is rheumatoid arthritis or not.

Intractable arthritis of the hip joint has, in dogs as in human beings, been overcome by major surgery involving removal of the top of the femur and replacement of the ball part of the ball-and-socket joint with a plastic prosthesis. Several such operations for the relief of painful arthritis have been carried out on dogs – more in the USA than elsewhere.

Synovitis is the name given to any inflammation of the membrane lining a joint cavity. It may be acute, sub-acute, or chronic.

Generally this is not a separate condition but occurs during the course of rheumatism, rickets, gout (in poultry), severe sprains and bruises, and in a variety of specific infections such as brucellosis, swine erysipelas, tuberculosis. Tubercular joint disease often produces a chronic synovitis in the neck bones of the horse, which leads to an arthritis later.

Conditions such as wind-galls, curb, bog spavin, etc., are really only synovitis that have become chronic, or are complicated with other pathological conditions.

The synovial membrane becomes inflamed, thickened, and secretes an excessive amount of fluid into the joint. As a result the joint becomes hot, swollen, and painful. The animal goes lame in greater or lesser degree according to the extent of the inflammation. When at rest, the joint is usually kept flexed with the toe of the affected leg just resting on the ground. If it is a simple condition, such as a mild sprain, these symptoms last for a few days and then gradually pass off. In more severe cases, such as in joint-ill, there may be pus formation, septicaemia, and death. In the chronic type the swelling persists. The animal is able to use its limb as usual, but the blemish of

the accumulated fluid in the cavity does not disappear (*e.g.* bog spavin, wind-galls, etc.).

Open joint is a condition in which a direct communication has been formed between the inside of the joint and the outside.

The seriousness of an open joint is not so much due to the initial injury as to the danger of infection. This may cause tissue destruction within the joint, and even lead to a fatal SEPTICAEMIA.

The most striking signs of open joint are, in the first place, the excessive degree of pain that seems out of all proportion to the visible amount of damage that has been inflicted; secondly, the great amount of swelling that is usually seen; and thirdly, the discharge of a thin, straw-coloured or blood-stained sticky synovia which has a tendency to coagulate around the skin opening.

Veterinary advice should be sought at once. The best outcome, and the lowest infection rate, were obtained in the horses which were treated surgically, and with antibiotics, within 24 hours of injury. (Almost a third of the injuries were not recognised until the joint became infected.)

Fifty-four per cent of the horses survived and many returned to 'athletic performance.' (Gibson, K. T. & others. *JAVMA* (1989) **194** 398.)

Dislocations (*see* DISLOCATIONS).

Bursitis, an inflammation of a bursa, commonly occurs in the region of a joint. The prominences of the hock, elbow, knee, stifle, etc., are protected by bursae – lined on their insides by synovial membrane. These sometimes become inflamed and lead to the formation of fluctuating swellings which have a tendency to become chronic. Capped elbow, capped hock, and hygroma of the knee, are of this nature.

(*See also* OSTEOARTHRITIS, MAST CELLS, OSTEOCHONDROSIS, RHEUMATISM.)

JOULE. A derived SI unit of metabolisable energy. (*See* CALORIES *and* STARCH EQUIVALENT, which it replaced; *also* SI UNITS.)

JUGULAR VEINS carry the blood back to the chest from the head and anterior parts of the neck. The *jugular furrow* is the groove between the trachea and the muscles of the neck, in the depths of which lies the jugular vein.

K

K88 ANTIGEN. This· is possessed by certain strains of *E. coli* which cause diarrhoea in piglets during their first few days of life. (*See* E. COLI and BACTERIAL ADHESIVENESS.)

K VALUE. This is used as a measure of the insulating value of building materials such as glass fibre, wood.

K, VITAMIN. This is necessary for the formation of PROTHOMBRIN. (*See under that heading, also* CLOTTING OF BLOOD, DICOUMAROL, SWEET VERNAL, WARFARIN, and VITAMINS.)

KALA-AZAR or DUMDUM FEVER. A human disease caused by LEISHMANIA (which see.)

KALE contains a factor which gives rise to goitre if fed in large amounts, without other foods, over a long period. Haemoglobinuria sometimes follows the grazing of frosted kale by cattle, which may suffer anaemia without showing this symptom. The illness can be serious, resembling POST-PARTURIENT HAEMOGLOBINURIA, and may result in sudden death. The frothy type of bloat may also occur in cattle eating excessive quantities of kale – especially, it seems, during wet weather, and when no hay is fed as well. There is some evidence to suggest that the feeding of large quantities of kale may lead to low conception rates, and to mastitis. (*See also* BLOAT.)

It should be added that kale anaemia and haemoglobinuria are by no means always associated with *frosted* kale, but merely with an excessive (probably over 40 lb per cow per day) intake of kale. The symptoms of kale anaemia include lassitude and rapid breathing and pulse-rate.

'KANGAROO GAIT' in ewes, both in New Zealand and the UK, appears to be associated with diseases of the radial nerves, which causes difficulty in advancing the front feet. When made to move rapidly, they do so with a bounding gait. (Duffel, S. J. & others, *Veterinary Record* (1986), **118**, 296.)

KAOLIN, or CHINESE CLAY, is a native aluminium silicate, which is used as a protective and astringent dry dusting powder. Kaolin is sometimes given internally as an adsorbent in intestinal disorders. Mixed into a paste with glycerine and some antiseptic, it is applied to acute sprains of tendons, etc. 'Antiphlogistine' is the name of a proprietary kaolin poultice.

KARYOTYPE. This is, roughly speaking, a plan showing an animal's chromosomes. In technical terms, a karyotype is a presentation of the metaphase chromosomes characteristic of an individual animal or species. (*See* CYTOGENETICS.)

'KEBBING' (*see* Enzootic Abortion of Sheep).

KED. *Melophagus ovinus*, the sheep ked, is wingless, and lives on the wool and skin of the sheep. It is much larger than any of the lice, being a quarter of an inch long. It can easily be distinguished from the ticks by its tripartite body. It is a dark brown colour with a sharp biting proboscis. The nearly mature larvae are laid on the wool and they at once pupate. The pupa may remain in the wool or fall to the ground. The young hatch in 19 to 24 days, and the females start to deposit larvac in 12 to 23 days after emergence, and lay a larva every 9 days. The fly can live for about 12 days away from the sheep: while the pupa can live for 6 weeks on the ground. The whole life-cycle may be completed on the sheep within 1 month.

The sheep ked can cause severe anaemia if present in large numbers, and also leads to a damaged fleece. Shearing aids control, which is achieved by means of a sheep dip.

The ked may attack men while shearing and inflict a very painful bite.

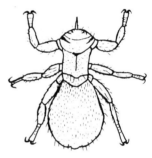

Melophagus. × 4.

KEMPS. Coarse hairs, the presence of which reduces the value of a fleece.

'KENNEL COUGH' is a convenient term for those outbreaks of respiratory disease, distinct from canine distemper, which are troublesome in boarding kennels and dog pounds.

Usually only the upper air passages are involved in Kennel Cough, the chief symptom being a fit of coughing which is aggravated by exercise or excitement. The cough is a harsh, dry one. It has to be differentiated from infestation with TRACHEAL WORMS.

CAUSES. *Bordetella bronchiseptica* is the principal cause. Other organisms involved are the canine parainfluenza virus (CPI), a canine herpes virus, two adenoviruses, a reovirus; also a mycoplasma. Bacterial secondary invaders may complicate the syndrome.

PREVENTION. Vaccination, which can be by application of nasal drops rather than an injection, is advisable a fortnight before a dog is taken to a show or left in boarding kennels. The intranasal live *Bordetella bronchiseptica* vaccine is 'Intrac' (Mycofarm).

KENNEL LAMENESS. A colloquial term for lameness arising from a nutritional deficiency, such as may occur in a dog fed entirely on dog-biscuits. (*See* RICKETS.)

'KENNEL SICKNESS'. A colloquial name used in the USA for outbreaks of salmonellosis, the symptoms of which may include pneumonia and convulsions. (*See also under* SALMONELLOSIS.)

KERATIN is the substance of which horn and the surface layers of the skin are composed. It is a modified form of skin which has undergone compression and toughening. It is present in the hoof of the feet of animals, in claws, horns, and nails.

KERATITIS (*see* EYE, DISEASES OF).

KERATOCOELE is a hernia through the cornea. (*See* EYE, DISEASES OF.)

KERATOMA is a horn tumour affecting the inner aspect of the wall of the hoof.

KEROSENE poisoning (*see* PARAFFIN).

KETONE BODIES arise from acetyl osenzyme A. They are not normal intermediates in the degradation of fatty acids, but are formed by special reactions to serve, together with free fatty acids, as a readily oxidisable fuel of oxidation in various tissues when the supply of glucose is restricted. The mild forms of ketosis, *e.g.* of starvation or of low carbohydrate diets, or of mild diabetes, are physiological processes. 'The severe forms of ketosis of the diabetic coma or of the lactating cow are connected with the high rates of gluconeogenesis which occur under these conditions. Oxaloacetate, which is an intermediate in gluconeogenesis, is diverted from the tricarboxylic acid cycle to gluconeogenesis, owing to the high activity of the enzyme converting it to phosphopyruvate. The liver compensates the loss of energy from a reduced rate of the tricarboxylic acid cycle by an increased rate of oxidations outside the cycle. The main reaction of this type is the oxidation of fatty acids to ketone bodies. These arise grossly in excess of needs, as a by-product of reactions which satisfy the requirements for energy.' – (Prof. Sir Hans Krebs.)

Ketonuria is the term applied to the presence of these bodies in the urine. (*See also* ACETONAEMIA.)

Ketoacidosis. A condition leading to diabetic coma. (*See* DIABETES.)

KETOSIS (*see* ACETONAEMIA).

KEY-GASKELL SYNDROME (*see* FELINE DYSAUTONOMIA).

KHAT. This plant (*Catha edulis*) contains two compounds – cathine and cathinone – which are both structurally related to amphetamine. This was stated by Dr A. J. Goudie of Liverpool University.

Chewing of khat leaves, popular in Arabia and East Africa, appears to be on the increase in the UK.

Addicts esteem khat for the euphoria and extra energy which it provides, but over-use can lead to dangerous mental illness.

Veterinary surgeons in small-animal practice will need to be on the lookout for cases of khat poisoning in dogs and cats; as they already are for the effects of CANNABIS.

KICKING (*see* 'VICES').

KIDNEY WORM. (*Stephanurus dentatus*) is a parasite of **pigs.** Occasionally migration of the larvae in the spinal canal causes some degree of paralysis. The intermediate host is the earthworm. In the USA the advice is to breed from gilts only as a means of eradicating the parasite; anthelmintics so far not having proved effective.

(For the kidney worm of **dogs,** *see* DIOCTOPHYMOSIS.)

KIDNEYS are paired organs situated high up against the roof of the abdomen, and in most animals lying one on either side of the spinal column.

Horse. The kidneys of the horse differ from each other both in shape and position. The right has the outline of a playing-card heart, and lies under the last two or three ribs and the transverse process of the 1st lumbar vertebra, while the left is roughly bean-shaped and lies under the last rib and the first two or three lumbar transverse processes. They are held in place by the surrounding organs and by fibrous tissue, called the renal fascia. Each of them moves slightly backwards and forwards during the respiratory movements of the animal.

Cattle. The kidneys are lobulated, each possessing from 20 to 25 lobes separated by fissures filled with fat in the living animal. The right kidney lies below the last rib and the first two or three lumbar transverse processes, and is somewhat elliptical in outline. The left occupies a variable position. When the rumen is full it pushes the left kidney over to the right side of the body into a position slightly below and behind the right organ, but when it is empty the left kidney lies underneath the vertebral column about the level of the third to the fifth lumbar vertebra. It may lie partly on the left side of the body in this position in some cases.

Sheep. In the sheep the kidneys are beanshaped and smooth. In position they resemble those of the ox, except that the right is usually a little farther back.

Pig. In this animal the kidneys are shaped like elongated beans, and they are placed almost symmetrically on either side of the bodies of the first four lumbar vertebrae. They sometimes vary in position.

Dogs and cats. In these animals the kidneys are again bean-shaped, but they are thicker than in other animals, and relatively larger. As in most animals, the right kidney is placed farther forward than the left, the latter varying in position according to the degree of fullness of the digestive organs. In the cat the left kidney is very loosely attached and can usually be felt as a rounded mass which is quite movable in the anterior part of the abdominal cavity.

Structure. The organ is enveloped in a fibrous coat continuous with the rest of the peritoneal membrane, and attached to the kidney capsule. This capsule does not permit of much swelling or enlargement of the organ, and consequently any inflammation of the kidney is attended with much pain. On the inner border there is an indentation called the *hilus*, which acts as a place of entrance and exit for vessels, nerves, etc. Entering each kidney at its hilus are a renal artery and renal nerves; leaving the kidney are renal vein or veins, lymphatics, and the ureter. If the kidney be cut across there are two distinct areas seen in its substance. Lying outermost is the reddish-brown granular *cortex*, which contains small dark spots known as *Malphighian corpuscles.*

Within the cortex is the *medulla*, an area presenting a radiated appearance, whose periphery is of a deep red colour.

The kidney tissue contains many thousands of filtration units called *nephrons*. Each of these comprises the *glomerulus* (almost a spherical arrangement of capillaries on an arteriole); *Bowman's capsule*, the blind end of a proximal tubule which expands so as almost to surround the glomerulus; the *convoluted tubule* itself (with its loop of Henle); the distal convoluted tubule which leads on to an arched collecting tubule. The latter continues with a straight tubule in the cortex of the kidney, and on into the medulla, where papillary ducts are formed to take the urine to the pelvis of the kidney.

The Malpighian corpuscle, comprising the glomerulus and inner and outer layers of Bowman's capsule, is where most of the filtration of fluid from the blood occurs; but only a small percentage of this fluid is finally excreted as urine.

Function. The kidney's two main functions are the excretion of waste (and excess) materials from the bloodstream: and, secondly, the maintenance of the correct proportions of water in the blood, the correct levels of its chemical constituents, and the correct pH. (*See* HOMEOSTASIS.)

Blood pressure in the arteries determines pressure in each glomerulus, and has an important bearing on the quantity of fluid filtered from the blood.

For its controlling effect on the kidney, *see* ANTIDIURETIC HORMONE.

The proximal tubules reabsorb a high percentage of the water, sodium chloride and bicarbonate. The distal tubules reabsorb sodium, or exchange sodium ions for hydrogen, potassium or ammonium ions; determining thereby the pH of the urine.

The kidney also secretes the hormone ERYTHROPOIETIN and produces RENIN (which see). Additionally, the kidney converts vitamin D_1 into its active form.

KIDNEYS, DISEASES OF. These are particularly common in the dog, and must account for a high proportion of deaths in dogs and cats.

Exact diagnosis is based almost entirely upon macroscopic, microscopic, and chemical examination of the urine in the laboratory. Blood urea nitrogen (BUN) and serum creatinine concentrations are used to evaluate renal function in several species.

Nephrosis/nephrotic syndrome. This may be a stage in nephritis and involves damage to the tubules of the kidneys, resulting in defective filtering, so that albumin is excreted in the urine to the detriment of albumin levels in the blood. Oedema occurs.

Nephrosis may be caused by poisoning with the salts of heavy metals, and with various toxins; or it may follow certain other diseases. (*See also* MEMBRANOUS NEPHROPATHY.)

Acute nephritis is a rapid inflammation of the kidney tissues as a whole, or of the glomeruli and the secreting tubules only. The latter is much the more common among all animals. Since the diagnosis and symptoms of each are clinically the same, and as their differentiation is only possible by microscopic examination after death it will suffice to describe the commoner type only.

Dogs. Acute and sub-acute nephritis is often associated with LEPTOSPIROSIS (which see), especially with *L. canicola* infection; it may follow the Nephrotic Syndrome, and may co-exist with Distemper or Canine Virus Hepatitis. A predisposing cause is often, it seems, exposure to cold, wet conditions, which lower the animal's resistance and so exacerbates any existing infection.

Symptoms may include depression, loss of appetite, thirst, vomiting. The back may be arched, and there may be stiffness. There is fever, and sometimes ulcers are present in the mouth.

Lambs. Acute kidney failure was diagnosed by clinical and autopsy means in 39 flocks served by six Veterinary Investigation Centres.

Forty-eight lambs of 12 different breeds or crosses were investigated. The mean age of affected lambs was 38 days; 21 lambs were aged seven to 28 days, while only eight were older than two months. Mortality in clinically affected lambs was almost 100 per cent, with no response to various treatments.

FIRST-AID. The animal needs rest, warmth, and light food. Reliable proprietary foods can be obtained for kidney disease cases. Barleywater instead of plain water is often advisable. (*See under* NURSING.)

TREATMENT includes the use of antibiotics. If there is much vomiting, normal saline may be necessary.

Chronic nephritis may follow the acute form, or it may arise insidiously. One attack of nephritis is always likely to render the dog more susceptible to subsequent attacks, and chronic nephritis is common in middle-aged and old dogs. In some cases of this disease RUBBER JAW may be present. Sometimes, despite treatment, kidney failure occurs and there are symptoms as described under 'STUTTGART DISEASE'.

Kidney failure may follow either chronic *interstitial nephritis* (involving some degree of fibrosis), which often results from leptospiral nephritis; or from *glomerular disease* (glomerulonephritis). Clinically, the two conditions are virtually indistinguishable.

Cattle. Kidney disease may also be associated with LEPTOSPIROSIS (which see), and may be a sequel to various other infections. *Corynebacterium renale* attacks the kidneys, and abscesses of these organs are not uncommonly found in cattle. (*See also* PYELITIS *and* PYELONEPHRITIS *below.*) Some poisons may damage the kidneys.

Symptoms in cattle include stiffness, an arched back, often the passing of small amounts of blood-stained urine, a poor appetite. Rumination may cease.

However in non-acute cases symptoms may not be noticed, and the existence of nephritis discovered only after death. A survey carried out at a Dublin abattoir in 1979–80 showed that of 4166 cattle, 4·2 per cent had kidneys rejected under EC export regulations. The rejection rate was 7·7, 1·7, 2·2, and 28 per cent for cows, bullocks, heifers and bulls, respectively; the most common reason being focal interstitutial nephritis (60 per cent). Other lesions included cysts (26 per cent), pyelonephritis, pigmentation, amyloidosis, and glomerulonephritis. (M. L. Monaghan & J. Hannan. *Vet. Record* (1983), **113**, 55.)

Horses. Nephritis may be a complication of influenza and other infections; may follow dosing with substances such as turpentine, cantharides; or follow contusions (arising from blows, falls) in the lumbar region; or feeding with mouldy or otherwise contaminated fodder. (*See also* PYELO-NEPHRITIS *below.*)

In the horse, symptoms of kidney disease may be somewhat vague, but in severe cases there is usually evidence of pain, stiffness in the gait, a poor appetite, often fever, and urine is passed as described above for cattle. Oedema may involve abdomen, chest, and legs.

Cats. Kidney disease is, generally speaking, likely to result in a poor appetite, loss of weight, dullness, thirst. Intermittent vomiting may occur. The cat may become pot-bellied, due to *ascites*.

However, a cat with chronic nephritis may live to old age, seemingly able to enjoy life still. There is likely to come a time, however, when the kidneys fail, and uraemia occurs.

If a cat is losing protein in its urine, the need is for a high-protein diet; but with chronic nephritis, a low-protein diet is usually indicated. For this purpose, Pedigree Petfoods' canned 'Nephritis Diet (intended for dogs) can be adjusted to feline taste by the addition of a little Marmite and warm water, A. S. Nash, of the University of Glasgow's veterinary faculty, has suggested. (*See also* 'PRE-SCRIPTION DIETS'.)

B. vitamins and diuretics are used in treating the nephrotic syndrome. (*See also* L-GLYCERIC ACIDURIA)

Other animals. Causes, symptoms, and treatment (antibiotics, sometimes diuretics) are in general similar. Vomiting may occur in the pig. (*See also* AVIAN NEPHRITIS.)

Purulent nephritis, or 'suppurative nephritis', is a condition in which one or both kidneys shows abscess formation. All species may be affected. It is caused by pus-producing (pyogenic) organisms,

which may gain access to the kidneys either by the blood-stream – when the term *pyaemic nephritis* is used, or by the ureters from the bladder – when the condition is *pyelonephritis. Pyelitis*, meaning pus in the pelvis of the kidney, is used to indicate abscess formation in the pelvis only, and generally precedes the more severe form of pyelonephritis. It may be associated with stone formation (renal calculus).

Pyelonephritis is generally preceded by an attack of inflammation of the bladder, vagina, or uterus. It is commonest in cows and mares after parturition when the genital tract has become septic, but it is seen in all females under similar circumstances. It is not so common in male animals. Generally only one kidney is affected, and the animal exhibits pain when turned sharply to the affected side, and tenderness when that side is handled.

Pyelitis shows symptoms that are practically the same as those of pyelonephritis, except when due to renal calculus. In such cases it causes an obscure form of colic, and small amounts of blood-stained urine are passed at frequent intervals.

Stone in the kidney. A calculus or stone may sometimes form in the pelvis of the kidney as the result of the gradual deposition of salts from the urine around some particle of matter that acts as a nucleus. (*See* UROLITHIASIS, CALCULI.)

Parasites of the kidney include *Dioctophyma* in the dog, and occasionally *Eustrongylus gigas* in horses, dogs, and cattle, the larvae of *Strongylus vulgaris* in colts, *Stephanurus dentatus* in pigs, and the cystic stages of certain tapeworms in the ruminants, are of most importance. (*See also* DIOCTOPHYMOSIS, *and* LEPTOSPIROSIS.)

Tumours of the kidney include carcinoma (mainly in dogs and cattle) and the usually benign nephroblastoma in pigs, puppies and calves. In cats lymphosarcoma of the kidney is common.

Hydronephrosis. In this condition the kidney may enlarge, owing to an obstruction. (*See* HYDRONEPHROSIS in the alphabetical section.)

Injuries of the kidney are not common, owing to the great protection that the lumbar muscles provide. They may be lacerated or bruised as the result of traffic accidents in the dog. Slips or falls in the hunting field may cause similar injuries. The kidney may be shattered and death from internal haemorrhage occurs, or in less severe cases the haemorrhage takes place below the capsule and the blood is passed in the urine. If only one kidney is affected, and provided the bleeding is not great, the other hypertrophies and acts for both.

KIMBERLEY HORSE DISEASE, or WALK-ABOUT DISEASE, occurs in the Kimberley district of W. Australia, and has a seasonal incidence – January to April (*i.e.* 'wet season'). Horses of all ages are susceptible.

CAUSE. Whitewood (*Atalaya hemiglauca*) taken voluntarily or fed when food is scarce.

SIGNS. Anorexia, dullness, wasting, irritability, biting other horses, and gnawing at posts. Yawning is a marked and almost constant sign.

Then muscular spasms lead to a phase of mad galloping in which the horse has no sense of direction and is uncontrollable. Gallops become more frequent but less violent, and gradually merge into the walking stage – slow, staggering gait, with low, stiff carriage of the head. The horse may walk about for hours, with a mouthful of unchewed grass protruding from its lips. (*See also* BIRDSVILLE DISEASE.)

'KINKY-BACK'. The colloquial name for a condition in broiler chickens involving distortion of the sixth thoracic vertebra. It is the cause of lameness and sometimes paraplegia. It appears to be of hereditary origin, perhaps influenced by growth-rate.

KIRSCHNER-EHMER SPLINT. Used in treating fractures in the dog and cat. It has transverse pins which are driven into parts of a long bone on either side of the fracture, and which are then held in position by an external clamp.

'KITCHEN DEATHS' (*see* CARBON MONOXIDE *and* 'FRYING PAN' DEATHS).

KLEBSIELLA. It was suggested that *Klebsiella pneumoniae* was an important cause of infertility in the thoroughbred **mare** but *see* EQUINE GENITAL INFECTIONS.
In the dog. Klebsiella infection may cause illness clinically indistinguishable from distemper, and may therefore account for some of the suspected 'breakdowns' following the use of distemper vaccines.
In the sow. The infection may result in acute mastitis. Both piglets and sow may die.

KLEIN'S DISEASE (*see* FOWL TYPHOID).

KNEE is the name, wrongly applied, to the carpus of the horse, ox, sheep, and pig. This joint really corresponds to the human wrist and should not be called 'knee', but custom has ordained otherwise. (*See* JOINTS.)

KNOCKED-UP SHOE is one in which the inner branch is hammered laterally so as to increase its height but decrease its width. There is one nail-hole at the inside toe, and four or five along the outside branch. The shoe generally has a clip at the toe and the outside quarter, and may have a small calkin on the outside heel.

It is used for horses given to brushing, cutting, or interfering with their hind feet.

KNOCKED-UP TOE. A term used in racing greyhound circles to describe a type of lameness associated with the digits. It sometimes yields to rest but may require surgical treatment (even amputation of the third phalanx).

KNUCKLING OF FETLOCK simply means that the fetlock joints are kept slightly flexed forwards above the hoof, instead of remaining extended.
Knuckling of the fetlocks in calves of the Jersey, Ayrshire, and Friesian breeds is an inherited defect which can sometimes be corrected by a minor surgical operation.
Occasionally foals are born with their fetlocks knuckled, but, like many other deformities of a similar nature, the condition gradually disappears as the muscles of the young animal obtain their proper control of the joints which they actuate. In older horses the two chief conditions that are responsible for knuckling are: (1) thickening and contraction of the tendons or ligaments behind the cannon; and (2) chronic foot lameness, such as is produced by ringbones, navicular disease, chronic corns, etc. The horse assumes the position of partial flexion of the fetlock apparently in order to ease the pain he feels in one or other of these structures, and as the result of the relaxation of the tendons, shortening occurs, and it finally becomes impossible to straighten out the joint. (*Note.* For descriptive purposes the word 'flexion' here means a bending backwards of the lower section of the limb from the fetlock joint – the cannon remaining stationary. Otherwise confusion between 'flexion' and 'extension' of the fetlock might occur.)

KUPPFER'S CELLS. Present in the liver, these are phagocytic.

KYASANUR FOREST FEVER is a disease of man and monkeys, occurring in Mysore, and resembling Omsk Fever. The causal virus is transmitted by the tick *Haemaphysalis spinigera*, and believed to have been brought by birds from the Soviet Union.

KYPHOSIS is a curvature of the spine when the concavity of the curve is directed downwards. It is sometimes seen in tetanus, rabies, etc., and is a symptom of abdominal pain in the dog.

L

L-CARNITINE. A vitamin of the B complex present in meat extract and needed for fat oxidation. In human medicine it is claimed to improve exercise tolerance; and so might have a potential use in racehorses.

L-FORMS OF BACTERIA. Those which can survive without a true cell wall. L-forms of staphylococci and streptococci have been recovered from cases of mastitis, and they are completely resistant to antibiotics such as penicillin which interferes with bacterial cell-wall formation.

LABIAL. Relating to the lips.

LABILE. Unstable. Thermo-labile – unstable in the presence of heat.

LABIUM is the Latin word for lip or lip-shaped organ.

LABORATORY ANIMALS. Since January 1990 it has been illegal to use non-purpose bred animals for scientific experiments.

LABORATORY TESTS. These include the (serum) Agglutination Test (*see* AGGLUTINATION), Complement Fixation Test (*see* COMPLEMENT), Milk Ring Test, Rose Bengal Test, Coombs Test (all for BRUCELLOSIS), California and Whiteside Tests, and White Cell Counts (all for MASTITIS). The Fluorescent Antibody Test (for rabies, etc.) is described under IMMUNOFLUORESCENT MICROSCOPY. Rothera's test is used for suspected acetonaemia. (*See also* COGGIN'S TEST *and* ELISA.)

LABOUR (*see* PARTURITION).

LABURNUM POISONING. All parts of the plant, whose botanical name is *Cytisus* – root, wood, bark, leaves, flowers, and particularly the seeds in their pods – are poisonous, and all the domestic animals and birds are susceptible.
SIGNS. The toxic agent is an alkaloid called *cystine*, which produces firstly excitement, then unconsciousness with incoordination of movement, and finally convulsions and death.
In the horse, when small amounts have been taken, there is little to be seen beyond a staggering gait, yawning, and a general abnormality in the behaviour of the animal. With larger doses there may be sweating, excitement, collapse, convulsions, coma and death.
In cattle and sheep, which are more resistant than the horse, the rumen becomes filled with gas, the limbs become paralysed, the pupils are dilated, the animal becomes sleepy, and later, salivation, coma, and convulsive movements follow each other. Fatal cases in these animals are not common; the symptoms may last for several days and then gradually pass off.

In the dog and pig, which vomit easily, the irritant and acrid nature of the plant causes free vomiting, and usually the animal is enabled to get rid of what has been eaten before the symptoms become acute. However, this is not always so. One dog, after 24 hours' mild diarrhoea following repeated chewing of a low-lying branch, suddenly collapsed and died. In another case, a stick which had been cut from a laburnum tree three months previously, was thrown for a dog to retrieve, and caused fatal poisoning after being chewed.
FIRST-AID. Very strong black tea or coffee that has been *boiled* instead of infused may be given as a drench.

LABYRINTH (*see* EAR).

LACOMBE. A lop-eared pig from Alberta, Canada. Breeding: Danish Landrace 51 per cent, Chester White 25 per cent, Berkshire 24 per cent. (The Chester White comes from Pennsylvania, and originates from eighteenth-century imports.) The import of Lacombes into the UK was sanctioned in 1966.

LACRIMAL, or LACHRYMAL relates to tears, to the gland which secretes these, and to the ducts of the gland.
Lachrymation. This term is often used to describe an excess of tears, as a result of a blocked duct or conjunctivitis, etc.

LACTATION depends directly upon the fact that if the milk is not regularly removed the secretion will cease. It reaches its maximum duration in the cow and goat which are milked by human agency for the production of milk for consumption. By this artificial method the duration of lactation and the quantities of milk have been enormously increased.
The definition of a lactation is now 305 days, commencing from calving and ending when the cow ceases to be milked at least twice a day and this is in line with other European records. The period for butterfat sampling continues to be from the fourth day after calving.
To produce 2000 gallons of milk the cow must secrete over 9½ tons of milk from the mammary gland, *e.g.* roughly about twelve or fourteen times the weight of her whole body. That remarkable British Friesian cow, Manningford Faith Jan Graceful, which died at the age of 17½, gave a life-time yield of 145 tons, 14 cwt, 85 lbs; and her highest 365-day yield – with her third calf – was 3829·5 gallons. A Jersey has, in 361 days, given over 2666 gallons (1157·46 lbs butterfat). An Ayrshire, Theale Maude 12th, established a world breed record in giving 20,112 gallons milk (7371 lbs butterfat) in 12 lactations, and was still milking. Another Ayrshire has produced over 3295 gallons at 3·73 per cent butterfat in 365 days.

(*See* MILK YIELD, LICKING SYNDROME, MAMMARY GLAND, MILK, WEANING; *also* section on Dairy Breeds of Cattle, *under* CATTLE, BREEDS OF.)

LACTATION, ARTIFICIAL. The artificial induction of lactation may be brought about by means of hormones. For example, barren, anoestrus ewes have been rendered good foster-mothers to lambs by a single dose of 40 mg stilboestrol diproprionate in oil. (*See also under* SPAYING.)

LACTATION TETANY (*see* HYPOMAGNESAEMIA, ECLAMPSIA, HYPOCALCAEMIA, and 'LAMBING SICKNESS').

LACTESCENT SERUM, or plasma, is milky in appearance because of high levels of triglyceride. Especially if fasted, patients are at risk of developing acute pancreatitis and gastro-enteritis (dogs) and skin eruptions (cats.)

LACTIC ACID (*see* MILK). Excessive production of lactic acid in the rumen – such as occurs after cattle have gorged themselves with grain – is a serious condition, and is followed by absorption of fluid from the general circulation (with consequent dehydration), ruminal stasis, and often death. (*See* BARLEY POISONING.)

Lactic acid is produced in muscle by the breakdown of glycogen. (Oxidation of lactic acid provides energy for the recovery phase after a muscle has contracted.)

After strenuous exercise, excess of lactic acid can lead to CRAMP (*see* MUSCLE, Action) and possibly to AZOTURIA.

LACTOSE. Sugar of milk. Lactose in cow's milk has a commercial value, and the Milk Marketing Board has stated that 'cows with low lactose production often have higher mastitis cell counts, so this information should be of real benefit in deciding culling policy.' (*See* SUGAR.)

LAKES (*see* ALGAE POISONING, LEECHES).

LAMB CARCASE REJECTION on inspection at abattoirs. Causes include 'MILK-SPOT LIVER', CYSTICERCOSIS, LIVER FLUKE.

LAMB DYSENTERY is an infectious ulcerative inflammation of the small and large intestine of young lambs, usually under 10 days old, and characterised by a high mortality.
CAUSE. *Clostridium welchii*, type B. This organism is one of the gas gangrene group. After birth the lamb runs every risk of getting infection from its mother's udder, from the soiled wool of the hind quarters, or from the soil itself.
SIGNS. In the acute type nothing seems to be wrong with the lambs at night, but in the morning two or three are found dead. If symptoms appear during the day, lambs are seen to become suddenly dull and listless; they stop sucking. If forced to move, they do so stiffly. Later, the faeces become brownish-red in colour (sometimes yellow), semi-liquid, and are often tinged with bright red blood. After a few hours in this state,

the lamb becomes unconscious and dies. In less acute forms, the lamb may live for 2 or 3 days.
PREVENTION. Two methods: The newly-born lamb is injected as soon after birth as possible, and not later than 12 hours, with lamb dysentery antiserum. This gives it a passive immunity enduring long enough to protect throughout the dangerous period – generally about 2 weeks. Alternatively, ewe vaccination is carried out, so that the lamb will be protected by antibodies in the colostrum. (*See also under* VACCINATION.)

LAMB SURVIVAL RESEARCH (*see* SHEEP BREEDING).

LAMBING DIFFICULTIES. Abnormality of the fetus, or its malpresentation, accounts for a high proportion of 'difficult lambings'. The failure of the cervix to dilate is another frequent cause of difficulty, which can usually be overcome by a veterinary surgeon. (*See* 'RINGWOMB'; *also* VAGINA, RUPTURE OF.)

LAMBING, LAMBS (*see under* SHEEP BREEDING).

LAMBING SICKNESS IN EWES, which is also called parturient hypocalcaemia, or milk fever in ewes, is a condition similar to milk fever in cows. The symptoms and treatment are the same. It may be mistaken for Pregnancy Toxaemia or Louping Ill. (*See* 'MOSS ILL'.)

LAMELLA is a small disc of glycerin jelly containing an active drug for application to the eye. It is applied by inserting within the lower lid. The four official lamellae are those containing atropine, cocaine, homatropine, and physostigmine.

LAMENESS consists of a departure from the normal gait, occasioned by disease or injury situated in some part of the limbs or trunk, and is usually accompanied by pain. In simple cases lameness is not difficult to diagnose; but in obscure cases, and in those instances where more than one limb is affected, it may be extremely difficult for any one, professional or otherwise, to determine where the lameness is, and to what it is due.

It is important to remember that lameness in cattle, sheep, and pigs may be the first symptom of FOOT-AND-MOUTH DISEASE.
CAUSES OF LAMENESS. The main causes are given below, according to animal.

Cattle: foul-in-the-foot, fluorosis, laminitis, mucosal disease, and 'milk lameness'.

Lameness in cattle is of great economic importance to the dairy farmer. The pain arising from several forms of lameness can reduce a cow's milk yield to a significant extent. Economic loss can go beyond this, however, since premature culling and cost of replacement often have to be taken into account also. A 1977 survey, carried out by the Institute for Research on Animal Diseases, Compton, of 1823 herds showed that the annual incidence of lameness was about 5½ per cent.

About 88 per cent of this lameness was due to foot lesions, with foul-in-the-foot predominating; closely followed by abscess formation at the white line, and by ulceration of the sole.

A foreign body, such as a stone or piece of broken glass, lodged between the claws of the hind feet, was a very common cause of lameness. In winter mud at near freezing temperatures is apt to lodge there too, predisposing to foul-in-the-foot.

Results of another survey, involving 262 farms participating in a dairy herd health and productivity service operated by the Royal (Dick) School of Veterinary Studies, University of Edinburgh, was published jointly by the University and Dalgety Spillers in 1981. Records showed that 'an astonishing 25 per cent of cows were treated for lameness, and one per cent culled because of it, in 12 months.'

James Kelly and David Whitaker, members of the veterinary team responsible for the service, emphasised that faulty feeding of high-yielding dairy cows often predispose to laminitis or coronitis, resulting in chronic, often incurable, lameness. They cited as faults: excessive steaming up, major changes of diet at calving, heavy feeding after calving, large single cake or barley feeds, and very acid silage.

On the subject of buildings and their maintenance, in relation to lameness, Kelly and Walker issued a reminder that rough concrete surfaces can abrade the sole of the foot, as can worn slats; and that bad cubicle design can also result in lameness. (*See also* FOOTBATHS).

Dairy cattle. Some 25 per cent become lame every year; but for those kept in straw yards the figure was only 8 per cent, and there were no cases of solar ulceration.

The highest incidence of the latter is found where the cows are in cubicles – a situation for 90 per cent of cows in the west of England (*Veterinary Record* editorial. July 29th 1989.)

Sheep: Footrot. (*See under* DIPS AND DIPPING).

Pigs: Bush foot, foot-rot, swine erysipelas; also a biotin deficiency.

In all species fracture of a bone may be the cause; or injuries to joints, ligaments, tendons or muscles.

Dogs (*see* BRACHIAL PLEXUS, INTERDIGITAL CYST).

Horses. The following remarks refer especially to the horse, but they are to a great extent applicable to the other four-footed animals.

SIGNS OF LAMENESS. The most characteristic and easily seen feature of practically all forms of lameness is abnormality in the manner of nodding the head, either at the walk or the trot. Normally, the horse's head rises and falls to the same extent at each step, and, in lesser measure, the point of the croup (i.e. the highest part of the hindquarters) follows the same course. If a horse be made to walk alongside a blank wall, the head is seen to describe a wavy line against the wall, the undulations of which are equal, provided the rate of the gait is uniform. In a lame horse these undulations become unequal.

FORE-LIMB LAMENESS. The withers of a horse which is lame in one of its two fore-legs, rise when the lame leg is on the ground, and fall when the sound leg comes to earth. And this rising and falling is transferred along the rigid bar of the neck to the head. Accordingly, when a horse is lame in this way, its head is said to 'nod' heavy on the sound leg, and rise on the lame leg.

HIND LIMB LAMENESS. The croup rises when the lame leg is on the ground, and falls when the sound limb is there. But the croup is connected by a rigid bar, passing over a fulcrum (the withers), with the head. It will be seen, therefore, that any rising of the croup will cause a lowering of the head, since the spinal column acts as a lever working over a fulcrum. In the horse which is lame on one of its hind limbs, therefore, the head falls when the croup rises, that is, when the lame leg is on the ground; it rises when the sound leg is on the ground. In other words, it behaves in a manner opposite to its behaviour when the lame limb is situated in front; the diagonally opposite hindleg is indicated.

OTHER SIGNS. The noise made by the lame limb falling to the ground is always less than the noise made by the sound limb, for obvious reasons. The lame limb may be lifted higher than the sound one during the walk, as in cases of sandcrack at the toe (often called 'symptomatic stringhalt' when affecting a hind limb), or, more often, it is not lifted so high (in most cases of pain in joints or in flexor tendons). On soft ground the footprint made by the lame leg is never so deep as that made by the sound leg, although this fact is not of great practical importance. In most lamenesses of the hindmost pair of limbs, the point of the haunch (external angle of the ilium) is carried higher on the same side as the lameness exists. This is most pronounced in lamenesses which involve the joints in greater pain when they are flexed. The raising of the pelvis on the same side as the lameness enables the foot to clear the ground during the stride with a lessened amount of flexion than would otherwise be the case. Finally, there may be some peculiarity of the swing of the lame limb through the air. It may be carried outward (abducted), or it may be carried too near to the other limb (adducted).

DETERMINING THE LAME LIMB. The observer should see the horse walked away from him, towards him, and then past him at right angles. The horse should then be trotted in the same way. If he watches the head carefully, he will see how it is nodding, and as soon as he gets the rhythm of the nods he should immediately commence nodding his own head at the same rate. When he is sure that he is nodding in time with the horse's head, he should at once drop his eyes to the horse's forefeet, and determine which fore-foot comes to the ground when the nod of his head is downwards. Having decided which fore-leg corresponds with a downward nod of the horse's head, he can state that the horse is lame either on the opposite foreleg, or else the hind leg of the same side. He should now attempt to decide whether the lameness is in the anterior pair of limbs or in the posterior pair. To do this it is necessary to observe

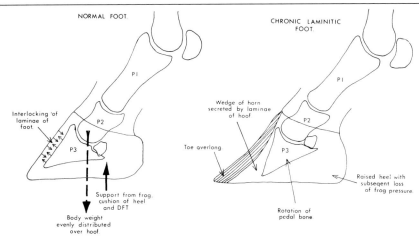

Diagnostic representation of forces involved in pedal bone rotation.

carefully, in which pair of limbs there is some discrepancy in movement, either a long or short step, a lighter noise, adduction or abduction (seen from in front and behind only), increased or diminished flexion, etc. By the aid of these rules practically all simple single-leg lameness can be determined. Where there are two or more limbs affected it is very much more difficult. The services of a veterinary surgeon should be obtained to diagnose the situation of the lesions and their extent and nature.

(*See also* RICKETS, LAMINITIS, HORSES, BACK TROUBLES IN; LIGAMENTS, BRUCELLOSIS.)

LAMINECTOMY. A surgical treatment for fracture of the dorsal arch of a vertebra.

LAMINITIS IN HORSES. This has 'traditionally been defined as inflammation or oedema of the sensitive laminae of the hoof. However, recent work suggests that there is only a transitory inflammation, followed by congestion of the laminae,' stated Mr C. M. Colles and Dr L. B. Jeffcott, of the Animal Health Trust's Equine Research Station. (*Veterinary Record.* (1977), **100,** 262.)

Laminitis is most common in ponies, and in fat or unfit horses. Sometimes all four feet are affected, sometimes only the fore feet; and occasionally only the hind feet or one foot.

CAUSES OF LAMINITIS.

1. Excess carbohydrate intake ('grain overload').
2. Post parturient metritis septicaemia.
3. Toxaemia – associated with enteritis, colitis X (exhaustion shock) and endotoxin shock.
4. Management and type – concussion in unfit horses or susceptible animal (*e.g.*, fat pony).
5. Unilateral leg lameness putting excess strain on contra-lateral limb.
6. High level corticosteroid administration.
7. Fatty liver syndrome.
8. Other suggested factors:
   (a) Hypothyroidism.
   (b) Allergic-type reaction to certain medication (*e.g.*, anthelmintics, oestrogens and androgens).
   (c) High oestrogen content of pasture.

Laminitis should always be regarded as a serious disease, whether it arises secondarily during the course of a generalised illness, or whether it occurs independently of any other recognisable disease.

Intense pain results from acute laminitis, either from inflammation of the sensitive laminae or from changes in the circulation of the blood within the hoof. Prompt treatment is needed to relieve this pain, and to try to prevent permanent damage to the foot. In severe cases of laminitis, separation of the sensitive and horny laminae may occur, and any subsequent infection may put the horse's life at grave risk.

SIGNS. Acute, subacute and chronic forms of laminitis are recognised. Symptoms, especially in acute and subacute laminitis are both general, affecting the whole body, and local.

In acute laminitis the body temperature often rises to 104–106°F, breathing becomes rapid, and the pulse rate likewise (80–120 per minute). Pain may cause the horse to tremble, and profuse sweating may occur. Depression, a facial expression suggestive of pain felt, loss of appetite, and a reluctance to stand or move, together with an unnatural stance are other symptoms. Visible mucous membranes are often bright red, the pupils dilated.

If lying on the ground, the horse will be extremely reluctant to rise; and if standing will maintain the same position, and grunt or groan if forced to take a step.

The affected feet feel hot to the touch, especially at the coronet, and a bounding pulse in the digital arteries can be felt or even seen.

Tenderness is evident immediately any pressure is applied to the affected feet. The appearance of blood, or blood-stained exudate, at the coronary bands is usually followed by death within 24 hours or so.

Each time the foot with laminitis is lifted from the ground, it is snatched up and held for a few moments as if contact with the ground was painful; later it may be rested out in front of the horse with the heel only on the ground. When two feet are affected it is always either the fore pair or the hind pair; diagonal feet are rarely or never attacked. If the fore-feet are involved the horse stands with these thrust out well in front of him, resting on the heels as much as possible, while the hind-feet are brought up under the belly in order to bear as much of the body weight as possible.

In the chronic form, which often follows the acute, laminitis presents a slowly progressive change in the shape of the foot. The toe becomes more and more elongated, the heels and the pasterns become vertical, rings appear around the coronet and move slowly downwards as the horn grows, and a bulge appears in the concavity of the sole.

The line drawings, reproduced by courtesy of the Editor of the *Veterinary Record*, and of Mr Colles and Dr Jeffcott, show both the stance of the horse with laminitis of the fore feet only, and also the rotation of the pedal bone which may take place during or after the acute stage.

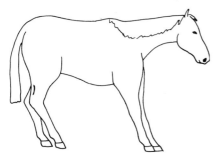

Laminitic stance – forelegs thrust forward, hindlegs drawn under the body and weight taken on heels.

TREATMENT. The above authors recommend blocking of the digital nerves with a local anaesthetic. This gives immediate relief from pain, enables the horse to stand and walk normally, and has a beneficial effect on the blood circulation of the foot. For the relief of pain acetylpromazine is also recommended, and this drug tends to reduce blood pressure. Phenylbutazone is another drug which has been used, and similarly corticosteroids. Warm or hot water applications to the feet are now regarded as preferable to hosing with cold water.

Green food in small amounts is good, and a little hay should be supplied.

In chronic cases the shoeing is of great importance and special surgical shoes may be needed. (*See also* HOOF REPAIR.)

LAMINITIS IN CATTLE. Laminitis has been encountered in both adult and young cattle. For over 50 years, overfeeding with barley has been regarded as a likely cause, and more recently the disease has been described among cattle 4½ to 6 months old in 'barley beef' units.

Excessive steaming up, a change of diet at calving, large single concentrate feeds (especially of barley), overfeeding in the early stages of lactation, and acid over-fermented silage have been cited as causes by Kelly and Whitaker. (*See under* LAMENESS.)

Laminitis in the cow is rarely the acute disease seen in the horse, but rather a milder, more insidious condition. 'A general tenderness of all

four feet develops, usually soon after calving. This stage may go unnoticed. It may be followed sooner or later by more clearly recognised chronic secondary foot problems such as ulceration of the sole, separation of the wall from the sole, and horizontal cracks in the wall.' Infection usually complicates such conditions.

LAMPAS. A swelling of the mucous membrane of the hard palate of the horse immediately behind the arch of the incisor teeth in the upper jaw. It is often seen about the time when the permanent teeth are cutting through the gums, *i.e.* at 2½, 3½, and 4½ years, and for a short time afterwards. It is erroneously thought that it is the *cause* of a falling off in condition which naturally occurs when the teeth are cutting; it is really rather an *effect*. It was the custom to lance 'lampas' in many parts of the country; this occasions unnecessary pain and discomfort to the horse, and if the incision is made towards one side instead of in the middle line there is a serious risk of wounding the palatine artery on that side.

LAMZIEKTE is botulism of cattle in South Africa which occurs as an enzootic in animals on phosphorus-deficient areas of the veldt. During winter lack of phosphorus leads grazing cattle to chew the bones of animals (often cattle) that have died, in an endeavour to take phosphorus into the body to make good the deficiency. This condition of bone-eating (oesteophagia) is actually only the result of a craving for minerals. Where the animals whose skeletons are left on the veldt, harboured in their alimentary canals, the *Clostridium botulinum*, this organism invades the carcase, and both it and its toxin are present in the decomposing remains.
PREVENTION. The researches of Sir Arnold Theiler and the workers at Onderstepoort showed that the best means of preventing lamziekte is to feed sterilised bone meal to cattle during the winter months in areas which are naturally deficient in phosphorus. (*See* BOTULISM.)

LANTANA POISONING of cattle and sheep has occurred in Australia and New Zealand. *L. camara* is the species commonly involved; especially the red-flowered variety. It causes light sensitisation, with exudative dermatitis of teats and vulva. Deaths have occurred due to it.

LAPARASCOPY. The use of optical instruments for viewing the interior of organs such as the bladder, the interior of joints for signs of arthritis, etc, and for avian sex determination.

LAPAROTOMY means surgical opening of the abdominal cavity. The incision is either made in the middle line of the abdomen, or through one or other of the flanks.

LAPINISED. This term is applied to a virus which has been attenuated by passage through rabbits. An example is afforded by lapinised swine fever vaccine.

LARKSPUR POISONING. Of the several varieties of Larkspur, most of which occur in America in the ranges of the West, where they cause great loss to cattle owners, only one species is commonly found in Great Britain – *Delphinium ajacis*. The seeds are the most dangerous parts of the plant, although the leaves have proved fatal when fed experimentally. Horses and sheep are not so susceptible as cattle. The active principles are four in number, viz. *Delphine, Delphisine, Delphinoidine*, and *Staphisagrine*, and of these the first three are highly poisonous.

SIGNS. Salivation, vomiting, colicky pains, convulsions, and general paralysis.

LARYNGITIS (*see* LARYNX, DISEASES OF).

LARYNX is the organ of voice, and also forms one of the parts of the air passage. It is placed just between, and slightly behind, the angles of the lower jaw. Externally it is covered by the skin, by a small amount of fibrous tissue, and sterno-thyro-hyoid muscles.

Structure. The *cricoid* cartilage is shaped somewhat like a signet ring and connects the rest of the larynx with the first ring of the trachea. To its upper part are attached the arytenoids and the posterior horns of the thyroids. A crico-tracheal membrane unites it to the trachea, and a crico-thyroid membrane unites it to the thyroid cartilage. The *thyroid* cartilage possesses a body which in man forms the protuberance known as 'Adam's apple'. The *epiglottis* lies in front of the body of the thyroid and curves forwards towards the root of the tongue; it is shaped somewhat like a pointed ovate leaf. The *arytenoids* are situated one on either side of the upper part of the cricoid to which they are attached. (For functions, *see under* VOICE.)

LARYNX, DISEASES OF (*see also* ROARING, WHISTLING, COUGHING).

Laryngitis is an inflammation of the larynx, but particularly of the mucous membrane which lines its interior. It is often associated with pharyngitis or with bronchitis and tracheitis, when it is usually due to the spreading of inflammation from one of these neighbouring structures.

In the **horse** it may occur during influenza. (*See also* LATHYRISM.)

SIGNS. In ordinary cases there is a cough, difficulty in swallowing, pain on pressure over the larynx, extension of the head to relieve pressure on the throat (a condition that is aptly described in popular terms as 'star gazing'). A wheezing or roaring sound accompanies breathing if membranes become so swollen as to interfere with respiration. A slight rise in temperature and pulse-rate accompanies the milder forms, but when influenza is present, or if other specific diseases arise, the signs of fever are more distinct. Uncomplicated laryngitis usually lasts from a week to about a fortnight. Occasionally complications, such as roaring or whistling, follow recovery from the initial disease.

FIRST-AID. It is advisable to isolate all cases of laryngitis in a loose-box or other building, especially those arising in newly purchased animals, on account of the risk of contagious disease developing. (*See* NURSING.)

Wounds of the larynx are not common, owing to its comparatively sheltered position in the body, but *see under* DRENCHING for a danger associated with the use of a drenching gun in pigs and sheep.

Foreign bodies (*see* CHOKING).

Laryngeal paralysis in horses. The abnormal inspiratory sound called 'Roaring'.

The usual cause was for long regarded as vibration of the slackened vocal folds on one or both sides of the larynx, due to paralysis of the muscles which move the arytenoid cartilages outwards.

Research by Dr W. R. Cook at the Animal Health Trust's equine research station provided findings in support of the hypothesis that the incurable laryngeal paralysis is a hereditary disease transmitted by a simple recessive factor (AHT report 1978.)

A large number of respiratory diseases may give rise to a temporary roaring due to inflammation and thickening of the mucous membranes lining the larynx. GUTTURAL POUCH DIPHTHERIA (which see) may have a permanent effect.

TREATMENT. The traditional Hobday operation entailed the vocal fold being encouraged to adhere to the wall of the larynx out of the path of the entering stream of air, by stripping the lining membrane from a little pouch which lies between the vocal cord and the laryngeal wall. Tracheotomy was an alternative: in this, a metal tube is inserted into the trachea at a lower level than the larynx, so that air is able to enter and leave through the tube instead of through the larynx. Tracheotomy is of most use in race-horses and hunters affected with roaring.

Roaring constitutes an unsoundness.

Dr C. J. Hillidge has emphasised that abnormal inspiratory noises during exercise, particularly in young horses which may have pharyngitis and laryngitis, should not be taken to indicate one-sided paralysis of the larynx. Similarly, normal respiratory sounds at exercise should not be regarded as implying soundness of the upper respiratory tract.

Idiopathic left-sided paralysis of the larynx was present in 4 of 169 horses on a thoroughbred breeding farm, i.e. 8·3 per cent.

Laryngoplasty has been re-introduced for the treatment of roaring, especially in those horses not required to perform at high speeds.

The operation involves securing the arytenoid cartilage in a lateral position, using prostheses to prevent intrusion of the arytenoid cartilage and vocal cord into the lumen of the larynx.

Asynchronous movement of the arytenoid cartilages was observed in 94 horses at rest (55·6 per cent), 86 of which were considered as normal after exercise.

Conversely, synchronous movement of the arytenoids was noted when at rest in six of the 14 horses diagnosed as having laryngeal hemiplegia after exercise. An abnormal inspiratory noise during exercise was detectable in 11 of these 14 horses, but not in the remainder. (Hillidge, C. J., *Veterinary Record* (1986) **113**, 535).

Poisoning. Four two-year-old thoroughbreds suffered an acute gastrointestinal illness shortly after being dosed with contaminated mineral oil.

Three weeks later they had developed bilateral laryngeal paralysis. Two of the horses died during severe bouts of dyspnoea six and eight weeks later, and a third was put down. In these horses there was a severe loss of myelinated fibres from both recurrent laryngeal nerves. The fourth horse had bilateral pharyngeal paralysis two years later. The acute clinical signs and delayed neurological effects were typical of ORGANOPHOSPHORUS POISONING. (Duncan, I. D. & Brook, D., *Equine Veterinary Journal* (1985) **17**, 228.)

LASER. An acronym for Light Amplification by the Stimulated Emission of Radiation.

Lasers emit beams of intense, monochromatic, non-dispersing light. They are used in the veterinary treatment of soft tissue injuries, making healing more rapid. Laser·beams have also been used instead of needles in acupuncture, and for ophthalmic and other surgery. Operators must wear protective glasses to protect their eyes.

LASSA FEVER. This disease occurs in West Africa, and is caused by an arenavirus first isolated in 1969. In man the infection is likely to prove fatal. The virus has been isolated from the rat *Mastomys natalensis*, which (possibly with other rodents) acts as a reservoir of infection.

LATERAL CARTILAGES are rhomboid plates of cartilage which are attached, one on either side, to angles of the third phalanx (*os pedis*) of the foot of the horse. They extend above the coronet sufficiently to be felt distinctly at the heels and for a certain distance in front of this. In old age they often become ossified in their lower parts. When they ossify in their upper palpable margins the name 'side bone' is applied to the condition. In certain cases they may become injured from treads or tramps by neighbouring horses or from the other foot, and the cartilage, being poorly supplied with blood, undergoes necrosis. (*See* SIDE-BONES, QUITTOR, FOOT OF HORSE.)

LATEX (natural rubber). Hypersensitivity to this can result in contact urticaria, respiratory symptoms, and shock.

The main source of the allergens is the wearing of rubber gloves during surgery.

Even a vaginal examination can result in an anaphylactic reaction in atopic people.

In the rubber-growing areas of Malaysia the ingestion of latex by cattle, *e.g.* from buckets left by rubber-tappers, is a 'frequent occurrence,' I. Fatimah and others stated (*Vet. Record* (1983) **113**, 89). They described two fatal cases after 9 and 14 litres, respectively, had been taken. The latex was from the tree *Hevea brasiliensis.* Rumentotomy brought a temporary improvement in both bulls, but they died, despite supportive treatment, 11 days after ingesting the latex.

Latex agglutination test. This can be used for measuring the concentration of IgG$_1$ in the plasma of newborn calves. The commercial test reagent (Ab-Ag Laboratories, Ely) is prepared by coating polystyrene latex beads with antibodies against bovine IgG$_1$.

LATHYRISM, or LATHYRUS POISONING, is caused by feeding upon one of the various 'Mutter peas' – *Lathyrus sativus* principally, and *L. cicera* and *L. clymenum*, less frequently. The latter are found in samples of field peas grown in South Europe and North Africa, while *L. sativus* is imported from India mainly. They are poisonous to all the domesticated animals, but seem specially dangerous for horses. Many outbreaks have been recorded, and in most the percentage of deaths has been high, sometimes as much as 50 per cent of the affected.

Symptoms of poisoning may not appear until the lapse of as much as 50 days after the peas cease to be used as a food-stuff. The cause of lathyrism was shown in 1952 or thereabouts to be the high selenium content of the plants. (*See* SELENIUM.)
SIGNS. Usually become visible when the animal is put to work or exercised. Typically, the chief symptoms are those of paralysis of some part of the body – usually the hind-limbs and the recurrent laryngeal nerve. This latter gives rise to the condition known as 'roaring', and unless quickly relieved the horse will die from asphyxia. In some instances the symptoms are so sudden in their onset that the horse drops while in harness and is unable to rise. In less severe cases there is staggering and swaying of the hindquarters, great difficulty in breathing, a fast, weak pulse, and convulsive seizures. The paroxysms may pass off in a few minutes, or the horse may collapse and die.
TREATMENT (*see* LARYNX, DISEASES OF).
The antidote is ascorbic acid, added to the diet.

LAUDANUM (*see* OPIUM).

LAUREL (Laurus) POISONING. The leaves of laurel shrubs and trees (Family: *Lauraceae*) contain CYANOGENETIC CLYCOSIDES which cause poisoning by HYDROCYANIC ACID. (*See under those headings.*)

LAVAGE. The process of washing out the stomach or the intestines. In gastric lavage a double-way tube is passed down into the stomach either through the mouth or by way of the nose, and water or some medicinal solution is poured or pumped through one channel in the tube, and after a time escapes by the other, carrying with it the contents of the stomach in small amounts. (*See also* ENEMA.)

LAW, THE, relating to the veterinary profession and veterinary practice, scientific research, domestic pets, farm animals, wild animals, zoos.

1991 legislation included the following:
Badgers Act. This makes it an offence to damage, destroy or obstruct a sett, disturb badger in a sett, or put a dog into a sett.
Badgers (Further Protection) Act. This legalises euthanasia of a dog, and disqualification of its owner from keeping a dog in future, after the offending dog has killed, injured or taken a badger, or the dog's owner has ill-treated or dug a badger out of its sett.
Blue-eared Pig Disease Order 1991.
Breeding of Dogs Act 1991. This extended

powers under the 1973 legislation, which permitted local authorities to inspect only those premises already licensed, or those for which a licence application had been made. Under this new Act the Council or a veterinary surgeon could apply to a magistrate for a warrant to enter and inspect the premises. Obstruction becomes a criminal offence.

Dangerous Dogs Act 1991. This requires that certain breeds (pit bull terrier, Japanese tosa, fila brasileiro, dogo argentino) must not be taken out unless on a lead, muzzled, and by someone at least sixteen years old.

Owners of these dogs were given until November 30th to register them with the police, and either comply with the exemption scheme or arrange for euthanasia carried out by a veterinary surgeon.

To comply with the exemption scheme owners must take out third-party insurance, arrange for the animal to be neutered, and to be identifiable by a tattoo and a microchip. The dog must also be kept under escape-proof conditions.

Earlier legislation
Animal Boarding Establishments Act 1963.
Animal Health Act 1981 consolidated the Diseases of Animals Acts of 1953, 1950, and 1975.
Animals (Scientific Procedures) Act 1986. This replaced the Cruelty to Animals Act of 1876.
Breeding of Dogs Act 1973.
Coal Mines Act 1911.
Dangerous Wild Animals Act 1976. (*See under that heading.*)
Deer Act. This consolidates previous Acts of 1963 and 1980.
Disease of Animals (Waste Food Order) 1973. This makes it an offence for producers to feed, intentionally or inadvertently, poultry carcase material to livestock on their premises. Litter should be examined for carcases before spreading on to pasture, ensiling or drying.
Diseases of Animals Act 1950. This covers the NOTIFIABLE diseases.
Diseases of Fish Act. This lists the nine or so NOTIFIABLE diseases.
Docking and Nicking Act 1949 (re Horses.)
Endangered Species Act 1982.
Export of Animals (Protection) Order 1951.
Food Safety Act 1990 'covers the whole of the food chain from retailers back to primary producers' – Sir Derek Andrews, MAFF.
Fresh Meat Export (Hygiene and Inspection) Regulations 1987.
Infectious Diseases of Horses Order 1975.
Injured Animals Act 1907.
Ionising Radiation Regulations 1985.
Medicines Act 1968. Veterinary Surgeons in the UK are limited to supplying prescription-only medicines (POM) for animals under their care and not to the public at large.
Movement and Sales of Pigs Order 1975.
Pet Animals Act 1971.
Ponies Act 1969.
Protection of Animals (Anaesthetics) Act 1964.
Riding Establishments Act 1939.
Slaughter of Animals Acts 1933 and 1954.
Slaughter of Poultry (Licences) Regulations. These cover premises.

Transit of Animals (Road and Rail) Order 1975.
Veterinary Surgeons Act 1966.
Veterinary Surgeons 1966 Act Amendment Order. This permits a veterinary nurse to carry out any medical treatment or any minor surgery to a companion animal, provided that the latter is under the care of a registered veterinary surgeon who has authorised the treatment.
Welfare of Animals at Slaughter Act. This amends Acts of 1974 and 1980, and covers the formal training, examination, and licensing of slaughtermen, codes of practice relating to welfare, both in slaughterhouses and knackers' yards.
Welfare of Pigs Regulations. These prohibit the tethering of pigs or keeping them in a stall or pen which does not meet minimum space requirements.
Zoo Licensing Act 1981. Of 150 zoos inspected following the passing of the Act, only five were refused a licence; and in those cases it was public safety considerations rather than the quality of animal care which brought about the refusal.
Zoonoses Order 1975.

Note
Health & Safety at Work Act.
(**Laboratory Animals.** Since January 1990 it has been illegal to use non-purpose-bred animals in scientific experiments.)

(*See also* EUROPEAN COMMUNITY (EC).) ☞

LAXATIVES (*see* SENNA) which has been recommended for pregnant sows; DIHYDROXYANTHRAQUINONE, useful in all domestic animals, including horses; EPSOM SALTS, but of doubtful efficacy in ruminants; GLAUBER'S SALTS, but they may have ill effects in pigs. (*See also* PARAFFIN, **medicinal.**)

LD$_{50}$ value is a statistical estimate of the number of mg of a given poison per kg of bodyweight required to kill 50 per cent of a large population of test animals. The LD value of a compound may refer to oral administration or to application to the skin.

LEAD POISONING.
Acute form of lead poisoning.
Cattle. This is very common in cattle which have eaten paint, licked out discarded paint tins, or licked newly painted railings, etc., or eaten tarpaulins. It is frequently fatal and many cattle are unnecessarily lost each year from this cause. Cows have also been fatally poisoned after licking lead-rich ash from a burnt-down shed; and after eating silage contaminated by an old battery broken up by a forage harvester; also by eating roofing material from an old railway carriage.

In another instance cows were poisoned after eating haylage made from grass in a field which had been used for clay-pigeon shooting. The haylage contained small particles of clay pigeons and lead shot. The cows in the high-yielding herd of 115 Holsteins began to lose their appetite, became dull, had diarrhoea. A few developed stiff and swollen joints. Many became incoordinated in their movements. Also there were 25 stillbirths or abortions.

Appropriate treatment brought some improvement, but 21 cows either died or had to be slaughtered.

A 24-volt lead battery was discarded but unfortunately scooped up with straw being added to a 'complete diet' in a feeder box. The result was that 55 heifers died; some rapidly, some after ataxia, head pressing, teeth grinding and convulsions. (Source: A 1991 Veterinary Investigation Service report.)

Dogs are sometimes poisoned through eating paint scrapings where a room is being redecorated, or after licking out a paint tin.

Cats. In one case, old lead primer was stripped by means of an electric sander, which dispersed particles of the primer so that the air soon contained a toxic amount of lead. One cat and an infant suffered lead poisoning as a result.

Pigs. Experimental work in the USA (1966) showed that pigs can consume, without showing any symptoms at all, a daily dose of lead which would rapidly kill a cow.

Geese. Ten lead pellets can kill a goose.

SIGNS. Nervous signs are an important feature of lead poisoning, and may include excitement, ataxia, blindness, paresis, and convulsions.

Cattle may bellow, charge around, and at intervals press their heads against a wall or other fixed object.

Abdominal pain, sometimes with constipation followed by diarrhoea, are other signs; also anaemia in chronic or subacute cases.

In horses 'roaring' (laryngeal paralysis) may be a sign, together with carpal swelling, and posterior paralysis.

TREATMENT. The treatment of lead poisoning was revolutionised by the introduction of the chelating agent, calcium di-sodium adetate, which converts inorganic lead in the tissues into a harmless lead chelate which is excreted by the kidneys. The drug must be given intravenously. In chronic cases, potassium iodide is given 3 or 4 times daily to hasten the elimination of the lead salt from the system. (*See also* CHELATING AGENTS.)

DIAGNOSIS of lead poisoning is usually made by estimating the lead content of the liver.

A DIFFERENTIAL DIAGNOSIS must take into account other possibilities such as hypomagnesaemia, encephalitis, acetonaemia, listeriosis, and poisoning by other substances.

Chronic lead poisoning has occurred as a result of flaking paintwork in dog kennels, and also in the proximity of former lead-mining sites. Four out of five sheepdogs, in an Australian incident, became agitated after working sheep satisfactorily for some 20 minutes. They left the work area and retreated to the underside of a vehicle or to a kennel.

The behavioural effects of lead poisoning in dogs may also include hysteria or aggressiveness.

LEECHES (Class Hirudinea, within Phylum Annelida, segmented worms).

They have strong muscular suckers; the anterior one surrounding the mouth which, in several species, contains saw-like teeth used to pierce the skin of the host. Leeches secrete a substance to prevent clotting of the host's blood, on which they feed, and cause a severe anaemia which is sometimes fatal.

Leeches live in ponds, streams, and on damp vegetation.

Limnatis nilotica is found in North Africa and Southern Europe. It reaches a length of 10 cm. The ventral surface is dark; but on the dorsal surface are six longitudinal stripes on a brownish-green background. It cannot penetrate skin, but on being taken in with water by men and animals, it attaches itself to the buccal mucous membrane. They produce constant small haemorrhages, which sometimes cause a serious anaemia.

L. africana and species of *Haemadipsa* are active in West Africa and in the tropical forests of Asia and South America, respectively.

Haemadipsa zeylanica occurs in Asia and lives on land. It is a clear brown colour with a yellow lateral stripe on each side and a greenish dorsal stripe. It has five pairs of eyes and three teeth. It lives in damp weather on the lower vegetation. They are small forms, about an inch long, but are very serious pests. The bite is painless but, as they occur in such enormous numbers, very deadly. They attack all vertebrates, and many different species of mammals have been killed by them through sheer loss of blood.

Two cases of infestation of dogs with *Diestecostoma mexicanum* have been reported from Honduras. In the non-fatal case, a catheter was passed through the inferior nasal meatus and a 50-ml capacity syringe containing chloroform water attached. The solution was injected slowly while the catheter was revolved. Over seventy leeches emerged after treatment.

In Nepal Dr S. N. Mahato found that leeches could be removed and killed by ivermectin. First water 'is sprinkled on to the nose' of the parasite, which makes the leeches protrude. They are expelled within three hours.

Ivermectin can also be applied in the form of nasal drops.

LEGIONELLA PNEUMOPHILA. This organism, first discovered in 1976, can tolerate hot water, and is spread by aerosols of it. People, cattle, sheep, horses, pigs, goats, dogs and cats all are at risk of pneumonia caused by this infection.

LEGISLATION (*see* LAW, THE).

LEGUME POISONING. This may occur when certain legumes are fed raw, and can result in death. Both navy beans (*Phaseolus vulgaris*) and jack beans (*Canavalis ensiformis*) contain a heat-sensitive toxin which can weaken the animal's resistance to coliform and other bacteria. Heat treatment of the beans renders them safe. (*See also* LATHYRISM, LUPINS, POISONING, INFERTILITY.)

LEISHMANIA. A genus of protozoon parasites. Each appears as a round or oval body with a micro- and a macro-nucleus.

Leishmaniasis is of considerable importance in man, but not in animals other than the dog.

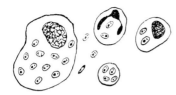

Leishmania as seen in spleen cells.

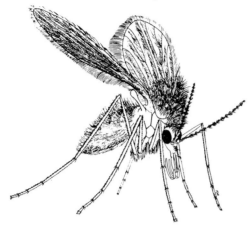

A female phlebotomine sandfly, the vector of leish-maniasis. Reproduced with permission from *The Leishmaniases: Report of Who Expert Committee*, WHO technical Report Series, no. 701, WHO, Geneva, 1984.

Cutaneous leishmaniasis, or 'oriental sore' is seen in Iran, India, parts of Africa, and South America, and is caused by *Leishmania tropica*. Visceral leishmaniasis, called also kala-zaar or 'dum-dum fever', occurs in the coastal countries of the Mediterranean, and is caused by *Leishmania donovani*. (At least five other species, and several sub-species, are recognised.) Both forms are diagnosed by laboratory examination. A third form, affect-ing mucous membrane of mouth and nose, is caused by *L. brasiliensis*, and has a poor prognosis.

SIGNS in the dog include wasting, enlarged lymph nodes, keratitis and/or conjunctivitis, and alopecia or dermatitis.

Leishmaniasis also affects cats, causing skin ulcers, nodules, and fistulae.

TREATMENT. When undertaken, this has been by intravenous injection of 10 cc of a 1 per cent solution of tartar emetic. The outlook for in-fected dogs is poor, especially as relapses often follow treatment. (*See* SANDFLIES.)

There have been several reports of dogs imported into the UK having this disease. Canine leishmaniasis has recently been found in the USA. Dogs are an important source of human infection in many regions.

LENS of the eye (*see* EYE).

'LENSES,' CONTACT, made not of the old, hard material but of a softer, hydrophilic type, have been used in horses, dogs and cats with keratitis and/or penetration of the cornea. Such

'lenses' can act more or less as a bandage for the cornea, and promote healing by reducing trauma from inflamed eyelids and so reducing pain. Ointment and eye drops can be still used. The 'lens' can be removed at the end of a week or so. (J. Tammeus & others. *JAVMA* (1983) **182,** 286.)

The effect of bright light on the retina of a racing greyhound's eye caused a lack of speed. This improved after a *tinted* contact lens had been fitted. (Ling, T. *JAVMA* (1986) **188,** 65).

LEPTOMENINGITIS means inflammation of the inner and more delicate membranes of the brain and spinal cord.

LEPTOSPIRA. This genus comprises two species: a pathogenic one, *L. interrogans*; and *L. biflexa*, which is found in surface water and is regarded as a saprophyte. Leptospires are SPIRO-CHAETES (which see).

LEPTOSPIROSIS. Infection with *Leptospira*.

LEPTOSPIROSIS IN CATTLE. This is an important infection which can give rise to a generalised illness, to mastitis, or to abortion. Jaundice may be one of the symptoms and, in the case of mastitis, discoloured milk. (*See* MASTITIS.) The leptospires tend to localise in the kidneys. Abnormal milk is a dominant symptom. Abor-tion due to leptospirosis is not uncommon. For example, in 1975 MAFF reported that in one outbreak three out of eight heifers aborted after being in-calf for eight months. In a 150-cow herd, five aborted, and in another herd nine out of 170 aborted, from this cause.

'A total of 406 cattle sera collected at the Edin-burgh abattoir from animals of 63 different herds in various parts of Scotland, the north of England and Northern Ireland were tested against the fol-lowing Leptospira serotypes: *ictero-haemorrhagiae, canicola, pomona, bratislava, ballum, sejroe, grippotyphosa,* and *bataviae; saxaebing* and *hardjo* were included when testing the last 80 cattle sera. The results of these tests revealed that 260 (64 per cent of the total) sera had agglutinins to one or more of these 10 sero-types.' (*Veterinary Record*, June 3, 1967.)

Cattle are the maintenance hosts of *L. hardjo*, which is a cause of leptospiral MASTITIS (which see) and also important from the public health aspect.

Leptospirosis of calves has been seen both in the UK (due to *L. icterohaemorrhagiae*) and over-seas (due to other *leptospires*). In Queensland an acute fever with jaundice and haemoglobinuria has been known in calves for many years. It is rapid in onset and death occurs within a few hours to 4 days after the appearance of symptoms; dull-ness, temperature 104° to 107°, dark red urine, pale and yellow visible mucous membranes. *L. pomona* was demonstrated in kidney sections on post-mortem examinations. Recovered calves continue to excrete *leptospires* for up to 3 months. Infection may occur through inhalation of drop-lets of infected urine splashing on concrete, or as a result of insect bites.

In the USA, where the important species are

L. pomona, *L. grippotyphosa*, and *L. sejroe*, abortion is reported to be the main symptom of leptospirosis in cows. In Illinois, a survey covering over 23,000 animals showed 14 per cent to be affected.

In Kenya, outbreaks of acute illness due to infection with *L. gryppotyphosa* have been reported in cattle, sheep, and goats. Jaundice is a symptom in some 30 per cent of cases, and death has followed within 12 hours of symptoms being observed. Snuffling, coughing, and holding down of the head are other symptoms. In cows, milk yield is reduced and is red in colour or otherwise abnormal. Urine varies from red to black. Temperature may rise to 105 degrees Fahrenheit.

In Europe, the above, *L. pomona* and *L. canicola* have been isolated.

CONTROL. A vaccine was introduced by the Wellcome Foundation in 1983 and claimed to be the first effective means of immunising cattle against infection by *L. interrogans* serovar *hardjo*, which causes a drop in milk yield, abortion, and premature calving. A Tasman vaccine also became available in 1983.

WILD ANIMAL HOSTS. After an outbreak of abortion associated with *Leptospires* in Scottish cattle, wild mammals were examined. *Leptospires* were isolated from 22/108 rats, 3/49 mice and 1/3 hedgehogs; voles, mice and shrews were found to be infected on the farm where the leptospiral abortion had been diagnosed. Contamination of pastures by the urine of wild mammals may play a part in the spread of leptospirosis in cattle.

Public health aspects. Cowmen working in milking parlours have become infected with leptospirosis as a result of the splashing of infected cows' urine on concrete. Inhalation of a resulting aerosol is one means of transmission. Leptospires can penetrate abraded skin and intact mucous membrane – another mode of infection.

Infection with members of the Hebdomadis serogroup was described by W. A. Ellis and others (*Vet. Record* (1976) **99**, 368) as 'the most commonly diagnosed leptospiral infection of man in Britain.' This serogroup includes *L. hardjo* and *L. sejroe*, which also cause mastitis in cows.

Two genotypes have been recognised: *hardjo bovis* and *hardjo prajitno*; 'the latter being less common but more pathogenic.' (Dr W. A. Ellis.)

Seventy-two cases of human leptospirosis, of which seven were fatal, were confirmed in the British Isles in 1981. In 30 cases the patient's occupation was associated with farming. Nine of the patients became infected through immersion in polluted water. Illness due to Hebdomadis serogroup infection was generally less severe than that due to *L. icterohaemorrhagiae*. (*British Medical Journal* (1982) **284**, 1276).

L. hardjo causes an influenza-like illness which can be severe and last several weeks. In rare instances there may be meningitis, kidney failure, and death.

In New Zealand cowmen with high titres were on farms where, apparently, there was active *L. hardjo* infection of 2- and 3-year-old cattle. Conventional measures for protecting milkers from contact with infected urine appeared to be ineffective, and it was concluded that herd vaccination of cattle was the only means of protecting dairy farm workers. (*New Zealand Veterinary Journal* (1982) **30**, 73.)

In 1986 about 6 per cent of dairy farmers in New Zealand and Australia had antibodies to *L. hardjo*.

LEPTOSPIROSIS IN DOGS. Jaundice in dogs caused by *Leptospira icterohaemorrhagiae* is dealt with under JAUNDICE, LETPOSPIRAL, OF DOGS. This organism also causes jaundice (Weil's disease) in man, and illness (with or without jaundice) in a number of domestic animals, including pigs and calves. Monlux showed in 1948 in the USA that of 100 rats used in a survey, 55 had leptospira in the kidneys, and that 23·07 per cent of the farm rats and 49, or 66·2 per cent, of the dump rats harboured leptospira in those organs. (The incidence of the leptospira in the rat varied with the location of the dump. Nearly all the rats obtained in one area were positive. If there is plenty of food, rats will migrate very little.) Similar surveys in the UK have shown 37·6 per cent rats infected.

In a Glasgow survey it was found that 40 per cent of dogs had at some time been infected with *Leptospira canicola* (the cause of Canicola Fever in man), which is 2 or 3 times more common as a parasite in dogs than *L. icterohaemorrhagiae*. The parasite is the cause of much of the acute and sub-acute nephritis in younger dogs, especially between November and April.

SIGNS of infection with *L. canicola* are very variable. There may be loss of appetite, depression, and fever alone, or together with *marked thirst* and *vomiting*, loss of weight, and sometimes a foul odour from the mouth. In a few cases there is jaundice. Ulceration of the tongue may occur. Collapse, coma, and death may supervene. (*See* 'STUTTGART DISEASE'.)

The symptoms first described above are related to leptospiral invasion of the bloodstream. This may be followed by invasion of, and damage to, the kidneys. This primary nephritis may be followed later by chronic interstitial nephritis, kidney failure, uraemia, and death.

TREATMENT. Penicillin has been used with considerable success in the early stage of *L. canicola* infection. Once the kidneys have been damaged, however, treatment is as for nephritis. In severe cases – where the 'Stuttgart' syndrome or symptoms of uraemia are evident, the animal dies, as a rule, despite all treatment. (*See* KIDNEYS, DISEASES OF; URAEMIA, NURSING, HEART, DISEASES OF.)

PREVENTION. Single and multiple vaccines are available. (*See* MATERNAL ANTIBODIES.)

Most of the dogs which recover from leptospirosis excrete the organisms in the urine for long periods (sometimes 4 to 18 months). This obviously makes control of the disease difficult.

LEPTOSPIROSIS IN HORSES is usually a mild disease, though sometimes fatal in foals; but *see* PERIODIC OPHTHALMIA.

LEPTOSPIROSIS IN PIGS. Cases of leptospiral jaundice in piglets due to *L. icterohaemorrhagiae* and also to *L. canicola* have been reported in the UK.

Symptoms in pigs include loss of appetite, fever, jaundice, and – in some cases – death. Pigs which have recovered excrete *leptospires* for some time afterwards. Indeed, infection in a herd may persist for years, with risk to human health. Sows may abort.

L. canicola can survive for 12 days in naturally infected pig kidneys kept in a refrigerator. (*See* CANICOLA FEVER, which pigmen may contract from pigs.)

L. pomona and *L. interrogans hardjo* may cause leptospiral abortion. *L. australia*, which in the UK has many free-living carnivore hosts, also infects pigs.

LEPTOSPIROSIS IN SHEEP. 'In Britain leptospirosis is not a recognised disease of sheep,' stated S. C. Hathaway of the Central Veterinary Laboratory in 1982: though MAFF serological surveys had shown evidence of infection. In Northern Ireland the infection was demonstrated in aborted, stillborn and weak lambs, by culture, immunofluorescence and fetal serology, from nine out of 42 flocks investigated during the 1980 and 1981 lambing seasons. Three serogroups were implicated: Hebdomadis, Australis, and Pomona. (W. A. Ellis & others. *Vet. Record* (1983) **112**, 291).

Clinical leptospirosis in sheep and goats in other countries has been characterised by either (a) abortion; or (b) an acute, often fatal disease, with symptoms of jaundice, fever, and haemoglobinuria.

LESION meant originally an injury, but is now applied to all changes produced by diseases in organs or tissues.

LET-DOWN OF MILK (*see* MILKING).

LETHAL FACTORS (*see* GENETICS).

LEUCINE. One of the essential amino-acids.

LEUCO- or **LEUKO-** is a prefix meaning white. **LEUKO-** is the spelling recommended currently by the EC.

LEUKAEMIA (or LYMPHOSARCOMA) is a malignant disease – a form of cancer – involving lymphoid tissue especially. It occurs in all the domestic animals in which, as opposed to man, there is commonly but not invariably no increase in the number of lymphocytes in the bloodstream (an 'aleukaemic leukaemia'). Accordingly, lymphosarcoma is the better name.

In one form there may be a large tumour mass at the site of the thymus. Usually, many lymph nodes are involved, with enlargement of the spleen and infiltration of the liver. Tumours may occur in almost any organ.

SIGNS. Enlargement of superficial or of mesenteric lymph nodes, depression, emaciation, anaemia, often diarrhoea.

In the dog, death commonly follows after 3 weeks, but the duration of illness varies from 1 to over 60 weeks.

Leukaemia is the commonest malignant disease in the cat in Britain, and is caused by a virus. (*See* FELINE LEUKAEMIA.)

(For the disease in cattle, *see also under* BOVINE ENZOOTIC LEUKOSIS.)

TREATMENT. All attempts at treatment have been unsuccessful.

LEUKOCYTES are white cells found in the blood and lymphoid tissue. (*See* BLOOD, LYMPHOCYTES, INFLAMMATION, PHAGOCYTOSIS, WOUNDS, IMMUNE RESPONSE.)

LEUKOCYTOSIS is a temporary increase in the number of white cells in the blood. It occurs after a feed, during pregnancy, after exertion, and when the temperature is elevated. It is seen during infections, when neutrophils will be numerous; though in some infections monocytes will be more numerous than normal for a time. In parasitic infestations and some allergic reactions, eosinophils increase in number.

Leukocytosis is seen in some cases of poisoning, *e.g.* by potassium chlorate, phenacetin.

The usual proportion of red cells to leucokytes in the blood of the healthy mammal is about 1000:1.

In true leukaemia there is an abnormal increase of leukocytes in the blood – some being of abnormal shape. Myeloblasts may predominate in the final stages of leukaemia. (*See* LEUKAEMIA.)

LEUKODERMA means a condition of the skin and hair when areas become white as a result of injury or disease. It is seen on the backs of horses that have worn badly fitting saddles and collars, when it is called 'saddle-mark' and 'collar-mark', and after ringworm.

LEUKOMA. The presence of an opaque patch or spots on the surface of the cornea. (*See* EYE.)

LEUKOPENIA. A condition in which the white blood cells are less numerous than normal. It occurs during the course of several diseases, *e.g.* swine fever, leptospirosis of cattle. (*See* FELINE ENTERITIS.)

LEUKORRHOEA. A chronic vaginal discharge, generally of a whitish or greyish colour. It is a symptom of vaginitis or of metritis. (*See* UTERUS, DISEASES OF, 'WHITES'.)

LEUKOSIS (*see* BOVINE ENZOOTIC LEUKOSIS, LEUKAEMIA, *and below*).

LEUKOSIS IN TURKEYS. Two distinct forms of leukosis infection are now recognised in this country and have caused serious and widespread economic loss among turkey flocks:

(a) *Lymphoproliferative disease* (*LPD*) affects turkeys from 9 weeks of age and can cause a mortality of 1 per cent a week. It is characterised by sudden death of birds in good condition with gross enlargement of the spleen and tumours in the liver, lungs and elsewhere. The causative agent of LPD is suspected to be an oncovirus unrelated to recognised avian viruses of this group.

(*b*) *Reticuloendotheliosis Virus (REV) Infection* can be distinguished clinically from lymphoproliferative disease by the fact that it is associated with a diarrhoea which frequently affects turkeys between 8 to 10 weeks of age. This is followed by the development of tumours resulting in mortality of up to 20 per cent. The most consistent *post-mortem* finding has been a large leukotic liver. The causative agent is a RE Virus which can be replicated in tissue culture. Experimental work shows that viraemia develops within 2 weeks of infection and antibodies persist for the lifetime of infected birds.

LEUKOVIRUS. This genus of viruses includes the Rous sarcoma virus, feline leukaemia virus and fowl sarcoma virus.

LEVAMISOLE. An isomer of TETRAMISOLE, and a broad-spectrum anthelmintic. It can be administered by injection or in the feed. Levamisole is also of value in stimulating the bodily defence mechanisms, when these have been depressed by, for example, viral infections, or by *Brucella abortus*. Any reduction of T-lymphocytes is apparently restored to normal, and phagocytosis increased, among other immuno-stimulant effects. (*See* ANERGY.)

In dogs levamisole is used mainly to treat heartworm infections. Its side-effects (vomiting, diarrhoea, loss of appetite) can be reduced by giving it with or after food. (Watson, A. D. J. *Res in Vet. Sci.* (1988), **45**, 411.)

LEYS, NEW. Cattle grazing these are, generally speaking, more prone to Hypomagnesaemia than when on permanent pasture. Clover-rich leys are also conducive to Bloat, unless precautions are taken.

LICE. Two distinct families of lice are found on the domestic animals; the sucking lice and the biting lice. All the fowl lice belong to the latter family. The lice are wingless insects which undergo a direct development. The egg is laid on the body, glued to a hair or feather, and the young louse is, except for size, identical with the adult. There is no pupal stage, although several moults take place. The sucking lice belong to the order SIPHUNCULATA.

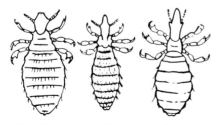

Sucking Lice. × 10. (Left, *Haematopinus*; centre, *Linognathus*; right, *Solenopotus*.)

The biting lice belongs to the order MALLOPHAGA. The mouth parts are very different from those of the sucking lice. They cannot suck blood, and the mouth parts consist of a pair of mandibles on the ventral side of the blunt head. In this order, as in the last, all the mammalian hosts, except the horse, has its own species.

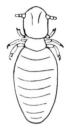

Biting Louse. × 15. (*Trichodectes*.)

Horses. Only one species of sucking louse is found on the horse, called *Haematopinus asini*. Two species of closely related biting lice are also found: *Damalinia equi* and *D. pilosus*. Sucking lice are more generally found at the base of the mane and tail, while the biting species are commonly on the lower parts of the body. They cause poorness of condition, itching, and loss of hair.

Cattle. Sucking lice include *Haematopinus eurysternus*, *H. tuberculatus*, and *Linognathus vituli*. In addition, one species of biting louse occurs, *Damalinia bovis*. The sucking lice are found mainly on the head and shoulders, the biting lice on any part of the body. They cause itchiness and scratching which may produce thickening of the skin, and cause mange to be suspected.

A fourth species of sucking louse, *Solenoptes capillatus*, is found in the UK, New Zealand, etc., but is not very common.

Sheep. *Haematopinus ovillus* (on the body), *Linognathus pedalis* (on the foot), and *L. africanus* are sucking lice. *Damalinia ovis* is a biting louse.

Goats. *Linognathus stenopsis*, and *L. africanus*, attack the goat. Biting lice include *Damalinia caprae* and *D. limbata*.

Pigs. *Haematopinus suis*, a large species causing intense pruritus, which seriously interferes with fattening. Young pigs have been known to die from the loss of blood and the extensive irritation. The lice are usually found near the ears, inside the elbows and on the breast.

Dogs and cats. Important species include: a sucking louse, *Linognathus setosus*, and a biting louse, *Trichodectes canis*. The latter is an intermediate host of *Dipylidium caninum*.

Poultry. All the lice affecting birds are biting lice, and include *Menopon gallinae*, *Goniodes gallinae*.

Lice can cause a severe anaemia in young animals especially.

CONTROL involves two applications of a suitable insecticide at a 7 to 10-day interval; repeated if necessary. Permethrin is suitable for dogs and cats.

For larger animals, sprays or dips, or ivermectin by injection may be used. (*See* IVERMECTIN, BHC, FLEA-COLLARS, AEROSOL SPRAYS, BATHS—Cats.)

'LICK GRANULOMA'. A tumour-like mass of granulation tissue which forms as a result of the incessant licking of a wound, ulcer, or even unbroken skin – in which case there may be a local neuritis causing itching of the spot, and so accounting for the licking.

TREATMENT. An Elizabethan collar may be necessary to prevent the dog's access to the part. A corticosteroid may be used. In long-standing, intractable cases cryosurgery is usually the recommended treatment, but American experience suggests that two or three applications may be necessary, but that the owner is not always willing to persevere. (For a similar condition in cats, see EOSINOPHILIC GRANULOMA.)

'LICKED BEEF' is that which shows greenish or yellowish tracks made by the larvae of warble-flies, with the formation of 'butcher's jelly'. This is of importance in food inspection.

'LICKING SYNDROME'. This is the name for a condition in which cattle tend to lick each other, or each other's urine, or the soil, in an attempt to obtain the extra salt they need, and is a sign of sodium deficiency. This occurs, in the absence of salt licks or the provision of sufficient salt in the feed, on sodium-deficient pastures which, according to ADAS surveys in the south of England, may amount to 50 per cent. A cow giving 5 gallons of milk loses nearly 1½ oz of sodium chloride in its milk each day, and – the ARC has stated – the cow has only 3 oz of salt in her body which can safely be used to balance this loss if the supply of salt in the diet is inadequate.

Dr P. Robart stated that urine-drinking was seen in yarded cows, even when given free access to salt and magnesium, in France. The habit disappeared once the herd gained access to spring pasture. Having drinking troughs placed too close together, or too few of them, in the yards led to dominant cows preventing others from approaching the sources of water and salt. (See under SALT LICKS, SODIUM DEFICIENCY, HAIR BALLS, METABOLIC PROFILES.)

LIEN is the Latin name for the spleen.

LIGAMENTS are strong bands of fibrous tissue that serve to bind together the bones forming a joint. They are cord-like in some instances, flat bands in others, and sheets in the case of the joint-capsule which surrounds a joint. (See JOINTS.)

Desmitis of the fetlock annular ligament was diagnosed in 30 horses which had been lame for a long time and which had chronically distended digital flexor tendon sheaths, or plantar annular ligaments. The ligament was cut longitudinally in 25 of the horses and 16 returned to full work without difficulty and one became sound after a second operation. None of the five untreated horses returned to work. (Verschooten, F. & Picavet, T.-M., *Equine Veterinary Journal* (1986) **18**, 138.)

LIGAMENTUM ARTERIOSUM. The fibrous remains of the *Ductus arteriosus* of the fetus. It connects the left pulmonary artery to the arch of the aorta.

LIGHT, INFLUENCE OF. Adequate light is necessary for maximum fertility. This applies to poultry (see under NIGHT-LIGHTING), to bulls – too often kept in dark places – and sheep, etc. (*See also* LIGHTING, RICKETS, VITAMIN D, TROPICS.)

LIGHT SENSITISATION implies a predisposing factor, such as the eating of a particular plant, which has the effect of making certain cells in the animal's body *abnormally* sensitive – for the time being – to light. Strong sunlight is then capable of causing serious and extensive damage, with a good deal of distress.

In Australia this trouble is frequently caused, in cattle, sheep, and pigs, through eating St John's wort. Elsewhere overseas, clover and buckwheat are often responsible. Occasional cases of light sensitisation occur even in the United Kingdom. To give an example, a British Friesian heifer was discovered in obvious distress. Over nearly all the white parts the skin was dead and had partly sloughed off. Appropriate treatment, which included temporary confinement in a darkened loose-box, was followed by a rapid recovery. Bog Asphodel and rape cause light sensitisation in sheep in Britain, where pigs have also been affected (probably by St John's wort). In New Zealand, where the condition is called Facial Eczema, moulds have been incriminated. In Britain another plant involved is the GIANT HOGWEED.

It is the white, pigment-free skin which suffers. Thus, some breeds of live-stock are never troubled with light sensitisation, while white or partly white cattle are susceptible. Similarly, grey and pie-bald horses in the USA and elsewhere are sometimes affected.

Light sensitisation is associated with disfunction of the liver, and the presence of porphyrins in the bloodstream. It also occurs in some cases of PORPHYRIA.

LIGHTING OF ANIMAL BUILDINGS. Various kinds of glass substitutes have been put on the market, which are reputed to allow the ultraviolet rays of natural sunlight to pass through without appreciable absorption.

Adequate light is necessary to prevent rickets, and to ensure maximum fertility in poultry and other animals. *Continuous* light, however, may have harmful effects. (*See under* NIGHT LIGHTING.)

Artificial lighting of poultry houses is now a common practice. (See NIGHT LIGHTING.). Red light is used in many broiler houses and in some laying houses in order to reduce cannibalism.

LIGHTNING STROKE. Cattle, sheep and horses, are most often affected. (*See under* ELECTRIC SHOCK.)

'LIMBERNECK'. An old, colloquial name for some of the symptoms seen in cases of botulism in poultry: a loss of power of the muscles of the neck, wings, and legs, affected birds first being dull and inactive. (See BOTULISM.)

LIMING OF PASTURES. If this be carried out *to excess* it can, according to André Voisin, lead to a deficiency in copper in the grazing animal and so bring about infertility (which see). Manganese deficiency is likewise a sequel when the soil becomes too alkaline. Cattle should be kept away from downwind of liming operations or eye inflammation (conjunctivitis and keratitis) may result.

LIMOUSIN. A pure beef breed noted for high liveweight gains, high killing-out percentages, and freedom from calving difficulties. Its import from France was sanctioned in 1970.

LINEAR ASSESSMENT OF DAIRY COWS.
(*See* conformation *under* PROGENY TESTING.)

LINER, TEAT-CUP. In selecting milking machinery equipment, one should avoid any liner with a hard mouthpiece.

LINGUATULA SERRATA (*see* MITES, PARASITIC.)

LINIMENTS, or EMBROCATIONS are preparations for external application, generally rubbed in. They are usually of an oily nature, poisonous, and should never be kept with medicines that are used internally. *E.g.* 'A B C liniment' consisted of aconite, belladonna, and chloroform, mixed together and used for painful muscular conditions, strains and sprains.

LINSEED. The flax plant (*Linum usitatissimum*). After extraction of linseed oil from the seeds, the residue is made into linseed cake for feeding to horses, cattle, and sheep.

Linseed poisoning. The flax plant contains a cyanogenetic glycoside in small amounts. An enzyme in the flax can act on the glycoside, with production of hydrocyanic acid. The enzyme is not always destroyed in the process of making linseed cake. Boiling for 10 minutes destroys the enzyme and renders linseed safe. However, linseed cake should be fed dry and not made into a mash with warm water—a dangerous practice owing to the formation of hydrocyanic acid. Linseed poisoning is not common. (*See also under* DIET – Fats; and NURSING.)

LIPASE. A fat-splitting enzyme found in the pancreatic juice.

LIPIDS. Fatty substances. Simple lipids are esters of fatty acids and alcohol, and include fats (esters of fatty acids and glycerol). Compound lipids contain, in addition to fatty acid and alcohol, carbohydrate or nitrogen or phosphoric acid, for example.
'**Protected lipids**' are those encapsulated in a protein envelope, which is then treated with formaldehyde. Because of their high energy value, fats and oils and their fatty acids seemed worth including in cattle feed supplements; and 'protected lipids' offered the possibility of avoiding the disturbance of normal rumen metabolism likely to occur with free fats being present in the rumen. 'Protected lipid' supplements are being widely used, but are not yet altogether trouble-free.

LIPOMA is a tumour mainly composed of fat. These are liable to arise almost anywhere in the body where there is fibrous connective tissue, but are especially common below loose skin. They are occasionally seen in the abdominal cavity, where they develop in connection with the peritoneum, and sometimes encase the bowel and obstruct its function or attain a large size. (*See* TUMOUR.)

LIPOPROTEIN. A complex of cholesterol, triglycerides, phopholipids, and apoproteins. An excess of lipoprotein in the blood, **hyperlipoproteinaemia**, occurs in some cases of diabetes, hypothyroidism, metabolic disorders and inherited disease.

LIPS are musculo-membranous folds which in the horse are covered on the outside with fine hairs, among which are longer, stouter tactile hairs, while some heavy draught horses have a 'moustache' on their upper lips; on the inside the lips are covered by mucous membrane which is continuous with that of the mouth generally. In the horse they are extremely mobile, and the upper lip especially contains a very dense plexus of sensory nerves which serve tactile purposes. In the ox the lips are thick and comparatively immobile. The middle part of the upper lip between the nostrils is bare of hair and is termed the muzzle. It is provided with a large number of tiny glands which secrete a clear fluid in health, which keeps the part cool and moist. Within the lower lip are numbers of horny papillae; its free margin is bare, but the under part of it is covered with ordinary and tactile hairs. The sheep possesses no hairless muzzle, but has a distinct 'philtrum' instead. The lips are thin and mobile. In the pig the upper lip is thick and short and is blended with the snout or nasal disc, while the lower is thin and pointed. (*See also* HARELIP.)

LIQUID FEEDING of dairy cows in the parlour enables them to eat up to 15 lb of concentrates in 7 minutes.

LIQUID PARAFFIN, MEDICINAL (*see under* PARAFFIN for its use as a laxative).

LISTERELLOSIS (*see* LISTERIOSIS).

LISTERIOSIS. A disease caused by *Listeria monocytogenes* which attacks rodents, poultry, ruminants, pigs, horses, dogs, and man. It causes encephalitis and abortion in cattle and sheep, and has to be differentiated from RABIES.

From studies carried out in Michigan, it appears that the infection in cattle and sheep occurs primarily in winter and early spring. Its duration is short in some cases, but as long as 10 days in others; generally much less in sheep than in cattle. The disease in sheep 'could easily be confused with ketosis or with the effects of overeating'. In cattle, the infection may be confused with rabies or poisoning. The affected animal is seen to keep aloof from the rest of the herd, and is later unable to stand without support. If walked, it usually moves in a circle. The head may be held back to one side, with salivation and a nasal discharge. Paralysis of one side of the face may occur. Some cows become violent in the terminal stages and bellow.

In one English outbreak, 12 out of 15 calves died between April and August, at 3 to 7 days old, from septicaemia. There was severe keratitis and conjunctivitis, (*L. monocytogenes* is recognised as one cause of IBK), extreme dejection, and distressed breathing.

Listeria is also a cause of IRITIS in cattle feeding at silage clamps. (*See* SILAGE.)

There is also a septicaemic form in adult cattle and sheep, which shows itself by depression, fever, weakness, and emaciation.

Pigs may have swelling of the eyelids, encephalitis, paralysis, or occasionally septicaemia.

Listeriosis is a rare cause of abortion in mares, and a common cause in other animals. Listeriosis is an important cause of abortion in goats.

Infection may be spread by urine, milk, faeces, an aborted fetus, and vaginal discharges.

Terramycin has given good results in treatment in a few reported cases which were not too advanced.

FOR PREVENTION OF THE DISEASE IN SHEEP a Bulgarian vaccine gave promising results during a field trial in Norway. (Gudding, R. & others, *Veterinary Record* (1985) **117,** 89.) (*See also* AVIAN LISTERIOSIS.)

LITHIASIS, the formation of calculi and concretions in tissues or organs, *e.g.* cholelithiasis means the formation of calculi in the gall-bladder. (*See also under* CALCULI, UROLITHIASIS.)

LITHIUM antimony thiomalate has been used by injection to remove multiple warts.

LITHONTRIPTICS are substances which are reputed to have the power of dissolving stones in the urinary system. (*See* HYALURONIDASE.)

LITHOTOMY is the operation of opening the bladder for the removal of a stone.

LITHOTRITY is an operation in which a stone in the bladder is broken into small fragments and removed by washing out the bladder with a catheter.

LITTER (*see* DEEP LITTER *and* BEDDING).

LITTER, OLD. Broiler chicks reared on previously-used litter may, as a result of the ammonia fumes, develop a severe inflammation of eye-surfaces and eye-lids. In one house, 3000 broilers were affected. The birds cannot bear to open their eyes, and appear obviously dejected. Mortality is generally low, but the trouble is a serious one for all that.

LITTER SIZE (PIGS). In Britain the average is between 9 and 10 born alive; mortality 0·84. (Meat & Livestock Commission, 1987). Earlier figures (PIDA) showed that an average of 2·2 pigs per litter died between birth and 8 weeks old. A litter of 34 has been recorded.

LIVER is a solid glandular organ lying in the anteriormost part of the abdomen close up against the diaphragm. Its colour varies from a dark red-brown in the horse to a bluish-purple in the ox and pig; it is soft to the touch though it is rather friable in consistency, and it constitutes the largest gland in the body.

Functions include the excretion of bile, the storage of glycogen and of iron, the breaking-down of old and worn-out red blood cells, and the breaking down of toxic substances and of waste substances from the tissues of the body. From the liver urea and uric acid find their way into the blood-stream and are excreted from the body in the urine by the kidneys. In animals except those of the horse tribe, the bile is collected in the *gall-bladder*, the bile-duct before passing to the small intestine, where it assists the pancreatic juice in the digestion of food after a meal.

Shape. There are probably few organs which vary so much in shape as the liver, not only in different animals, but in different individuals of the same species. Its general outlines only will be given here. *In the horse* it lies obliquely across the abdominal surface of the diaphragm, its highest and most posterior part being at the level of the right kidney. It possesses a strongly convex diaphragmatic surface which is moulded into the concavity of the diaphragm, and a posterior or abdominal surface which lies in contact with the stomach, duodenum, and right kidney, each of which organs forms a depression in the liver substance. It is only incompletely divided into three lobes in the horse. Lying mainly in the right lobe on its abdominal surface is the 'porta' of the liver, where the portal vein and hepatic artery enter and from whence the hepatic duct (bile-duct) emerges. Part of the posterior vena cava passes through the liver substance, whose blood it eventually drains. The liver is held in position by the pressure of other organs and by six ligaments. These are: the coronary, which attaches it to the diaphragm; the falciform, from the middle lobe to the diaphragm and abdominal floor; the round, to the umbilicus; the right lateral, to the costal part of the diaphragm; the left lateral, to the tendinous part of the diaphragm; and the hepato-renal or caudate, to the right kidney.

Cattle. The liver lies mainly to the right of the middle line through the body, and its long axis is directed downward and forward. Its diaphragmatic surface fits into the concavity of the right part of the diaphragm, and its posterior surface is very irregular. It presents impressions of the two main organs with which it comes into contact – the omasum and reticulum. There is only one distinct lobe – the caudate. There is no left lateral ligament, and the round ligament is only found in the calf. A gall-bladder is present; it is situated partly in a slight depression on the posterior surface of the liver, and partly on the abdominal wall.

Sheep. The bile duct joins the pancreatic to form a common duct instead of opening separately as in other animals. *In the pig* the liver is large, very thick, and very much curved. It lies in the anterior part of the abdominal cavity, occupying the whole of the anterior hollow of the diaphragm and more to the right than to the left side of the body. It has four main lobes. *In the dog* the liver is very large, being about 5 per cent of the whole bodyweight, and possesses six or seven lobes. The gall-bladder is buried almost completely in the space between the two parts of the right central lobe, only a very small portion of it being visible from the outside.

Minute structure. The liver is enveloped in an outer capsule of fibrous tissue with which is blended the hepatic peritoneum. The hepatic artery, portal vein, and bile-duct divide and subdivide. Between the rows of liver cells also lie fine bile capillaries which collect the bile discharged by the cells and pass it into the bile-ducts lying around the margins of the lobules. The liver cells are amongst the largest cells of the body, and each contains one large nucleus. With careful special staining methods there can also be seen tiny passages or canals, passing into the cells themselves; some of these communicate with the bile-duct, and others with the ultimate branches of the portal vein. After a mixed meal many of the liver cells can be seen to contain droplets of fat, and granules of glycogen (animal starch) can also be determined. In addition to the cells above described, there occur at intervals along the walls of the sinusoids in a lobule stellate cells which represent the remains of the endothelium from which the capillary-like sinusoids are developed. They are known as 'Kupfer's cells'.

LIVER, DISEASES OF. One of the commonly known signs of liver disturbance is jaundice – a yellow coloration of the visible membranes, which is considered under JAUNDICE. The presence of gall-stones which is a complication of some liver diseases, is treated under GALL-BLADDER, DISEASES OF.

Hepatitis, or inflammation of the liver may be either acute, suppurative (in which abscesses are formed), or chronic.

Acute inflammation is produced by viruses, bacteria or poisons (of bacterial, vegetable, animal, or mineral origin), from the intestines, and it is sometimes caused by the migration of parasites through the liver. The symptoms are pain on pressure over the abdomen, an elevation of temperature, suppression of the appetite, a disinclination to move, and often diarrhoea or constipation in the later stages. (*See also* CANINE VIRUS HEPATITIS.)

Chronic inflammation accompanies many diseases among animals, the commonest probably being infestation with liver-flukes, but it may also be present as a result of tuberculosis. Poisoning may be responsible. (See, for example, RAGWORT which gives rise to **cirrhosis**, which see.)

SIGNS include a gradual loss of condition, irregular appetite, a staring coat, and a general unthriftiness; often oedema.

Abscess formation is due to the entrance into the liver of pus-forming organisms, and is usually secondary to some disease, *e.g.* tuberculosis. In the USA liver abscesses are found in about 8 per

cent of all cattle slaughtered, and they are common in 'barley beef' animals in the UK. The lesions consist of abscesses in the substance of the liver. Symptoms are vague and diagnosis is often impossible, (but *see* HAEMOGLOBIN REACTIVE PROTEIN).

Fatty liver (*see* 'FATTY LIVER SYNDROME' of cattle and poultry, *and also* CEROIDOSIS).

Liver/kidney syndrome (*see under* this heading).

Tumours include adenoma, carcinoma, haemangioma (*see* CANCER). Benign tumours may give rise to passive congestion, biliary obstruction with jaundice, or they may cause degeneration. (*See under* TUMOURS.)

Parasites (*see* LIVER FLUKES, HYDATID DISEASE, HORSE BOTS, 'LIZARD-POISONING' in cats).

Rupture of the liver is by no means rare among old animals, especially dogs and cats. It may result from a blow, kick, run-over accident, fall, or from violent struggling, when the liver is diseased. Even a small wound in such a vascular organ as the liver, is likely to prove fatal. (*See also* 'MILKSPOT LIVER' of pigs and sheep; *also called* WHITE SPOT.)

Rupture of the liver in lambs, aged one to three months, was found to be the cause of sudden death. The liver surface was covered with haemorrhagic tracts made by migrating metacestodes of *Taenia hydatigena* (*see* TAPEWORMS).

In a survey covering a period of 12 years, the Thurso Veterinary Investigation Laboratory found that liver rupture in neonatal lambs from 16 farms exceeded 8 per cent.

Woolliams, C. & others had in 1983 noted a trend for rupture to increase with inbreeding. (*Journal of Agricultural Science* **100**, 553).

LIVER-FLUKES are parasitic flat worms which infest the livers of various animals, especially sheep and cattle. They may cause severe illness and even death.

Liver-flukes may increase the susceptibility of the host animal to *Salmonella* infection. (*See* SALMONELLOSIS.)

Life-history of a typical fluke. The egg is usually passed to the exterior in the faeces of the host and under suitable conditions, chiefly of moisture and warmth, a small ciliated larva, called a 'miracidium', hatches from it. This larva, which is unable to feed and will die within some hours unless it finds a suitable host, gains access to the liver or some other special organ by actively penetrating the skin of an appropriate snail – usually a specific snail for any one parasite. In the snail's tissue it develops into a sac-like sporocyst which, by a process of budding from the internal lining of cells, gives rise to a number of elongated 'rediae'. Each redia is a simple, cylindrical sac-like organism which gives rise, by budding of cells, either to another generation of 'daughter rediae' or to 'cercariae'. The cercaria, which resembles a miniature tadpole in general form, leaves the snail and, after leading a free existence in water or on wet vegetation for a short time, comes to rest on grass or other objects, loses its tail and becomes encysted within a protective covering and remains in this state until it is swallowed by the final host, in which it becomes a sexually mature fluke.

Fasciola hepatica. This is the common 'liver-fluke' of sheep. (Other hosts are cattle, goats, pigs, rabbits, hares, horses, dogs, man, beavers, elephants, and kangaroos.) It is shaped more or less like a leaf, about 1 in long, but considerable variations exist, and elongated forms are found. It has been recorded from most herbivorous animals and from man; but it is in cattle and sheep that it is of most importance. It is generally found in the bile-ducts of the liver, but may be found in other organs.

The life-history is typical, the intermediate host being various species of *Limnaea* snails. Cercariae may be swallowed with drinking water or encysted on grass.

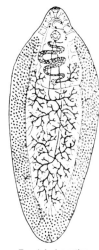

Fasciola hepatica.

Infestation, sometimes called 'Fluke Disease', results in anaemia and hepatitis. (*See also* 'LIVER ROT'.)

Fasciola gigantica. A parasite of cattle, sheep, and wild animals in the tropics and sub-tropics, and more pathogenic than *F. hepatica.*

Fascioloides. This genus contains only one species, *F. magna,* the large American liver-fluke. In general anatomy, this species resembles the common liver fluke, but differs from it in its larger size (up to 4 in).

Its larger size and its tendency to form cysts in the liver substance (not in the bile-ducts) make it a more formidable parasite. The cysts may become abscesses, and may be found in the spleen and lungs.

Dicrocoelium. This genus is small and semi-transparent, the common species, *D. lanceatum,* being about ½ in long. It occurs in all herbivores and in man. It is less serious a pest than *F. hepatica.* It is carried by various land snails; a second intermediate host – the ant – is required; the ants being eaten by the grazing animal. Infestation of a heifer with *D. dendriticum* was reported in Ireland in 1960. This species has similar

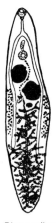 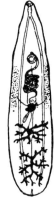

Dicrocoelium.   *Clonorchis.*

hosts and a world-wide distribution. *D. hospes* occurs in Africa. Netobimin kills the flukes.

Clonorchis. *Clonorchis sinensis* is a common fluke of carnivores, pigs, and man in Asia. It is a small form.

The first part of its life-history is on general lines, the molluscan intermediary being a species of *Bythinia.* The sporocysts give rise directly to cercariae which escape and encyst on various freshwater fish. Infection to mammals is by eating infected fish which are either uncooked or imperfectly cooked.

Closely related flukes are found in the liver of dogs in North Europe and North America. (*See also* 'SALMON POISONING'; 'LIZARD POISONING' in the cat.)

INCIDENCE OF LIVER-FLUKES. Cattle and sheep on half the farms in the UK are infested with liver-flukes, according to a survey made by ICI. 'Cattle are the major victims.' Of 37,338 cows surveyed, 40 per cent had fluke-infested livers, while 17 per cent of heifers and steers (over 160,000) were positive. A diminution of milk yield can be an important result of fluke infestation in dairy cattle.

Among ewes, 13 per cent of nearly 78,000 surveyed were found positive in the ICI survey, and 5 per cent of lambs (over 299,000 surveyed) were positive.

The map overleaf shows the UK incidence of liver-fluke, based on this survey, the results of which were published in 1974.

CONTROL MEASURES. To be effective they require a planned campaign rather than a single battle or weapon. In the sheep, infestation does not lead to subsequent immunity, and this fact gives very little hope of an effective vaccine (similar to the irradiated huskworm larvae vaccine) ever being produced. Not until 1971 was there any drug to kill all young, immature flukes within the body, and it is these which on their mass migrations through the liver can damage it so severely that sudden death inevitably follows.

However, it is claimed that diamphenethide kills all stages of the liver-fluke, including those 3 days old and upwards. A dose is given as soon as the outbreak is detected, and a further dose 4

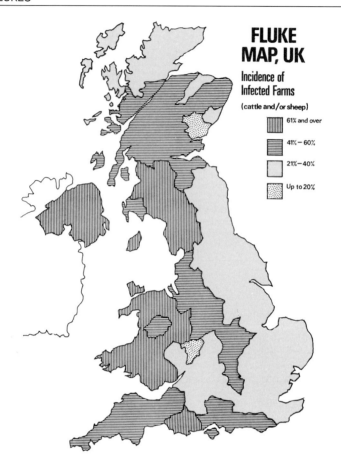

FLUKE MAP, UK

Incidence of
Infected Farms

(cattle and/or sheep)

▦	61% and over
▤	41% – 60%
▢	21% – 40%
▨	Up to 20%

weeks later. It is claimed to be safe for lambs and pregnant/in-milk ewes.

Drugs used against liver flukes include NITROXYNIL, CLOSANTEL, and RAFOXANIDE.

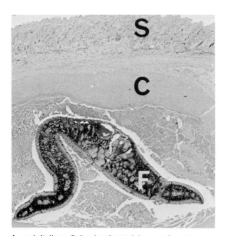

An adult liver fluke implanted in a subcutaneous pocket in a rat. This technique showed that the rat gained thereby immunity to adult flukes without the complication of liver damage, and was part of the research carried out at the ARC's Institute for Research on Animal Diseases, Compton, into possible means of immunising cattle against liver flukes.

In the UK over 60 per cent of our cattle and 80 per cent of our sheep are kept in the main fluke areas.

While sheep farmers are mostly fully alive to the fluke problem, it is suggested that most cattle farmers are not. Moreover, it is pointed out that on farms where mixed grazing is practised, it is a waste of time and money to dose only the sheep and not the cattle.

Profit margins in beef production have been improved by a combined anti-fluke attack, using routine dosing of the cattle together with a chemical spray (Frescon) on pasture to kill the host snails. In trials 18-month-old beef animals finished 25–30 days earlier than controls, giving an additional margin of £4–5 per head through savings in feed alone. Returns were further increased by better carcase grading.

An 8 per cent drop in milk yield has resulted from low-grade infestations in dairy cattle, and it is claimed that autumn and winter dosing of dairy cattle helps to improve, or at least maintain, milk quality levels.

A vaccine against Black Disease – in which spores of one of the gas-gangrene group of organisms are stimulated into activity by young flukes in the liver – can prevent deaths from the resulting toxaemia. Against the live-flukes themselves, routine dosing is essential on all farms where they are likely to occur.

Drugs in use have included: nitroxyril, oxy-clonazide, rafoxanide.

Land drainage is still high on the list of control measures.

The use of snail killers is a recommended part of the campaign against fluke disease, but not a snag-free method. It is so easy to miss small areas inhabited by snails, and this applies even when using a knapsack sprayer – the only possible method of spraying if the land is too wet, as it often is, is to take a tractor. Snail killers can be unpleasant to work with. The cheapest is sodium pentachlorophenate. N-trityemorpholine is expensive per acre but has the advantages of being relatively harmless to stock, so that grazing need not be delayed for a fortnight as after copper sulphate dressings or pentachlorophenate. All are poisonous to fish.

Running ducks over snaily land is not among the official recommendations but it might prove of some value. A few farmers have tried it in the past. In Zambia years ago a large-scale duck-rearing scheme was introduced in areas flooded by the River Zambesi as a method of fluke disease and bilharzia control. Hoof-prints, where the soil is exposed, are favourite habitats of the snails. (*See also under* ANTS.)

Public health. Watercress is the chief source of infestation. Illness is most marked during migration of immature flukes. Eosinophilia is a pointer to aid diagnosis; eggs may not appear in the faeces for 12 weeks.

Symptoms in the human patient include: urticaria, jaundice, enlarged and tender liver, and eosinophilia. (R. Reshef & others. *British Medical Journal* (1982) **285**, 1243.)

Cats (*see under* 'LIZARD POISONING', PANCREAS).

LIVER/KIDNEY SYNDROME OF CATS. This illness resembles leptospirosis in the dog, but this infection has not been proved to be the cause.

LIVER/KIDNEY SYNDROME OF POULTRY affects birds usually 2 to 3 weeks old. Symptoms may not be observed – or there may be depression for a day or two; occasionally trembling or paralysis of legs. Mortality: 1 to 5 per cent. The whole carcase may have a pink tinge. The liver is pale, swollen, and fatty. The kidneys may be very swollen. (*See also under* FATTY LIVER.)

The syndrome has to be differentiated from Toxic Fat disease, Gumboro disease, and Infectious avian nephrosis.

LIVER ROT is the popular name for the condition resulting from mass migration of immature liver flukes. (*See* LIVER-FLUKES.)

LIVER, RUPTURE OF (IN FOWLS) (*see* HAEMORRHAGIC DISEASE).

LIVESTOCK PRODUCTION (*see* BEEF CATTLE HUSBANDRY, DAIRY HERD MANAGEMENT, TROPICS, *and under* PIGS *and* SHEEP).

'LIZARD POISONING' IN CATS. This term is applied to infestation with the liver-fluke *Platynosomum concinnum*, which has been reported from South America, the Caribbean Islands, Malaysia, the USA and, more recently, Nigeria. The life cycle of the parasite involves a large land snail, a crustacean, and lizards, frogs, and probably other amphibians and reptiles. Symptoms in the cat include listlessness, fever, jaundice, diarrhoea, vomiting, and emaciation; but sub-clinical infestations also occur.

LLAMAS. These belong to the order Camelidae, which includes also Alpaca, Guarnaco, and Vicugna.

Imports of llamas from South America are banned owing to the risk of their infection with foot-and-mouth disease. They have, however, been imported from Sweden, Holland, and Poland.

Mr and Mrs Gerald Walker, of Maplehurst Llamas, Horsham, Sussex, UK, sold 27 lots within two hours at the Royal Show – an average price being £3,255 per animal.

LOBE is the term applied to the larger divisions of various organs, such as the lungs, liver, and brain. The term *lobar* is applied to structures which are connected with lobes of organs, or to diseases which have a tendency to be limited to one lobe only, such as 'lobar pneumonia'.

Lobules are divisions of a lobe. The term *lobular* is applied to disease which occurs in a scattered irregular manner affecting lobules here and there, such as 'lobular pneumonia'.

LOCAL   ANAESTHETICS   (*see   under* ANAESTHESIA, ANALGESICS).

LOCAL IMMUNITY (*see under* IMMUNE RESPONSE, ORIFICES, *and* SECRETORY IgA).

'LOCK-JAW' (*see* TETANUS).

'LOCO WEED'. Legumes oxytropis and astragalus in the USA produce a chronic contracted front-leg condition in lambs born to ewes which ate just insufficient of the plant to cause abortion. Five of 26 pregnant mares seen eating *Astragalus mollisimus* subsequently aborted, and 10 produced foals with various limb deformities in New Mexico. (C. Wayne and L. F. James *JAVMA* (1982) **181**, 255.)

LOOSE-BOXES. The best type has well-built brick walls lined on the inside to the roof with cement-plaster finished off smooth. The floor is of cement-concrete, grooved to facilitate the draining away of fluids and to provide a foothold, and the corners are rounded off with fillets of cement. The only fittings inside are hay-rack, water-bowl, and manger, of iron, and rather larger than in the stall of a stable, so that cattle as well as horses may use them; in some cases one or two rings, to which animals may be tied, are provided. One or more windows, high up out of reach of the animals' heads, should be included, and the door should always be made in two halves, so that horses with respiratory diseases may be able to stand with their heads out of the box, and so obtain a plentiful supply of fresh air. Wherever possible, loose-boxes should be built with a southerly aspect, so that the disinfectant action of sunlight may be taken full advantage of, whenever sick animals are housed in the box.

LORDOSIS is an unnatural curvature of the spine, so that the concavity of the spine is directed upwards. It is seen in tetanus, and sometimes in rabies.

LOUPING-ILL is a paralytic disease of sheep, transmitted by *Ixodes ricinus*, the tick commonly present on hill pastures. It occurs in western Scotland, the North of England, and the Northwest of Ireland. It has a definite seasonal incidence, most cases occurring between March and June, and between September and October, and only a few sporadic cases are met with at other times of the year. All breeds of sheep are susceptible. It has been recorded as affecting pigs, horses and deer and also **dogs**, in which the signs were: fever, nystagmus, hyperaesthesia, and sometimes a tetanus-like rigidity. In two cases bitches had whelped five weeks previously, and eclampsia was at first suspected.

Cattle. On upland grazings where ticks abound, louping-ill has, of recent years, become of economic importance in cattle. The animals become dull and uninterested in food, walk in an unnatural way, sometimes with their heads down, and occasionally become excited.

Horses. An outbreak of louping-ill in a group of four **horses** was reported from Eire in 1975.

Pigs. The first naturally occurring outbreak in pigs was reported only in 1980 by Mr Colin Bannatyne, of the West of Scotland Agricultural College's veterinary investigation centre, and colleagues. Ten out of 16 piglets became severely affected with the disease when about six weeks old. They showed nervous symptoms, were either reluctant to move or wandered aimlessly and pressed their heads into corners. Of the three worst cases, two failed to survive transport to the VI Centre, and the third – being in a state of convulsions – was killed on arrival there. Of the remainder, five more died and two recovered.

Those piglets had been housed in a covered pen with a concrete run considered to be tick-proof; and the louping-ill virus was probably transmitted through the feeding of uncooked carcases of lambs which had died on the farm after showing symptoms suggestive of louping-ill.

In another outbreak, pigs six to eight months old died of louping-ill after being allowed free range on tick-infested pasture.

Dogs. Louping-ill may also occur in dogs.

CAUSE. A flavivirus. This is transmitted by the bites of infected ticks (adult or nymphal). The virus primarily multiplies in the blood, and in certain cases invades the central nervous system at a later stage in the infection.

It would appear that accessory conditions favour such invasion, *e.g.* tick-borne fever, a disease also transmitted by the *I. ricinus.* The periods when outbreaks of the disease are commonest correspond with the first and second tick crops during the year.

The ticks can survive, in the absence of sheep and cattle, on deer, rabbits, hares, voles, field mice, grouse, etc., and these animals may act as host of the virus.

SIGNS. Two forms of the disease are recognised: viz. an acute and a sub-acute form. In the *acute form* the symptoms may appear in from 4 to 6 days after the sheep are infested with the carrier ticks. The sheep becomes uneasy, lies down and rises frequently during the day. Its temperature ranges between 104° and 107°F during the next week or 10 days, and it develops nervous symptoms. At first, it is merely more timid and more easily frightened than usual; later, the muscles of the jaws and neck begin to twitch and quiver, and there may be frothing at the mouth. It staggers when made to move rapidly or turn suddenly, and as the disease becomes firmly established it may be seen taking short spasmodic jumps, rising apparently from all four feet at the same time, and landing upon all four feet again. In this way an affected sheep can usually be easily noticed among a flock when the sheep are being driven or collected by a dog. In more advanced stages the animal becomes paralysed, unable to stand, and often has its head drawn round over its fore flank. Unconsciousness quickly appears, and the animal dies a short time afterwards.

In the *sub-acute type* the sheep is seen taking very high steps with its fore-legs; it holds its head very high, and sometimes carries it to one side (often the left); the pupils are dilated, and the expression of the sheep is one of extreme fear when caught. It may attempt to feed, but actually eats very little. Tremblings of the muscles, staggering and falling, and sometimes paralysis of one or more groups of muscles, are seen. As times goes on the sheep loses condition. If not fed by hand it dies from starvation.

Recovery from one attack confers a degree of immunity, which may last for life. (*See also* TICK-BORNE FEVER).

PREVENTION. Control measures should aim at the eradication of the infecting ticks from grazing lands. This is not easy, as the tick can live under rough herbage without access to the living sheep for as long as one year.

Sheep. A vaccine against louping-ill, developed at Moredun, gives a degree of immunity equal to that resulting from a natural infection within 7 to 10 days of infection. Vaccination of ewes confers protection in their lambs. Inoculations are carried out in spring prior to the season when ticks become active.

Cattle. Investigations on hill farms where louping-ill is a problem have shown that cattle play an important part in the maintenance of virus. **Hill cattle** as well as sheep therefore should be vaccinated, not only for their own protection, but to reduce the transfer of virus to the ticks which are the only agents passing on the infection each year.

Public health. Shepherds, farmers, and slaughterhouse workers—as well as veterinarians—may become infected. The main symptom is fever. Meningoencephalitis has been recorded, and has soemtimes proved fatal.

LUBRICANTS. The type of lubricant used in pellet mills and other forms of machinery for processing animal feeding-stuffs may be of the greatest importance. Lubricants containing chlorinated naphthalene compounds and used on such machines may give rise to Hyperkeratosis in cattle eating the food so contaminated by the minutest quantity of lubricant.

LUCERNE. A valuable leguminous plant (*Medicago sativa*) for fodder and forage. Lucerne-hay is highly valued for the feeding of horses if of good quality. (It is of little value when most of the leaf has been lost, or it is dusty or mouldy.) Lucerne is also a valuable crop for cattle, but for precautions and dangers, *see* BLOAT; *also* NUTRI-TIONAL MUSCULAR DYSTROPHY under MUSCLES, DIS-EASES OF.

LUGOL'S SOLUTION. A solution of 50 gm iodine and 100 gm potassium iodide in distilled water to 1000 cc.

LUING. A beef breed evolved by Messrs Cadzow from Beef Shorthorn and Highland cattle, and named after the island. Colour: red with a touch of gold; or roan; or white. There are a breed society and herd book. Recognised by Secretary of State, Scotland, 1965.

LUMBAR is a term used to denote either the struc-tures in or disease affecting the loins, that is, the region lying between the last rib and the point of the hip, from one side of the body to the other. There are lumbar vertebrae, lumbar muscles, etc.

LUMEN. The space inside a tubular structure, such as an artery or intestine.

LUMINAL, or PHENOBARBITONE (*see* BARBITURATES).

'LUMPY SKIN DISEASE'. This affects non-indigenous cattle in parts of Africa. A discharge from the eyes and nose, lameness, and salivation may be observed – depending upon the site of nodules which sometimes involve mucous mem-brane as well as skin.

Oedema may occur, and involve the genital or-gans, udder, dewlap, and limbs. Sloughing of skin may occur. Exotic cattle may die.

The disease is caused by the Neethling pox virus; and a modified sheep-pox vaccine is used.

'LUMPY SKIN DISEASE, PSEUDO-'. This is characterised by the formation of raised plaques on the skin, which exude a discharge and then ulcerate; and by fever. The cause is the bovid herpes-virus-2, which also cause mammillitis of cattle.

LUMPY WOOL, or WOOL ROT, is caused by a bacterium which attacks the sheep's skin during wet weather, causing irritation and the formation of a hard yellowish-white scab about ⅛ inch thick. Healing soon occurs and the wool continues to grow, carrying the hard material away from the skin as a buff or brownish zone in the wool. Severe infection may lead to loss of wool.

The bacterium causing this dermatitis is *Der-matophilus dermatonomus*. (*See also* DERMA-TOPHILUS and STREPTOTHRICOSIS.)

In America, this disease has been treated by defleecing with cyclophosphamide and the use of streptomycin and penicillin.

LUNG FLUKES (*Paragonimus* genus). These flukes are plump oval forms. The flukes infect the carnivores, pig and man. Generally two flukes are found together in a cyst in the lungs. The presence of the flukes cause bronchitis, and consolidation of portions of the lung. Lesions resembling tuber-culosis may be developed. The flukes are found in America and Asia. Eggs are coughed up, swal-lowed, and passed out with the droppings. The cercariae develop in snails, and afterwards escape and encyst on freshwater crabs or cray-fish. These are eaten, and the adult flukes develop in the body. Treatment with niclosamide and al-bendazole appear to be effective against *P. ke-llicotti*, which causes coughing and sneezing in cats. For the pancreatic fluke of cats, *see* PANCREAS.

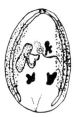

Paragonimus.

LUNG WORMS (*see* PARASITIC BRONCHITIS, WORMS, DONKEYS).

LUNGS. These two organs are, of course, con-cerned with respiration, in which carbon dioxide is exchanged for oxygen. The air breathed in is warmed before reaching the lungs via the AIR PAS-SAGES (which see).

Blood is carried to the lungs by the pulmonary artery, which divides and subdivides into tiny capillaries which lie around the walls of the air cells.

Functions. Apart from their main function of gas exchange (*see* AIR), the lungs can release hista-mine, metabolise noradrenaline, and inactivate prostaglandins – to give a few of the examples of their 'pharmacokinetic activity' quoted by Dr H. M. Pirie at the 1976 BVA congress. Local im-mune mechanisms also operate in the lungs. 'Not only is antibody present on the mucous surfaces of the bronchi, such as secreted IgA, but it may be found in the peripheral part of the lung, where IgG, transuded or formed locally, may be present.'

Lung is composed of very highly elastic tissue which consists of multitudes of tiny sacs arranged at the terminal parts of the smallest of the bron-chioles, and which collapse when the balance of pressure between the air in the sacs and on the

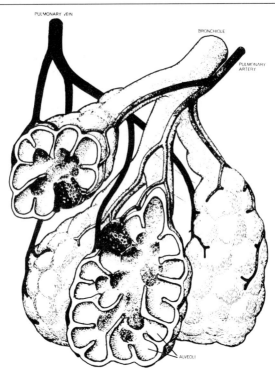

Relationship of alveoli to terminations of pulmonary artery and pulmonary vein. (From *Surface Tension in the Lungs* by John A. Clements. Copyright © 1962 by Scientific American, Inc. All rights reserved.)

outside of the lung surface is disturbed. Thus a lung shrinks to about one-third of its normal size when removed from the chest cavity.

Horses. The lungs occupy the greater part of the thoracic cavity, and are accurately moulded to the walls of the chest and to the other organs contained within it. The right is considerably larger than the left, owing to the presence of the heart, which lies mostly to the left side of the middle plane of the cavity. In the equidae the lung is not divided into lobes as it is in some of the other animals. The apex is that portion which occupies the most anterior part of the chest cavity, and just immediately behind it is the deep impression for the heart. Behind this again, and a little above it, is the 'root' of the lung, which consists of the blood-vessels entering and leaving the lung, lymph vessels, nerves, the bronchus, and here also are situated the bronchial lymph nodes. In cross-section each lung is somewhat triangular in shape, with one of the angles rounded. The rounded angle lies in the uppermost part of the chest, alongside the bodies of the thoracic vertebrae, and the more acute of the remaining angles lies along the floor of the chest.

Cattle. The lungs are thicker and shorter than in the horse, and there is a greater disproportion in size – the right weighing about half as much again as the left. They are divided into lobes by deep fissures. The left has three lobes, and the right four or five. The foot in each case is almost immediately above the impression for the heart. The apical lobe (*i.e.* the most anterior of the right lung) receives a special small bronchus from the trachea direct.

Sheep. The lungs show but little lobulation.

Pigs. The left lung is like that of cattle, but the right lung has its apical lobe very often divided into two parts. Otherwise there are no great differences. Three bronchi are present, as in cattle.

Dogs. The lungs are thicker than in either the horse or ox in conformity with the more barrel-like shape of the chest. There is no cardiac impression in the left lung. Each has three large lobes, but the right has a small extra mediastinal lobe, and there may be one or more accessory lobes in either lung.

Colour. In the perfectly fresh lung from a young unbled animal the colour of the lung is a bright rose-pink, with a glistening surface, the pleural membrane, but in the lungs of older animals there is usually a certain amount of deposit of soot, dust, etc., which has been inhaled with the air and collected in the lymph spaces between the air cells. In an animal which has been bled the lung is of a pale pink, owing to the lesser blood content. In the case of pit ponies, town dogs, and other animals which have breathed a comparatively impure atmosphere, the lungs show a greater or lesser degree of pigmentation, so that the colour of the normal lung may vary from a slate-blue to black.

Connections. The lungs are firmly anchored in position by their roots to the heart and trachea, and by the pleura to a longitudinal septum running vertically from front to back, called the 'mediastinum' (*see* PLEURA). The pulmonary artery, carrying impure blood to the lungs, divides into two large branches after only a very short course. Each of these branches enters into the formation of the root of the lung, and there begins to divide up into a very large number of smaller vessels. These subdivide many times until the final capillaries are given off around the walls of the air-sacs. From these the blood, after oxygenation, is carried by larger and larger veins, till it eventually leaves the lung by one of the several pulmonary veins. These number six or seven or more, and leave the lungs by the roots. In addition to the blood carried to the lung for aeration a small bronchial artery carries blood to the lung substance for nutritive purposes. This accompanies the bronchi and splits into branches corresponding to the small bronchi and bronchioles. The lymph vessels in the root of the lungs are very numerous, and are all connected with the large bronchial glands for this part.

Minute structure. The main bronchial tube, entering the lung at its root, divides into branches, which subdivide again and again, to be distributed all through the substance of the lung, till the finest tubes, known as 'bronchioles' or 'capillary bronchi', have a diameter of only about $\frac{1}{100}$th of an inch. In structure, all these tubes consist of a mucous membrane surrounded by a fibrous sheath. The larger and medium bronchi have plates of cartilage in the fibrous layer, and are richly supplied with glands secreting mucus, which is poured out on to the surface of the lining membrane and serves to keep it moist. The surface of this membrane is composed of columnar epithelial cells, provided with little whip-like processes known as 'cilia', which have the double function of moving any expectoration upwards towards the throat, and of warming the air as it passes over them. The walls of the bronchial tubes are rich in fibres of elastic tissue, and immediately below the mucous membrane of the small tubes is a layer of plain muscle fibres placed circularly. To this muscular layer belongs the function of altering the lumen of the tube, and, consequently, its air-carrying capacity. It is a spasmodic contraction of the muscular layer that produces the characteristic expiratory 'cough' of true asthma.

The smallest divisions of the bronchial tubes open out into a number of dilatations, known as 'infundibula', each of which measures about $\frac{1}{20}$th of an inch across, and these are covered with minute sacs, variously known as 'air-vesicles', 'air-alveoli', or 'air cells'. An air cell consists of a delicate membrane composed of flattened plate-like cells, strengthened by a wide network of elastic fibres, to which the great elasticity of the lung is due; and it is in these thin-walled air cells that the respiratory exchange of gases takes place.

The branches of the pulmonary arteries accompany the bronchial tubes to the farthest recesses of the lung, dividing like the latter into finer and finer branches, and ending in a dense network of capillaries, which lies everywhere between the air vesicles, the capillaries being so closely placed that they occupy a much greater area than the spaces between them. The air in the air vesicles is separated from the blood only by two most delicate membranes, viz. the wall of the air cell and the wall of the capillary, and it is through these walls that the respiratory exchange takes place.

LUNGS, DISEASES OF. The chief of these, **pneumonia**, is described under that heading. (*See also under* PLEURISY, EMPHYSEMA, TUBERCULOSIS, MAEDI/VISNA, CALF PNEUMONIA, EQUINE RESPIRATORY VIRUSES, ENZOOTIC PNEUMONIA OF PIGS, CONTAGIOUS BOVINE PLEUROPNEUMONIA, PARASITIC BRONCHITIS, PULMONARY ADENOMATOSIS, etc.)

Congestion of the lungs. This is the preliminary stage of several types of acute pneumonia. It also occurs in disease of the left side of the heart. 'FOG FEVER' of cattle is another condition in which congestion of the lungs is seen.

'Hydrostatic congestion' of a lung is apt to occur if an animal, which cannot stand, lies for too long on one side. Regular turning of the animal on to its other side is a necessary nursing procedure.

Pulmonary oedema. This may occur during pneumonia (some forms), in disease of the left side of the heart, and (in cattle) in 'FOG FEVER', and in PARASITIC BRONCHITIS of cattle and sheep.

An acute and usually rapidly fatal oedema of the lungs occurs in animals exposed to smoke in a burning building; the animal almost literally 'drowns' in its own blood serum. (Administration of oxygen can be tried if an animal has been rescued before severe lung damage has been caused.)

Poisoning by PARAQUAT, and ANTU result in oedema of the lungs. (*See also* DIPS and DIPPING, ELECTROCUTION.)

Pulmonary emphysema (*see* 'FOG FEVER').

Pulmonary haemorrhage (*see* RACEHORSES).

Allergic alveolitis. Inflammation of the alveoli of the lungs of cattle exposed to mouldy hay or straw contaminated with micro-organisms such as *Thermopolyspora polyspora*, and resembling 'farmer's lung'. (*See* 'FARMER'S LUNG.)

Tumours of the lung are usually of metastatic origin, *i.e.* they are secondary growths which have started from another centre in the body, being carried to the lung tissue either by the blood- or lymph-stream. (*See* CANCER.)

Gangrene of the lung may be a complication of, or a sequel to, pneumonia, and is usually fatal. It is characterised, by the presence of a foul-smelling, usually rusty-red, and almost always very copious discharge from both nostrils, in addition to the other symptoms of pneumonia. It is commonest in the horse as a sequel to ordinary pneumonia, and in other animals it may occur when the pneumonia has been produced through faulty drenching. (*See* PNEUMONIA.)

Collapse of the lung. The lungs are so resilient, in consequence of the elastic fibres throughout their substance, that if air be admitted within the pleural cavities the lungs immediately collapse to about a third of their natural size. Accordingly, if the chest wall is wounded and air gains entrance through the wound (pneumothorax), the lung collapses. After the wound has healed, and provided no complications occur, the elasticity is restored as the air is absorbed. (*See* PNEUMOTHORAX.)

Torsion of a lung lobe, usually the right cardiac lobe, is seen rarely in dogs and cats; causing dyspnoea, pulmonary oedema, and death. The lobe may become twice its normal size and blackish. (Williams, J. H. & Duncan, N. M. *J. S. Afr. V. A.* (1986) **57**, 35).

Wounds of the lung are serious on account of the air admitted through the chest wall, which leads to collapse; and the haemorrhage, and the difficulty of checking it. The lung may be wounded by the end of a fractured rib pointing inwards. (*See* 'FLAIL-CHEST'.)

Parasites of the lungs. Liver flukes are sometimes found in the lungs of cattle and sheep; lung flukes attack cats, dogs, pigs, and man in the Far East and the United States. Other parasites include LUNGWORMS. (*See also* HEARTWORMS for pulmonary Dirofilariasis.)

LUPINS, POISONING BY. Lupins of different species have often been found to cause poisoning of sheep; sometimes of horses, cattle, and goats.

Poisoning by lupins is of two kinds: (1) due to alkaloids within the plant producing a nervous disease; and (2) due to infestation of the plant with a fungus which produces a toxin affecting the liver. This second type of poisoning is known as **lupinosis,** is usually chronic, and produces loss of appetite and weight, jaundice, cirrhosis of the liver, oedema of the head, ascites and death. A few animals do recover but seldom thrive well afterwards.

In the United States of America great loss among sheep flocks has been occasioned by feeding on lupins animals not accustomed to them. The alkaloids are present chiefly in the seeds.

Poisoning by the alkaloids gives rise to symptoms which include loss of appetite, laboured breathing, excitement, convulsions, and death from respiratory paralysis. There is no jaundice or cirrhosis of the liver, and animals which recover are likely to do so completely.

LUPUS ERYTHEMATOSUS. An autoimmune disease of dogs and cats which occurs in two forms: (1) the cutaneous or *discoid* form, and (2) the *systemic* form.

The *discoid* form is characterised by symmetrical lesions on face, nose, and ears. Alopecia, loss of pigment, erythema, and a scaliness may be seen. Exposure to sunlight worsens the condition.

The *systemic* form affects many tissues and organs. Autoantibodies against platelets, red and white blood cells may be present; with antibodies also in joints, kidney, skin, and other organs. Symptoms include bilateral polyarthritis, fever, muscle pain, enlarged lymph nodes, and sometimes nervous symptoms.

Prednisolone is used in treatment.

(For further information *see* the paper by David Bennett, *In Practice*, May 1984).

LUTEINISING HORMONE (LH). A secretion of the anterior lobe of the pituitary gland. LH controls the development of the corpus luteum and its production of progesterone. In the male animal, LH stimulates secretion of testosterone by the testicle.

LUTEOLYSIS. Regression of a *corpus luteum.* Two factors appear to be involved in luteolysis in most domestic animals; one being prostaglandin F_2a and the other being follicular oestrogen synthesis. It has been suggested that PGF_2a is the normal luteolytic compound, and that it is transferred from the non-gravid uterus to the ovary by some form of counter-current distribution between the uterine vein and ovarian artery. While the actual route for PGF_2a transfer is in some doubt its physiological role is certain.

'A number of procedures for inducing luteolysis in domestic animals have been used. These range from the squeezing out of an established *corpus luteum* by rectal palpation in cattle, to the use of oestrogens. Although these methods are used in cases of infertility, their use in routine synchronisation has not been widely advocated, prostaglandins being preferred.' (Dr J. M. Chesworth, 1975.)

LUXATION (*see* DISLOCATION).

LYME DISEASE. This was first recognised in Connecticut, USA, in 1975; the source of infection being Ixodes ticks on deer, apparently.

The disease occurs both in the UK and other EC countries; in adults as well as in children. CAUSE: *Borrelia burgdorfei.* (*See* BORRELIA.) SIGNS: Blurred vision, lethargy, headaches, arthritis. In a few cases meningitis or encephalitis or myocarditis result.

Lyme disease in dogs has been reported in the UK, other EC countries, the USA and Australia.

LYMPH is the fluid which circulates through the lymphatic spaces of the animal body. It is a colourless fluid, containing less protein but otherwise similar to, the blood-plasma. It also contains *lymphocytes.*

Lymph nourishes the tissues and returns waste products from them back into the blood-stream. There are certain tissues which are not provided with a blood-supply at all, *e.g.* the cornea of the eye, cartilage, horn, etc., and in them the lymph is the only nourishing medium.

The lymph is derived in the first place from the blood-stream, of which the watery constituents exude through the fine walls of the capillaries into the tissue spaces. After meals, lymph from the small intestine may be milky in appearance due to contained fat. (*See also* LYMPH NODES, LYMPHOCYTES.)

The term 'lymph' was also applied to the material which collects in the vesicles of cow-pox and was used for vaccination.

LYMPH NODES. Formerly called Lymph Glands, these are situated on the lymphatic vessels, act as filters, and have an important role in body defence by producing lymphocytes. (*See also* RETICULOENDOTHELIAL SYSTEM, IMMUNE RESPONSE, LYMPHOCYTES, PLASMA CELLS.)

LYMPHADENITIS Inflammation of lymph nodes.

LYMPHADENOMA (*see* HODGKIN'S DISEASE).

LYMPHANGITIS. Inflammation of the lymphatic vessels.

In horses three infective forms occur; (1) EPIZOOTIC LYMPHANGITIS (caused by a yeast); (2) ULCERATIVE LYMPHANGITIS (bacterial); and (3) GLANDERS (bacterial). (*See under these headings.*)

The non-infective LYMPHANGITIS used to be called 'Monday morning disease'; often being seen in horses after a weekend of no work and a protein-rich diet.

SIGNS. Fever, lameness in one or more legs, with enlarged and tender lymph nodes. Later, doughy swellings which pit on pressure, may affect the whole limb.

The appetite is lost for a day or two, but the horse is usually very thirsty. Under appropriate treatment, the severity of the symptoms abates in 2 or 3 days' time, or sooner; and although lameness still persists, perhaps for as long as a week, the general appearance of the horse rapidly improves. The horse is usually able to resume work in from 10 days to a fortnight.

Recurrences are likely, resulting in some permanent thickening of the limb.

TREATMENT. Antihistamines may be tried. Antibiotics may be necessary; also diuretics to help reduce the swelling, and phenylbutazone, or some other analgesic, to reduce the pain.

In the 1970s it was stated that lymphangitis occurred in about 20 per cent of French cavalry horses, with between 7 and 9 per cent being affected annually. 'If treated early, when the oedema is barely visible,' Dr Benazet stated, 'the recovery period is considerably reduced; and in some cases the horses can resume work after only five days.' He used the anti-inflammatory agent

alpha-chrymotrypsin, either by intramuscular injection or as tablets given by stomach tube.

LYMPHATICS are the vessels which convey the lymph through the body. (*See* LYMPH.)

LYMPHOCYSTIS. A viral disease of fishes, which may give rise to whitish nodules on the cornea of the eye.

LYMPHOCYTE. Lymphocytes in mammals are of two main classes: thymus-derived, called T-cells; and B-cells derived from bone marrow. Unlike polymorphonuclear leukocytes and monocytes, the white cells in this group have cell surface receptors for antigen, and they are not involved in phagocytosis.

T cells do not secrete antibodies and act directly on foreign cells. B cells divide rapidly to form plasma cells which secrete antibodies. (*See under* BLOOD, B-CELLS, IMMUNE RESPONSE, RECEPTORS.)

'A much simplified scheme of the relationship between antigens and some of the lymphoid cells of the body is shown below. Natural immunity is conferred by the natural secretions of the body surfaces. If these surfaces are penetrated, scavenger cells (macrophages) attempt to engulf and destroy the antigens. Macrophages have a central role in immunity and if they are successful no further effects of antigen may be detectable. The activity of macrophages is increased if the antigen is coated with specific antibodies. Macrophages are also attracted to areas where antigen is concentrated by soluble factors secreted by certain sensitised lymphocytes.' (With acknowledgements to Dr M. R. Williams and Dr R. Halliday, and to the 1976 Report of the A R C's Animal Breeding Research Organisation).

Large granular lymphocytes are a type of T-lymphocytes, stated to have a prominent role in modulating normal immune responses, and in eliminating virus-infected and transformed cells. H. W. Reid and others suggested that infection of these cells by the malignant catarrhal fever agent

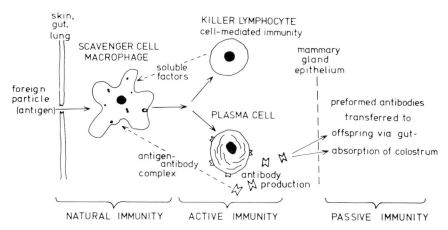

Relationships between antigen and lymphoid cells illustrating the many stages at which antigen can be destroyed. If antibodies are formed they may be passed on from mother to young.

was the essential initial step in precipitating the disease. (*Veterinary Record* (1984) **114**, 582.)

'A large pool of migrating lymphocytes is continuously being shuffled between the spleen, the lymph nodes, and the gut-associated lymphoid tissue' (W. L. Ford), with the blood serving as the channel for this redistribution. (*See also* LYMPHOKINE.)

LYMPHOCYTIC CHORIOMENINGITIS. A virus disease of mice transmissible to human beings, in whom it may give rise to fever, headache, pain in muscles and occasionally, death from meningo-encephalitis. (*See Lancet*, Aug. 2, 1975, p. 216, for human outbreaks of LCM in Germany and the USA arising from infected hamsters.) Dogs may act as symptomless carriers.

LYMPHOID LEUKOSIS of chickens is a form of cancer caused by an RNA virus, and begins in the bursa of Fabricius. 'Lymphoid leukosis is a malignancy of the bursal (B) system of lymphocytes' (*see Vet. Rec.*, May 17, 1975).

LYMPHOKINE. Secreted by T-lymphocytes, and formed when sensitised cells react with antigen, lymphokines can attract other lymphocytes and monocytes, modify vascular permeability and activate macrophages. In man they are believed to play an important role in the production of rheumatoid arthritis.

LYMPHOSARCOMA (*see* LEUKAEMIA; *also* FELINE LEUKAEMIA, BOVINE ENZOOTIC LEUKOSIS, CANCER).

'LYNX' COMPUTER. The measurement of cellular and chemical components of blood is widely used in the diagnosis and monitoring of disease in human beings and domestic animals. Haematological and biochemical analyses are also increasingly used in the conservation and care of captive and free-living wild animals. In the past, however, the interpretation of the results in non-domestic species has been hindered by the paucity and inaccessibility of species-specific reference data.

IBM-compatible software has been developed so that quantitative and qualitative haematological and biochemical reference data for over 500 species of mammals, birds and reptiles can be made readily accessible to veterinary surgeons. The Lynx software makes it possible to retrieve these data at different taxonomic levels (species, genera, families, orders and classes) and to select data by age and sex. Notes describing the variations in blood cell morphology observed in healthy individuals of each species are included in the database. The user's own data can also be entered. (Bennett, P. M. & others. *Veterinary Record* (1991) **128**, 496.)

LYSINE is a very important amino acid. Synthetic lysine is added to pig feeds (concentrates) both to improve performance and to avoid using so much protein. (*See* AMINO ACIDS.)

LYSIS has two meanings: the *gradual* ending of a fever (as compared with *crisis*); and the destruction of a cell by an antibody.

LYSOSOMES are structures within the cytoplasm of a cell, are surrounded by a membrane, contain enzymes, and may carry out a digestive function for the cell, getting rid of bacteria, etc.

Lysosomal storage disease. These are due to genetically determined deficiences of specific enzymes; and are common in some breeds of dogs and cats.

An accumulation of *lipofusin*, and its related pigment *ceroid*, is a feature of some lyosomal storage diseases. (*See* CEROIDOSIS.)

LYSSA is another name for rabies. (*See* RABIES.)

M

MACAW-WORM FLY. This is a parasite of cattle and other animals in Central America. It is another name for the warble-fly *Dermatobia homini*. (*See* FLIES.)

'M & B. 693'. Sulphapyridine, one of the sulphonamide drugs (which see).

MACROCYTE is the term applied to an unusually large erythrocyte especially characteristic of the blood in some forms of anaemia.

MACROPHAGE. A former monocyte (type of white blood-cell) which has migrated into the tissues and become larger. (*See under* BLOOD, INFECTION.)

MACULES are spots or stained areas of the skin or of mucous membrane, usually brownish, red, or purple in colour.

MADNESS IN DOGS (*see* RABIES, ENCEPHALITIS, MENINGITIS).

MAEDI/VISNA. A slowly progressive disease of sheep and goats, first recognised by Dr G. Gislason in Iceland in 1938 or 1939, and believed to have been introduced into that country by karakul sheep imported from Germany. Iceland is now free from the disease, following two eradication programmes, but Maedi occurs in the UK, continental Europe, North America, Africa, and Asia.

Although maedi/visna has never been recorded in Australia, a retrovirus was isolated from goats there and shown to produce antibodies indistinguishable from those produced by meadi/visna virus in goats.
CAUSE. A lentivirus.
Maedi is the Icelandic word for dyspnoea, and the disease is a type of pneumonia with a very long incubation period – one to three years or even more. An early sign is dyspnoea; after physical exertion the breathing becomes very rapid and shallow. Later, breathing becomes difficult even when the animal is at rest, and death often follows.
Visna is a name applied to the same viral infection when the brain or spinal cord rather than the lungs are involved. Demyelination occurs.
DIAGNOSIS can be confirmed by microscopical examination of the tissues and by isolation of the virus. There is also an ELISA test.

MAFF is used as an abbreviation for Ministry of Agriculture, Fisheries and Food.

MAGGOTS which have fed on carcases contaminated by *Clostridium botulinum* may contain a dose of toxin lethal to birds. This has caused deaths among domestic poultry, wild birds, and on game farms in the UK.

In 1974 the London Zoo lost 37 birds from botulism arising from a batch of *commerically bred* maggots.

MAGGOTS IN SHEEP. In many parts of the world certain dipterous flies may lay their eggs on the wool of sheep during summer, and the eggs hatch into maggots which either live on the surface of the skin or burrow down into the subcutaneous tissues. They cause great loss from wasting of flesh, destruction to fleeces, and sometimes result in the death of the affected sheep. The green-bottle flies (*Lucilla caesar* and *L. sericata*, in Great Britain, and *L. macellaria*, both North and South America) are those responsible for this condition. (*See under* MYIASIS *and* FLIES.)

'MAGIC MUSHROOM POISONING'. This is caused by psilocypin, a hallucinogen present in *Psilocybe semilanceate* and *Panaeolus foenisecii*.
SIGNS: Aggressiveness, ataxia, nystagmus and salivation plus a body temperature in excess of 42°C were noted in a **dog** by Mr A. P. Kirwan, who practises in Lancashire. Recovery followed on day 3. (*Veterinary Record* (1990) **126**, 149.)

Aggressiveness in a normally docile **pony**, which had been grazing in a field where 'magic mushrooms' were growing in profusion, was seen in Mid Glamorgan. (Same source.)

MAGNESIUM is a light white metal which burns in air with the production of a brilliant white flame, leaving a white powder as a residue. The salts of magnesium used as drugs are the oxide, carbonate, and sulphate. There is a heavy oxide, known as 'magnesia ponderosa', a light oxide called 'magnesia levis', a heavy carbonate, and a light carbonate. Both the oxides and the carbonates are antacids and slightly laxative. The sulphate of magnesium is commonly called 'Epsom salts'. (For blood magnesium, *see under* HYPOMAGNESAEMIA.)
USES. Magnesia, whether light or heavy is usually prescribed for foals, calves, and dogs when these require a mild antacid and laxative. The sulphate of magnesium is a saline purgative. (*See under* LAXATIVES.)

Calcined magnesite is used as a top-dressing for pastures in an attempt to prevent hypomagnesaemia (about 10 cwt per acre). For cattle, a daily dose of 2 oz calcined magnesite is considered to be of great value in the prevention of hypomagnesaemia, but it should be fed only during the 'danger period'. This is because prolonged feeding of magnesium salts is apt to accentuate any latent phosphorus deficiency and may lead to 'milk lameness' or similar conditions.

A mixture of magnesium acetate solution and molasses has been used, being available on a free-choice basis to cattle from ball feeders placed in the field.

Magnesium oxide. Too high a level in concentrate feeds for lambs and calves has led to urolithiasis. (*See under* URETHRAL OBSTRUCTION.)

MAGNETS have been used to treat traumatic reticulitis and prevent traumatic pericarditis in cattle. (*See under* HEART, DISEASES OF.)

MAINE-ANJOU. A French dual-purpose breed of cattle. Colour: red and white, and roan.

MAIZE (*see* PHYTIN, SILAGE).

MAJOR HISTOCOMPATIBILITY SYSTEM. One of the chromosomal regions controlling immune responses. Dr R. L. Spooner at the Animal Breeding Research Organisation, Edinburgh, demonstrated association between MHC type in cattle and their resistance to mastitis, thus raising the possibility of selecting for AI bulls which pass on resistance.

Dr Ian Tizzard has commented: 'Histocompatibility antigens are inherited through a set of genes known as the Major Histocompatibility Complex (MHC). Every animal possesses its own unique set of Histocompatibility antigens.'

Class I genes code for antigens that provoke the rejection of foreign grafts. Antigens of this class are of the cell surface type, located on all nucleated cells, and concerned with cell recognition.

Class II antigens.

Class II cell surface antigens are located mainly on B cells, and concerned with regulation of the immune response.

Class III antigens, located in serum protein, and regulate complement activity. (See COMPLEMENT). (Tizzard, I., *Veterinary Medicine* (1986) 574.)

MALACHITE GREEN. A dye used in the treatment of external fungal and protozoal infections of fish, and for the control of proliferative kidney disease. (Alderman, D. T. & Clifton-Hadley, R. S. *Veterinary Record* (1988) **122**, 103.)

MALACIA. Softening of a part or tissue in disease, *e.g.* osteomalacia or softening of the bones.

MALARIA (*see under* MONKEYS).

'MALARIA OF BIRDS' (*see under* PLASMODIUM).

MALATHION. An organic phosphorus insecticide used for the control of external parasites in cattle. It is relatively safe since it is detoxified by the mammalian liver – unless another organic phosphorus compound, which destroys the relevant enzyme, is absorbed at the same time. (*See* POTENTIATION, INSECTICIDES.)

Malathion is also used on crops, and at least 24 hours should be allowed between spraying and grazing.

MAL DE CADERAS, or MALADIE DE CADERAS, is a trypanosome disease of the horse, occurring in Brazil, the Argentine, Bolivia, and Paraguay, being most serious in the latter country. It is caused by the *Trypanosoma equinum.* Suramin or quinapyramine is used in treatment.

MAL DE PLAYA. A form of poisoning in cattle by a plant *Lantana camara.*

MAL DU COIT, or MALADIE DU COIT (*see* DOURINE).

MALE FERN. The growing point of Male Fern may attract cattle on bare pasture, and lead to poisoning. In Scotland 61 out of 68 head of beef cattle were involved in this way, with 45 wholly blind, 10 partly blind, and 21 recumbent. All recovered within a week except for 4 cows and 4 calves, which remained completely blind. One cow was additionally recumbent and was destroyed. (*See also under* FERNS.)

MALEIC HYDRAZIDE. A growth retardant used on grass verges which has caused non-fatal gastritis in small animals.

MALFORMATION (*see* DEFORMITIES).

MALIGNANT APHTHA OF SHEEP (*see* ORF).

MALIGNANT CATARRHAL FEVER (*see* BOVINE MALIGNANT CATARRHAL FEVER.)

MALIGNANT JAUNDICE OF DOGS (*see* BILIARY FEVER).

MALIGNANT OEDEMA (*see* GAS GANGRENE).

MALIGNANT STOMATITIS (*see* CALF DIPHTHERIA).

MALIGNANT THEILEROSIS OF SHEEP AND GOATS. A tick-borne disease caused by the protozoan parasite *Theileria hirci*, and occurring in E. Europe, the Middle East, Egypt, and Sudan. SIGNS include high fever, constipation, glandular enlargement, pale anaemic mucous membranes with later jaundice and death; but the disease may be very mild in animals with some locally acquired immunity.

MALLEIN TEST is a method of testing for the presence of glanders in a horse. (*See* GLANDERS.)

MAMMARY GLAND, or UDDER.

Structure.

Mare. The mammary glands are two in number, situated in the inguinal region.

Cow. The udder has four glands or 'quarters'. A strong septum divides the two right-hand glands from the two on the left side, but there is no such demarcation between fore and hindquarters on the same side of the body.

The structure of the gland is similar to what is seen in the mare, being composed of lobes and lobules, held in position by fibrous tissue, and sending ducts down into an irregular milk sinus. This latter is large, and partly divided into compartments by folds of mucous membrane. From it leads one large lactiferous duct down the teat to

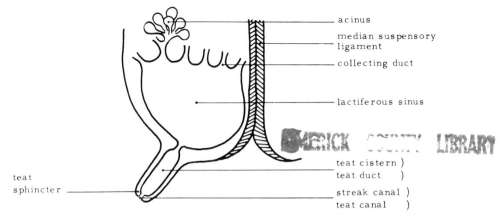

acinus

median suspensory ligament

collecting duct

lactiferous sinus

teat cistern)
teat duct   )

teat sphincter

streak canal)
teat canal   )

A diagram showing one half of the cow's udder, and the median suspensory ligament which separates the two halves. (With acknowlegements to Smith Kline & French Ltd.)

its apex, which possesses a sphincter muscle of almost two-fifths of an inch in width.

Ewe. There are two mammary glands, each of which has a single teat. They are situated in the inguinal region, as in the mare and cow.

Sow. The mammary glands number twelve in most sows (although a few have more), and are arranged in two rows reaching from just behind the level of the elbows along the abdomen to the inguinal region. As a rule, the glands which are situated towards the middle of the series are the best developed and secrete the most milk. Each teat has two ducts as a rule.

Bitch. As in the sow there are two rows of glands along the lower line of the abdomen. They are usually ten in number, but in the smaller breeds there may only be eight, and in the larger breeds there are sometimes twelve. The teats each possess from ten to twelve tiny lactiferous ducts.

Secretion of milk. This is a continous process, initiated at parturition or before by the hormone prolactin (from pituitary gland) and another from the thyroid. A number of other hormones may be involved, both in stimulating and in maintaining secretion of milk.

Milk accumulates in the alveoli, upper channels, and milk cisterns; the rate of secretion decreasing as internal udder pressure rises.

Milk 'let-down' in the cow, associated with the hormone oxytocin, is referred to under MILKING.

Colostrum is the name given to the first milk that is secreted by the udder.

(The importance of the newly born of any species of animal getting a supply of colostrum-containing first milk, soon after it is born, is explained under COLOSTRUM.)

(For other information concerning milk, *see* MILK.)

Conditions affecting the milk yield of cows.
(1) *Breed.*
(2) *Temperament.* There is no doubt that a placid but not sluggish, alert but not highly nervous, cow makes the best milker.
(3) *Health.* It is, of course, necessary that a cow should be in good general health if the best results are to be obtained from her.

(4) *Age.* A cow in good health improves in her milk-yield up to her seventh or eighth year, and remains at a high level until her tenth or twelfth year. The milk of a young cow is much richer in fats and solids than that of an aged animal, so that the ideal position in a herd is to have enough young stock to counteract any possible deficiency in those substances from the milk of the old cows.
(5) *Lactation.* A cow yields the greatest amount of milk between the sixth and eighth week after calving; thence she gives a smaller amount each day till about the three-hundredth day, when she goes dry. Cows give best results when their lactation period does not exceed 8½ to 9 months, *i.e.* when they are dried off about 8 weeks before they are due to calve, having settled in-calf at the first (*See also* PROGENY TESTING, RATIONS.)

MAMMARY GLANDS, DISEASES OF.

Mastitis, or inflammation of the udder. All the domestic animals are liable to the disease, but it is commonest in the cow, ewe, and goat. (*See* MASTITIS IN THE COW.)

Abscess formation. Penicillin or sulpha drugs are indicated. (*See* ABSCESS. Specific abscesses are considered under ACTINOMYCOSIS, TUBERCULOSIS, etc.)

Tuberculosis of the udder. (*See* TUBERCULOSIS.)

Tumours include papillomas, fibro-adenomas, and adenocarcinomas. Some tumours of the bitch's mammary glands appear to be hormone-dependent and contain oestrogen receptor protein. Of 2,075 malignant tumours in bitches reported by 14 veterinary schools in the USA and Canada, 1,187 were histologically malignant, 557 benign, and 331 in the 'malignancy not determined' category. (W. A. Priester, National Cancer Insititute, Maryland, USA.) In cats, mammary carcinoma is twice as common in the Siamese breed as in all other breeds combined. (*See* TUMOURS, CANCER.)

Hypertrophy of the mammary glands in the cat has been recorded both in pregnant queens and in neutered females treated with megestrol acetate for 14 months to five years. The condition has to be differentiated from neoplasia.

Wounds and injuries of the udder and teats are commonest in the cow and sow, owing to greater pendulousness than in other animals.

All wounds of the udder and teats are serious on account of the danger of infection and the development of mastitis.

TREATMENT. As a first-aid treatment wounds of the teats and udder should be washed with warm water and an antiseptic, dry sulphanilamide powder afterwards being applied.

When a teat has been torn or injured so that milk escapes from the canal it is usually difficult to get the fistula, so formed, to heal until the cow goes dry. An operation is usually necessary to obtain healing. This procedure necessitates the cow remaining dry for at least 2 months. In some cases a cow with a fistula is better turned out to grass at once, and made to rear calves until her milk flow ceases, when she can be taken in and undergo the operation.

Eruptions on teats may be specific, such as are seen during outbreaks of foot-and-mouth disease, cow-pox, malignant catarrhal fever, rinderpest, etc. (*See* VIRAL INFECTIONS OF COWS' TEATS.)

Many teat sores, however, are caused through 'chapping', or 'cracking' of the delicate skin of the teat. (*See under* MASTITIS.)

Warts on teats (*see* WARTS).

Teat obstructions. Difficulty in milking may be caused by stricture of the sphincter, milk clots or (rarely) calculi in the teat canal, or by the presence of warty growths inside the canal. The latter condition is considered under WARTS.

MAMMILLA is the Latin term for the nipple.
Mammilitis. Inflammation of the nipple. Bovine herpes mammilitis is a recognised disease which can also affect the skin of the udder.

MAN. Maximum recorded age: 120 yrs. In the USA a man reached a height of 8 ft 11 ins (but died at the age of 21.)

In the UK a height of 7 ft 9 ins has been recorded. (*Guinness Book of Records.*)

MANDELIC ACID. A urinary antiseptic, effective in *acid* urine.

MANDIBLE is the bone of the lower jaw. (*See* JAW.)

MANDIBULAR DISEASE (*see* SHOVEL BEAK).

MANGANESE is a trace element. Insufficiency of it in the pasture herbage may cause infertility in cattle, e.g. in Devon and Cornwall, UK.

In New Zealand, on one farm, 32 calves were born with very shortened limbs and enlarged joints. They had been sired by four bulls. Owing to a dry season, the cows had been fed large quantities of apple pulp and corn silage, both of which contained very low levels of manganese. (Valero, G. & others. *New Zealand Veterinary Journal* (1990) **38**, 161.) (*See* TRACE ELEMENTS, 'SLIPPED TENDON'.)

MANGE. Sarcoptic mange occurs in man (when it is known as Scabies), the dog, cat, cattle, pigs, sheep, horses, etc. Psoroptic mange in the sheep is known as SHEEP SCAB. (For types of mange, causal mites, and treatment, *see under* MITES, PARASITIC.)

MANIOC. An ingredient of some compound animal feeds which has been found unsafe for turkeys. (*See* CASSAVA.)

MANNOSIDOSIS. The most widely recognised lysosomal storage disease of cattle, especially of Aberdeen Angus. It is due to a deficiency of the enzyme mannosidase.

β-**mannosidosis,** an inherited disorder of glycoprotein metabolism, has been identified in goats, and is rapidly fatal. Signs include inability to rise from a recumbent position, carpal contractures, pastern joint hyperextension, a dome-shaped skull, and deafness. (Kumar, K. & others. *Veterinary Record* (1986) **118**, 325.)

MANURE HEAPS. It is important to prevent grass growing near these and to fence them, as such herbage tends to become heavily infested with Husk parasites and constitutes a menace to cattle. Pig manure can be a source of *trichomoniasis* in cattle. (*See also* SLURRY.)

'MARBLE BONE' DISEASE (*see* OSTEOPETROSIS).

MARBURG DISEASE (*see* MONKEYS).

MAREK'S DISEASE. This contagious disease of domestic poultry was first described in Austria–Hungary in 1907. It was first recorded in America in 1914, and in Great Britain in 1929, and spread widely.

Formerly called Fowl Paralysis, this disease had, before the advent of vaccination against it, become the most economically important disease of poultry in many countries, in terms of fowl mortality, carcase condemnation, and lost egg production.

'As a result of vaccination, losses from Marek's disease have been reduced by more than 80 per cent.

'Marek's disease is essentially a neoplastic, leukaemia-like disease, primarily affecting the thymus-dependent system of lymphocytes.' (N. L. Payne, *A R C Research Review* (1976) **2**, 56.)

Dr Payne referred to two main sequels to infection: firstly, replication of the virus; and, secondly, infection and neoplastic transformation of thymus-derived lymphocytes leading to the development of tumours.

At least two forms of Marek's disease are recognised: the **classical form,** in which paralysis – to a varying degree – is the outstanding feature; and an **acute leukosis form,** in which lymphoid tumour formation is the main feature, with nervous symptoms less in evidence.
CAUSE. A Herpes virus.
SIGNS. The 'classical' form affects birds commonly between the ages of 3 and 4 months, but cases have been recorded in broilers a little over 3 weeks old, and also in birds over a year

old. It is frequently noticed that certain strains of birds are affected, in-contact birds of a different parentage remaining healthy. Affected birds may show lameness of one or both legs. This lameness becomes progressively worse, and general paralysis results. A common attitude for an affected bird to adopt is to lie about with one limb extended in front and the other extended behind. In spite of this the bird appears alert and will feed if placed beside a supply. Drooping of wings may be noted. In some cases the tip of the wing may touch the ground. Eye lesions may be seen.

In the acute form of Marek's disease, birds as young as 6 to 8 weeks may be affected. Loss of appetite and depression are noticeable; and tumours can often be palpated – these involving abdominal organs, muscles, skin, and sometimes the comb. Paralysis is not the predominant characteristic of this form of the disease.

MORTALITY. The mortality varies, but in birds 6 to 8 weeks old may exceed 20 per cent. It is difficult actually to arrive at a satisfactory figure as this disease may co-exist with others, *e.g.* coccidiosis, tapeworm infestations, tuberculosis, vitamin deficiency, etc.

CONTROL MEASURES. On the disease being diagnosed, all affected birds should be destroyed as soon as the first symptoms are observed. The disease is always introduced to a farm by the purchase of fresh stock, either in the form of eggs, day-old chicks, or adult birds.

Control measures consist in careful selection of the source of fresh stock.

Both the fowl tick, *Argas persicus*, and the Darkling beetle, can harbour the virus of Marek's disease.

VACCINES. A live attenuated Marek's virus vaccine may be used, or a (HVT) vaccine made from a non-pathogenic virus isolated from turkeys.

Dr Payne has stated that, although successful, MD vaccines – while preventing clinical disease – do not prevent a persistent infection, and so vaccinated birds may still be a source of infection to other birds.

MARES, INFERTILITY IN (*see under* EQUINE GENITAL INFECTIONS).

MARIE'S DISEASE (*see* HYPERTROPHIC PULMONARY OSTEOPATHY).

MARIJUANA (cannabis) poisoning has occurred in dogs in the USA as a result of being given home-made sweet biscuits containing the drug. Symptoms include acute depression, retching or vomiting, and a staggering gait. The dogs may be ill for 36 to 48 hours, and vomiting may be frequent. Besides vomiting, muscular tremors, and weakness one other dog showed incontinence, ataxia, leant against objects and then sank to the floor.

MARKETS. A common source of infection. (*See under* SALMONELLOSIS.) In the UK covered accommodation must be provided for dairy cows in milk, calves, and pigs, in accordance with the Markets (Protection of Animals) (Amendment) Order, 1965.

Animals suffering from a notifiable disease must not be exposed for sale in a market. (*See* DISEASE OF ANIMALS ACT.)

'MARMITE DISEASE'. A form of dermatitis encountered in piglets 3 days old and upwards. (*See* 'GREASY PIG' DISEASE.)

MARROW. The soft substance that is enclosed within the cavities of the bones. Yellow marrow owes its colour to the large amount of fat contained in it, while red marrow is of a highly cellular structure. Formation of the red blood-cells (erythrocytes) takes place in the marrow, as also that of the blood platelets (thrombocytes). The marrow is also the source of lymphocytes (B-cells), monocytes, and other leucocytes. (*See* BLOOD, *also* MYELOCYTES.)

MARSH MARIGOLD POISONING. The Marsh Marigold, or 'King cup' (*Caltha palustris*) has occasionally been the cause of poisoning, and is similar in its effects to BUTTERCUP POISONING (which see).

MASHAM. The cross resulting from a Blackface ewe × a Wensleydale ram.

MAST CELL is a type of connective tissue cell. (*See* under BLOOD – *Basophils.*) (*See also* REAGINIC ANTIBODIES.)

MAST-CELL TUMOURS of the skin had previously been regarded as both malignant and ultimately fatal in cats. However, in 14 cases none of the tumours metastasised to lymph nodes or viscera, none recurred at a previous excision site, and none caused death. (Buerger, R. G. & others. *JAVMA* (1987) **199**, 144.)

MASTITIS. Inflammation of the udder. (*See* MAMMARY GLAND, DISEASES OF, for mastitis in animals other than the cow.)

MASTITIS IN THE COW. Inflammation of the udder, involving either the secreting cells of the mammary glands, or its connective tissue, or both.

Subclinical mastitis. Mastitis may be unaccompanied by obvious symptoms. This form commonly reduces milk yields by 10 per cent or so, and is consequently of great economic importance. 'Approximately one cow in three in Great Britain was affected with subclinical mastitis,' Mr C. D. Wilson stated at the 1980 BVA Congress.

Simple tests have been used to detect the presence of an abnormally high content of white cells in an ordinary-looking sample of milk, and so indicate the presence of mastitis. Once it is known that it exists, bacteriological tests can be used to identify the organisms responsible and to determine the best treatments. Sometimes an excess of white cells (over 500,000 per ml) in the milk is the result of inflammation due to trauma and not to infection. Thus, the California or Whiteside Test

Cell count ranges (cells/cc)	Estimate of mastitis problem	Estimate of milk production loss per cow per year
Below 250,000	Negligible	—
250,000–499,000	Slight	42 gallons
500,000–749,000	Average	74 gallons
750,000–999,000	Bad	169 gallons
1,000,000 and over	Very bad	197 gallons

(With acknowledgements to Beecham Laboratories Ltd.)

may draw attention to a faulty milking machine or bad milking technique.

The mastitis situation in a herd can be monitored on a monthly basis by laboratories operating electronic cell counters. The **table** shows the ranges of white cell counts.

The **graph**, reproduced with acknowledgements to the Milk Marketing Board shows the spread of mastitis in an autumn calving herd.

Mastitis tends to rise as the winter progresses and falls when the cows first go out to grass. The cell counts rise again in July and August chiefly because of the high proportion of the cows nearing the end of their lactation. Cell counts and mastitis levels fall again in September when some of the older cows are being culled and first calf heifers are coming into the herd. Mastitis levels rise again through the winter period.

Clinical mastitis should be regarded as a herd problem.

ACUTE. Shivering may usher in the attack. Later, there is a rise in temperature, fast, full pulse, short, quick respirations, an uneasy appearance. The animal paddles with her feet, but is usually afraid to lie on account of the pain occasioned to the udder. She refuses food, and rumination is in abeyance. When the udder is examined it is found that one (or more) quarter is swollen, tense, reddened, and very painful to the touch; the cow may stand with her hind legs straddled apart.

'SUMMER MASTITIS' (often involving gangrene of the udder) usually occurs either in heifers or in dry cows; but occasionally in cows just after calving. It is caused by *Corynebacterium pyogenes* often in association with other pathogenic bacteria, e.g. *Peptococcus indolicus*.

'Summer mastitis' is something of a misnomer, in that, while it is most common in July and August, it is also common in January and February.

If the gangrene affects a large part of the quarter, or when more than one quarter is attacked, the condition of the cow is serious in the extreme.

The animal may stand aloof from the rest of the herd, sometimes paddles with her hind feet, and is obviously in pain. On examination the trouble is soon located to the udder, where hardness – but not necessarily swelling – of a quarter is detected. Foul-smelling pus (grey, greenish-yellow, or blood-stained) is present.

Treatment. Promptly call in the veterinary surgeon who may administer antiserum, toxoid and sulpha drugs, and succeed in saving the animal's life, though use of the quarter is usually lost.

Prevention. The injection of long-acting antibiotic prior to turning out, repeated every 3 weeks during summer. (In maiden heifers and in-calf heifers, this procedure may be difficult and not always practicable. Care is needed to avoid both teat damage and the introduction of pathogenic bacteria.)

Give such protection against flies as is practicable.

SUB-ACUTE MASTITIS. The disease runs a course not unlike that of the acute form, but the symptoms appear much more slowly. There is a greater difficulty in milking, the first drawn milk often containing little clots and always large numbers of shed epithelial cells, and later, as a gradually increasing pain and swelling in the affected quarter, accompanied by an alteration in the colour of the milk to yellowish, yellowish-grey. The amount of milk decreases. As a rule, appetite remains normal, pulse and breathing are unaltered, and if there is any rise in the temperature it is slight.

CHRONIC MASTITIS shows little general constitutional disturbance, and an almost complete absence of pain, a slowly progressing increase in

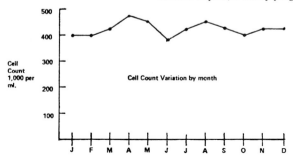

Cell Count 1,000 per ml.

Cell Count Variation by month

J F M A M J J A S O N D

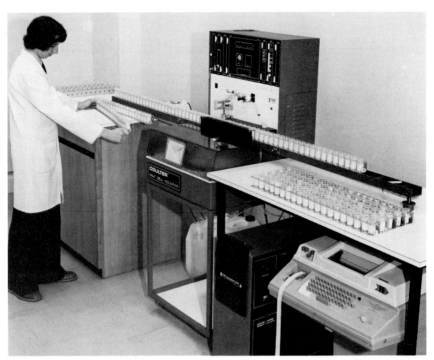

Mastitis control. All dairy herds in the UK have a cell count carried out to aid in the control of subclinical mastitis. (MMB photo)

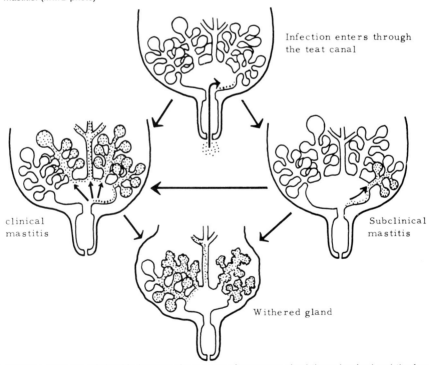

Infection enters through the teat canal

clinical mastitis

Subclinical mastitis

Withered gland

The diagrams show the relationship between the amount of mammary gland tissue involved and the form of mastitis which results. (With acknowledgements to Smith Kline & French Ltd.)

the density of the gland, a diminution in the secretion of milk, and a gradual *increase* in the size of the affected quarter or quarters.

Chronic mastitis with increase in udder size is one of the characteristics of tuberculosis of the udder.

It is estimated that over 700 cases of tuberculoid mastitis occur in Britain each year, and are almost invariably caused by the introduction of antibiotics into the teats before cleaning them.

Pathological changes in the udder may render any antibiotic ineffectual; and ARC research at Compton, by Drs N. Craven and J. C. Anderson, has shown that one problem is the **survival within phagocytes of staphylococci, where they are protected from the lethal action of most antibiotics.** (*See* PHAGOCYTOSIS.) 'One antibiotic which does kill intracellular staphylococci is rifampicin, but bacterial resistance to it is easily acquired.'

Antibiotics can more economically be used when the cow is in the dry period. Long-acting antibiotics can then be given without aggravating the problem of antibiotic residues in milk. (*See under* MILK.)

Bacterial mastitis. At the 1980 BVA Congress Mr C. D. Wilson stated that *Staphylococcus pyogenes* was the most common pathogen, with *Streptococcus agalactiae, S. uberis* and *S. dysgalactiae* next in that order.

Earlier it had been reported that mastitis due to *S. agalactiae* had almost disappeared from many areas, though L-forms of this organism were still proving troublesome. In one large dairy unit of 500 cows, over 700 cases of clinical mastitis occurred within 3 months – 95 per cent of the cases being due to L-forms of *Streptococcus agalactiae* (*see* L-FORMS).

Of other streptococci, *dysgalactiae* is seldom a serious problem; *uberis* is more resistant.

In a survey of five herds, *Streptococcus uberis* was found to be the major pathogen associated with **dry-cow** mastitis.

COLIFORM OR 'ENVIRONMENTAL' MASTITIS has become increasingly prevalent in recent years, and is common during the winter. This infection of the udder is often long-lasting, and the cow is ill with it, so that its economic effects may be greater than with streptococcal or staphylococcal mastitis. Many outbreaks have been linked with cold, wet weather; damp bedding, sawdust, and muddy conditions underfoot when strip-grazing kale, etc. The above conditions would appear to favour the entry of *E. coli* through the teat canal, but the organism may also reach the udder via the bloodstream in cattle which are scouring – often after a sudden change of diet – as a result of an active *E. coli* gut infection.

'Experimentally, severe cases of coliform mastitis can be produced only in early lactation following the stress of calving – a situation commonly prevailing in naturally occurring field cases.' (Source: IRAD, Compton). *See* COLIFORM.)

LEPTOSPIRAL MASTITIS. The existence of this form of mastitis was confirmed in 1976 by Dr W.

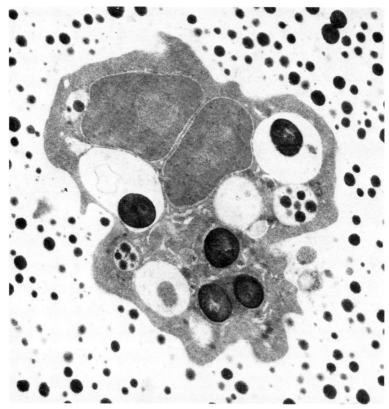

In bovine mastitis, as in other inflammations caused by microorganisms, neutrophils, a type of white blood cell (*leukocyte*), migrate from the blood into the inflamed tissue as the first line of defence. In this electron micrograph (magnification × 7000) a neutrophil or phagocyte is shown to contain five staphylococci. (*See* PHAGOCYTOSIS.) Reproduced by courtesy of the Agricultural and Food Research Council.

A. Ellis and colleagues at the Veterinary Research Laboratories, Stormont, where *Leptospira hardjo* was isolated from the milk and blood of cows with clinical mastitis. In one outbreak involving half a herd of 140 cows, over a 2-month period, symptoms included a sudden drop in milk yield, flaccid udders ·with all four quarters affected, thickish and sometimes blood-stained milk, fever (a temperature of up to 106°F), and quickened breathing and pulse rates. 'The illness in individual cows lasted from one to four days.' (*See* LEPTOSPIROSIS.)

Among other bacteria which may cause mastitis are *Bacillus subtilis*, which has been isolated from washing water, header tank, and teat-cup liners; *Pseudomonas*; and *Chlamydia*. *Campylobacter jejuni* has also caused mastitis.

MYCOPLASMAL MASTITIS occurs in Britain and many countries overseas, and may prove resistant to antibiotics. In an outbreak in North Wales over a 5-week period half a herd of 115 cows became infected, and 14 had to be sold for slaughter. The milk was at first brownish in colour. The mastitis was rapid in onset, producing a hard swollen quarter which was neither hot nor tender; and the cows showed little sign of general illness. 'Unlike other forms of mastitis, there was a rapid spread to other quarters of the udder,' A. B. Davies and E. Boughton of MAFF reported in the *Veterinary Record*. The first isolation of *Mycoplasma californicum* from cows with chronic, incurable mastitis in the UK was made in 1982; 10 years after its first isolation in California. Other species include *M. bovigenitalium*.

Viral mastitis has been associated with Vesicular Stomatitis and Infectious Bovine Rhinotracheitis.

Mycotic mastitis. Over 25 species of fungi have been incriminated. The worst of these is called *Cryptococcus neoformans* and it can cause outbreaks of mastitis severe enough to lead to cows being slaughtered.

Algal mastitis. A UK outbreak of severe indurative mastitis in newly calved cows, from which *Prototheca zopfii* was isolated, was reported. (Spalton, D. E., *Veterinary Record* (1985) **116,** 347). (*See* ALGAE.)

Man-to-cow-infections. Occasionally, mastitis in cattle arises from infection by human beings. The kind of streptococci which can give rise either to a severe sore throat or to scarlet fever can result in an outbreak of mastitis in a dairy herd, and several such outbreaks have been reported in various countries. The pneumococcus, a cause of human pneumonia, has been isolated from the udders of cows with streptococcal mastitis in Essex, Bedfordshire, and other counties; the source being the cowman's throat. *Campylobacter jejuni* has also been transmitted from man to cow. (*See under* MILK-BORNE DISEASE for SALMONELLOSIS, *Corynebacterium ulcerans*, etc.)

The spread of infection. Evidence has accrued that infection enters by way of the teat and that it can easily be spread from cow to cow by milker's hands or the cups of the machine, but apparently less easily by the latter method. Udder cloths and towels are also commonly infected. It has also now been shown that in an infected herd a large proportion of sores or chaps harbour organisms, and these may be a source of infection of the udder itself in the same cow or another. It has been shown also that the skin of the teats and the milker's hands may remain infected from one milking to another, and that in a heavily infected herd. The skin of the cow's body, milker's clothes, floor, partitions, etc., become contaminated and may remain so for considerable periods.

Treatment. Proper treatment depends upon a correct diagnosis and the use of suitable antibiotics in adequate dosage, introduced into the udder with aseptic precautions so as not to introduce further (and perhaps more virulent) infection. Adequate dosage is important as otherwise strains of resistant organisms may arise. In some cases sulphanilamide may be used. (*See* ANTIBIOTIC RESISTANCE.)

The control of mastitis. An important aid is **Teat-dipping.** 'The teat-dip, first adopted by a veterinary surgeon in 1916, has proved to be the most important procedure in the hygiene system,' is the view of F. K. Neave of the NIRD. He compares the method favourably with the pasteurisation of teat-cups 'which does nothing to prevent infection of the teat canal'. The liquid mainly used for teat-dipping is an iodophor – a type of disinfectant containing iodine but extremely mild in its effect upon the tissues. Good results can also be obtained with hypochlorite teat-dips containing 1 per cent available chlorine.

In rotary parlours with automatic cluster removal equipment and only one operator, teat-dipping is often impracticable and teat- spraying (probably less effective) the only alternative.

A second recommendation is the wearing by the cowman of smooth rubber gloves, which can be dipped in disinfectant before the udder is washed. They represent a partial solution of the problem created by the fact that hands cannot be sterilised.

Warm water sprays may be used for udder washing, and disposable paper towels for drying. The latter obviate cross-infections from udder cloths. (*See also* SPONGES.)

If warm water sprays are not available, wash udder (if very dirty) with plain warm water first, then with, *e.g.* ICI Udder Wash.

It is significant that in herds with a low incidence of mastitis, udder washing is avoided in 40 per cent and practised only in 11 per cent (but *see* **sediment in milk** *under* MILK).

Questions which the farmer must ask himself are as follows:

(1) Is the cowman capable of handling the cows properly, and keen to do so?

(2) Are the vacuum gauges and cup liners kept correctly adjusted?

(3) Is hand stripping avoided?

(4) If a disinfectant is used, is it used at the correct strength?

(5) Are there disposable paper towels?

(6) Are there any old, chronically infected cows in the herd which do not respond to treatment and would be better disposed of?

(7) Is fly-control being practised in the milking parlour?

(8) Is attention being given to the 96-hour rule regarding the withholding of milk from a cow after calving, whether treated with antibiotics or not? (MMB's *Milk Producer* (1991).)

Rough inexpert milking and stripping predispose to mastitis. With machine milking the use of a badly designed teat-cup liner, for instance, or leaving the cups on an empty quarter may lead to trouble. (*See under* MILKING MACHINES for faulty use of these leading to mastitis.) Bruising is an important predisposing cause, and for this reason cows should never be hurried, especially before milking, as the udder may be injured. This applies particularly to older cows in which the udder is large and pendulous. Chilling must be avoided, and also chapped teats. The latter should be left dry after milking. Even the smallest injuries and sores on the teats should be carefully attended to, since the germs which gain entry to these so often gain entry to the udder later.

The routine use of the strip cup is helpful. If flecks or clots are seen in the milk, segregate the cow(s) if practicable, and – in any case – milk after the others. When a strip cup is used care should be taken to see that neither the handle nor the fingers become a source of infection to clean cows. Use the cup *before* the udder is washed.

DRY-COW THERAPY. It has been shown in large-scale field experiments that the best time to treat cows to eliminate infection from the udders is during the dry period. Particularly with staphylococcal infection, there is a better chance (Mr C. D. Wilson has stated) of removing infections at this time than during lactation, and better results are achieved when cows are treated in the subclinical phase of the disease rather than during a clinical attack. Treatment during the dry period not only eliminates most of the existing infection; it also prevents most of the new infections from occurring during the dry-period, including 'summer mastitis'. Another advantage is that there is no problem of milk being contaminated with antibiotic(s), provided that a cow is dry for 6 weeks or longer. It is advisable to treat *all* cows. Preparations containing cloxacillin have proved very effective. Teat dipping of dry cows is also useful in preventing Summer Mastitis.

CONTROL MEASURES SUMMARISED (with acknowledgements to Beecham Laboratories Ltd).

(1) *Records.* Keep all details of cell-count figures on a monthly basis and use these to monitor the incidence of mastitis in the herd. Record also details of milking machine testing and maintenance.

(2) *Milking machines.* Have machinery tested regularly and thoroughly at least once a year. At each milking check the vacuum pressures, pulsation rates, air bleeds and liners. Remember that machines are used 730 times a year and faulty machines can lead to a mastitis build-up.

(3) *Teat dipping and hygiene.* Use an effective iodophor-plus-lanolin teat dip on each quarter as the cluster is removed. Wear smooth rubber gloves for preference, use the fore-milk cup before washing the udders with clean, running water. Use clean paper towels – not a dirty cloth – to dry the udders.

(4) *Dry-cow therapy.* The farmer's veterinary surgeon will not only advise generally on mastitis control, but will also recommend the appropriate treatment at the end of lactation. This will include the infusion of a specially formulated, long-lasting antibiotic into each quarter, to destroy residues of infection and to counter new infections in the dry period.

(5) *Treatment.* Clinical mastitis can occur at any time and will need prompt attention immediately by the veterinary surgeon who can advise the correct treatment during lactation.

(6) *Culling.* Any cow which has several attacks of clinical mastitis in a lactation endangers the rest of the herd. Records of treatments and responses will identify those cows with recurring cases in one lactation and show which should be culled from the herd.

The cow's own protection. 'Pathogens invading the mammary gland of the cow are subjected to non-specific resistance factors at two levels, either in the teat canal or in the mammary gland itself. The teat canal acts as a mechanical barrier, but in addition invading pathogens within the canal are subjected to the activity of antimicrobial fatty acids and cationic proteins. Pathogens breaching these barriers are then subjected to the defences of the mammary gland itself. In the early stages of infection there is a considerable increase in somatic cells in the milk which is associated with an increased resistance to infection. During the early stages of the inflammatory reaction the invading pathogens are exposed to the action of neutrophils, locally produced humoral factors and proteins from the systemic circulation which pass into the mammary gland. These serum factors include the immunoglobulins, complement units and other antimicrobial proteins.' (Dr K. G. Hibbitt and Dr A. W. Hill, *Report for 1977* of the IRAD, Compton.)

Breeding for resistance to bovine mastitis may be possible in the future. (*See* MAJOR HISTOCOMPATIBILITY.)

MASTITIS IN EWES. A vaccine, for the prevention of mastitis caused by *Staphylococcus aureus*, was introduced in 1988.

MASTITIS IN GOATS. The same bacterium caused gangrenous mastitis in 150 goats. Treatment with terramycin was successful in the early and intermediate stages; but the late stage of the disease could be treated successfully only by surgery. (Abu-Samra, M. T. & others. *Cornell Veterinarian* (1988) **78**, 281.)

MASTOCYTOMA. A type of tumour which is common in the dog and involves skin and subcutaneous tissue; occasionally muscle. A mastocytoma may be malignant. It contains numerous MAST CELLS (which see). In cattle this tumour is also regarded as potentially malignant.

MATERNAL ANTIBODIES. The function of these in protecting the offspring from infections encountered by the dam is referred to under COLOSTRUM (which see). The immunity so produced is a temporary one, and wanes, so that the timing of vaccination is crucial (*see* DISTEMPER); for if carried out while the level of antibody is significant, vaccination will fail. (*See also* MEASLES VACCINE, CANINE PARVOVIRUS.)

MAXILLA (*see* SKULL).

MEADOW SAFFRON POISONING. The Meadow Saffron, (as distinct from the autumn crocus, *Colchicum autumnale*), a common inhabitant of meadows, hedge bottoms, and woodland areas in England and Wales, is a cause of poisoning among horses and cattle. Pigs may sometimes eat the bulbous root (corm) and suffer, but sheep and goats are resistant. All parts of the plant are poisonous, both when green and when dried in hay, but the toxicity varies at different times of the year. Cases of poisoning are usually seen in the spring, when the leaves and seed-vessels are produced, and then again in summer and autumn (from August to October), when the flowers are formed.

The poison is present in largest amounts in the seeds and corms; it is called *Colchicine*, and is cumulative in its action.

SIGNS. When only small quantities have been taken there is loss of appetite, suppression of rumination, profuse dribbling of saliva, and diarrhoea. The excretion of acrid colchicine by the kidneys cause irritation in the urinary bladder, and induces the animal to pass urine in small amounts almost as soon as it is formed. Blood may be present in both the urine and the milk of dairy cows.

Abortion is common in pregnant cows and heifers.

When large amounts have been eaten the symptoms include ataxia, abdominal pain, and death may occur in from 16 hours to 4 days.

The plant should be eradicated from pastures in the autumn when its striking pale purple crocus-like flowers can be easily seen. The bulbs should be dug out or cut with a hoe.

MEAL FEEDING IN PIGGERIES. This can result in a very dusty atmosphere under some circumstances, causing coughing and a feeling of tightness in the chest in people working there, and to a sometimes false assumption that the pigs are coughing because of Enzootic Pneumonia.

MEASLES (*see under* MONKEYS *and* MEASLES VACCINE).

'MEASLES' IN BEEF (*see* CYSTICERCOSIS, TAPEWORMS).

'MEASLES' IN PORK (*see* CYSTICERCOSIS, TAPEWORMS).

MEASLES VACCINE. An attenuated measles virus vaccine was developed for use in the dog to give protection against distemper. (*See also under* DISTEMPER.)

Forney, Bordt and Theodore (1967) reported a series of experiments which demonstrated a limitation on the use of measles vaccine. 'This limitation is due to the fact that puppies born of bitches vaccinated with measles virus may possess sufficient maternally acquired measles antibodies to interfere with their response to vaccination with measles virus. Such puppies would be expected to become susceptible to canine distemper in a manner similar to non-vaccinated puppies.'

MEAT (*see* PALE SOFT EXUDATIVE MUSCLES, HORSEMEAT, DOGS' DIET, and below).

MEAT, CURED. For some years, stated the A F R C, the microbiological stability and safety of cured meats, and the composition of curing solutions, have exercised the minds of authorities and traders. 'The absence of *Cl. botulinum* spores from pork and pork products cannot be guaranteed.' In addition to its bacteriostatic role, nitrite is considered by the meat industry to be essential for good colour and flavour development. However, the possible formation in cured meat products of carcinogenic nitrosamines has led to a demand for a drastic reduction in the amount of nitrite used. The A F R C's Meat Research Institute is carrying out further investigation.

MEAT, DARK. Dark cutting beef is possibly the single biggest cause of loss to beef processors. It is caused by a deficiency of glycogen in the muscles of an animal at slaughter which prevents the normal decrease in pH post mortem. As a result there is an increase in enzyme activity which uses up the oxygen which would normally convert the dark myoglobin into pink oxymyoglobin and the meat appears dark; it also tends to be dry because of the higher water binding capacity of muscle protein at higher pH. The stores of glycogen are depleted principally by muscular exhaustion and stress, and these two factors must be avoided in the 48 hours before slaughter in order to minimise the risk of dark cutting beef. (Cooke, M. E., *Meat Hygienist* (1986) **49**, 24.) (*See also* PALE, SOFT EXUDATIVE).

Glycogen in the livers of pigs was assayed within 20 to 30 minutes of death. From previous data, the relationship between liver glycogen concentration and fasting time was used to predict how long the pigs had been without food. Of the 1873 pigs, three-quarters had been fasted for more than 8·1 h, half for more than 18·7 h and one quarter for over 30·8 h before slaughter. Long fasting times are associated with a reduction in carcase yield and an increase in the incidence of dark, firm, dry (D F D) meat. In addition, fasts of 12 h or more have been associated with increased aggression between pigs. (Warris, P. D. & Bevis, E. A. *British Veterinary Journal* (1987) **143**, 354.)

MEAT HANDLERS' occupational hazards include β-haemolytic Lancefield group streptococci (which can infect cattle, sheep, pigs, chickens). People involved in the slaughter of these animals may be exposed to ringworm and impetigo, and any cuts on their hands may become infected. (Barnham, M. & Neilson, D. *Epidemiology & Infection* (1987) **99**, 257.)

(*See also under* ZOONOSES, e.g. ORF, LOUPING-ILL, TUBERCULOSIS.)

(*See also* ANTHRAX, RABIES.)

MEAT INSPECTION REGULATIONS. The Fresh Meat Export (Hygiene and Inspection) Regulations 1987 specify the requirements for the production, inspection, cutting, storage and transport of fresh meat for export or for sale for export to the European Community. These regulations do not refer to exports to non-EC countries; but do refer to meat inspection in the UK.

The Slaughterhouses (Hygiene Amendment) Regulations 1987 make the skinning of the heads of goats and sheep mandatory only if intended for human consumption – as is the case with the export regulations.

Ante-mortem inspection of animals became compulsory in non-exporting countries on January 1st 1991. (*See also* FOOD INSPECTION.)

MEAT, KNACKER'S is to be avoided for the feeding of pet animals unless sterilised. (*See* MEAT STERILISATION, EARS AS FOOD.) Unsterilised meat may be infested with viable hydatid cysts, be infected with anthrax or tuberculosis. Even if it is cooked by the pet owner before use, it may contaminate hands, cooking utensils, etc., and thereby be a danger to public health. (*See also* SALMONELLOSIS, E. COLI, BOTULISM, AUJESZKY'S DISEASE, and HORSE-MEAT.)

MEAT SCRAPS, BONES can be a source of foot-and-mouth disease or swine fever infections. (*See* SWILL.) (*See also last two paragraphs of section* TUBERCULOSIS.)

MEAT (STERILISATION) REGULATIONS, 1969. These require all knacker meat to be sterilised before being supplied to owners of pets, kennels, etc. In 1982 new controls on the trade in meat, unfit for human consumption, came into force. If not sterilised, meat must be stained; likewise offal. Poultry meat is exempt. The colouring agent used is black PN or brilliant black BN.

MEATUS is a term applied to any passage or opening, *e.g.* external auditory meatus, the passage from the surface to the drum of the ear.

MECKEL'S DIVERTICULUM, of human pathology, apparently has a veterinary equivalent – a finger-like projection from the small intestine, recorded as a congenital abnormality in the dog.

MECONIUM. Faeces present in the rectum of a newborn animal. They should in all cases be discharged soon after birth. In the first milk of the dam there is a natural purgative for this purpose. (*See also* ILEUS.)

MEDIASTINUM is the space in the chest which lies between the two lungs. It contains the heart and the great vessels, the gullet, the extremity of the trachea, the thoracic duct, the phrenic nerves, as well as other structures of lesser importance.
PNEUMOMEDIASTINUM. The presence of air in the mediastinum, following damage to lung alveolar tissue near its root. In other cases the trauma may be of a more serious nature; for example, escape of air from a damaged trachea, or rupture of the oesophagus. A swelling of a dog's whole face and neck due to subcutaneous emphysema may follow pneumomediastinum; the air tracking upwards. It may take weeks before the swelling totally disappears, but the condition is seldom serious unless trachea or oesophagus are damaged. (Houlton, J., *In Practice* (July 1986) 157.)

MEDICINES ACT, 1968, was designed to control many aspects of manufacture, testing and marketing of medicines for human and animal use. In particular, its aim was to bring safety standards up to those already enforced by the leading companies. The Act required wholesalers, importers and manufacturers to obtain licences. (*See also* VETERINARY PRODUCTS COMMITTEE.)

The Act authorises which medicines may be sold to the public on a veterinary prescription. (*See* POM). 'Additional requirements now exist under the Animal Health & Welfare Act, 1984, concerning products for incorporation into animal feeding-stuffs.' Kidd, A. R. M. (1986. BVA Congress).

MEDICINES (LABELLING OF MEDICATED ANIMAL FEEDING STUFFS) REGULATIONS, 1973. These set out the detailed particulars required on labels of containers or packages of medicated animal feeds. The Medicines (Labelling) Regulations, 1976, covered the labelling of containers and packages for medicinal products, and were amended in 1977.

MEDITERRANEAN FEVER. A tick-borne disease of cattle and the water-buffalo, occurring in SE Europe, Africa, and Asia, and caused by *Theileria annulata*.
SIGNS. Fever, loss of appetite, a discharge from eyes and nose, anaemic pallor of mucous membranes, constipation followed by diarrhoea. Survivors recover very slowly.

MEDITERRANEAN SPOTTED FEVER. A human disease.
CAUSE: *Rickettsia conori*, transmitted by a dog tick.
SYMPTOMS: fever, nausea, vomiting, headache, muscle pain, and a rash.

MEDULLA OBLONGATA (*see* BRAIN).

MEDULLARY CAVITY. Marrow cavity of bones.

MEGA- and MEGALO- are prefixes denoting largeness.

-MEGALY. An abnormal enlargement; *e.g.* of the spleen (which may attain four or five times its normal size in *e.g.* babesiosis (Redwater) in sheep).

MEGAOESOPHAGUS implies usually a pathological enlargement of the oesophagus, such as may be seen in FELINE DYSAUTONOMIA and 'FLOPPY' LABRADORS.

MEGESTROL ACETATE. The active ingredient

of Glaxo's 'Ovarid', an oestrus-suppressant widely used in cats and dogs. It is also used empirically in the treatment of feline miliary dermatitis (eczema). Contra-indications are cats with diabetes or genital disease. It is recommended that it be given for up to 18 months. Prolonged dosage or overdosage may adversely affect the uterus or result in hypertrophy of the cat's mammary glands. (*See also* OESTRUS SUPPRESSION, DIABETES.)

MEIBOMIAN GLANDS. These are minute and situated in the eyelids. Inflammation may develop around an eyelash, and later there may be suppuration with the formation of a stye.

MEIOSIS, or reduction division, occurs during the formation of ova in the female and of spermatozoa in the male, and reduces the number of chromosomes by one half, to the haploid number.

MELAENA. The passing of dark tarry faeces, usually due to bleeding from the stomach or small intestines. The blood undergoes chemical changes as the result of the action of the digestive juices, which produce large amounts of sulphide of iron.

MELANOMA. A tumour containing the black pigment melanin, which is present in hair, etc. Melanomas are potentially malignant, and not uncommon in old horses that have been grey and are turning whiter.

Of three horses treated in the USA with cimetidine, an H_2 histamine antagonist, two had melanotic tumours which had begun to increase rapidly in both size and numbers over the past six and 27 months, respectively.

During the treatment, which lasted for two months to one year, the number and size of the melanomas decreased by 50 to 90 per cent.

In the third horse a slower development had occurred, and treatment was being continued at a lower dosage. (Goetz, T. E. & others. *JAVMA* (1990) **196**, 449.)

MELANOTIC is the adjective from MELANOMA.

MELATONIN. A hormone secreted by the PINEAL BODY (which see).

MELIA (Dhrek). The fruits and leaves of this Asiatic tree, *Melia azedarach*, are poisonous to farm livestock. Abnormal gait, trembling of hind limbs, paresis, and abdominal pain have been reported in the pig.

MELIOIDOSIS. A disease resembling glanders, caused by *Pseudomonas pseudomallei*, and occurring in rodents – occasionally in human beings and farm animals – in the tropics. Diagnosis: 'whitmorin' test. In man, chloromycetin is used in treatment. Cases have occurred in Germany, and in 1975 a suspected outbreak led to closure of a zoo in Paris.

MEMBRANA NICTITANS (*see* NICTATING).

MEMBRANES (*see* PLACENTA, BRAIN, MENINGES, MUCOUS MEMBRANES, SEROUS MEMBRANES, etc.).

MEMBRANOUS NEPHROPATHY. A progressive disease of the kidneys of dogs and cats, affecting the glomeruli, and leading eventually (sometimes after several years) to kidney failure. Most cases in the cat are first seen when showing the nephrotic syndrome. There is persistent excretion of protein in the urine, too little protein in the blood, and subcutaneous oedema and/or ascites. (*See* KIDNEYS, DISEASES OF.)

MENAPHTHONE (*see* VITAMIN K).

MENINGES (*see* BRAIN, SPINAL CORD, PIA MATER).

MENINGIOMA. A tumour affecting the meninges, and perhaps the commonest brain tumour in the cat.

MENINGITIS. Inflammation affecting the membranes covering the brain (cerebral meningitis), and spinal cord (spinal meningitis), or both (cerebrospinal meningitis). When the outer membrane is affected the condition is called 'Pachymeningitis', and when the inner membrane is it is known as 'Leptomeningitis', although clinically it is not often that these distinctions can be determined, for inflammation readily spreads from one to the other.

CAUSES. Meningitis frequently develops in association with virus or bacterial diseases of animals, such as rabies, tuberculosis, swine erysipelas, distemper.

In lambs it may be caused by Pasteurella haemolytica, in pigs by *Streptococcus suis* or Encephalomyocarditis virus. (*See* GID, TAPEWORMS.) It may be produced through an external injury which fractures the skull and allows entrance to organisms, or it may appear during the course of other head injuries in which there is no fracture. It accompanies most cases of encephalitis caused by viruses.

SIGNS. As a rule the first signs are those of restlessness and excitement. The animal moves about in a semi-dazed fashion, and stumbles into or against fixed objects. Neighing, bellowing, squealing, and barking, apparently at nothing, may be noticed, and at times the animal exhibits a wild frenzy. After an attack of delirium or frenzy the animal becomes dull and quiet; the head hangs, the eyes stare, the expression is vacant. Other symptoms, such as turning in circles, falling over, rolling along the ground, turning forward and backward somersaults, resting the head upon any convenient fixed object, such as a loose-box door, lying curled up in an unusual attitude, etc., may be seen in some cases. Paralysis of one side of the body (hemiplegia), of both hindlimbs (paraplegia), or of a group of muscles, is not infrequent in the smaller animals.

TREATMENT. Absolute quiet in a dark place is advisable pending professional advice.

Dogs. A form of spinal meningitis occurs in which bony tissue is laid down in the spinal canal towards the posterior part of the vertebral column. It is called 'chronic ossifying pachymeningitis' as a consequence. It mainly affects old dogs, and only causes inconvenience when severe. It may lead to complete paralysis of the hind limbs, accompanied by incontinence of urine and faeces.

In all animals in which meningitis follows injury, the skull should be examined for fractures.

MENINGOENCEPHALITIS EOSINOPHILICA OF PIGS. This is characterised by death of the cells in the grey matter of the brain in front of the *corpora quadrigemina*, and by thickening of the blood vessels around which are found considerable numbers of eosinophils.

Symptoms include: walking in circles, pressing the head against a wall, champing of the jaws, convulsions.

The cause, or a cause, is considered to be salt poisoning.

MENINGOCELE. A congenital defect: the protrusion of meningeal membrane through an abnormal opening in the skull or spinal column.

The defect occurs in calves, foals, puppies, kittens, piglets, etc; and it is also a human abnormality.
TREATMENT is surgical.
SIGNS. The owner of a calf stated that it was born with a 'tumour' which it repeatedly damaged and caused to bleed.

On admission to the department of large-animal surgery, University of Utrecht, in the Netherlands, a red soft mass of tissue, which pulsated in rhythm with the heart, was seen.

The meningocele was surgically removed, under general anaesthesia, and the skin sutured.

Three months later the owner reported that the calf was doing well, and showing no sign of any abnormal behaviour. (Back, W. & others. *Veterinary Record* (1991) **128**, 569.)

MENISCUS is a crescentic fibro-cartilage in a joint.

MEPACRINE HYDROCHLORIDE. An antimalarial drug which has been used in the treatment of coccidiosis in cattle.

MEPYRAMINE MALEATE. An antihistamine which is given by the mouth, by intra-muscular injection, or applied to the skin as a cream. Used in the treatment of laminitis, azoturia, urticaria, etc. (*See* ANTIHISTAMINES.)

MERCUROCHROME. An antiseptic, and a stain for spermatozoa. It is a proprietary name of a preparation of merbromin. and is an organic compound of mercury.

MERCURY, also known as QUICKSILVER, and HYDRARGYRUM, is a heavy silver-coloured liquid metal. In this form it was once used as an ingredient of ointments and even purgative powders.

The salts of mercury are of two varieties: mercu*ric* salts, which are very soluble and powerful in action; and mercur*ous* salts, which are less soluble and act more slowly and mildly. Mer-

curic salts are all highly poisonous; organic compounds less so. In strong solution they may be caustic, and in weaker solutions are irritant, the biniodide having been used as a blister.

Biniodide of mercury, or red iodide of mercury, made up into an ointment, formed the base of the common 'red blister'. With this and other mercury dressings, it is essential that care be taken, for the drug may enter the system by absorption from the skin, or by the animal licking itself.

Mercury poisoning Preparations of mercury have, with the possible exception of calomel as a laxative, given way to safer and more effective drugs. Consequently, mercury poisoning is now far less common than it was.

However feeding dressed seed corn has led to the death of pigs and cattle.

Three out of 17 bullocks and heifers died after being given seed barley, treated with phenyl mercuric acetate, as part of their feed. The deaths were sudden; the autopsy findings multiple and extensive haemorrhages. Gastro-enteritis, ataxia, and renal failure (often associated with mercury poisoning) did *not* occur. (Boyd, J. H., *Veterinary Record* (1985) **116**, 443.)

In Japan, the eating of fish with a high mercury content led to an outbreak of illness, with nervous symptoms, in cats.

Acute poisoning results in vomiting, diarrhoea, and abdominal pain; with death from shock. (Cattle may show only the first symptom.) Stomatitis and salivation may also occur. Severe purgation occurs in the smaller animals, together with signs of acute abdominal pain. Lips and mouth may become white.

Chronic mercury poisoning (mercurialism). Salivation; swelling of tongue, which bleeds readily; loosening of the teeth. Nervous signs may develop; e.g. ataxia, blindness.
FIRST-AID: Give white of egg.
ANTIDOTE: A CHELATING AGENT such as Dimercaprol.

A human case. The mercury from a broken thermometer, spilt on a carpet, led to severe illness in a 33-month-old girl. Symptoms included loss of appetite, sensitivity to light, eczema, sweating and scaling palms. Improvement followed two weeks' treatment with a chelating agent: 'Dimaval'.

Dental amalgam is another source of mercury vapour.

MERCURY, POISONING BY DOG'S. Both Dog's Mercury (*Mercurialis perennis*) and Annual Mercury (*Mercurialis annua*) are poisonous especially when seed-bearing. Cows are most often affected. Animals may not show symptoms until from 7 to 10 days after the plants are first eaten.
SIGNS. Diarrhoea. Urine is passed frequently, accompanied by painful straining, and is of a blackish or blood-red colour, as is the diarrhoea. Other signs are severe anaemia and semi-coma. Deaths have occurred.
FIRST-AID. The animal should be given strong black tea or coffee.

MESENCEPHALON is the mid-brain connecting the cerebral hemispheres with the pons and cerebellum.

MESENTERY is the double layer of peritoneum which supports the small intestine.
MESENTERIC HERNIA (*see* HERNIA).

MESH GRAFTS (*see* SKIN GRAFTING).

MESOCOLON is the name of the fold of peritoneum by which the large intestine is suspended from the roof of the abdomen.

MESOMETRIUM is the fold of peritoneum running from the roof of the abdomen to the uterus. It consists of two layers, between which run the blood and lymph-vessels, and the nerves to the uterus, and it acts as an elastic suspensory ligament supporting the uterus in position. During pregnancy it gradually stretches under the weight of the fetal contents, but retracts again after parturition under normal conditions.

MESOSALPINX is the suspensory ligament of the oviduct.

MESOTHELIOMA. A tumour developing from the mesothelium covering membrane surfaces.

MESOVARIUM is the suspensory ligament of the ovary.

MESULPHEN. A parasiticide which allays itching, used in cases of sarcoptic mange.

METABOLIC. Relating to metabolism.

METABOLIC PROFILE TESTS. To quote a paper given by Dr J. M. Payne and colleagues at the Institute for Research on Animal Diseases, Compton, 'modern farming imposes severe strains on the metabolism of dairy cows. Every effort is made to secure high yields at minimum cost. This is likely to increase, because high yielding cows are advantageous both in terms of financial return and in efficiency of protein conversion. New types of feed and unconventional methods of husbandry are also likely to be employed, thus adding to the strain and possibly introducing hidden dangers to the metabolic health of the animals. The metabolic profile test was devised to help meet this situation.'

The method depends on the fact that *imbalances between feed input and production output are reflected in abnormal concentrations of key metabolites in the blood.* The test appears to be of most value in (a) monitoring optimum input/output balances in apparently normal dairy herds; and (b) as an aid in diagnosing basic nutritional inadequacies in herds suffering from production disease problems.

As a first step in devising the test it was necessary to establish 'normal' values, and this was provisionally achieved by analysing 2400 blood samples from 13 dairy herds. The second step involved carrying out routine metabolic profile tests in 50 dairy herds. In many of these, abnormalities were detected which could be associated with actual or potential production disease problems. If necessary, a change of diet was recommended, and the effects of this monitored by repeated tests.

Haemoglobin levels were low in herds sampled at the end of the winter indoor period, but rose steeply when cows were turned out to pasture in the spring. 'This was so marked as to suggest that in some herds animals were saved from clinical anaemia only by the spring grass!'

Low blood sugar levels were associated in one herd with a severe and unexplained ketosis (acetonaemia) outbreak; but the effects of somewhat ham-handed over-correction in another herd led to secondary ketosis, following supplementation with a mixture of brewer's grains, sugar beet pulp and rolled barley. Two herds with low blood sugar showed few clinical problems, but many cows failed to come on normal heat in winter – a situation remedied by supplements.

Serum urea concentrations tended to be low on conventional indoor winter rations, but high in herds grazing highly fertilised pastures. The latter gave rise also to high concentrations of inorganic phosphate and potassium in the blood.

A dramatic example of low serum magnesium was shown in one herd where the farmer thought that his cows were dying from calving injuries. Magnesium supplements in the diet overcame the trouble. The detection of low serum magnesium levels may, of course, be valuable in the prediction of impending outbreaks of clinical hypomagnesaemia. Indeed, in one herd – apparently clinically normal – two animals died of grass tetany before the supplementation recommended after testing could become effective.

The dietary intake of sodium may be too low. For example, in an experiment 30 cows grazing known sodium-deficient herbage licked surrounding objects, each others' coats and even urine. This craving disappeared when sodium supplements were given.

Too little blood albumin was a feature in some herds on low-cost, low-protein diets. Cows on highly fertilised pastures tended to have high blood albumin levels.

Until recently, the number of blood samples involved would have been far too great for the metabolic profile tests to be applied on anything but a small, laboratory scale; but now new automatic analytical equipment together with a computer allow a rapid and large-scale analysis and interpretation of data.

As time goes on the 'normal' values may need revision, and trace elements and other metabolites may be included in the test which, it is hoped, will 'be of value in providing a link between the veterinary surgeon and the dairy farmer in the application of modern preventive medicine'.

But the test must be carried out in a carefully planned and standardised manner, under veterinary supervision. In other words, it is not a 'do-it-yourself' procedure, with a few samples at random taken from a dairy herd and sent through the post for testing.

METABOLISABLE ENERGY (ME) is defined as the energy of food less the energy of faeces, urine and methane. The unit of ME replaced – under metrication – the starch equivalent for calculating the composition of livestock rations. ME is measured in joules (an SI unit) instead of calories. The ME energy requirement for maintenance of a dairy cow is about 60 million joules or 60 megajoules (MJ) per day.

METABOLISM includes all the physical and chemical processes by which the living body is maintained, and also those by which the energy is made available for various forms of work or production. The constructive, chemical, and physical processes by which food materials are adapted for the use of the body are collectively known as *anabolism*. The destructive processes by which energy is produced with the breaking down of tissues into waste products is known as *catabolism*. Basal metabolism is the term applied to the amount of energy which is necessary for carrying on the processes essential to life, such as the beating of the heart, movements of the chest in breathing, chemical activities of secreting glands, and maintenance of body-warmth. This can be estimated when an animal is placed in a state of complete rest, either by observing for a certain period the amount of heat given out from the body or by estimating the amount of oxygen which is taken in during the act of breathing and retained.

METABOLITES. Any product of metabolism.

METACARPAL region is the part of the limb lying between the carpus, and the phalanges or digits, and in the horse is commonly called the region of the 'cannon' on account of the comparatively straight tubular form of the large or third metacarpal bone. There are three bones here, of which the central or third is the largest, and the inner (second) and outer (fourth) are rudimentary. In the ox there are two large metacarpals fused together; the sheep is similar; the pig has four separate from each other, and the dog possesses five bones in this region.

METAL DETECTOR. This instrument is put to veterinary use sometimes to confirm a tentative diagnosis of a metal foreign body in the reticulum.

METALDEHYDE POISONING has been encountered in the **dog** and **cat** following the eating of 'Meta' tablets used for killing garden slugs. Symptoms may include: excitement, vomiting, muscular tetany, nystagmus in the cat, partial paralysis, and stupor. The animal should be kept quiet in the dark pending veterinary aid, when anaesthesia may be required. Professor E. G. C. Clarke recommends pentobarbitone sodium, 10–30 mg/kg intravenously or intraperitoneally; or acetyl promazine, 0·5 mg/kg by intramuscular injection.

Metaldehyde poisoning has occurred also in horses, cattle, sheep, and birds.

Cattle. An estimated 2 lb of slug pellets sufficed to kill 6 calves which had broken into a store shed. In another incident, 10 suckler cows were found dead in a field. In a third case, 3 out of 5 milking cows died after consuming, between them, about 20 lb of slug pellets.

Symptoms in these cows included: a staggering gait, profuse salivation, scouring, partial blindness, and hyperaesthesia. Later, muscular spasms were observed.

Horses. A hunter died after showing similar symptoms (but without diarrhoea or partial blindness) after helping itself from a pile of pellets spilled in a field and not cleared up.

METAPHASE. 'The phase of mitosis or meiosis in which the chromosomes are maximally contracted and their longitudinal division into chromatids has been completed' (Hare, W. C. D., *et al J. Small Anim. Pract.* (1966) **7,** 575).

METAPLASIA is described as 'the change of one kind of tissue into another; also the production of tissue by cells which normally produce tissue of another sort.'

METASTASIS and 'metastatic' are terms applied to the process by which a malignant tumour spreads to distant parts of the body, and gives rise to secondary tumours similar to the primary. Thus a sarcoma in some part of the abdomen may spread to the thorax by pieces of tumour or clusters of cells breaking away from the parent growth, and being carried by the blood-stream to the lungs, etc., and setting up new sarcomatous growths there. (*See* CANCER.)

METATARSAL is the name given to the bones and structures lying between the tarsus or hock and the digit of the hind-limb. It corresponds to the metacarpal region in the fore-limb, and has a somewhat similar arrangement of bones.

METHAEMOGLOBIN is a modification of haemoglobin, the red pigment of blood; the iron being in the form of ferric rather than ferrous sulphate.

Some methaemoglobin is normally present in the blood; but various poisons can increase the amount found in blood, and sometimes in urine after administering large doses of certain drugs, such as acetanilid, and also in some diseases. Chemically, methaemoglobin is the same as oxyhaemoglobin, except that it cannot part with its oxygen so readily as the latter.

METHANE (MARSH GAS) has the chemical formula CH_4. Large quantities (up to 250 litres per day) may be formed in the rumen of the healthy cow. The gas is inflammable. (*See* SLURRY.)

METHIOCARB. A snail-killer used in agriculture. Poultry and other animals must be kept away from treated areas for at least a week.

METHONIUM COMPOUNDS block impulses in sympathetic ganglia and are employed in arterial hypertension, *e.g.* Hexamethonium.

METHOPRENE (*see under* FLEAS, Control).

METHYCILLIN. A semi-synthetic penicillin resistant to penicillinase.

METHYL is the name of an organic radicle whose chemical formulae is CH_3, and which forms the centre of a wide group of substances known as the methyl group. For example, methyl alcohol is obtained as a by-product in the manufacture of beet-sugar, or by the distillation of wood; methyl salicylate is the active constituent of oil of wintergreen; methyl hydride is better known as marsh gas.

METHYLATED SPIRIT is a mixture of rectified spirit with 10 per cent by volume of wood naphtha, which renders the spirit dangerous for internal administration. (*See* ALCOHOL.)

METHYLENE BLUE, given intravenously at a dose of 10 mg/kg of a 4 per cent solution, is an antidote to nitrate poisoning, and also to chlorate poisoning. In cats it was formerly used as a urinary antiseptic but gave rise to HEINZ-BODY ANAEMIA.

METOESTRUS is the period in the oestrous cycle following ovulation and during which the corpus luteum develops.

METRIC SYSTEM (*see under* EQUIVALENTS, TABLES OF).

METRITIS (*see* UTERUS, DISEASES OF).

METRONIDAZOLE. Useful against anaerobic bacterial infections, and also GIARDIASIS.

MEUSE-RHINE-IJSSEL (MRI). A dual-purpose breed of cattle from Holland, with good milk yields and high butterfat. Its import was sanctioned for the Shorthorn Society in 1970.

MICE (*see* LYMPHOCYTIC CHORIOMENINGITIS *and* RODENTS). Polyoma viruses of mice and mouse hepatitis virus are other infections important in laboratory mice; also ECTROMELIA (Mouse Pox). (*See also* PETS.)

MICRO- is a prefix meaning small.

MICROCEPHALY is abnormal smallness of the head.

MICRON. 0·001 mm, the unit of measurement in microscopical and bacteriological work. Its symbol is μ.

MICRO-ORGANISMS (*see* BACTERIA, VIRUSES, MYCOPLASMA, RICKETTSIA, CHLAMYDIA, FUNGAL DISEASES, etc).

MICROPHTHALMIA. An abnormal smallness of the eyes, accompanied by blindness. In piglets it is believed to be associated with a Vitamin A deficiency.

MICROSCOPE. The ordinary microscope with oil-immersion lens gives magnification up to 1500 diameters. (*See also* ELECTRON MICROSCOPE.)

MICROSPORUM. A group of fungi responsible for ringworm.

MICTURITION. The act of passing urine.

MIDDLINGS (*see* WEATINGS).

MIDGES, BITING. Species of *Culicoides* are of veterinary importance in connection with Sweet Itch in horses, and also with the transmission of viruses to farm livestock; *e.g.* the virus of Blue-tongue, and that of Epizootic Haemorrhagic Disease (EHD) of deer.

MIGRAM. A disease of sheep on the Romney Marsh. The cause is unknown, but one line of investigation is into a possible association with blue-green algae in the dykes.

Symptoms include trembling and muscular incoordination. In one incident in 1983 MAFF reported that 150 out of 260 lambs collapsed while being driven to new pasture.

MIL is a contraction for millilitre, equal to one cubic centimetre of fluid.

MILIARY is a term, expressive of size, applied to various disease lesions which are about the size of a millet seed, *e.g.* miliary tuberculosis, feline miliary dermatitis.

MILK.

Composition. Cow's milk is a very valuable food substance as it contains all the essential food constituents, *viz.* proteins, carbohydrates, fats, and vitamins, in addition to a considerable percentage of mineral matter. The most important protein in milk is casein; it is present in a state of partial solution. Carbohydrates are represented by the milk-sugar or lactose which is dissolved in the liquid portion of the milk. They, along with the fat which occurs as spherical globules, are heat and energy-producing substances. The mineral matter consists, to a very large extent, of compounds of lime and phosphorus. These substances are the essential constituents of bone.

The percentages of the main constituents of milk vary considerably, particularly as regards the percentage of fat, which alters most; the following are average figures:

	Per cent
Protein	3·40
Milk-sugar	4·75
Fat	3·75
Mineral matter	0·75
Water	87·35
	100·00

In the young growing animal muscle and bone are being formed rapidly. Hence the food of the young must be adequately provided with protein and mineral matter in particular. Milk, since it

APPROXIMATE COMPOSITION OF MILK PRODUCTS

	Water	Proteins	Fats	Sugar	Ash
Separated milk	90·0	3·7	0·2	4·9	0·8
Skimmed milk	90·0	3·6	0·8	4·6	0·8
Butter milk	91·0	3·3	0·5	3·4	0·6
Cream (thin)	64·0	2·8	30·0	3·5	0·5
Cream (thick)	39·0	1·6	56·0	2·3	0·4
Whey	93·0	0·9	0·2	4·8	0·5

APPROXIMATE COMPOSITION OF MILK OF DIFFERENT ANIMALS

	Water	Proteins	Fats	Sugar	Ash
Mare	90·5	2·0	1·2	5·8	0·4
Cow	97·4	3·4	3·8	4·8	0·8
Ewe	81·9	5·8	6·5	4·8	0·9
Goat	84·1	4·0	6·0	5·0	0·8
Sow	84·6	6·3	4·8	3·4	0·9
(Human)	(87·4)	(2·1)	(3·8)	(6·3)	(0·3)

contains considerable quantities of both of these constituents, and vitamins, is an excellent food for growing animals; but not a complete one – it will not provide adequate iron in the piglet (*see* SOW'S MILK) or adequate magnesium in the calf.

Legal standards. In Great Britain, under the 'Sale of Food and Drugs Act', milk containing less than 3 per cent of butterfat, or less than 8·5 per cent of non-fatty solids (*i.e.* proteins, sugar, and ash), is deemed to be not genuine (until or unless the contrary is proved) by reason of either the addition of water or the abstraction of some of the fatty or non-fatty solids. (See SOLIDS-NOT-FAT.)

The specific gravity of cow's milk varies between 1·028 and 1·032. The greater the fat content the lower the specific gravity because fat is lighter than water and solids, bulk for bulk.

The reaction of the milk of the herbivorous animals is generally approximately neutral, while that of the carnivorous animals is acid.

Bacteria. In 1982 the Milk Marketing Board introduced the 'total bacterial count (TBC)' test. This is applied once weekly to samples of milk collected from each supplier. Average results over one month determine the payment band for the milk; as shown in the **table.**

Band	Average number of micro-organisms in each ml	Milk price adjustment
A	20,000 or less	+0·2 ppl
B	above 20,000 and up to 100,000	nil
C	above 100,000 and up to 250,000*	−0·4 ppl
D	above 250,000**	−1·2 ppl

* provided at least two results are greater than 100,000 organisms per ml

**provided at least two results are greater than 250,000 organisms per ml

(*see also* MILK-BORNE DISEASE and PASTEURISATION.)

Sediment in milk. Milk containing sediment has been the subject of prosecutions under the Food and Drugs Act, 1955. Milk and Dairy Regulations 1959 require that before milking is begun, all dirt on or around the flanks, tail, udder and teats of each cow shall be removed, and the udder and teats shall be kept thoroughly clean during milking. Additionally, milking must be carried out in a good light (daylight or electric light); and no dusty material may be moved during or within half an hour before milking.

In order to minimise contamination of milk during milking, the cow's udder should be sprayed or wiped with a disposable towel wrung out of water containing a disinfectant, and the hands of the milker should be thoroughly washed before the milking of each cow (preferably in water containing a disinfectant). (*See* MASTITIS IN THE COW for recommended procedure.)

Lactic acid is produced by the action of bacteria on lactose – the result being sour milk – and is also present in sour cream and yogurt.

White blood-cells in milk. 'A cow with a healthy udder should not be producing milk with a white cell count regularly in excess of 500,000 per ml.' (L. H. Aynsley and J. M. Buol, *Veterinary Record*, April 3, 1965.) An excess of white cells, as indicated by the California Milk Test, for example, makes the milk undesirable for human consumption. The cause is subclinical mastitis due to (*a*) trauma, defective milking machine or technique; or (*b*) infection; (*c*) or both. (*See* MASTITIS IN THE COW.)

Antibiotics in milk. A 1961 survey showed that in Great Britain 11 per cent of the supplies of milk which were tested contained antibiotics. The most common one (90 per cent) was penicillin. Fortunately, results of tests carried out by MMB creameries in 1964 indicated that the incidence of antibiotic residues in milk approximately halved during the intervening period.

For a number of years concern over the presence of antibiotic residues in milk has been expressed by the medical profession, as well as by the manufacturers of cheese and yoghourt. Some people are allergic to antibiotics, and if they drink milk containing them they may suffer severe effects, *e.g.* a troublesome rash and a period off work. It has also been feared that the continual consumption of small quantities of antibiotic may result in people becoming sensitised, later undergoing a severe reaction when given that antibiotic by their doctor. A third danger is the development of organisms resistant to antibiotics, which could possibly give rise to illness not responding to antibiotic treatment.

The sale conditions for the Milk Marketing Board, stipulate that 'a producer shall not deliver any milk produced from a cow that shows any symptom of disease of the udder, or is undergoing treatment of the udder by chemotherapy including the use of antibiotics, or produced from a cow which has undergone any such treatment unless he believes that sufficient time has elapsed since such treatment to avoid the presence of antibiotics in milk'.

Abnormal changes in colour are not infrequent. A red colour in milk may be due to blood, if it is present when the milk is drawn from the udder and does not increase on keeping. Red, blue, and yellow colours may develop in milk on keeping, and are due to certain forms of bacterial activity. Very often abnormal odours or flavours, such as the flavour of turnips, are due to other types of bacterial action. (*See* MASTITIS.)

Chlorophenol taint. Most milk producers are aware that strong-smelling disinfectants can taint milk, and accordingly store them well away from the dairy or parlour. They are usually phenol or cresol based, and it is when they come into contact with chlorine, the active element in hypochlorite solution used for sterilising milking equipment, that they produce chlorophenols.

These do not have to come into direct physical contact with the milk, but can be absorbed from the atmosphere by any exposed milk surface, particularly in the bulk tank.

Chlorophenol only has to be present in milk at a concentration of one part in a thousand million to taint it. At this low concentration it cannot be smelt, and unless taste testing is carried out at the receiving dairy or creamery, the contaminated milk can reach the consumer without being detected. By the time the taint has been discovered by the consumer, many thousands of pints of milk may well have been affected.

Accordingly neither creosote nor products containing phenols should be used where they may come into contact with teats and udders by indirect means; e.g. on woodwork of buildings, or in the disinfection of cubicle beds, cowsheds, loose boxes, and collecting yards. (Source: the Milk Marketing Board's *Milk Producer*.)

Plants affecting the milk. A large number of plants affect milk or milk secretion in animals eating them, and very often the real cause of unusual tastes or odours in the milk is some common wild plant. Some plants give milk a characteristic taint or odour (such as garlics), and others alter its colour; some decrease the total secretion and others lessen the fat content; a few alter the colour and character of butter made from the milk, and one or two, whose poisonous

principles are excreted by the mammary gland, render the milk actually poisonous. (*See* BRACKEN.)

Dioxins in milk. Unacceptably high levels of dioxin were found in milk received by the Milk Marketing Board from two farms in Derbyshire in 1991. (This milk was subsequently collected separately and disposed of in a sewage plant.)

The World Health Organisation has recommended a 'Tolerable Daily Intake' for dioxins of 0·01 nanogrammes per kilogramme of milk.

MILK ALLERGY IN COWS. This may develop especially in the Channel Islands breeds, in cows which have become sensitised to the alpha-casein in their own milk. If milking is delayed, they may develop clinical signs of a type 1 hypersensitivity, e.g. dyspnoea, drooling of saliva, urticaria in an otherwise bright animal. The withdrawal of milk results in an almost immediate remission of these symptoms. (Drs Alasdair Wiseman & Hugh Pirie, *In Practice*.)

MILK, ABSENCE OF, in the mammary glands following parturition, is discussed under AGALACTIA, and SOW'S MILK, ABSENCE OF.

MILK-BORNE DISEASE. Various infections may be transmitted to people through unpasteurised or defectively pasteurised milk. (*See* BRUCELLOSIS, SALMONELLOSIS, Q FEVER, for examples.)

Seventy-seven per cent of 233 reported outbreaks of communicable disease attributed to milk and dairy products in England and Wales between 1951 and 1980 were associated with unpasteurised or defectively pasteurised milk. (N. S. Gailbraith & others. *British Medical Journal* (1982) **284**, 1761).

After August 1983, when compulsory pasteurisation was introduced in Scotland, outbreaks of milk-borne salmonellosis fell to eight affecting 46 people; as compared with 14 outbreaks affecting 1090 people in the previous three years. (Howie, J., *British Medical Journal* (1985) **291**, 422.)

Campylobacter jejuni, present in unpasteurised or incompletely unpasteurised milk, led to 13 outbreaks of human enteritis. In another, 1984, outbreak 18 people were ill with the same disease; infection being traced back to milk from a producer-retailer's herd of 34 cows. No further cases were reported following the imposition of a heat treatment order on the retailer.

Corynebacterium ulcerans was diagnosed as the cause of sore throat in a patient from a community that drank raw milk. The source of this was a herd in which eight cows were infected with this organism; while a ninth cow was found to be an intermittent excretor of it. (Hart, R. J. C., *Journal of Hygiene* (1984) **92**, 161.)

Goat's Milk, if unpasteurised, may be a source of various infections transmissible to people. (*See* BRUCELLOSIS—*Br. melitensis*; Q FEVER; CHLAMYDIA; LOUPING-ILL; TOXOPLASMOSIS; YERSINIOSIS; TUBERCULOSIS.

'MILK FEVER', is a metabolic condition – mainly hypocalcaemia of milk cows, milk goats,

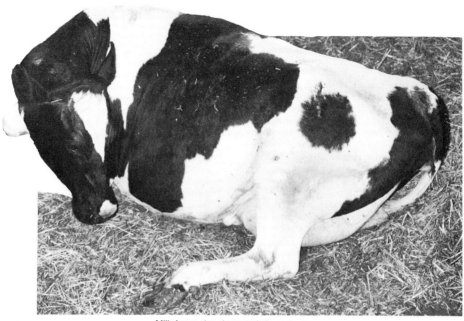

Milk fever: the characteristic posture.

and sometimes of ewes, bitches, and cats in which there is a partial or complete loss of consciousness, paralysis of the hindquarters, and sometimes paralysis of other parts.

In the hill ewe the condition is colloquially known as MOSS-ILL (which see). Hypocalcaemia also occurs in lowland ewes.

'Milk fever' would appear to be one of the diseases that is to some extent traceable to artificial methods of management. It is most frequently, though not exclusively, met with in heavy milking cows, of the essentially dairy breeds. Animals in good condition, liberally fed, and getting only a minimum of exercise, are more often affected than are those under opposite conditions of management. It is commonest between the third and fifth calving, and animals having had an attack are liable to a repetition when they next calve. A few cases occur some hours before calving, but the majority take place within 3 days subsequent to parturition.

Some cases occur up to 4 weeks after calving, but, as a rule, delayed cases are mild, though they take longer to recover. It is more common after easy parturition than after a difficult one, though this rule has many exceptions. However, subclinical milk-fever may be associated with dystokia (see CALVING, DIFFICULT).

Experimental work has shown that a cow in full lactation not infrequently secretes daily in her milk about twelve times the amount of calcium present in her blood. As all the calcium salts in the milk have to come from the bloodstream, it follows that the blood calcium must be replaced about twelves a day. Should anything go wrong with the 'mechanism' controlling the calcium supply for the blood, then symptoms of hypocalcaemia or 'milk fever' begin to appear.

Research has suggested that the calcium-controlling 'mechanism' is a very complex one, involving all the endocrine glands and both the sympathetic and parasympathetic nervous systems.

It must be added that blood samples have shown that as well as a shortage of calcium in the blood, there may be too little phosphorus and either too much or too little magnesium. This accounts for the differing symptoms in what is collectively called 'milk fever'.

Lowering the blood magnesium, experimentally, decreased the ability of cows to mobilise calcium; and P. A. Contreras & others (*Research in Veterinary Science* (1982) **33**, 10) concluded that even a mild hypomagnesaemia at calving might increase the likelihood of milk fever.

The level of CORTISOL (which see) in the plasma of cows during milk fever is significantly higher than in normal cows.

SIGNS. The animal at first shows a certain amount of excitement. She paddles with her hindfeet, stares around in a somewhat fearful manner, may bellow, and if tied attempts to break loose. The pupils are dilated. After a time she staggers on her feet, loses balance, and falls to the ground. When down she may make one or two efforts to rise, but after struggling for a time she gives it up and remains quiet. In very many cases a characteristic position is assumed. The cow lies on her brisket, head turned round over one shoulder (often the left), and the muzzle pointing to the stifle.

The breathing becomes deep and slow, pulse is fast but weak, the extremities of the body grow cold, the temperature falls to 4 or 5 degrees below normal, and death may follow coma.

Whereas formerly the mortality was 90 per cent or so, it has been reduced to less than 5 per cent in cases that are treated.

DIFFERENTIAL DIAGNOSIS. In countries where rabies is present, this disease may be mistaken for milk fever – especially as the position in recumbency, with the head turned to one side, resembles the milk fever posture.

In Britain cases of what were treated as milk fever did not respond to treatment with calcium borogluconate, and were found to be nutritional myopathy associated with low vitamin E and selenium intakes. (Reluctance to move, stiffness, and recumbency were the symptoms, and some deaths occurred. (M. Gitter and R. Pepper, *Vet. Rec.* (1978), **103**, 24.)

TREATMENT. The intravenous or subcutaneous injection of calcium borogluconate solution with or without magnesium (*see also* UDDER INFLATION).

When a deficiency of blood phosphorus complicates 'milk fever', and this does not completely respond to calcium treatment, phosphorus in the form of 3 oz of sodium acid phosphate may be given by mouth twice daily.

PREVENTION. Milk fever which, according to the University of Leeds, affects 30 per cent of cows over 6 years old and must cost UK farmers at least £5m a year, has proved a difficult disease to prevent. Vitamin D supplementation at a high level has been advocated in the past, but the dose has to be given night and morning for between 3 and 7 days before calving; and results have not been all that might be desired. Vitamin D_3 is slow-acting, since it has first to be converted by liver and kidney to another compound, and results with D_3 have been somewhat disappointing. More promising is a compound known as $1a$-OH D_3. This has the advantage over vitamin D_3 that it is converted by the liver directly to the desired $(1a \; -25(OH)_2D_3)$ and therefore acts more quickly. Studies at the ARC's Institute for Research on Animal Diseases continued (1978) to evaluate this method of prevention, which may involve a single injection 24 hours before the expected calving is due.

Dr D. Pickard has, in small-scale trials at Leeds, 'reduced milk fever by a factor of four'. Encouraged by the results, he arranged larger-scale trials with the co-operation of other dairy farmers.

Dr Pickard's method is to feed in-calf cows with a minimum intake of essential mineral calcium throughout the dry period towards the end of pregnancy. Calcium in the feed is then stepped up sharply, 'i.e. when the cow needs it most'.

The lower calcium intake seems to make the cow's metabolism more receptive to a high dose given 2 to 3 days before calving.

'MILK LAMENESS'. This is a translation of the Swedish name for a condition encountered in high-yielding dairy cattle, and characterised by hip lameness. During one stage they assume a characteristic posture.

Some unthriftiness and sluggishness of movement may be observed in the herd. Animals stop frequently to rest.

The cause of 'milk lameness' is a deficiency of phosphorus in the blood-stream, and – since hip lameness may have several causes – blood tests are necessary in order to confirm a diagnosis.

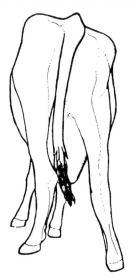

'Milk lameness' – the characteristic posture.

In a Scottish outbreak, recovery soon followed the feeding of sterilised bone-flour in small amounts. It seemed that the cows had been unable to acquire sufficient phosphorus from unsupplemented grazing, although the phosphorus-content of the herbage was probably normal.

Lameness associated with a blood-phosphorus deficiency is, of course, well known in many parts of the world – subjected either to drought or to high rainfall – where the soil or herbage are deficient in phosphorus.

MILK RING TEST, THE, for brucellosis, is a valuable method of detecting infected herds of dairy cattle. It has been recommended that a sample of milk for ring-testing should be from not less than 15 or more than 150 cows. The test is of no value in detecting the disease in individual animals.

Occasionally, as with most biological tests, false positives or false negatives are given. Colostrum, or milk from a cow with mastitis, will sometimes affect the accuracy of the test adversely.

The test is used in many countries to assist in disease-eradication programmes.

'MILK SCALD' around the mouths of pail-fed calves may be a bacterial dermatitis caused by DERMATOPHILUS which produces Lumpy Wool or Wool-Rot in sheep.

MILK SINUS is the chamber situated at the base of each of the teats in the cow (and in other animals), into which the milk tubules discharge their milk, and from which the teat canal leads to the tip of the teat. (*See* MAMMARY GLAND.)

'MILKSPOT LIVER' is a name given to pigs' livers showing whitish spots or streaks of fibrous tissue, the result of chronic inflammation caused by the larvae of the roundworm *Ascaris suum.* A similar condition may occur in lambs which have been grazing fields or fodder crops to which pig

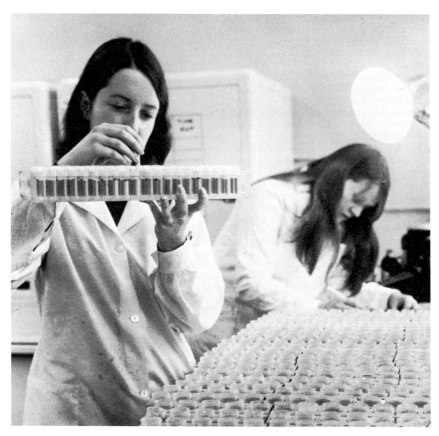

'The milk ring test being carried out on samples of milk at the Milk Marketing Board's Veterinary Research Unit, Worcester, for the diagnosis of herd brucellosis.

slurry has been applied. On one Scottish lowland farm this led to the condemnation of 70 per cent of lambs' livers at the local abattoir in two successive years. (*See* LAMB CARCASE REJECTION.)

Migrating larvae of *Toxocara canis* and *T. cati* may also cause 'milkspot liver' in pigs.

MILK TEETH (*see* DENTITION).

MILK, UNPASTEURISED (*see* MILK-BORNE INFECTIONS).

MILK YIELD. Before the 1939–45 war, the average yield of dairy cows in Britain was about 560 gallons, and total production in England and Wales was about 1000 million gallons. The average yield in 1960 was in the region of 750 gallons per cow, with nearly 1900 million gallons total production in England and Wales. In recorded herds, cows averaged 926 gallons in 1960–1, heifers 792 gallons. National average for 1969 was about 815 gallons, and for 1977 in the region of 1000 gallons for England and Wales. (*See Table on page 381.*)

Daily milk yield: at Olympia during the 1960 Dairy Show, an Ayrshire cow gave over 13½ gallons in the 24 hours. Expressed in pints, the yield of the 1962 supreme champion (British Friesian) was 91 in 24 hours. (For other figures *see under* LACTATION.) (*See also* STRESS.)

Butterfat: In 1969 a Guernsey cow gave 16,371 lb milk at 10·16 per cent butterfat in 305 days.

Milk production: 'A cow producing 5,000 litres of milk and a calf valued at £200 is as good as one giving 6,000 litres and a calf valued at £130 – and requires 1,000 litres less quota to achieve the same gross margin,' stated Dr F. Gordon of the Agricultural Research Institute, Hillsborough. (MMB 1989).

(*See also* PROGENY TESTING, RATIONS.)

MILKER'S NODULE. Human infection with pseudo-cowpox. (*See under* TEATS, COW'S, INFECTIONS OF.)

MILKING (*see also under* MASTITIS *and under* MILKING MACHINES). At milking time the 'milk letdown' mechanism begins to operate; it is actuated by the hormone 'oxytocin' which is secreted in the posterior pituitary gland and which is released into the blood-stream on the receipt of a nervous stimulus. This stimulus may be caused by the rattling of milk pails, the placing of food in the manger, the washing of the udder, etc.

MILKING MACHINES. Their action simulates that of the sucking calf. The teat orifice is opened and milk withdrawn by means of a partial

MILK YIELD FOR RECORDED HERDS
England and Wales by breed

Recording Year	Milk Yield		Butterfat		Protein	
	1987–8	1988–9	1987–8	1988–9	1987–8	1988–9
	kilograms		percent by weight			
Ayrshire	5 184	5 260	3·96	3·92	3·32	3·29
British Friesian	5 751	5 800	3·89	3·86	3·22	3·20
British Holstein	6 443	6 483	3·86	3·82	3·16	3·14
Brown Swiss	5 779	5 799	3·77	3·66	3·40	3·40
Dairy Shorthorn	5 006	5 175	3·71	3·67	3·27	3·26
Dexter	2 347	2 308	4·17	4·08	3·38	3·45
Guernsey	4 224	4 275	4·68	4·66	3·56	3·54
Jersey	3 978	4 047	5·34	5·31	3·82	3·80
Red Poll/British Dane	3 994	4 228	3·65	3·78	3·32	3·29
Simmental	3 999	4 306	4·00	3·87	3·31	3·32
South Devon	3 522	3 575	4·01	4·01	3·61	3·52
Mixed and Others	5 724	5 766	3·88	3·84	3·21	3·19
All Breeds	5 707	5 758	3·91	3·88	3·23	3·21

Recording year is 12 months ending September.
Results for certain breeds may be based on a very small number of herds.

MILK YIELD for RECORDED HERDS
United Kingdom by country

Recording Year	England and Wales *a*	Scotland *b*	Northern Ireland *b*
	kilograms		
1989	5 758	5 775	5 783

Data refer to herds (in Official Schemes only) recorded for the full recording year and animals completing qualifying lactations within the recording year; figures are averages per lactation not averages per year.
a Recording year is 12 months ending September.
b Recording year is calendar year.

vacuum applied to the outside of the teat. As continuous vacuum would restrict circulation of the blood in the teat, cause pain, and inhibit milk ejection, the vacuum is applied intermittently by means of a pulsator.

The basic principles of machine milking are, in fact, vacuum and pulsation, and the way in which these are applied to the teat in the teat-cup assembly.

For maintenance of a healthy udder, what is required first, is a strong stimulus to 'let-down', followed by rapid milking. As soon as the machine ceases to milk, the udder should be stripped and the machine removed. In practice, attention to this involves the cowman not having too many units to cope with, or other tasks to perform.

Milking machines can be made to milk faster by increasing the degree of vacuum, increasing the pulsator rate, or by widening the pulsator ratio. If, however, the cowman already has more to do than he can manage, a faster milking can result only in prolonged attachment. The milking routine must be re-organised to avoid this – or mastitis will follow.

A liner with a hard mouthpiece is likely to cause trouble. One of the best, and also the cheapest, types consists of a straight rubber tube with a metal inserted to form one end into a mouthpiece.

In one herd badly affected with mastitis, a change from slack, wide-bore liners to the narrow-bore stretched type resulted in a spectacular improvement.

C. D. Wilson, of Weybridge, once pointed out: 'A fallacy which has died hard is that leaving milk in a cow predisposes to mastitis. More harm is done to a cow by pulling on four quarters for milk contained in only one, than by leaving a pound of milk in the udder.'

Investigation has shown that the slow milker is almost invariably the cow with a small teat orifice. If it is not practicable to cull such an animal, the milking machine pulsation ratio may, with advantage, be altered. At 60 pulsations per minute, and at 15 inches of mercury, a ratio of 4:1 (*i.e.* the liner being opened for four times as long as it is closed) will reduce milking time – *especially with slow milkers* – without hurting her, or adversely affecting the stripping yield.

Common faults in milking machines are: incorrect vacuum level, or vacuum fluctuations, blocked air bleeds, unsuitable pulsation rate, and faulty liners. Such faults can lead to MASTITIS. Regular, skilled maintenance of milking machines is therefore all important.

During a survey among 71 farms participating in a mastitis control scheme, 95 per cent of the milking machines were found to be faulty. The

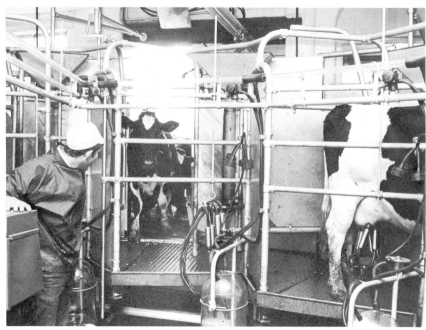

Milking in a rotary herringbone parlour.

importance of this is shown by another survey, of a small number of herds with a serious mastitis problem, in which cell counts were carried out before and after machine testing and adjustment. It was found that cell counts fell by about 25 per cent following the first annual test, and by about 15 per cent following the second annual test. **This shows that the correction of milking machine faults really can achieve something worthwhile, whether measured in cow health or farmers' profits.**

The fitting of shields in teat-cups was hailed as an advance in 1988; but in 1986 ball-valve milking clusters had been found to exclude air from the multi-valve claw, producing flooding of the liners ('hydraulic milking') that was gentler to the teats than conventional milking. (R. J. Grindal, AFRC's Compton Laboratory.)

MILKING PARLOURS (*see under* DAIRY HERD MANAGEMENT).

MILLING MISTAKES (*see* MONENSIN).

MILLIPEDES. In the USA *Narceus annularis* is the intermediate host of a large, white 'thorn-headed' worm *Macracanthohyncus ingens*, which has caused diarrhoea (and sometimes mild dysentery) in dogs. Other definitive hosts are: raccoons, black bears, skunks, foxes, moles.

MINERALOCORTICOIDS (*see* ADRENAL).

MINERALS (*see under* PHOSPHORUS, CALCIUM, FLUOROSIS, TRACE ELEMENTS, METABOLIC PROFILES, SODIUM DEFICIENCY).

MINIMAL DISEASE PIGS. Those reared free from certain infections. (*See also* SPF.)

MINK, DISEASES OF. These include distemper (caused by the virus of canine distemper), botulism, salmonellosis, tuberculosis, paralysis due to a vitamin B deficiency, mastitis, metritis, and paragonimiasis. A vaccine against botulism is available. Transmissible Mink Encephalopathy (TME). (*See* ALEUTIAN DISEASE.)

MITES, PARASITIC. (including **Mange mites**). **Drugs to kill them (Acaricides).**

Name of drug	Effective against
BHC (banned in the UK)	Sheep scab & 'Dairyman's itch'
Ivermectin	Sheep scab & Ear mange
Rotenone	Mange
Benzyl benzoate	Mange & Ear mange
Piperonyl butoxide	Mange
Selenium disulphide	Chicken mites & others

Types of mite. The following genera are important. All are minute, and under favourable circumstances just visible to the naked eye.

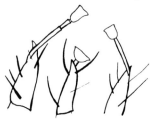

Legs of mange mites. (Psoropt, Choriopt, Sarcopt.)

SARCOPTES, with one species, *S. scabiei*, and numerous varieties. These mites live in the skin of mammals.

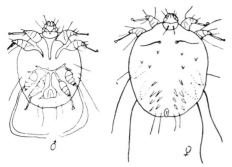

Sarcoptes. × 70.

NOTOEDRES is a closely allied genus found on carnivores.

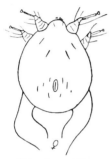

Notoedres. × 70.

OTODECTES is found in the external ear.

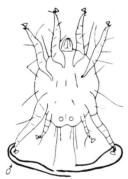

Otodectes. × 70.

CHORIOPTES (Symbiotes). One species is known, *C. equi*, with numerous varieties.

PARASITUS CONSANGUINEUS. A mite which normally feeds on small arthropods, round-worms and their eggs. It is found in dung, compost, spilt grain, etc. An opportunist infestation of a recumbent cow was reported, and the white mites swarmed over a veterinary surgeon's clothing. (Garry, J. W. *Vet. Record* (1989) **125** 18.)

PSOROPTES.

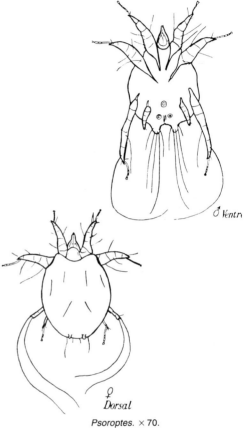

♂ *Ventr*

♀ *Dorsal*

Psoroptes. × 70.

CNEMIDOCOPTES, found in birds. They resemble the first genus.

Mange in the horse. In this host four varieties of mange occur.

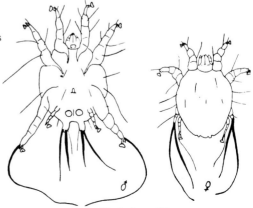

Chorioptes. × 70.

SARCOPTIC MANGE. In this type the parasites burrow into the epidermis and make treatment difficult. The disease commences by the hair dropping out in patches with the formation of papules and an intense continuous itching. The hair becomes thin and broken, and abrasions are present. The skin is hard and folded. Emaciation is progressive, and death may occur from exhaustion. The disease especially attacks the thin-skinned area, and under the harness, where the skin is thickened and the lesions are diffuse, but seldom hairless. It reaches its height in spring, and is at an ebb in late summer and autumn. Diagnosis is by demonstration of the parasite. It is the most serious form, and in Britain is a notifiable disease.

Treatment. Gamma BHC is undoubtedly one of the most efficient mite killers but its use in the UK is banned. The organo-phosphorus compounds, diazinon and fenchlorphos are also effective. For the best results they should be applied by dipping or as saturating sprays, and for the sarcoptic manges particularly, two or more treatments may be necessary at intervals of 10 to 14 days.

PSOROPTIC MANGE. Two varieties of this genus occur on the horse, one in the ear and one on the skin. The lesions on the skin are localised at first, and usually start near the dorsal line where the hair is long. The patches are generally barer than in sarcoptic mange. The parasites bite the epidermis, but do not penetrate the skin. The serum which exudes forms a scab in which the parasites live. The disease is **notifiable** in Britain. Treatment is on similar lines to the last species. It is important to remember the presence of parasites in the ear, and to treat this part of the body also.

CHORIOPTIC OR SYMBIOTIC MANGE is usually confined to the legs or root of the tail. It is not notifiable. It causes great itching, stamping, and rubbing of one leg against the other. Papules, scabs, and even ulcers may be found. Treatment is similar to the last.

DEMODECTIC MANGE (*See* illustration and description *and also* **Mange in fowls** on p. 385.)

Mange in cattle.

SARCOPTIC MANGE is common in Britain and America and is the cause of 'dairyman's itch'. It is usually found on the head and neck, but may occur on any part of the body. Bulls are particularly liable to this form of mange.

CHORIOPTIC MANGE is usually confined to the base of the tail, but may spread.

PSOROPTIC MANGE, causes debility, failure to thrive, and reduced liveweight gain.

Psoroptic mange is an important disease of feedlot cattle in the USA, and was once the most prevalent form of cattle mange in Britain, where it is now seldom seen.

An outbreak in this country, in a beef herd comprising 306 animals, was described in 1984 by Linklater and Gillespie. The infected areas of skin were thickened and scabby, with blood and serum oozing from the lesions. These extended along the back and down the sides. Ivermectin (Ivomec; MSD Agrovet) by injection proved highly successful.

Mange in sheep.

SARCOPTIC MANGE is usually confined to the head, and is seldom found on the woolly parts of the body. It tends to become more generalised in the goat.

CHORIOPTIC MANGE, caused by *Chorioptes bovis*, occurs in horses as well as cattle and sheep, and can be serious, especially in housed sheep overseas, and it is not uncommon in the UK. Of 130 sheep received from South Wales at Weybridge 33 per cent were found infested. Lesions occur on the pasterns and interdigital spaces.

PSOROPTIC MANGE or 'SHEEP SCAB', occurs on all parts of the body covered with wool and in the ears. The life-cycle is typical, and can be completed in 13 to 16 days. The progress of the disease is in consequence very rapid. It is one of the worst of sheep diseases, and is notifiable in Britain.

Itching is usually the first symptom of the disease, and should be investigated *at once*. The skin becomes thickened and even ulcerated, the wool becomes detached and the sheep becomes emaciated. The itching causes the animal to rub itself against fences, and detaches the scab. This further spreads the disease, and permits secondary infections of the wound by bacteria.

Treatment is usually by means of double dipping at an interval of about 8 to 12 days, but which depends on local circumstances. In Britain a dip sanctioned by the Ministry of Agriculture must be used. If a commercial dip is used, it should be purchased *only* from a well-known firm and used exactly as directed.

Prevention (*see* IVERMECTIN).

THE 'ITCH-MITE' OF SHEEP. *Psorergates ovis*, which occurs in Australasia, Africa, and North and South America, has not, so far, been found in Britain. This mite causes thickening of the skin and scurf formation. The growth of the wool fibre is affected and the fleece is further damaged by rubbing.

Mange in pigs (*see above in this entry under* 'Parasitus Consanguineus').

SARCOPTIC MANGE starts on the head and gradually spreads all over the body, especially attacking the thinner skin. There is intense itching, the hair falls out, and the skin becomes covered with scab or with wart-like projections. It is found in the UK and America.

Treatment. Improved liveweight gains have followed treatment of sarcoptic mange. (*See also* IVERMECTIN.)

Mange in dogs and cats.

SARCOPTIC MANGE in the dog generally starts on the muzzle and spreads backwards. The animal should be clipped and bathed with green soap. It may then be treated with phosmet. If the infection is generalised treat one-half of the body one day, and the other half after 2 or 3 days.

NOTOEDRIC MANGE in cats is similar to the last form in dogs. It is intensely irritating. It affects face, ears; occasionally legs and external genitalia. Now very rare in the UK.

Benzyl benzoate may prove toxic to cats and so one of the sulphur preparations or piperonyl butoxide is recommended.

OTODECTIC OR AURICULAR MANGE in dogs and cats. *Otodectes* is the most frequent cause of irritation in the ears. It causes scratching and shaking of the ear.

The eggs and larvae are very resistant, and survive under treatments which kill the adults.

First-aid. Cat-owners may be able to provide a little temporary relief by means of a few drops of cooking oil, which will help to soften waxy deposits and kill some mites. A few drops of warm, soapy water (*not* dish-washing detergent liquid!) may achieve the same result. However, professional advice should be obtained without delay.

Owners should not poke around with cotton-wool wound round an orange stick or tweezers; as the wool will slip off, and the skin of the external ear canal is then likely to be abraded, or even the ear-drum punctured.

Professional treatment consists in the use of ear-drops containing an effective mite-killer, plus an analgesic to reduce the irritation caused by the mites.

In neglected cases, or those complicated by bacterial or fungal infections, where a painful, suppurating condition is present, antibacterial or anti-fungal drugs must be used.

(*See* DEAFNESS, *and* EARS, DISEASES OF; *also* HAEMATOMA.)

DEMODECTIC MANGE. Cigar-shaped mites invade the hair follicles, causing the hair to fall out in patches.

Demodectic mange (also known as Follicular or 'Black Mange') is most common in dogs.

Signs. Two types of demodectic mange in dogs have been described: (1) the *squamous* type, in which the skin becomes scaly, wrinkled, and ringworm-like in appearance (and sometimes mistaken for ringworm); and (2) the *pustular* type in which secondary bacterial infection occurs. This is always very serious, and constitutes an illness as well as a mere skin disease, since the dog suffers from toxaemia. Indeed, sometimes euthanasia becomes the only humane course, especially when extensive areas of skin are involved.

Cause: Demodex canis.

Treatment is made difficult by the fact that the mites are sometimes living at a depth difficult to reach. However, IVERMECTIN is effective.

Diagnosis is made or confirmed by the examination of skin scrapings under a microscope.

Cattle, goats, sheep, pigs, horses and hamsters are all susceptible to infestation by the respective species named according to their hosts.

DEMODECTIC/FOLLICULAR MANGE in the dog.

Demodex folliculorum is considered identical with *D. canis.* It may be present without causing symptoms.

Demodex canis, the cause of 'Follicular' or 'Black Mange' in dogs, is the most important species. The disease is apparently caused by a *Staphylococcus* introduced by the mite. The disease may assume a pustular or a squamous form. In the latter the skin is usually pigmented and the hair falls out in patches. It is generally chronic. In the pustular form the skin becomes reddened,

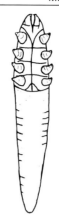

Demodex canis. × 150.

hair falls out in tufts, pustules appear, a toxaemia sets in, and the animal becomes emaciated and may die. There is little puritus, but the dog has a characteristic smell.

The disease often appears in the dog when 8 to 12 months old, usually first on the head, around the eyes and nose, and on or near the feet.

Treatment is not always satisfactory. The parasite lives in a very protected position and is difficult to reach. (*See* also IVERMECTIN.)

Mange in goats is caused by *D. caprae*, and characterised by palpable nodules or pustules without loss of hair. The disease usually starts on face, neck, and shoulders. Rotenone has proved successful in treatment. (*See also* IVERMECTIN.)

Mange in fowls.

'DEPLUMING SCABIES' in fowls is caused by *Cnemidocoptes laevis*, which lives at the base of the feathers, and so irritates the fowl that it pulls them out. The stumps left may be seen to be surrounded with crusts.

The affected spots and surrounding areas may be treated with IVERMECTIN.)

'SCALY LEG' is caused by *Cnemidocoptes mutans.* The feet and legs become enlarged and crusted. The birds may become very lame and even lose a toe. Destruction of infected birds combined with rigorous disinfection is the most common method of eradication. If this procedure is not convenient, the scab should be removed with soap and water, the leg dried, and one of the preparations mentioned above used. This should be repeated in 3 or 4 days.

Cage birds may suffer from this infestation. *Cnemidoeoptes pilae* causes 'scaly face' and 'tassel foot'.

DERMANYSSUS GALLINAE is the chicken mite

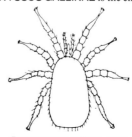

Dermanyssus gallinae. × 35.

of Europe and North America. It is whitish to red in colour. The complete life-cycle takes about 7 to 10 days.

The mite lives exclusively on blood. It is nocturnal in its habits, living in crevices during the day. It can live thus for 4 months or even longer without food. It is only found on birds when feeding. It causes a severe anaemia in poultry.

Eradication of the mite must be thorough. All wooden structures must be disinfected. A painter's blow lamp is very useful for cracks. An insecticide, Sevin, is of use.

Although primarily a parasite of fowls, this mite will attack horses and other mammals, causing much irritation, with the eruption of papules and the formation of scabs. The mite, as it feeds only at night, may be overlooked as the cause of the disease. The proximity of fowls suffering from the mite may give a clue.

ORNITHONYSSUS SYLVIARUM, the northern fowl mite which is also common in Britain, causes scab formation, soiling of the feathers and thickening of the skin around the vent. In contrast to the chicken mite, this parasite remains on its host.

In Israel allergic rhinitis and bronchial asthma have been caused by this mite among poultry farmers.

LIPONYSSUS BURSA, the tropical 'fowl mite', replaces the last species in the warmer parts of the world. Unlike it, however, this species is found on the fowls and in the nest. It may feed during the day. It also lays eggs and moults on its host. The symptoms are similar. Dusting the bird and nest with sulphur is recommended.

Other mites

HARVEST MITES. The so-called 'harvest mite' or 'chigger' is the larva of a species of *Trombidium*. It is microscopic in size, blood-red in colour, and in shape resembles a tick. The mite burrows under the skin of man and various animals, especially the dog and cat, and engorging with blood appears as a red spot in the centre of an inflamed area. In 2 or 3 days the spot becomes a blister and ultimately a scab which falls off. The spot is extremely itchy. (*See* HYPERSENSITIVITY.)

The nymphs and adults are free-living.

FORAGE MITES are occasionally parasites of the horse which live normally in the forage. They may cause considerable damage to the skin, but are usually easily killed.

FLOUR MITES. These can cause loss of nutrients in stored animal feeds (*see under* DIET), and can also be parasitic on animals, causing dermatitis. For such a case in horses, *see* FLOUR MITE INFESTATION.

CHEYLETIELLA. Two members of this genus are of some veterinary importance in Britain, viz., *C. parasitivorax* and *C. yasguri*. These mites infest dogs, cats, foxes, rabbits, hares. In the dog they are most frequently found on the nape of the neck, and down the back. Redness of the skin and intense itching may be caused – the latter symptom occurring in man also. Three dressings, at 5-day intervals with derris or pyrethrum, are recommended; for cats, selenium sulphide.

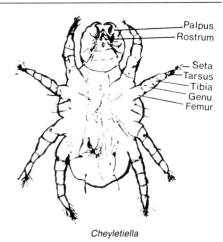

Cheyletiella

NOSE MITES. (*See* CANINE NASAL MITES, *and below.*)

LINGUATULA SERRATA. This parasite has a flat body shaped somewhat like a tongue, but grooved. It is without appendages, apart from two pairs of hooks at its anterior end. The adult lives in the nasal passages of dogs, cats, and foxes, and is up to 2 cm in length.

The eggs are expelled from the nose by sneezing; they may also be swallowed and excreted in the faeces. Sheep, cattle, and rabbits swallow the eggs and become intermediate hosts.

After the eggs hatch in the stomach, larvae migrate to the mesenteric lymph nodes, and encyst either there or in organs such as the liver, lungs, or kidneys.

The life cycle is completed when the final host eats viscera containing the infective nymphs.

CAT FUR MITE (*Lynxacarus radooskyi*). This has a pair of flap-like appendages which enable it to cling to a hair-shaft. It causes scurfiness, especially along the cat's back; and is present in the USA, Australia, Fiji, Hawaii.

HOUSE-DUST MITE. *Dermatophagoides pteronyssinus* can cause allergies in people and pets.

MITOCHONDRIA (*see* CELLS).

MITOSIS. The usual process of cell reproduction. Hence MITOTIC RATE. Mitosis gives each of the new cells the same number of chromosomes as possessed by the dividing cell, *i.e.* the diploid number. (*Compare* MEIOSIS.)

MITRAL VALVE is the left atrioventricular valve of the heart, which is so-called because of its supposed likeness to a bishop's mitre. Disease of the mitral valve is a common condition in the dog. (*See* HEART.)

MOIST GRAIN STORAGE, using propionic acid as a preservative (*see* MUSCLES, DISEASES OF – Nutritional Muscular Dystrophy).

MOKOLA VIRUS. This was first isolated from shrews in Nigeria, and is rabies-related. It has caused the deaths of cats in Zimbabwe, where rabies vaccine has been found ineffective against Mokola virus. The latter infection has also proved fatal in humans.

MOLAR TEETH (*see* DENTITION).

MOLECULAR BIOLOGY. The study of the structure and function of biological molecules; especially nucleic acids and proteins.

MOLLITIES OSSIUM (*see* OSTEOMALACIA).

MOLLUSCICIDE. A snail killer. (*See under* LIVER FLUKES.)

MOLYBDENUM. This trace element is commonly present in soil and pasture grasses, and is beneficial except when it occurs in excessive amounts – such as in the 'teart soils' of central Somerset, and of small areas of Gloucestershire and Warwickshire. Here 'molybdenosis' causes scouring in ruminants, especially cattle. The scouring is worse from May until October when the grass contains most water-soluble molybdenum. Staring coats, marked loss of condition and evil-smelling faeces are observed in affected cattle. A daily dose of copper sulphate (2 grammes for adults and half this for young stock) obviates or remedies the trouble.

Molybdenosis may occur also as the result of aerial contamination of pasture in the vicinity of aluminium-alloy and other factories, and of oil refineries. In an outbreak in 1960 near the Esso Refinery at Fawley, younger cattle showed a marked stiffness of back and legs, with great difficulty in getting to their feet and reluctance to move – in addition to diarrhoea.

If an animal is receiving extra molybdenum in its diet, it is likely to need extra copper. Levels of molybdenum which interfere with copper metabolism also inhibit the synthesis of B_{12}, the cobalt-containing vitamin, by the rumen microflora.

MONENSIN SODIUM. This is produced by fermentation of a strain of *Streptomyces cinnamonensis*, and is licensed in the UK as a growth promoter for cattle (*see* ADDITIVES) and as a coccidiostat for poultry.

Monensin resulted in the death of 9 out of 84 beef cattle which had received twelve times the recommended dose. All the cattle lost their appetite and had diarrhoea. Autopsy findings included multiple haemorrhages and oedema of the right side of the heart.

In another incident 9 out of 40 calves died following accidental overdosage with monensin.

Monensin toxicity has also been recorded in horses, chickens, turkeys.

Poisoning has also been reported in dogs given a proprietary dog food contaminated with monensin still present in a silo previously used. (*See also* IONOPHORES.)

MONGOOSES are vectors of rabies in South Africa, Central America, West Indies, and India.

MONILIA. A group of yeast-like organisms.

MONILIASIS is a disease due to the yeast-like fungus *Candida albicans*. In humans it follows, in some cases, the use of certain antibiotics.

The disease occurs in turkeys and fowls, in other domestic animals, including dogs and cattle, and it must be borne in mind when using antibiotics. A high temperature, loss of weight, and oedema of the lungs may result.

Nystatin has been used – successfully, it is claimed – in the treatment of turkeys with moniliasis.

MONKEYS belong to the order *Primata* which includes about 200 species; ranging in size from the tree shrew, weighing about 100 g, to the gorilla, weighing up to 275 kg.

Two sub-orders are recognised: New World monkeys; and Old World monkeys, apes, and man. (Sainsbury, A. W.; Eaton, B. J.; and Cooper, J. E. *Veterinary Record* (1989) **125** 640.)

MONKEYS, ANAESTHETISING. Ketamine is recommended.

MONKEYS, DISEASES OF. These include:

(1) Infection with Herpes Simian B virus. This is easily transmitted to people bitten by monkeys (or perhaps to people merely handling monkeys with B virus lesions), and is of the greatest importance, as an encephalitis or encephalomyelitis is produced in man, with death as the usual outcome. This infection should be suspected in monkeys showing vesicles on the lips, tongue, inside of the cheeks, or on the body. The vesicles burst and give rise to ulcers and scab formation. Occasionally, affected monkeys have conjunctivitis and a thick discharge from the nose.

(2) Tuberculosis. This is generally the miliary form, due to the human type of tubercle bacillus. Symptoms include: loss of weight, of appetite, dullness; sometimes cough and rapid breathing.

(3) Pneumonia (unconnected with tuberculosis). A monkey that is coughing and sneezing can be assumed to be seriously ill. Death from pneumonia can occur within 24 hours, and affect a high proportion of any group of monkeys.

(4) Dysentery due to *Shigella* organisms. This is a common cause of death among laboratory monkeys.

(5) Phycomycosis.

(6) Marburg disease, which can be fatal both in monkeys and man, has been seen in laboratory workers in contact with blood and tissues of Vervet monkeys. *Symptoms*: headache, fever, muscular pain, prostration, diarrhoea and vomiting, with epistaxis and vomiting of blood.

(7) Rabies.

(8) Monkey Pox. This is an apparently rare disease of monkeys. The virus was first isolated in 1958 in a monkey colony in the Statens Seruminstitut, Copenhagen. Cases of presumed monkey pox (resembling human smallpox) in man occurred in Africa in 1970.

Since the world-wide eradication of smallpox, monkeypox has become the most important orthopox virus infection of man. Yet, despite a recent increase in the number of cases reported, human monkeypox remains 'a rare sporadic disease.'

(9) Yellow fever. (*See under separate entry under* YELLOW.)

(10) Measles. This was reported in (1975) in 11 colobus monkeys imported into the U K. No rash was seen; symptoms comprised a nasal discharge, conjunctivitis, cough, facial oedema, and pneumonia. All died. Diagnosis was by laboratory means. (*Vet. Rec.* (1975) **97**, 392).

(11) Malaria. Fulciparum malaria has occurred in owl monkeys.

(12) *Yersinia enterocolitica* infection. (*See also* KYASANUR FOREST FEVER.)

(13) Leptospirosis.

(14) Simian sarcoma virus.

(15) Toxoplasmosis.

(16) Infectious hepatitis.

(17) Jaundice and blindness (temporary) have been caused by lead poisoning as a result of cage bars being painted with lead-containing paint. A chelating agent was used with success.

(18) An outbreak of disease caused by an Ebola-related filovirus and by simian haemorrhagic fever occurred at an American quarantine station in monkeys imported from the Philippines. 'This was the first case in which a filovirus had been isolated from non-human primates.' (Jahrling, P. B. *Lancet* (1990) **335** 502.)

(*See also* PETS.)

MONKSHOOD POISONING (*see* ACONITE).

MONOCHLOROACETATE POISONING has occurred in cattle, sheep, and other animals. Sodium monochloroacetate is a contact herbicide.

MONOCLONAL ANTIBODIES (*see* GENETIC ENGINEERING).

MONOCYTE. A type of white blood-cell. (*See under* BLOOD.)

MONOCYTOSIS (*see* PULLET DISEASE).

MONOPLEGIA means paralysis of a single limb, or part. (*See* PARALYSIS.)

MONORCHID. This term is commonly used by dog-breeders to mean an animal in which only one testicle has descended into the scrotum. Such an animal is correctly called a unilateral cryptorchid; the term Monorchid being reserved for the animal with a single testicle (a far rarer condition).

Under Kennel Club rules, a dog which has not both testicles in the scrotum cannot be entered for show; but there is as yet no ban on the registration of dogs sired by a cryptorchid.

Cryptorchidism is an inherited condition (though it has been claimed that feeding rats on a biotin-deficient diet caused their testicles to return to the abdomen after 2 or 3 weeks), but the precise mechanisms of inheritance has not yet been determined.

MONOSACCHARID is the term applied to a sugar having six carbon atoms in the molecule. Among monosaccharides are glucose, galactose, levulose, etc.

MONOTOCOUS. Normally producing only one offspring at birth, as compared with a litter of, for example, puppies.

MONSTERS or grossly deformed young are occasionally born to all species. Haemolytic disease, for example, is responsible for abnormal piglets. (*See also under* TERATOMA, BULL-DOG CALVES, GENETICS.)

'MOON BLINDNESS' (*see* PERIODIC OPHTHALMIA.)

MORAXELLA. Outbreaks of conjunctivitis and keratitis are often associated with *M. bovis* infection, a gram-negative bacterium found in pairs or short chains. For a time *Moraxella bovis* was known as *Haemophilus bovis.* (*See under* EYE, DISEASES OF.)

MORBIDITY, PROPORTIONAL. e.g. 'morbidity is 60 per cent' in a given group of animals with reference to a particular disease.

MORBILLIVIRUSES. These include the viruses of canine distemper, rinderpest, *peste de petits ruminants*, and human measles. (*See also* SEALS.)

MOREL'S DISEASE. This affects sheep and is caused by a Gram-positive micrococcus. The disease bears some resemblance to caseous lymphadenitis, with abscesses in subcutaneous tissue and intra-muscular fascia, and has been reported in France and Kenya.

MORLAM. A strain of sheep bred at Beltsville, USA. The best ewes have given 6 lambs in 2 years; lambs being born in September, January, and May – an 8-month breeding cycle.

MORNING GLORY. The pink or reddish flowered *Ipomoea muelleri* is said to have caused losses of up to 7000 sheep on some sheep stations in Western Australia. There is a loss of condition, and after a time forced exercise gives rise to a swaying, incoordinated gait, and knuckling of the hind feet, with panting when the animal is driven a few yards.

MORPHINE is the chief alkaloid of opium. Given to the dog by hypodermic injection it causes vomiting and a period of excitability which makes it unsuitable for use in euthanasia. It may, however, be indicated for pain relief following accident or surgery. In the horse morphine may produce great excitement and is contra-indicated.

MORTAR EATING by cattle may be regarded as an indication of a mineral-deficient diet – probably it is calcium and magnesium which the animals are seeking.

MORTIERELLA. A genus of fungi. *M. wolfii* is the most frequent cause of mycotic abortion in cattle in New Zealand, and has been isolated in the U K from cases of abortion, from one of mastitis, and from the diseased liver of a calf.

MORULA. In the cow, some 5 days after fertilisation of the egg, the embryo comprises a minute spherical group of 30–60 cells, inside a transparent shell, known as the morula from its mulberry-like appearance.

MOSAIC. An animal having one or more cell populations with different KARYOTYPES (which see) which have originated from a single zygote as a result of mutation or mitotic loss, etc. (*See* CYTOGENETICS.)

MOSAICISM (*see under* ERYTHROCYTE MOSAICISM).

MOSQUITOES (*see under* FLIES).

'MOSS-ILL'. A colloquial name for hypocalcaemia (*see under* MILK FEVER) in hill ewes. It is seen mainly in the mature ewe, and during the weeks preceding and following lambing. It often follows within 12 to 48 hours of a move to fresh pasture.
SIGNS. Stilted gait, abnormally high carriage of the head, muscular tremors – particularly of the lips in the early stages – recumbency, coma.
TREATMENT. Calcium borogluconate by subcutaneous injection.

MOTH BALLS (*see* NAPHTHALENE POISONING).

MOTHS, PARASITIC. In tropical Africa, Asia, and America, a small moth *Arcyophora longivalvis* feeds on the secretions of the eyes of cattle; its long proboscis being able to reach under the cow's third eyelid (nictitating membrane). After sunset these moths fly out from their daytime woodland cover and alight on cows' faces. Several moths may be seen feeding from the same eye at the same time, and they are apparently attracted to eyes which are already inflamed. During the daytime the cattle's eyes are visited also by numerous flies, which transmit bacteria, worms, and other infective agents causing eye disease. As a result of their feeding habits, the proboscis of the moth becomes contaminated and transmits infection to other cattle.

Arcyophora patricula also frequents eyes, and so do some African hawkmoths. Their hosts include elephants, horses, pigs, cattle, as well as man.

In Malaya Hans Banziger found blood-feeding moths. Some of these take blood from wounds already inflicted, or they take surplus blood left on the skin surface by mosquitoes. Banziger also found what one might call a vampire moth – *Calpe eustrigata* – which can, with its proboscis, penetrate human or animal skin in order to obtain blood.

MOTOR is a term applied to those nerves and tracts in the brain and spinal cord that have to do with the impulses which pass from the higher nerve centres to the muscles causing movement. (*See* NERVES.)

MOULDY FOOD (*see* DIET *under* PALATABILITY, *and* FOXY OATS, *also* MYCOTOXICOSIS). Mouldy hay

or straw can lead to farmers' lung, and to abortion in cattle. (*See* ASPERGILLOSIS, *and also* SWEET VERNAL.)

'MOUNTAIN SICKNESS'. A disease of cattle kept at high altitudes in N. and S. America. Local cattle are affected to an extent of only 1 per cent or so; recovery is unusual. Death occurs from congestive heart failure, after symptoms of depression, oedema of the brisket, and distressed breathing on light exertion. There may also be pulsation of the jugular vein.

MOUSE (*see* MICE, RODENTS).

MOUTH, DISEASES OF. The mouth being one of the few internal cavities which can be examined by direct vision, its examination affords valuable evidence in some cases of disease, *e.g.* in anaemia, jaundice, cyanosis (and *see* TONGUE).

Inflammation of the mouth is known as *Stomatitis*, and that of the gums as *Gingivitis*.

Conditions of the mouth. As a rule the symptoms that lead one to suspect that the mouth is diseased are as follows: salivation and difficulty in feeding in all animals; 'quidding' in the horse; smacking of the lips, in cattle particularly; rubbing the mouth along the edge of the trough, floor, etc., or pawing at it with the front feet, and much working of the jaws. Dogs may occasionally hold their mouths open, especially when a piece of bone or other substance becomes fixed between the teeth, and this symptom is also present in rabies. (*See also* FELINE CALICIVIRUS, FELINE STOMATITIS, RANULA.)

Deformities of the mouth occasionally occur in all animals. (*See* CLEFT PALATE. Jaw deformities are referred to under TEETH and, in the case of cattle, under ACTINOMYCOSIS.)

Ulceration. The presence of ulcers in the mouth may be associated with foot-and-mouth disease, swine vesicular disease, mucosal disease of cattle, cattle plague (rinderpest), blue-tongue; and sometimes with Orf in sheep, feline enteritis, and kidney failure/leptospirosis in dogs.

In 'calf diphtheria' a whitish false membrane may cover part of the inside of the mouth. 'BROWN MOUTH' (which see) may be accompanied by necrosis. A bluish discoloration may be seen after asphyxia or in blue-tongue.

Gingivitis. The gums may become inflamed (and often ulcerated) as a result of the diseases mentioned above, of cutting teeth, diseased teeth, and the deposition of tartar in the dog and cat. Actinobacillosis gives rise to abscesses on the gums and tongue, lining of the cheeks, etc. (*See also* FELINE GINGIVITIS.)

Tumours in the mouth are sometimes seen. Warty growths, scattered over the mucous membrane of the whole of the cavity of the mouth are not uncommon in young dogs. In addition to papillomas, fibromas, squamous cell carcinomas and malignant melanomas may occur. (*See also* EPULIS, a non-malignant gum tumour often difficult to remove.)

Oral tumours were removed from 100 dogs by

mandibulectomy or maxillectomy. For basal cell carcinomas and squamous cell carcinomas these techniques gave one year survival rates of 100 and 84 per cent, respectively. However, the prognosis for sarcomas was not so good; the tumours recurred in 32 per cent of cases and metastases developed in 27 per cent of cases; the one year survival rates for fibrosarcomas, osteosarcomas and malignant melanomas were 50, 42 and 0 per cent, respectively. (White, R. A. S. *Journal of Small Animal Practice* (1991) **32,** 69.)

High-energy ionizing radiation gives good penetration of bone, and 'is indicated for tumours of the mouth which it is not practicable to treat by surgical excision.' (Dobson, Jane M. & White, Richard. *In Practice* (1990, July, p. 135).)

Wounds and injuries. In the majority of cases mouth wounds do not prove serious after any foreign bodies have been removed, for the whole cavity is so well supplied with blood-vessels that healing is always rapid. Haemorrhage may be alarming at first, but, unless a larger artery has been severed, it soon ceases. Large tears in the mucous membrane or in the skin of the lips or cheeks, should be sutured. Antiseptic mouth washes should be applied afterwards. When the wounding has been severe an animal will often refuse to eat solid food, and may require to be fed on liquids for a few days. Plenty of water should always be provided for drinking purposes. (*See also under* TONGUE, SALIVATION, TEETH.)

MOVEMENT OF PIGS ORDER 1973 was drafted to control the movement of swill-fed pigs in order to reduce the incidence of Swine Vesicular Disease.

MUCILAGE is prepared from acacia or tragacanth gum, and is used as an ingredient of mixtures containing solid particles in order to keep the latter from settling as a deposit. It is also a demulcent.

MUCIN (*see* MUCUS).

MUCOPURULENT. Containing a mixture of mucus and pus.

MUCOMETRA (Hydrometra). An uncommon condition in cats in which the uterus becomes filled with fluid. It is usually discovered at hysterectomy; but can be diagnosed in advanced cases by an ultrasound scan. (van Haaften, D. & Taverne, M. A. M. *Veterinary Record* (1989) **124,** 346.)

MUCOPOLYSACCHARIDOSIS VI. A rare genetic defect which deforms both children and cats, lacking an enzyme which breaks down mucopolysaccharides.

A feline case was treated at Colorado State University, using bone marrow from a healthy female Siamese cat, transplanted into a crippled 2-year-old male cat with the same parents but from a different litter.

The transplant was successful, and the recipient's face 'is less deformed, appetite better; eyes clearer,' commented Dr Peter Gesper and Dr Mary Thrall. (*JAVMA* (1984) January 1st issue.)

MUCORMYCOSIS. Infection with *Rhizopus microsporus* is a cause of death of piglets under a fortnight old. The organism has been isolated from stomach ulcers in piglets which, before death, showed symptoms of vomiting and scouring. In many cases Moniliasis was also present. Abortion in cattle has been attributed to mucormycosis.

MUCOSAL DISEASE (*see* BOVINE VIRUS DIARRHOEA).

MUCOUS MEMBRANE lines many hollow organs, the air passages, the whole of the alimentary canal and the ducts of the glands which open into it, the urinary passages, and the genital passages. (*See* MUCUS, BRUSH BORDERS, IMMUNE RESPONSE.)

MUCUS is the slimy secretion derived from mucous membranes, such as those lining the nose, air passages, stomach, intestines, etc. Mucus is composed of a substance called *mucin*, water, and cells cast off from the surface of the membrane, white blood-cells, particles of dust, etc.

Under normal circumstances the surface of a mucous membrane is lubricated by only a small quantity of mucus. Excessive mucus secretion is the familiar accompaniment of nasal catarrh. (*See also* PREGNANCY DIAGNOSIS.)

MUCUS AGGLUTINATION TEST. This is used in the diagnosis of VIBRIO FETUS INFECTION in cattle (which see).

MUD, MUDDY GATEWAYS (*see* 'POACHING').

'MUD FEVER'. An old name for *Dermatophilus* infection in horses forced to stand for long periods in mud, or wet deep litter. It was common in the 1914–18 war. Lesions occur on limbs and abdomen. (*See also under* 'GREASY HEEL'.)

'MULBERRY HEART' causes death in pigs. It is a faulty diet for the pregnant sow which can lead to mulberry heart being caused in the newborn piglet; whereas after weaning the cause is usually lack of vitamin E and selenium supplements in the weaner/grower ration. The disease is mainly one of pigs between three and four months old.

The main thing to note about the disease is that it is preventable.

Symptoms include lack of appetite, shivering – especially of shoulders and hindquarters. The fore-legs may be splayed in an effort to maintain balance, and the snout may be rested on the ground. A sitting-dog posture may be assumed. Black spots on buttocks, ears, etc., may be seen on many pigs in the herd. Temperature is subnormal. Distressed breathing may be observed. Death usually follows within 12 hours of the onset of symptoms. Occasional survivors are usually blind and unsteady on their legs. (*See also under* HEART, DISEASES OF.)

Post-mortem findings: oedema of the pericardium and epicardial haemorrhages.

MULE. The common definition of a mule is the sterile offspring of a jack donkey and a mare.

However, recent scientifically authenticated reports from both China and the USA have supported ancient folklore—to the effect that a female mule is sometimes fertile.

'Red Dragon', now (1986) a 4-year-old fertile female mule appears to have inherited a mixture of both horse and donkey chromosomes; and is technically a chimera rather than a hybrid.

The American report concerns a female mule mated to a jack donkey, and which produced a colt foal. This, on karyotyping, has proved chromosomally to be a mule. (Totaliser *Veterinary Record* (1985) **117,** 676.)

In the context of **sheep**, 'mule' is a most imprecise term; indeed, a colloquial expression varying according to period, locality, and changes in breeding policy.

The following crosses have all been referred to as a 'mule':

Border Leicester ram × Blackface ewe, Border Leicester or Hexham/Leicester ram × Swaledale or Swaledale/Blackface ewe, Blueface Leicester ram × Swaledale or Blackface ewe (though this cross is now known as the North Country mule).

MULE'S OPERATION. This involves the removal of a fold of skin from the crutch of Merino sheep and is carried out by Australian sheepmen for the control of blowfly strike. Mulesing is a synonym.

MULTIPLE SUCKLING (*see under* NURSE COWS).

MULTIPLE VACCINES (*see under* VACCINATION).

MUMMIFICATION OF FETUS sometimes occurs after resorption of fluid from the placenta and fetus following the death of the latter. It is not uncommon in dairy cattle. In sows, it has been reported following Aujeszky's disease and swine erysipelas. In ewes, it may be associated with toxoplasmosis and enzootic abortion. A mummified fetus, remaining in the uterus longer than the normal gestation period, will lower a cow's productivity. (Cloprostenol can be used to abort the mummified fetus in many instances.) Mummification may also occur in the bitch and cat.

MUMPS is another name for parotiditis or inflammation of the parotid glands at the base of the ears and at the back of the angle of the lower jaw. (*See* PAROTIDITIS.)

Antibodies against the human mumps virus have been detected in the blood-serum of dogs.

A 1956 survey revealed that 38 out of 209 apparently healthy country dogs in Pennsylvania had at some time been exposed to human mumps infection. Mumps was confirmed in a Labrador bitch in Middlesex, UK, in 1975. Symptoms included loss of appetite, depression, and greatly enlarged and painful submaxillary lymph nodes.

'MUNGA'. The African name for the grain of the bulrush millet, *Pennisetum typhoides.* The grain, when parasiticised with ergot, has in Rhodesia caused agalactia in sows without other symptoms. A heavy piglet mortality resulted.

MURINE TYPHUS. A disease of rodents caused by a rickettsia, which is transmissible to people, in whom it has been known to cause death in some cases.

MURMUR (*see* HEART).

MURRAY GREY. An Australian beef breed, originating from a roan Shorthorn cow and an Angus bull. A first consignment of 50 reached the UK in 1973. The breed is noted for its size, docility, and easy calving.

MURRAY VALLEY ENCEPHALITIS. Caused by a mosquito-borne flavivirus, this disease occurs in Australia and New Guinea. It affects wild birds. In children it may cause fever, vomiting and encephalitis, sometimes with a high mortality.

MUSCLE. Muscular tissue is divided into three great classes, *Voluntary muscle, Involuntary muscle* and *Cardiac muscle*, and of these the first only is under the control of the will, the two latter working automatically. Voluntary muscle is often called 'Striped' or 'Striated', because under the microscope each muscle fibre shows very distinct cross striping, while involuntary muscle does not, and is consequently often called 'Unstriped', 'Non-striated', or 'Plain'. Cardiac muscle is striated in an imperfect manner, is not under the control of the will, and has a specialised arrangement of its fibres.

Structure of muscle. *Voluntary muscle* forms the chief clothing of the skeleton, and is the red flesh forming beef, mutton, pork, etc., of the food animals. The voluntary muscles are arranged over the body, the majority of them being attached to some part of the bony or cartilaginous skeleton, and are called 'skeletal muscles'. Each has an *origin*, from the stable part of the skeleton to which it is attached, which is succeeded by a *fleshy belly*, the motive part, and an *insertion* into the part of the skeleton which it moves. When contraction occurs, the insertion is brought closer to the origin, and this is known as the *action* of the muscle. In some muscles, such as the brachyaphalic running from the shoulder to the base of the skull, either attachment may be alternately origin or insertion, depending upon which part of the skeleton is fixed at the time.

Each muscle is enclosed in a sheath of fibrous tissue, known as the 'fascia' or 'epimysium', and from this partitions of fibrous tissue, known as 'perimysium', run into the substance of the muscle, dividing it into small bundles of 'fibres'. A muscle fibre is about 1/500th of an inch thick, and of varying length. If the fibre be cut across and examined by the microscope, it is seen to be further divided into 'fibrils'. Within the sarcolemma lie numerous nuclei belonging to the muscle fibre, which was originally developed from a single cell. To the sarcolemma, at either end, is attached a minute bundle of fibrous tissue fibres, which unites the muscle fibre to its neighbour or to one of the connective tissue partitions in the muscle, and by means of these connections the fibre produces its effect upon contracting. The sarcolemma is pierced by a nerve fibre, which breaks up upon the surface of the muscle fibre into a complicated 'end-plate', and by this means each muscle fibre is brought under the guidance of the central nervous system, and the discharge of energy which produces muscular contraction is controlled.

Between the pillar-like muscle fibres run many capillary blood vessels. They are so placed that the contractions of the muscle fibres empty them of blood, and thus the active muscle is ensured of a continually changing blood-supply. None of these capillaries, however, pierce the sarcolemma surrounding the fibres, so that the blood does not come into direct contact with the fibrils themselves. They are nourished by the lymph which exudes from the capillaries and bathes the outside of the sarcolemma, passing into the fibrils by a process of osmosis. The lymph circulation is also automatically varied, as required, by the muscular contractions. Between the muscle fibres, and enveloped in a sheath of connective tissue, lie here and there special structures known as 'muscle spindles'. *Involuntary muscle* forms the greater part of the walls of the hollow organs of the body, such as stomach, intestines, bladder, etc., and the walls of the blood-vessels, ducts from glands, the uterus and Fallopian tubes, the urethra, ureters, the iris and ciliary muscle of the eye, the 'dartos' tunic of the scrotum, and is associated with the skin and hair follicles. The fibres are smaller than those of voluntary muscle. Each is pointed at the ends, has usually one oval nucleus in the centre, and a delicate sheath of sarcolemma enveloping it. The fibres are grouped in bundles, much as are the striped fibres, but they adhere to one another by a cementing material, not by tendon bundles found in voluntary muscle.

Cardiac muscle is a specialised form of involuntary muscle in which the fibres are provided with numbers of projections, each of which is united to a similar projection from an adjacent cell, so that the whole forms an intricate network or meshwork of fibres instead of an arrangement of bundles. Each fibre possesses a large nucleus which is more or less central in position.

DEVELOPMENT OF MUSCLE. All the muscles of the developing animal arise from the central layer (mesoblast) of the embryo, each fibre taking origin from a single cell. Later on in life muscles have the power both of increasing in size, as the result of use, for example in race-horses and greyhounds and other animals that are trained to be fit, and also of healing themselves after parts of them have been destroyed by injury or removed surgically. This occurs by development of certain cells called 'myoblasts' in the same way as muscle is formed in the growing embryo. Unstriped muscle as well as striped muscle can take part in this increase in size, as witness the development of the muscular wall of the uterus during pregnancy. In this case not only do the numbers of muscle fibres increase, but each becomes three or four times its previous size. The fully pregnant uterus increases its weight about 20 times what it is when empty, and in the course

of a month to 6 weeks after parturition decreases again in weight and size.

Action of muscles. A nerve impulse originates in some part of the brain or spinal cord, either as the result of volition or as a reflex, passes down the fibres of the motor nerve to the muscle, where a series of complex chemical reactions occur. The source of energy for muscular contraction is adenosine triphosphate (ATP). When this is split into adenosine diphosphate (ADP) and phosphoric acid, energy becomes available. For subsequent resynthesis of ATP from ADP, creatine phosphate (CP) is converted to creatine plus phosphoric acid; oxygen from the bloodstream being required.

(These are but two of many complex reactions, involving several enzymes.) (*See also* LACTIC ACID.)

During strenuous exercise, more oxygen may be needed than is readily available, leading to the so-called 'oxygen debt', which results in panting. This **'oxygen debt'** can be partly offset as the muscle makes use of another chemical reaction, involving the conversion of glycogen to lactic acid.

Fatigue. The accumulation of this acid in the muscles causes the stiffness of fatigue, which has been defined as 'a decrease in capacity for work caused by work itself'. In large quantities lactic acid in the muscles can lead to cramp.

After exercise, lactic acid is either eliminated as carbon dioxide and water, or converted in the liver back to glycogen.

The importance of a sufficient period of rest for animals which have been called upon for great exertion, such as in hunting or racing, is obvious.

Muscle tonus is the state of partial contraction of a muscle by virtue of which it is ready for work at all times. Tonus is specially evident in the plain muscle fibres present in the walls of the arteries, and it is owing to it that such striking and rapid changes in the amount of the blood in a part can occur. If the inhibitory fibres (called 'vasodilators') in the arteries are activated an immediate increase of blood takes place, while if the stimulating fibres (called 'vasoconstrictors') are acted upon, the muscle fibres in the walls contract, the calibre of the vessels is decreased, and the blood-supply is lessened.

CONDITION is that remarkable state into which horses and other animals can be brought by care in feeding, general management, and carefully regulated work, which is the highest pitch of perfection to which muscles can attain. It is a potential quality not possessed by all animals, and, even when attained, does not last for long periods. In the process of training it is possible by overmuch enthusiasm to produce a condition of 'staleness', in which speed or staying power diminishes, but recovery from which follows a period of rest. Condition consists in a gradual education of the muscles of the skeleton, of the heart and respiratory organs particularly, as well as of the body generally, so that they will sustain fatigue with greater and greater facility.

All superfluous fat is removed from the body, the volume of the muscles is increased, their elasticity, tone, responsiveness to stimuli, power of contraction, and blood-supply are heightened; the respiratory system is made to accommodate itself to the oxygenation of vastly greater amounts of blood in a shorter space of time than normally; the heart muscle, the main pump of the circulation, hypertrophies, and the walls of the smaller arteries, the secondary pumps of the circulatory system, are keyed up to the highest state of responsiveness to local requirements. In the production of all this lies the art of the trainer.

EQUINE AND CANINE ATHLETES. The speed and stamina of the thoroughbred and the grey-hound are due to the fact that both animal species can increase, during exercise, their packed cell volumes to between 60 and 70 per cent. Together with large increases in the heart's output, the result is much larger increases in effective blood flow to the muscles than occurs in humans. In the fit thoroughbred, resting heart rates of 25 to 30 beats per minute can be increased to between 240 and 250; and in the greyhound, heart rates below 100 can be increased to 300 beats per minute. Both species also have large hearts for their bodyweight. Approximately 57 per cent of the greyhound's liveweight is due to muscle, as compared with 40 per cent for most other mammals. (Snow, D. H. *Proceedings of the Nutritional Society* (1985) **44**, 267.)

MUSCLES, which are collectively and popularly known as the 'flesh' of an animal, comprise the voluntary muscles, and amount to over one-third the weight of the whole body in an average animal of ordinary condition. The total number of voluntary muscles is over 700 in the horse, and more than this in some of the other domesticated animals, so that they cannot all be described here. Each voluntary muscle is named, its blood- and nerve-supplies are mentioned, and its shape, relations, and actions are considered in works on Comparative Anatomy, to which reference must be made for further details.

Generally speaking, muscles which cause a joint to bend are called 'flexors', those which straighten a bent joint are 'extensors', one which carries a limb farther away from the middle line of the body than previously is an 'abductor', one which has the opposite action is an 'adductor', and one which causes a segment of a limb to revolve is a 'rotator', or 'supinator', or a 'pronator', according to its position. A sphincter is usually involuntary, but a few are voluntary; they cause a contraction of the ring-like opening which they circumscribe. Many muscles have an insertion distant from their fleshy part (called the 'fleshy belly') by means of a tendon which is composed of fibrous tissue strands.

MUSCLES, DISEASES OF. Atrophy of muscles may occur as the result of inaction, diminished blood-supply, or nerve injuries, as well as from malnutrition.

INFLAMMATION of muscle, or MYOSITIS, may arise as the result of injury through kicks, blows, falls, etc. It also frequently arises as the result of a sprain or strain in the limbs. Occasionally it may be associated with partial or complete rupture.

Signs. The part affected usually becomes swollen and is painful on manipulation. The muscles affected are held relaxed, and if in a limb the foot is rested. When handled, they contract and become hard to the touch, and upon occasion they may crackle or be oedematous. When resulting from external injury there is usually some sign of this on the covering skin, but when due to strain no external lesions may be seen. Occasionally, after injury, an abscess may develop in the affected muscle, but much more frequently there is *Haematoma*.

ATROPHIC MYOSITIS. This has been described in the dog. The cause is unknown, but possibly damage to the fifth nerve due to over-extension of the temporo-mandibular joint.

Signs. Inability to eat solid food or to lap, atrophy of the jaw muscles, very little voluntary movement of the jaws, and any attempt to force the jaws apart is resisted.

With careful nursing, recovery takes place naturally in a high proportion of cases after 3 to 6 months. (*See also* 'STIFF-LIMBED LAMBS'.)

EOSINOPHILIC MYOSITIS. A disease of dogs, especially Alsatians, in which there is hardening of the muscles of mastication and of the temporal muscles. The dog assumes a foxy appearance. The nictitating membrane is in evidence. There may be tonsilitis. The cause is unknown; the outlook grave. Diagnosis may be confirmed by blood smear.

ISCHAEMIC CONTRACTURE. A disease of muscles due to failure of their arterial supply. There is necrosis and the muscle is replaced by fibrous tissue which contracts or shortens. The condition has been reported in the dog.

NUTRITIONAL MUSCULAR DYSTROPHY. This is most common in beef cattle, but is occasionally seen in dairy cattle also. In calves and lambs it is often called 'White Muscle disease'. Muscular dystrophy also occurs in foals and pigs. It may prove fatal.

Cause. Animal feeds deficient in selenium (a trace element) or vitamin E, between which there is a complex relationship. Crops grown on selenium-deficient land may give rise to nutritional muscular dystrophy unless concentrates are fed as well or unless the diet is supplemented with vitamin E. This vitamin is sometimes adversely affected by the use of proprionic acid as a preservative in the storage of moist barley.

A vitamin E deficiency may also be brought about by giving cod-liver oil in conjunction with rations low in vitamin E, such as dried skim milk powder, for research has shown that the inclusion of cod-liver oil in the diet leads to a striking increase in their requirements of vitamin E. The disease may also be associated with poor quality food, such as the mainly turnip and oat straw diet fed to pregnant cows during the winter in Scotland. Deterioration of food in storage, and especially of those containing unsaturated fatty acids may be associated with the condition.

High rates of application of fertilisers containing sulphates may inhibit absorption of selenium from the soil by plants, which in turn can lead to a deficiency in grazing animals. Lucerne, clover, and beans all contain an unidentified antagonist to vitamin E: another point to bear in mind when considering supplementing the diet.

Signs. Muscular dystrophy takes three forms so far as symptoms are concerned. The most dramatic form occurs when the heart muscle is involved – causing a heart attack which is usually followed by death within minutes or hours.

When the muscles of the back and legs are affected, the animal prefers to remain lying down, rises with difficulty, and walks slowly and stiffly. The third form is seen when the chest muscles are affected. Exaggerated compensatory movements are then made by unaffected muscles in order to maintain breathing.

The more severely affected cattle may pass dark reddish-brown urine, resulting from the presence in it of myoglobin. This symptom accounts for another name for the condition – 'Paralytic Myoglobinuria'.

Prevention. Give the cow and calf vitamin E, or alternatively plenty of good quality silage.

'Small amounts of selenium will prevent the muscular dystrophy of cattle in north Scotland, a disease which is also prevented by relatively large amounts of ϕ-tocopherol. The farms concerned were on soils derived from arenaceous sands of old red sandstone origin, which suggests that on comparable soils dietary deficiency of selenium might also occur. Such deficiency might well be masked by an adequate tocopherol intake as instanced by the absence of the disease on farms in the Moray Firth area, which feed rations containing silage and green fodder and its limitation to those feeding turnips and straw, a ration which provides about one-tenth of the tocopherol of silage rations.'

Selenium supplements are useful; but there have been many cases of poisoning due to overdosage in farmers' home-mixes. (*See* CONCENTRATES.)

BACK MUSCLE NECROSIS (*see under* this main heading for a disease of pigs).

MUSCULAR RHEUMATISM is a form of myositis which attacks dogs and pigs especially, although horses and cattle are also affected. Certain animals seem to have a susceptibility to this trouble.

Causes include exposure to cold, draughts, and dampness, insufficient protection against changes in the weather, standing for long periods in rainy weather, and insufficiency of bedding (especially in piggeries and kennels).

The affected muscles are found tense and quivering, and manipulation of them causes such excruciating agony that the smaller animals often scream with the pain when the parts are handled, and the larger animals may grunt or moan. Sometimes voluntary movements in the part of the animal itself excites the same distress. The muscles of the neck, shoulders, and abdominal wall are those most often affected in all animals; the muscles of the lower jaw are frequently affected in dogs; and the condition may attack almost any of the muscles of the body. When the loins are affected the condition is called *lumbago*,

and when the croup and thigh are involved it is known as *sciatica*.

Massage of the affected muscles with some mild liniment, such as soap liniment, hot applications, exercise, and warmth are necessary outwardly, and internally salicylates or phenylbutazone may be given.

CRAMP of the muscles is common in animals that are not in a fit condition when they are worked or exercised. (*See under* CRAMP, *and also* SCOTTIE CRAMP.)

PARASITES are sometimes met with in the muscles (*see* TRICHINOSIS, GIARDIASIS).

TUMOURS are occasionally met with.

SHIVERING, STRINGHALT. For these two muscular diseases of horses, *see under* those headings. (*See also* MYASTHENIA, MYOTONIA, MYOGLOBINURIA.)

MUSCULAR DYSTROPHY (*see* MUSCLES, DISEASES OF).

MUSCULAR RELAXANTS are drugs, other than anaesthetics, which produce relaxation or paralysis in voluntary muscle, such as does curare. They are sometimes used in conjunction with a general anaesthetic, since a larger dose of the latter is usually required to obtain muscular relaxation than to abolish pain; and large doses of some anaesthetics can give rise to poisoning. Muscular relaxants can, however, only too easily be misused, and should be reserved for the specialist anaesthetist.

'MUSHY CHICK' DISEASE. Omphalitis. (*See under* this heading.)

MUSTARD POISONING. The dried ripe seeds of *Brassica nigra* and *Brassica alba* ground together. The former contains a glycoside called 'sinigrin', the latter contains one name 'sinalbin', while both contain a quantity of an enzyme named 'myrosin' which, in the presence of cold or lukewarm water, converts the two glycosides into the volatile oil to which the action of the mustard is due. Cattle have died as a result of white mustard seed being swept off the floor of a barn on to pasture. Symptoms included: walking backwards and in circles, profuse salivation, and curvature of the spine. (Acute gastro-enteritis also occurs.)

MUSTY FOOD should not be used for animals food. It is very unpalatable; and a small quantity can spoil a large amount of food. It is not easily digested, and may lead to serious digestive upsets. There is also a risk of ASPERGILLOSIS (*see* MOULDY FOOD).

MUTATION. A permanent change in the characteristics of bacteria or viruses. This is the usually implied, though not exact meaning. (*See also* GENETICS.)

MUTILATION. This term is used in a veterinary sense as meaning any operation affecting the sensitive tissue or bone structure of an animal other than for therapeutic purposes. (*See* FARM ANIMAL WELFARE COUNCIL.)

MUTING OF DOGS. This involves a surgical operation under general anaesthesia, when the vocal cords are completely excised. It was performed during the 1939–45 war on army dogs. Legally the operation is permissible (UK) in peacetime and may be the only alternative to euthanasia where complaints have been made about a dog's excessive barking.

MUTTER-PEA POISONING (*see* LATHYRISM).

MUTUALISM is the association of two species as a mutually beneficial partnership.

MUZZLE, TAPE (*see under* RESTRAINT, DOG).

MYALGIA. Pain in a muscle.

MYASTHENIA GRAVIS. A disease of muscles seen in dogs and cats, and occurring in both a congenital and an acquired form.

The former, less common, has been diagnosed in puppies from six to eight weeks old and showing muscular weakness exacerbated by exercise.

The acquired form is regarded as an immune-mediated disease in which there is an impairment of neuromuscular transmission.

Apart from the muscular weakness, there may be difficulty in swallowing, vomiting, urinary incontinence, and depression. (*See also* MEGAOESO-PHAGUS. *under* MEGA-.) Diagnosis can be made with the aid of prostigmin, which gives relief within the hour. Relapse may follow treatment with prostigmin.

MYCOBACTERIUM. A genus of acid-fast, Gram-positive, non-motile bacteria in the form of slender rods. Species include: *M. tuberculosis, M. johnei, M. leprae* (the cause of leprosy); and *M. intracellulare* and *M. xenopi*, both of which may cause a tuberculoid infection, resembling avian TB in pigs, chickens, mice. *M. phlei* is the timothy-grass bacillus.

MYCOPLASMA. An infective agent distinct from bacteria as well as from viruses. In size they resemble a large virus and they are filterable, but they can be cultured on artificial media.

Mycoplasma mycoides was isolated from cattle with pleuro-pneumonia in 1898; *M. agalactiae* from goats in 1923. Since then other species of mycoplasma have been found in man, dogs, pigs, fowls, turkeys, rats, and mice. The species most commonly associated with disease in the turkey and chicken are *Mycoplasma gallisepticum, M. meleagridis* and *M. synoviae*. Several other species such as Iowa 695 with have also been found associated with disease in these birds while *M. anatis* has been isolated from an outbreak of sinusitis in ducks.

In goats *M. mycoides* causes CONTAGIOUS CAPRINE PLEUROPNEUMONIA, as well as septicaemia and mastitis.

Mycoplasma bovis, first isolated in the USA in 1962, has caused severe respiratory disease in the UK. It also causes mastitis.

M. canadense was first reported in the UK in 1978, and causes abortion in cattle; and *M. californicum* causes mastitis.

In many parts of the world, even where contagious bovine pleuropneumonia has been eradicated, mycoplasmal diseases are of considerable economic importance. They include mastitis, arthritis, bone disease, and keratitis. In cattle, *M. bovigenitalium* is a cause of abortion and mastitis.

Mycoplasma hyosynoviae was found by the Cambridge V.I. Centre to be the cause of lameness in a 220-sow breeding unit. The pigs frequently adopted a 'dog-sitting' posture; and areas of hyperaemia on the hams were a guide to the stockman.

Mycoplasmas are also important as contaminants of cell cultures used for vaccine production. (*See also under* 'KENNEL COUGH'.)

MYCOPLASMOSIS. A mycoplasma infection. (*See above and* CONTAGIOUS BOVINE PLEURO-PNEUMONIA, VULVO-VAGINITIS, ENZOOTIC PNEUMO-NIA OF PIGS, SINUSITIS, INFECTIOUS BRONCHITIS OF POULTRY, MASTITIS.)

MYCOSIS, MYCOTIC INFECTIONS are diseases due to the growth of fungi in the body. Among the commonest are ringworm, sporo-trichosis, aspergillosis. Mycotic mastitis is important in dairy cattle, and 26 or more species of fungi are involved. (*See also* RHINOSPORIDIOSIS, FUNGAL DISEASES, SPORIDESMIN.)

MYCOTOXICOSIS. Poisoning by toxins produced by fungi. (For examples of such toxins, *see* ERGOT OF RYE, AFLATOXIN, OCHRATOXIN A, ZEAR-ALENONE, SPORIDESMIN, T_2 TOXIN, FUSARIUM, PENI-TREM, *and under* FESCUE, RYE GRASS.)

When, in farm animals, a change of feed leads to depressed output, or to symptoms of illness, poisoning by fungal toxins may be suspected. However, a 1973–4 survey by the Central Veterinary Laboratory, UK, led to a report (*Vet. Rec.* (1975) **97**, 275) to the effect that 'Most suspect rations contained fungal toxins in amounts too small for chemical detection. When detected, the toxins could not be confidently linked with the onset of illness.'

However, there is 'proof of occasional outbreaks of aflatoxicosis, ergotism, and zear-alenone (F_2) intoxication' in the UK.

In one outbreak two cows became dull and feverish, with bleeding from mouth and eyelids, and died within 48 hours. Other cows became ill, some with diarrhoea. About 60 members of this Friesian herd had bleeding eczema-like lesions of both black and white skin of udder and abdomen. A third cow died later and two had to be slaughtered. The final tentative diagnosis was fungal poisoning, after examination of mouldy barley (containing many potentially poisonous fungi) which formed 87 per cent of a supplementary concentrate ration. Similar haemorrhages and deaths from this cause have been reported in the USA. (D. A. Dyson and J. B. H. Reed. *Vet. Rec.* (1977) **100**, 400.)

MYDRIASIS. An excessive dilation of the pupil of the eye. Drugs which are given when dilation is required for diagnostic purposes are called *mydriatics*. (*See also* ATROPINE.)

MYELIN is the white fat-like substance forming a sheath round myelinated nerve-fibres.

MYELITIS is a condition in which destructive changes occur in the spinal cord. It usually follows upon viral infections. Paralysis of a muscle or of groups of muscles may occur; there may be twitchings or spasms of muscles; the penis may hang from the prepuce; the bladder and rectum become unable to retain their contents, and finally a form of paraplegia often occurs. The paralysis may gradually pass forwards; the sensation is lost in the skin of the loins, then of the back, and later the fore-legs become unable to support the weight of the body. Occasionally the condition disappears spontaneously, but the majority of cases end fatally. (*See also* OSTEOMYELITIS.)

MYELOCYTE. A bone-marrow cell, from which white cells (basophils, neutrophils and eosinophils) of the blood are produced. They are found in the blood in certain forms of leukaemia.

MYELOGRAPHY. Radiography of the spinal cord. (*See* SPINAL CORD, DISEASES OF.)

MYELOID. Cells similar to those found in bone-marrow. (*See* LEUKOSIS COMPLEX.)

MYELOMA (*see under* GENETIC ENGINEERING).

MYELOPROLIFERATIVE DISEASES. These develop as the result of the abnormal proliferation of bone-marrow cells, both within and outside the medullary cavity of bones.
SIGNS: Fever, weight loss, anaemia. A veterinary examination will reveal enlargement of both spleen and liver.
   In cats the feline leukaemia virus (FeLV) is often a complicating factor.

MYIASIS. The presence of larvae of dipterous flies in tissues and organs of the living animal, and the tissue destruction and disorders resulting therefrom. In sheep blow-fly myiasis is commonly known as 'strike'. The condition may occur in cats. (*See* FLIES *and* 'STRIKE', *also* UITPEULOOG.) Cyromazine, administered in capsules, has been used to protect sheep against *Lucillia cuprina*.

MYOCARDITIS (*see* HEART, DISEASES OF, *and below*).

MYOCARDIUM. The heart muscle. Disease of this can lead to congestive heart failure, which is characterised by congestion of the veins, with a tendency towards liver enlargement and ascites. It results from pathological changes in the heart muscle rather than from disease of the coronary artery or heart valves, and is seen in the giant breeds of dogs, *e.g.* Great Dane, Irish Wolfhound. Symptoms include loss of appetite, lethargy, accelerated heart beat, irregular pulse

and, in the later stages, ascites. Death occurs within days or weeks. Dilation of auricles and ventricles is seen at autopsy.

Myocarditis, or inflammation of the heart muscle, is referred to under HEART, DISEASES OF, but it should be added that epidemics of myocarditis have been seen in puppies 5–16 weeks old in Britain, Australia, and the USA. Spaniels, Boxer crosses, Alsatians, Scottish terriers and Poodles are breeds in which sudden death has occurred – puppies dropping dead a moment after eating or playing – no premonitory symptoms having been noticed. (*See* CANINE PARVOVIRUS INFECTION.)
In cattle, for the effect of Nutritional Muscular Dystrophy, *see under* MUSCLES, DISEASES OF.)

MYOCLONIA CONGENITA (*see* TREMBLING of pigs).

MYOCLONUS (*see* CANINE DISTEMPER *and* EPILEPSY.)

MYODYSTROPHIA OF LAMBS (*see* 'STIFF-LIMBED LAMBS').

MYOGLOBINURIA. The presence of muscle pigment in urine. It occurs in azoturia. In cattle, for example, it occurs during muscular dystrophy. (*See* EQUINE MYOGLOBINURIA, MUSCLES, DISEASES OF.)

MYOMA is a tumour which consists almost totally of muscular tissue. They are rare in animals, and when encountered are generally found in the wall of the uterus.

MYOPATHY. Non-inflammatory degeneration of muscles, such as may occur in muscular dystrophy.

MYOSIN. A contractile protein present in muscle, along with *actin*. Their interaction is controlled by calcium.

MYOSIS means an unusual narrowing of the pupil.

MYOSITIS means inflammation of a muscle. (*For* EOSINOPHILIC MYOSITIS *and* ATROPHIC MYOSITIS *see also under* MUSCLES, DISEASES OF.)

MYOTICS are drugs which contract the pupil of the eye, such as eserine and opium.

MYOTONIA. A difficulty or delay in muscle relaxation after muscular effort; also a type of muscular dystrophy. Myotonia was the diagnosis in a case involving a 9-month-old Cavalier King Charles Spaniel, which could not withdraw its tongue into its mouth. The tongue protruded from the left side of its mouth. Eating and drinking were rendered difficult. It was considered that the condition was not inherited in this case. Replacement of muscle fibres by fat was the main finding. (Jones, B. R. & Johnston, A. C., *New Zealand Veterinary Journal* (1982) **30**, 119.)

MYSOLINE. An anti-convulsant drug used in the treatment of epilepsy. A side-effect of this drug may be thirst, polyuria resulting in urinary incontinence, in the dog.

MYXOEDEMA (*see* THYROID, DISEASES OF.)

MYXOMA is a tumour consisting of imperfect connective tissue, set in a mucoid ground substance. (*See* TUMOURS.)

MYXOMATOSIS, INFECTIOUS. A disease of rabbits caused by a virus. Hares are occasionally affected also, but not domestic animals. The disease has a very high mortality rate when introduced into a country, but later the virus may become less potent or the survivors more resistant. Myxomatosis appeared in wild rabbits in Kent and Sussex in October 1953, and spread rapidly throughout most of Britain. Symptoms include: conjunctivitis, 'gummed' eyelids, swelling of the nose and muzzle, and of the mucous membrane of the vulva and anus. Orchitis is caused in the male. Emaciation, fever, and death follow. The disease is transmitted by the rabbit flea and, mechanically, by thistles.

MYXOVIRUS (*see* VIRUSES).

N

NAGANA is an unscientific but convenient name for trypanosomiasis transmitted by tsetse flies (*Glossina* species) in Africa. The trypanosomes involved are: *T. vivax, T. uniforme, T. congolense, T. brucei, T. simiae,* and *T. suis.* (*See* TRYPANOSOMIASIS.)

The symptoms of 'Nagana' include anaemia, intermittent fever, and (except in pigs, in which the disease may be very acute) a slow, progressive emaciation. In both horses and dogs the eyes may be affected, as shown by corneal opacity. Horses often have oedema affecting the limbs and abdomen. Cattle may abort.

The drug quinapyramine is (among others) used in treatment.

The koodoo, hyena, and bush-buck, as well as other wild animals, act as reservoirs of the infection.

NAIL BINDING. (*See* INJURIES FROM SHOEING.)

NAILS, or CLAWS. A claw contains a matrix with blood-vessels, nerves, etc., from which it grows and is nourished. Lying within the matrix is the bone of the terminal phalanx of the digit, which gives the nail its characteristic form in the different animals. When not in use in the carnivora they are retracted by ligaments in an upwards direction; this is more marked in cats, where the nail may almost disappear, than in dogs.

NAILS, DISEASES OF. The nails of cats and dogs sometimes become torn or broken through fighting or accidents. Sometimes only the tip is injured, and the matrix higher up is undamaged; in such cases a fine pellicle of horn covers the tip until such a time as the horn has grown down from above, and the whole nail is not shed. In other cases infection occurs, causing great tenderness of the part.
ingrowing nails occur upon the 'dew claws', on the insides of the paws of dogs. These more or less rudimentary digits do not touch the ground, and are consequently not subjected to wear from friction. The nails grow, and owing to their curve eventually penetrate the soft pad behind them. Where actual penetration has occurred the nail should be cut short and an antiseptic dressing applied. It is customary for owners of sporting and other dogs to have the dew claws removed during puppyhood to avoid future trouble of this nature. Amputation of dew claws can be carried out in the adult under anaesthesia.
Onychomycosis, or a fungus infection of the claws, is a not uncommon condition in cats, and is of public health importance as a reservoir of ringworm transmissible to children. (*See* RINGWORM.)

NAIROBI SHEEP DISEASE is an acute infectious fever of sheep and goats, caused by a bunyavirus, and occurs in eastern and southern Africa. The virus is transmitted by ticks.

Signs. Imported sheep usually show an acute febrile disturbance within 5 or 6 days after being infected by the ticks. This lasts for up to 9 days and then a fall in temperature occurs and other clinical symptoms appear. Death may take place a day or two later, or a second rise in temperature may be shown, death or recovery following. There is rapidity and difficulty in breathing, a mucopurulent nasal discharge and green watery diarrhoea, which may contain mucus or blood. The genital organs of ewes are swollen and congested and abortion may occur in pregnant ewes.

Immunity. In the great majority of cases, recovery confers a strong and lasting immunity. This is also possessed by sheep in areas where the infection is endemic.

NANOGRAM. This unit of measurement is equivalent to one part per thousand millions.

NANOMETRE (nm). A unit of measurement used in virology. One nm equals one millionth of a millimetre.

NAPHTHALENE POISONING might arise from the ingestion of moth-balls. In the dog, it has been shown experimentally to give rise to haemolytic anaemia. (In children, poisoning from moth-balls gives rise to 'port-wine coloured' urine.) Another symptom is cataract. Chlorinated naphthalenes have been identified as one cause of HYPERKERATOSIS in cattle; and tear stains may be a symptom of this type of poisoning.

NARCOLEPSY. This has been recorded in dogs, and American veterinarians have suggested that it may be partly genetic in origin. A case was recorded (P. G. Darke & V. Jessen. *Vet. Record* (1977) **101,** 117) in the UK in a 3-year-old Corgi which sometimes collapsed when taken for his first walk of the day, or offered food. Often yawning and a vacant expression would precede a sudden drop from a standing position to a sitting one or a lying one. No excitement, salivation, or convulsions were seen, and at other times the dog was active and mentally alert; and he was easily aroused after he had collapsed. Electroencephalograms supported the diagnosis.

NARES is the Latin word for the nostrils.

NASAL BOT FLY (*Oestrus ovis*) larvae are serious parasites of sheep. (*See* FLIES.)

NASAL DISORDERS (*see* NOSE, DISEASES OF).

NASO-PHARYNX. The upper part of the throat lying posterior to the nasal cavity.

NATAMYCIN. An antibiotic used for the treatment of ringworm in cattle. Application can be made with a knapsack sprayer. (*See* RINGWORM.)

NATIONAL OFFICE OF ANIMAL HEALTH LTD. (NOAH). Founded in 1986, to represent those UK companies which manufacture animal-health products licensed under the Medicines Act. NOAH currently represents 56 companies which in 1990 had combined sales worth more than £188.9 million. Address: 3 Crossfield Chambers, Gladbeck Way, Enfield, Middlesex EN2 7HF. Publication: *The Safe Storage & Handling of Animal Medicines.*

'NATURE' (*see under* OEDEMA).

NAVEL-ILL (*see* JOINT-ILL).

NAVICULAR BONE is the popular name for the sesamoid of the third phalanx of the horse. It is a little boat-shaped bone, developed just above the deep flexor tendon, and serves, as do all sesamoid bones, to minimise friction where the tendon passes round a corner of another bone. It enters into the formation of the 'coffin-joint', between the second and third phalanges of the digit. It is of great importance in deep punctured wounds of the foot when these are situated towards the heels, for, when damaged, its surface becomes inflamed, the inflammation spreads to the coffin-joint and may produce incurable lameness.

NAVICULAR DISEASE is a chronic condition of inflammation affecting the horse's navicular bone and its associated structures. The fore-feet are usually both attacked, though the condition may arise in only one of these, or in the hind-feet (rarely). Ulceration of the cartilage first and later of the bone on the surface over which the deep flexor tendon plays, may sometimes be seen at autopsy.

CAUSES. These are still a matter of hypothesis rather than certainty, and controversy persists. Some authors have referred to increased vascularisation of the navicular bone; while a paper (C. M. Colles and J. Hickman, *Equine Veterinary Journal* (1977) **9**, 150) suggests that ischaemia may be responsible, leading to pain and, if at least two of the distal arteries be occluded, to chronic lameness. A consistent finding in horses lame as a result of navicular disease was, stated Mr Colles (*Vet. Record* (1980) **107**, 434), occlusion of the main artery and progressive arterial thrombosis, with a resulting area of ischaemic necrosis and cavitation of the navicular bone.

Another view is that the disease is not caused primarily by ischaemia and subsequent necrosis, but is a consequence of bone remodelling due to altered pressure from the deep flexor tendon and increased load on the caudal part of the foot; the condition not being irreversible unless secondary lesions such as adhesions and bony spurs have developed. Special shoeing to alter the load on the navicular bone is recommended. (Ostblom, L. & others, *Equine Veterinary Journal* (1982) **14**, 199.)

SIGNS. Navicular disease usually develops so slowly that the owner has considerable difficulty in remembering exactly when the first symptoms were noticed. In fact, little or no importance may be attached to the almost characteristic 'pointing' of one or both fore-feet, because 'he has *always* done that'. 'Pointing' consists of resting the affected foot (or feet) by placing it a short distance in advance of the other when standing in harness or in the stable. When both feet are affected, each is alternately pointed. Later, the horse may go lame or be tender on his feet at times, but with a rest he generally becomes sound again. As the disease advances, he may either start off in the mornings stiff and become better with exercise as he warms to his work, or may become lame as the day goes on. Sooner or later, however, there comes a time when he will go permanently 'pottery', or 'groggy'. The length of the stride decreases and there is difficulty in advancing the feet, as to suggest that the shoulder is the seat of the lesion. When made to turn, the horse pivots round on the fore-feet instead of lifting them, and when made to back, drags the toes. If the wearing shoe of such a horse is examined it is usually found to be more worn at the toes than at the heels. In fact a 'groggy' horse may wear his shoes quite thin at the toes before the heels show much sign of wear at all. In the final stages the horse becomes distinctly lame and unfit for work. When observed in the stable he is noticed to be continually shifting from one foot on to the other, and the resting foot is placed well out in front.

TREATMENT must aim at the relief of pain and improvement of the local blood circulation. A formulation of Warfarin intended for human use has been given in their feed to horses, but the dosage requires great care – with overdosage there is a danger of haemorrhage. Warfarin treatment was effective, Mr Colles said, in about 75 per cent of cases of navicular disease.

In Australia, in order to avoid the potentially dangerous side-effects of warfarin therapy, trials were made with a vasodilator, isoxuprine hydrochloride, to improve the blood supply to the navicular bone. Results were encouraging but not conclusive.

Before the advent of Warfarin therapy it was customary to perform the operation of neurectomy, which consists of section of the plantar or median nerve of the limb. In a favourable case, following operation, the horse becomes apparently sound, although the diseased condition is still at work in the bone. No pain is felt, and the horse is fit for light work at slow paces. The feet require constant attention to ensure that no stones, nails, etc., lodge in the hoof, for even when these inflict serious damage the horse still goes sound, not feeling the pain.

NAVY BEANS may cause death if fed raw. (*See* LEGUME POISONING.)

NEAR EAST ENCEPHALITIS. An alphavirus infection of horses, donkeys; less frequently of cattle and sheep. Convulsions/paralysis may follow fever and precede death. (*See* EQUINE ENCEPHALITIS *and* BORNA DISEASE.)

NECK. Its main function is to support the head. Both the mouse and giraffe have seven cervical vertebrae, as do most mammals.

The weight of the head is supported by the powerful *ligamentum nuchae*, which takes the strain off the muscles; thereby avoiding fatigue. In the horse the ligament extends from the spines of the withers to the posterior of the occipital bone of the SKULL (q.v.)

NECROPSY (*see* AUTOPSY).

NECROSIS. Death of cells or of a limited portion of tissue.

NECROSIS (BACILLARY), or NECRO-BACILLOSIS (*see* CALF DIPHTHERIA).

NECROTIC ENTERITIS. A condition of unweaned and older pigs, characterised by scouring.

The lesions are in the caecum and ileum. (*See also under* ILEUM.)

CAUSE. *Clostridium perfringens* (*C. welchii*). Cold, damp, dirty surroundings appear to predispose to Necrotic Enteritis. (*See* PORCINE INTESTINAL ADENOMATOSIS.)

NECROTIC ENTERITIS IN CHICKENS. This has been reported in Australia, among broilers, associated with *Clostridium perfringens* and probably some defect in nutrition.

NECROTIC STOMATITIS (*see* CALF DIPHTHERIA).

NEGRI BODIES are comparatively large, rounded inclusion bodies which can be demonstrated by staining with Seller's stain, among others, and are found in the brains of dogs and other animals which have died of rabies. The cerebral cortex, Ammon's horn, and the Purkinje cells of the cerebellum are the main sites to examine. Negri bodies are not present in cases affected with 'fixed virus'. The diagnosis of rabies once depended upon their demonstration in the affected animal. (*See* RABIES.)

NEISSERIA. Spherical, Gram-negative bacteria, some of which are associated with eye infections.

NEMATODE is a general term applied to the parasitic *Nemathelminthes*, which include the round worms, as distinct from the *Platyhelminthes*, or flat worms. (*See* WORMS.)

'NEMATODE POISONING'. In the USA larvae of *Anguina agrostis* on Chewing's fescue in immature hay has caused an outbreak of poisoning in cattle. Symptoms include knuckling of the fetlocks, head tucked between the forelegs, recumbency, convulsions, and death.

NEMATODIRUS. Parasitic worms of sheep (and calves in the case of *N. battus*). (*See* WORMS.)

NEMBUTAL (PENTOBARBITONE) (Sodium ethyl/ methylbutyl barbiturate). A white crystalline powder, soluble in water, and used for its narcotic and anaesthetic effects.

First used as a general anaesthetic in veterinary surgery in America in 1931, nembutal was brought to the notice of the veterinary profession in the United Kingdom by Professor J. G. Wright, who studied and improved the technique of its administration.

Nembutal has been used to produce anaesthesia in all the domestic animals including the fowl, but it is not recommended for horses, calves, or sheep. For anaesthesia in the dog and cat, however, nembutal is very extensively employed, and is usually given by the intravenous route – a method which permits of varying depths of anaesthesia being obtained and the avoidance of overdosage. The drug may also be given by intra-peritoneal injection or by mouth; narcosis being then slower in onset (8 to 20 minutes), and occasionally preceded by some degree of excitement, while the dose has to be an estimate calculated on the basis of bodyweight.

Deep anaesthesia with nembutal may last for an hour, being followed by 2 to 7 hours of narcosis. (*See* ANAESTHETICS, EUTHANASIA.)

NEOARSPHENAMINE. A drug effective against BLACKHEAD OF TURKEYS.

NEOMYCIN. An antibiotic obtained from *Streptomyces fradiae*. It must not be given by injection, owing to resulting kidney damage. Its action closely resembles that of streptomycin. A topical spray of this antibiotic has caused profound deafness in children. (*See* DEAFNESS.)

NEONATAL diseases are those of the newborn.

NEOPLASM means literally 'a new growth', and is applied to tumours in general.

NEOSPORUM CANINUM. This parasite was discovered in Norway in 1984, and later recognised in Sweden, USA, Australia, and the UK in 1990. CAUSE: A protozoan, named as above, and resembling *Toxoplasma gondii*. Congenital infection occurs in cattle, dogs, and cats. SIGNS: Ataxia, a fleeting paralysis, nystagmus. Meningitis appears in some cases. (Dubey, J. P. & others. *Veterinary Record* (1990) **126**, 193).

NEPHRECTOMY is the name given to the operation by which one of the kidneys is removed. (*See* KIDNEY, DISEASES OF.)

NEPHRITIS (*see* KIDNEY, DISEASES OF; LEPTOSPIROSIS).

NEPHROLITHIASIS. The presence of a stone (calculus) in the pelvis of the kidney.

NEPHRON (*see* KIDNEYS).

NEPHROPTOSIS (*see* KIDNEY, DISEASES OF.)

NEPHROSIS. This is a disease of the kidneys, involving damage to the tubules. It leads to albuminuria and often to oedema. (*See also* KIDNEYS, DISEASES OF).

NEPHROSIS, INFECTIOUS AVIAN. A disease of chickens. (*See* GUMBORO DISEASE *and* INFECTIOUS BURSAL DISEASE.)

NEPHROTIC SYNDROME (*see* NEPHROSIS).

NEPHROTOMY. Surgical incision into a kidney.

NERVES. The basic unit of the nervous system is the *neuron*, comprising a cell with at least one projection. Bipolar neurons have one long projection, the *axon*, and one short branching projection, the *dendrite*. A typical neuron (multipolar) has several dendrites but usually only one axon (nerve fibre).

Dendrites conduct nerve impulses towards the nerve cell, axons conduct away from it.

A synapse is a point or area where one neuron is able to make contact with another; the contact being between the axon of one neuron and a dendrite of another neuron, or between the axon of one neuron and the cell of another neuron. Any neuron may synapse with axons or dendrites of several other neurons.

Nerve fibres may be *myelinated* or *unmyelinated* (*see* MYELIN). Some nerve fibres (axons) convey impulses to brain or spinal cord from skin or sense organ, and are termed *sensory* or *afferent*. Their impulses are passed, through connecting links or interneurons, to *motor* or *efferent* nerves from brain or spinal cord (*but see* Spinal Reflex under SPINE functions).

Nerve impulses are dependent upon the permeability of cell membranes. There is a potential difference of about 70–80 millivolts between the inside and the outside of an axon – the inside being the negative. This is owing to the fact that in a resting state the cell membrane is permeable to $K(+)$ and $Cl(-)$ ions, but not to $Na(+)$ ions. Stimulation of the nerve results in the membrane becoming permeable to the sodium ions, which flow in causing the inside of the axon to carry a positive electrical charge instead of a negative one. A so-called depolarisation wave is set up, 'self-perpetuating', along one neuron after another. A single nerve fibre can send about 1000 separate impulses per second.

ACETYLCHOLINE (which see) is released by somatic nerve fibres at synapses between neurons on either side of ganglia and also at the junction of motor nerve endings and voluntary (striated) muscle. Acetylcholine is released also at synapses by parasympathetic nerve fibres. NORADRENALIN is released at synapses of sympathetic nerve fibres, and at their junction with smooth (unstriated) involuntary muscle fibres.

NERVES, INJURIES TO. Continued or repeated severe pressure upon a nerve trunk may be sufficient to damage it and result in paralysis; severe bruising in which a nerve is driven against a bone with considerable force may produce paralysis or inflammation of the nerve; a nerve may be severed along with other tissues in a deep wound; fracture of a bone, such as the first rib, may produce rupture of any nerves that lie upon or near to it; and other accidents may also involve the nerves

of the part. A nerve may sometimes be injured at its origin before it leaves the brain or spinal cord by haemorrhage. (*See also under* IMMUNISATION.)

SIGNS. Sometimes, it is not until after a wound has healed that the injury to the nerve becomes obvious. In 'radial paralysis', or in other cases where large and important motor nerves have been damaged, the resulting paralysis of the muscles they supply is seen at once. (*See* RADIAL PARALYSIS.) Atrophy of muscles results.

(*See* FACIAL PARALYSIS for another example of a nerve injury.)

A tumour, such as a neurofibrosarcoma or (in the cat) a lymphosarcoma, may press upon or infiltrate the brachial plexus causing progressive lameness and pain. (*See* BRACHIAL.) Another tumour is a NEUROMA.

If a nerve is cut, the distal part undergoes Wallerian degeneration.

Neuritis (*see separate section* NEURITIS).

NERVOUS SYSTEM (*see* CENTRAL NERVOUS SYSTEM).

NERVOUS SYSTEM, DISEASES OF (*see* BRAIN, DISEASES OF; ENCEPHALITIS; BOTULISM; CHOREA; DISTEMPER; CANINE VIRAL HEPATITIS; TETANUS; RABIES; SPINAL CORD; LISTERIOSIS; etc.).

NETTLE-RASH (*see* URTICARIA).

NEURECTOMY is an operation in which part of a nerve is excised. The operation is sometimes performed to give relief from incurable lameness in the horse but only a few months' work may be gained.

NEURILEMMA is the thin membranous covering of nerve-fibres.

NEURITIS means inflammation affecting nerves or their sheaths. It is often accompanied by pain (NEURALGIA), sometimes by spastic paralysis. Causes include virus infections, allergies, malnutrition, and poisoning, as well as physical injuries. (*See* NEUROMA, NERVES, INJURIES TO, *and under* IMMUNISATION.)

NEUROGLIA. A fine web of tissue and branching cells which supports the nerve-fibres and cells of the nervous system.

NEUROMA means a tumour connected with a nerve, generally of a fibrous nature and very painful.

NEURON is a single unit of the nervous system, consisting of one nerve-cell, with all its processes. (*See illustration overleaf and also* NERVES.)

NEUROTROPIC VIRUS is one which shows a predilection for becoming localised in, and fixing itself to, nerve tissues. The best known of these is that of rabies. Rabies virus enters the body through torn nerve-fibres at the seat of an injury, such as a bite, and, growing along them, eventually reaches the spinal cord and brain. Other neurotropic viruses are those of louping-ill in sheep, and Borna disease in horses and cattle.

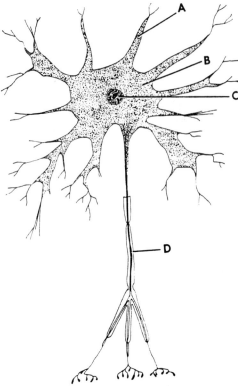

A typical neuron: A – dendrites, B – nerve cell body, C – nucleus, and D – axon. (After Francis, *Introduction to Human Anatomy*, courtesy of C. V. Mosby Co.)

NEUTERING (*see* CASTRATION and SPAYING; *also* VASECTOMY).

NEUTROPENIA. A reduced number of neutrophil granular leukocytes in the blood.

(In human medicine, most cases are attributed to the direct toxic effect of certain antibiotics, *e.g.* penicillin and the cephalosporins, or to immune-mediated mechanisms. With this type of blood dyscrasia patients are at serious risk of an overwhelming infection.)

NEUTROPHIL. A type of white blood-cell which can migrate into the tissues and engulf bacteria, etc. (*See under* BLOOD, ABSCESS.)

'NEW FOREST DISEASE' (Infectious Bovine Keratitis). A painful eye condition which can lead to blindness if neglected. (*See* EYE, DISEASES OF.)

NEW FOREST FLY. A blood-sucking fly, found in many parts of Britain. *Hippobosca equina* attacks horses and cattle. It deposits larvae (not eggs) in the soil. When disturbed, it makes a characteristic sideways movement. (*See* FLIES.)

NEWCASTLE DISEASE. A NOTIFIABLE infectious febrile disease of chickens, turkeys, ducks, pigeons and wild birds. In people the only sign of infection is usually conjunctivitis.
CAUSE. A paramyxovirus.
SIGNS. Listlessness and a reduced egg yield. There may be a discharge of mucus from the nostrils. The eggs may be misshapen and soft-shelled.

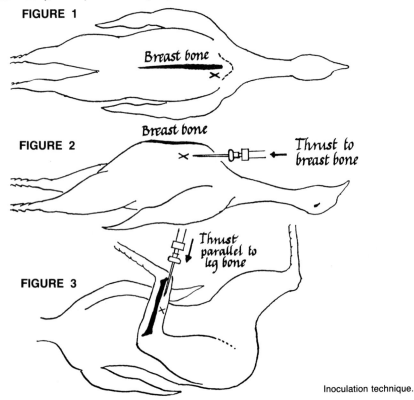

FIGURE 1

Breast bone

FIGURE 2

Breast bone

Thrust to breast bone

FIGURE 3

Thrust parallel to leg bone

Inoculation technique.

The signs may remain mild, but in most outbreaks they change to those of a serious illness, with the onset of diarrhoea, difficult breathing through an open beak, and twitching of the head and neck – a preliminary indication of ENCEPHALITIS (which see). A high mortality rate is to be expected.

CONTROL. Inactivated vaccine. Live vaccines include: the Hitchner B1 and La Sota. These vaccines are *not* administered by injection, but as described later. La Sota is not recommended for birds under 28 days old, except under veterinary advice. (*See* CROWS.)

*Inoculation technique.** Needles and hypodermic syringes must be sterilised.

With young stock, 10 to 20 days old, the greatest care is necessary because the amount of muscle is small. There are two sites of injection to consider:

(a) *Breast muscle*. This is a relatively safe site for injection of the small bird. The needle must be introduced from the head end of the bird into the breast muscle about ¼ inch to the side of the point of the breast bone as shown in Figure 1. The vaccinator must locate the point of the breast bone with the thumb of his left hand and use it as a guide. It is important to make sure that the thrust of the needle is always parallel to the line of the breast bone so that no damage is done to the chest of the bird. (Figure 2.) The bird must be held with the breast region uppermost so that the vaccinator can approach the bird with plenty of room.

(b) *Leg muscle*. Injection is best carried out into the back of the chick's leg in the mid line above the point where the feathers begin. (Figure 3.) The vaccinator should grasp the leg himself while the bird is held upside down with the legs towards him. It is important to introduce the needle carefully and parallel to the bone; otherwise damage may again be brought about since important nerves and blood-vessels pass in this region.

Adult birds may be injected at any one of three sites: (a) Breast muscle; (b) Leg muscle; (c) Behind the head. In these older birds there is a larger mass of muscle to inject into, but care is still very necessary. Birds in batteries are best injected into the leg muscle simply by carefully pulling the leg through the feeding gap. Adult turkeys are normally vaccinated behind the head.

Where the actual vaccination is being carried out by a visiting contractor or teams of vaccinators, the farmer should insist upon the highest standards of hygiene for their clothes, their persons, and their instruments.

It will sometimes happen that vaccination will be carried out in a flock in which, unknown to the owner, some of the birds are in the incubation stage of the disease. In other words, although no symptoms of illness will be shown by those birds, people handling them can become heavily contaminated with the virus of Newcastle disease – on their hands, face, clothes, boots, vaccine bottles, and cartons. It follows, of course, that unless they begin the next day's work with fresh bottles of vaccine, with boiled syringes and

needles, and freshly laundered overalls, caps, and Wellington boots disinfected, a vaccinating team can carry such infection on to the next farm. This is important because it takes birds 10 to 14 days to acquire immunity following inoculation. (At least 2 inoculations needed.)

It is preferable for farm staff to carry out vaccination, if practicable, rather than rely on outside help.

In the human being, Newcastle disease virus may cause conjunctivitis and an influenza-like illness.

Administration of live vaccines. These vaccines are in a freeze-dried form and have to be dissolved in water before use. They can cause stress and therefore should be given only to healthy, vigorous birds. Administration can be by individual dosing or by mass methods:

(1) eye dropping – suitable all ages including day-old
(2) beak dipping – suitable day-olds only
(3) spraying – suitable day-olds only*
(4) in drinking water† – suitable over 3 days old

'NEWMARKET COUGH' (*see* EQUINE INFLUENZA, COUGH).

NIACIN. (Nicotinic acid). One of the vitamin B group, present in most animal feeds, and produced in the digestive system from tryptophan. With maize feeding, a niacin deficiency may occur. A R C research has suggested that niacin supplements would benefit dairy cows, as synthesis of the vitamin in the rumen may not be sufficient. as was thought to be the case in the late 1970s. In dogs a niacin deficiency causes 'BLACK TONGUE'. (*See* SHEEPDOGS, VITAMINS.)

NICKING. this is defined in the Docking and Nicking of Horses Act, 1949, as 'the deliberate severing of any tendon or muscle in the tail of a horse'. The practice is illegal.

NICOTINE POISONING has killed cattle dressed with nicotine against warbles, and may also arise from the old practice by shepherds of dosing with tobacco against parasitic worms.

NICOTINIC ACID (*see* NIACIN).

NICTITATING MEMBRANE. The 'third eyelid' or haw, consists of a plate of cartilage covered with conjunctiva, and having lymphatic tissue and the Harderian gland. Often pigmented, the membrane is always prominent in breeds of dogs such as the Bloodhound and St. Bernard. In other breeds of dog, and in the cat, its protrusion across part of the eye may indicate general debility if bilateral; other causes include the presence of a foreign body, ulceration, a nerve injury, occasionally a tumour.

Nictitating membrane protrusion and diarrhoea syndrome was studied at the Department

---

*Operators must wear a face mask and goggles.
†Adequate trough space essential – additional temporary drinkers needed – deprive of water 1 or 2 hrs beforehand.

*With acknowledgements to Glaxo Laboratories Ltd.

of Veterinary Medicine, University of Bristol. Fifty cats with the syndrome were compared with nine cats with diarrhoea only and 17 healthy cats. A novel torovirus-like agent was isolated from 11 cats, including seven of those showing the syndrome. (Muir, P. & others. *Veterinary Record* (1990) **127**, 324.)

'NIGHT BLINDNESS' (*see* PROGRESSIVE RETINAL ATROPHY *under* EYE, DISEASES OF, *and also under* NYCTALOPIA).

NIGHT LIGHTING is now commonly practised in poultry houses, using 40-watt lamps to give a 14-hour day, or 1500-watt lamps for three 20-second exposures a night. The object is increased egg production during the winter months, and the effect is due not merely to the provision of extra feeding-time, but also to the influence of light indirectly on the ovaries. However, an investigation carried out in conjunction with the ADAS into eye abnormalities in turkey breeding flocks, leading to blindness, showed that the cause was continuous artificial light. Seventy per cent of poults showed symptoms after 5 weeks of this, and it was proved that it was the continuity and not the intensity of the light which was doing the damage.

NIGHTSHADE POISONING. The Nightshades comprise: Garden or Black Nightshade (*Solanum nigrum*), Woody Nightshade or Bittersweet (*Solanum dulcamara*), and Deadly Nightshade or Belladonna (*Atropa belladonna*). (*see* GARDEN NIGHTSHADE, BITTERSWEET, and ATROPINE POISONING).

NIGROID BODIES are black or brown irregular outgrowths from the edges of the iris of the horse's eye. (*See* IRIS.)

NIKETHAMIDE (*see* CORAMINE).

NIPPLES. Infection and necrosis of sows' nipples is not uncommonly caused by *Fusiformis necrophorus*, and may lead to the death of piglets from starvation. (*See* MAMMILITIS.)

NISIN. An antibiotic of bacterial origin. It has potential use against two pathogens which contaminate human and animal food, and is a product of genetic engineering.

NIT. Egg of louse or other parasitic insect.

NITRATE POISONING (*see* NITRITE POISONING).

NITRITES are salts which, in excess, convert haemoglobin into methaemoglobin, and may cause death from lack of oxygen. (*See* NITROSAMINES *and below*.)

NITRITE POISONING. Poisoning as a result of eating plants with a high potassium nitrate content is common in some of the western parts of the USA. The nitrate is reduced to nitrite by substances within the plant under certain climatic conditions, and when such a plant is eaten the

nitrite is rapidly absorbed from the digestive system and converts haemoglobin into methaemoglobin. This is incapable of giving up its oxygen to the tissues and as a result the animal dies.

Sodium nitrite is used for curing meat and has found its way into swill, causing fatal poisoning in pigs. The main symptoms observed were vomiting, squealing, and distressed breathing. Nitrite poisoning has also occurred, in piggeries with poor ventilation, from condensation dripping down. It may arise, too, in grazing animals where nitrogenous fertilisers have been spread during dry weather, or before rain has had time to wash it all in. This could be called nitrate poisoning, but the nitrate itself has a fairly low toxicity, being converted into the poisonous nitrite. The nitrate content of heavily fertilised plants may increase the animal's intake of nitrates.

The Worcester VI Centre reported acute poisoning in 13 cows after they had been brought into a shed. An hour or two later, two were dead, two were dying and nine were very distressed, showing dyspnoea, salivation, cramping pains and head pressing. Their blood was dark brown. The local hospital made up a 4 per cent solution of methylene blue within 15 minutes, following advice from the centre, and when each cow was injected intravenously with 500 ml the response was dramatic and reminiscent of that seen in the successful treatment of milk fever with calcium. Sequelae of this event were abortion in two of the cows and a change in temperament, normally quiet cows becoming wild.

The source of the nitrate was believed to be straw bedding contaminated with fertiliser from broken bags.

Fatal nitrite poisoning of pigs has occurred following the use, for drinking purposes, of rainwater containing decaying organic matter.

SYMPTOMS include signs of abdominal pain, sometimes diarrhoea, weakness and ataxia, dysnoea, rapid heart action and, especially, cyanosis. Convulsions, coma, and death may follow.

TREATMENT consists of methylene blue intravenously, and ascorbic acid. (*See* NITROSAMINES.)

NITROFURANS. A group of drugs developed in the USA during the 1940s, and including Nitrofurazone, Furazolidone, and Nitrofurantoin (for urinary tract infections). They are effective against a wide range of bacteria; some against protozoa and fungi. It is thought that they interfere with the carbohydrate metabolism of micro-organisms.

NITROGEN (*see* AIR). For **liquid nitrogen** *see* CRYOSURGERY, ARTIFICIAL INSEMINATION, FROZEN EMBRYOS.

Nitrogen dioxide. A reddish-brown heavy gas with an offensive odour. This is formed by oxidation, on exposure to air, from the colourless nitric oxide. The latter appears to be the chief oxide of nitrogen produced in the early stages of silage-making.

Nitrogen dioxide poisoning occurs in man ('silo-fillers' disease'); and in cattle and pigs housed close to silos.

SIGNS. Dyspnoea, cyanosis, muscular weakness and, in piglets, vomiting. (McLoughlin, M. F., *Veterinary Record* (1985) **116**, 119.)

NITROPHENIDE POISONING, characterised by paralysis, has occurred in pigs fed medicated meal intended for poultry and containing nitrophenide as a treatment for coccidiosis.

NITROSAMINES. They are very powerful chemical carcinogens. They cause cancer of specific organs irrespective of the route of administration. Some nitrosamines can be formed from nitrite and secondary amine or amide in the acid stomach contents of animals. Nitrites used as food preservatives, and high levels of nitrates in drinking water, can be carcinogens.

NITROTHIAZOLE. The drug 2-amino-5-nitrothiazole is effective in controlling Blackhead in turkeys (by preventive medication).

NITROUS OXIDE. This anaesthetic is not very much used in veterinary practice but, where it is, there is a need for good ventilation, as it interferes with vitamin B metabolism and, in a pregnant anaesthetist, may bring about a miscarriage.

NOAH (*see* NATIONAL OFFICE OF ANIMAL HEALTH).

NOCARDIOSIS. Infection with *Nocardia asteroides* in cattle, dogs, cats, and man. It is a saprophytic inhabitant of the soil and belongs to the genus actinomycetes. It was formerly classified as a fungus but is now regarded as a bacterium. It has occasionally been isolated from the udders of cows affected with mastitis, and has been reported as the cause of 'incurable mastitis' in an outbreak on a Texas farm. Involvement of the liver and mesentery, with marked loss of condition, thirst, and some diarrhoea – calling for euthanasia – has been recorded in the dog in Britain. Pleuropneumonia, occasionally also a skin infection, may result from Nocardia in dogs and cats.

NODE (*see* LYMPH NODES).

NODULAR PANNICULITIS. An inflammatory reaction involving subcutaneous fat, and characterised by nodules which burst. Abscesses and sloughing may occur. (*See* AUTOIMMUNE DISEASE, of which the above is an example, occurring in dogs.)

NOISE (*see* STRESS).

NORADRENALIN. A hormone secreted by the adrenal gland medulla (*and see* NERVES).

NORMAL SALINE, or PHYSIOLOGICAL SALINE, is a solution of sodium chloride in sterile distilled water, which is isotonic with the strength of this salt in the blood-stream, that is about 0·9 per cent for mammals. (*See also* DEHYDRATION, DEXTRAN.)

NORMOBLAST is a red blood cell which still contains the remnant of a nucleus.

NORTHERN FOWL MITE. This can infect canaries as well as poultry, and has caused allergic reactions in poultrykeepers in Israel. (*See* MITES.)

NORWEGIAN SCABIES. ☛

NOSE AND NASAL PASSAGES. The 'nose' of an animal, which is more often termed the 'muzzle', or 'snout', according to the species, serves two important functions. It forms the outermost end of the respiratory passage, and it lodges some of the end-organs of the sense of touch.

Horses. Externally, the rims of the nostrils are built up on a basis of cartilages covered over by a fold of delicate skin possessing long tactile hairs. The cartilages are not complete laterally, thereby allowing the nostrils to become greatly distended during occasions of emergency. Situated at the upper and outer part of each nostril there is a pouch-like sac which opens into the nostril at one end, but is blind at the other. This is often called the 'false nostril'. Lying just within the entrance to the nasal passages about an inch or so inside each nostril is the lower-most opening of the lacrimal duct carrying tears secreted by the lacrimal gland of the eye. *Internally*, each nostril, and the nasal passage to which it gives access, is completely divided from the other by the *septum* of the nose and its associated structures. This is composed partly by the vomer bone, and partly by a wall of cartilage which is continuous with the cartilages of the nostrils. The walls of each passage are lined by mucous membrane which is reflected on to the two turbinated scroll-like bones that are found in the passage, and this membrane, being well supplied with blood, and being continually moist from the secretion of its mucin glands, serves to warm and moisten the incoming air before it passes to the lungs, and to extract the larger particles of dust, soot, etc., that the air picks up, by causing them to adhere to its sticky surface. The entrance to the air sinuses of the skull leads out from the posterior part of each passage, the mucous membrane lining the sinuses being continuous with that of the nose. (*See* SINUSES OF SKULL.) The end-organs of the sense of smell are scattered throughout the nasal mucous membrane in the upper parts particularly. The olfactory nerves from the brain, which pass out of the cranial cavity into that of the nose by way of the ethmoid bone, are distributed to these end-organs. Posteriorly, the nasal passages lead into the pharynx.

Cattle. The nostrils, situated on either side of the broad expanse of moist hairless muzzle, are smaller and thicker than in the horse. No false nostril is present, and the opening of the lacrimal duct is not visible.

NOSE AND NASAL PASSAGES, DISEASES OF.

Catarrh. Inflammation of the nostrils is called RHINITIS, and may accompany ordinary catarrhal inflammation of the nasal passages such as occurs in cases of distemper in the dog, and of other febrile illnesses; the symptoms often resembling those of a human 'cold in the head', with a discharge from the nostrils which is at first clear and colourless, later becoming thick and yellowish green. Horses and cattle often snort and shake their heads; dogs sneeze. Conjunctivitis may accompany the nasal catarrh.

In horses, the presence of ulcers in the mucous membrane with a punched-out appearance may indicate GLANDERS. For a specific condition in the pig, see RHINITIS, ATROPHIC.

PARASITES, such as larvae of the sheep nostril fly; *Linguatula* or leeches in dog or cat, may cause a discharge from one or both nostrils.

A discharge from **one nostril** only may in the dog, for example, indicate the presence of a FOREIGN BODY such as a grass awn; or there may be a fungal infection (*e.g.* ASPERGILLOSIS) which may follow local injury or tumour formation. Another possible cause is an abscess at the root of a tooth, with pus collecting in the maxillary sinus and escaping through the naso-maxillary opening.

TREATMENT. Nasal catarrh should be considered contagious. The animal should be isolated accordingly, and attention paid to comfort, ventilation, and suitability of food, as discussed under NURSING OF SICK ANIMALS. Symptoms of other diseases must be looked for, especially when the temperature is high, and a professional diagnosis should be obtained. The nostrils should be kept moist and pliable by rubbing small quantities of Vaseline around their rims daily, after sponging away discharges.

Diseased conditions of the turbinated bones or of the molar teeth call for surgical measures for their correction; parasites in the nasal cavities must be expelled (*see* MITES); and if other foreign bodies are present they must be removed.

Haemorrhage from the nostrils may be due to injuries which cause tearing or laceration of the mucous membrane; it may occur during violent exertion, such as racing or hunting with horses not in maximum condition; it may be associated with ulceration, congestion, tumour formation, or other diseased condition of the nasal mucous membrane; it may be due to fracture of a horn core in cattle and sheep, the blood entering the nose from the sinuses of the skull; in horses it may be seen in GUTTURAL POUCH DIPHTHERIA; and see 'BLEEDER HORSES'.

When the haemorrhage is only slight, little more than keeping the animal quiet, and applying douches of cold water to the bridge of the nose, will be required. A thin trickle of blood coming from one nostril only can be disregarded, as it will generally cease of its own accord. When the bleeding is very profuse, and there may be danger of collapse more drastic measures are needed. Where only one nostril is affected it should be plugged with swabs of cotton-wool enclosed in gauze, and so arranged that some of the gauze is left outside the nostril to allow of removal some hours afterwards. In other cases, where both nostrils are affected, injections of normal saline containing adrenaline, into each nostril may be carried out; or both nostrils may need to be

plugged after first having performed tracheotomy. These measures must be undertaken by a veterinary surgeon.

Tumours include polyps, especially in the cat; and adenocarcinoma in dogs and other animals.

Among other conditions in which the nose or the nasal passages are affected may be mentioned: fungal infections, tumours, mucosal disease, malignant catarrh, glanders, urticaria, purpura haemorrhagica, strangles, and influenza (*see* these headings, *also* INFECTIOUS GRANULOMA, RHINOSPORIDIOSIS, RHINOTRACHEITIS).

NOSOCOMIAL. Hospital-acquired. Human nosocomial infections, usually associated with medical or surgical interventions, affect about 5 to 6 per cent of hospital patients; i.e. about two million people in the USA alone, resulting in some six million excess hospital bed-days. About 1 per cent of the victims die. (Professor John M. Last, University of Ottawa, *World Health Forum* (1985) **62**, 135.)

NOSTRIL (*see* NOSE).

NOSTRIL FLIES, or the *Oestridae*, are members of the class of two-winged flies, whose larvae are parasitic in the nasal cavities, and in the air sinuses of the skull, of sheep. (*See* FLIES.)

NOTIFIABLE DISEASES are those which, when they break out upon farm premises, must be notified to the police or government department concerned. In Great Britain these diseases are:

Africa Horse Sickness
Anthrax
Aujeszky's disease
Bovine spongiform encephalopathy (BSE)
Bovine tuberculosis
Cattle plague (Rinderpest)
Contagious pleuropneumonia
Dourine
Enzootic bovine leukosis
Epizootic lymphangitis
Equine contagious metritis
Equine infectious anaemia
Equine encephalomyelitis
Foot-and-mouth disease
Fowl Pest
Glanders
Parasitic mange (horses)
Rabies
Sheep pox
Sheep scab
Swine fever
Swine vesicular disease
Teschen disease

(*See under* DISEASES OF ANIMALS ACT, for duties and responsibilities of animal-owners.)

Also notifiable are diseases of fish listed under FISH, DISEASES OF. ☛

NOTOEDRIC MANGE (*see under* MITES).

NOXYTHIOLIN. A drug useful where antibiotic-resistant organisms contaminate a wound. (*See* WOUNDS. last paragraph.)

NSAIDS. Non-steroidal anti-inflammatory drugs. Both their therapeutic and side-effects were described, together with their uses in dogs and cats, by Lees, P. & others. *Journal of Small Animal Practice* (1991) **32**, 183.

NUCLEAR MEDICINE. Involves the use of unsealed radioisotopes for diagnosis and therapy. (*See* RADIOISOTOPES.)

NUCLEAR WEAPONS (*see under* RADIOACTIVE FALL-OUT).

NUCLEIC ACIDS (*see* DNA and RIBONUCLEIC ACID (RNA)).

NUCLEIN is a protein substance containing phosphorus derived from the nuclei of cells.

NUCLEOTIDES (*see* RADIOISOTOPES.)

NUCLEUS means the central body in a cell which controls its activities. (*See* CELLS.)

NURSING OF SICK ANIMALS. The advent of qualified professional VETERINARY NURSES (which see) has been of great benefit to practising veterinary surgeons especially those engaged in small-animal practice and to their patients; and has facilitated measures for intensive care.

Nursing of small animals at home. The following notes are offered to owners. If your dog or cat has an infectious disease, nursing will have to be undertaken at home, since veterinary hospitals usually cannot accept such cases owing to the risk to other patients.

In other cases, after initial veterinary treatment, it is often preferable to have the animal at home for nursing. There is likely to be less stress for it is not sent or kept away from its familiar surroundings.

Accordingly, the following notes are offered to owners on the subject of home nursing.

A dog or cat which is ill, or recovering from an operation or accident, tends to seek solitude and require peace. Continual fussing and interference, however well meant, are to be avoided. (This is something which has to be impressed on children.)

Fresh air, warmth, and an absence of bright lights and noise (such as those emanating from a TV set) are desirable. A patient with eye inflammation, tetanus, or some other nervous system disorder, needs protection from bright light.

In many cases, it is helpful to put down old newspaper, which can be burnt after use. If a dog cannot go outside, a box of earth or ashes, or the material sold for cat trays may be useful too. An extra sanitary tray will be needed for an ill cat under these circumstances.

Constipation may be a problem. A little 'sardine oil' may be taken voluntarily. (Remember that a cat straining ineffectually over a litter tray may be trying to pass urine and not faeces.)

Temperature-taking often forms a part of animal nursing. Buy a clinical thermometer with a stout, stubby end, and lubricate the latter before passing it into the rectum. Cooking oil will serve for this purpose.

An improvised jacket, with holes for the front legs is useful in cases of bronchitis or pneumonia.

Never omit to wipe away the discharges from the eyes and nose of an ill animal.

It is sometimes difficult to keep an ill dog or cat clean. Any hair or fur which becomes soiled should be cut away, and the part washed.
FEEDING.

'Prescription diets'. These are specially formulated by Drs Mark L. Morris and Don D. Lewis to aid in the treatment of various canine and feline disorders, and are available both in canned or dry form – to be prescribed by veterinary surgeons.

Human invalid foods are often useful. Complan is an example. Build-Up (Carnation Foods) and Proteinaid (Veterinary Drug) are comparable veterinary specialities.

Do not force solid foods on a sick animal which, if suffering from a digestive upset, is usually better off without solid food for a day or two. (*See also under* VOMITING – last paragraph.) Variety is important in feeding the sick.

During convalescence the animal may be tempted to eat by offering small quantitites of warmed food such as meat jelly, minced liver or rabbit, or sardine.

Nursing of horses. The affected horse should be removed from its stall in the stable and placed in isolation. It should have plenty of bedding, be provided with clean water, and if the weather is cold it should be clothed with a rug. In cases where the horse is unable to stand, a specially thick straw bed should be given, and one or two bags filled with straw, or bales of hay, are useful to prop it up in an upright position on the breast. Horses that are down must be turned over on to the other side twice or thrice daily. The rectum and bladder may require evacuation artificially, if it does not occur naturally. If bed sores appear, they should be dressed twice daily with surgical spirit, and more bedding should be supplied. In respiratory diseases the most important factor in nursing is the adequate provision of fresh air. Small feeds should be offered several times daily, and when a horse refuses one type of food it should be offered another. Whenever the breathing is faster than normal drenching should be avoided.

Nursing of cattle. Isolate in a loose-box. Calves should be shut alone in a pen. The same conditions as to bedding, clothing, water, ventilation, etc., apply to cattle as well as to horses. Patient kindly treatment, the avoidance of all unnecessary fuss and haste, and a gentle firmness are essential.

A sick cow which refuses hay from a new ley will often eat hay from old pasture. Molasses may add palatability to food otherwise rejected; so may a little salt.

NUTRITION, FAULTY can lead to disease and losses of farm animals. Examples are nutritional muscular dystrophy (*see under* MUSCLES, DISEASES OF); blindness as a result of vitamin A deficiency (*see* EYE, DISEASES OF); poisoning by excessive fluorides in the diet (*see* FLUOROSIS); an all-muscle meat diet can lead to CANINE and FELINE JUVENILE OSTEODYSTROPHY. (*See also* 'ANGRY CAT POSTURE'.)

NUTRITIONAL MYOPATHY (*see* MUSCLES, DISEASES OF; PARALYTIC MYOGLOBINURIA; SUDDEN DEATH).

NUTTALLIA is the name given to a genus of piroplasms which cause biliary fever in horses in many parts of the world. There are two forms involved – *Babesia* (*Nuttallia*) *equi*, which is the smaller and more important, and *B.* (*Nuttallia*) *caballi*. Each is transmitted by one or more ticks. (*See* BABESIOSIS.)

'NUVAN TOP' (Ciba-Geigy's aerosol spray formulation contains 0·2 per cent dichlorvos and 0·8 per cent fenitrothion; for use against fleas, lice and other parasites on dogs and cats.

NUX VOMICA is the seed of the *Strychnos nux-vomica*, an East Indian tree. It has intensely bitter taste. The medicinal properties are due to two alkaloids – *strychnine* and *brucine*, which the plant contains. Brucine has an action similar to, though much weaker than, strychnine. (*See* STRYCHNINE.)

NYCTALOPIA or night-blindness. (*See* EYE, DISEASES OF.)

NYMPHOMANIA is associated with pathological changes, often of a cystic nature, in the ovaries. Hormone treatment may be tried under veterinary advice; or removing the ovaries by surgical measures, as early as possible after the erotic symptoms have made their appearance. (*See* OVARIES, DISEASES OF; HORMONE THERAPY.)

NYSTAGMUS is a condition in which the eyeballs show constant fine jerky movements of an involuntary nature.

O

OAK POISONING. Both the acorns and the leaves of the oak (*Quercus* sp.) may be dangerous when eaten by stock, but the leaves are usually harmless unless eaten in large quantities. In a Northumberland outbreak, however, in a herd of 40 Galloways, 6 cows died and 4 aborted. A taste for oak buds was acquired early in the year when trees were felled and keep was scarce. Felling went on until September, when symptoms (fever and scouring with blood-stained faeces) were first shown after one cow had aborted and died.

It is when there is a scarcity of food in pastures towards the end of very dry summers that symptoms of poisoning occur. The animals most affected are young store cattle.

Horses have been poisoned through eating either oak leaves or acorns.

It is well known that both pigs and sheep can eat acorns in small quantities without ill effects.
SIGNS. **Ruminants** that have eaten many acorns become dull, cease feeding, lie groaning, and appear to be in considerable pain. At first, there is severe constipation accompanied by straining and colicky pains, cessation of rumination, weakness of the pulse, and a temperature below normal. Later, small amounts of inky-black faeces are passed, and a blood-stained diarrhoea sets in. Great prostration is seen, and the animals die in from 3 to 7 days when large amounts have been eaten. In chronic cases there is always great loss of flesh, and death does not take place till weeks or months after the beginning of the symptoms.

Horses may not show signs of pain. The poisoned animal becomes weak and dull, has a subnormal temperature, may discharge food and saliva from its nostrils, show head-pressing, mouth ulcers, have reddish-brown urine, ataxia and convulsions.

Autopsy findings include a uraemic smell from the carcase, oedema and haemorrhages, and kidney lesions.
TREATMENT. Cattle should be given long hay. The animals should be made comfortable, plenty of bedding being provided. During convalescence, the animals require liberal feeding to make up the loss of flesh they have sustained.

OATS (*see* CEREALS, DIET; *and* HORSES, FEEDING OF).

OBESITY is an important condition in the dog, and may arise from over feeding, or an unsuitable diet, or from a hormone imbalance. Obesity is often associated with, and may predispose to, heart disease, arthritis, and some skin and respiratory disorders, as well as intolerance of heat. Old dogs need less carbohydrate and more protein in the diet.

Obesity is also a problem in cats, especially those which accept meals in two different households (*and see* OESTRUS SUPPRESSION).

OBSTETRICS (*see* PARTURITION, CALVING).

OCCIPUT is the uppermost posterior part of the head where it meets the neck. The occipital bone lies in the part of the skull which forms the occiput, and can be felt as a hard bony plate in most animals. Some of the neck muscles are attached to the occipital bone, and the powerful ligamentum nuchae, which is the main supporting structure of the head and neck, is inserted into the prominence that can be felt between the ears.

OCCUPATIONAL HAZARDS (*see* COWMEN, SHEPHERDS, ORF, PIGMEN, MEAT HANDLERS, ZOONOSES IN UK VETERINARIANS, NITROGEN DIOXIDE, SPOROTRICHOSIS, SALMONELLA, BUBONIC PLAGUE).

OCHRATOXIN A is a fungal toxin sometimes found in stored feeds and originating from *Penicillium viridicatum*, for example. Poisoning in pigs may result in thirst, enlarged kidneys, and polyuria. (*See* MYCOTOXINS.)

ODONTOMA is a tumour arising in tissues which normally produce teeth. They are encountered in horses and cattle in association with the roots (usually) of teeth, where they may appear either as rounded or irregular masses attached to an otherwise normal tooth (sometimes making extraction extremely difficult), or they may occur as large, irregular, solid masses replacing the greater part of a normal tooth and causing a swelling on the side of the jaw. They are usually extremely dense and difficult to cut.

A so-called 'temporal odontoma' is a tumour, not uncommon in horses, about the size of a bantam's egg occurring in connection with the temporal bones. These tumours generally have an opening to the surface of the skin just below, or just in front of, the base of the ear. They contain one or two large, or many (sometimes over 100) small, imperfectly formed teeth enclosed in a single fibrous capsule.

OEDEMA is an accumulation of exudate in one or more of the body cavities, or beneath the skin.

A normal, physiological form of oedema affecting the region of the mammary glands occurs in cows and mares shortly before parturition, and disappears within a day or two afterwards.

Otherwise, oedema is a pathological condition. When affecting tissue spaces immediately below the skin, it is usually due to a local disturbance of circulation or it may arise through weak heart action, and is not uncommon following debilitating diseases or in old age. Oedema of the lungs occurs in an animal exposed to smoke in a burning building, parasitic bronchitis and as the result of an allergy (*e.g.* milk allergy, and SWEET-POTATO POISONING). Oedema involving the brisket or under the jaw may be a sign of severe liver-fluke infestation in sheep or cattle. (*See also* PARAQUAT.)

Oedema affecting the abdomen is also known as *ascites* and may give rise to a visible swelling or 'pot-bellied' appearance. It is seen in cases of tuberculosis in the dog and cat especially, and may also result from disease of heart, liver or kidneys, and sometimes accompanies diabetes. It may be associated with parasites such as liver-flukes.

Excessive fluid in the chest is also known as *hydrothorax*, which may be associated with, for example, chronic pleurisy.

Oedema is a symptom rather than a disease, and accordingly treatment must be directed at the cause. If due to parasites, the appropriate anthelmintic must be used. Heart tonics may be indicated, or diuretics, or both. 'Tapping' the chest, *i.e.* aspiration of the fluid, may be indicated but will not alone effect a permanent improvement. If tuberculosis is diagnosed, immediate destruction on public health grounds is called for. (*See also* BOWEL OEDEMA.)

OEDEMA, MALIGNANT (*see* GAS GANGRENE).

OESOPHAGEAL GROOVE. Reflex closure of this groove is desirable when administering certain drugs as otherwise they pass into the rumen instead of the abomasum. Copper sulphate solution is used as a closure stimulant.

OESOPHAGOSTOMIASIS. Infestation with *Oesophagostomum* worms. In calves, there is a reduced intake of food for several weeks; anaemia, and diarrhoea. In goats, peritonitis has been recorded in India. In pigs, these worms may be important in the causation of NECROTIC ENTERITIS (which see). Third-stage larvae of these (and also *Ostertagia*) worms have been found clinging to psychodid flies cultured from pig faeces. Larvae have also been recovered from flies caught near a field in which pigs were grazing. It is possible that rats may also transmit larvae from farm to farm. (*See also* THIN SOW SYNDROME *and under* ROUNDWORMS.)

OESOPHAGOTOMY. A surgical operation involving incision of the oesophagus for removal of a foreign body, etc.

OESOPHAGUS. Passage from throat to stomach. Food passes down from the mouth to the stomach by the process of PERISTALSIS (which see).

Oesophagus, diseases of. In the tropics stricture of the oesophagus in dogs and cats is caused by *Spirocerca lupi* larvae.

Stricture has also followed anaesthesia in people and cats; the suggested cause being a reflux of gastric fluid causing oesophagitis. Signs may appear as long as 50 days after the anaesthetisation.

A balloon oesophageal dilator has been used to relieve some cases of stricture. (*See also under* CHOKING.)

OESTRADIOL and OESTRONE are hormones

secreted by the ovary (interstitial cells and Graafian follicles) which bring about oestrus and, in late pregnancy, stimulate development of the mammary gland. The early conceptus synthesises oestrogens. In dairy cattle these are secreted in the whey fraction of the milk as oestrone sulphate – (*See* PREGNANCY DIAGNOSIS TESTS.)

OESTRIN (*see* HORMONES).

OESTROGENS. Hormones, either of natural origin or prepared synthetically, which have the effect of inducing oestrus. (*See under* HORMONES.) Pasture oestrogens may cause infertility and sometimes abortion. (*See* INFERTILITY *and* HORMONES IN MEAT PRODUCTION, *and under* OESTRADIOL.)

OESTRUS. 'Season', or 'Heat', is the period during which the female shows desire for the male, and during which oestrogens from the Graäfian follicle are circulating in the blood-stream. Oestrus precedes, or may coincide with, ovulation – rupture of the follicle and release of the ovum which passes into the top of the Fallopian tube. (*See* OVULATION, PHEROMONES.)

The oestrous cycles in animals vary in different species and in different breeds, and to some extent in different individuals.

Mare. She is a polyoestrous animal with a breeding season during spring and summer. 'In the British Isles most mares first show normal oestrous cycles in mid-April, the frequency of ovulation is greatest in late July, and oestrous cyclical activity is at its lowest in early February. In the northern hemisphere the arbitrary covering season from mid-February to mid-July does not fully coincide with the natural breeding season and most non-pregnant mares are thereby condemned to a restricted period of little more than two months in which ovarian activity is sufficient to provide opportunities for conception.' (Dr W. R. Allen, *Vet. Rec.* (1977) **100,** 68.)

During the oestral period the mare behaves unusually. She may become irritable or sluggish, and is easily tired. Her appetite is capricious and she may lean against the stall partition when in the stable. If her flanks are accidentally touched she may squeal or kick. The clitoris is frequently raised and there is usually a discharge of some amount of slimy mucus from the vulva. Urine may be passed at frequent intervals. She shows a strong desire for the society of the male – even occasionally for that of the usually scorned gelding. Occasionally hysteria may be seen when the animal becomes quite unmanageable.

Cow. The oestrous cycle is controlled by complex interactions among higher brain centres, the hypothalamus, anterior pituitary gland, ovary and uterus. Higher brain centres mediate responses to light, temperature, pheromones, and other stimuli which exert their effects through the central nervous system. The most important hormone, in regulating the oestrous cycle, is gonadotrophin-releasing hormone (GnR H). (Britt, J. H., North Carolina University.)

OESTROUS TABLE

Animal	Time of year	Periodicity of Oestrus	Duration	First occurrence after parturition
Mare	Feb. to July	21 days (14 to 28 days or more)	2 to 8 days	3 to 12 days; service on 9th day often successful
Cow	All year; most intense midsummer	20 days (16 to 24 days or more)	4 to 24 hours	30 to 60 days (see below)*
Ewe	End of Aug. till Jan., depending on breed and district	16 to 17 days (10 to 21 days)	1 to 2 days	(See below)†
Sow	Oct. to Nov. and Apr. to June	21 days (15 to 30 days)	1 to 3 days	8 weeks after farrowing, or 1 week after weaning of litter
Bitch	Usually Dec. to Feb., and in spring	Once only during each period	9 to 18 days	(See below)‡
Cat	Jan. onwards for 8 to 10 months (if unmated) Oestrus may recur every 2 or 3 weeks.		7 to 14days	

* In the cow that is suckling a calf it is seldom that oestrus occurs until after weaning, when its appearance is somewhat variable, but often on 3rd to 12th day.

† With the exception of ewes of the Dorset Horn breed, which comes into season twice a year, and can rear two crops of lambs per year, sheep only show season in the autumn. It depends upon the breed as to how soon the rams may be put out with the flock. Generally speaking, the more low-lying the district and the milder the climate the earlier the ewes come into season; thus Suffolks are served from August till the end of September, and lamb from January till March. Mountain breeds are served from November till January, and lamb in April, May, and June.

‡ The bitch usually comes in season twice a year, but great variation takes place with the smaller toy breeds. Bitches of the Basenji breed (and a few individuals of other breeds) have only one 'heat' period per year.

She mounts her fellows or stands to be mounted by them. She may bellow and race about with tail raised, or break out of a field in search of a bull. In other instances, signs are so slight as to be missed by the cowman. (See OESTRUS, DETECTION OF.) Both cows and heifers in milk usually give less milk during the oestral period than in the intervals. (See CALVING, EARLIER, INFERTILITY.)

Goat. Rapid side-to-side and up-and-down tail movements may be seen. the animal is restless and bleats. Oestrous occurs every 19–21 days during the autumn, and lasts 12–48 hours.

Sow. The sow becomes torpid and lazy, and when asked to move often grunts in a peculiar whining manner. If housed with others she behaves like the cow – mounting or being mounted. The vulva is usually distinctly swollen, and there is sometimes a blood-stained discharge. Oestrus in the sow lasts up to 60 hours and

ovulation begins at 34 to 50 hours after its onset, the process taking up to 5 hours. The sow will accept service between 15 and 35 hours after the onset of oestrus, with the optimum at 25 to 35 hours.

Bitch. She wanders away from home unless confined, and the odour of her blood-stained vaginal discharge attracts male followers. As bleeding from the vulva is slight in some bitches, especially at their first oestrus, owners should watch for swelling of the vulva. During the 7–9 days of *pro-oestrus*, the bitch will flirt with a dog but not accept him. Usually it is only during the last week of 'heat' that the bitch will accept the dog, usually between the 10th and 12th days.

Cat. The signs may suggest pain and/or a strong desire to have her back and flanks rubbed or scratched. She will roll over and over on carpet or floor, rub herself against furniture, etc., and emit little pleased mews.

THE SEXUAL CYCLE

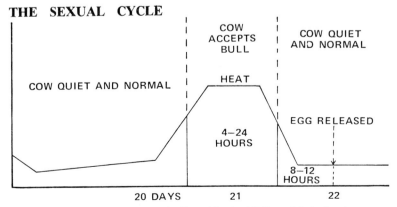

(With acknowledgements to the East of Scotland College of Agriculture.)

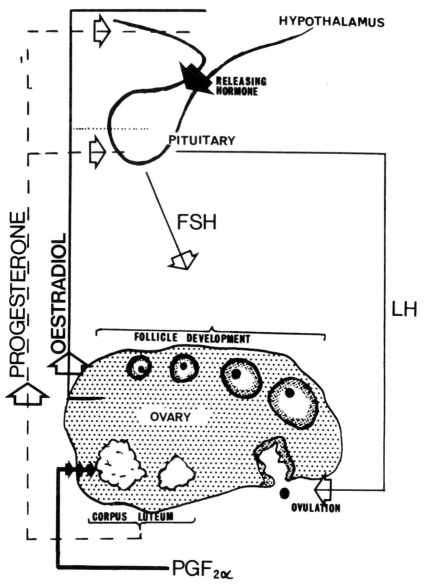

Endocrine interactions controlling normal oestrous cycle. (With acknowledgements to Dr J. M. Chesworth.)

The first oestrus may be expected between the ages of six and eight months. However, it may occur as early as 3½ months, or occasionally be delayed until the queen is about a year old.

OESTRUS, DETECTION OF, IN COWS.
Especially in winter, detection of oestrus is not as easy as might be thought. Studies in the USA suggest that where cows are watched 4-hourly round the clock, the efficiency of heat detection should be around 95 per cent, but in a herd where cows are seen only twice per day, the percentage is likely to drop to around 74 per cent.

These figures would appear to be over-optimistic, however. In Britain Dr D. B. Harker, of ICI, has stated that the average oestrus detection rate among dairy farmers is about 55 per cent. This is a gloomy figure when one considers that 'the

average calving figure of our four million dairy cows is 30 days longer than experts say it should be, with each of these days representing a net waste of about £1'. (1980 figure.)

Part of the problem is that while 'bulling lasts 12 hours on average it may last only one hour; and as to the timing, 50 per cent of the displays occur at night. Moreover some cows may stand only once in 20 minutes; others will stand only for favourites; and some aggressive cows mount other cattle at a crowded trough in order to induce them to move aside to create a space.'

Sometimes a cow is seen to mount another from the front. This is valuable evidence of oestrus, but it is important to remember that it is the riding cow which is bulling, not the one underneath.

The importance of pin-pointing heat dates cannot be over emphasised. Only by record

HOURS

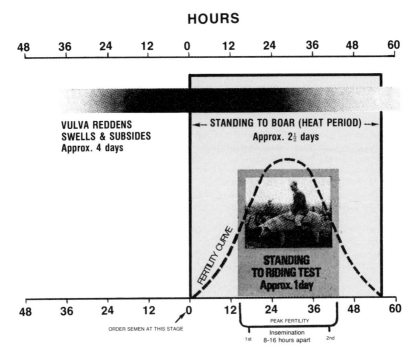

A guide to insemination time (with acknowledgements to the MLC).

keeping is it possible to identify animals that are not coming in heat at the normal time; in addition to those which are cycling (coming in heat) irregularly. Delay in seeking veterinary advice may lead to delay in conception.

As an aid to herd management, a VASECTOMISED (which see) bull may be used, or a heat detection device may be placed on a cow's back, liberating a dye when she is mounted. ICI's Tel-Tail paste can prove especially helpful in avoiding missed oestrus. 'This can account for 10–16 per cent of

sub-fertility even in well managed herds' – Professor Lamming. (*See* *also* 'CONTROLLED BREEDING'.)

OESTRUS, SUPPRESSION OF. Bitches and cats may be prevented from coming 'on heat' by oral dosing with the synthetic equivalent of a naturally occurring hormone, *e.g.*, MEGESTROL ACETATE.)

The latter is marketed by Glaxo under the name 'Ovarid', and is widely used. To quote the

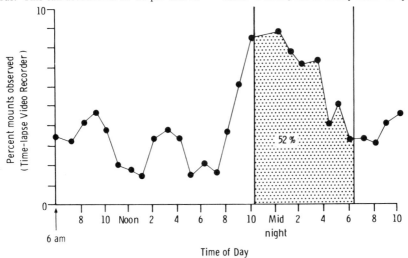

D.B. Harker. Adapted from Hurnik and others (1975): Applied Animal Ethology 2, 55-68

Oestrus in the cow. Mounting activity over 24 hours. Composite of 2880 cow-days. (36 adult Holstein cattle.) With acknowledgements to Dr J. Frank Hurnik, University of Guelph, Canada, and to Dr D. B. Harker of ICI's Animal Health Department.

manufacturers, 'The vast majority of cats can be safely medicated with Ovarid, but some are not suitable candidates, *e.g.* those with genital disease or diabetes.'

As owners cannot tell by glancing at it whether a cat has diabetes or not – nor metritis, for that matter – some cats being dosed with Ovarid will be receiving it against the manufacturers' advice. The latter also states that Ovarid may be given for '*up to* 18 months'. So owners using it for longer will again be acting against advice.

Two possible side-effects from overdosage or prolonged dosage are mentioned by the manufacturers; one involving the uterus, the other being hypertrophy of the mammary glands. The latter is not a serious condition, and the glands are likely to return to their normal size after dosing has ceased.

When dealing with colonies of semi-wild cats, Ovarid can be useful as a stop-gap measure to spread the cost of spaying over a period. Ovarid can also be of service when a stray cat has been rescued and found to be in poor condition, and in need of care and good feeding before it can attain a state of health sufficient to withstand anaesthesia and spaying.

Some progestogens can cause pathological changes in the uterus, induce abnormal levels of growth hormone, suppress cortisol levels, and possibly increase the risk of mammary tumours. So in some cases spaying may be preferable. (Evans, J. M. *J. Small Animal Practice* (1988) **29**, 535.)

OFFALS (*see* WEATINGS).

O.I.E. (*see* ORGANISATION INTERNATIONALE DES EPIZOOTIES).

OILFIELD HAZARDS, POISONING. In the USA about 500 cases of suspected poisoning by oilfields wastes are investigated each year at the Oklahoma animal disease diagnostic laboratory. 'Most of these cases present the potential for litigation,' Dr William C. Edwards commented.

Hazards arise from the ingestion by cattle of petroleum hydrocarbons, salt water, heavy metals, chemicals stored on site, and rubbish such as discarded soda bags. A quantity of lead-based pipe-jointing material is used, and also chemicals to treat the mud which lubricates the drilling bit.

Signs of poisoning include weight loss and unthriftiness. A differential diagnosis has to take into account the possibility of internal parasites, faulty nutrition, or other causes of debility; but standard analytical methods make it relatively easy to detect the ingested poisons.

The presence of petroleum in lung tissue and in rumen contents is frequently confirmed. Liver and kidney lesions may be found. (Edwards, W. C., *Veterinary Medicine* (1985) **80**, 98.)

OILS are divided into *fixed oils*, which are of the nature of liquid fats, and are derived by expression from nuts, seeds, etc., and *volatile* or *essential oils*, which are obtained by distillation. Examples are the oils of aniseed, cajaput, eucalyptus, peppermint, and turpentine. (*See also* PARAFFIN.)

OILSEED RAPE. Horses grazing in fields adjacent to this crop are at risk of developing respiratory disease.

OLAQUINDOX. The active ingredient of ICI's growth promoter Fedan. (*See* ADDITIVES.)

OLDENBURG. A breed of sheep native to the Hamburg Marshes, West Germany. Fleece weights up to 14 lb and lambing percentages of 170–80 are claimed.

OLFACTORY NERVE, or the NERVE OF SMELL, is the first of the cranial nerves.

OLIGURIA. A diminution in the amount of urine excreted. (*See* URINE.)

OLLULANUS (*see* WORMS in cats).

OMASUM, or 'Many-plies', is the name given to the third stomach of ruminants. It is situated on the right side of the abdomen at a higher level than the fourth stomach and between this latter and the second stomach, with both of which it communicates. From its inner surface project large numbers of leaves or *folia*, each of which possesses roughened surfaces. In the centre of each folium is a band of muscle fibres which produces a rasping movement of the leaf when it contracts. One leaf rubs against those on either side of it, and large particles of food material are ground down between the rough surfaces, preparatory to further digestion in the succeeding parts of the alimentary canal.

Studies at the ARC's National Institute for Research in Dairying have shown 'massive exchanges of water and solutes in the omasum of the steer. The organ appears to be the main site of magnesium absorption, and it is probably here that the cause of clinical hypomagnesaemia should be sought.'

OMENTUM is a fold of peritoneum which passes from the stomach to some other organ. There are several such folds, but the most important is that which passes to the terminal part of the large colon and the beginning of the small colon, and which is called the **great omentum.** This does not run direct to the colon from the stomach, but forms a loose sac occupying the spaces between other organs in the abdomen. In health, there is always a considerable amount of fat deposited in the folds of the great omentum, and this, in the ox, sheep, and pig forms part of the suet of commerce.

In the dog the great omentum lies between the abdominal organs and the lower abdominal wall, and acts as a kind of protective bed which supports the intestines, etc.

OMPHALITIS. 'Navel ill.'

OMPHALITIS OF BIRDS. Infection of the yolk sack, by bacteria found in the alimentary canal and on the skin of the hen, leads to the death of embryos and chicks. These bacteria may be relatively non-pathogenic elsewhere than in the yolk. The disease occurs where hygiene is bad, and takes two forms: 'Mushy Chick' disease (with deaths occurring up to 10 days after hatching), and a true omphalitis or 'navel ill'.

OMPHALO-PHLEBITIS means inflammation of the umbilical vein. It occurs in young animals and is commonly present in the early stages of navel ill.

OMSK FEVER. The cause of this is related to the Russian Spring–Summer Virus (which see), but is more serious in its effects and is spread by the tick *Dermacentor pictus.*

ONCHOCERCIASIS. Infestation with worms belonging to the class *Onchocerca*. (See ROUND WORMS.)

ONCOGENE. A gene associated with tumour formation. (See CANCER.)
   The determination of the protein encoded by the *ras* oncogene has helped to explain how genes of this kind cause cancer.
   The *ras* protein is part of the system on the cell surface that transmits signals from growth factors in the interior of the cell. In its mutated, oncogenetically coded form, the signal is locked in the 'on' position, so causing unrestrained growth. (*BMJ Science* (1988) **239**, 63.)

ONCOGENIC. Giving rise to tumour formation.

ONCOLOGY. The study of tumours.

ONCORNAVIRUSES are those which give rise to tumours; e.g. the feline leukaemia virus, the Rous sarcoma virus. (See CANCER, RETROVIRIDAE.)

ONDIRI DISEASE (*see* BOVINE INFECTIOUS PETECHIAL FEVER).

ONION POISONING. The toxic effects of onions have been seen in cattle, sheep, horses and dogs.
   The toxic principle is a pungent volatile oil, n-propyl disulphide. This gives rise to Heinz bodies, and red blood cells which contain them are removed by the reticulo-endothethelial system; giving rise to anaemia.
SIGNS. Inappetance, tachycardia, staggering, jaundice, haemoglobinuria, collapse, and sometimes death.

'ONTARIO ENCEPHALITIS'. A disease of piglets, as young as 4–7 days, ending in a fatal encephalitis, and caused by a virus. (See ENCEPHALOMYELITIS, VIRAL, OF PIGS.)

ONYCHETOMY. De-clawing.

ONYCHIA is an inflammation affecting the nails or claws of animals. (See NAILS, DISEASES OF.)

ONYCHOMYCOSIS. Infection of the claw with a fungus. In cats *Microsporum canis* Bodin infection is not uncommon. (See RINGWORM.)

OOCYTE. An immature ovum.

OOPHORECTOMY (*see* SPAYING.)

OOPHORITIS is another name for ovaritis or inflammation of an ovary.

OPEN JOINTS (*see* JOINTS, DISEASE OF).

'OPENING THE HEELS' means the cutting of the horn at the angles of the heels of the horse's foot, by which the continuity between the horn of the wall and of the bar on either side of the foot is destroyed. It is performed by some blacksmiths and owners in the hope that it will allow the heels to expand and so produce a 'fine open foot'. Actually, the operation results in an interference with the shock absorptive mechanism of the foot, and eventually produces *contraction* of the heels. It is by no means to be recommended. (See FOOT OF HORSE.)

OPHTHALMIA means inflammation of the whole of the structures of the eye, but is sometimes restricted to mean keratitis. Contagious Ophthalmia is caused by *Richettsia conjunctivae* in sheep, and by *Moraxella bovis* in cattle. Verminous ophthalmia also occurs in cattle. (See EYES, DISEASES OF.)

OPHTHALMOSCOPE is an instrument used for the examination of the back of the eye.

OPIOIDS. Endogenous opioids in the central nervous system, the *encephalins* and *endorphins*, are able to modify the perception of pain.

OPISTHOTONOS is the position assumed by the back-bone during one of the convulsive seizures of tetanus, and also sometimes seen during epileptiform convulsions and strychnine poisoning. The spinal column is markedly arched with the concavity facing upwards away from the lower parts of the body, so that the head is drawn backwards, and the tail and hind parts of the body are pulled forwards. The condition is due to the spasmodic contraction of the powerful muscles lying above the vertebral column. (*See also* 'BERENIL' poisoning.)

OPIUM is the dried milky juice of the unripe seed-capsules of the White Indian Poppy – *Papaver somniferum*. Good opium should contain about 10 per cent of *morphine*, the chief alkaloid and active principle. It also contains other alkaloids, the most important of which are *codeine, narcotine, thebaine, papaverine, apomorphine.*
   The preparations of opium used in veterinary medicine are now virtually nil, but have included the following: (1) Powdered opium, which is the dried juice powdered, contains about 9·5 per cent to 10·5 per cent morphine. (2) Tincture of opium, or 'laudanum', consists of the powder treated with distilled water and alcohol, and contains about 1 per cent of morphine. (3) Opium extracts, one dry of 20 per cent morphine, and one liquid of 3 per cent morphine, as well as a fluid extract which contains about 5 per cent morphine. (4) Compound tincture of camphor, or 'Paregoric'. (5) Compound ipecacuanha powder, or 'Dover's

Powder', contains 10 per cent of opium. (6) Gall and opium ointment, containing 7·5 per cent of opium, is used as an astringent ointment. (7) Compound tincture of morphine and chloroform which contained morphine, chloroform, dilute prussic acid, as well as Indian hemp and capsicum, is similar to the proprietary mixtures which are called 'Chlorodyne'. Morphine, codeine, apomorphine, heroin, and dionin are also preparations from or derivatives of opium. (*See* MORPHINE.)

OPSONINS. Substances present in blood serum which facilitate the engulfment of bacteria (and other foreign proteins) by certain white cells. (*See* PHAGOCYTOSIS.)

OPTIC NERVE is the second cranial nerve running from the eye to the base of the brain. It conveys the sensations of light that are received by the retina, and registers them in the optic centres of the brain. (*See* EYE, VISION.)

ORBIT is the eye socket.

ORBITAL GLAND (*see* HARDERIAN GLAND *and* EYE, DISEASES OF).

ORCHARDS. Animals grazing in orchards may run the risk of poisoning if fruit-trees have recently been sprayed with copper or lead-arsenate insecticides or fungicides. Orchards, like paddocks, sometimes become a reservoir of parasitic worm larvae. (*See* PADDOCKS; *also* ALCOHOL POISONING.)

ORCHITIS. Inflammation of the TESTICLE.

'OREGON MUSCLE DISEASE'. This occurs in turkeys and chickens. The breast muscles become necrotic and greenish. The cause is possibly an inherited abnormality affecting the blood vessels.

ORF. A disease of sheep, cattle, and goats which has a very wide distribution and many names. Among its numerous designations are the following: 'Ulcerative stomatitis'; 'Contagious pustular dermatitis'; 'Contagious ecthyma'; 'Necrobacillosis of sheep'; etc.

It is enzootic in the Border counties of England and Scotland, but outbreaks may arise in any county in Great Britain, as well as in Germany, France, Austria, the United States of America, and other sheep countries. It was described as long ago as 1745.

The disease attacks sheep of all ages, sexes, and breeds; and kept under all conditions of management. It very frequently attacks lambs just before or after weaning, or after docking or castration, and from them it may spread to the teats of the ewes. In other cases it is common among gimmers until they are one year old.

CAUSES. Essentially a Parapoxvirus; but secondarily *Fusiformis necrophorus* (*Fusobacterium*). The virus is needed to produce pox-like lesions first, which the necrosis organism then invades.

SIGNS. In the milder form of the disease vesicles, followed by ulcers, appear on the lips – especially at the corners of the mouth. Sometimes healing takes place uneventfully; in other cases verrucose masses form and persist. The animal loses weight.

In the severe form the inside of the mouth becomes involved in most cases, and in addition other parts of the body such as the vulva and the skin of the face, legs, tail, etc. A greyish-black crust often appears which, if removed, leaves a raw, angry-looking surface.

Sheep with lesions on the head frequently rub their muzzles on their fore-feet, or scratch at their heads with their hind-feet. In this way the feet and legs often become affected. Abscesses may form in the region of the coronet. The sheep becomes extremely lame, so much so that it is frequently unable to put the affected leg to the ground, and hobbles about on three legs. If both fore-feet are affected – which is commonly the case – the animal may be observed feeding from a kneeling position. In severe cases the horn separates from the sensitive structures below, large quantities of foul-smelling thick pus are produced, and the hoof may be shed. The space between the claws, and the parts around the front and sides of the coronets, are the commonest situations of the lesions.

Less commonly the external genitals of both male and female are affected. (*See also* BALANOPOSTHITIS on page 441.)

TREATMENT. As soon as a case of orf appears among a flock of sheep it should be isolated at once. Isolated sheep that are already affected usually do best when they can be shut up indoors, given hand feeding, and provided with clean dry litter. A dressing is applied over the raw ulcerated area and around its margin. Crystal violet is very suitable as a dressing, and antibiotics are useful in treatment.

On farms previously heavily infected, and where orf was very common on the feet, passing the whole of the sheep through a foot-bath at 3-weekly intervals has resulted in a complete disappearance of the disease. (*See* FOOT-BATHS FOR SHEEP.)

Infected sheep after recovery should not be put out with the healthy flock until 2 weeks after the lesions have healed, and it is always advisable to dip them first.

The shepherd, or the attendant who treats the affected sheep, should ensure that he does not carry infection from one sheep to another by contamination of his clothes or hands. He ought always to wash in some disinfectant immediately after attending to cases of orf, since his hands and arms may become affected with orf. Indeed, orf is well recognised as an occupational hazard of shepherds.

CONTROL. A vaccine is available.

Orf in the dog. An outbreak of orf in a pack of hounds was reported in 1970 (*Veterinary Record*, **87,** 766), and was characterised by circular areas of acute inflammation, with a moist appearance, ulceration and scab formation.

Public health. Between 1975 and 1981 there were

344 laboratory reports of patients with Orf lesions in Britain. Contact with live sheep or lambs was reported 142 times. In 49 cases the people affected were abattoir workers, butchers, or domestic meat handlers. The possible source in 36 patients (including 13 milkers) was contact with cows or calves. Sixteen patients were farmers; seven were veterinary surgeons or veterinary students. (Communicable Disease Surveillance Centre. *British Medical Journal* (1982) **1**, 1958).

Severe mouth lesions have been successfully treated by DIATHERMY and CRYOSURGERY (which see).

ORGANELLES (*see* CELL).

ORGANIC DISEASES, as distinct from 'functional diseases', are those in which some actual alteration in structure takes place, as the direct result of which faulty action of the organ or tissue concerned, follows.

ORGANISATION INTERNATIONALE DES EPIZOOTIES (OIE) was set up in 1924 following the realisation that joint action between countries was necessary to control contagious animal diseases especially when animals were being transported in large numbers over considerable distances.

ORGANO-CHLORINE POISONING (*see* CHLORINATED HYDROCARBONS).

ORGANO-PHOSPHORUS POISONING. This may arise from contamination of crops, or other food material, with organic-phosphorus insecticides such as dimethoate, schradan, parathion, or dimefox.

For a case of laryngeal paralysis arising from organo-phosphorus poisoning of racehorses, *see under* LARYNX, DISEASES OF.
TREATMENT. Atrophine sulphate given intravenously or intra-muscularly, and repeated in 30 minutes. Barbiturates may be needed to control excitement. Oxygen for distressed breathing and gastric lavage are recommended in the human subject. In the latter, PAM has been recommended as an antidote to parathion and other insecticides in this group – in conjunction with atropine.

ORIFICES, IMMUNITY AT. Dr K. G. Hibbitt has referred to the defence mechanisms, directed against the invasion of pathogenic bacteria, which exist in the natural orifices of the body. For example, research at Compton led to the isolation of a number of cationic proteins from the keratin of the teat canal's lining, and these have been shown to inhibit the growth of mastitis strains of staphylococci and streptococci. These proteins, which are soluble in distilled water and carry a positive electrical charge, were shown to inhibit the growth of two strains of *Staphylococcus aureus* and one strain of *Streptococcus agalactiae*. The proteins in very low concentration caused a 50 per cent mortality in the test bacterial cultures.

The secretions of the uterine cervix of the cow during oestrus also contain cationic proteins which possess antibacterial activity against staphylococci. In the laboratory these proteins were shown also to inhibit growth of *Brucella abortus*.

The anionic proteins from the cervical mucus, however, showed no inhibitory action on the bacteria. This difference 'suggested that the killing of the bacteria was preceded by an electrovalent binding of the positively charged cationic protein on to the negatively charged surface of the bacteria', and this has proved to be the case.

Antibacterial cationic proteins have also been isolated from cells normally present in cow's milk, and research has shown that synthesis of these proteins can be stimulated. Induction of a mild sterile mastitis by the injection of *E. coli* endotoxin through the teat canal led to increased numbers of neutrophils in the milk from which was extracted cationic proteins with a higher antibacterial activity.

ORNITHOSIS. The name for *Chlamydia psittaci* infection in birds other than those of the parrot family, in which it is called Psittacosis. (*See* CHLAMYDIA.)

In the UK ornithosis is common in pigeons.

ORTHOPOX VIRUSES. This genus contains those pox viruses genetically and antigenetically related to smallpox virus. (*See* VIRUSES table.)

OS. The Latin word for a bone. Examples: *Os cordis*, a bone (one of two) present in the hearts of cattle; *Os penis* in the dog.

OSSIFICATION means the formation of bone tissue. In early life the bones are represented by cartilage or fibrous tissue, and in these, centres appear in which the cells undergo a change and lime salts are deposited. This process proceeds until the areas or centres meet each other, and the tissue is wholly converted into bone. When a fracture occurs, the bone unites by ossification of the blood-clot which forms between the broken ends of the bone. (*See* FRACTURES.) In old age, ossification takes place in parts where normally there are cartilages found, such as in the larynx, in the rib-cartilages, in the scapular cartilages, etc., and these parts lose their normal elasticity and become easily broken. (*See* SIDE-BONES.)

OSTEITIS or OSTITIS (*see* BONE, DISEASES OF).

OSTEOARTHRITIS/OSTEOARTHROSIS. In human medicine, the name Osteoarthrosis is now preferred, and 'emphasises the currently held view that this is a degenerative rather than an inflammatory disease'. (L. E. Glynn, *Lancet*, March 12, 1977.) 'The primary disturbance is generally regarded as occurring in articular cartilage, and as resulting from a combination of ageing and mechanical factors.' An alternative hypothesis is that it begins in the synovial lining cells.

OSTEOCHONDRITIS. Inflammation of bone

and cartilage. (*See* HIP DYSPLASIA.) Osteochondritis dissecans is characterised by separation of a piece of articular cartilage which, together with a small piece of underlying bone, forms a loose body within a joint.

OSTEOCHONDROSIS. This is similar in some respects to Osteochondritis, and may be a more accurate description in cases where there is no inflammatory response to the changes in bone and cartilage. There may be necrosis of bone and separation of splinters or flaps of articular cartilage. A hereditary basis for the condition has been recorded in man, horse, dog, and pig.

In young horses, the most frequently diagnosed conditions are *osteochondrosis dissecans* and a subchondral bone cyst. These are two separate entities, though often bracketed together under the osteochondrosis syndrome. Severe lameness may be caused by the former, and surgical treatment needed. (Animal Health Trust.)

OSTEOCLASTS. Cells which aid the breakdown or resorption of excess bony tissue, laid down following fractures, as part of the repair process.

OSTEODYSTROPHIC diseases (*see under* BONE, DISEASES OF). An example is **Osteodystrophia fibrosa**, a nutritional disease caused by mineral or vitamin deficiencies, occurring in cats, dogs, horses, goats, and pigs. In goats lesions may be confined to the jaws, in which there is rarefaction and softening of the bone.

OSTEOMALACIA is the equivalent of rickets occurring in the adult animal. The bones become softened as the result of the absorption of the salts they contain. The cause of the disease is obscure, but it appears to be more common in pregnant females than in other animals, and it may be associated with a deficiency of vitamin D and/or phosphates. (*See* VITAMINS.)

The most serious feature is the deformity which occurs in the softened bones, owing either to the weight of the body or to the pull of the muscles upon them. When the deformity is located in the pelvis of the dam, great difficulty is often experienced at the birth of the young animal, and fractures of this part are not unknown.
TREATMENT: Give vitamin D and good nourishing food with an adequate phosphate content.

OSTEOMYELITIS. Inflammation and infection of the bone-marrow. It is sometimes a complication of atrophic rhinitis of pigs and of actinomycosis of cattle. (*See* BONE, DISEASES OF.)

OSTEOPENIA. A reduction in the body's bone tissue.

OSTEOPETROSIS, or MARBLE BONE DISEASE is characterised by thickening of the legs of poultry. (*See* illustration.)

OSTEOPHAGIA means bone eating, and is a symptom shown by sheep and cattle in certain parts of South Africa which are deficient in phosphorus and sometimes in calcium in soil and herbage. (*See* LAMZIEKTE.)

Deer living wild in forests where there is a similar deficiency, as in many parts of the Scottish Highlands, exhibit osteophagia by chewing and actually eating portions of shed antlers. Sheep exhibit similar tendencies in the same areas.

OSTEOPOROSIS is a rarefying condition of bones which lose much of their mineral matter and become fragile and often deformed. It occurs in OSTEOMALACIA and OSTEOFIBROSIS.

OSTERTAGIASIS. Infestation with species of Ostertagia worms, which produce gastroenteritis. It is seen in calves and lambs. This is an important disease in Ireland. (*See* WORMS, FARM TREATMENT.)

OSTRICH (*Struthio camelus*). There has been a revival of interest in ostrich farming. Ostrich meat is low in cholesterol, and fetches good prices; as do the feathers. The round, melon-sized eggs are marketable.

Ostriches pass urine – unique in a bird.

The shaded areas of the drawing show sites suggested for the administration of 'Immobilon' by PROJECTILE SYRINGE (which see).

An ostrich can run at a speed of 40 m.p.h.

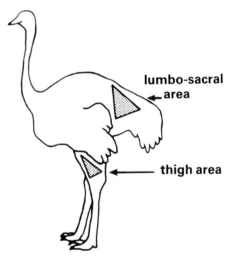

Darting sites suggested for ostriches

OTITIS means inflammation of the ear. (*See* EAR, DISEASES OF.)

OTODECTES. Mites which cause ear mange in dogs and cats. (*See* MITES.)

OTORRHOEA means a discharge from the ear. (*See* EAR, DISEASES OF.)

'OULOU FATO'. A form of rabies occurring among dogs in parts of Africa, and probably Asia also. People are rarely bitten, epidemics are uncommon, infected dogs may show either no symptoms, or transient symptoms followed by recovery. Repeated attacks prove fatal, however.

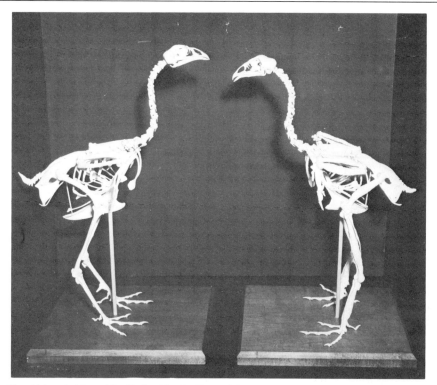

Two chicken skeletons at the Regional Poultry Research Laboratory at East Lansing, Michigan. One (left) is the skeleton of a 216-day-old normal White Leghorn cockerel. The other is the skeleton of a 202-day-old White Leghorn cockerel affected with osteopetrosis, a disease that causes an enlargement and hardening of the bones. (With acknowledgements to USDA, photograph by Madeleine Osborne.)

'OVARID' (see MEGESTROL ACETATE under OES-TRUS, SUPPRESSION OF).

OVARIES. They are suspended in a fold of peri-toneum from the roof of the abdomen, called the 'mesovarium'. In the *mare* they are situated in the abdomen, lying a little below and behind the kid-neys, usually in contact with the muscles of the lumbar region. Each possesses a groove which gives the organ a shape not unlike a bean, and which is called the *ovulation fossa*. It is into this groove that the ripe ova escape from the ovary, and it is the only part covered by germinal epi-thelium in the mare. In the *cow* the ovaries are oval in outline and possess no fossa. Each is situated about half-way up the shaft of the ilium of the corresponding side of the body. The ovaries of the *sow* are usually situated in a position simi-lar to those of the cow, but their position changes somewhat after breeding has occurred. They are studded upon the surface with irregular promi-nences, so that the organs present a mulberry-like appearance, and are enclosed in a 'purse' of peri-toneum. In the *bitch* the ovaries are situated in close proximity to, if not in actual contact with, the kidneys of the respective sides.

Structure. Each ovary is composed of a stroma of dense fibrous tissue in whose spaces are numer-ous blood-vessels, especially towards the centre. On the surface of the organ is a layer of *germinal epithelium* from which arise the *Graäfian follicles*. These vary very much in size: when young they are

microscopic, and lie immediately under the outer surface, but as they grow older they become more and more deeply situated, and finally, as ripening occurs, they once more come to the surface. Growth or ripening of a follicle occurs following stimulation of the ovary by the follicle-stimulating hormone (FSH) from the pituitary gland. The follicle produces, also as the result of FSH, oestrogens which prepare the uterus, Fallopian tubes and vagina for the other pro-cesses of reproduction. In a ripening Graäfian follicle there is one (rarely two) of the essential female germ cells, called an *ovum*. This is situated at the pinnacle of a mass of cells which project inwards from the inner surface of the follicle, and which is known as the *cumulus*.

Function. When the follicle is ripe, a process known as *ovulation* occurs, in which the outer sur-face wall of the follicle ruptures and liberates the contained ovum, which escapes from the ovary. The ovum is caught by the oviduct, and either fertilised or passed on through the female system to the outside. The cavity of the Graäfian follicle fills up afterwards with spindle-shaped cells, under the influence of the luteinising hormone (LH) from the pituitary. (LH becomes more plentiful as FSH becomes less so) and the struc-ture is called the CORPUS LUTEUM or yellow body.

If an ovum is fertilised, resulting in pregnancy, the corpus luteum persists and secretes proges-terone, a hormone necessary for the maintenance of pregnancy.

If the animal does not become pregnant, the corpus luteum breaks down and disappears. (Occasionally, however, it fails to do so, and may then cause infertility in the dairy cow especially.) (*See also under* CYSTS and below for cystic ovaries – leading often to NYMPHOMANIA.) (*See also* OESTRUS and diagram under UTERUS.)

OVARIES, DISEASES OF. In cystic degeneration large cavernous cysts appear in the substance of the organ, and fill with fluid. For a time there are no definite symptoms shown, but after the cysts attain considerable size the animal begins to exhibit signs of fretfulness and excitability. As time goes on these symptoms increase in violence until in the mare, in which the condition is quite common, it usually becomes dangerous to work her. Upon the slightest provocation, and often with no provocation at all, the mare starts to kick. After her bout of kicking is over she resumes her normal behaviour, but another attack may come on at any time afterwards.

Cysts are also met with in cows where they may be associated with sterility, and in bitches where they are frequently present along with tumour formation in the mammary glands. They are recognised in America as a common cause of sterility in gilts; heat periods being irregular and the clitoris becoming enlarged. Hypoplasia of the ovaries may also occur.

(*See* NYMPHOMANIA; *see also under* INFERTILITY.)

OVARIO-HYSTERECTOMY. Surgical operation for removal of the uterus and ovaries. This is carried out in the dog and cat in cases of pyometra, and following dystokia where a recurrence is feared. It is the usual technique for spaying, especially of cats to prevent the birth of unwanted kittens. (*See also* SPAYING.)

OVARIOTOMY. Surgical operation for removal of a diseased ovary. (*See also* SPAYING.)

OVERGROWN FOOT is one in which the horn of the wall all the way round has continued to grow downwards and outwards, without any compensatory wear along its lower edge. A horse with overgrown feet, which may arise either from too long periods between successive shoeings, or from living on marshy land where the unshod foot gets no wear, is unable to walk correctly. The frog does not reach the ground, the toe is too long, and the heels are too high, so that the normal anti-concussion mechanism of the foot is thrown out of action. The condition predisposes to the occurrence of sprains and contractions of tendons, upright pasterns, and splitting of the horn, with the production of sandcracks as a consequence. Horses' feet that are shod should have the shoes removed at least once a month, and the growth since the last shoeing should be removed by rasping the lower edge of the wall. Young colts, running out at grass, should have their feet properly reduced at least once during every two months or so. Overgrown foot is of importance in cattle and sheep, and in animals confined in 'zoos'.

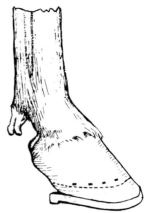

Overgrown hoof, showing how much should be cut away at the next shoeing.

OVERLYING by the sow is one cause of PIGLET MORTALITY (which see) and can be prevented by the use of farrowing crates, rails, and the roundhouse. It should be remembered, however, that an ill piglet is more likely to be crushed by the sow than a healthy one; and it has been shown that after one hour in an environmental temperature of 35° to 40° a piglet becomes comatose. (*See under* ROUNDHOUSE for an effective means of preventing overlying.)

OVERSTOCKING. This term refers both to the cruel practice of exposing in a market cattle in urgent need of milking (with the object of obtaining better prices for animals with impressive udders); and also to an excess of grazing animals on a given acreage of pasture. (*See* STOCKING RATES.)

OVIDUCT (*see* FALLOPIAN TUBES, SALPINGITIS, EGG-BOUND, PROLAPSE OF OVIDUCT).

OVINE ENCEPHALOMYELITIS. Louping ill.

OVINE ENZOOTIC ABORTION (*see* ABORTION, ENZOOTIC, OF EWES).

OVINE EPIDIDIMYTIS. Brucellosis of sheep, important in Australia and New Zealand, and caused by *Brucella ovis*. (*See* RAM, BRUCELLOSIS.)

OVINE INTERDIGITAL DERMATITIS (OID). This has been described in foot-rot free flocks in Australia, and is caused by *Fusiformis necrophorus*. (*See also* 'SCALD' *and* 'SCAD'.)

OVINE KERATOCONJUNCTIVITIS (OKC). The name for a group of infectious eye diseases of sheep. (*See also* EYE, DISEASES OF.)

OVINE LEUKOPENIC ENTEROCOLITIS (*see* 'BORDER DISEASE').

OVULATION. In the mare, cow, ewe, sow, and bitch, ovulation has no relation to coitus; whereas in the cat, ferret and rabbit it is coitus that determines the onset of ovulation. (*See under* OVARIES *and* OESTRUS.)

OVUM is an egg cell. (*See* EMBRYOLOGY, OVARY, TRANSPLANTATION.)

OXYGEN (*see* OZONE, AIR, RESPIRATION).

Cylinders of oxygen are essential items of equipment for anaesthesia. They are fitted with a pressure gauge and a reducing valve. A flowmeter is incorporated in the anaesthetic circuit. (*See* ANAESTHESIA).

Oxygen is used in the treatment of animals rescued from burning buildings and suffering from the effects of smoke inhalation.

Hyperbaric oxygen is that used at high pressures (*e.g.* 3 atmospheres) for the treatment of carbon monoxide poisoning; and it has also been used for gas gangrene in a dog.

Oxygen embolism is a potential danger when hydrogen peroxide is syringed into a deep wound.

'OXYGEN DEBT' (*see* MUSCLES, action of).

OXYTETRACYCLINE. An antibiotic. (*See* TETRACYCLINES.)

OXYTOCIN. A hormone, secreted by the posterior pituitary gland, and also by the *corpus luteum*, which actuates the 'milk let-down' mechanism; and also stimulates contraction of the muscles of the uterus.

OXYURIS is another name for the thread worm, which possesses a long finely-tapered tail. (*See* ROUNDWORMS.)

OZAENA is a chronic inflammatory disease of the nasal passages. (*See* NOSE, DISEASES OF.)

OZONE. The chemically highly reactive allotropic form of oxygen, ozone (O_3). As a constituent of the upper atmosphere it forms a layer which protects us from excessive exposure to ultraviolet radiation from the sun. Ozone may be the main constituent of smog, and Los Angeles is reputed to have the highest exposure to ozone in the world. 'In southern England, during several days in 1971, oxidant, mainly O_3, was found in excess of 10 p.p.h.m. compared with the 2–5 p.p.h.m. present during the day in clean air and virtually none at night.

'Ozone has been described as the most hazardous of all the gaseous air pollutants because of its long-term association in laboratory animals with emphysema, lung cancer, accelerated ageing, increased neonatal deaths, decreased litter size, teratogenesis, and jaw anomalies. In animals exposed to ozone the mortality from lung infections is increased.' (*Lancet*, Nov. 29, 1975.)

P

PACEMAKERS (Cardiac). In 1981 B. Bigler and others reported the successful use of a pacemaker in a 2-year-old dachshund bitch, which had a history of loss of consciousness after exercise. ECG showed a grade 3 atrio-ventricular block. A unipole electrode was inserted into the right ventricle from the jugular vein, and sutured into the subcutaneous tissue of the neck. The pacemaker took over as soon as the batteries were connected, to give 72 heart beats per minute (as compared with 15 to 25 previously).

In America in 1983 John D. Bonagura and others reviewed the cases of 11 dogs treated by implantation of a pacemaker for bradycardia caused by various pathological conditions. Eight of the 11 dogs died from 'complications' arising from day 1 to 35 months after surgery. The other three dogs were alive and well.

In the UK pacemakers have been used with success in dogs. (Bigler, B. & others, *Schweizer Archiv fur Tierheilkunde* (1981) **123,** 545.) (Bonagura, J. D. & others *JAVMA* (1983) **182,** 149.) (*See* CREMATION.)

Eighteen dogs and one cat were fitted with cardiac pacemakers; at the necks of the dogs and at the abdominal wall of the cat. In subsequent operations the pacemaker was enclosed in a dacron pouch. Clinical signs were relieved in all cases, and these animals subsequently lived for more than 18 months. (Darke, P. G. B. & others. *J of Small Animal Practice* (1989) **30,** 491.)

PACHECO'S DISEASE. Caused by a herpesvirus, this killed 8 out of 60 parrots imported into Britain in 1983.

PACHYMENINGITIS means inflammation of the dura mater of the brain and spinal cord. (*See* MENINGITIS.)

PACINIAN CORPUSCLES (*see under* TOUCH, SKIN).

PACKED CELL VOLUME (*see under* BLOOD).

PADDOCKS. These often become reservoirs of parasitic worm larvae – a point for animal owners to bear in mind. Paddocks need 'resting' for 12 months or grazing by a different species of animal periodically.

Paddock grazing is a system of grassland management in which a given area of land is divided into a number of paddocks by fences and used for what André Voisin described as 'Rational Grazing'.

In Britain, on farms costed by ICI, paddock grazing of dairy cows has given very good financial results. The system should be set up on an area of grassland as near to the farm buildings as possible, allowing 1 acre for every 2 cows; *e.g.* 21 acres for a 42-cow herd. This area is then divided into 21 paddocks each of 1 acre, over which the herd should circulate in about 3-weekly intervals; one day's grazing per paddock being ideal. Paddocks should be squarish rather than long and narrow, and well supplied with water. A 21-acre cutting block should yield the bulk fodder for the winter, and each acre must therefore produce enough silage for 2 cows, *i.e.* 14 tons.

Fertiliser, especially nitrogen, is the key to the success of this system, and must be applied regularly, throughout the grazing season. After the first graze, grass growth may be such that the farmer may have to take full silage cuts from a number of paddocks without grazing, so that the cows could circulate in a shorter cycle over a fewer number of paddocks. The cut paddocks would come back into the grazing system at a time when grass is slightly less abundant. Topping will be needed at least once in the early part of the season, and should be done without delay after the cows have left the paddock. (*See also under* PASTURE MANAGEMENT.)

The two-sward system involves the use of paddocks for grazing and of separate areas of grassland for conservation.

In order to reduce STRESS (which see) among sheep in paddocks, Stephen Williams recommends surrounding a system of paddocks by solid hedges and filled-in gates. 'The hedges are A-shaped and leafed to the ground and deflect noise upwards when they are alongside roads. In full leaf, they are high enough and solid enough to give perfect privacy for the sheep units they enclose. Various types of fences, hedges, and walls for subdividing the area into paddocks have been examined and, quite certainly, the open type wire fence is superior, even essential. Lambs like to keep their dams in view and are much more likely to forage in the forward paddock better and more widely if they can do this.'

PAIN. (For relief of pain, *see* ANALGESICS, ANAESTHESIA.) Because an animal does not cry out, or show signs of restlessness, it should not be assumed that it is not in pain. Pain can be a cause of aggressiveness.

PAINT (*see* HOUSE DECORATING, LEAD POISONING, CAGE BIRDS).

PALATABILITY (*see under* DIET).

PALATE is the partition between the cavity of the mouth below, and that of the nose above. It consists of the *hard palate* and the *soft palate*. The hard palate is formed by the bony floor of the nasal cavity covered with dense mucous membrane, which is crossed by transverse ridges in all the domesticated animals. These ridges assist the tongue to carry the food back to the throat. The hard palate stretches back a little beyond the last molar teeth in animals, and ends by becoming continuous with the soft palate. This latter is formed by muscles covered with mucous membrane, and acts as a sort of curtain between the cavity of the mouth and that of the pharynx. In most animals it is short, and will allow food to be regurgitated back into the mouth, but this is not the case in the horse. In that animal it is long, and forms a division so arranged that food material can only pass from the mouth to the pharynx, and not in the reverse direction. It is owing to this anatomical peculiarity that the horse is not able to vomit through his mouth. Material brought up from the stomach must pass out by way of the nostrils. In race-horses, distressed breathing may arise as the result of inflammation or partial paralysis of the soft palate, which may be linked with paresis or paralysis of the vocal cords. Partial resection of the soft palate has been carried out as treatment for this latter condition. (*See* GUTTURAL POUCH DIPHTHERIA.)

Prolonged Soft Palate is a recognised inherited abnormality of the short-nosed breeds of dogs, *e.g.* Boxers, Bulldogs, Pekingese, Pugs, Cocker Spaniel. It makes breathing difficult at times, with snoring or even loss of consciousness resulting. An operation to correct the condition is often very successful.

Severe injury to the hard palate is not uncommonly seen in cats which have fallen from a height, and suturing may be required.

Palatine arterial haemorrhage. This occurred on three occasions in a 15-year-old cat. The source was found to be a 1-mm lesion overlying the right major palatine artery. The bleeding was stopped by means of electro-cautery. (Wildgoose, W. H. *Veterinary Record* (1990) March 17th issue.)

PALE SOFT EXUDATIVE MUSCLE (PSE) is a condition in pig meat associated with an abnormally rapid fall in muscle pH after slaughter, pH 6·0 being a level below which carcases are likely to show PSE. The incidence of this condition, which reduces the value of the carcase, is high in the Piétrain breed, and geneticists suggest that PSE is likely to become more common as a correlated response to selection of British breeds for lean meat. Apart from breeding, PSE is associated with pre-slaughter stress arising from transport, conditions in the lairage, and the method by which pigs are moved to the stunning point. 'Any situation which is likely to stress a pig could cause rapid conversion of glycogen to lactic acid soon after slaughter while the carcase is still warm,' states the MLC. (*See* PORCINE STRESS SYNDROME.)

Dark firm dry meat (DFD) is a condition which 'appears to occur if muscle glycogen reserves are depleted before death, as a result of some form of stress, so that only a small reduction in muscle pH is possible after slaughter.... Recently some interest has been shown in feeding sugar as a liquid to pigs in the lairage prior to slaughter to replace depleted glycogen reserves, and thereby produce meat with a lower ultimate pH. Such meat would then be less likely to be DFD in nature.' (MLC, 1975.)

PALO SANTO TREES. The leaves, fruit, and seeds cause poisoning in cattle in South America. Signs include tympany, depression, and convulsions.

PALPEBRAL. Relating to the eye-lids.

PAM. Pyridine-2-aldoxime methiodide. This has been recommended as an antidote to be given intravenously in parathion poisoning, in addition to treatment with atropine.

PAN- is a prefix meaning all or completely.

PANCREAS, is partly an endocrine gland, producing hormones; and partly an exocrine gland, producing the pancreatic juice for digestive purposes.

The pancreas is situated in the abdomen, a little in front of the level of the kidneys and a little below them. When fresh it has a reddish cream colour.

The pancreatic juice is secreted into the small intestine to meet the food which has undergone partial digestion in the stomach. The juice contains alkaline salts and at least nine enzymes, *e.g. trypsin*, which carries on the digestion of proteins already begun in the stomach; *amylase*, which converts starches into sugars; *lipase*, which breaks up fats; and a substance that curdles milk. (*See* DIGESTION.)

The pancreas also has groups of cells, the islets of Langerhans. (*See* INSULIN, DIABETES, GLUCAGON, HORMONES.) Here alpha-cells produce GLUCAGON, and beta-cells produce INSULIN.

PANCREAS, DISEASES OF. These include DIABETES, inflammation, suppuration, atrophy, tumour formation, etc. (*See* INSULINOMA.)

Acute necrotic pancreatitis has been reported in obese dogs.
SIGNS: Abdominal tenderness or pain. Hyperglycaemia and shock may follow.

Exocrine pancreatic insufficiency in dogs has three main causes: congenital hypoplasia, degenerative pancreatic atrophy, and chronic pancreatitis.
SIGNS include a ravenous appetite, loss of weight, fatty faeces, and a dry scurfy coat.

Atrophy of the pancreas is the most common form, and is seen especially in the German shepherd dog. Cimetidine was found to be highly effective in treatment. (Pilsworth, R. C. & Lehner, R. P., *Vet. Record* (1986) **119**, 240.)

Parasites which may be found in the pancreatic ducts include *Toxocara canis* and, in cats in America, the pancreatic fluke *Eurytrema procyonis*. The latter may interfere with the gland's exocrine function to a great extent. Fenbendazole is effective against the fluke.

PANCREATITIS (*see above*).

PANCYTOPENIA. A reduction in the number of red cells, white cells, and platelets in the blood; usually due to a bone-marrow dyscrasia.

'PANJET'. An injector, for local anaesthetics mainly, which does away with the need for a hypodermic needle, and uses spring-compressed air to produce a fine jet which penetrates the skin. Localised surface anaesthesia can be achieved quickly, and permits painless suturing or incision.

For fish-marking, it is used to inject a dye. (Wright Health Group Ltd., Dundee).

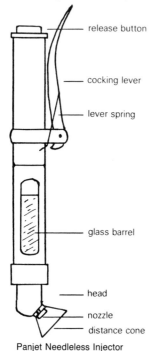

release button

cocking lever

lever spring

glass barrel

head

nozzle

distance cone

Panjet Needleless Injector

PANLEUCOPENIA. Feline Infectious Enteritis.

PANNICULITIS (*see under* NODULAR).

PANNUS (*see* EYE, DISEASES).

PANOSTEITIS (*see under* CANINE).

PANSTEATITIS (*see* STEATITIS).

PANTOTHENIC ACID (*see* VITAMINS).

PANZOOTIC means a disease which affects all animals in an area.

PAPAIN. An enzyme extracted from the pawpaw (custard apple) and used to tenderise meat.

PAPER. Waste paper has been incorporated in ruminant diets with apparent success as a roughage.

In one trial, waste paper from an office was ground through a hammermill and incorporated in sheep rations at levels of 15, 30 and 45 per cent replacing equal amounts of chopped hay. At the 45 per cent level, paper was the only roughage in the diet and urea was added to balance the nitrogen at the various levels of paper addition.

Dry-matter consumption of 15 and 30 per cent paper rations was equal to the control, and the ration containing 45 per cent paper was eaten at about 95 per cent of the control consumption. (Nishimuta, J. F., and others (1969), *J. Anim. Sci.*, **29**, 642.)

However, some samples of paper crumble have been found to contain 500 ppm of lead instead of the expected 50 ppm.

Shredded paper has been used as a bedding material. (*See* BEDDING.)

PAPILLA. A small projection.

PAPILLOMA (*see* WARTS, *and below*; *also* VIRAL INFECTIONS, TUMOURS). In some animal species a papilloma may, through the action of sunlight, lead to a squamous cell carcinoma.

PAPILLOMA VIRUS group includes viruses infecting cattle, sheep, goats, horses, dogs, rabbits, etc.

PAPULE. A pimple.

PARA- is a prefix meaning near, aside from, or beyond.

PARACENTESIS. (*See* ASPIRATION.)

PARACETAMOL (acetaminophen). An analgesic. Poisoning has arisen in cats dosed by their owners with this drug (which is chemically related to phenacetin). Symptoms include cyanosis and facial oedema. Acetylcysteine, given orally, is an antidote.

PARAFFIN is the general term used to designate a series of saturated hydrocarbons. The higher members of the series are solid at ordinary temperatures, some being hard and others soft. Lower in the scale comes petroleum, which is liquid at ordinary temperatures. Naphtha, petroleum spirit, and hydramyl, are members of the series lower still, which are very volatile bodies, and finally lowest comes methane or marsh-gas.
USES. Internally, only **medicinal** liquid paraffin is used; it is a gentle laxative, but has the disadvantage that it is liable to become tolerated by the system and lose its effect when given continually as a routine laxative. It was given in old dogs liable to impaction after eating bones. It should not be given regularly as it is said to absorb vitamin D and may cause rickets. Externally, the hard and soft paraffins are used in the preparation of various ointments and lubricants. They are not absorbed to the same extent as the animal fats, and are therefore not so suitable for the basis of a drug which requires to be absorbed so that its action may be made use of.

Kerosene (the paraffin sold for use in stoves and lamps) has no place in animal medicine, either as an external dressing for the skin or given internally. Poisoning is likely to result from either use. (*See also* KEROSENE POISONING.)

PARAFILARIA. A genus of filarial worms. *P. bovicola* causes serious skin lesions in cattle in several parts of the world. (*See* FILARIASIS.)

PARAGLE FLY (*see* FLIES).

PARAGONIMIASIS. Infestation with lung flukes of *Paragonimus* species in dogs, cats, foxes, mink. (*See* LUNGFLUKES.)

PARAINFLUENZA 3 VIRUS. Infection with this is widespread in sheep in the UK; and the virus is also one cause of CALF PNEUMONIA and of respiratory diseases in the horse. (*See* EQUINE RESPIRATORY VIRUSES.) *Parainfluenza 5* infects the dog, and may be associated with 'KENNEL COUGH'. (*See also* INFLUENZA.)

PARAKERATOSIS. The name applied to a scaly, elephant-like skin. The condition has been seen in pigs suffering from a zinc deficiency following, *e.g.* a 'diet of maize, lucerne, limestone, and Aureomycin'. It occurs in pigs fed dry meal *ad lib.*, and gradually clears up when a change to wet feeding is made. It often begins with a red pimply condition of the skin on the flanks, abdomen, etc. Thin, dry yellowish or greyish scales may be seen on the skin, which later becomes thickened. It responds to small doses of zinc sulphate. (*See* CALCIUM SUPPLEMENTS.)

Inherited parakeratosis has been reported in calves of Friesian descent, and although a zinc supplement proved successful in treating the encrusted skin of head, neck and limbs, the lesions returned after cessation of the supplement. (O'Brien, J. K., *Vet. Rec.* (1986) **119**, 205.)

PARALDEHYDE. A narcotic.

PARALYSIS, in its widest sense may mean loss of nerve control over any of the bodily functions, loss of sensation, and loss of the special senses, but the term is usually restricted to mean loss of muscular action due to interference with the nervous system. When muscular power is merely weakened, without being lost completely, the word *paresis* is often used.

Various terms are used to indicate paralysis distributed in different ways. (*See* HEMIPLEGIA, PARAPLEGIA, QUADRIPLEGIA.)

Paralysis should be regarded rather as a symptom than as a disease by itself.

Varieties. Paralysis is usually looked upon as being due to cerebral, spinal, or peripheral causes.

Cerebral paralysis. Conditions resulting from brain lesions, such as encephalitis, tumour formation, fracture of the skull with depression of a portion of bone, haemorrhage, etc., are accompanied by severe general or local paralysis, either of the whole body (when death usually follows very rapidly), or of one side (hemiplegia).

Paralysed limbs when examined are found to be flaccid, with the muscles totally relaxed, and passive movements are not resisted. Sensations of pain may be felt, however, and an indication that sensation is not destroyed is shown by raising the head, or struggling with the sound limbs when a pin-prick is made in a paralysed part.

In cases of cerebral haemorrhage the seizure is sudden; while in encephalitis there is usually some co-existing disease, such as influenza, distemper, etc., and the brain symptoms develop as a complication; or the encephalitis may be the result of a primary viral infection, such as equine encephalitis or rabies; with fracture and depression there is an immediate loss of power, just as when an animal is stunned.

Spinal paralysis or paraplegia is most often due to fracture of, or severe injury to, the vertebrae. (*See separate entry* PARAPLEGIA.)

In complete paralysis death usually takes place in from 12 to 48 hours after the injury. (*See* SPINE AND SPINAL CORD, DISEASES AND INJURIES OF; INTERVERTEBRAL DISC; *and*, for horses, *under* COMENY'S *and* EQUINE VIRAL PNEUMONITIS.)

In *Peripheral paralysis* there is usually some injury to a nerve trunk, some lesion of the nerve-endings in the muscle fibres. (*See* SUPRASCAPULAR PARALYSIS and RADIAL PARALYSIS.)

Brachial paralysis results from road accidents, collisions, stake wounds. *Gluteal paralysis* is very uncommon. Wasting of the muscles of one hindquarter and a tendency to carry the limb out to one side occur. '*Paralysis of the sciatic nerve*' causes a loss of power in all the muscles of the thigh except those situated above and to the front of the stifle joint, *i.e.* the quadratus group. The limb hangs loosely and the animal jerks it forward when attempting to walk; although the stifle is advanced the hock and the fetlock remain flexed and the front of the foot comes to the ground.

When there is severe injury to the side of the thigh from a fall, kick, or other similar cause, *paralysis of the external popliteal nerve* (common peroneal) may occur; it results in an inability to extend the foot or flex the hock. When the horse is made to walk the limb is drawn out backwards into a position resembling that seen in dislocation of the stifle, but the fetlock is flexed instead of being fully extended. The limb is then carried a short distance forward and the foot comes to rest upon the ground on its anterior face instead of on the sole. In '*crural paralysis*' (paralysis of the femoral nerve) the quadriceps muscles above the stifle, which normally extend that joint, are paralysed. When weight is put upon the limb the stifle sinks to the level of the hock or below it, all joints are flexed, and there is a peculiar drop of the hindquarter on the same side. (*See also* PARAPLEGIA.)

PARALYSIS IN THE DOG (*see also* DISTEMPER, BOTULISM, THROMBOSIS OF THE FEMORAL ARTERIES, SPINE – diseases of; TICK PARALYSIS, LEAD POISONING, RABIES, RACOON BITE, ORGANOPHOSPHORUS POISONING.)

Aid. A 'k-9 cart' can be the alternative to euthanasia for some paraplegic dogs. The trolleys are available from Poplar Farm, Oxford Road, Oakley, Nr. Aylesbury, Bucks. HP18 9RQ.

PARALYTIC MYOGLOBINURIA (*see* MUSCLES, DISEASES OF under Nutritional).

PARAMETER. Normal levels of values, *e.g.* of calcium in the blood-stream of a particular species of animal.

PARAMPHISTOMIASIS. A disease caused by rumen flukes of the genus *Paramphistomum*. (*See* RUMEN FLUKES).

PARAMYXOVIRUSES. *See* Paramyxovirus parainfluenza 3 virus in the Table under EQUINE INFLUENZA. Two paramyxoviruses infecting dogs are the canine distemper virus, and canine parainfluenza virus/S V 5; and a third was isolated in 1985 from a puppy dying from haemorrhagic enteritis. This third virus was named Glasgow 491. Dr L. Macartney and colleagues were making further studies to ascertain whether it is implicated in canine disease. (Macartney & others *Veterinary Record* (1985) **117**, 205.) (*See also* PIGEONS, and NEWCASTLE DISEASE.)

PARAPHIMOSIS. A constriction preventing the penis from being withdrawn into the prepuce. This is not uncommon in the dog, and is serious, for gangrene may occur unless relief is afforded. As a first-aid measure, swab the penis with ice-cold water. Surgical interference under anaesthesia may be necessary. The use of hyaluronidase in normal saline, by injection, has been recommended.

For paraphimosis in horses and cattle *see under* PENIS, ABNORMALITIES OF.

PARAPLEGIA. Paralysis of the hindlegs. It may be accompanied by paralysis of the muscles which control the passage of urine and faeces to the outside. (*See* PARALYSIS.)

It is seen following accidents involving injury to the spine – frequently in the dog knocked down by a car – and may also be associated with 'Disc' lesions. A rare cause is thrombosis of the femoral arteries. In the dog, this may occur suddenly – the animal playing one minute, and collapsing with a yelp the next. Absence of pulse in the femoral arteries assists a diagnosis. (*See also under* THROMBOSIS, COMENY'S.)

PARAPOX VIRUSES (*see* table under VIRUSES).

PARAQUAT. This herbicide has caused fatal poisoning in man. Poisoning in the dog gives rise to lung oedema, congestion and consolidation; also kidney damage.

Paraquat was detected in the urine of 2 out of 5 dogs showing acute respiratory distress, leading to cyanosis after 4 days' illness. Three of the dogs died, and euthanasia was resorted to with the others. (*Vet. Rec.* (1975) **97**, 370.)

In New South Wales, a dog died and a cat recovered (partially if not completely); the latter animal had been seen eating grass from a lawn of

---

PARASITES AND PARASITOLOGY

Anaplasmosis   20
Arachnida   28
Babesiosis   40
Balantidium   45
Biliary Fever (*see* BABESIOSIS)   45, 98, 193
Bladder-worms   613
Blood flukes (*see* SCHISTOMIASIS)   523
Blood parasites of cattle (U K)   62
Blow-flies (*see* FLIES)   226
Bots (*see* FLIES)   228
Canine babesiosis   98
Chicken mites (*see* MITES)   385
Coccidiosis   122
Cysticercosis (*see* TAPEWORMS)   570
Ear Mange (*see* EAR, DISEASES OF)   180
East Coast Fever   181
   (*see* THEILERIOSIS)   582
Fleas   223
'Flesh' flies (*see* FLIES)   226
Flies   224
Flour mites (*see* MITES)   382
   (*see* FLOUR MITE INFESTATION)   233
Flukes   234, 348, 353, 515
Forage mites (*see* MITES)   386
Fungal diseases   251
Gadflies (*see* FLIES)   225, 228
   (*see* WARBLES)   638
Giardia (*see* GIARDIASIS)   263
Globidiosis   264
Gnats (*see* FLIES)   224
'Green-bottle' flies (*see* FLIES)   227
Haemobartonella   273
Harvest mites (*see* MITES)   386
'Hookworms' (*see* ROUNDWORMS)   514
House flies (*see* FLIES)   225
Husk and Hoose (*see* ROUNDWORMS)   427, 513
Jaundice, malignant (*see* CANINE BABESIOSIS)   98
Ked, Sheep   327
Leeches   340
Leishmaniasis   340
Lice   344

Linguatula (*see* MITES)   386
Liver flukes   348
Lung flukes   353
Lung worms   428, 511, 513, 514
Mange, mites (*see* MITES)   382
Midges   375
Mites   382
Mosquitoes (*see* FLIES)   225
Myiasis (*see* FLIES)   226
Nematodes (*see* ROUNDWORMS)   510
Red-water fever   494
Ringworm   505
Roundworms in the Horse   510
Roundworms in Ruminants   512
Roundworms in the Pig   513
Roundworms in the Dog and Cat   514
Roundworms in Poultry (*see* GAPES)   253
Rumen flukes   515
Sarcocystis   522
'Scaly Leg' (*see* MITES)   385
Schistosomiasis   523
'Screw-worm' Fly   525
Sheep Nostril Fly (*see* FLIES)   229
Sheep Scab (*see* MITES)   384
Strongyles (*see* ROUNDWORMS)   511
   (*see* STRONGYLES)   559
'Summer sores'   562
Tapeworms in the Dog and Cat   570
Tapeworms in the Horse   570
Tapeworms in the Pig   570
Tapeworms in Ruminants   570
Texas Fever   581
Theileriosis   582
Ticks   584
Toxoplasmosis   592
Trichomoniasis   597
Trypanosomiasis   601
Tumbu flies (*see* FLIES)   227
Warble flies (*see* FLIES)   228
   (*see* WARBLES)   638

which the weedy areas had been treated with undiluted Gramoxone (20 per cent paraquat). In both animals vomiting was a symptom, as well as distressed breathing. (*Vet. Rec.* (1976) **98**, 189.)

Cyanocobalamin has been suggested as an antidote for small animals; though it is generally held that no effective antidote exists.

Complete recovery was achieved for a dog taken to the University of Dublin's veterinary clinic, with a history of weakness, and rapid breathing over the previous six hours.

The animal's condition deteriorated, despite intensive treatment. Nursed at home, the patient was seen at the clinic daily. On the fifteenth day came improvement. Although still breathing through its mouth, respirations were down to 120 per minute. It was seven weeks before they had come down to 60.

The patience and perseverance of both owner and clinic staff were rewarded, for when seen again six and eighteen months later the dog was well and fully active again. (O'Sullivan, S. P. & others. *J. of Small Animal Practice* (1989) p. 361.)

PARASITISM is the association of two organisms, one of which (the parasite) benefits by nourishing itself at the expense of the other (the host) but without normally destroying it.

The following types of parasitic relations are recognised: 1 (*a*) ectoparasites, which live on the host; and (*b*) endoparasites, which live within the body of the host; 2 (*a*) accidental parasites, which are normally free-living animals but may live for a certain period in a host; (*b*) facultative parasites, which are able to exist free or as parasites, *e.g.* blowfly larvae; and (*c*) obligatory parasites, which are completely adapted to a parasitic type of life and must live in or on a host, *e.g.* most parasitic worms; 3 (*a*) temporary or transitory parasites, which pass a definite phase or phases in their life history as parasites and during which time the parasitism is obligatory and continuous, *e.g.* botflies, ticks; (*b*) permanent parasites, which always live for the greater part of their life as parasites, *e.g.* lice, tapeworms, coccidia, etc.; and (*c*) periodic, occasional, or intermittent parasites, which only visit the host for short periods to obtain food, *e.g.* bloodsucking flies, fleas; 4 (*a*) erratic parasites, which occur in an organ that is not their normal habitat, *e.g. Fasciola hepatica* in the lungs; (*b*) incidental parasites, which, exceptionally, occur in an animal that is not their normal host; they are incidental only in this first host, *e.g. Dipylidium caninum* is incidental in man; and (*c*) specific parasites, which occur in a particular species of host or group of hosts, *e.g. D. caninum* is specific for dogs and cats.

PARASITIC DISEASE, NATURE OF. The scientific name of a parasitic disease is formed by adding '*osis*' or '*iasis*' to the generic stem; *e.g. strongylosis* is the disease caused by the genus *Strongylus* in the horse and *Leishmaniasis* is the disease caused by the genus *Leishmania* in man and dogs. If more than one closely related genus is implicated the termination '-*id*' is sometimes added to the stem of the type genus of the group, before the usual termination; *e.g. strongylidosis* is the disease caused by the strongylid (or strongyle-

like) worms in the horse.

Parasitic diseases are seldom caused by one or a few specimens, but as a rule depend on mass infestations. There are exceptions to this, however, as one *Ascaris* may obstruct the bile-duct with fatal results. Parasites, with few exceptions, do not spend all their lives in the animal body, but always require to spend a certain proportion of their life-cycle outside the host. They may cause damage to the host in the following ways:

(1) By abstraction of nourishment properly belonging to the host, *e.g.* many of the intestinal worms;

(2) By mechanical obstruction of passages or compression of organs, *e.g.* gapes (in chickens), hydatid, etc.;

(3) By feeding on the tissues of the host, *e.g.* blood-sucking worms or flies;

(4) By production of toxins with varying effects;

(5) By actual traumatic damage, *e.g.* by piercing and destroying skin (ticks, mites, flies, etc.), by depositing eggs in the tissues (lung-worms), by migrations of larvae (*Ascaris* and *Trichinella*), by clinging to surfaces by means of sharp hooks (tapeworms), and in many other ways;

(6) By facilitating the entrance of bacteria; *e.g.* stomach worms in pigs allow the entrance of *Fusiformis necrophorus* (the necrosis bacillus);

(7) By transmitting diseases for which they act as intermediate hosts; *e.g.* ticks and babesiosis, etc.;

(8) By causing inflammatory or neoplastic reactions in the invaded tissues; *e.g.* pneumonia, gastritis, fluke adenomata in the liver, and so on. These are only some of the more obvious methods of injuring the host. Apart from the loss due to actual deaths, the depreciation in value of hides, meat, milk, and work is enormous, and, although less spectacular than a bacterial epizootic, the loss is more constant, and in the aggregate is probably even greater than the loss due to bacterial diseases. (*See under* BRAIN for parasites which migrate to the brain.)

PARASITES AND DISEASE. For details, see indexed list on page 426.

PARASITES AND IMMUNITY. 'Parasite antigens are a potent stimulus for antiparasite antibodies of the IgE class' (*see* IMMUNOGLOBULINS), 'and parasite infection can potentiate a pre-existing IgE response to an unrelated antigen.' (*Lancet*, April 24, 1976.)

Examples of the effect of parasitism on the immune response are given under CANCER and ALLERGY, respectively.

PARASITIC BRONCHITIS. This occurs in cattle, sheep and goats, and on account of the husky cough produced, the disease is, in the UK, commonly called 'Husk' or 'Hoose'.

Although of greater economic importance in calves, nevertheless the cost of an outbreak in a dairy herd may be very high – not so much as a result of deaths (which do occur in adult cattle) but on account of reduced milk yields and the need for extra feed. Marshy land and mild, wet weather both favour the parasites, as does overstocking.

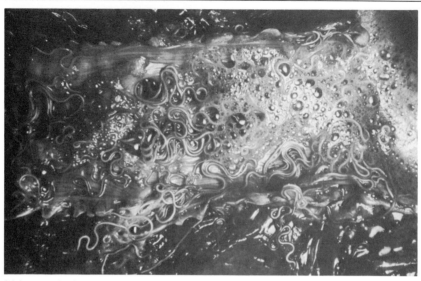

Adult worms in the air passages of a calf's lungs. In a heavily infected animal several thousand lungworms may be present.

CAUSE. In cattle the lungworm *Dictyocaulus viviparus* is the important species. (*See* LUNGWORMS.)

'Workers at Glasgow university have defined infection with the parasite into five phases: penetration, prepatent, patent, post patent, and reinfection. In all but the first phase oedema and emphysema can be found.

Parasitic bronchitis normally affects cattle in their first grazing season. Affected animals experience a drop in the saturation level of oxygen in their blood to 70% even before clinical signs become apparent. In clinical cases the percentage may be reduced to 30.' (G. Oakley, I C I.)

Spread of the worm larvae is assisted by their rocket-like propulsion by the fungus *Pilobolus*, which is found in faecal deposits on pasture. The worm larvae are projected along with the fungal spores, often between 10 a.m. and noon.

SIGNS. The characteristic husky cough is a symptom in the milder cases, but in acute cases may be absent, with the main symptom being *dyspnoea* (laboured breathing). In calves, death may occur from actual suffocation due to masses of worms obstructing the air passages, or it may result from general debility or pneumonia. In adult cattle pneumonia, with *Corynebacterium*

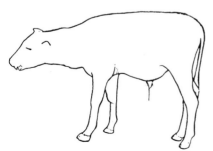

In a case of parasitic bronchitis, the neck is held extended and there may be continual coughing and/or distressed breathing.

pyogenes acting as a secondary invader. Oedema of the lungs may occur, and cause death.

PREVENTION and TREATMENT (*see under* WORMS, FARM TREATMENT AGAINST).

PARASITIC GASTRO-ENTERITIS OF CATTLE. This is an insidious and economically important disease, and the cause of death in many calves and yearlings. It is now known that the output of worm eggs in the faeces does not bear any constant relation to the number of worms present. It rises to an early peak and then declines, and is not a reliable guide to the degree of infestation.

CAUSE. Infestation with various species of round-worms, none of them much above one inch in length. (*See under* ROUNDWORMS.)

SIGNS. A gradual loss of condition; a harsh, staring coat; sometimes, but not always, scouring; pale mucous membranes; progressive weakness and emaciation. In adult cattle, which acquire a high degree of resistance (only broken down when under-feeding, chilling, pregnancy, or massive contamination of pasture occurs), no symptoms may normally be shown, but nevertheless the animal's efficiency is lowered.

TREATMENT. Dosing should not be delayed until the stock are weak.

PREVENTION. Calves should be dosed once with an efficient anthelmintic in mid-July and moved to pasture which has not been grazed that season by other cattle. Dose again in the autumn. (*See* WORMS, FARM TREATMENT AGAINST, 'CLEAN' PASTURE.)

PARASITIC GASTRO-ENTERITIS OF SHEEP. It is likely that outbreaks in early lambs in March and April are the result of over-wintered larvae. In one experiment, worm-free lambs were turned on to a pasture – 'rested' during the winter – in the spring and became infested with 12 species of gastro-intestinal worms.

SOME OF THE EFFECTS OF PARATHYROID HORMONE AND CALCITONIN, THE TWO MAJOR HORMONES CONTROLLING THE REGULATION OF BLOOD CALCIUM

	Parathyroid hormone	Calcitonin
Mode of Action	Separate fast and slow components. Increases cell membrane permeability. Activates adenyl cyclase enzyme systems.	Uncertain.
Effect on Kidney	Increases P excretion by decreasing tubular reabsorption. Decreases Ca excretion by increasing tubular reabsorption. Increases Na excretion by decreasing tubular reabsorption.	Increases Ca, P, Na, and K excretion. Decreases Mg excretion.
Effect on Intestine	Increases Ca, P and Mg absorption.	? Decreases P absorption. Decreases volume and acidity of gastric juice.
Effect on Bone	Increases resorption. Stimulates osteoclast and osteocyte activity. Inhibits formation. Suppresses osteoblast activity.	Inhibits resorption.
Resultant effect on Blood Calcium	Elevated.	Diminished.

(With acknowledgements to Mr D. Bennett, B Sc, B Vet Med, and to the *Veterinary Record*.)

TREATMENT and PREVENTION. Routine use of, *e.g.* Tetramisole. (*See* WORMS, FARM TREATMENT AGAINST, 'CLEAN' PASTURE.)

PARASITIC TRACHEOBRONCHITIS (*see* TRACHEAL WORMS).

PARASYMPATHETIC NERVOUS SYSTEM is one division of the Autonomic nervous system; the other division being the Sympathetic. (*See* AUTONOMIC NERVOUS SYSTEM, CENTRAL NERVOUS SYSTEM.)

PARATHION is chemically diethyl-*para*-nitrophenyl-thiophosphate and is used for agricultural purposes to destroy aphis and red spider. In man and domestic animals it is a cumulative poison which readily enters the system through inhalation, by the mouth or by absorption through the skin. Animals should not be allowed to graze under trees sprayed with parathion for at least 3 weeks. In man symptoms of poisoning include headache, vomiting, and a feeling of tightness in the chest. Later there is sweating, salivation, muscular twitching, distressed breathing and coma. (*See* PAM *and* ORGANO-PHOSPHORUS POISONING.)

In animals copious salivation and lachrymation, twitching, and increased intestinal movement are shown. Cattle are apparently tolerant of parathion, being able to break it down chemically.

The danger of spray drift, and the risk to dogs and cats wandering in sprayed areas, are obvious.

PARATHYROID GLANDS are small structures situated either wholly within, or upon the surface of, the thyroid gland. Their secretion, the *parathyroid hormone*, is important in the control of the level of blood calcium. Insufficiency of this hormone leads to muscular twitchings or tremors or, in more severe cases to convulsions. (*See* TETANY.) The hormone also controls phosphate excretion via the urine. See table above.

Hyperparathyroidism in dogs. Of 21 dogs with primary hyperparathyroidism, 20 had a parathyroid adenoma and one had a parathyroid carcinoma. The most common clinical signs were polydipsia/polyuria, listlessness, muscular weakness and inappetence. The only consistent biochemical abnormality was persistent hypercalcaemia (12·1 to 19·6 mg/100 ml). The external parathyroid tumours, found in nine of the 19 dogs which underwent surgery, were easily removed; internal parathyroid tumours were removed by thyroidectomy. (Berger, B. & Feldman, E. C. (1987) *Journal of the American Veterinary Medical Association* **191**, 350.)

Primary hyperparathyroidism in a cat. A 12-year-old cat showed clinical signs of lethargy, reluctance to move and pain along the back. Radiological examination revealed multifocal lesions, particularly in the skeleton. There was bilateral parathyroid hyperplasia but no evidence of neoplastic change. Histological examination revealed that a large proportion of bone had been resorbed and replaced by fibrous connective tissue and that osteoclasts were numerous. It is suggested that hyperparathyroidism should be considered in the differential diagnosis of conditions involving skeletal pain and lethargy in the cat. (Blunden, A. S., Wheeler, S. J.

& Davies, J. V. (1986) *Journal of Small Animal Practice* **27**, 791).

PARATUBERCULOSIS. A synonym for JOHNE'S DISEASE.

PARATYPHOID (*see* SALMONELLOSIS).

PARENCHYMA is a term now reserved for the functional cells of an organ, as opposed to its supporting, connective tissue (interstitial) cells. In a gland the parenchyma is the mass of secreting cells; in the lung, similarly, the parenchyma comprises the cells concerned with respiration, not the fibrous supporting tissue.

PARENTERAL (administration of a substance) other than via the digestive system, *e.g.* by injection.

PARESIS means a state of slight or temporary paralysis, also called 'fleeting paralysis'. (*See* MILK FEVER, NUTRITIONAL MUSCULAR DYSTROPHY, LEAD POISONING, PARALYSIS, GUTTURAL POUCH DIPHTHERIA.)

PARIETAL is the term applied to anything pertaining to the wall of a cavity; *e.g.* parietal pleura, the part of the pleural membrane which lines the wall of chest.

PARONYCHIA is inflammation near to the nail. (*See* RINGWORM.)

PAROTID GLAND is one of the salivary glands. It is situated just below and behind the ear on either side, in the space between the angle of the jaw and the muscles of the neck. From its base commences a duct, the parotid duct, or *Stenson's duct*, which in the horse runs within the border of the mandible for a distance, and then turns round its rim to the side of the face in company with the external maxillary artery and vein, and ends by opening into the mouth opposite the anterior part of the third upper cheek tooth; in other animals it runs straight across the face instead of along the lower jaw bone.

The salivary glands are composed of collections of secreting acini held together loosely by a certain amount of fibrous tissue, but they do not possess a distinct capsule. (*See* SALIVARY GLANDS.)

PAROVARIUM is the name of rudimentary structures situated near the ovary, which are the remnants of the Wolffian bodies. The name Paroöphoron is also used. These structures are often the seat of cysts in the young adult. (*See* OVARY.)

PARROTS (*see* PSITTACOSIS, *also* BIRDS, IMPORT OF; *and* PACHECO'S DISEASE).

PARTHENOGENESIS. Birth from a virgin. This is a common method of reproduction among animals which have no backbone. It implies the division of an ovum, and its development into an embryo, 'by itself'; that is to say, without a sperm being in any way involved. Its occurrence has been reported in connection with the eggs of cat, ferret, and turkey. Living rabbits have been born to virgin does. It is now believed that, exceedingly rarely, parthenogenesis leading to the birth of young may occur under natural conditions; both in the rabbit and in other mammals.

PARTRIDGES (*see* GAME BIRDS, MORTALITY).

PARTURIENT PARESIS (*see* MILK FEVER and 'DOWNER COW' SYNDROME).

PARTURITION is the expulsion of the fetus (and its membranes) from the uterus through the maternal passages by natural forces, and in such a state of development that, in domesticated animals at least, though not in the Marsupials, it is capable of independent life. The process is called 'foaling' in the mare, 'calving' in the cow, 'lambing' in the ewe, 'kidding' in the goat, 'farrowing' in the sow, and 'whelping' in the bitch. It is more likely to proceed successfully without than with human interference in the great majority of cases. It is not to be understood that human assistance should never be offered; there are many occasions when the judicious application of traction to a limb, or to the head and neck, will greatly assist the delivery of the foal or calf and relieve the dam of a considerable amount of suffering. (*See* CALVING, DIFFICULT for information on traction.)

The forces of expulsion. The powers by which expulsion is achieved are exerted by the plain muscle of the wall of the uterus in the first place, and, secondly, by contraction of the walls of the abdomen which raises the intra-abdominal pressure.

Stages in parturition. Although the act is really a continuous one it is customary to divide it into four stages: (1) The Preliminary Stage; (2) The Dilatation Stage; (3) The Expulsion of the Fetus Stage; (4) The Expulsion of the Membranes Stage.

(1) **THE PRELIMINARY STAGE** may occupy some hours or even days. The udder swells, becomes hard and tender, and a clear waxy fluid material oozes from the teats or may be expelled by pressure of the hand. The external genitals become swollen, enlarged, and their lining is reddened. A vaginal secretion appears. The abdomen drops and becomes pendulous. The quarters droop and the muscles and ligaments of the pelvis slacken. The animal separates itself from its fellows if at pasture, if at liberty, it seeks a remote or an inaccessible place in which to bring forth its young, and some, such as the sow, bitch, and cat, prepare a bed or nest.

(2) **DILATATION OF THE CERVIX STAGE** merges with the preceding. – Restlessness is evident. The mare paces around the loose-box (often with tail raised); and perhaps lying down and rising again several times. Sweating occurs under the mane and tail, and soon over most of the body.

During the second stage of labour, the mare is usually lying down on her side, and in some cases a mare will show symptoms of colic, *i.e.* kicking at the belly, turning and gazing at her flanks, or wandering round in an aimless fashion. Meanwhile the labour pains have been getting more and more powerful and the intervals between them shorter. The pulse is quickened, and the breathing rapid. When a pain has passed the animal calms down and remains so till the next takes place. After a variable time – from about ½ to 3 hours – the 'water-bag' appears at the vulva. It is tense and hard during a pain, but becomes slack and flaccid in the intervals. It is found to be empty at first, but the fore feet of the young animal can be felt in it later. At this time the cervix is fully dilated, and the third stage follows without any appreciable break in the sequence of events.

(3) **EXPULSION OF THE FETUS STAGE.** In this stage the severity of the pains is greatest, and the auxiliary muscles of the abdomen assist in the contractions. The animal may remain standing, may lie down in the recumbent position, or may alternately lie and stand. The back is arched, the chest expanded, and the muscles of the abdomen become board-hard with each labour pain. The animal may groan, or squeal or even scream with each effort. Frequently the rectum forcibly discharges its contents and the urinary bladder does likewise. At each contraction the 'water-bag' protrudes farther and farther from the vulva until it finally ruptures in its most dependant part. There is a rush of fluid from the uterus to the outside and the animal has a period of ease. Then fore-feet, and the muzzle lying behind and over them, appear at the vulva, forming a kind of cone which dilates the softer tissues of the genital canal. In the larger animals the feet come first, but in the **carnivora**, where the head is large, the head precedes the fore feet, which are tucked against the young animal's chest and sides. When the head has cleared the vulva there is usually another pause, which allows the tissues to become accustomed to the great distension, and prepares them for the still greater distension and strain that is soon to follow. The thorax and shoulders are now in the pelvis of the dam, and are driven slowly through it by the most powerful and painful of the contractions that occur during the process. As this part of the fetus reaches the outlet of the pelvis there is generally a more energetic and painful effort than all the others – which pushes the fetal trunk to the outside. This culminating effort may cause the **bitch** or **cat** to cry out.

Sometimes the **foal's** umbilical cord does not rupture, in which case the mare will usually gnaw through it, and so liberate the foal. It sometimes happens that a foal is born completely enveloped in its membranes; in such instances unless assistance is at hand to free the foal it will be rapidly suffocated.

In **cows** the umbilical cord is much shorter and it ruptures before the hind legs of the calf have passed to the outside. Owing to the cotyledonary attachment of the placenta the membranes are seldom born along with the calf. In the smaller animals, especially in the sow, bitch, and cat, the young are frequently born in their membranes, and these are licked away and cleared from the young by the dam,

the umbilical cord being broken or bitten through in the process.

(4) EXPULSION OF THE MEMBRANES STAGE, or the 'delivery of the afterbirth', may occur with, immediately following, or not for some considerable time after, the production of the young in an animal.

Very soon after the young animal is born the uterus contracts and becomes smaller – a process known as 'Involution' – so that its capacity is decreased. The attachment between the membranes and the mucosa of the uterus is loosened and the placenta is separated from the uterus. These contractions also serve to force the membranes to the outside through the wide open cervix.

With the **mare**, owing to the diffuse and not very intimate adherence between the uterine mucous membrane and the placental membrane, the separation and the discharge of the envelopes are soon accomplished. In fact, if these are retained for more than a very few hours (4 or 6 or so), serious results are probable, but retention of the membranes is rare in the healthy mare.

In the **cow**, the attachment is limited to the surfaces of the cotyledons and is very close, and where the shrinkage in the uterine wall (*i.e.* involution) does not tend greatly to upset the intimacy of the adhesion, the calf is not born in its membranes, and retention of these is more common. They are generally discharged within a few hours of the birth of the calf, but the time varies.

Animals which produce more than one young at a time generally discharge the membranes of each at the same time as or soon after it is born, with the exception of the last of the litter, whose membranes are occasionally retained in the extremity of one horn of the uterus.

In animals that are really uniparous (*i.e.* produce only one fetus at a birth but which have been modified by breeding so that they often produce two or more young, such as the sheep and goat) the membranes of the first twin come away with the second, and those of the second are expelled after it has been born.

Early discharge of the membranes is very desirable, because so long as they remain in position they are likely sources of infection to the uterus, and they prevent that organ from returning to normal. After they have been evacuated the involution of the uterus becomes more and more complete, until in a few days it has shrunk to less than half its former size. It never decreases to its original virgin size.

The **mare** should have been housed in the 'foaling-box' for a month or so previously, so that she shall feel quite at home (*see* PREGNANCY), and the ventilation, warmth, bedding, cleanliness, etc., should be as near an approach to the ideal as circumstances will allow. If possible, the **cow** should calve in a separate loosebox. **Ewes** lamb out in the open and do quite well, but if the weather be cold or stormy, or if the ground is very wet, it is better to provide a 'lambing-pen', especially with Lowland breeds which have not the same hardiness as the mountain varieties. **Sows** should on all occasions have a pen to themselves, for if other pigs are present the little pigs will most probably be eaten as soon as they are born.

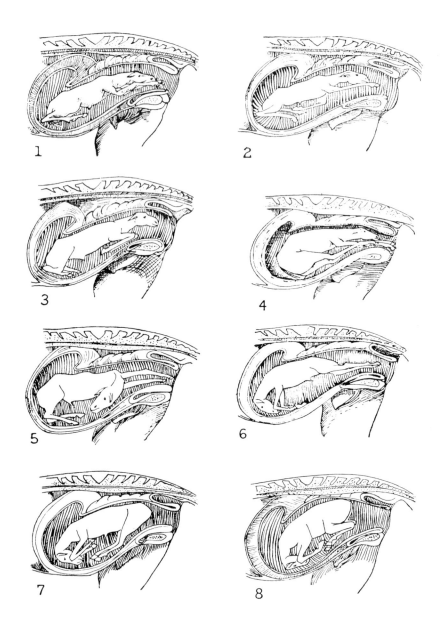

Different varieties of presentations of the foal.

1. Normal anterior presentation – nose and both fore-feet in passage.

2. Anterior presentation with one fore-limb retained completely. This should be brought forward by hand, or by passing rope round flexure of knee.

3. Anterior presentation with both fore-limbs retained at the knees, corrected as in No. 2.

4. 'Dog-sitting' presentation – nose and all four limbs presenting. The two fore-limbs should be corded and the hind-limbs repelled or pushed back.

5. Anterior presentation with head and neck retained. Delivery may often be effected by strong traction on fore-limbs in foal, the head being pressed into the soft abdomen. In calf, owing to the short neck, this is not usually possible. Where possible, fore-limbs should be corded, pushed back, and the head brought round by the hand or by hooks and cords.

6. Posterior presentation. Successful delivery often possible if the birth is speeded up by strong traction to avoid suffocation (see text).

7. 'Breech presentation'. Delivery difficult, foal nearly always dead. Cords in front of the foal's stifles and round buttocks may be applied if mare is large and foal is small, but usually necessitates amputation of one or both hind-limbs.

8. 'Thigh and croup presentation'. Cord round hocks may be successful in converting this into an ordinary posterior presentation. Quarters must be strongly repelled after hocks are corded.

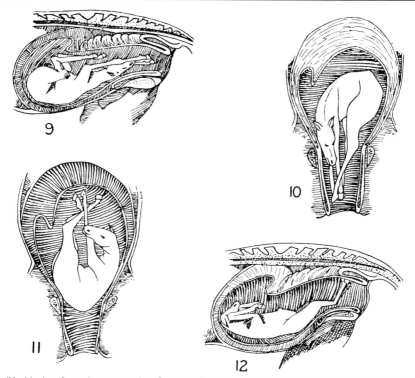

9. 'Upside-down' anterior presentation. Occasionally delivery may be effected without adjustment, but assist-ance is always necessary. Removal of one or both fore-limbs, with or without head and neck, often essential.

10. Ventral transverse presentation. This and No. 11 are the two worst positions in which foal can lie. Each case must be treated differently. Fore- or hind-limbs may be pushed back or brought forward according as they lie back in the passage or advanced. Removal of the foal in portions, a limb at a time, is often necessary.

11. Dorsal transverse presentation. Foal usually requires to be bisected and each half removed separately.

12. 'Upside down posterior presentation.' Delivery may be possible as soon as limbs have been adjusted, or amputation or version may be carried out.

When the act has begun the attendant may re-quire to soothe and quieten the dam if she becomes very excited, but beyond this the pros-pective mother should be left alone for some time. If all is going well the 'water-bag' will soon appear and later burst. No hard-and-fast rule can be laid down, but if the fore-legs and nose of the fetus do not appear in from 10 to 20 minutes in the mare, and in double that period in the cow, a simple examination should be made by the at-tendant to ensure himself that the presentation is a normal one. After washing hands and arms in Dettol or Cetrimide solutions, and thoroughly lubricating them with a vaginal lubricant, he should gently insert his hand into the posterior genital passage and explore whatever presents it-self to his hand. The two fore-feet should be dis-tinguishable in that part of the passage that lies lowermost when the dam is standing. Above them and slightly behind, the nose and mouth should be felt. These structures are often covered with fetal membrane, but in a normal case can be located with difficulty. In such cases as this nothing further need be done in the meantime; the dam will probably produce her young quite normally, and any attempts at assistance will only irritate and perhaps exhaust her.

It may happen, however, that one or both of the fore-legs may be missing, or that the nose cannot be found. On introducing the arms still farther

these parts can sometimes be discovered, and, by gentle pulling or readjustment, can be brought into the normal position. Before the process of parturition has advanced very far abnormal pos-itions of the fetus can be comparatively easily corrected, and serious trouble from subsequent jamming may be avoided. If all efforts at correc-tion prove futile, a veterinary surgeon should be called in, seeking skilled assistance, for the longer the dam is allowed to exert useless labour pains with the fetus in a position impossible for delivery, the more she will exhaust herself, the longer and the more difficult will be the act of parturition, and the less chance of survival will remain to the young animal.

Upon comparatively rare occasions none of the foremost positions of the body can be felt, but the two hind-feet or legs (distinguishable by the difference between knees and hocks), and perhaps the tail of the young animal, are discovered. This is a posterior presentation, and as the head is the last part of the fetus that will be born, respiration cannot begin until birth is complete, and the risk of suffocation is great. Accordingly, it is necess-ary to attempt to hurry the whole process and a veterinary surgeon should be called.

Attention to offspring. As soon as the young animal is born and free from the maternal pas-sages, it is absolutely essential to ascertain that the fetal membranes are not obstructing its mouth or nostrils. It generally gives one or two spasmodic gasps or struggles, and then begins to breathe. Each respiration is shallow and weak at first, but in a very few minutes the breathing settles down to the normal.

Suspended animation. Occasionally, foals and calves are born in a state of suspended animation, and ARTIFICIAL RESPIRATION (which see) will be needed.

The umbilical cord is, according to work carried out by the Equine Research Station, Animal Health Trust, best not interfered with.

'As a consequence of early severance of the cord the new-born foal is commonly deprived of 1000 to 1500 ml of placental fetal blood, whereas under 'natural' conditions the amount concerned is probably well under 200 ml.

'It is suggested that apart from the possibility that specific illnesses might sometimes be precipitated by this blood loss, the general interests of the animal are better served when they are allowed to retain the blood, as they almost always do under natural conditions.

'Since the umbilical cord has a point at which it will rupture normally after a period during which mother and foal rest, and since haemorrhage from either end of the severed cord is then extremely rare, it is suggested that the cord requires no human attention after a normal birth.

'Largely because it is not possible to state a time at which the transference of blood from the placenta is complete we would prefer that severance of the cord be left entirely to natural processes. We do not believe that the umbilical cord requires any human attention whatsoever provided it is allowed to break at the correct place and time (generally by the movement of the mare). Under normal circumstances there is no risk at all of haemorrhage from the vessels in the navel stump, their retraction occurs in a way which is virtually impossible after cutting and provides an effective seal against both bleeding and (almost certainly) infection. It is difficult to imagine a worse procedure than leaving a substantial 'meaty' mass of umbilical cord at the navel as happens so commonly after cutting the cord with scissors. This provides an ideal medium for the passage of micro-organisms whose entrance to the abdominal portions of the umbilical vein and arteries are not hindered in any way by the 'sterile' piece of tape so frequently used to 'tie off' the stump. Almost as undesirable a procedure is the application of strong antiseptics (notably iodine) destructive as they are to tissue with which they come in contact.'

Other advice. If a young mare, for instance, does not at once begin to dry and cleanse her foal, a little salt rubbed over its coat may induce her to do so. Should the mother refuse to perform this office, the offspring must be dried with a towel, cloth, wisp of hay, etc., so far as is possible.

Suckling. The first suck is of great importance. Within about half an hour the young of the domesticated animals are usually able to stand on their feet – although they are shaky at first – and as soon as they master this feat they make endeavours to reach the teat. The first milk contains a mild natural purgative, and it is essential that the newly born should obtain some of this as soon as possible. Colostrum promotes a secretion from the intestinal glands and stimulates peristalsis, so that the débris and black, gummy, faecal material (called 'meconium') that has been lying in the bowels of the foal is evacuated and the way prepared for the digestion of food. When a dam dies before the foal obtains any of her first secreted milk, it is necessary to supply a substitute for the colostrum, such as castor oil and milk, or melted butter and milk.

Attention to the dam. Where parturition has been easy and normal the dam rapidly recovers from her trying experience, and may be up on to her feet within a few minutes of the discharge of the fetus. It is usually better to allow her to remain lying as long as she wishes while attentions are being paid to her offspring. It is good practice to offer a drink of warm barley-water or thin oatmeal gruel containing a tablespoonful of common table-salt, as soon after the act as convenient. Her system has undergone a considerable shock, and has lost quantities of fluid which should be replaced. The larger animals may require a rug if the weather is at all cold. In from 6 to 3 hours or thereabout a pailful of bran mash and a little hay should be given.

When the dam is very exhausted by her labour it is necessary to administer stimulants. If the birth of the young was difficult, and when the passages have been exposed to considerable strain by ropes and traction, it is advisable to apply hot fomentations to the external genital organs. Afterwards the parts must be covered with a warm and dry blanket, sewn in position on to the rug or a surcingle, to prevent any chilling. The loose-box must be warm yet well ventilated, and the mare should be encouraged to lie and rest as much as possible.

Subsequent management. No oats or concentrated food-stuff should be given to the dam for the first 2 days after parturition; her rations should consist of water, bran mashes, and hay or green food given three times daily. After that time a gradually increasing amount of crushed oats and cut hay or chaff may be added to the mash daily, until at the end of a week or 10 days she is back on to her usual diet. Gentle exercise is as necessary for the foal or calf as it is for their dams, and if the weather be suitable the dam and her progeny should be allowed out on to a sheltered meadow for an hour or so twice daily, after the first 3 or 4 days following the birth of the young. This period is gradually increased until in 2 weeks' time the pair may be left out from 9.0 a.m. till 5.0 in the evening, or even may be allowed to sleep out all night if the weather permits. In this connection it should be remembered that cold dry nights are much less harmful than those that are wet or foggy. Young animals of all species withstand dry cold very much better than wet cold, and it is inadvisable to allow foals or calves less than a month old to sleep out on a wet or marshy meadow. A useful method is to erect a covered-in shed in a corner of the meadow, containing a feeding-trough and well littered with straw, into which both dam and her offspring may retire whenever they wish. The amount of hand feeding which the dam receives must be judged according to circumstances. If the grass is rich and well forward, one feed of oats and hay may be sufficient after the first 3 or 4 weeks, but it is always better to err on the safe side and keep the dam in good general condition, for much of the subsequent quality of the off-spring depends upon the start in life that it receives through its mother's milk, and if she herself is in poor condition her milk will be inferior.

If it be not too severe, the mare may work for half a day at a time when the foal is from 2 to 3 months old. When the mare is at work the foal should be shut in a loose-box with a mate if possible, and given freshly cut green clover or lucerne. It is very important to avoid allowing a hungry foal to suck its mother when she is in a heated or sweating condition, for serious attacks of indigestion and diarrhoea are frequent results of such an indiscretion. If the mare returns to the stable hot and sweating – as she will when the weather is warm and before her condition is hardened – she should be given a feed of oats and a little hay and allowed to stand in a loose-box or stall for an hour until she has cooled down, before the foal is let out with her.

The general principles given above for the larger domestic animals are applicable to the smaller ones.

PARTURITION, DRUG-INDUCED is a technique used in some cases of debility of the dam in late pregnancy, where there is some abnormality associated with the pregnancy, to avoid dystokia in the cross-breeding of dairy cows for beef production, and for programming the date of parturition. In a trial in Denmark induced calving, using corticosteroids (dexamethasone), resulted in 73 per cent of treated cows calving within 4 days. Stillborn calves averaged 16 per cent; retained placenta 34 per cent.

In a small trial in Australia, 15 cows tested with dexamethasone trimethyacetate, between 240 and 252 days after conception, calved 24 days prematurely (range: 14 to 32 days). There were no calving problems but their calves were lighter at birth and at 12 weeks. Treated cows returned earlier to oestrus, had shorter periods of calving to conception, and had less subclinical mastitis during the first 2 weeks of lactation. (Bailey, L. F., et. al., Aust. vet. J. (1973) **49**, 557.)

Premature parturition was induced in 709 cows and heifers three to eight months pregnant. Most received I/M injection with 10 ml dexamethasone (2·2 mg/kg and 1 mg/ml phenylproprionate and sodium phosphate ester respectively) though two and three doses had to be given to 240 and 12 animals respectively. About half the cattle required treatment for retained fetal membranes while 184 of the 709 calves died before four weeks of age. Induction of calving had no apparent effect on the incidence of dystokia, post-calving fertility or on milk production. (Allen, J. G. and Herring, J. (1976) Aust. vet. J., **52**, 442.)

In sows, prostaglandin analogues are used to cause regressions of the *corpora lutea* of pregnancy and so reduce the concentration of circulating progesterone, thereby imitating one of the hormone changes that precede the onset of normal parturition. Give 3 to 5 days before the expected farrowing date, parturition was induced within 26 hours. The method, when perfected, should enable farrowings to be grouped within the working hours of a 5-day week. (*See also* 'CONTROLLED BREEDING'.)

PARVOVIRUS. This has been associated with infertility in the sow, and a cause of mummified fetuses and small litter size. (*See* VIRUSES, Classification Table, CANINE PARVOVIRUS INFECTION, *and* FELINE INFECTIOUS ENTERITIS.) ☞

PAS is the abbreviation for para-aminosalicylic acid, a drug which has been used in the treatment of tuberculosis in zoo animals.

PASSAGE (pronounced as in French) is a bacteriological term meaning the passing of a strain of organisms through a series of animals to decrease or increase virulence. For example, passage of cattle plague virus through goats is done to reduce its virulence for cattle, and is a technique used in the production of cattle plague vaccine.

PASTERN. The name given to the first (long) and second (short) phalanges of the fore-limb, and to the joint so formed.

PASTEURELLA. A genus of bacteria, which are small, ovoid, Gram-negative, bipolar staining. Both non-motile and motile species occur, and they are aerobic or facultatively anaerobic. For the diseases they cause, see following entries.

PASTEURELLOSIS OF CATS (*see* YERSINIOSIS and BUBONIC PLAGUE; *see* BITES for human infection with *Pasteurella multocida*, formerly known as *P. septica*.

A survey by P. E. Curtis and G. E. Ollerhead, University of Liverpool, indicated that *P. multocida* can readily be recovered from the throats of cats on poultry farms, and that some cat strains are of similar virulence for chickens as a strain which has caused deaths in adult turkeys. The cat itself harbours *P. multocida* as one of its bacterial flora.

It is unlikely that cats have an important role in outbreaks of pasteurellosis in poultry. (*Veterinary Record* (1982) **110**, 13.)

PASTEURELLOSIS OF CATTLE. This includes HAEMORRHAGIC SEPTICAEMIA (*see under* that heading) of cattle and buffaloes in the tropics; SHIPPING FEVER ('Transit fever') of the American feedlots and elsewhere; and another pneumonia occurring in Europe.

In calves, *Pasteurella haemolytica* serotype A1 may be the primary pathogen. (Serotype A2 and *P. multocida* may also be isolated). Symptoms include a nasal discharge, a respiratory rate of 60 to 100 per minute, and a temperature of up to 107°F.

(*See* CALF PNEUMONIA for viruses which may be involved, and for synergism between Pasteurella and Mycoplasma.)

The pneumonia is fibrinous in type, and this is seen also in older cattle; *P. haemolytica* or *P. multocida* often being found in large numbers.

PASTEURELLOSIS OF DUCKS. Caused by *Pasteurella anatipestifer*, this is a disease of considerable economic importance in ducklings, with a mortality sometimes as high as 70 per cent. Less acutely infected birds may shake their heads or draw their heads close to their bodies. Sulphadimidine has been used in treatment.

PASTEURELLOSIS OF SHEEP is caused occasionally by *Pasteurella multicocida* but far more commonly by *P. haemolytica*, and sub-clinical infection may develop into pneumonia if parainfluenza III virus is present too.

P. haemolytica biotype A causes enzootic pneumonia; while biotype T is mainly associated with septicaemia. Both may be isolated from cases of arthritis. *P. haemolytica* also causes mastitis in ewes, and meningitis – especially in lambs.

Young sheep are liable to die from the acute septicaemic form, while older ones show a slower type of the disease, in which the pneumonic lesions predominate.

SIGNS. The acute cases are ushered in by high temperature, great dullness and nervous depression, difficult respirations, muscular tremors, followed by rapid collapse and death in from 1 to 3 days.

In the less acute cases, similar but slightly milder symptoms occur. These are accompanied by a discharge from the eyes and nose, loss of appetite and absence of rumination, with signs of pneumonia or pleurisy.

DIAGNOSIS. The acute form may be confused with anthrax or Braxy.

IMMUNISATION. Improved vaccines containing several strains of *P. haemolytica* are available; also a combined clostridial and pasteurella vaccine. A serum has also been prepared. (*See also* PNEUMONIA IN SHEEP.)

PASTEURELLOSIS IN MAN. *Pasteurella multocida* is a commensal organism in the mouth and nasopharynx of many animals. In humans, superficial infections of the skin and mucous membranes, such as corneal, oral or leg ulcers and infections of compound fractures, conjunctivitis or sinusitis and panophthalmitis may result from animal bites or scratches. In these infections *P multocida* is likely to have been acquired when saliva from the animal contacted injured tissue. Pasteurella organisms may also invade the body via the respiratory system or, less commonly, via the alimentary tract and skin lesions. The most commonly seen internal infections of *P multocida* are associated with chronic obstructive lung disease. A third category of infection is suggested: septicaemia and bacteraemia in patients with chronic disease, especially chronic liver disease. Underlying disease may predispose to pasteurellosis in man; it was associated with carcinomas in 11 patients in one hospital. *P. multocida* may be

acquired as a result of handling raw poultry carcases. Small domestic pets may be carriers of *P. multocida*. Internal infections may derive from farm animals; in one study 27 of 37 patients with internal infection lived on farms. Other *Pasteurella* species that affect animals rarely occur in man. (Carter, G. R. *Veterinary Medicine/Small Animal Clinician* (1984) **79,** 629.)

In the UK there were reports of 3699 cases of human pasteurellosis during the period 1975 to 1986. Eighty-six per cent of these were skin infections; two-thirds due to dog bites; a quarter due to cat bites. In a small proportion of cases meningitis and septicaemia were complicating factors. (Young, S. E. J. *PHLS Microbiology Digest* **5,** 4.)

PASTEURISATION OF MILK.

High temperature pasteurisation consists in heating the milk for 10 or 20 minutes at a temperature of $167°F$ ($75°C$). This is sufficient to render harmless the germs of enteric and scarlet fever and diphtheria, and also bacteria which give rise to summer diarrhoea in children. It also affords a considerable measure of protection against tuberculosis.

Low temperature pasteurisation consists in maintaining the milk for at least half an hour at a temperature between $145°F$ and $150°F$ ($63°$ to $65°C$). This has the effect of considerably reducing the number of bacteria contained in the milk and very greatly delaying souring and similar changes. This procedure is sufficient for the sale of milk as 'pasteurised milk' in England. (*See also* ULTRA HIGH TEMPERATURE TREATMENT.)

Unpasteurised milk (*see* MILK-BORNE INFECTIONS).

PASTURE 'CLEAN'. It was widely assumed that resting a pasture heavily contaminated with parasitic worm larvae of sheep or cattle for 4 to 6 weeks during dry, cold weather, will render it safe for grazing by susceptible stock. This is a dangerous assumption, for such larvae can survive on pasture rested for a whole winter.

Professor James Armour and colleagues at the department of veterinary parasitology, University of Glasgow, reported their finding of clinical parasitic bronchitis ('Husk'), due to the lungworm *Dictyocaulus viviparus*, and gastro-enteritis due to *Osertagia ostertagi*, in young cattle grazing aftermath pasture in late summer. In one instance, worm-free calves, previously housed, were grazed on a hay aftermath in August and developed signs of parasitic bronchitis within three weeks. Calves on pasture lightly infested with *Ostertagia* 'were effectively treated with an anthelmintic and transferred to a silage aftermath in late July. A marked increase in 3rd-stage larvae numbers on the aftermath occurred within the first week, and clinical signs of type I ostertagiasis were observed four weeks later.'

'In both instances the aftermath pastures had not been grazed since the previous autumn, and the interval between entry to the aftermath and clinical or other evidence of infection precluded the possibility of the calves being responsible for cycling of the infection.'

Such findings suggested the existence of a reservoir of infective larvae in the soil persisting from previous grazing seasons. 'Preliminary observations on core samples of soil from permanent cattle pastures in the Glasgow area revealed that *Ostertagia* 3rd-stage larvae were regularly present, and lungworm 3rd-stage larvae occasionally present, over the 12-month period August 1978 to July 1979.'

Research in the USA has shown that if *Ostertagia* eggs are buried to a depth of 12·5 cm under pasture, or beneath 15 cm of soil in the laboratory, 3rd-stage larvae develop and migrate vertically through the soil. 'Whether this migration occurs independently under natural conditions, or requires the aid of transport hosts such as earthworms, is not yet definitely known,' the Glasgow research workers commented; but these findings suggest that the concept of 'clean' pasture is now less credible than ever before. However, the good husbandry rule of keeping young stock off pasture previously grazed in the same season by adult stock is, obviously, still worth applying as a means of avoiding even worse outbreaks. (J. Armour and others. *Vet. Rec.* (1980) **106**, 184.)

PASTURE, CONTAMINATION OF. This may occur in the vicinity of smelting works (*see under* FACTORY CHIMNEYS), or as the result of droplets of chemical sprays being carried by the wind to adjoining fields. (For a list of chemical sprays, *see under* WEEDKILLERS *and* INSECTICIDES.) Contamination may also occur as the result of atomic fall-out. (*See* RADIOACTIVE FALL-OUT.) Bacterial contamination is exemplified by the presence of anthrax spores. (*See under* ANTHRAX.) Resting pasture for 3 weeks provides a measure of control of foot-rot; the organism responsible being unable to survive for more than a fortnight. For contamination by worm larvae, *see* PARASITIC BRONCHITIS, GASTROENTERITIS, and preceding section. For contamination by organic irrigation *see under* SLURRY. *See also* BASIC SLAG, FERTILISERS.

The average cow defaecates about 12 times daily and each pat weighs about 2·5 kg; in a 180 day grazing season, she will put about 5 tons of faeces (containing about 1500 lb dry matter) on to the pasture. (*See* DAIRY HERD MANAGEMENT.) (For contamination by slurry applications, *see* SLURRY and 'MILKSPOT' LIVER; *also* SOIL-CONTAMINATED HERBAGE.)

Contamination of pasture may occur during FLOODING (which see) and, in a sense, when ticks are left behind by a batch of cattle infected with piroplasms; the ticks then infecting other cattle put on to that land (*see* RED-WATER FEVER).

PASTURE MANAGEMENT is of the greatest importance in relation to diseases such as Bloat, Hypomagnesaemia, Parasitic Gastro-Enteritis and Bronchitis. (*See under these headings; also under* DEEP-ROOTING PLANTS, TOPPING, *and* WILTING.) Controlled grazing is effected by means of an electric fence. (*See* STRIP-GRAZING *and under* PADDOCKS.)

It is important that heavy application of nitrogenous and potash fertilisers to grassland should be made at the right time, or animals grazing there will be exposed to a greatly increased risk of hypomagnesaemia. (*See also* BASIC SLAG poisoning.) (*See also* HOOF-PRINTS.)

The sudden (and harmful) change of diet which may occur when stock are turned out in the spring, or brought off pasture into yards for the winter, are discussed below.

In spring, it is a mistake to turn calves straight out on to grass. This means a sudden change from protein-poor food to the rich protein of the early bite, and the resulting effect upon the rumen will set them back. It is wise to get them out before there is much grass for a few hours each day; let them have hay and shelter at night to protect them from sudden changes of weather. Hypomagnesaemia, too, is far less likely under these circumstances.

Before yarding cattle in the autumn, it is wise to make a gradual change from sugar-poor autumn pasture to things like roots, and to accustom them to concentrates. Otherwise digestive upsets are very likely to occur.

It should be borne in mind that *Trichostrongylus axei* is a parasite common to cattle, sheep, goats, and horses, and grazing one species of animal after another in a field could give rise to a very heavy contamination with this one parasite.

Prompt removal of faeces from pasture has been found effective in reducing the worm burden, and practicable where acreage is small, labour cheap, or racehorses are concerned. It has been advocated for horse pasture by Dr Rupert Herd, Ohio State University's College of Veterinary Medicine, and is practised in Cairo.

Use of goats in sheep grazing systems. Recent work has shown that goats prefer to graze plant species not readily eaten by sheep and also that, given the choice, goats will discriminate against plant species such as clover which are important and beneficial in sheep production systems. The introduction of goats can benefit the sheep stock by helping to prevent the degeneration of the improved areas and by keeping the indigenous vegetation in a more productive and nutritious state, while at the same time not competing with the sheep for the more valuable plant species. (*Hill Farm Research Organisation.*)

Other aspects of pasture management are referred to under the following headings: PASTURE CONTAMINATION; BRACKEN; RAGWORT; FOX GLOVES; WORMS, FARM TREATMENT AGAINST; EXPOSURE; STRESS; POACHING; BEEF CATTLE HUSBANDRY; SHEEP BREEDING; SILAGE; FOG FEVER; HAY, STOCKING RATES, TOPPING.

Grass varieties. Professor P. T. Thomas has commented that plant breeding for improved pastures is in its infancy as compared with that for the agronomically less complex arable crops. The potential for improvement is therefore great, though difficult to quantify.

Of course, mere yield (whether annual or seasonal) is only one of four criteria useful in judging a new variety. Its persistency, palatability and nutritive value are important criteria, too; for a high-yielding variety may be contra-indicated if animals lose weight on it, as they do with one variety of Phalaris tried some years ago. Then again one must consider the effect which the system of grassland management has, and how varieties will stand up to a given system. Professor Thomas drew attention in the *Journal of the RASE* to the fact that with regular defoliation, perennial rye-grass yields more than Italian ryegrass; whereas with infrequent cutting, Italian ryegrass yields more.

'We have long regarded Britain as being essentially a ryegrass country, but these studies indicate clearly that for future systems of farming at high production we should be considering more seriously a species like tall fescue, whose biological potential is known to be very high, and whose reaction to intensive systems of defoliation is favourable.'

Differences between the grazing habits of beef and dairy cattle may have their effect, he observes; and a 'poachability table' is needed for grass varieties.

Horses. Pasture grasses and herbs recommended by the Animal Health Trust, after preliminary trials, for horses are classified as under:
Desirable species
Perennial Ryegrasses, Sceempter, Melle, Petra, Midas, S.23 and S.321, Timothy S.50 and S.48, Cocksfoot S.143, Crested Dogstail, Wild White Clover, Dandelion, Ribgrass, Chicory, Yarrow, Burnet, Sainfoin.
Probably useful (turf species which are also palatable).
Tall Fescue Alta. Canadian Creeping Red Fescue. Smooth Stalked Meadow Grass. Rough Stalked Meadow Grass.
Best excluded
Perennial Ryegrass S.24. Creeping Red Fescue. Brown Top. Meadow Foxtail. Red clover.

PATELLA is the bone that lies at the front of the 'stifle joint', and is called the 'knee-cap'. It lies in the tendon of the large extensor muscles of the joint, just above and in front of the true femorotibial joint. It is roughly pyramidal in the horse, with the apex of the pyramid pointing downwards. It is dislocation of the patella that constitutes the condition known as 'slipped stifle'. (*See* BONES.)

Dislocation of the patella (Patella luxation) may occur as an inherited abnormality in certain breeds of dogs, *e.g.* Boston Terriers, Boxers, Bulldogs, Cairn Terriers, Chihuahuas, Wire Fox Terriers, Griffons, Pekingese, Maltese, Papillons, Pomeranians. Poodles, Labradors, Scotch Terriers, King Charles Spaniels.

Indications for surgery of the canine stifle are congenital medial luxation and rupture of the anterior cruciate ligament.

Congenital patellar luxation occurs also in cats, rendering them unable to walk normally or jump.

PATENT DUCTUS ARTERIOSUS. An abnormality in which the *ductus arteriosus*, between the aorta and the pulmonary artery, fails to close at or shortly after birth. This condition has been recognised in the puppy, and gives rise to a characteristic murmur on auscultation; and also in cattle and cats. (*See* LIGAMENTUM ARTERIOSUM.)

PATENTED ANIMALS. Reuters reported that the USA government had awarded the first patent of this kind in 1988. It covered a mouse strain, bred at Harvard University, and containing a single human gene 'that makes it develop tumours after exposure to very small amounts of carcinogens. The patented animals are expected to be useful in testing new chemicals.'

PATHETIC NERVE is the fourth nerve arising from the brain and controlling the superior oblique muscle of the eye.

PATHOGENIC: disease-producing.

PATHOGNOMONIC is a term applied to those signs or symptoms of a particular disease which are characteristic of that disease, and on whose presence or absence the diagnosis depends.

PATHOLOGICAL SPECIMENS, POSTING OF. Specimens must be sent by letter post only, and marked 'Pathological Specimen'. They should be enclosed in a waterproof receptacle, *e.g.* a sealed polythene bag, and this should be surrounded with plenty of cotton-wool or sawdust, or other absorbent material in a strong box. For further information, *see* the Post Office Guide.

PATHOLOGY is the science which deals with the causes of and the changes produced in the body by disease.

PAZONE is the proprietary name of Nitrovin, a growth promoter. (*See* ADDITIVES.)

PEAS, MUTTER (*see* LATHYRISM).

'PEAT SCOURS' is a name given in Australasia and Canada to molybdenum poisoning in grazing cattle. (*See* MOLYBDENUM.)

PECK ORDER. This is the equivalent in poultry of the order of precedence described under BUNT ORDER.

PEDICULOSIS is infestation with lice.

PELLAGRA (*see* BLACK TONGUE).

PELLETS (*see* CUBES).

PELVIS is the posterior girdle of bones by which the two hind-limbs are attached to the rest of the skeleton. It is composed of two ilia, two pubes, and two ischia, united together by fusion into a basin-shaped whole (*see* BONES). Strictly speaking, it includes the sacrum and the coccygeal vertebrae. The two 'haunch bones' are the external angles of the ilia; the 'croup' is composed of the internal angles of these bones along with the spines of the sacrum; and the 'points of the buttocks' are the tuberosities of the two ischia. The pelvis is spoken of as having an 'inlet', formed by the brim of the pubes, and an 'outlet' posteriorly. In the living animal the outlet is occupied by the soft tissues forming the perineal region, except for the anus in the male and the anus and vulva in the female. The deep notch between the sacrum and the haunch bone is closed by the sacro-sciatic ligaments, upon which lie the gluteal muscles which give the quarters their shape. The pelvis varies' in the two sexes: in the female it is broader from side to side, and deeper from above downwards, than in the male; this difference being chiefly necessary to allow of the act of parturition.

The contents of the pelvis are the rectum and urinary bladder in both sexes (except in the dog, where the urinary bladder is abdominal in position). In the male there is in addition the prostate gland and the seminal vesicles around the neck of the bladder and the beginning of the urethra; while the female pelvis contains the vagina, uterus, their appendages, and perhaps the ovaries.

PEMPHIGUS. A type of bullous autoimmune disease seen in dogs. Various forms have been described, *e.g. P. vulgaris*, in which lesions affect the mucous membrane lining the mouth, and the junction with the lips, giving rise to ulcers. Sometimes the pads of the feet are affected. *P. erythematosis* is characterised by crusty lesions on and around the nose, and elsewhere on the face.

In *P. vegetans* alopecia and pruritus follow pustules which ulcerate on the body and extremities. (*In Practice* May 1984.)

PENIA. A suffix meaning too few, less than normal. (*See* LEUKOPENIA for an example.)

PENICILLIN. The first of the antibiotics, discovered by Sir Alexander Fleming in 1929. Benzyl penicillin is the sodium or potassium salt of the antimicrobial acids produced when the moulds *Penicillium notatum* or *Chrysogenum* (or related species) are grown under suitable conditions.

Purified penicillin salts occur as a white crystalline powder, readily soluble in water. Their therapeutic potency is expressed in International Units.

Following injection into the animal body, penicillin is rapidly absorbed and diffused in the blood-stream throughout the body, being excreted by the kidneys. It is non-poisonous even in large doses and is effective against:

Staphylococci, causing local pyogenic inflammation as primary or secondary infections.
Haemolytic streptococci, usually causing localised infections either primary or secondary.
Streptococcus equi, causing strangles in horses.
Streptococcus agalactiae causing
*Streptococcus dysgalactiae** mastitis
*Streptococcus uberis** in cattle.
B. anthracis, causing anthrax.
Clostridium chauvoei, causing blackleg in cattle.
Corynebacterium renale, causing pyelonephritis in cattle.

* To a slight extent.

Erysipelothrix rhusiopathiae, causing swine erysipelas.
Actinomyces bovis, causing actonoymycosis.
Leptospira canicola, causing leptospirosis in dogs.

Penicillin is of some value in the treatment of wounds and for the prevention of sepsis in surgery.

It is of great importance that penicillin should be used in full doses; otherwise there is a risk of strains of bacteria resistant to penicillin being developed. The *minimum* dosage for systemic administration is 2000 units per 5 lbs body-weight or, in the large animals 50,000 units per 1 cwt.

'The long-established benzyl penicillin has the following shortcomings: (1) It is unstable in acids, and therefore cannot be given orally. This consideration, however, is of little importance in the veterinary field. (2) Organisms which produce penicillinase, and these are not uncommon, are resistant to benzyl penicillin. (3) It is active against only a narrow range of organisms. Semisynthetic penicillins were developed to overcome these drawbacks. Firstly, Phenethicillin potassium was developed as a penicillin stable in acids and which is an improvement on the older acid stable penicillin Phenoxymethylpenicillin, because after oral administration it gives twice as high a level in the blood. It is slightly resistant to penicillinase and is used in the veterinary field mainly in the treatment of mastitis involving susceptible strains of streptococci and staphylococci. Secondly, Methicillin; the main feature of methicillin is that it is resistant to penicillinase; it can, however, be given only parenterally. Methicillin should never be used in the treatment of infections caused by organisms susceptible to benzyl penicillin, since it is much less potent and may give rise to strains of organisms which show a penicillin resistance which is not due to the production of penicillinase. Moreover, methicillin actually stimulates the production of penicillinase. Thirdly, Cloxacillin; this penicillin is resistant to penicillinase, is stable in acids, but induces the production of penicillinase. Fourthly, Ampicillin; this is a most important introduction, because it is a penicillin active against both Gram-positive and Gram-negative organisms. It is useful particularly in the treatment of tetracycline-resistant coliforms, strains of *Proteus* and *Pseudomonas*, *Salmonellae*, *Shigellae*, and *Pasteurellae*. It is not resistant to penicillinase, and is acid stable.

'Benethamine penicillin is a long-acting preparation, given by intramuscular injection as an insoluble suspension from which benzyl penicillin is slowly released. Benzathine penicillin has the same properties as benethamine penicillin, but is acid stable and can therefore be given by mouth to dogs and cats.

'While these long-acting preparations of penicillin eliminate the necessity for frequent administration, they do, however, present the risk of inducing resistant strains because they must by their nature provide a lower level of penicillin in the tissues for a long period after their administration has terminated. This feature should be borne in mind when using them.' (Professor F. Alexander.)

PENICILLIN IN MILK (*see* PENICILLIN, SENSITIVITY TO).

PENICILLIN, SENSITIVITY TO. People handling penicillin suffer a risk of sensitisation, shown by skin lesions. In a limited survey, 4·3 per cent nurses working under local health authorities had become sensitised to one or more antibiotic. Some have had to abandon their profession. The same risk obviously applies to veterinarians. There is danger in the use of milk containing penicillin (*e.g.* milk from quarters of the udder treated for mastitis), especially in people sensitised to penicillin. Extremely severe skin lesions, and accompanying illness, have been caused in this way among farmers and others. A similar risk applies in the case of other antibiotics. (*See also under* MILK.) Hypersensitivity to penicillins has been recorded also in cattle and other animals, including cats.

PENICILLINASE. A penicillin-destroying enzyme produced by certain bacteria, *e.g. E. coli.*

PENIS is attached by roots (*crura*) to the ischial arch of the pelvis. From the roots extends the body of the penis along the interior of which runs the urethra, for the passage of urine and semen. Erection of the penis depends upon the increased flow of blood into the spongy, erectile tissue in the body of the penis, and simultaneous decrease in relative outflow from the veins, partly as a result of contraction of the *ischiocavernosus* muscles. The bull, ram and boar each have a sigmoid or S-shaped curve in the penis. On erection this curve is straightened. The penis increases in length but not much in girth. In the stallion and dog, in which the penis is straight, erection brings an increase in girth to a greater extent. The *Os penis* in the dog is a grooved bone within the *glans penis*, which is the terminal portion of the penis (except in the boar). The shape of the *glans* differs in the other species as regards shape. The penis of the cat is a frequent site of urethral obstruction owing to its very small diameter. Sand-like deposit, a calculus, plug of organic and crystalline deposit, or a grass seed may cause blockage. In some cases manipulation of the penis may allow the passage of urine, otherwise the use of a catheter may be tried or cystotomy undertaken. (*See* UROLITHIASIS, FUS).

PENIS and PREPUCE, ABNORMALITIES AND LESIONS. These include the following conditions:

Phimosis. A narrowing of the orifice of the prepuce, preventing normal protrusion of the penis. Congenital phimosis is occasionally seen in dogs, cats, and horses. It can be corrected surgically.

Paraphimosis. A condition in which the penis cannot be retracted into the prepuce. This is not uncommon in the **dog**, and is potentially serious unless quickly relieved owing to interference with

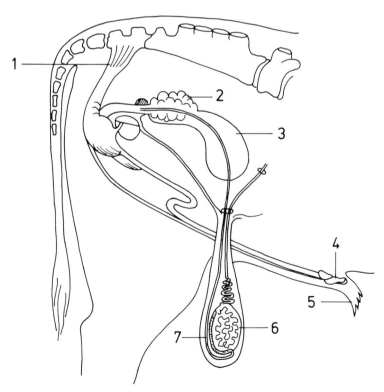

Genitalia of the bull: **1** muscle which controls penis; **2** vesicles which store semen; **3** bladder; **4** penis; **5** sheath which covers penis; **6** testicle; **7** epididymis.

the circulation. As a first-aid measure, swabbing the penis with ice-cold water may prove helpful, but professional aid under anaesthesia is usually needed to avert gangrene.

Prolapse of the penis due to paralysis is seen in bulls which have rabies, and also as a chronic condition in Zebu **cattle** (*Bos indicus*) and occasionally in breeds of UK origin.

Horses. Prolapse of the penis may follow use of acepromazine (to effect relaxation of the retractor muscles so that swabbing can be undertaken for contagious equine metritis). In six cases involving protrusion, oedema, and paresis of the penis, four of the horses had received acepromazine with etorphine hydrochloride, and two had received the former drug along with others. 'It is recommended that following the use of neuroleptic drugs a check should always be made to ensure that penile retraction is taking place as the effects of medication wear off. If not, treatment should be started without delay.' (Pearson, H. & Weaver, B. *Equine Veterinary Journal* (1978) **10**, 85.)

Priapism. A persistent erection of the penis unassociated with sexual stimulation. (*See also entry under that main heading.*)

Balanitis. Inflammation of the *glans penis*.

Posthitis. Inflammation of the prepuce.

Balanoposthitis. In this both the penis and the prepuce are affected. One example is an enzootic form, called 'Pizzle Rot' or 'Sheath Rot', of sheep (especially Merinos) in Australia. *Corynebacterium renale* is the primary cause.

A herpes virus also causes balanoposthitis in cattle and sheep. Amputation of the prepuce close to the prolapsed and infected area has given good results in bulls.

An infectious balanoposthitis (also known as Ulcerative Dermatosis) of sheep may affect not only the penis, prepuce, and vulva but also the face, feet, legs; and has to be differentiated from ORF. It occurs in Europe, South Africa. In lambs mortality may be up to 30 per cent.

Cause. A virus.

Tumours of the penis include warts (papillomas) and also, in dogs, infective granulomas. (*See* VENEREAL TUMOURS).

Traumatic lesions include injury to the penis from a kick by the cow or mare at service, or when a bull proves too heavy for a heifer. There is usually an accompanying haematoma. Trauma may also result in adhesions at the sigmoid flexure. In dogs a fracture of the *os penis* may occur as the result of being hit by a car.

Spiral deviation of the penis occurs in bulls. Service is prevented if deviation occurs *before* insertion of the penis; but it may also occur afterwards. (In the USA deviation of the penis is sometimes deliberately produced surgically in teaser bulls.)

PENITREM A. A mycotoxin. It was isolated from mouldy cream cheese in a refrigerator, and given to a dog which became very ill with ataxia, muscular tremors, and opisthotonos. The mould was identified as *Penicillum crustosum*.

PENTASTOMIASIS. Infection with the nymphs of the pentastomid *Armillifer armillatus*; the adults of which infest snakes in Africa and Asia.

The disease has been recognised in man, dog and cat.

SIGNS: Abdominal or thoracic oedema.

Infection occurs through drinking water contaminated by the eggs or eating a snake.

DIAGNOSIS: In human medicine this is based on the radiographic appearance of calcified nymphs. (Moens, Y. & Tshamala, M. *Veterinary Record* (1986) **119**, 44.)

PENTOBARBITAL SODIUM. A narcotic and anaesthetic. (*See* NEMBUTAL.)

PEPSIN is an enzyme found in the gastric juice which digests proteins.

PEPTIDES are composed of two or more amino acids, and represent an intermediate stage in the digestion of protein. **Polypeptides** are proteins composed of several amino-acids linked by the peptide grouping CH–CO–NH–CH.

Synthetic polypeptides have potential uses as vaccines; *e.g.* against foot-and-mouth disease.

PEPTOCOCCUS indolicus. A gram-positive bacterium which is sometimes a complicating factor in CASEOUS LYMPHADENITIS of sheep and 'summer mastitis' in cattle.

PERCHERIES. A system of housing for laying hens which is stated to combine some of the benefits of free range with most of the efficiency of cage systems. 'We house 22 birds per sq. metre, with 15 cm of perch space per bird,' stated Sue Tucker, deputy director (poultry) at Gleadthorpe Experimental Husbandry Farm, England.

PERCUSSION is a method of making an examination of the deeper parts of the body by means of striking the area overlying such organs, either with the fingers of one hand or with an instrument known as a 'plessor', in such a way as to give out a note. According to the degree of dullness or resonance of the note, an opinion can be formed as to the state of consolidation of air-containing organs, the presence of abnormal cavities, the dimensions of solid or air-containing organs when these lie adjacent to each other, the presence of fluid in various parts, etc. Percussion is practised along with auscultation of the parts, and by considering the net results a fairly accurate estimation of the conditions can be given. (*See* AUSCULTATION.)

PERFORATION is one of the serious dangers attached to the presence of ulcerating conditions in the stomach and bowels. When a perforation of one of these hollow organs takes place in the peritoneal cavity, multitudes of bacteria, much ingesta, mucus, and other putrescible materials escape and set up peritonitis. (*See* PERITONITIS.) The immediate signs are a collapse of the patient, with, later, collections of gas or fluids in the abdominal cavity. It is not uncommon to observe vomiting in the horse when the stomach ruptures and the contents escape into the abdominal cavity; this is one of the very rare times when the horse is seen to vomit, and it is important accordingly.

PERFORMANCE TESTING. A method of comparing strains or breeds of, *e.g.* beef cattle, by studying liveweight gains over a stated period with given rations. (*See also* PROGENY TESTING.)

PERI- is a prefix meaning round or about. Examples: pericardium, the membranous sac enclosing the heart; perianal abscess.

PERICARDITIS. Inflammation of the pericardium.

Traumatic pericarditis is common in cattle as a result of swallowing pieces of wire, nails, etc. (*See* HEART DISEASES.)

PERICARDIUM is the smooth lubricating membrane which surrounds the heart. (*See* HEART.)

PERINEUM is the region lying between the anus and the genital organs in the male, and lying between the anus and the mammary region in the female of the horse, ox, sheep, goat, and pig. In bitches and cats the female genital organs lie lower than in other animals and in them the perineum lies between the anus and the vulva.

Rupture of the perineum sometimes occurs in the cow at calving, when the fetus over-distends the vulva. Suturing, under local anaesthesia, is usually required.

PERIODIC OPHTHALMIA. Specific ophthalmia, or 'moon blindness', is a condition of the eyes of horses, due to inflammation of the uveal tract (especially of the iris and ciliary body) which is characterised by a remarkable tendency to recur time and time again.

CAUSES. These are still in doubt, but it is known that leptospirosis is one. Some two to eight months after acute leptospirosis, periodic ophthalmia appears in up to 45 per cent of the horses affected. Leptospires have been isolated from eye lesions over long periods.

SIGNS. In the first stage a horse is found one morning with the eye-lids on one side half-closed; tears run from the eye down the face, and any effort to examine the eye is resented. Bright light is avoided, and the eyeball appears sunken in the socket. There is usually a certain amount of inflammation of the conjunctiva, and the deeper parts of the eye are also seen to be inflamed. The temperature is seldom much above normal. The iris gradually loses its lustre, and appears of a dully yellow colour; the fluid in the anterior chamber of the eye (aqueous humour) becomes thick and turbid-looking; and the cornea becomes blurred. This period of inflammation may last up to 10 days, after which it gradually disappears and the eye returns to practically its normal appearance. Repeated attacks are apt to occur. Total blindness may follow and/or lesions of the retina. Periodic ophthalmia is common in Europe, the USA, and Asia.

PERIODONTAL (*see* TEETH, DISEASES OF).

PERIOPLE (*see* FOOT OF THE HORSE).

PERIOSTEUM is the membrane surrounding a bone. The growth of a bone in its thickness is due to the action of the cells of this membrane forming fibrous tissue in which lime salts are deposited. (*See* BONE.)

PERIOSTITIS means inflammation on the surface of a bone affecting the periosteum. (*See* BONE, DISEASE OF.)

PERISTALSIS is the characteristic movement that takes place in the tubular organs of the body, such as the intestines, oesophagus, and the ureters. The movement is somewhat similar to the motion of a worm during progression, when viewed from the outside. It consists of firstly a slight dilatation of the calibre, associated with a small amount of shortening in length, then a vigorous contraction follows, the contraction taking place in a longitudinal as well as a transverse direction. The result is that the food material which is contained at any particular part is squeezed, mixed, and propelled forwards. In some parts of the bowel a reverse action takes place, by which the food is forced back towards the mouth. This is called 'reverse peristalsis' and is seen particularly in the small intestines. (*See* INTESTINES.)

PERITONEUM is the membrane lining the abdominal cavity, and forming a covering for the organs contained in it. That part lining the walls of the cavity is called the 'parietal' peritoneum, and that part covering the viscera is known as the 'visceral' peritoneum. Between the two is a film of lubricating liquid.

In structure the peritoneum consists of a dense, though very thin and elastic, fibrous membrane covered, on its inner side, with a smooth glistening layer of plate-like epithelial cells. Here and there between the cells are minute openings (stomata), each of which communicates with a lymphatic vessel, so that the fluid in the cavity is constantly being drained away into the general lymphatic circulation.

PERITONITIS means inflammation of the peritoneum. It may be either localised to one part or generally diffused.

Acute peritonitis. CAUSES. The direct cause of acute peritonitis is nearly always the invasion of the membrane by micro-organisms. It is very rarely primary, but usually occurs through a wound in the abdominal wall, in the stomach or intestines, uterus, bladder, etc., or through the spreading of inflammatory conditions from one or other of these parts, or from some other area of the body. It may follow castration, when the infection gains entrance by the inguinal canal. Peritonitis may occur during the course of anthrax, acute tuberculosis, etc.

SIGNS. These include restlessness and signs of distress and pain. Horses and cattle usually remain standing, but the smaller animals lie almost continually. The temperature is raised by from 3 to 6°F, and the pulse is quick, small, and wiry. Faeces and urine are usually retained and lead to further complication, and vomiting in dogs is common. Pressure over the sides of the abdomen is painful, and the animal usually 'boards' the muscles of the abdomen, and may groan or grunt. As the disease progresses fluid may be thrown out into the cavity in great quantities, leading to ascites. (*See* OEDEMA *and* PARACENTESIS.)

TREATMENT. Operative treatment and drainage may be undertaken.

Antibiotics and/or sulpha drugs may be given by injection. Hot fomentations to the abdomen relieve the acute pain. The prognosis is seldom good.

Chronic peritonitis. CAUSES. Slowly forming abscesses in the liver of the ox, tuberculous lesions in the peritoneal cavity, foreign bodies in the reticulum of the ox, etc.

SIGNS. There may be slight attacks of pain at times, but very often it is only after death that the condition is discovered. Ascites and a gradual loss of condition may be seen.

TREATMENT. This will vary according to the nature of the infection, the presence of systemic disease, or of adhesions.

PERMETHRIN. (*See* INSECTICIDES, FLIES.) Excessive applications to cats can induce hyperaesthesia, with excitement, a staggering gait, muscular twitching, and occasional collapse.

PERNICIOUS ANAEMIA, or SWAMP FEVER, also called equine pernicious anaemia, is another name for the anaemia that affects horses in certain parts of America. (*See under* EQUINE.)

PERONEAL is the name applied to the muscles, nerves, etc., that lie on the outer or fibular side of the hind-limb.

PEROSIS (*see under* 'SLIPPED TENDON').

PERTHE'S DISEASE. This name is given to a deformed condition of the head of the femur met with in children aged 3 to 8 years old. It simulates tuberculosis of the joint. The name is also applied to a similar condition recognised (by means of X-ray examination only) in the dog. The animal is noticed to be lame. The condition may clear up spontaneously within 6 months, but during that time drugs to relieve pain are indicated.

PERVIOUS URACHUS is a failure on the part of the umbilicus to close at or before birth. In the condition, which is also popularly called 'leaky navel', there is a continual dribbling of urine and serum from the navel.

Before birth the urinary bladder is in direct communication with the fluid in the allantoic sac, and the fetal urine which is formed escapes into this sac, thus preventing over-distension of the bladder. Immediately before the young animal is born, this communication is narrowed down to only a very small passage, and at birth it is either already closed, or it has practically ceased to function as a means of escape for the urine. With the tying of the umbilical cord, or with the shrinkage that follows exposure of this structure to the air, the urachus, which hitherto has connected the bladder with the outside of the animal's body, becomes quite impervious in the normal animal, and the urine now escapes by the urethra or natural passage to the outside. In pervious urachus this closure does not take place, and there is a continual dribble from the region of the umbilicus. The fluid tends to blister the skin of the surrounding area, and causes considerable discomfort, besides being very unsightly. Surgical treatment is necessary.

PESSARIES are compounds of drugs made up with a basis of coco butter and some antiseptic element, which are used for introduction into the natural cavities of the body so that they may dissolve and liberate their active substances slowly. They are mainly used for the uterus and for the teat-canals of the mammary gland. In some instances pessaries are made with dry powders of the active antiseptics filled into gelatine capsules. (*See* SYNCRO-MATE.)

PESTIVIRUS (*see* BOVINE VIRUS DIARRHOEA, BORDER DISEASE, SWINE FEVER, EQUINE VIRAL ARTERITIS).

PET ANIMALS ACT 1971 covers the licensing of pet shops, and the conditions under which animals are kept there and offered for sale.

PET FOODS. These now come under the Feeding Stuffs (Sampling and Analysis) Regulations 1982, to conform with EC directives. (*See also* DIET, DOGS' DIET, CAT FOODS, etc.)

PETS, CHILDREN'S and EXOTIC. For information on the breeding, care, diseases and treatment of mice, rats, rabbits, hamsters, guinea pigs, gerbils, reptiles, fish, birds, and monkeys, the reader is referred to the British Small Animal Veterinary Association's 'Manual of the care and treatment of children's and exotic pets'. (*See also under* CAGE BIRDS, MONKEYS, HAMSTERS, GUINEA-PIG, FERRETS, AMERICAN BOX TURTLES, TORTOISES, VIETNAMESE POT-BELLIED PIGS and ANAESTHETICS.)

PETECHIAE are small spots on the surface of an organ or the skin, generally red or purple in colour and resembling flea-bites. They may be minute areas of inflammation, or they may be small haemorrhages. (Petechial fever is another name for PURPURA HAEMORRHAGICA.)

PETHIDINE. An analgesic (pain reliever) used for dogs and cats.

PETRI DISH. A shallow circular glass dish with lid in which bacteria are grown on a solid medium.

PEYER'S PATCHES. In sheep these have a function analogous to that of the bursa of

Fabricius in birds. This investigation of jejunal Peyer's patches (JPP) and ileocaecal Peyer's patches (IPP) showed that, in JPPs, there are big interfollicular T-cell areas but IPPs contained mainly B-lymphocytes. Germinal centres of JPPs had about 40 per cent IgM positive cells and, in IPPs, about 80 per cent of these cells were present. (Larsen, H. J. & Landsverk, T., *Research in Veterinary Science* (1986) **40,** 105.) (*See also under* INTESTINES).

pH. A symbol used to express acidity or alkalinity; pH7 being neutral, a higher figure being alkaline and a lower figure being acid.

PHAGE (*see* BACTERIOPHAGE).

PHAGOCYTOSIS is the process by which the attacks of bacteria upon the living body are repelled and the bacteria destroyed through the activity of the white blood-cells other than lymphocytes. Bacteria coated with antibodies are phagocytosed more efficiently. Recent research has shown that influenza viruses inhibit, *in vitro*, phagocytosis by human polymorphonuclear leucocytes. (*Lancet*, Feb. 7, 1976, p. 283.) (*See* B-LOOD, IMMUNE, INFECTION, ABSCESS, IN-FLAMMATION.)

In 1981 the ARC referred to the ability of many bacteria to survive within phagocytes in mammary tissue, where staphylococci are protected from the lethal action of most antibiotics used in treating bovine mastitis. 'Some antibiotics do penetrate the cells but fail to kill bacteria because of the intra-cellular conditions and the dormancy of entrapped organisms.' The situation may then arise where the staphylococci live longer than the phagocytes, so that when the latter die and disintegrate the staphylococci are released, with potential for further mastitis-production.

PHALANX is the name given to each of the main bones below the metacarpal and metatarsal regions. There are three in each limb in the horse, six per limb in the ox, twelve in the pig, and fourteen in the dog. In general each of the digits possesses three phalanges, but the first digit in each foot of the dog has only two as in the thumb and great toe of man. The horse has now only one functional digit left in each of its limbs.

'PHALARIS STAGGERS'. A condition seen in Australia and New Zealand among cattle and sheep grazing on pasture dominated by *Phalaris tuberosa*. Cattle may show stiffness of the hocks and dragging of the hind legs. Similar symptoms are shown in sheep, with the addition of excitability, muscular tremors, and head nodding in the early stages. Dr D. J. Richards has stated: 'It is thought that phalaris contains a specific nervous system poison which is normally destroyed in the digestive passage of the animal but, where there is a deficiency in cobalt, the destruction of the poison is impeded and the symptoms occur. Provision of oral cobalt seems to stimulate the growth of organisms in the digestive system which in turn destroy the toxin.'

PHANTOM PREGNANCY (*see* PSEUDO-PREGNANCY, *also* 'CLOUDBURST').

PHARMACOGNOSY. The science of crude drugs.

PHARMACOKINETICS. The study of the movement of drugs within the body, including absorption, distribution, and excretion. (For an example *see* LUNGS – Functions.)

PHARMACOLOGY. The science of drugs, and especially of their actions in the body.

PHARMACOPAEIA is an official publication dealing with the recognised drugs and giving their doses, preparations, sources, and tests. Most countries have a pharmacopaeia of their own, that of Great Britain being known as the *Pharmacopaeia Britannica*, or often called the 'BP'. In the United States the official publication is the *United States Pharmacopaeia*, often called the 'USAP'.

PHARYNGITIS means inflammation of the pharynx. It often accompanies catarrhal inflammation in adjoining areas, viral infections, and tonsillitis.

PHARYNX is an irregularly funnel-shaped passage situated at the back of the mouth, common both to the respiratory and digestive passages. It acts as the cross-roads between these systems. Into its upper part open the two 'posterior nares', by which air enters and leaves the nasal passages during respiration. Below is the opening from the mouths, known as the 'fauces'; while lower still is the entrance to the larynx – the 'glottis'. Situated

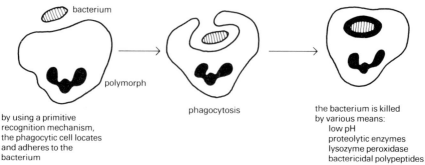

bacterium

polymorph

phagocytosis

the bacterium is killed by various means:
low pH
proteolytic enzymes
lysozyme peroxidase
bactericidal polypeptides

by using a primitive recognition mechanism, the phagocytic cell locates and adheres to the bacterium

Non-specific immunity: phagocytosis.

most posteriorly is the beginning of the oesophagus, and on either side are the openings of the Eustachian tubes, communicating with the middle ear. (*See* EAR.)

The walls of the pharynx are composed of muscles which are the active agents of swallowing, along with a sheet of fibrous tissue known as the pharyngeal aponeurosis. On the inside they are lined with mucous membrane which is continuous with that of the several cavities which open into it.

Pharyngeal injuries. Sixty-five dogs were treated for penetrating wounds of the pharynx. Recent wounds resulted in dysphagia, pain, pyrexia and local cellulitis; longstanding wounds led to discharging sinuses of the head, neck or cranial thoracic region. Pieces of wood were removed from 37 dogs, and they recovered. No foreign body was found in 18 dogs whose clinical signs resolved after treatment of the wounds. Four dogs died shortly after the injury from major oesophageal tears which resulted in mediastinal contamination. In six dogs, the discharging sinuses persisted, although no foreign body was recovered at surgery. (White, R. A. S. & Lane, J. G. (1988) *Journal of Small Animal Practice* **29,** 13).

PHEASANTS (*see* GAME BIRDS, MORTALITY).

PHENACETIN (*see* ANTIPYRINE).

PHENAZONUM (*see* ANTIPYRINE).

PHENOBARBITONE (*see* LUMINAL).

PHENOGROUPS. Blood groups in the B system of cattle occur in numerous fixed groupings termed phenogroups. Some of these are unique to particular breeds. They are particularly valuable in detecting incorrectly stated parentage.

PHENOL (CARBOLIC ACID). A tar derivative, related to the cresols and, like them, used in disinfectant preparations, but not suitable (1) where animals may come into contact with them, as absorption through the skin—leading to poisoning—readily occurs; (2) in the proximity of milk. (*see* MILK, **chlorophenol taint.**)

Phenol is a corrosive poison when swallowed, giving rise to shock, convulsions and death; and cats especially may be fatally poisoned as a result of absorption of phenol compounds through the skin.

FIRST-AID consists in the administration of milk and raw white of egg. The skin (in cases where the phenol or cresol compounds have come into contact with it) should be washed with soap and water.

PHENOL-PHTHALEIN is a substance much used as an indicator in the testing of urine, gastric juice, etc., being colourless in an acid and a brilliant red in an alkaline medium. It is also sometimes given to dogs as a mild purgative. Phenolsulphone-phthalein has been used as a test for the excretory powers of the kidneys; a known amount is injected into a muscle and the urine is tested by comparison of its colour with that of known standards during the next few hours. Phenoltetrachlor-phthalein is a coal-tar derivative used to estimate the functional power of the liver.

PHENOTHIAZINE. A pale greenish-grey powder which darkens on exposure to light and is practically insoluble in water. In the body it is oxidised to colourless compounds which are excreted in the urine, and on exposure to air are converted to a red dye.

Phenothiazine is an anthelmintic, at one time widely used in farm animals against a variety of parasitic roundworms; but it has been superseded by more modern drugs. (*See* WORMS, FARM TREATMENT AGAINST.)

TOXICITY. Young animals are more susceptible than older ones; sheep are more resistant than horses. Lambs under one month old, in-lamb ewes, or young foals should not be dosed with phenothiazine. In the horse cases of idiosyncracy have been reported, and overdosage has led to haemolytic anaemia. (The reddish colour of the urine should not be confused with haematuria.) In cattle, symptoms of poisoning have been reported as dullness, weakness of the hindquarters, prostration, and coma. In calves exposed to bright sunlight following the administration of phenothiazine, a form of light-sensitisation and keratitis may occur, even in the UK.

PHENOTYPE. In heredity this refers to all the individuals showing the same characters. The term can also mean the individual resulting from the reaction between genotype and environment.

PHENYLALANINE. One of the essential amino acids.

PHENYLBUTAZONE. An analgesic for the relief of pain, associated with inflammation of joints and muscles. It apparently acts as an analgesic via the central nervous system, while its anti-inflammatory effects have been attributed to reduced capillary permeability. (Colin Vogel, *Vet. Record* (1981) **108,** 248.) It is not a steroid. Phenylbutazone can be given orally or intravenously. It is often used for chronic arthritis and associated bone disease. Withdrawal of the drug before a horse competes in international events is necessary.

PHENYTOIN SODIUM. An anti-convulsant drug.

PHEROMONE. A chemical substance produced by one individual which affects the behaviour or physiology of another. The most obvious mammalian example is the odour which attracts the dog to the bitch ready for mating. In pregnant mice the odour of a strange male regularly causes fetal resorption. Two compounds in the breath of a boar will stimulate a gilt or sow to display mating behaviour.

PHIMOSIS, or PHYMOSIS (*see under* PENIS AND PREPUCE, ABNORMALITIES AND LESIONS).

PHLEBITIS means inflammation of a vein.

PHOCID DISTEMPER. This caused a high death rate among seals in European waters in 1988; and there is evidence that it also caused outbreaks of distemper in farmed mink and in dogs. (Blixen-krone-Moller, M. & others. *Veterinary Record* (1990) **127**, 263).

PHOLEDRINE SULPHATE. A drug which raises the blood-pressure, and is used in cases of heart failure after pneumonia or bronchitis and shock.

PHONATION (jargon). Voice production, *e.g.* barking in the dog.

PHOSGENE. This gas, first produced experimentally by John Davy in 1812 by the combination of carbon monoxide with chlorine in the presence of sunlight, has the formula $COCl_2$. Phosgene has a characteristic smell of musty hay, and is ten times more toxic than chlorine. The gas in the presence of water is converted into carbon dioxide and hydrochloric acid, and it is the latter which damages the lung tissues, giving rise to pulmonary oedema. Horses usually die between the seventh and twenty-fourth hour following exposure to the gas. Birds are highly susceptible. The gas may be liberated from chloroform, carbon tetrachloride, and paint strippers in the presence of heat. Still-births and heavy piglet losses followed the feeding in the USA of mouldy, weevily grain which had been fumigated with a mixture containing carbon tetrachloride.

PHOSPHATES are salts of phosphoric acid, and as this substance is contained in many articles of food, in bone, the nuclei of cells, as well as in the nervous system, quantities are continually excreted in the urine. (*See also under* PHOSPHORUS.)

PHOSPHORESCENCE of meat is a luminous condition due to the organism *Photobacterium phosphorescens*. The meat is apparently unchanged during the daytime, but in the dark it glows with a yellowish light. Fish, especially herring, show this condition normally, but sausages, pork and occasionally beef may also exhibit the phenomenon. It is not associated with unwholesomeness.

PHOSPHORUS itself is not used in medicine, but is usually given in the form of one or other of the glycerophosphates, or hypophosphites of sodium, potassium, calcium, magnesium, or iron. Preparations are used with calcium and dextrose in the treatment of 'Milk Fever'.

PHOSPHORUS DEFICIENCY. This is seen in rickets, 'milk lameness', post-parturient haemo-globinuria, and may complicate 'Milk Fever'. (*See under these headings and infertility*.)

PHOSPHORUS POISONING may occur in the dog and cat, either through puppies eating matches, or from animals gaining access to rat poison made with phosphorus.
SIGNS. When an animal has been poisoned by phosphorus there is acute abdominal pain, vomiting, intense thirst, diarrhoea, and great dullness. The material vomited may be green in colour and is often luminous in the darkness. Collapse rapidly follows, and the animal dies in a few hours. Or, where less has been taken, death may not occur for 2 or 3 days. Where small amounts are taken over a considerable period of time, there is fatty degeneration of the liver and kidneys, increasing loss of condition, jaundice, and extreme weakness.
FIRST-AID. An emetic should be given at once, so soon as the symptoms appear, such as sulphate of copper (bluestone). This induces vomiting, gets rid of the majority of the phosphorus, and renders inert what remains. In 15 minutes another dose dissolved in water as before should be given, and this should be repeated every quarter of an hour till four doses have been given. In all cases, *white of egg, milk, oils, and fatty substances* must be avoided, for these dissolve the phosphorus and render it able to be absorbed with greater rapidity. (*See also* ORGANO-PHOSPHORUS POISONING, which arises from contaminations with certain farm chemicals.)

PHOTOPHOBIA means a condition in which an animal, suffering from inflammation in the eye, objects to a strong light.

PHOTOSENSITISATION (*see* LIGHT SENSITISATION).

PHRENIC NERVE is the nerve which is concerned in supplying the diaphragm. It arises from the fifth, sixth, and seventh cervical spinal nerves, passes through the thoracic cavity, and ramifies in the muscular part of the diaphragm.

PHTHIRIASIS. Infestation with lice of the genus Phthirus.

PHTHISIS, or PHTHYSIS means wasting, and was generally applied to tuberculosis affecting the lungs. (*See* TUBERCULOSIS, PNEUMONIA.)

PHYCOMYCOSIS. A group of fungal infections by species of *Absidia, Mucor, Rhizopus*, etc., which affects the lymph nodes, and may give rise to loss of weight and tumour-like (granulomatous) swellings. It may affect the lungs and intestines. A monkey died from systemic phycomycosis in the UK after loss of appetite, depression, and laboured breathing.

PHYLLOERYTHRIN. A substance formed in the rumen from chlorophyll by bacterial digestion. Some is absorbed and excreted in the bile, but when the liver is damaged in any way the phylloerythrin may reach the peripheral circulation and give rise to Light Sensitisation.

PHYMOSIS (*see* PENIS AND PREPUCE, ABNORMALITIES).

PHYSIOTHERAPY. In the UK some veterinary practices already use the services of qualified physiotherapists for the treatment of selected cases of disease in animals; and there was, in 1986, the likelihood that such collaboration would be extended. The opinion of the RCVS and the Chartered Society of Physiotherapists is that some physiotherapists should specialise in animal work, rather than that veterinary surgeons should specialise in physiotherapy. There was concern in both organisations that some racehorse owners employed unqualified manipulators.

PHYSIS. The parts of a bone which are involved in its increase in length, i.e. the Growth Plate. (*See* BONE, Growth.)

PHYSOSTIGMINE, ESERINE, is a preparation derived from the ripe seeds of *Physostigma venenosum*, a tree from West Africa. Eye drops containing physostigmine sulphate are used to contract the pupil and lessen intra-ocular pressure: and, alternated with atropine, it has been used for adhesions of the iris, following iritis.

PHYTIN. A substance present in oatmeal, maize meal (and in other cereals) antagonistic to calcification of bone, and thus a rickets-producing factor.

PIA MATER is the membrane that closely invests the brain and spinal cord. (*See* BRAIN, SPINAL CORD.)

PICA. 'Depraved' appetite. (For causes, *see under* APPETITE.)

PICORNAVIRUS (*see* FELINE CALICIVIRUS DISEASE; VIRUSES).

PICROTOXIN. Used in veterinary medicine principally as an antidote to barbiturate poisoning.

PIETRAIN. This Belgian breed of pig dates from about 1920, but the Breed Society was formed in the 1950s. There is uncertainty as to the origins of the Piétrain, but it is thought that it stems from old native stock crossed with English breeds such as the Berkshire, Tamworth, and Wessex, and with the French breed Bayeux.

There is still some lack of uniformity within the breed, but a constant feature is the extreme development of the hams – perhaps the result of a mutation such as is believed to have occurred in a strain of Devon cattle. The Piétrain is white with large black spots. It is a pork pig which gives high killing-out and lean-meat percentages, but it is slow growing and has, in comparison with Large Whites and Landrace, a somewhat high food conversion ratio.

The boars attain a weight of between 550 and 650 lb; sows 600 lb. The sows are usually quiet and docile. Litter-size is smaller than that expected in the UK. Pale-muscle disease and heart failure are by no means rare in this breed, of which there are now many in the UK. (*See* PORCINE STRESS SYNDROME, PALE SOFT EXUDATIVE MUSCLE.)

PIG, THE, as seen by research workers: The fastest-growing of the domestic animals, prone to heart troubles and disease of the arteries, greatly affected in body by mental stress.

PIG CARCASES, REJECTION OF. The causes of rejection of carcases and viscera among 1·3 million pigs slaughtered in seven abattoirs in 1980 was analysed. A total of 2556 (0·2 per cent) whole carcases and parts of 25,583 (2·0 per cent) carcases were rejected. The principal causes of rejection of whole carcases were pneumonia, pleurisy, peritonitis and fever; for parts of carcases, abscesses and arthritis. The main reason for rejection of liver, heart and lungs were 'milk spot', pericarditis and pneumonia, respectively. The variation between abattoirs in the amount of meat and viscera rejected was very large and economically significant. Hill, J. R. & Jones, J. E. T., *British Veterinary Journal* (1984) **140,** 558.)

PIG, EXTERNAL PARASITES OF THE. Half the bacon pigs examined at an abattoir were found to have external parasites – mange mites, lice, or forage mites; and a recent survey made at the Department of Veterinary Medicine, University of Edinburgh, suggests that 20 per cent of pedigree pigs and piggeries in Britain are infested with sarcoptic mange mites.

The itchiness and scurfiness of many infested pigs are attributed to the results of dry feeding or of a zinc deficiency, but pig breeders would be wise not to be in too much of a hurry to make this assumption.

A proper investigation by a veterinary surgeon would not merely pay for itself, but could effect a big saving; for mange can have an important effect upon food conversion ratios. Moreover, mange can actually kill piglets – and lead to stunting of others which do not succumb.

It is recommended that, once buildings have been cleared of the infestation, each new intake of pigs should be sprayed. (*See also* IVERMECTIN.)

PIG HEALTH SCHEME. This came into force in 1968, and was confined to the élite and accredited herds of the Meat and Livestock Commission's Accreditation Scheme, and to candidate herds. The owners of these herds were offered free veterinary advice on disease control and eradication, and a free quarterly visit of inspection by a ministry veterinary officer or his own veterinary surgeon. By means of these 'routine herd inspections, the examination of disease incidence, the use of readily available *post-mortem* data and by ensuring that expert advice is acted upon, the health scheme should make it possible to reduce significantly losses through disease' – Dr D. R. Melrose.

Pig Health Control Association is a private enterprise mainly concerned with spreading knowledge of enzootic pneumonia in pigs, and with setting standards for herds claiming freedom from diseases. (*See also under* HEALTH SCHEMES.)

PIG-MEAL, SURPLUS. Pig breeders who rear cattle and sheep should be wary of feeding surplus pig-meal to those animals unless it is definitely known that the meal does *not* contain a copper supplement. Sheep are very easily poisoned by repeated dosage of a copper supplement well tolerated by pigs, and the death of a heifer was reported after 5 months of supplementary feeding on pig-meal. Conversely, poultry meal medicated with nitrophenide against coccidiosis, should never be fed to pigs. It has caused paralysis.

PIGMENTATION, LOSS OF. This mostly affects Siamese cats. Eyelids, foot-pads, etc., are altered, with resultant exclusion from cat shows.

PIG POX (*see under* POX).

PIGLETS. Normal piglets were obtained from hatched blastocysts frozen at −196°C. (Kashiwazaki, S. & others. *Veterinary Record* (1991) **128,** 256.)

PIGS.

History. Domesticated pigs are believed to be the descendants of the native European Wild Pig. (*Sus scrofa*) with probably an admixture of the blood of the closely related Asiatic species (*Sus vitatus*).

The pigs of this country, during early historic times and up till the seventeenth century, were practically pure descendants of the European wild pig; characterised by long and rather narrow bodies and long snouts, and strong bristles of a rusty colour.

During the eighteenth and early nineteenth centuries there were introduced into Britain considerable numbers of pigs belonging to a markedly different type, which originated at a very early date in China and South-Western Asia. This type, variously known as the Siamese or Chinese, and given the specific designation of *Sus indicus*, was of smaller size than the native stock; short-legged and round-bodied, with a short dished snout and a coat of soft hair. Its most marked economic characteristics were its early maturity and tendency towards rapid fattening. At the same time it was both less hardy and less prolific than the native type. The Chinese type was not long preserved in a pure state in Britain, but was widely employed for crossing with the native sorts, and it seems certain that all of our modern breeds have been influenced to a greater or lesser extent by the infusion of this Eastern blood. The influence is most clearly to be seen in the smaller and earlier maturing breeds such as the Middle White and the Berkshire, while it is least apparent in breeds such as the Tamworth and Wessex.

British breeds of pigs have included nine main breeds:

White breeds
The Large White
The Middle White
The Welsh
The British Landrace

Black and Black-and-White Breeds
The Large Black
The British Saddleback
The Gloucester Old Spots
The Berkshire

Red Breed
The Tamworth

Breeds of pigs in the UK (1988 figures)

Breed	Litter notifications	Herd book entries
Large White	11,081	5,854
Landrace	6,701	3,205
Welsh	1,404	695
Duroc	238	220
Hampshire	87	101
Gloucester Old Spots	244	273

Most favoured crosses
Large White × Landrace; Large White or Landrace × LA/LW; Duroc × LW/LA.
(National Pig Breeders' Association).

Chinese Meishan pigs
These, stated the A F R C in 1989, can rear an average of 14 to 16 piglets, compared with 10 to 12 from Western breeds. Meishans reach sexual maturity when three months old.

Backed by five major breeding companies and the L T I, the A F R C Institute of Animal Physiology, Edinburgh, is seeking to identify the genes responsible for the Meishan's prolificacy.

Foreign breeds. Pigs imported into the U K for commercial use and breeding trials, crossing purposes, etc., include: Duroc, Hampshire, Lacombe, Piétrain, Poland, China.

The Vietnamese pot-bellied pig is becoming popular as a pet, and has been imported for that purpose. It is, however, subject to the Movement & Sale of Pigs Order 1975.

It is only within the last 100 years or so that any particular care has been devoted to pig-breeding in Britain. Before 1884, when the National Pig Breeders' Association was formed, there were no herd books, and pure breeds, in the modern sense, can hardly be said to have existed. Even in the case of the Berkshire, which is frequently mentioned by old writers as far back as the eighteenth century, it is clear that the old type was rather variable in its characteristics, and was in the main quite unlike the breed that now goes under this name.

In Britain there is, to quote Mr J. White, Chief Livestock Officer, M L C, 'a place in the industry for breeders who will specialise in producing high quality first-cross females for sale to commercial breeders.

'It is a great mistake to think that any cross-bred pig will give better results than any pure bred, or that by crossing pigs one gets a bonus in all the economic characters. Strangely, hybrid vigour results in improvement in those characters which are very weakly inherited, and not at all in the characters that are highly inherited. So far as food conversion ratio and carcase quality are concerned, a cross-bred pig will give about the average of the two parents. For this reason it is very important to know that the pure bred animals used in producing the first-cross are of the highest possible quality. It is in such things as numbers born and reared that one can expect improvement from cross-breeding.'

LEADING HYBRIDS include the Camborough female, and the Cotswold.

Breeding. (*See* GENETICS – HERITABILITY OF CERTAIN TRAITS.)

Boars may be used for breeding at from seven to nine months according to size and development. Oestrus occurs, in females that are in good thriving condition, at all seasons of the year, except when the animal is pregnant or nursing. The period of gestation is about 16 weeks; the time allowed for nursing varies from 7 to 12 weeks, and oestrus generally recurs within 10 days, and very commonly on the third or fourth day, after the litter is weaned. The whole breeding cycle is thus completed in from 24 to 28 weeks, and it is possible to arrange for sows to produce two litters a year regularly throughout their breeding life. Some pig farmers, by means of early weaning, managed to obtain three litters in little over a year; but early weaning, and so-called 'piglet batteries' are sometimes accompanied by unacceptable losses. The normal breeding life is 5 or 6 years, but exceptionally good breeders are sometimes kept much longer, and 12 years or more is not unknown.

PIG MANAGEMENT and DISEASE. From a veterinary viewpoint, outdoor pig rearing has advantages; namely, fresh air, exercise, and the availability of grass (and soil) which can minimise any deficiencies of vitamins or trace elements. (The outdoor piglet will not need iron injections to avert anaemia, but may still need a vitamin A supplement in autumn and winter.)

The disadvantages are that, especially in the bleaker parts of the country, piglets in arks on grassland may not thrive during the winter; also, where sows and their litters share an enclosure, there may be some savaging by sows of other sows' piglets.

Straw-bale 'houses' have much to be said for them. They provide excellent insulation and hence warmth, and can be burnt after use – which obviates the need for disinfection.

Fattening pigs, if properly fed indoors, make better liveweight gains than those outside. They are however utterly dependent upon the feed provided, having no opportunity to graze or scavenge. Should the feed be deficient in trace elements or vitamins, their health will suffer.

Pregnant sows thrive best when allowed free access to grassland and the opportunity for exercise, but see PADDOCKS for the danger of contamination of pasture by parasitic worm larvae, unless precautions are taken.

Housing. Pig housing, varying from simple wooden huts and arks to costly and elaborate controlled environment buildings, naturally has an important bearing on health. The type and quality of building materials can be important as well as the design of the building. Abrasive concrete can lead to injuries and abscesses, resulting in lameness. (*See* CONCRETE.)

Straw bedding is the ideal from a health angle. It can keep the pigs warmer, improve liveweight gains, obviate boredom (a possible cause of tail-biting), and reduce stress. (*See* BEDDING.)

Recommended temperatures for pigs are given under the separate heading HOUSING. With controlled-environment buildings, precautions must be taken against the effects of power-cuts. It is useful to have a tractor-pto generator for such emergencies. These may arise during both winter and summer, and be due not to a district power-cut but to fuses blowing in the building itself. In the summer of 1983, for example, fuses blew during a thunderstorm, and 'fail-safe' ventilators failed to operate, with the result that 500 pigs inside that building died of heat-stroke. (MAFF veterinary investigation service report.)

As pigs are particularly susceptible to the

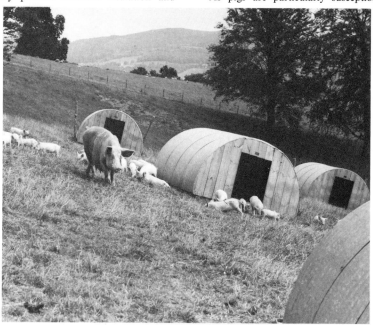

Arks for outdoor pig keeping. (*Pig Farming*.)

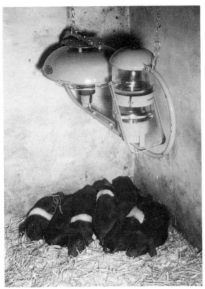

Infra-red electric lamps are commonly used in creeps. Here is an oil-burning alternative.

effects of water deprivation, precautions must be taken to ensure that water pipes do not freeze, and that the levers of automatic drinkers are not too stiff for piglets to manage. (*See under* WATER for other dangers).

Feeding stalls prevent greedy and aggressive sows from obtaining more than their fair share of feed, leaving others under-nourished. However, confinement of sows in stalls (other than for feeding only) deprives the animals of any opportunity for the slightest exercise, and they are unable to move away to escape any cold draughts. Stress results (*see* 'THIN SOW SYNDROME'.)

Stress (which reduces bodily resistance to infection) may also occur at times when pigs are moved from one building to another, or when litters are first mixed. Accordingly, Dr D. W. B. Sainsbury strongly advocated the use of farrowing-to-finish pens.

However, relatively few fatteners breed their own pigs. Bought-in pigs are best kept away from other stock on the farm for 3 or 4 weeks. Dr Sainsbury has commented: 'My impression is that pigs do much better at this period if they are kept as far away from their dung as possible, and this is one reason why slatted floors and floor feeding rarely work at this stage.

'A popular way of achieving good accommodation at this time is to provide a simple covered straw yard allowing about 10 sq. ft per pig of total area preferably with part of the area 'kennelled' to give a warm sleeping area. If the latter is raised and dark it will usually be kept clean, and the dung placed in the lighter and lower strawed area. Suitable sized groups are of 25–30 weaners and a lean-to yard will be as cheap a method of housing as any, particularly with *ad lib.* feeding from large hoppers.

'An alternative procedure is required by the farmer who cannot use straw or other bedding and there are a number of designs of kennel-type pens

with covered or uncovered yards where the muck can be readily cleared away, sometimes with tractor or squeegee, sometimes with a hose to wash it down a drain. An essential of this system is to have pigs in small and separated groups perhaps no more than 20 to a pen.

'After the conditioning period, the usual practice is to finish the pigs under more intensive conditions. This often involves keeping pigs in litterless pens and there is little doubt that this is the type of environment that can be conducive to tail biting and cannibalism.'

Ventilation – at pig level – becomes all the more important in such circumstances. 'Railed or Weldmesh pen fronts or sides are often preferred as they allow a much better circulation of air in a low-roofed building in particular. Their advantages do not stop there. Many farmers find that it is difficult to get the younger pig dunging in the passage rather than the pen. A sure help is a gate of Weldmesh or of bars, as a new group will appear to follow the habits of its older companions on the other side of the gate.'

It should be added that it is wise to have separate sections or units which can be cleaned and disinfected between batches.

The age for weaning piglets is usually 5–7 weeks. Where for any reason the sow is not wanted for breeding again immediately, the period of suckling may be extended by an additional week or two. In countries with a severe winter climate, where only spring litters are satisfactory and where consequently only one litter per annum is bred, the last course is that normally followed. (For early weaning, *see under* WEANING.)

It has been found that it is not normally advisable to put pigs into the finishing house until they are at least 32 kg in weight, and most feeders continue the weaner-pool system until this weight is reached.

Feeding. Many unsatisfactory results are directly attributable to badly balanced rations. (*See* CONCENTRATES.)

The growing pig needs at least ten amino acids in order to form body proteins. It is advisable to provide vitamins A and D also – and this applies not only to pigs indoors, receiving little or no greenstuff or sunshine; but also to sows at pasture, where the grass often provides insufficient vitamin A. Vitamin E is also important. The vitamin is best added as a special preparation according to the manufacturer's recommendations. (*See* ADDITIVES, RATIONS, COPPER SUPPLEMENTS, SOW'S MILK.)

Floor feeding, Dr D. W. B. Sainsbury has commented, has a connection with vices. If pens are dirty and the food goes on top of this muck a scouring, uncomfortable pig can be the result – and it does not seem to take long for the other pigs to set about the weakened individual. Also if ventilation is bad, the dust from meal fed on the floor can appear to induce coughing and fractiousness – in pig and even in pigmen – which is an intolerable state of affairs.

A virtually automatic system of liquid feeding *via* pipelines is not uncommon in large, modern

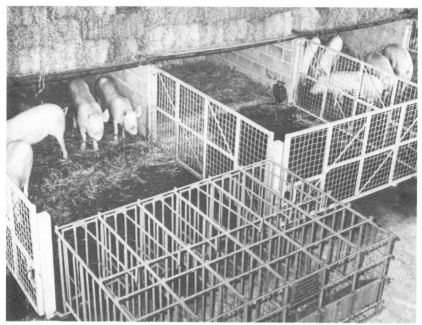

Sowyards with individual feeding stalls. (*Pig Farming.*)

piggeries. Dry meal may be delivered from hoppers in pre-arranged quantities and at set intervals by means of a time-switch.

Experiments have shown that dry-fed pigs took 10 days longer to reach bacon-weight and 0·2 lb more food for each 1 lb liveweight gain, as compared with wet feeding.

Good results have been obtained by feeding moist barley from a Harvestore tower silo.

A method practised at Harper Adams College is for weaners to be brought into the fattening house at 8 weeks old, and there they have meal from self-feeders. At 100 lb liveweight, the *ad lib.* feeding ceases, and the pigs are trough-fed daily. Water is run into the trough (from a conveniently placed tap) and the meal is placed on top, being mixed with the water by the pigs themselves. They are given as much as they will clean up in 20 minutes, subject to limit of 7 lb per head per day. (*See* RATIONS.)

Aspects of pig husbandry having a bearing on health and disease problems, and of economic importance to the farmer, are given under the following headings:

ADDITIVES, ARTIFICIAL INSEMINATION, 'BABY PIG DISEASE', BEDDING, BUNT ORDER, CASTRATION, CONDENSATION, 'CONTROLLED BREEDING', CONTROLLED ENVIRONMENT HOUSING, COPPER, COPPER POISONING, CREEP FEEDING, DIET, DISINFECTANTS, 'DRENCHING', DRESSED SEED CORN, DRIED GRASS, FARROWING CRATES, FARROWING RATES, FLY CONTROL, GENETICS, HEAT STROKE, HOUSING, INFERTILITY, INJECTIONS, INTENSIVE LIVESTOCK PRODUCTION, LAMENESS. LIGHTING, MEAL FEEDING, MUMMIFICATION OF FETUS, NIPPLES, NITRITE POISONING, NOTIFIABLE DISEASES, OESTRUS, OVERLYING, PARASITES, PIGLET ANAEMIA, PIGLET MORTALITY; PIGS, WORMS IN; POISONING, RATIONS, ROUNDHOUSE, SALT POISONING, SENNA, SLURRY,

SOW STALLS, SOW'S MILK, STILLBORN PIGS, STRESS, SWEATHOUSE SYSTEM, SWILL, TAIL BITING, TAIL SORES, 'THIN SOW SYNDROME', TRACE ELEMENTS, TROPICS, VENTILATION, VITAMINS, WATER, WEANING, WHEY FEEDING, WORMS, FARM TREATMENT AGAINST.

PIGS, DISEASES OF (*see under the following headings:* AGALACTIA; ANAEMIA; ANTHRAX; AUJESZKY'S DISEASE; BRINE POISONING; CLOSTRIDIAL ENTERITIS; ENCEPHALOMYELITIS OF PIGS; ENZOOTIC PNEUMONIA; EPERYTHROZOÖN; GASTRIC ULCERS; HAEMOLYTIC DISEASE; HEAT STROKE; LEPTOSPIROSIS; LISTERIOSIS; MANGE; MASTITIS; MENINGOENCEPHALITIS; MILK FEVER; MULBERRY HEART; NECROTIC ENTERITIS; OEDEMA OF THE BOWEL; PERICARDITIS; POST-PARTURIENT FEVER; PYELONEPHRITIS; RHEUMATISM; RHINITIS, ATROPHIC; SALMONELLOSIS; SWINE DYSENTERY; SWINE ERYSIPELAS; SWINE FEVER; SWINE FEVER, AFRICAN; SWINE INFLUENZA; TAIL SORES; TALFAN DISEASE; TESCHEN DISEASE; TOXOPLASMOSIS; TRANSMISSIBLE GASTROENTERITIS; TRICHINOSIS; TUBERCULOSIS. *See also* BACK MUSCLE NECROSIS; EPIDEMIC DIARRHOEA; FOOT-ROT; GLASSER'S; 'GREASY PIG' DISEASE; HAEMORRHAGIC GASTRO-ENTERITIS AND WHEY FEEDING; OESOPHAGOSTOMIASIS; PITYRIASIS; PNEUMONIA; POLIOENCEPHALOMALACIA; PORCINE INTESTINAL ADENOMATOSIS; PORCINE STREPTOCOCCAL MENINGITUS; PORCINE ULCERATIVE SPIROCHAETOSIS; SWINE VESICULAR DISEASE; VOMITING AND WASTING SYNDROME; WORMS, TREATMENT AGAINST *and headings under* **Porcine.** *See also* 'BLUE-EAR' DISEASE.)

(For causes of death among unweaned pigs, see list of diseases, etc., given under PIGLET MORTALITY. *See also* PIG CARCASES, REJECTION OF.)

PIGS, NAMES GIVEN ACCORDING TO AGE, SEX, etc. The naming of pigs at various times in their life, and according to their age, sex, etc., varies in different areas; the following gives the most usual names:

Store Pig – a pig between the time of weaning and being fattened.

Hog – a male pig after being castrated.

Stag, Steg, or *Seg* – a male castrated late in life.

Gilt or *Yelt* – a female intended for breeding purposes, and up to the time that she has her first litter.

Boar, Bran, or *Hogg* – an uncastrated male.

Sow–a breeding female after the first litter.

PIGS, SALE OF. In the UK this is subject to the Movement & Sale of Pigs Order 1975.

PIGS, SEDATION OF. Sedation is useful to prevent fighting after the mixing of litters or re-grouping of pigs; to 'cure' fighting after it has broken out; to make the aggressive sow accept her litter; to facilitate castration, nose-ringing, detusking, etc. Among drugs used for this purpose is Azaperone, an ingredient of 'Stresnil' and 'Suicalm', claimed to be virtually non-toxic, and short-acting.

Precaution. There is a risk of damaging the sciatic nerve when making intra-muscular injections into the hindlegs of pigs; and it is therefore advisable to inject into the neck muscles, just behind the ear.

CASE HISTORIES: Within one to eight weeks of an injection of an antibiotic into the ham of one hindleg of 180 4-week-old piglets, 150 had developed paralysis of that leg.

In another group of 380 5-week-old piglets, 30 per cent had become paralysed within 10 days, and 30 per cent had died from complications such as septicaemia and pneumonia – 'probably due to necrosis of the foot.' (Van Alstine, W. G. & Dietrich, J. A. *Compendium of Continuing Education* (1988) **10**, 1329.)

PIGS, TRANSPORT OF. The use of containers for the transport of pigs can reduce the risk of infection being carried on to a purchaser's farm. One crate can hold a complete litter group, and keep the pigs from coming into contact with the sides and floor of the lorry – which are often not properly cleaned and which can seldom or never be sterilised.

PIGEON-EYED. (For this term, as applied to the horse, *see under* CONFORMATION DEFECTS.)

PIGEON POX VIRUS is probably a modified form of the fowl pox virus. It has a low pathogenicity for the fowl, and has been used to immunise the latter against fowl pox.

PIGEONS in cities may constitute a hazard to public health, since many are infected with ornithosis. Some harbour *salmonellas*, and *Cryptococcus neoformans* has been isolated from pigeon droppings (but never from pigeons). Grain soaked in the narcotic chloralose has been successfully

tried as bait; loss of consciousness beginning 10 minutes or so after eating the bait.

Dieldrin is highly poisonous to pigeons. (*See also under* GAME BIRDS.)

In Scotland a herpes virus has been isolated from racing pigeons, and gave rise to conjunctivitis, rhinitis, and malaise.

In 1981 a highly contagious viral disease causing high morbidity but low mortality spread through racing pigeons in Europe. The virus belongs to the avian paramyxovirus sero group 1. The clinical signs include watery droppings, polydipsia and neurologic signs ranging from ataxia and tremor of the head and neck, to torticollis varying from slight head tilt to carriage of the head upside down. The most important differential diagnosis is salmonellosis. Good immunity against the disease can be acquired by subcutaneous vaccination with an inactivated oil adjuvant vaccine for Newcastle disease in poultry. Adult pigeons should be vaccinated after moulting and before breeding and young pigeons should be vaccinated four weeks before racing. (Lumeij, J. T. & Stam, J. W. E. *Veterinary Quarterly* (1985) **7**, 60.)

One vaccine, Paramyx 1 (Glaxo Animal Health) is licensed for use in pigeons in the UK for the prevention of PMV1 infection.

Ornithosis occurs in young racing pigeons, the symptoms including diarrhoea, conjunctivitis, nasal discharge. (*See* CHLAMYDIA.)

'One-eyed cold' is a pigeon-fancier's term for keratitis, often accompanied by nasal discharge, in one eye.

Mycoplasmal infections include *M. columborale, M. columbinum*, and *M. columbinasale*; though the pathogenicity of these is in doubt.

Pigeon pox is associated with vesicles around the beak and eyes, and with hard growths – which, if on the feet, may cause lameness.

'Canker' may give rise to a 70 per cent mortality and is caused by *Trichomonas gallinae* which affects the liver and alimentary canal.

Salmonellosis is often fatal in recently hatched birds, and in adults may cause diarrhoea, distressed breathing, swollen joints, lameness, dropped wing, loss of weight.

Parasitic worms, especially capillaria, may cause huddling, loss of weight and anaemia. (*See also* CLAY PIGEONS, and SPEEDS OF ANIMALS.) ☛

PIGLET ANAEMIA. A common cause of pre-weaning losses among housed pigs.

CAUSE. The disease is associated with a deficiency of iron, and is aggravated by cold and damp. (A deficiency of copper and cobalt may sometimes also occur, it has been suggested.)

SIGNS. Dullness, a pale whitish skin, scouring, and sometimes exaggerated heart-beats.

TREATMENT. Turn sow and litter out to grass. Give an iron and copper preparation sold for the purpose.

PREVENTION. If outdoor rearing is not desired, give a suitable iron preparation (with cobalt and copper, preferably) at 7 days of age. (A solution made by dissolving 2 oz of commercial iron pyrophosphate in 1 pint of water is effective; a quarter of a teaspoonful being given daily for 4 or 5 days.)

Place a fresh turf in the farrowing house. Acute iron poisoning, often leading to death within 24 hours, sometimes follows the injection or oral dosing of normally used iron preparations. To prevent this it is advisable to wait until the piglets are a week old when this danger is less; it is also wise to ensure that gilts' rations contain adequate vitamin E.

The intramuscular injections of iron dextran to prevent piglet anaemia are sometimes followed by ham abscesses – the result of broken-off needles or failure to clean the skin adequately before making the injection. Recent research at the AFRC's Institute for Research on Animal Diseases, Compton, has shown that unweaned piglets eat a significant amount of their dam's dung, and that if the sow's diet is supplemented with 2000 mg iron per kg dry matter, it is possible to prevent piglet anaemia; since the dung will then contain enough iron to protect the piglets.

Supplements of calcium carbonate fed to fattening pigs from weaning onwards can cause iron deficiency, shown by reduction in blood haemoglobin concentrations and rates of live weight gain. This effect is especially marked in litters with low weaning weights, probably because their reserves of iron are generally lower. Iron injections or dosing at weaning will overcome these harmful effects.

A secondary anaemia, due to blood-sucking lice, must be borne in mind.

PIGLET MORTALITY. Causes include: Aujeszky's Disease, 'Baby Pig' Disease, Piglet Anaemia, Haemolytic Disease, Leptospiral Jaundice, *E. coli* infections, Streptococcal Meningitis, Swine Erysipelas, Swine Fever, Trembling, Enzootic Pneumonia, Glasser's Disease, Talfan Disease, Atrophic Rhinitis, and transmissible Gastro-enteritis (TGE); also overlying by the sow. (*See also under* ILEUM for another form of enteritis *and* DYSENTERY I; GASTRIC ULCERS *and* MUCORMYCOSIS; LISTERIOSIS; PERICARDITIS; DERMATOSIS; SPLAYLEG.) *Chlamydia psittaci* is another cause of piglet mortality. A list of diseases which affects pigs usually after weaning is given under PIGS, DISEASES OF.
Normal piglets were obtained from hatched blastocysts frozen at −196°C. (Kashiwazaki, S. & others. *Veterinary Record* (1991) **128,** 256.)

PIGMEN. Occupational hazards of people handling pigs include Erysipeloid (the human form of SWINE ERYSIPELAS infection); PORCINE STREPTOCOCCAL MENINGITIS; (SWINE VESICULAR DISEASE has been transmitted to laboratory workers, but there appear to be no reports of farm workers becoming ill); LEPTOSPIROSIS. (*See under* these headings.)

PILOBOLUS. A fungus often present in bovine faeces on pasture, it acts as a disperser of lungworm larvae, by means of a 'rocket-like' effect.

PILOCARPINE. The chief use is in the treatment of impaction or stoppage of the intestines. It is also the antidote to atropine poisoning. Pilocarpine constricts the pupil and is used to reduce intra-ocular pressure in cases of glaucoma.

PILUS. An American name for bacterial FIMBRIA (which see). For **sex pilus,** *see under* PLASMIDS.

PINEAL BODY is a small structure situated in a deep recess of the mid-brain. Its function is not known, but it occupies a position similar to the third eye in certain reptiles. The pineal body is often regarded as an endocrine gland, probably concerned with growth and development. After puberty the pineal body degenerates.

'PINING' (or 'PINE') was a term formerly used to describe any progressive loss of condition in sheep, but nowadays – together with 'vinquish' – it is usually reserved for cobalt deficiency. This occurs in many parts of the world, is known as Bush Sickness in New Zealand, and has been reported in areas of Scotland, Northumberland, Devon, and North Wales, where tracts of land are cobalt deficient. (*See under* COBALT.)

'PINK-EYE' is the colloquial name for infectious keratitis of cattle caused by *Moraxella* (*Haemophilus*) *bovis*; and also for Equine Viral Arteritis.

'PINK TOOTH'. The colloquial name for congenital PORPHYRIA in South Africa.

PINNA. The major part of the external ear, supported by the conchal cartilage.

PIPERAZINE compounds are used in the treatment of roundworm infestations in dogs, cats; also in pigs, poultry, and horses. They are of low toxicity and can be given in wet or dry food.

PIROPLASMS are protozoon parasites of the red-blood cells and the cause of numerous tick-transmitted diseases. They include *Babesia* and *Theileria*. (*See* BABESIOSIS.)

PITANGUEIRAS. A breed of cattle; $\frac{5}{32}\frac{3}{16}$ Red Poll and $\frac{5}{8}\frac{3}{16}$ Guzera (itself originally a Red Poll Brahman) developed in Brazil with Red Poll semen from the UK.

PITCH POISONING. This has occurred with fatal results in pigs after eating clay pigeons, and after contact with tarred walls and floors of pig pens. The symptoms are: inappetence, depression, weakness, jaundice, anaemia.

PITUITARY GLAND is a small oval body up to an inch in diameter, attached to the base of the brain and situated in a depression in the upper surface of the sphenoid bone called the *Sella turcica.*

The gland is connected to the Hypothalamus, which partly controls the pituitary gland. The latter has two main parts or lobes, and its main function appears to be the control of other endocrine glands.

The anterior lobe produces several hormones. One of these, the growth hormone (STH) has an important effect on protein metabolism. Lack of this hormone causes or contributes to dwarfism. *Somatotrophin* (STH hormone) controls body growth, including fetal growth in pregnant females.

ACTH (adrenocorticotrophin) stimulates the cortex of the adrenal gland. TSH stimulates the thyroid.

Pituitary gonad-stimulating hormones include LH (luteinising hormone), FSH (follicle stimulating hormone), and *prolactin* which is associated with lactation. (For the functions of LH and FSH *see under* LUTEINISING and FOLLICLE STIMULATING, respectively.)

When hypertrophied in the young the gland causes gigantism in which a great increase in size occurs. Hypertrophy or increased function in adults results in acromegaly, in which there is a sudden growth of extremities of the body. If it be atrophied, injured, or removed in the young creature, growth ceases, and a condition of infantilism results. In this there is a pronounced lack of development of ovaries and testes and of secondary sex characters, together with deposition of fat, and a general sluggishness and lack of development. In the male there is a tendency towards reversion to female characteristics, but the opposite effect in the female is not observed. Anterior lobe extract is used to correct such atrophic conditions. (*See also* TWINNING.)

The posterior lobe secretes two important hormones: (1) *vasopressin*, which is also known as the *antidiuretic hormone* or *ADH*, being concerned with water loss from the body. Lack of ADH gives rise to *Diabetes insipidus*. (2) *Oxytocin* acts on the muscular wall of the uterus causing contraction, *e.g.* during birth. It also acts on the mammary gland and is sometimes known as the 'let-down hormone' in connection with the release of milk.

Pituitary tumours in 8 dogs were found to be carcinomas in two of them, and adenomas in five. SIGNS: lethargy, pacing, circling, head-pressing, and partial paralysis affecting all four limbs.

Death occurred in from two weeks to 13 months. (Sarfaty, D. & others. *JAVMA* (1988) **143**, 854.)

PITUITRIN. An injection prepared from the posterior lobe of the pituitary gland, and containing two distinct fractions; one affecting the blood-vessels and the other the uterine muscle. These fractions are named the 'pressor' and 'oxytocic' principles, respectively. Pituitrin is used in cases of uterine atony, uterine haemorrhage, pyometra, intestinal atony, and in cases of shock and collapse following severe injury or operation.

In the horse, pituitrin may produce inhibition of the smooth muscle of the gut, and fatal constriction of the coronary vessels. In human and veterinary medicine, the whole extract is no longer used because of the fear of 'pituitrin shock'; the oxytocic fraction only being employed. (*See* HORMONES, ENDOCRINE GLANDS.)

PITYRIASIS is a bran-like eruption that appears on the surface of the skin. *Pityriasis rosea* was recorded in 72 out of 120 litters sired by a certain Landrace boar. Lesions resembled ringworm, were red, and lasted 10 weeks.

'PIZZLE ROT'. A disease mainly of Merino sheep in Australia. (*See under* BALANITIS.)

PLACENTA is the technical name for the afterbirth. Strictly speaking, placenta means the medium by means of which the mother nourishes the fetus.

Structure. It is composed of three fetal membranes: (1) the chorion, which is the outermost, is a strong fibrous membrane, the outer surface of which is closely moulded to the inner surface of the uterus. The chorion has villi which are vascular projections inserted into the crypts of the uterine mucous membrane.

(2) the allantois is the middle membrane. It develops early in embryonic life as an outgrowth from the hindgut, and insinuates itself between the other two membranes. That part of the allantois remaining inside the abdominal cavity of the fetus forms the urinary bladder in after-life, and, until the time of birth, is in direct communication with the extra-fetal portion by means of the urachus—that part passing through the umbilicus. Fluid secreted by the kidneys of the fetus and passing to the urinary bladder gains exit to the allantoic cavity which is outside the fetus until just before the time of birth, when the communication is occluded.

(3) the amnion, which is continuous with the skin at the umbilicus (navel), and completely encloses the fetus but is separated from actual contact with it by the amniotic fluid, or the 'liquor of the amnion', which in the mare measures about 5 or 6 litres (*i.e.* 9 to 10½ pints).

This 'liquor amnii' forms a kind of hydrostatic bed in which the fetus floats, and serves to protect it from injury, shocks, extremes of temperature, allows free though limited movements, and guards the uterus of the dam from the spasmodic fetal convulsions which, late in pregnancy, are often vigorous and even violent.

At birth it helps to dilate the cervical canal of the uterus and the posterior genital passages, forms part of the 'waterbag', and, on bursting, lubricates the maternal passages. (*See* PARTURITION.)

At birth, the membranes should be discharged from the uterus with or soon after the young animal, but it is not uncommon to find their expulsion delayed for a variable time, depending upon the species and the individual. Immediately after the birth of the young animal the uterus contracts to a size smaller than when pregnant with the result that the attachment between fetal envelopes and maternal uterus is severed to a greater or lesser extent. Afterpains follow, similar to those of normal labour, but less severe, with the object of expelling the membranes.

In the mare, with a scattered and slight attachment, the afterbirth separates rapidly and is soon expelled; indeed, not infrequently the foal is born still enveloped in, or attached to, its membranes. These appear as a complicated mass of pinkish-grey tissue, plentifully supplied with blood, and often possessing little bladderlike pockets of amniotic or allantoic fluid.

If in 6 hours the placenta has not been discharged naturally, measures should be taken to effect its prompt removal, for the mare is very susceptible to metritis.

In the cow, where the attachment is cotyledonary, the fetal membranes may be expelled at any time during the first 6 hours after calving, or not for 1 or 2 days, without any serious consequences. Retention occurs frequently.

In those animals which normally produce multiple offspring at a birth—ewe, sow, bitch, and cat—as each fetus is born the corresponding membranous envelope either accompanies or else immediately follows it. The exception to this otherwise almost invariable rule is in the case of the last fetus to be born, that fetus which occupied the extremity of one or other horn of the uterus; the envelopes of this, the youngest member of the family, are sometimes retained, and may occasion a mild or severe metritis, until such time as they are expelled.

The bitch, cat, sow, cow, and even the mare eat the membranes.

The placenta is a source of **hormones**, which may stimulate milk production or involution.

Equine fertility studies by Dr W. R. Allen have shown that the **'placental barrier'** (which protects the fetus from being rejected by the mother) can prevent rejection of a fetus even of a different species. As mentioned at the end of TRANSPLANTATION OF MAMMALIAN OVA (embryo transfer), this was achieved, despite the horse having 64 chromosomes per cell. It is Dr Allen's view that breakdown of the placental barrier may be one of the causes of early abortion in the mare.

Retained placenta is one of the undesirable sequels of parturition. Retention of the fetal membranes is commonest in the cow. Normally, the membranes should be expelled in from ½ to 4 or 5 hours after the birth of the calf, but owing to the intricate corlyedonary attachment in cattle, they are often retained for long periods. (*See* PARTURITION.)

SIGNS. A portion of the fetal membranes hangs from the lips of the vulva attached to what remains inside the cavity of the uterus. The exposed portion may measure only a few inches, or be a large mass reaching to the cow's hocks. In some cases there is no membrane visible externally, but there is an odour of decomposition evident.

During the first day after calving the membranes in an ordinary uncomplicated case are fresh, slimy, and pinkish in colour. There is no objectionable smell, and the cow is not distressed. After the second day the external portions undergo decomposition; the colour becomes greyish; an offensive chocolate-coloured discharge makes its appearance and soils the hindquarters and tail of the cow. She stands with her back arched, frequently switches her tail and paddles with the hind-feet.

Masses of semi-dissolved membrane, looking like pieces of wet cobweb, are passed out at intervals, and can be found behind the cow along with quantities of greyish foul-smelling discharge; the mucous membrane of the vagina is inflamed, and the cow resents having her hindquarters examined.

It is certainly not advisable that a mass of decomposing fleshy material should be allowed to hang from a cow's uterus for a longer time than is absolutely necessary, but too hasty attempts at removal may be followed by infertility or even death.

In modern practice stilboestrol injections have largely displaced manual removal, with its attendant risks. Manual removal consists of introducing the hand and arm which have been previously cleansed as far as possible by thorough washing in an antiseptic solution, and a subsequent rinsing in strong salt and water. The membranes should not be removed until they can be displaced *without difficulty, and without distress to the cow.* Each cotyledon is grasped as it is reached, and the adherent membrane is peeled off from its surface with the fingers and thumb. At the same time gentle traction should be exerted upon the protruded membranes from the outside.

After removal it may be advisable to douche out the uterus with a suitable antiseptic solution, and to introduce one or more uterine pessaries (*see* section 'Metritis', UTERUS, DISEASES OF).

In the sow and bitch the membranes that are liable to be retained are those belonging to the fetus that is born last, which occupied the extremity of one or other of the horns of the uterus, but the condition is rare in each of these animals.

It is most advisable that owners of animals which have retained their afterbirth after parturition should seek veterinary advice.

PLAGUE (*see* CATTLE PLAGUE, AVIAN PLAGUE, BUBONIC PLAGUE).

PLANTAR. At the back of the hind-limb.

PLANTAR CUSHION is the dense fibro-fatty rubber-like structure which lies immediately above the frog in the foot of the horse, and is one of its most important anti-concussion or shock-absorbing mechanisms. (*See* FOOT OF HORSE.)

PLANT JUICE. At grass drying plants, when mechanically de-watering forage before drying, a rich green juice is expressed. Under the auspices of the AFRC, the National Institute for Research in Dairying, and the Rowett Institute found the juice to be a new source of protein concentrate comparable with fish meal in value.

From six tons of fresh material, such as lucerne or grass, 2½ tons of this plant juice is squeezed out.

Using plant juice presents some problems, as it is very unstable, due to enzyme action. It must be heated to about 85°C to stabilise the protein, and some chemical preservative is also added.

The easiest way to use the juice is to include it in liquid pig feed. Whey and skim milk tankers should be able to cope with this liquid.

PLASMA is the fluid portion of the blood.

PLASMA CELLS. Larger than lymphocytes, with dark-staining granules in the nucleus, plasma cells are found in the lymph nodes, and are concerned with antibody production. (*See diagram under* LYMPHOCYTES.)

PLASMA SUBSTITUTES (*see* DEXTRAN, GELATIN).

PLASMIDS are genetic structures which many species of bacteria possess in addition to their chromosomes, and which, like the chromosomes, determine the inheritance of various properties. Since plasmids are not essential to cell growth, the cell may gain or lose them without lethal effect. Some plasmids can unite with chromosomes; these are called episomes. All episomes are plasmids but not all plasmids are episomes.

Plasmids were defined (*Lancet*, 1976) as 'Circular lengths of DNA which behave as viruses with a restricted range of host bacteria, and which are replicated in step with the organism.' (*See also* 'Genetic Engineering' *under* GENETICS.)

Infectious (self-transmissible) plasmids are found in Gram-negative rods. In addition to genes coding for specific properties (*e.g.* R-determinants coding for antibiotic resistance) these plasmids also possess other genes which code for the production of sex pili by which conjugation with a recipient cell is made possible. Non-transmissible plasmids, also found in Gram-negative rods, lack the genes necessary for self-transfer; for these plasmids to be transferred the cell must first be infected with a sex-factor from another cell. Other plasmids have never been transferred by conjugation.

In Gram-positive organisms, plasmids may be transduced from one cell to another by bacteriophages.

PLASMODIUM GALLINACEUM. *Plasmodium gallinaceum* causes 'bird malaria' in poultry imported into Sri Lanka and India, with death following quickly upon symptoms of fever, congestion of the comb. Local birds have immunity.

P. durae causes death in turkey poults similarly in Kenya.

'Malaria of birds' is a group of almost worldwide infections which include *Haemoproteus* and *Leucocytozoon* as well as *Plasmodium*.

PLASTER CASTS (*see* SPLINTING MATERIALS.)

PLASTIC BAGS, SHEETING. Cattle have died following ingestion of plastic bags discarded on grazing land. In some instances the material is digested and does not cause an obstruction.

PLASTIC 'BONES'. A fractured scaphoid in the right hind-leg of a racing greyhound has been successfully replaced by a plastic replica of a scaphoid bone. For a further use of plastics, *see under* HOOF REPAIR.

PLATE CULTURE. The growing of bacteria in a medium contained in a Petri dish which gives a large surface.

PLATELETS, or thrombocytes, are described under BLOOD (which see).

PLATING is the cultivation of bacteria on flat plates containing nutrient material. The term is also applied in surgery to the method of securing union of fractured bones by screwing to the sides of the fragments narrow metal plates which hold them firmly together whilst union is taking place.

PLEURA is the membrane which covers the external surfaces of the lungs and lines the inside of the chest walls. (*See* LUNGS.)

PLEURAL CAVITY. In normal healthy animals, this is merely a potential cavity; since between the pleura lining the chest and the pleura covering the lungs there is normally a thin film of fluid. Surface tension holds the one surface to the other, as does a drop of water between two small plates of glass.

PLEURISY, or PLEURITIS. Inflammation of the PLEURA (*see above*), which may occur as a complication of pneumonia, of 'shipping fever' in cattle, and in cases of tuberculosis and other infections; occasionally from a chest wound.

Friction between the inflamed surfaces gives rise to pain each time the animal breathes, and the breathing is changed in character, *i.e.* there is minimal movement of the chest walls, and extra effort by the abdominal muscles, which appear to be doing all the work. The line of the rib cartilages often stands out prominently, giving rise to what has been called the 'pleuritic ridge'. Other symptoms include fever, dullness, and what is often described as a 'hacking' cough; sometimes a rasping sound due to friction may be heard.

After 12 to 48 hours the painful stage of pleurisy may be followed by an effusion of fluid. This ends friction and so pain.

In the horse the quantity of fluid may amount to 10 gallons, and in the dog to 3 pints. Removal of this fluid becomes necessary if respiration is seriously impaired by it.

Sometime the fluid is purulent, a condition known as Empyema. Sometimes there is very little effusion, and the condition remains one of 'dry pleurisy'.

A complication of pleurisy is that adhesions sometimes occur, and persist, between the parietal and visceral pleura. (*See also the next two entries.*)
TREATMENT. Pleurisy is one of those conditions in which professional advice is highly desirable in the early stages, and reliance should not be placed on first-aid. It may be necessary to withdraw fluid from the chest, to administer an appropriate antibiotic; and it is important to establish the presence or absence of tuberculosis. (*See also* NURSING.)

PLEURODYNIA means a painful condition of the chest wall. It is a symptom of pleurisy; it may be due to fractures of the ribs; it is sometimes seen in tumours affecting the chest wall, and it is commonly recognised by pressing the fingers into the spaces between the ribs in intercostal rheumatism.

PLEURO-PNEUMONIA means a combination of pleurisy with a pneumonia. Acute pneumonia is often accompanied by some amount of pleurisy, which is largely responsible for the painfulness which accompanies pneumonia. (*See* CONTAGIOUS BOVINE PLEURO-PNEUMONIA, PNEUMONIA.)

PLEXUS is a network of nerves or vessels, *e.g.* the brachial and sacral plexuses of nerves and the choroid plexus of veins within the brain.

PLUMBISM is another name for chronic lead poisoning. (*See* LEAD POISONING.)

PMS. Pregnant Mare's Serum.

PNEUMOCYSTIS PNEUMONIA, one of the most serious diseases of human AIDS patients, has been found in dogs, cats, rodents, and primates.

PNEUMOGASTRIC or VAGUS NERVE is the tenth cranial nerve. This nerve is remarkable for its great length, and for the attachments which it forms with other nerves and with the sympathetic trunks. It arises from the side of the medulla, passes out of the skull, runs down to the jugular furrow of the neck, where, along with the sympathetic, it accompanies the carotid artery to the entrance to the chest. From this point the right and left vagi differ from each other in their course. They both pass through the chest cavity, giving branches to the pharynx (which run up the neck again), to the heart, bronchi, oesophagus, etc. Each nerve then splits into two parts and the two upper branches fuse with each other to form the dorsal trunk, the lower branches behaving similarly to form the ventral trunk. These two branches now pass through the diaphragm, with the oesophagus, into the abdominal cavity, and end by giving branches to the stomach, duodenum, liver, and various ganglia near by.

PNEUMOMYCOSIS. A fungal infection of the lungs.

PNEUMONIA, may be defined as inflammation of lung tissue.

Pneumonias have been classified in various ways; *e.g.* according to the area or tissue involved, or according to lesions, or causes.

Lobar pneumonia is that in which a whole lobe is involved; in lobular pneumonia the inflammation is less localised, more patchy. Bronchopneumonia is that in which the inflammation is concentrated in and around the bronchioles leading from the bronchi. Pleuropneumonia, as the name suggests, involves the pleural membranes as well as the lung itself. Interstitial pneumonia affects the fibrous supporting tissue of the lung rather than the parenchyma though consolidation of the latter can then occur. (*See also* LUNGS, DISEASES OF for lesions.)

Pneumonia, which can be acute or chronic, may – as mentioned above – also be classified according to causes; *e.g.* viral, mycoplasmal, bacterial, mycotic, parasitic and non-infective. It must be borne in mind, however, that infections may be mixed and changing (*see* INFECTION AND RESPIRATORY DISEASE IN PIGS for an explanatory diagram.)

Pneumonia may arise from a primary viral infection, with complications caused by secondary bacterial invaders, as in canine distemper. Some viruses and bacteria depend upon each other, as explained under SYNERGISM. The infection may be a very mixed one; *e.g.* in ENZOOTIC PNEUMONIA of pigs. Bacterial pneumonia may be acute, *e.g.* KLEBSIELLA infection, or of a chronic suppurative type, *e.g.* TUBERCULOSIS.

The **main effect of pneumonia**, whether through the presence of exudate in the bronchioles and alveoli, or destruction of areas of lung by abscess formation or consolidation or hepatisation, is that the normal exchange of carbon dioxide for oxygen is impaired and impeded. The animal has to struggle to obtain sufficient oxygen.

SIGNS. With less oxygen available to the red blood cells (and hence to the organs and tissues) at the normal respiratory rate, the animal accordingly needs to breathe faster. This increased respiratory rate (*tachypnoea*) is therefore a main symptom. The breathing may also become laboured and painful (*dyspnoea*). Fever is usually present, with accompanying dullness and loss of appetite (but *see under* CALF PNEUMONIA for an exception to this). There is often a cough, though this is not an invariable or attention-catching symptom.

Viral pneumonia. In cattle, an acute exudative pneumonia may develop in some cases of Infectious bovine rhinotracheitis (*see* RHINOTRACHEITIS.) Bovine syncytial virus is another important pathogen, causing coughing, oedema of the lungs, consolidation and emphysema. (*See also* CALF PNEUMONIA.) In horses, pneumonia in young foals may be caused by Equine herpesvirus 1. (*See also* SWINE PLAGUE.)

Mycoplasmal pneumonia. An example of this is fully described under CONTAGIOUS BOVINE PLEUROPNEUMONIA – a disease not present in the UK. *M. bovis* and *M. dispar* are primary pathogens in the UK. The latter may cause CALF PNEUMONIA (which see) of a mild type except for the harsh cough. (*See also under* MYCOPLASMA.)

Bacterial pneumonia. Bacterial toxins may have an important additional effect in this. In cattle *Pasteurella haemolytica* can be a primary cause of pneumonia, as well as a secondary invader. In horses *Corynebacterium equi* causes a suppurative broncho-pneumonia in foals, and in adult horses a suppurative pneumonia may also occur during the course of Strangles.

Streptococcus pneumoniae, and *Staphylococcus aureus* are other important secondary invaders of damaged lungs.

Parasitic pneumonia. This may be an extension of PARASITIC BRONCHITIS (which see) in calves, caused by the lungworm *Dictyocaulus viviparus*. Autopsy findings include dark red consolidation of some lung lobes. In pigs, lungworms (*Metastrongylus*) are also a cause of pneumonia.

Mycotic (fungal) pneumonia is caused by Aspergillus species, and also by *Candida albicans* (*see* MONILIASIS.) The latter may be associated with oedema of the lungs, both in mammals and birds, and may follow the use of certain antibiotics. (*See also* PHYCOMYCOSIS.)

Allergic pneumonia (*see* 'FARMER'S LUNG' which affects cattle also.)

Non-infective pneumonia can result from the action of certain poisons; e.g. PARAQUAT, ANTU, and phenolic sheep dips (*see* DIPS); and from aspiration pneumonia. The latter may result from milk 'going the wrong way' in bucket-fed calves, and also from medicines administered to animals by stomach tube passed in error into the trachea instead of the oesophagus (a fortunately rare occurrence!) Aspiration of vomit is another example.

Non-infective pneumonia quickly becomes infective, as micro-organisms take advantage of the inflamed mucous membranes. The animal becomes suddenly dull, uninterested in food, feverish, and may show signs of chest pain. Death can be expected within 72 hours, and autopsy findings may include areas of necrosis and abscess formation.

Treatment of pneumonia. Heart stimulants, the administration of oxygen, and possibly diuretics in the case of oedema, may be indicated. Appropriate antibiotics, sulpha drugs, trimethoprim may all be of service. The one golden rule in the treatment of pneumonia in all animals is: '*Do not drench*'. Medicines should be administered by injection, in the food, or perhaps as an electuary. (*See also* NURSING.)

PNEUMONIA IN CALVES (*see* CALF PNEUMONIA).

PNEUMONIA IN CATS. Bronchopneumonia can be a complication of feline viral rhinotracheitis in young cats.

In older cats tuberculosis is still sometimes a cause of disease of the lungs, though with nearly all milk now pasteurised in EC countries, feline TB is no longer at all common. It can, however, result from a cat eating TB-infected prey.

A granulomatous pneumonia is caused, rarely, by *Corynebacterium equi*. Theoretically, a stable cat would be more prone to it.

PNEUMONIA IN HORSES. Anaerobic bacteria were isolated from pleural fluid or tracheobronchial aspirates obtained from 21 of 46 horses with bronchopneumonia. *Bacteriodes oralis* and *B melaninogenicus* were the species most commonly isolated (nine and five horses, respectively). Other *Bacteriodes* species were cultured from 12 animals and *Clostridium* species from eight. A putrid odour was associated with the pleural fluid and, or, breath of nearly two-thirds of the horses from which anaerobes were isolated. The prognosis was significantly poorer in cases with anaerobic infections, 14 of the 21 horses involved either died or were euthanased. (Sweeney, C. R., Divers, T. J. & Benson, C. E., *Journal of the American Veterinary Medical Association* (1985) **187,** 721.) (*See also under* FOALS, DISEASES OF).

Another cause is *Corynebacterium equi*, which can also infect cats.

PNEUMONIA IN PIGS. *Haemophilus parahaemolyticus* has been reported as a cause of severe pleuro-pneumonia in pigs in the USA, Argentina, Switzerland and the UK. (*See* RESPIRATORY DISEASE IN THE PIG.)

For the most common form of pneumonia in pigs (*see under* ENZOOTIC PNEUMONIA). (*See also* 'SWINE PLAGUE'.)

PNEUMONIA IN SHEEP. In Britain a disease which has spread much in recent years is pneumonia caused by *Pasteurella haemolytica*. This organism commonly lives in normal sheep, and causes disease only when the animal's resistance is weakened by bad weather, transport from one farm to another, movement from a poor to a richer pasture, or perhaps by a virus. In some outbreaks, where the disease takes an acute form, a sheep which seemed healthy enough in the evening may be found dead in the morning. Usually, however, the shepherd sees depressed-looking animals with drooping ears, breathing rather quickly and having a discharge from eyes and nostrils, and a cough. Death often occurs within a day or two. The last sheep to be involved in the outbreak tend to linger for several weeks, looking very tucked-up in the meantime, with a cough and fast breathing. A vaccine is available.

Another cause of pneumonia in sheep is *Chlamydia psittaci*. (*See also* HAEMORRHAGIC SEPTICAEMIA, which occurs in the tropics) and PARAINFLUENZA 3 VIRUS, MAEDI/VISNA.)

PNEUMOTHORAX means a collection of air in the pleural cavity which has gained entrance through a wound in the chest wall. (*See* LUNGS, DISEASES AND INJURIES OF.)

Pneumothorax is not uncommon in the dog which has fallen out of a window, or been run over or hit by a car. Distressed breathing and cyanosis are, following an accident, suggestive of pneumothorax.

Mild cases may be accompanied by mild symptoms, and spontaneous recovery may occur. Severe cases may die. Treatment includes aspiration of the air. (*See also* COLLAPSE OF LUNG *under* LUNGS, DISEASES OF.)

Simple pneumothorax. In such cases, 'the leak may be caused by sudden *non-penetrating trauma* to the chest wall which momentarily raises the intrathoracic pressure. If this occurs against a closed glottis, then alveolar tissue may rupture. In many cases the leak will be small, but in others sufficient air will enter the pleural cavity to cause marked dyspnoea.' (Houlton, J. *In Practice*, July 1986, 157).

Open pneumothorax is caused by a penetrating wound of the chest wall, resulting in an immediate and total collapse of the lung. 'Air can be heard entering the chest wound at each respiratory effort.' There is severe dyspnoea.

Tension pneumothorax may develop following an open pneumothorax, or when a small bronchus ruptures, and air accumulates in the pleural space during inspiration but is not expelled during expiration. The mediastinum is apt to be displaced from the midline, partially collapsing the remaining functional lung.

PNEUMOVIRUS. A cause of rhinotracheitis in turkeys and chickens. An ELISA test is available for diagnosis.

'POACHING'. Especially on heavy land, with high stocking rates, wet weather can bring serious poaching problems. (See DAIRY HERD MANAGEMENT.) At gateways deep mud, in winter often at near freezing temperatures, can lead to foul-in-the-foot and mastitis.

PODODERMATITIS (see FOUL-IN-THE-FOOT).

POIKILOCYTE is a malformed red blood cell found in the blood in various types of anaemia.

POIKILOTHERMIC. 'Cold-blooded'. The rate of metabolism of such an animal varies with its environmental temperature.

POISONING. This usually results from the poison being swallowed. In a few instances poison may be taken in through a wound of the skin, or even through the unbroken skin, e.g. phenol preparations. Malicious poisoning is most frequently carried out against dogs and cats, although horses and ruminants also sometimes suffer, but the nefarious practice of poisoning an opponent's animal is, in the civilised countries, fortunately very rare.

The use of poison to control vermin – rabbits, foxes, rats, mice, etc. – is a hazard, for when the poisoned bait is accessible to domesticated animals, cases of poisoning in them may result. It should be remembered that the exposure of such poison above ground constitutes a punishable offence.

The constituents of common and commercial rat-poisons are mentioned under RAT-POISONS (which see).

Many cases of poisoning result from the careless use of sheep-dips, paints, weed-killers, insecticides, which, either in powder, paste, or solution, are left about in places to which animals have access. Cattle are notoriously inquisitive, and will lick at anything they find, sometimes with fatal consequences.

It is perhaps not widely enough realised that cattle seem to like the taste of lead paint – one heifer helped herself to a whole pint of it – and that very small quantities spattered on the ground can kill several beasts. Even the contents of old, discarded paint tins can be lethal. In one instance, children found such tins and scraped out the residue on to pasture, killing five yearlings. In another instance, cattle licked out old paint tins on a rubbish dump in a pit to which they found their way. A recently-painted fence is also a danger; and it is worth while getting a farm-worker to clear up behind any plumber using red-lead.

Thirsty cattle will drink almost anything. Diesel oil and a copper-containing spray liquid have each caused death in these circumstances. Salt poisoning is certainly no myth, and pigs should never be kept short of drinking water.

Some insecticides, such as TEPP and Parathion, are totally unsuitable for use on livestock. Fatal poisoning of a herd of cattle sprayed with

TEPP has been reported from Texas. A farmer in Ireland used aldrin as an orf-dressing, and killed 105 out of 107 lambs. Fatal poisoning of cattle has also occurred through the application to their backs of a carbolic-acid-arsenic preparation against flies. (See also HERBICIDES, WEEDKILLERS.)

Near factories and chemical works, grass etc., may become impregnated with fluorine compounds, copper, lead, or other metals and lead to chronic poisoning of any animals grazing near by. The same thing applies in orchards after spraying of fruit-trees. Pasture may be contaminated by spray-drift or dusting operations, particularly from the air, and the chemicals used may cause poisoning. This applies also to other treated green crops which animals may eat. DDT and BHC and other insecticides (used in home and garden) of the CHLORINATED HYDROCARBON group may poison birds, cats and dogs. (See also ORGANO-PHOSPHORUS POISONING, FARM CHEMICALS, and FLUOROSIS.)

The use of pitch (the poisonous ingredient of clay-pigeons) or coal tar on the walls and floors of piggeries is a cause of poisoning. Some wood preservatives cause Hyperkeratosis.

Poisoning may result from indiscretion on the part of owners or attendants in the use of patent or other animal medicines, or from the administration to animals of tablets, etc., intended for human use, e.g. paracetamol, caffeine.

Dogs and cats may also be poisoned by gaining access to unsecured medicines (pills, tablets, etc.) intended for human use. For home and garden hazards to pet animals (including cage birds) see under CARBON MONOXIDE, 'FRYING PAN DEATHS', ANTIFREEZE, CREOSOTE, LEAD POISONING, METALDEHYDE, BHC POISONING, BENZOIC ACID POISONING, WARFARIN, DDT, HOUSE PLANTS, HOUSE DECORATING. If one considers dogs out for walks, one should add DIELDRIN, PARAQUAT, FARM CHEMICALS. As regards **dog and cat foods**, poisoning has resulted from biscuit meal made from corn dressed with dieldrin, from stored food contaminated by rats' urine containing warfarin, from aflatoxins, and from horse-meat containing barbiturates or choral hydrate. In the cat, food containing benzoic acid as a preservative has caused poisoning. (See also CAGE BIRDS.)

Fodder poisoning. Excess of fodder beet may cause scouring in both pigs and cattle, and the after-effects may be serious. In sows just farrowed the milk supply may almost disappear. Beet tops have caused the deaths of cattle when given unwilted, and even when wilted they should be strictly rationed. Kale and rape must likewise be used sparingly and not constitute an animal's sole diet; hay in particular being necessary in addition. Deaths have occurred in horses and cattle restricted to rye-grass pasture. Sheep have been fatally poisoned by feeding them surplus pig-meal containing a copper supplement; a heifer likewise. Pigs have been poisoned by giving them medicated meal intended for poultry and containing nitrophenide against coccidiosis. Which all goes to show that medicated feeds are by no means always interchangeable between different species of livestock since there are genetic differences between them as regards susceptibility to poisoning; depending in part upon possession or absence of some enzyme which can readily de-toxify the poison. (*See* GROUNDNUT MEAL.)

The use of surplus seed corn for pig-feeding has led to fatal poisoning – the mercury dressing having been overlooked! (*See* DIELDRIN *for poisoning from seed dressings; and* FLOOR SWEEPINGS; *also* MONENSIN.)

Hay contaminated with foxgloves or ragwort is a source of fatal poisoning. Silage contaminated with ragwort has similarly caused death. Silage contaminated with Hexoestrol has caused abortion. (*See under* HORMONES IN MEAT PRODUCTION.)

Poisonous plants growing in pastures, in swampy or marshy places, in the bottoms of hedges, on waste land and in shrubberies and gardens, are other very fruitful sources of poisoning. In the early spring, when grass is scarce, and when herbivorous animals are let out for the first time after wintering indoors, the tender succulent growths attract them, often with serious consequences. Similar results may be seen during a very dry summer when grass is parched. (*See* BRACKEN.)

Clippings from shrubs, especially from yew, rhododendrons, aconite, boxwood, lupins, laurel, laburnum, etc., should never be thrown 'over the hedge', because in some of these the toxic substances are most active when the clippings have begun to wither, and animals are very prone to eat them in this condition. It is a safe rule to regard all garden trimmings as unsafe for animals, with the exception of vegetables, such as cabbages, turnips, etc. (*See under separate headings e.g.* ACONITE, BITTERSWEET, FOXGLOVE, HEMLOCK, LABURNUM, POTATO, RAGWORT, WATER DROPWORT, YEW, LOCOWEED, etc.)

SIGNS. The symptoms of each of the more common poisonous agents are given under their respective headings.

It must be emphasised that the symptoms of some illnesses are the same as those of some poisons, and *vice versa*. For example, not only vomiting and diarrhoea but also cramp, fever, rapid breathing, convulsions, hysteria, jaundice, salivation, blindness, and deafness are common to both. A professional diagnosis is therefore important.

Irritant poisons produce acute abdominal pain, vomiting (when possible), purging, rapidly developing general collapse, and often unconsciousness, perhaps preceded by convulsions.

Narcotics produce excitement at first, unsteady movements, interference with sight; and later, stupor and unconsciousness appear; coma, with or without spasmodic or convulsive movements, supervenes, and death occurs in many cases almost insensibly.

Narcotico-irritants produce symptoms of irritation in the first place, and later, delirium, convulsions, and coma.

As a general rule poisoning should be suspected when an animal becomes suddenly ill, soon after feeding; when put out to pasture for the first time in the season; after dipping; or when a change of food has recently taken place. Newly purchased animal feeds may be followed by an outbreak of illness, and such results point to the inclusion of some harmful substance. Fungal poisoning may occur as a result of mouldy barley, etc.

FIRST-AID. In suggesting simple first-aid measures, it should be emphasised that they necessarily differ from – and are likely to be less effective than – those the veterinary surgeon will take. It should be realised, too, that against some poisons there are no effective antidotes.

Where it is suspected that poisoning has arisen from use of some proprietary product, take the container (or the label from it) to your veterinarian (or write down name of manufacturer and product) so that he may ascertain the chemical ingredients and, if necessary, consult the manufacturers as to the recommended antidote.

If it is suspected that poisoning may have resulted from a skin dressing, wash this off with warm soapy water to prevent further absorption. (*See for example,* CARBOLIC ACID POISONING.)

Where a poison is believed to have been taken by mouth, give an **emetic**.

Emetics which may be safely used are – pig, a dessertspoonful of mustard in a cupful of water; dog, a strong salt solution (ordinary household salt), or a crystal of washing soda; cat, the latter.

To hinder absorption in the horse, ox, or sheep, strong black tea or coffee which has been *boiled* may be given. These substances, all of which contain tannic acid or tannates, are useful against vegetable poisons.

To counteract the effects of irritants, use demulcents (olive oil, milk, milk and eggs, or liquid paraffin). Yellow phosphorus is an exception to this rule; oily substances favour its absorption and must be avoided; copper sulphate should be given instead. Against narcotics, stimulants are needed; *e.g.* strong coffee or black tea, given by the mouth as a first-aid measure.

Advice on poisons. In the UK veterinary surgeons may obtain information and advice concerning poisonous compounds, and their antidotes, if any, from the National Poisons Information Service, New Cross Hospital, London.

Confirmation of poisoning. No matter how strong circumstantial evidence seems to be, it is always essential that a post-mortem examination be made, and that necessary samples of the stomach contents, portions of the liver and perhaps other organs, should be submitted to a qualitative and quantitative chemical examination by an analyst, before a suspected case of poisoning can be considered to be definitely proved. The necessity for this procedure is obvious when legal proceedings are contemplated. G.P.W.

POISONING BY SALMONELLA (*See* SALMONELLOSIS).

POLAND CHINA. A breed of pig from Ohio, USA. Colouring is black with six white points (feet, tip of noise and tail). Rapid growth and good meat production are characteristics of the breed.

POLIOENCEPHALOMALACIA. A disease of cattle, sheep, and pigs, characterised by oedema of the brain. It may affect up to 25 per cent of the stock, and up to 90 per cent may die in feedlots in North America. It appears similar to the effects of salt poisoning in pigs.

Muzzle twitching, opisthotonos, blindness, and inability to stand are symptoms observed in affected calves in Britain. (*See also* CEREBRO-CORTICAL NECROSIS which closely resembles the above or may be identical with it.)

The cause may be thiaminase-type-l-producing bacilli or clostridia.

POLIOMYELITIS OF PIGS. This disease is distinct from that of human beings and is possibly identical with TALFAN DISEASE.

POLL. The region lying between the ears and a little behind them.

'POLL EVIL' is an old, colloquial name sometimes incorrectly applied to any swelling in the poll region, but which should be reserved for a sinus following infection of some of the deeper tissues and giving rise to pus-formation. It may result from an injury which displaces a chip of bone from the atlas. Apart from this, and its situation, 'Poll Evil' resembles Fistulous Withers.
CAUSES. Self-inflicted injuries such as striking the poll against the top of a doorway, or falling backwards with the poll striking the ground; blows, such as from a whip-handle; bridle pressure.
Fusiformis necrophorus has been associated with some cases and may have gained entrance through damaged skin. It has been suggested that some cases may arise through infection without injury. *Brucella abortus* and the worm *Onchocerca reticulata* have each been found, and the former is now known to account for some cases of Fistulous Withers.
SIGNS. A painful swelling on one or both sides with, after a time, the appearance of one or more orifices exuding pus. The animal resents the part being touched and, if the *ligamentum nuchae* is involved, avoids downward movement of the head.
FIRST-AID MEASURES include the use of an antiphlogistine poultice and the placing of food at a level which the animal can reach without pain.
TREATMENT may necessitate the removal of any dead tissue and the surgical enlargement of any openings to allow free drainage. Antibiotics may be used to overcome the infection.

POLLED. Inherited hornlessness of an animal belonging to a normally horned breed, *e.g.* Hereford cattle. (*See* SCUR.)

POLLEN of oilseed rape has been linked to obstructive lung disease seen in horses at pasture.
Clenbuterol is recommended for treatment.

POLYARTHRITIS. Inflammation of several joints occurring simultaneously as in 'JOINT ILL' (which see.) In pigs a common cause is *Erysipelothrix rhusiopathiae*; but streptococci and staphylococci may also be involved. The disease is seen also in lambs, calves, and foals.

POLYCYTHAEMIA. A marked increase in the number of red blood cells. This disorder is seen, rarely, in dogs and cats.

POLYDACTYLY. A congenital defect in which an animal has an extra digit. Cattle, horses (rarely), dogs and cats may be affected.

POLYDIPSIA is excessive thirst.

POLYMELIA. A developmental disorder resulting in an extra limb or limbs.

POLYMORPH is a name applied to certain white cells of the blood which have a nucleus of varied shape. (*See* BLOOD.)

POLYNEURITIS means an inflammation of nerves or their sheaths occurring in different parts of the body at the same time. (*See* NEURITIS.)

POLYOESTROUS animals are those which have several oestrus cycles per year; the converse being *monoestrous*.

POLYP is a tumour which is attached by a stalk to the surface from which it springs. The term only applies to the shape of the growth and has nothing to do with its structure or to its nature. Most polyps are benign, but some may become malignant. They are generally of fibrous tissue in the centre covered with the type of local epithelium. In animals, the common situations where they are found are in the nostrils; in the vagina, where they sometimes interfere with successful copulation; and in the interior of the bladder.

POLYPLOIDY. The presence of exact multiples of the haploid number of chromosomes greater than the diploid number; *e.g.* triploidy, tetraploidy.

POLYRADICULONEURITIS idiopathic. A disease of dogs, and occasionally cats, affecting nerves.
SIGNS: weakness of the hindlegs, followed by paralysis of them within a few days. The forelegs then become involved. Hyperaesthesia of all legs occurs. Body temperature remains normal.

Muscle wasting occurs. Recovery is gradual. In one case a puppy was able to walk again after four weeks; but complete recovery took over six months.

POLYSACCHARIDES (*see* SUGAR).

POLYTOCOUS. Producing several offspring at birth, *i.e.* a litter.

POLYURIA is a condition in which a much greater amount of urine is passed than is usual.

Polyuria is also a symptom of diabetes, and it occurs in certain forms of inflammation of the kidneys, especially in the early stages of pyelonephritis affecting cows after calving, when infection has travelled into the bladder, up the ureters, and so into the kidney. (*See* INCONTINENCE; KIDNEY, DISEASES OF; URINE; STRESS.)

POLYVALENT VACCINE. One prepared from cultures of several strains of the same bacterial or viral species or from different species. A single vaccine can now protect against eight diseases.

POM. (UK readers: *see* PRESCRIPTION-ONLY-MEDICINES.)

PONDS. *Salmonella typhimurium* was isolated from marl ponds on a farm where the dairy herd had a reduced milk yield, fever, and dysentery. 'Fencing off the ponds to prevent access by the cattle stopped the outbreak immediately.' (Liverpool VIC report, 1976.). (*See also* LEECHES, ALGAE POISONING, COCCIDIOSIS, JOHNE'S DISEASE, BOTULISM.)

PONIES. (*See under* HORSES, BREEDS OF; HORSES, FEEDING OF.)

PONS, or PONS VAROLII, is the so-called 'bridge of the brain'. It is situated at the base of the brain in front of the medulla, and behind the cerebral peduncles, and appears as a bulbous swelling not unlike a small curved artichoke. It is mainly composed of strands of fibres which link up different parts of the brain.

POPLITEAL refers to a region that lies behind the stifle joint, and to the vessels, lymph glands, nerves, etc., lying in this region. It is protected laterally by the biceps femoris, posteriorly by the semitendinosus and the gastrocnemius, and internally by the gracilis and semitendinosus tendon; consequently it is seldom that its vessels or nerves are injured.

PORCINE CORONAVIRUS infection. This has become enzootic in the UK and some other EC countries. The virus has a close antigenic relationship with Transmissible Gastro-enteritis virus and is a cause of a non-severe pneumonia. (O'Toole, D. & others. *Research in Veterinary Science* (1989) **47** 23.)

PORCINE CYTOMEGALOVIRUS (PCMV) is a new name for Inclusion-body rhinitis virus, which can produce rhinitis and pneumonia in pigs.

PORCINE ENCEPHALOMYELITIS. (*See* TALFAN *and* TESCHEN.)

PORCINE ENTEROVIRUS ENGLAND/72 is the cause of SWINE VESICULAR DISEASE (which see).

PORCINE INTESTINAL ADENOMATOSIS. This disease of pigs is believed to be an infectious one, the bacterium involved being *Campylobacter*

sputorum subspecies *mucosalis*; although the lesions resemble a neoplasm with proliferating epithelial cells. (*See* L. Roberts, *et al., Vet. Rec.* (1977), **100,** 12.) Death may occur from necrosis of the altered epithelium of the intestine, sometimes with perforation. However, many cases may not be noticed, and failure to make satisfactory weight gains may be the only indication of its presence. (G. H. K. Lawson *et al., Vet. Record* (1981) **107,** 424.) (*See also* Proliferative Haemorrhagic Enteropathy under HAEMORRHAGIC GASTRO-ENTERITIS OF PIGS.)

PORCINE PARVOVIRUS. This can be a cause of fetal death and mummification, if infection occurs during the first half of the gestation period. An inactivated vaccine is available.

PORCINE STREPTOCOCCAL MENINGITIS. This was first recognised in fattening pigs in the UK as recently as 1975 (though in unweaned pigs in 1954). A national survey carried out by the Cambridge Veterinary Investigation Centre revealed 17 outbreaks in 1974, 52 in 1975, and 152 in 1976; most of the cases occurring in the south and east of England.

Streptococcus suis type I causes meningitis as a complication of septicaemia in the unweaned piglet. Symptoms include fever, loss of appetite, a tendency for the piglets to bury themselves in the litter, stiffness, and an unsteady gait. The ears may be drawn back and held close to the side of the head. An inability to rise and paddling movements of the hind legs precede death in many instances. Some pigs recover; others die from septicaemia associated with arthritis or pneumonia.

Streptococcus suis type II affected pigs mainly in the age bracket 8–16 weeks, but of late the age group principally involved is 4–8 weeks.

The death of a large pig in excellent condition is often the first sign of the disease. If symptoms are observed, they are similar to those already described for the unweaned pig. In untreated cases the illness is usually brief and fatal.

This streptococcal meningitis is 'primarily associated with the mixing and moving of young weaned pigs', and may affect from less than 1 per cent to over 50 per cent of pigs, depending on management factors, etc. Poor ventilation favours a higher incidence, which is seen more in imperfectly managed controlled-environment buildings than in old or converted fattening houses.

CONTROL MEASURES. So far, vaccination has not been very successful. Accordingly, control measures can be aimed either at eradicating the infection on the farm or, if this is considered impracticable, minimising losses. If weaners are being bought from different suppliers, it may be possible to discover which is the source of infection. On some farms, buildings could be emptied, disinfected, and re-stocked – avoiding buying from anyone known or suspected of having the disease on his premises. If carrier sows can be identified they should be culled.

R. S. Windsor referred to the use of penicillin in an eradication attempt. A single injection can be given to each pig on the farm, or long-acting penicillin treatment of breeding stock followed by treatment of individual sows as they go into the farrowing house. Two injections at a 96-hour interval have also been given on some farms. (*Vet. Record* (1977) **101,** 378.)

Public health. Pigmen should be warned of the risk to them, even though the risk is a small one.

Streptococcus suis type II was isolated from a case of meningitis in an abattoir worker by the public health laboratory, Cambridge. Seven of 10 cases of streptococcal meningitis occurring in Holland were associated with infection with the porcine streptococcus Group R. The other three isolates were similar but lacked the R antigen. All streptococci fell into the bacterial species provisionally named *Streptococcus subacidus.* Nine of the 10 patients had contact with pigs while the other person liked to eat raw meat. One of the affected people died of the disease. (Zanen, H. C. and Engel, H. W. B. (1975) *Lancet*, June 7, p. 1286.)

PORCINE STRESS SYNDROME (PSS). A group of symptoms, due to a single gene, occurring in some breeds of pigs, notably Dutch Piétrain, Belgian Landrace, German Landrace, and French Piétrain. Under stress, death from heart failure may occur suddenly. The syndrome is associated with PALE, SOFT, EXUDATIVE (PSE) MEAT (which see). The anaesthetic halothane can be used for on-farm testing of pigs to discover whether they are susceptible.

PORCINE ULCERATIVE SPIROCHAETOSIS. An infection believed to be present in the UK, and reported also in the USA, Australia, and New Zealand. Experimentally, injection of the spirochaetes has led to footrot, schirrhous cord, and ulceration of the skin.

PORCUPINE QUILLS. In some areas of the USA and Canada dogs require treatment as a result of rash encounters with porcupines. The North American porcupine uses its tail as a means of defence, leaving behind numerous quills; while if the dog attempts to bite a porcupine, the result may be a mouthful of quills, which stick in the tongue and cheeks.

In the UK free-living porcupines (Asiatic and African species) in both Devon and Staffordshire are, like mink and coypu, escapers, and have bred since gaining their freedom.

Removal of quills must be a very painful process, for they are barbed. American veterinary authorities nevertheless recommend that the owner should, if the dog will let him, remove quills as soon as possible as a first-aid measure, especially from the tongue and over the chest and abdomen, as deep penetration may occur with possible fatal injury involving internal organs. Quill removal should be completed under a general anaesthetic by a veterinary surgeon.

If there is delay, some quills will have disappeared from sight and, as they are not revealed by X-rays, no veterinary surgeon could guarantee 100 per cent removal. Some quills may work

themselves out through the skin in due course. One dog died after penetration of the pericardium by quills.

PORKER. In Britain, porkers weigh 100–190 lb (liveweight). 'Heavy Hog' weight is 260 lb.

PORPHYRIA (*see* BONE, DISEASES OF, *and* HEXA-CHLORO-BENZINE, *also under* ALUMINIUM TOXICITY with reference to the rat).

PORTAL VEIN carries to the liver the blood that has been circulating in many of the abdominal organs. It is unique among the large veins of the body in that on entering the liver it breaks up into a capillary network, instead of passing its blood into one of the larger veins to be carried back to the heart. It is formed by the confluence of the anterior and posterior mesenteric with the splenic vein in the horse, and by the union of the gastric and mesenteric radicles in the ox, and, from a point behind the pancreas and below the vena cava, it runs forwards, downwards, and a little to the right, to reach the *porta* of the liver. Here it divides and subdivides in the manner usual with an artery. (*See* LIVER for further course, and DIGESTION.)

The blood that is carried to the liver by the portal vein is that which has been circulating in the stomach, nearly the whole of the intestines, the pancreas, and the spleen.

POSOLOGICAL. Relating to dosage.

POSTHITIS (*see* PENIS AND PREPUCE).

POST-MORTEM EXAMINATION (*see under* AUTOPSY).

POST-PARTUM. Following parturition.

POST-PARTURIENT FEVER of sows occurs, as a rule, 2 or 3 days after a normal farrowing. The animal goes off her food, is slightly feverish, and apt to resent suckling by her piglets. The udder is hard; the hardness beginning at the rear and extending forward. A watery or white discharge from the vagina is not invariably present. The uterus may not be involved at all. Treatment by antibiotics and pituitrin is successful if begun early. (*See also* UTERUS, DISEASES OF.)

POST-PARTURIENT HAEMOGLOBINURIA. This disease is seen in high-yielding dairy cows in North America, two to four weeks after calving. A deficiency of phosphorus in the diet and/or consumption of rations containing cruciferous plants or beet products are among the causes. Mortality may reach 50 per cent. In New Zealand it is associated with copper deficiency, and mortality is low.

SIGNS. These are sudden in onset and include red-coloured urine, loss of appetite, and weakness. Faeces are firm. Breathing may be laboured. Death may occur within a few days.

TREATMENT. Blood transfusion, a suitable phosphate preparation intravenously, or bonemeal by mouth. (*See also under* KALE.)

POTASH, or POTASSA, is the popular name for carbonate of potassium.

Potash fertilisers are best not applied to pasture land in the spring shortly before grazing, owing to the increased risk of HYPOMAGNESAEMIA (which see).

POTASSIUM is a metal which, on account of its great affinity for other substances, is not found in a pure state in nature.

Potassium is a mineral element essential for the body. It helps to control the osmotic pressure of the fluid within cells. Its content in body fluids is controlled by the kidneys. (*See also under* AL-DOSTERONE, *and* PURGATION.)

Potassium salts are used in human and animal medicine, but as their action depends in general not upon the metallic radicle, but upon the particular acid with which each is combined, their uses vary greatly and are described elsewhere. Thus for the action and uses of potassium iodide *see* IODIDES.

All salts of potassium are supposed to have a depressing action on the nervous system and on the heart, but in ordinary doses this effect is so slight as to be of no practical importance. The corresponding sodium salts can be used if preferred. **For intravenous injections, however, potassium salts must not be used as they are liable to be rapidly fatal; sodium salts must be used instead.**

Potassium chloride, given intravenously, has caused both accidental deaths (when mistakenly used instead of sodium chloride), and has been used in malicious poisoning of a horse in the USA.

Potassium deficiency. This was diagnosed in six cats at the College of Veterinary Medicine, Colorado. They all showed an acute onset of weakness, loss of weight, a reluctance to walk, a stiff stilted gait. Their necks were bent downwards, and palpation was painful.
TREATMENT: Lactated Ringer's solution supplemented with potassium chloride by intravenous or subcutaneous injection; with further K supplementation by palatable elixirs. All recovered. (Dow, S. W. *JAVMA* (1987) **191** 1563.)

POTATO POISONING. The haulms are most dangerous just after flowering. Both the haulms and the tops contain varying quantities of *solanine*, an alkaloid, which is present to a dangerous extent in green and sprouting potatoes. When boiled, the alkaloid is dissolved out in the water, and does no harm.

There is some evidence that alkaloids of the solanine type – present in green and sprouting potatoes – can cause deformities in litters of piglets born to sows fed on such potatoes.

Rotting or mouldy potatoes have also caused poisoning.
SIGNS. Pigs have shown loss of appetite, dullness, exhaustion, watery diarrhoea, low temperature, and coma.

Cases on the continent of Europe have exhibited peculiar skin lesions. They occurred after the green haulms had been eaten by cattle, and consisted of eczematous ulcerated areas occurring on the scrotum of the male and the udder of the female. In addition, there were ulcers in the mouths of some animals, and blisters about the hind-limbs which suggested foot-and-mouth disease, except that considerable quantities of pus were produced.

The most constant symptoms appear to be loss of appetite, prostration or interference with movement, a weak pulse, a low or sub-normal temperature.

In North America, **sweet potato** (*Ipomea batatas*) poisoning may cause acute respiratory distress in cattle fed mouldy tubers; the fungus (*Fusarium solani*) causing toxin production by the potato itself.

POTENTIATE. To increase the effectiveness of two drugs by administering them together.

POTOMAC HORSE FEVER. This occurs in the USA, and has a seasonal incidence (May to October.)
CAUSE: *Ehrlichia sennetsu* or *E. risticii*.
SIGNS: In addition to fever there may be acute diarrhoea, sometimes abortion, leukopenia.

The vectors are mainly black flies of *Simulium* species.

The infection has been detected in farm cats.

POULTICES AND FOMENTATIONS are useful in all stages of inflammation to soothe the pain and promote resolution, or in the late stages, when pus is forming, to hasten the formation of an abscess.

Poultices include a mixture of kaolin and glycerin, made into a paste, incorporated with an antiseptic, and applied hot upon a piece of gauze or cotton-wool to the part. A proprietary preparation of this nature is on the market, made up in conveniently sized tins, containing directions for its use, which can be considered fully reliable and satisfactory for use by an owner instead of a poultice. It goes by the name of 'Antiphlogistine'.

Hot fomentations are usually made by cooling boiling water down to a temperature that can be easily borne by the bare elbow, wringing a piece of flannel or blanket out of the water, and applying it to the part.

POULTRY, DISEASES OF (*see under* ASPERGILLOSIS, AVIAN INFECTIOUS ENCEPHALOMYELITIS, AVIAN LISTERIOSIS, AVIAN PLAGUE, AVIAN TUBERCULOSIS, BUMBLE-FOOT, CAGE LAYER FATIGUE, COCCIDIOSIS, CRAZY CHICK DISEASE, *E. coli*, EGG-BOUND, FAVUS, FOWL CHOLERA, FOWL PARALYSIS, FOWL TYPHOID, GAPES, 'HAEMORRHAGIC DISEASE', MONILIASIS, NEWCASTLE DISEASE (Fowl Pest), OMPHALITIS, PULLET DISEASE, PULLORUM DISEASE, SALMONELLOSIS, SLIPPED TENDON, SYNOVITIS, 'TOXIC FAT DISEASE', GUMBORO, BRONCHITIS, NEPHROSIS, LIVER/KIDNEY SYNDROME, MAREK'S DISEASE).

POULTRY AND POULTRY KEEPING. These have, so far as large-scale production is concerned, undergone great changes in recent decades. Many of the older breeds and strains of poultry have given way to more efficient hybrids.

Increasingly there has been a move towards intensive production of layers or broilers in controlled-environment houses. Formulation of poultry foods for optimum production has advanced, too, and well-balanced proprietary compounds are extensively used.

Hybrids. The following have done well in Britain: Double-A1, Babcock 300, CH20, Honegger, Shaver 288, Sykes 3, SW20, Thornber 606, Sterling White Link.

Large-scale production. Information will be found under CONTROLLED ENVIRONMENT, HOUSING OF ANIMALS, BROILERS, INTENSIVE LIVESTOCK PRODUCTION, BATTERY SYSTEM, NIGHT LIGHTING, CANNIBALISM, DEEP LITTER, EGG YIELD, etc.

Hen yards are nowadays preferred to large pens for birds kept intensively, and are often adapted from old bullock yards. Protection from cold winds and rain is necessary. The high cost of straw is sometimes a disadvantage; gravel, shingle or sand from a beach, or clinker, may be used. The system is labour-saving and does not involve great capital expenditure.

Housing. Competitive broiler and egg production has now led to highly expensive (though economic) and elaborate buildings. The main features are described under CONTROLLED ENVIRONMENT HOUSING and HOUSING OF LIVESTOCK.

What follows relates to non-intensive housing where high capital expenditure is not possible or desirable.

Height. A very high house is apt to be cold and draughty, while a very low one is difficult to ventilate and troublesome to clean. From 6 ft 6 in to 7 ft at the highest point to 4 ft 6 in or 5 ft at the lowest should be allowed.

Ventilation. There must be good top ventilation. The amount to be given depends a good deal upon the situation and exposure. Houses of the open-fronted type may prove to be too draughty for exposed wind-swept districts. For such places a pitched roof is rather to be preferred to a lean-to. Dampness in a house may be due to faulty ventilation.

Light. The maximum amount of light and sunshine should be aimed at. Fowls will not shelter during the day in a dark house. Additional windows should be placed a few inches above the level of the floor, if possible at the east and west sides. This means that the floor will always be light, and the birds will always be encouraged to scratch for grain buried in the litter. (*See also* NIGHTLIGHTING.)

Litter. The floor should be covered to a depth of a foot or more with clean dry litter, such as straw. (*See* DEEP LITTER.)

Perches. These should measure 2 in by 2 in and have the edges on the upper surface smoothed off. They should be all on one level about 2 ft 6 in from the floor, and made to drop into sockets. About 6 or 8 in below the perches should be placed a removable dropping board. This keeps the floor clean and prevents upwards draughts. They must be cleaned regularly, and lightly sprinkled with sand or peat moss litter.

Nests are best placed on the same sides as the windows, so that the light does not shine directly into them.

Houses should be regularly cleaned and sprayed with disinfectant from time to time.

Runs. Fresh clean ground is very necessary. If birds remain too long in one place the ground becomes foul, and the egg-yield and the birds' health soon suffer. Where space permits (as on farms) the birds may be kept on free range in portable houses. When the ground round the house becomes dirty the house may be removed to another place. In this way the fowls always have clean land.

Hatching and rearing. The time to begin hatching depends on the breed, the strain, and the poultry-keeper's requirements. Quick maturing breeds, such as Leghorn, Ancona, and good laying strains of White Wyandottes, Rhode Island Reds, and Light Sussex, will, if properly fed and managed, lay at 5 or 5½ months, so that if pullets are wanted to lay in October, chickens should be hatched in March or April. It is generally considered that birds hatched early in the year have more natural vitality and mature more rapidly than those hatched later. Against this must be the fact that in very cold weather and in exposed districts the percentage of fertility may be low in the first two months of the year, and there may be heavy mortality in the rearing of the chickens unless adequate protection can be given. June or even July chicks may be brought on to lay if they are well fed. As soon as the days begin to get short, these late-hatched chicks should be fed by lamplight, otherwise they are not getting sufficient food to make their full growth. Where only a few chickens are to be raised, or where very special eggs are to be set, the hen is to be preferred to the incubator. It is sometimes difficult to get broody hens early in the season, and in such cases

Silkies make excellent sitters and mothers. They are small eaters, their eggs are of fair size, they lay a small batch, and then go broody almost irrespective of the season. A silkie hen can cover from 6 to 8 ordinary eggs.

Brooders. Bottled gas is much used nowadays for heating brooders, and has advantages over paraffin burners. Infra-red heating, especially the dull-emitter kind, is popular where reliable electricity supplies are available, and enables the chicks to be readily observed. (*See also* HAY-BOX BROODERS which enable the chicks to be kept for a shorter time in the rearing house.)

Rearing houses. These should be well ventilated but free from floor draughts, well lit by windows, and spacious enough. Allow half a square foot per chick up to a month old.

DRINKING WATER (*see under* CHICKS) must be constantly available.

TROUGH SPACE. Six lineal feet of trough space per 100 chicks should be provided until the birds are 3 weeks old; 10 feet per 100 chicks at from 3 to 6 weeks old; 12 feet at from 6 to 12 weeks old; 16 feet at from 12 to 16 weeks old, and 20 feet thereafter.

Bought-in stock. If buyers insist on 'Accredited'

stock, they can be almost certain of avoiding trouble from Pullorum disease (Bacillary White Diarrhoea) and from Fowl Typhoid.

When chicks are bought as day-olds, mortality should not exceed 3 per cent by the third week. Losses exceeding 5 per cent indicate the need for an investigation; and several dead chicks should be sent to a laboratory for a *post-mortem* examination.

Chick feeding. There is no longer support for the old idea that chicks must not be fed for the first 48 hours. It is better to feed day-olds on arrival (otherwise they pick at their bedding) and to allow them ample cold water. Feeding appliances must be of a good design and not placed in a dark spot where chicks may fail to find them.

Proprietary crumbs, or mash or meal, may be fed. Limestone grit and oyster shell should *not* be given with these. (*See under* GRIT.) Day-olds do not need this unless they are to be fed on grain or to be put on grass when very young. Grain should not be fed *ad lib.*, but rather as a twice-daily scratch feed, until chicks are about a month old.

The following materials have been used in poultry feeding:

Sussex ground oats.
Barley meal.
Maize meal, maize germ meal.
Wheat and millers' offals.
Rice bran.
Linseed cake meal.
Coconut cake meal.
Palm Kernel cake meal.
Sunflower cake meal.
White fish meal, Herring meal.
Meat meal.
Dried skimmed milk.
Dried buttermilk.
Dried whey.
Dried grass or lucerne meals.
Dried yeast.
Molasses.
Synthetic vitamins A, B_1, B_2, D_3, and E.
Concentrates of carotene.
Anti-oxidants.

Wet whey. The addition of this at 5 per cent was found to reduce the numbers of *Salmonella typhimurium* in the caecum of chicks. (De Loach, J. & others. *Avian Diseases* (1990) **34**, 389.)

Dirt, dampness, and overcrowding are the chickens' worst enemies. Coops and brooders should be moved constantly, so that the chickens have fresh clean ground to run on. After the birds have been removed from the rearing ground, the land should be dressed with burnt lime at the rate of 40 cwt to the acre. The cockerels should be separated from the pullets as soon as it is possible to differentiate them. The pullets need plenty of space both in their houses and in their runs. It is best to get them into their winter quarters by August or September and not move them again, as changes of all kinds are apt to check laying. As a preventative of soft-shelled eggs, 2 per cent steamed bone-flour or bone-meal may be added to the mash. Pullets should begin to lay in October or November if hatched in good time. Trap-nesting should be adopted wherever it is possible,

as it is important to find out the winter records of the pullets. A good winter record (for 4 months) is from 30 to 40 eggs, but birds of good strain, properly managed and fed, will produce up to 70 or 80 eggs. A good flock average for the year is 180, but there are, of course, instances of birds producing up to 300 eggs in their first year.

Feeding. Where fowls have access to good grass runs, and especially where these contain a fair proportion of clover, they can themselves correct any faults in a badly balanced ration, but birds on earth runs, or kept purely on the intensive system, are entirely at the mercy of the poultry-keepers, and their diet must be carefully considered. An excess or deficiency of any one substance in the ration may cause derangement of the digestive system of the bird, and so may affect egg-production. Birds, especially those kept in confinement, often suffer from a deficiency of some sort. **Modern carefully formulated proprietary foods have been developed to obviate all known deficiencies in housed birds.**

The amount which a fowl will eat must depend on the breed, the condition of the bird, whether she is laying or not, and the conditions under which she is kept. The bird's appetite is the best guide, but a rough rule is to allow about 2 oz of grain and 2 to 2½ oz of mash per bird per day. For a grain food a mixture of two parts oats and one part cracked maize may be recommended. The grain should be lightly buried in the litter, so that the birds have to work for it. The mash may be fed either wet once a day, or dry in hoppers, so that the fowls can help themselves. (*See under* RATIONS.)

POULTRY KEEPERS. The occupational hazards of people looking after poultry include: allergy to the Northern Chicken Mite (*see* MITES); conjunctivitis and/or an influenza-like illness from NEWCASTLE DISEASE virus. *See also* VENT GLEET, TUBERCULOSIS (avian), and SALMONELLOSIS.

POULTRY SLAUGHTER ORDER. An order under Section 29 of the Animal Health Act 1981 came into force in 1989, providing for the compulsory slaughter of poultry flocks where salmonella had been confirmed.

POULTRY WASTE, DRIED. This has been fed to beef cattle as part of their diet, especially in the USA. The product is very variable in its content – droppings being the main ingredient; but litter, feathers, broken eggs may also be present. From a veterinary point of view there may be dangers – high levels of copper or arsenic, for example, used in broiler diets; also high calcium carbonate levels. Crude protein content may vary from 15 to 35 per cent, crude fibre 12 to 35 per cent.

Feeding beef cattle with large quantities of this waste product has, in Israel, caused sudden deaths from heart failure. It was found that the broilers had been receiving a coccidiostat: either maduramycin or salinomycin. 'Some ionophores are well recognised as having a cardiotoxic potential.' (Pert, S. & others. *Veterinary Record* (1991) **129**, 35.)

Ensiled poultry litter, fed to cattle, proved to be a source of *Clostridium botulinum*, and caused botulism.

Producers intentionally or inadvertently feeding poultry carcase material to livestock on their premises commit an offence under the *Disease of Animals (Waste Food) Order* 1973.

The World Health Organisation (WHO) has pointed out that the feeding of poultry manure introduces the risk that people may acquire zoonoses, such as salmonellosis from cattle products; and that there is a danger of drugs and other chemicals fed to poultry accumulating as residues in cattle.

POX. The best known pox diseases, caused by Orthopox viruses, are Cow-pox and Smallpox (*Variola*). The latter disease was eradicated on a world-wide basis, WHO announced, in 1980. However, the other pox diseases are transmissible to human beings.

Some of the pox diseases are mild, whereas in others there may be a high fever, and even a high mortality.

These pox diseases are all contagious, and characterised by skin lesions. Typically these begin with small red spots followed by papules. Exudate causes these to become vesicles, and pus forms, so that the vesicles become pustules. These either burst or become dessicated, and the larger one may leave a pock mark which can be a deep lesion with permanent scarring.

Mucous membrane may be affected as well as skin. (In horses lesions may occur in the mouth; and in canaries lesions may be found only in the trachea.)

Public health. Human cases of cowpox are reported only rarely, and may be severe. However, mild or sub-clinical infections may occur, and the possibility of person-to-person infection has been suggested.

Cowpox (*Vaccinia***)** is now a rare disease in the UK. In the days of hand milking it was spread from cow to cow by that means (and also sometimes by milkers recently vaccinated against smallpox). Lesions appear on the teats and skin of the udder mainly, but the lips and perineal region may be affected too. Cow-pox is usually a mild disease, with slight fever, reduced appetite and milk yield. Cow-pox is transmissible to people, horses, dogs, sheep and goats. It was diagnosed in cats for the first time in the UK in 1978, but see CAT-POX below, as a different virus may be involved.

Pseudo-cowpox (Parapox) is a common disease of cattle, and affects man also. The papules tend to be larger than with COW-POX. A mild disease.

Cat-pox. This name has come to be preferred to 'Cowpox in cats', since evidence for the cow's involvement is questionable, and there is a greater likelihood that the infection comes from some small wild animal.

The pock may appear at the site of a bite, and several cases have occurred in cats known to be keen hunters. The siting of pocks on the lips or at the base of the claws further supports the idea that the infection comes from cats' prey.

Previously it was thought that catpox was not transmissible from cat to cat; but recent evidence from the Netherlands indicates that it can be, and that cat-to-human infection may also occur.

Catpox appears to be patchy in its geographical distribution, and not common.

Lesions in the cat vary from no more than a scabby condition along the back, in mild cases, to small red glistening areas of skin covered by scabs. White pus may be present. The paws become ulcerated in some cases; also lips and eyelids.

Buffalo-pox is a mild disease but one of economic importance. Similar to cow-pox, it is caused by an orthopox virus distinct from vaccinia virus. (The latter can also cause pox in buffaloes.)

Camel-pox is usually a mild disease, except in young camels in which a generalised form may prove fatal. Facial oedema and lip lesions occur in adult camels.

Sheep-pox. This is the most serious of the poxes affecting farm or domestic animals. Infection can occur through inhalation, direct contact, and probably the bites of insects or other parasites.

Symptoms include high fever, perhaps dyspnoea, salivation as a result of mouth lesions, a discharge from eyes and nose. Skin lesions follow in a day or two, and may cause intense irritation or pain, leading to self-mutilation. Areas of skin may slough off leaving deep ulcers. In peracute cases the mortality may be as high as 80 per cent; in mild cases a figure of 5 per cent is to be expected. White nodules may be found in many organs at autopsy.

In the UK sheep-pox is a NOTIFIABLE disease, and compulsory slaughter is the policy in the event of its introduction.

Goat-pox. In the tropics goats may suffer from Stone Pox or Goat Dermatitis; the symptoms of which are similar to those of sheep-pox; mortality varying from less than 10 per cent to over 50 per cent.

Ordinary goat-pox, which occurs in most parts of the world, is relatively mild, and if death occurs it is usually the result of a secondary bacterial pneumonia.

Horse-pox is usually a mild disease. Lesions may appear on the back of the pastern, hollow of the heels, and be confused with grease; or may involve the lips, mouth, nostrils, vulva. A painful stomatitis, with loss of appetite and salivation, may occur. Recovery may take two to four weeks. However in a few cases lesions may affect much of the body, the horse becomes debilitated, and young ones may die.

Swine-pox is usually mild. Lice may possibly spread the infection. (Cow-pox may also appear in pigs.)

Monkey-pox (*see under* MONKEYS.)

Pox in birds (*see* FOWL POX, PIGEON POX.)

PPR. 'Peste des petits ruminants' (small ruminants' plague) is a disease of goats and sheep, but not cattle, resembling Cattle Plague and occurring in West Africa.

PRECARDIAL or PRECORDIAL REGION is the region of the chest cavity that lies in front of the heart.

PRECIPITINS. Precipitating antibodies; *e.g.* to *Micropolyspora faeni* in 'farmer's lung'.

PREDNISOLONE. A corticosteroid which raises blood-sugar levels and has been used in the treatment of agalactia in sows. It can cause immunosuppression and exacerbate the effects of worm infestations (*e.g. Filaroides hirthi*, feline heartworms), and viral diseases such as CATPOX. (*See* CORTICOSTEROIDS, for reference to the treatment of Rheumatoid arthritis and other diseases.)

PREGNANCY and GESTATION. The uterus, the ovaries, and the whole of the tissues of the mother are influenced directly or indirectly during pregnancy, but the gross changes exhibited, with certain exceptions, subside quickly after the birth of the young. The minor alterations which persist throughout life, such as increased size of the mammary glands, enlargement of the uterus, and of the whole of the genital canal, are not generally obvious except after repeated breeding, and in from 4 to 6 weeks the dam has returned to normal to all intents and purposes, always excepting the flow of milk in the mammary glands. In most uniparous animals – producing one young at a time – the horn of the uterus which becomes pregnant greatly enlarges and becomes straightened out so as to be practically continuous with the body of the uterus, and the non-pregnant horn appears as a small appendage projecting from its side; in the multiparous animals, however, both horns usually carry a share of the number of the young, and both are consequently nearly alike in size. The pregnant horn (or horns) develop an intricate and very complete vascular system. The uterine arteries increase to a great size, and together they form a very perfect plexus in and around the wall of the uterus, thereby ensuring an even and regulated blood-flow for the needs of the young. As the organ gradually increases in size to accommodate its contents, the broad ligament, which supports it from the roof of the abdomen, increases in length and strength to allow the uterus to move farther and farther forward and downward in each animal, so that eventually it may occupy the greater part of the abdominal cavity. At the same time there is a very great increase in the muscular coat of the uterus. Not only do the individual muscle fibres greatly hypertrophy, but it appears that there is an increase in their numbers as well. The walls of the organ become firmer, stronger, and thicker, and better able to accommodate the extra weight of the young. The lining mucous membrane also shows well-marked changes. In those animals which have a diffuse placenta, *e.g.* mare and sow, the mucous membrane over the inside of the uterus is thickened, very vascular, and in it are found the crypts which receive the villi of the chorion (outermost fetal membrane). In the ruminants the characteristic cotyledons enlarge and multiply. These are mushroom-like elevations projecting into the lumen of the uterus, with crypts scattered over their convex crowns (cow), or over their concave crowns (ewe and goat). In the dog and cat, the zones where intimate connection between dam and fetal membrane occurs show a corresponding hypertrophy and increased vascularity.

Duration of pregnancy. This varies greatly in different species and to some extent in different individuals. Male feti are carried longer than females. Debility, weakness, or illness in the dam shortens the duration of pregnancy. (*See* TABLE *below*.)

A PROLONGED GESTATION PERIOD IN EWES in western Scotland was reported (Barlow, R. M. & others *Vet. Record* (1985) **117,** 124). Gestation periods extend up to eight months and, unless relieved of their fetuses surgically, the ewes usually die. Long hairy coats, skeletal deformities, and extensive liquefaction of the central nervous system are characteristic of the fetuses. The cause is unknown, but could be a toxic plant.

A similar syndrome occurs in south-west Africa, associated with feeding on the shrub *Salsola tuberculata* var *tomentosa*; and in the USA prolonged pregnancy in ewes has been linked to the plant *Veratum californicum*.

PERIODS OF GESTATION

Animal	Average period		Shortest period Young born alive	Longest period Young born alive
	Months (Calendar)	Days		
Mare	11	419	340	307
Ass	12¼	374	365	385
Cow	9	283 or 284	200	439
Ewe and Goat (Merinos)	5	144 to 150 (150)	135	160
Sow	—	114	110	130
Bitch	—	58–63	55	76
Cat	—	55–63	—	—
Elephant	2 years (nearly)		—	—
Zebra	13 months or over		—	—
Camel	45 weeks		—	—
Rabbit	32 days		—	—
Guinea-pig	63 days		—	—

PERIODS OF DEVELOPMENT DURING PREGNANCY

State of pregnancy		Mare	Cow	Ewe and goat	Sow	Bitch
I	Duration of period	14 days	14 days	14 days	14 days	10 days
	Length of fetus	Ovum $\frac{1}{12}$ in	Ovum $\frac{1}{12}$ in	Ovum $\frac{1}{15}$ in to $\frac{1}{20}$ in	Ovum $\frac{1}{15}$ in to $\frac{1}{20}$ in	Ovum $\frac{1}{15}$ in to $\frac{1}{20}$ in
	Stages in development	Fertilised ovum has reached uterus from oviduct				
II	Duration	3 to 4 weeks	3 to 4 weeks	3 to 4 weeks	3 to 4 weeks	10 days to 3 weeks
	Length of fetus	$\frac{1}{2}$ in	$\frac{1}{3}$ in	$\frac{1}{8}$ in	$\frac{1}{2}$ in	$\frac{1}{8}$ in
	Stages	Traces of fetus appear; head, body and limbs are discernible by end of this period				
III	Duration	5 to 8 weeks	5 to 8 weeks	5 to 7 weeks	4 to 6 weeks	3 to 4 weeks
	Length of fetus	$2\frac{1}{8}$ in	$1\frac{3}{4}$ in	$1\frac{1}{4}$ in	$1\frac{3}{4}$ in	1 in
	Stages	First indications of hoofs and claws visible as little pale elevations at ends of digits				
IV	Duration	9 to 13 weeks	9 to 12 weeks	7 to 9 weeks	6 to 8 weeks	5th week
	Length of fetus	6 in	$5\frac{1}{2}$ in	$3\frac{1}{2}$ in	3 in	$2\frac{1}{2}$ in
	Stages	Stomach well defined in foal, pig, and puppy; differentiation of four stomachs in ruminants at end of this period				
V	Duration	14 to 22 weeks	13 to 20 weeks	10 to 13 weeks	8 to 10 weeks	6th week
	Length of fetus	13 in	12 in	6 in	5 in	$3\frac{1}{2}$ in
	Stages	Large tactile hairs appear on lips, upper eye-lids, and above eye. Teats visible in female fetuses				
VI limbs	Duration	23 to 24 weeks	21 to 32 weeks	13 to 18 weeks	11 to 15 weeks	7 to 8 weeks
	Length of fetus	2 ft 3 in	2 ft	1 ft 2 in	7 in	5 in
	Stages	Eye-lashes well developed. A few hairs appear on tail, head and extremities of				
VII	Duration	35 to 48 weeks	33 to 40 weeks	19 to 21 weeks	15 to 17 weeks	9th week (8th in cat)
	Length	$3\frac{1}{2}$ ft	3 ft	$1\frac{1}{2}$ ft	9 to 10 in	6 to 8 in (kitten 5 in)
	Stages	Fetus attains full size. Body becomes gradually covered with hair, hoofs and claws complete, but soft				

Signs of pregnancy. When well advanced the typical signs of pregnancy are well enough known to the majority of livestock owners, and require no mention here, but in the earlier stages they are not always so clear, and for the first few weeks in the larger animal it is often difficult to diagnose pregnancy by clinical signs.

The chief changes and differences to be looked for are as follows:

Cessation of oestrus. In the majority of cases, but not in all animals, the female exhibits no desire for the male after conception occurs. There are many instances, however, when service is allowed until late on in pregnancy, and there may be all the usual signs of oestrus evident on each occasion. In such cases abortion of the fetus may occur, or no harm may result. When the *bull* refuses to serve a cow which is apparently in season it may be taken as a strong sign that she is pregnant.

Alteration in temperament. Vicious, troublesome, or easily excited mares generally become very much more tractable and quiet after conception, whereas if they are served and do not conceive they are frequently more intractable than previously. The same signs are sometimes seen in the cow.

Fattening tendency. In the sheep and the cow particularly, condition markedly improves during the first few weeks of pregnancy, but during the latter stages when the abdomen has increased in size the opposite effect is seen in all animals.

Easily induced fatigue. In the later stages, pregnant animals almost always show an increased desire to rest as much as possible.

Enlargement of the abdomen, which occurs in every direction, is a most important sign of pregnancy; it occurs at about the same rate as the rate of development of the young, which is greatest towards the end of the period. It descends or 'drops', the flanks become hollow, the spine appears more prominent, and its line tends to become flat or even concave in the thoracic and lumbar region, the muscles of the quarters appear to fall in, making the haunches and the root of the tail appear more prominent, and the pelvis tilts into a more vertical position.

Enlargement of the mammary glands commences very soon in pregnancy in those animals which are bearing young for the first time. The glands become larger, and firmer, and more prominent. *Increase in weight* is, of course, *a sine qua non* of normal pregnancy in a healthy well nourished animal. (*See* PREGNANCY DIAGNOSIS).

Care of the dam during pregnancy. In all species of animals exercise (or work) is essential if the vigour of the dam is to be retained, and if her circulatory, digestive, muscular, and nervous systems are to be maintained in a fit state for the strains they will have to withstand at parturition. Food is of great importance. No sudden changes in the ration should be made. It is better to give an extra feed each day rather then unduly to increase the quantities given at each feed. This avoids excessive distension of stomach and intestines which may lead to nausea and indigestion.

The mare should be treated as usual until the time that her abdomen begins to increase in size. During the last month an extra feed per day should be given, and if clover, or better lucerne, hay is available it should be given in preference to other kinds of hay. Lucerne, being rich in lime and magnesium salts, provides a plentiful supply of these for the mare's milk, as well as for the developing foal. During this last month it is well to allow the mare to sleep in the foaling-box, so that she may become accustomed to it, and settle better. The box should have previously been thoroughly cleaned out, its walls scrubbed with boiling water containing a suitable disinfectant, especially where joint-ill exists upon a farm. Where the climate is mild, mares may, with great advantage, be allowed to foal out of doors. The foal is often born during the night.

Food given should be gently laxative; for this purpose the addition of pulped roots, carrots, bran, or treacle to the food is good. (For further information see under PARTURITION.)

The cow is usually allowed to calve in a loose-box. (*See under* 'STEAMING-UP'.)

Ewes may either be kept out on the hill, or brought down to lower land, and housed in a lambing-pen during the last week or so of pregnancy, but otherwise little special attention is necessary. Chasing by dogs, crowding through gateways, and all other forms of rough treatment are to be avoided. Care is needed when catching. Heavy in-lamb ewes should not be turned up to have their feet dressed.

Sows greatly benefit from having access to an old pasture or paddock, where they will not be disturbed by other animals, and where they may take as much exercise as they desire. But at night they should have a clean, warm, dry bed to sleep on. Pregnant sows are best fed individually or in twos: otherwise some sows get more than their fair share, while others suffer from under-feeding. Wet, cold floors and cold, draughty premises predispose to mastitis and agalactia.

Bitches must be given regular exercise, and after the first month extra meals of protein-rich food, including a little liver once a week. An improvised whelping box is useful. (*See also* SUPERFETATION, BREEDING OF ANIMALS, PARTURITION, PREGNANCY DIAGNOSIS, etc.)

PREGNANCY COMPLICATIONS. In the mare these include twin foals (*see* ABORTION) and PREPUBIC TENDON RUPTURE. (*See also* ECTOPIC PREGNANCY, MUMMIFICATION OF FETUS, SUPERFETATION.)

PREGNANCY DIAGNOSIS TESTS. Among tests not involving use of laboratory animals is that for PROGESTERONE (which see). Pregnancy diagnosis in the cow, based on a radioimmunoassay technique for the detection of progesterone in a sample of milk, became a commercial proposition in 1974. The milk sample is taken 24 days after the last insemination.

In 1980 a new test, based on the measurement of oestrone sulphate in milk, was introduced after research at the AFRC's Institute of Animal Physiology, Babraham. The milk sample is taken 15 weeks or more after insemination. 'It is a convenient method of testing batches of cows to confirm that they are in-calf,' stated the Milk

Marketing Board, which was using both tests in 1981.

Real-time ultrasonic scanning. Diagnoses of pregnancy were made on 110 Hereford cross Friesian and 69 blue grey (white shorthorn cross Galloway) cows between 92 and 202 days after last service using a real-time ultrasonic scanning instrument with a 3·5 MHz rectal transducer. Of the 174 cows which subsequently calved, one was wrongly diagnosed as non-pregnant. Of the five cows which did not subsequently calve two were diagnosed as pregnant and may in fact have been pregnant at the time of scanning. The overall level of accuracy of pregnancy diagnosis was 98·3 per cent. In further trials with 16 Hereford cross Friesian and 16 blue grey cows scanned at regular intervals between 20 and 140 days of gestation, pregnancy was diagnosed with confidence from 30 days. (White, I. R. & others, *Veterinary Record* (1985) **117,** 5.)

In 1985 the MMB adopted an enzyme method of milk pregnancy testing, and supply kits for this purpose; the test taking about 45 minutes.

In Norway, a very accurate test for the early diagnosis of pregnancy in the sow has been evolved, based upon the quantity of oestrin in the urine. The test takes an hour and is expensive.

Ultrasonics are being used for pregnancy diagnosis in ewes – and also in sows. The method, adapted from the echosounder of marine application, has not the dangers for the fetus of X-rays and is claimed to be over 90 per cent accurate.

Vaginal biopsy is a technique now being applied to large pig herds on a commercial scale.

Pregnancy in the **bitch** cannot be diagnosed in the early stages. From 24 to 32 days is the best time for abdominal palpation; after 35 days pregnancy may be difficult to recognise by this means: though occasionally posterior fetuses can be felt at 45 to 55 days – when the fetal skeleton can be palpated. Auscultation of fetal hearts in the final week of pregnancy will differentiate pregnancy from pyometra and show that the fetuses are alive. Pregnancy has to be differentiated also from pseudo-pregnancy, ascites, adiposity, and diabetes mellitus.

Eighty-two bitches were examined for pregnancy using several different techniques. Abdominal palpation 26 to 35 days after mating was 82 per cent accurate in detecting bitches that would whelp and 73 per cent accurate in identifying those that would not do so. A-mode ultrasound was best used 32 to 62 days after mating and was 90 per cent and 83 per cent accurate in diagnosing pregnancy and non-pregnancy respectively. The better of the two Doppler ultrasound instruments that were used was 85 per cent and 100 per cent accurate in detecting pregnancy in the periods 36 to 42 days and 43 days to term respectively. It was completely accurate in detecting bitches which were not pregnant. (Allen, W. E. & Meredith, M. J., *Journal of Small Animal Practice* (1981) **22,** 609.)

Mares. Pregnancy can be diagnosed by means of the Enzygnost Serum Progesterone Test, which takes only 35 minutes. A test kit is available from Hoechst, and uses an improved enzyme immunoassay technique.

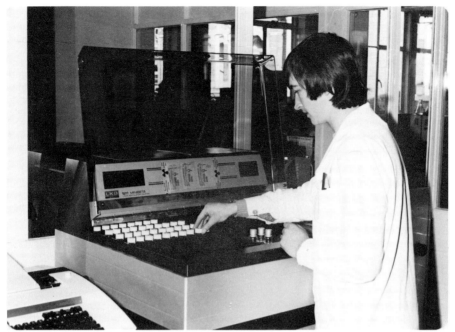

A pregnancy test for dairy cows, using the radioimmunoassay of oestrone sulphate (a hormone produced by the developing embryo), has been available to UK dairy farmers since October 1980. Milk samples are taken for testing at any time from 15 weeks of pregnancy onwards. One hundred per cent accuracy has been claimed for this test. (MMB photo.)

An ultrasonic scanner has been used for pregnancy diagnosis in mares. It has been possible to detect the presence of a developing fetus with great accuracy as early as 14 days after conception and this technique is particularly useful for the diagnosis of twin pregnancies.

PREGNANCY, ECTOPIC. The presence of a fetus (or more than one) inside the abdomen but outside the uterus. Many cases occur as the result of trauma; *e.g.* in a dog or cat struck by a car. The uterus is torn and the fetus becomes dislodged and undergoes mummification. The latter also occurs when a fertilised egg has 'gone the wrong way'; *i.e.* instead of taking the normal route down the Fallopian tube to the corresponding horn of the uterus, it develops outside the uterus.

PREGNANCY EXAMINATION of cattle is carried out by means of rectal palpation, but requires expert knowledge not only of anatomy but of physiology and pathology. It is not always a simple matter and an accurate diagnosis is not always achieved. The dangers of attempts by herdsmen and other untrained people to carry out such an examination include: rupture of the heart of the embryo calf; perforation of the rectum; and abortion due to malhandling of the ovaries. In the mare, rectal palpation is a common method of pregnancy diagnosis. (*See also* PREGNANCY – signs of, *and* PREGNANCY DIAGNOSIS.)

PREGNANCY, FALSE (*see* PSEUDOPREGNANCY *and* 'CLOUDBURST' (in goats)).

PREGNANCY, TERMINATION OF. With a

pregnant bitch or sow, for example, there are three possible outcomes: (1) she may have her litter; (2) she may abort; (3) resorption of the fetuses may take place. (*See* RESORPTION *and* MUMMIFICATION; PARTURITION, DRUG-INDUCED; *and* CLOPRESTONOL.)

If it is desired to terminate pregnancy in a bitch, a non-hormonal drug is available, namely DL 717-IT. This has minimal side-effects. (Oliva, O. and others, *Journal of Small Animal Practice* **28,** 223.)

PREGNANCY TOXAEMIA IN EWES. An acute metabolic disorder occurring during the last few weeks of pregnancy; or, perhaps it would be more correct to say, a number of disorders – one of which may be acetonaemia.

CAUSES. In the more typical outbreaks, ewes are generally in good bodily condition, are carrying twins or triplets *in utero*, or have a particularly large single lamb. They are on good rich grazing, seldom getting much exercise. Bad weather, *e.g.* a fall of snow, has often occurred previous to the outbreak. It has been claimed that the disease can be produced experimentally by a short period of starvation during advanced pregnancy, and that ewes which become fat during the first three months of pregnancy are especially susceptible.

SIGNS. The first symptoms are incoordination of movement, the animal lagging behind others when driven, stepping high, and often staggering and falling. In another hour or two the ewe lies down and can only be induced to rise with difficulty. She stands swaying and will fall or lies down again almost immediately. In general appearance she is dull, hangs her head, her eyes appear to be staring – owing to widely dilated pupils – and breathing is laboured or stertorous. Fluid may be copiously discharged from the nostrils. Acetonaemia may be present, giving rise to the characteristic odour from breath and urine. A comatose condition develops. Death occurs within 1 to 6 days.

PREVENTION. It has been recommended, that after the pre-tupping flush, ewes should be kept in store condition for the first 3 months of pregnancy.

TREATMENT. Ewes should be dosed at once with glycerine (2 tablespoonfuls) in water; or glucose (2 oz in ½ pint of warm water) or, preferably, glucose solution may be given intravenously. (See ACETONAEMIA.)

PREGNANT MARE'S SERUM (see PMSG under CONTROLLED BREEDING, and HORMONES).

PREMATURE BIRTH (see ABORTION and PARTURITION, and the table under PREGNANCY).

PREMEDICATION. Use of a drug or drugs before administration of a general anaesthetic. An analgesic will relieve pain in an animal awaiting surgery, and a tranquilliser will relieve anxiety and facilitate handling. Both effects may be obtained by the same drug. (See ANALGESICS, TRANQUILLISERS.)

PRE-MILKING (see under PREPARTUM MILKING).

PREMUNITION, is a term used in relation to the type of resistance shown by cattle, and possibly other animals against severe illness caused by trypanosomes. Animals which are premunised are *infected* with trypanosomes but are not *affected* by trypanosomiasis.

There are two types recognised: (a) Natural premunition, which occurs inside or in close proximity to a fly-belt, and (b) Artificial premunition, which results from the administration of a sub-sterilising dose of a trypanocidal drug. Unfortunately, it seems very probable that, at least in the majority of cases, natural premunition only gives protection against one local strain of trypanosomes, and cattle which are thus premunised against a local strain may succumb when exposed to infection with a different strain of the same species; if, for instance, they are moved out of one fly-belt to another. The occurrence of intercurrent diseases of other varieties may also lead to a breakdown in premunition. Similarly, artificial premunition can only be relied upon to protect against a single strain. (See also TSETSE-FLY.)

PRE-PARTUM MILKING. Milking a heifer or cow a few days before the birth of her calf. Where this is practised, the calf when born must be provided with colostrum from another cow.

PREPOTENCY. The ability of one parent, in greater degree than the other, to transmit a characteristic (e.g. high milk yield) to the offspring.

PREPUBIC TENDON, RUPTURE OF. A possible complication of pregnancy, especially in heavy mares. Diagnosis is difficult but the condition should be suspected whenever ventral oedema occurs suddenly in late gestation, and is associated with considerable pain (due to the trauma). The condition is usually fatal, and may be a cause of sudden death. (For a case report see P. G. G. Jackson, *Vet. Record* (1982) **111,** 38).

PREPUCE. Crystals on the hairs here in the calf are seen in some cases of UROLITHIASIS. (*See also* PENIS AND PREPUCE.)

PRESBYOPIA is the term used to indicate the changes that normally affect the eye in old age, quite apart from any disease. The most important of these changes is a diminution of the natural elasticity of the lens of the eye, resulting in an impaired power of focusing objects near at hand.

'PRESCRIPTION DIETS'. These are specially formulated by Drs Mark L. Morris and Don D. Lewis to aid in the treatment of various canine and feline disorders, and are available both in canned or dry form – to be prescribed by veterinary surgeons.

One of their 'Prescription Diets' is specially formulated for cats suffering from the feline urological syndrome (FUS).

PRESCRIPTION-ONLY MEDICINES. Under the terms of the MEDICINES ACT 1968 (which see), veterinary surgeons in the UK may supply Prescription-Only medicines (POM) only for animals or herds under their care; and not to the public at large.

PRESENTATION (see PARTURITION).

PRESSOR is the term applied to anything that increases the activity of a function, *e.g.*, a pressor nerve or pressor drug. Producing a rise in blood-pressure is its most common meaning.

PREVALENCE. This is defined as the number of cases of disease or infection existing at any given time in relation to the unit of population in which they occur. It is a static measure as compared with the dynamic measure INCIDENCE.

PREVENTIVE VETERINARY MEDICINE. This is the keynote of modern veterinary practice, and is of increasing importance in these days of intensive livestock husbandry and of very large units. (*See* HEALTH SCHEMES FOR FARM ANIMALS.)

PRIAPISM. Six cases of priapism in horses with subsequent protrusion, oedema and paresis of the penis after neuroleptanalgesia and anaesthesia were reported. Four of the six cases had received acepromazine with etorphine hydrochloride and two acepromazine with other anaesthetic agents. It is recommended that following the use of neuroleptic drugs a check should always be made to ensure that penile retraction is taking place as the effects of medication wear off. If it is not, treatment should be started without delay. (Pearson, H. and Weaver, B. M. Q. (1978), *Equine Veterinary Journal*, **10**, 85.) (*See also* PENIS.) (*See also under* PENIS, ABNORMALITIES.)

PRIMARY MOSAICISM is a sequel to fertilisation of an ovum by spermatozoa derived from the same zygote but having different chromosomes. (*See* ERYTHROCYTE MOSAICISM, GENETIC ENGINEERING.) Secondary mosaicism occurs in the FREEMARTIN.

PRIMATES. These include about 200 species, ranging in size from the tree-shrew, weighing about 100 g, to the gorilla, weighing up to 275 kg.
 Two sub-orders are recognised: New World monkeys; and Old World monkeys, apes, and man. (Sainsbury, A. W. & others. *Veterinary Record* (1989) **125**, 640.)

PRION. A self-replicating infectious protein. (For prion diseases, *see* SCRAPIE, BOVINE SPONGIFORM ENCEPHALOPATHY, TRANSMISSIBLE MINK ENCEPHALOPATHY.)

PRIVET POISONING is very rare, and occurs only when horses and cattle have free access to privet hedges, or break into gardens and shrubberies containing this common ornamental shrub. Privet – *Ligustrum vulgare* – contains a glucoside – *Ligustrin*, which causes loss of power in the hind legs, dilated pupils, slightly injected mucous membranes, and death in 36 to 48 hours.

PROBANG. A rod of flexible material designed to aid removal of foreign bodies from the oesophagus. (*See* CHOKING.)

PROBIOTICS. According to the original definition these are 'organisms and substances which contribute to intestinal microbial balance.'
 Successful probiotic micro-organisms do this through their ability to colonise the gut by adhesion to its wall, and by resistance to antimicrobial agents present in the environment.
 Dr Roy Fuller, of the AFRC, prefers to restrict the term to preparations containing live micro-organisms, such as yoghurt and some animal feed supplements.

PROCAINE HYDROCHLORIDE is used in solution as a local anaesthetic, and for epidural anaesthesia (which see). It is also known under the names of Novocain and Kerocain. A synthetic product, it is, generally speaking, as effective as cocaine (except for anaesthetising the cornea, for which cocaine is preferable) but far less toxic and safer to use, besides not coming under the Dangerous Drug Act regulations. It is often combined with adrenalin, in order to lessen haemorrhage during minor surgery.
 Given by intravenous injection, procaine hydrochloride has been used in cases of pruritus in dogs. Occasionally, relief from scratching lasts only a few hours, but in other cases it is reported that relief lasts several days, often until the cause has ceased to act.
TOXICITY. Excessive amounts of procaine

hydrochloride cause stimulation of the central nervous system. In the horse 5 mg per lb body-weight gave rise to nervousness (tossing of the head, twitching of the cars, stamping of the feet, snorting, or neighing), while muscular incoordination and convulsion follows larger doses. In the dog, 20 mg per lb caused salivation and vomiting, with muscular tremors and incoordination.
Procaine penicillin. The procaine salt of penicillin is often used, the concentration of penicillin in the blood remaining for a longer period, and the injection being less painful.
 However, procaine penicillin G can, under certain circumstances be toxic and even lethal to pigs. The toxicity can be potentiated by swine erysipelas. (E. Embrechts. *Veterinary Record* (1982) **111**, 314.)

PROCTITIS means inflammation or only irritation situated about the anus or rectum. It is a frequent symptom of the presence of parasitic worms in almost all animals.

PRODROMAL is a term applied to symptoms of a disease which are among the first seen but not necessarily characteristic.

'PRODUCTION DISEASE'. A name suggested to embrace all the syndromes hitherto classified as metabolic disease. ('They are all problems of high production ... and due primarily to imbalance between the rates of input and output of certain key metabolites. Such imbalances are common in modern farm husbandry because high production is frequently expected on diets which are not always suitable for the purpose.' Dr J. M. Payne.) (*See* METABOLIC PROFILES.)

PRODUCTIVITY is an unsatisfactory criterion of farm animal welfare, for animals that are lame or otherwise injured from their housing can give a profitable return. A better criterion is the ability of animals to express their full range of normal behaviour, and this can be established by studying farm livestock in a range of physically and socially varied environments. Key features which elicit important behaviour patterns can be identified by such studies and analogues of them can be incorporated into new housing systems which are more humane than most intensive livestock accommodation. These principles are illustrated by a description of the development of the Family Pen System for pigs. (Wood-Gush, D. G. M., *State Veterinary Journal* (1985) **39**, 26.)

PROESTRUS. The first phase of the oestrous cycle, when the ovary is producing hormones which bring about enlargement of uterus, oviducts, and vagina, and when the ovarian follicle containing the ovum is also increasing in size. (*See* OESTRUS.)

PROGENY TESTING. A method of assessing the value of, *e.g.* a bull as a sire, by examining the milk yield, etc., figures for an unselected sample of his daughters. Dam–daughter comparisons may show whether a high-yielding cow can transmit her capability to her progeny, but these comparisons are valid only under identical systems of feeding and management.

The standard Contemporary Comparison (CC) and Relative Breeding Value (RBV) began to be superseded in the UK in 1974 by the Improved Contemporary Comparison (ICC).

CC is defined as the weighted* mean difference between the daughter average yield and the contemporary average yield, and involves comparing the yields of daughters of *all* other bulls milking in the same herds at the same time.

RBV is calculated separately with respect to the herds in which the bull's daughters have been recorded, and also with respect to the breed average.

ICC is a modification of Cornell University's 'Direct comparison', and the reasons for its introduction have been explained by Sandy McClintock, the Milk Marketing Board's geneticist, as follows:

'To evaluate a bull in such a way that management effects are reduced, one must ask the question "how did the daughters of this bull compare with the daughters of other bulls managed in a similar way?" In other words, "were they better or worse (plus or minus)?" There are occasions when this question may give a misleading answer. For example, suppose we have a young bull which has just completed his progeny test who appears to be +50 gallons. A bull which completed his test at a different point in time and in a different area may also be +50 gallons but, because the contemporaries of the two bulls are unlikely to be of the same genetic standard, the two bulls may not be as "equal" as they appear. The new method relies on bulls which have been used in both areas and at both points of time in order to detect and take into account differences in the two groups of contemporaries.'

A second major change involves the definition of a contemporary. At present any heifers which complete lactations in a 12-month period in a particular herd are regarded as having had similar management. The ICC method will split each herd into three groups of contemporaries corresponding to spring, summer and autumn

*Weighting figures indicate reliability of the CC figures – the higher the weighting, the more reliable the CC. Weighting (W) is calculated as follows: W = (No. of daughters × no. of contemporaries) + (No. of daughters + no. of contemporaries).

calvers. The change should allow for the fact that these groups may be managed differently within a single milking herd.

'The effect of age at calving has been recognised for many years, and when culling decisions are being made on MMB-owned AI bulls, care has always been taken that the progeny tests have not been affected by calving age.' (There can be as much as 90 gallons difference between animals calving at 2 years and those calving at 3 years.) 'The intention is to correct all heifer records so as to eliminate the effect of age for use in ICC calculations.'

Conformation. It should be added that selection of proven bulls for the MMB depends not only on the production figures of the daughters, but also on an assessment of (as many as possible) daughters by an inspection panel consisting of pedigree and commercial breeders.

Qualities of commercial importance taken into account are size, temperament, ease of milking – plus appearance, dairy character, udder, legs, feet, etc. Gradings are Excellent, Very Good, Good Plus, Good, Fair and Poor.

Below is shown a summary for a particular bull which had 56 daughters inspected by a type assessment panel. It will be noted that all but two of his daughters were quiet, and over half of them were in the top three ratings. The score of 107 indicates that the fore udder was the best point when compared with the national average.

GENERAL CHARACTERISTICS		No.	%
Size	Large	21	38
	Medium	34	60
	Small	1	2
Temperament	Quiet	54	96
	Nervous	2	4
Ease of Milking	Satisfactory	55	98
	Hard	—	—
	Too Easy	1	2

LINEAR ASSESSMENT. While breed societies are continuing to use the 'scorecard' in an abbreviated form, many of them are doing so only to supplement the Linear Assessment method. This is widely used in the USA and Canada, and was officially adopted by the Milk Marketing Board of England and Wales in 1983.

'It does away with the idea of scoring against an ideal, makes no attempt to define good or bad, but simply describes where, between the

SCORECARD BREAKDOWN	Ex	VG	G+	G	F	P	Nat. Ave. Compar.
General Appearance	—	14	31	10	—	1	105
Dairy Character	1	24	26	4	—	1	102
Body Capacity	3	22	24	6	—	1	102
Mammary System	—	11	21	17	6	1	103
Fore Udder	—	14	22	13	6	1	107
Rear Udder	—	16	24	9	6	1	101
Legs and Feet	—	15	26	13	1	1	103
Rump	—	14	30	11	—	1	102
Final Rating	—	12	27	15	1	1	Nat. Ave. for each Character is 100

biological extremes for agreed traits, an individual animal comes.'

'The linear system identifies the point between the extremes at which an animal is felt to come by describing it numerically in the range 1 to 9.'

'Since the total number of single biological traits is very large, the most important ones have to be selected', to keep the total a manageable one.

A common set of 16 traits was agreed following discussions with the British Friesian Cattle Society and the Associated A I Centres. The traits are: Stature, chest width, body depth, angularity, rump angle, rump width, rear legs (side view), rear legs (rear view), foot angle, fore udder attachment, rear udder attachment, udder support, udder depth, teat placement (rear view), teat placement (side view), teat length.

Other traits which need recording, such as weak pasterns, teats not plumb, or high pelvis can be dealt with by means of a list of miscellaneous characteristics; and the Board's livestock staff will continue to collect information on beef shape, temperament and ease of calving.

'It would seem logical to use the same system to describe the progeny group. This can be done both diagrammatically and numerically.'

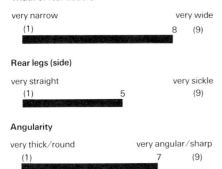

Width of rear udders

Rear legs (side)

Angularity

The progeny group illustrated in the diagram would have very high rear udders, legs about midway between very straight and very sickle, and would be rather sharper, cleaner cut animals than average, though not excessively so.' (MMB)

PROGESTERONE. A sex hormone from the *corpus luteum* and (in the pregnant animal) the placenta. It inhibits Follicle Stimulating Hormone (FSH) and action of oxytocin. (*See under* ENDOCRINE GLANDS.)

PROGESTIN. A proprietary brand of progesterone.

PROGESTOGENS. These drugs are used in 'CONTROLLED BREEDING' (which see) and have a progesterone-like action. A progestogen is administered over a period of time so that the established oestrous cycle is arrested at the point at which all *corpora lutea* have regressed. The removal of the progestogen then allows the continuance of reproductive activity. Examples of progestogens are:

Name	Synonymous
Megestrol Acetate	Ovarid
Medroxyproges- terone Acetate	MAP, Methyl acetoxy progesterone Veramix, Repromix, Provera
Flurogestone Acetate	FGA, Cronolone, SC9880 synchronate, Synchro- mate
Norgestomet	SC21009
Alphasone	DHPA

Their use can sometimes lead to diabetes in dogs and cats.

PROGLOTTIS. A segment, of an adult tapeworm, capable of reproduction.

PROGRESSIVE RETINAL ATROPHY. In the UK there is a joint scheme operated by the British Veterinary Association and the Kennel Club to reduce the incidence of this disease in any breed of dog; and certificates are issued to dog-owners. (*See* EYE, DISEASES OF.) The disease also occurs in some breeds of cats.

PROJECTILE SYRINGE. Fired from a crossbow, gun or blowpipe, this instrument is useful for immobilising and/or anaesthetising wild animals. The use of dart guns is, in the UK, restricted under section 5 of the Firearms Act 1968.

'Blowpipes and dart guns are short range – up to 40 yards only. They use a compressed air discharge system. They facilitate the treatment of dangerous or unapproachable animals with safety. They are often used to administer antibiotics, vaccines, and so are not purely for anaesthetics. Preparing and loading darts takes up to five minutes per dart.

'The difficulty in obtaining such useful equipment is mainly due to the fear of accidental injury to the public when etorphine (Immobilon; C-Vet) is used for capturing animals.' (Simon J. Adams, Doha Zoo, Qatar, *Veterinary Record* (1988) **122**, 567).

In America Pneu-Dart (Williamsport, Pennsylvania) have developed a blowpipe system that utilises the same impact-detonated darts as their rifles.

'We believe that the use of telescopic sights on capture rifles is an absolute necessity for distances greater than 40 to 50 metres,' commented Michael D. Kock & David A. Jessup, of the International Wildlife Veterinary Services, Orangevale, California.

'PROJECTILE VOMITING'. This term is used when the vomitus is thrown 2 or 3 feet from the body – a symptom of pyloric stenosis in the dog.

PROLACTIN. A hormone associated with lactation and secreted by the PITUITARY GLAND.

PROLAN A is a follicle-stimulating hormone obtained from the pituitary of the pig. PROLAN B is a leutenising hormone from pig and sheep pituitary glands.

PROLAPSE means the slipping down of some organ or structure. The term is applied to the displacements of the rectum and female generative organs, which result in their appearance to the outside.

The best plan is to seek professional assistance at once. (*See* UTERUS, DISEASES OF; RECTUM, DISEASES OF.)

PROLAPSE OF OVIDUCT. This condition is fairly frequently met with in fowls, particularly in birds which have been laying heavily. It is nearly always associated with some aberration from normal of the cloaca or oviduct, irritation resulting and causing the bird to strain. Occasionally it is seen after an endeavour to pass a large or malformed egg, yolk concretion, etc., and in cases known as 'egg bound'. It is also sometimes met with in cases of vent gleet. The prolapsed oviduct appears as a dark red swelling protruding from the vent. Other birds are attracted by the swelling and peck at it, frequently leading to evisceration and death. Treatment consists in removing the affected bird from the flock. The prolapse should be washed with warm water containing a mild antiseptic, and then gently pressed back into the abdominal cavity after first removing the egg or other foreign body, if the presence of such can be detected. It greatly aids return to have the bird held head downwards by an assistant.

PROLIFERATIVE HAEMORRHAGIC ENTEROPATHY in pigs (*see* HAEMORRHAGIC GASTROENTERITIS).

PROLONGED SOFT PALATE. An inherited abnormality of dogs. (*See under* PALATE.)

PROMAZINE HYDROCHLORIDE. An effective sedative and prenarcotic, administered to the dog by intravenous or intramuscular injection. (*See under* CHLORPROMAZINE.)

PROOESTRUS. A period in the oestrus cycle when the Graäfian follicles are increasing in size (*see* OVARIES) and the female reproductive organs are being prepared for possible pregnancy.

PROTETAMPHOS. A non-lindane containing compound approved as a sheep dip, and also for fly strike and control of keds, ticks and lice.

PROPHYLAXIS means any treatment that is adopted with a view to prevent disease.

PROPIONATE, SODIUM. A bacteriostatic and fungicide which has been recommended in the treatment of obstinate infections of the conjunctiva and cornea.

PROPIONIC ACID (*see* MUSCLES, DISEASES OF – Nutritional Muscular Dystrophy).

PROPOFOL. One of a group of alkyl phenols, it (Diprivan; ICI) is useful as an intravenous anaesthetic for dogs. Recovery from it is 'quiet and rapid – an advantage when the patient has to be returned to the owner's care with the minimum delay.' (Watkins, S. B. & others. *Veterinary Record* (1987) **120,** 326.)

'Rapinovet' (Coopers Animal Health) was found equally efficacious in trials involving 290 dogs and 207 cats.

PROPYLENE GLYCOL has been used in the treatment of acetonaemia in cattle.

PROSTAGLANDINS. A group of hormone-like compounds which can cause contraction of the uterus, lower blood pressure, have an effect on platelets, and lower body temperature.

Synthetic analogues of naturally occurring prostaglandins are used to bring about regression of the *corpus luteum* for control of oestrus.

Prostaglandins can cause local ischaemia at the intramuscular injection site, followed by diffuse swelling and emphysema.

In one case sloughing of skin and muscle occurred, and *Clostridium chauvoei* was isolated from the exudate. The mare became recumbent, and euthanasia was decided upon.

(*See* 'CONTROLLED BREEDING'; *also* PYOMETRA, CHRONIC METRITIS, RETAINED PLACENTA, *and* MISALLIANCE.)

A code of practice relating to the use of prostaglandins in cattle and pigs was agreed by the RCVS and the BVA in 1987.

PROSTATE GLAND is one of the accessory sexual glands that lies at the neck of the bladder in the male animal, and partly surrounds the urethra at that point. Hyperplasia is common, especially in dogs. When greatly enlarged not only does it interfere with the free passage of urine to the outside, but it may obstruct the passage of faeces. At times it causes a very troublesome incontinence of urine. Use of stilboestrol was helpful; otherwise operation of castration is necessary. When the testicles are removed the activity of the gland ceases and it undergoes atrophy.

Apart from this gradually occurring hyperplasia of the gland in dogs over 5 years old, enlargement may be due to an acute infection, when evidence of pain (with arched back and a stiff-legged gait) may be added to the symptoms. Cancer of the prostate is not rare in the dog; cysts sometimes occur. (*See also* BRUCELLOSIS.)

PROSTHESIS. An artificial replacement of a part of the body.

PROTECTION OF ANIMALS (ANAESTHETICS) ACT, 1954 (*see under the heading* ANAESTHETICS). (*See also under* LAW.)

PROTEIN CALORIES. A measure of the nutritional value of a food, not of a requirement by the animal.

PROTEIN CONCENTRATES. Products specifically designed for further mixing, at an inclusion rate of 5 per cent or more, with planned proportions of cereals and other feeding-stuffs either on the farm or by a feed-stuff compounder.

PROTEIN EQUIVALENT. This provides the measure of the value of a feeding-stuff, taking into account the protein content plus the non-protein nitrogen content, capable of being converted into protein by the animal's digestive system. It is expressed as a percentage. For example, the protein equivalent of linseed cake is 25 per cent; *i.e.* 100 lb of the cake is equivalent to 25 lb of protein and potential protein. The protein equivalent of grass silage is about 2 per cent; that of kale, 1·3 per cent.

PROTEIN, HYDROLISED. A mixture of amino-acids and simple polypeptides prepared by enzyme digestion of whole muscle. A valuable source of protein used in cases of shock, malnutrition, convalescence, fevers, chronic nephritis, etc. It may be given by mouth or injection.

PROTEIN SHOCK. A reaction following parenteral administration of a protein. (*See* ANAPHYLAXIS.)

PROTEINS are complex chemical compounds containing nitrogen, carbon, hydrogen and oxygen, found in every body tissue and living cell. Proteins are formed from (and convertible to) amino-acids. (*See* DIET.)

PROTEOGLYCANS. Proteins which are combined with a carbohydrate.

PROTEUS. A genus of bacteria. Proteus species are common pathogens affecting the urinary system of the dog.

PROTHROMBIN. A substance formed in the liver with the assistance of vitamin K, and essential for the clotting of blood.

PROTOPLASM (*see* CELL).

PROTOTHECOSIS. Poisoning by a colourless alga, Prototheca; possibly a mutant form of Chlorella, a green alga. (*See* MASTITIS.)

PROTOZOA. Single-celled organisms.

PROUD FLESH is the popular name given to the unhealthy granulations which sometimes arise perhaps around an inflamed ulcer, when a wound is greatly infected and the discharge copious, or at the edges of a sinus. It can be checked by the application of a caustic astringent. (*See* 'LICK GRANULOMA'.)

PROVEN SIRE is one having an adequate number of measured progeny. (*See* PROGENY TESTING.)

PROVENTRICULUS. The true, glandular stomach of birds. In it digestion is effected by hydrochloric acid and enzymes. (See diagram.)
Proventricular region of the horse's, and pig's, stomach is near the oesophagus and devoid of glands.

PROXIMAL is a term of comparison applied to structures which are nearer the centre of the body or the median line, as opposed to more 'distal' structures.

PrP. A protein found on the surface of neurons (nerve cells) and involved in the development of transmissible SPONGIFORM ENCEPHALOPATHIES, including BSE.

PRURITUS is the symptom of itching which is a prominent feature of most parasitic skin diseases, and of Aujeszky's Disease and Scrapie. (In human medicine an iron deficiency is recognised as one cause of pruritus.)

PRURITUS, PYREXIA, HAEMORRHAGIC SYNDROME. This was reported in cattle fed on citrus pulp, which was mouldy and contained citrinin. (Griffiths, I. B. & Done, S. H. *Veterinary Record* (1991) **129**, 113.)

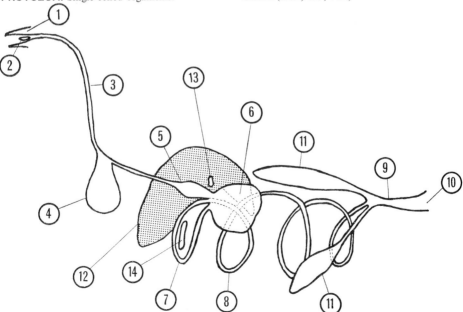

Proventriculus. Its position in the digestive tract of the fowl is indicated (5). Other numbers indicate beak and tongue (1 and 2); oesophagus (3); crop (4); gizzard (6); duodenum (7); small intestine (8); large intestine (9); cloaca (10); caeca (11); liver (12); gall bladder (13); pancreas (14). Reproduced with permission from the *UFAW Handbook on Care and Management of Farm Animals.*

PRUSSIC ACID (*see* HYDROCYANIC ACID).

PSAMMOMA is the name given to a small hard tumour of the brain.

PSEUDO-LEUKAEMIA. This is not a single entity but rather a group of diseases – all of which bear a close resemblance to leukaemia although there is no increase of white cells in the blood. Lympho-sarcomatosis is not uncommon in animals. The lymph nodes, spleen, and liver are usually enlarged in pseudo-leukaemia, and there is anaemia.

PSEUDOMONAS. A genus of bacteria. *P. pyocyanea* is a motile, Gram-negative rod, 1·5 to 3 μ long. It flourishes in suppurating wounds, and has been found in cases of otitis in the dog. It has also been reported as causing outbreaks of disease in turkey poults and other birds.

Chronic mastitis, with diarrhoea and wasting resembling Johne's disease, has been caused in cows by *P. aeruginosa*. This organism, often found in non-mains water supplies, is thought likely to be increasingly involved in mastitis in cattle. It appears to have an increased incidence during August, September and October. (*See* NOXYTH-IOLIN, WOUNDS; *also* MELIOIDOSIS.)

PSEUDO-PREGNANCY is a condition commonly seen in the bitch, but probably occurring in all breeding female animals to a lesser degree. In it the physical signs of pregnancy are exhibited in the absence of fetus or fetuses. The abdomen increases in size, the uterus becomes swollen and turgid, its walls are thickened, and in extreme cases mammary development may occur, and milk may be secreted. The bitch may actually make a bed.

In time, since no fetuses are present, the organs and tissues return to their normal state without the occurrence of parturition; heat returns, and successful breeding may occur subsequently.

The condition has been described as an intensification and prolongation of metoestrus. The essential feature is persistence of the *corpora lutea* in the ovaries.

The condition can – where necessary – be treated by injection of the appropriate hormone.

A Belgian veterinarian, L. A. A. Janssens, reviewed 442 cases of pseudo-pregnancy in a total of 142 bitches. Of these, 19 had only one pseudo-pregnancy, 31 had two, 54 had three, and 39 had four or more pseudo-pregnancies.

Instead of using a hormone treatment, he and his colleagues employed an ergot alkaloid, bromocriptin, which he deemed safer. It does have one side-effect, however—vomiting, but this can be successfully overcome with the anti-emetic metoclopramide.

A total of 81 per cent of pseudo-pregnancies responded to the new treatment, and 80 per cent of the behavioural or psychological problems were resolved. (Janssens, L. A. A., *Veterinary Record* (1986) **119**, 172.)

(*See* REPRODUCTION, BREEDING, 'CLOUD-BURST' of goats, etc.)

PSEUDO-RABIES. A name occasionally used for AUJESZKY'S DISEASE.

PSEUDO-TUBERCULOSIS (*see* YERSINIOSIS, CASEOUS LYMPHADENITIS).

PSITTACOSIS, or 'PARROT FEVER'. Illness in man and birds of the parrot family (including budgerigars and cockatiels) caused by *Chlamydia psittaci*. (*see* CHLAMYDIA).

PSOAS is the name of two muscles, *Psoas major* and *Psoas minor*, which lie along the roof of the abdomen immediately beneath the last two or three thoracic and the whole of the lumbar vertebrae, and stretch into the pelvis. The psoas minor is inserted in the *psoas tubercle* of the ilium, and the psoas major runs to the inner or lesser trochanter of the femur in common with the *iliacus* muscle. The action of these muscles is to bend the pelvis on the rest of the trunk, or if those of one side of the body are acting alone, to bend the posterior part of the trunk towards that side. The act of crouching preparatory to kicking is accomplished by these muscles and others, and they are largely concerned in the movements of galloping. Disease or injury, such as a severe sprain, is shown by a difficulty in walking both forwards and backwards, by a crouching appearance of the back, and by extreme difficulty in rising from the ground.

PSORIASIS is a chronic inflammatory skin disease with scurf formation.

PSOROPTIC MANGE of cattle (*see under* MITES).

PTOSIS means a drooping of the upper eye-lid due to paralysis of the third or oculomotor nerve, which actuates the muscle that raises the upper eyelid. It is commonly seen along with facial paralysis, which is due to paralysis of the facial nerve, and is commonest in the horse after accidents to the head. It may be so severe as to make vision difficult, and it only disappears gradually. Ptosis may be a symptom of GUTTURAL POUCH DIPHTHERIA.

PTYALIN is the name of the enzyme contained in the saliva, by which starchy food-stuffs are changed into sugars, and so prepared for absorption.

PUBERTY. Ewes, sows, and bitches may mate when only 6 or 7 months old; mares reach puberty at from 15 to 18 months old; heifers from 7 to 15 months old. In the cat oestrus may occur as early as 3½ months, or occasionally be delayed until the queen is about a year old. In the male, puberty commonly occurs at an age of 10–12 months, but here again there may be considerable variation. Some toms may reach puberty as early as six months, while others do not mate until their second spring.

PUBIS is the bone that forms the lower anterior parts of the pelvis. The pubes of right and left sides meet each other at the 'symphysis of the pubes', which in old age is no longer a separable union, bony fusion having taken place.

PUBLIC HEALTH (*see* MILK, FOOD INSPECTION; ANTIBIOTIC RESISTANCE, and information given under the main animal diseases communicable to people. *See also* SHEPHERDS, COWMEN, and PIGMEN for occupational hazards; and ZOONOSES.

PUFFER FISH (*see* TOADFISH poisoning).

'PULLET DISEASE'. A transmissible enteritis of pullets and turkey poults, first described in the USA in 1951. (*See also* 'VISCERAL GOUT'.)

Signs include loss of appetite, diarrhoea with watery or whitish evacuations and *sometimes* darkening of the comb. Birds appear drowsy. About 10 per cent die. The cause is a REOVIRUS.

PULLORUM DISEASE OF CHICKS (BACILLARY WHITE DIARRHOEA) has been virtually eradicated in the UK. It is an acute, infectious, and fatal disease of chicks, causing much loss during the first 2 weeks of life. Adult fowls, especially laying hens, act as 'carriers' and transmit infection through their eggs to the chick before hatching. They may also spread infection in their droppings.

CAUSE. *Salmonella pullorum*, which is found in the ovary and oviduct of carrier hens, which are birds which themselves contracted the disease when young, but which survived. The disease is a true 'egg-borne' disease, and since only one infected egg in a large number can, if it hatches successfully, infect many or most of the chicks in a batch, it can be realised that incubator hatching and artificial foster-mother and brooder rearing, where perhaps several hundreds may run together, is a very important factor in causing the disease to spread. With eggs hatched by hens the spread is of only small dimensions, since only a particular clutch can be infected from each infected egg.

In addition to direct infection from birds on the same farm, outbreaks have been traced to the use of 'clear' eggs from incubators used to add to chick food.

SIGNS. The symptoms are not very characteristic at first, but young chicks are noted to be uneasy, cheeping continuously in a weary manner, dull and generally unlike the normally alert, active young chick. Down is ruffled and the chicks are unsteady on their feet. Later, a yellowish or whitish diarrhoea occurs and the down feathering around the vent becomes gummed and sticky. However, in acute cases, no diarrhoea may be seen. Mortality may be low, though it can reach 50 per cent.

Lameness, with swelling of the hocks, is characteristic of chronic pullorum disease.

It should be noted that in spite of the name of this disease, diarrhoea is not a constant symptom in all outbreaks. Moreover, diarrhoea which is not distinguishable from that associated with this disease may occur from other causes, such as bad feeding or management. To reach an accurate diagnosis, laboratory examination of sick or dead chicks is necessary.

TREATMENT. In most cases it is not satisfactory to attempt treatment when an outbreak is confirmed. Fumigation with formaldehyde gas (generated by pouring commercial formalin on to potassium permanganate crystals) is effective for fumigating incubators and incubator houses.

PREVENTION. This can be achieved by testing

all birds, eggs from which are to be used for hatching, by the 'BWD Agglutination Test'.

The negatives are moved to fresh, clean ground and a second test a month later is desirable, and if further reactors are found, monthly tests are carried out until an all-clear pass is obtained.

The agglutination test can either be done with the co-operation of a laboratory, when samples of each bird's blood must be collected and sent away for test, or the 'rapid' test can be carried out on the farm itself.

GENERAL. There are some points of general importance regarding pullorum disease which should be kept in mind.

(i) Infection may be present on a farm without any signs of illness being seen among the 'carrier' birds, so that the appearance of the flock is of no guidance in establishing the presence of infection.

(ii) Eggs from 'carrier' hens do not always hatch into chicks which become clinically affected. The number of infected eggs varies from only 5 per cent to about 40 per cent of those laid by a carrier.

(iii) One blood test cannot be relied upon to clear an infected flock, and the reintroduction of infection from other sources must be constantly guarded against.

PULMONARY ADENOMATOSIS (jaagsiekte) is caused by Bovid Herpesvirus (*see* HERPESVIRUSES) and is a lung disease of adult sheep. First recognised in South Africa, it occurs also in the UK, Iceland, USA. In Britain, one East Anglian farmer lost 50 out of 200 half-bred ewes from jaagsiekte during 1958. The disease is probably widespread but subclinical in hill sheep in Scotland. The disease could assume considerable economic importance in intensively managed sheep.

The lungs gradually lose their normal tissue, breathing becomes laboured, and death follows emaciation after a few months.

It is thought that a second, oncornavirus, may act synergistically in producing this disease.

PULMONARY DISEASES (*see* LUNGS, DISEASES OF).

PULPY KIDNEY DISEASE attacks lambs between about 3 weeks and 18 weeks of age, particularly those which are thriving. The disease has been seen in lambs under a week old. It occurs in Britain, America, New Zealand, etc.

CAUSE. *Clostridium Welchii*, Type D.

SIGNS. As a rule the affected lambs are found dead without having previously been noticed ailing. Usually the lambs in the best condition are the first to be affected. The loss may be very heavy, especially with the larger earlier maturing breeds. Post-mortem examination shows striking changes in the kidney, which are different from those encountered in almost any other condition. They are soft in consistency, mottled in colour, and the cortex is jelly-like or almost semi-fluid. The liver usually shows haemorrhagic spots on its surface and is markedly congested. There may be diffusely scattered small haemorrhages over the peritoneal surface of other organs. In adult sheep the disease is known as Entero-toxaemia (which see), and the 'pulpy kidney' lesions are absent.

PREVENTION. It is recommended that immunity be maintained by autumn vaccination, with a second dose of vaccine in the spring, preferably about 10 days before lambing, unless the ewes are to be moved to a better pasture prior to lambing, when the second dose should be given before the move is made. These two doses should protect the ewe through the spring months and allow her to pass to the lamb *via* the colostrum sufficient antibodies to protect it for the first 8 to 12 weeks of life. That temporary immunity in the lamb should be converted to an active one by the use of vaccine.

PULSE. The forcing of blood from the heart into the elastic arteries of the systemic circulation brings about a pulsation in them. This may be better understood when it is remembered that the beating of the heart drives blood out from the left ventricle into an already full aorta, in which it is imprisoned by the closing of the aortic semilunar valves. To accommodate this extra blood the aorta dilates, and the blood already in it moves onwards throughout the course of the vessel, and through the larger branches to which it gives origin. The wave of dilatation also travels along the course taken by the blood, and is therefore distributed along all the larger arterial trunks. If the fingers be laid over any of these latter, which lie near the surface, a periodic thrill or 'pulse' can be felt, occurring about 35 to 45 times per minute.

The pulse-rate varies according to the state of the animal's health, being faster in fevers, and slower and weaker in debilitating non-febrile diseases; according to the age of the animal (faster in the very young and very old); according to the climate, bodily condition, and under other circumstances. During and immediately after exercise it is greatly increased, but in health it subsides rapidly subsequently. During sleep and unconsciousness it is slower.

The normal pulse-rates of the domesticated animals at rest are as follows:

	Per minute
Horse	36 to 42
Ox	45 to 50
Sheep }	70 to 80
Pig }	
Dog	90 to 100
Cat	110 to 120

and of certain other animals as follows:

	Per minute
Elephant	25 to 28
Camel	28 to 32
Buffalo	40 to 45
Reindeer	60 to 65
Mouse	130 to 150

If the above table is studied it will be seen that, roughly speaking, the smaller the bulk of the animal the faster the pulse. The same principle applies to animals of one species but of different sizes or of different breeds; *e.g.* the pulse of the Shire stallion is usually about 35 per minute, while that of the Shetland pony is 45 or more. These facts must be taken into account when counting the pulse of any given animal. (*See also under* HEART.)

PUPIL (*see* EYE).

PUPPIES, NEW-BORN, INFECTION IN (*see* FADING, TOXOCARA).

PURGATION is now recognised as involving dangers which include potassium depletion.

PURGATIVES. This is the age of laxatives rather than purgatives. The old drastic purgatives are obsolete; they tended to make the patient's condition worse. (*See* LAXATIVES.)

PURPURA HAEMORRHAGICA often occurs in a horse recovering from influenza or strangles, and is characterised by oedema of the head and also of the lower parts of the body. There may be kidney lesions.
CAUSE. The precise cause of purpura is unknown, but it is generally regarded as of an allergic nature.
SIGNS. Appear suddenly; often overnight. Swellings, very often the same on each side of the body, are found on the limbs, the breast, the eyelids, and almost always about the muzzle and nostrils. These swellings may be diffuse from the first, or they may begin as isolated circumscribed flat prominences which coalesce in the course of a day or more. And when pressed with the point of the thumb a little pit remains afterwards for some moments. Petechial haemorrhages are present in the nostrils (from which a blood-stained discharge is often seen) and on any mucous membrane.

The horse is dull, loses its appetite, moves stiffly and with difficulty, and if the swellings of the nostril are large, shows rapid and laboured breathing. Swollen lips may prevent a horse from feeding or drinking, swollen eye-lids may hinder or prevent vision, and a swollen sheath in the male may make the act of micturition difficult. The temperature usually remains between 102°F and 104°F; the pulse is soft, feeble, generally rapid, and may be very irregular.

The percentage of recoveries is not large in well-marked cases, and even where death does not occur, complete recovery takes a long time, and relapses are common. It is said that cases showing nervous complications *always* end fatally, and the same may be said of those with pneumonia.
TREATMENT. The most careful nursing and feeding are essential in all cases of purpura. (*See* NURSING OF SICK ANIMALS.) Good results often follow the intravenous injection of an antihistamine.

After apparent recovery the horse must have a long period of convalescence.

Purpura may, rarely, occur in cattle and dogs.

PUS. This thick, often yellowish fluid, found in abscesses and sinuses, and on the surfaces of ulcers and inflamed areas where the skin is broken, comprises blood serum, bacteria, white blood cells, and damaged tissue cells. (*See* ABSCESS, STREPTODORNASE, PHAGOCYTOSIS.)

'PUSHING DISEASE'. A colloquial name for poisoning of cattle by 'Staggers weed' (*Matricaria nigellaefolia*) in South Africa.

PUSTULE means a small collection of pus occurring in the skin, or immediately below it. (*See* ABSCESS.) 'Malignant pustule' is the name applied to the form that anthrax most commonly takes when it affects the human being.

PUTTY. Eating of this can result in lead poisoning. A discarded drum of putty thrown into a field led to 12 bullocks dying within 24 hours, and a further 40 required treatment. (VI Service report).

PYAEMIA. The presence of pus in the blood-stream.

PYELITIS means a condition of pus-formation in the kidney which produces pus in the urine. It is due to inflammation of the part called the *pelvis of the kidney*, which is connected with the ureter. The condition is commonest among cows after calving, when infection has reached the bladder, invaded the ureters, and has arrived at the pelvis of the kidney.

PYELONEPHRITIS. This term is used when both the pelvis and much of the rest of the kidney are involved, as described under PYELITIS.

CONTAGIOUS BOVINE PYELONEPHRITIS is a specific infection of cattle caused by *Corynebacterium renale*, giving rise to inflammation and suppuration in kidneys, ureters and bladder. As a rule, only one cow in a herd is attacked – though others may be carriers. The passage of blood-stained urine and abdominal pain are symptoms. Penicillin is useful in treatment. Otherwise, death may occur (sometimes after several weeks).

In the pig, an infectious pyelonephritis is caused by *C. suis.*

PYLORIC STENOSIS. This occurs as a rare congenital defect in the dog. Only liquid food can pass into the stomach. 'Projectile vomiting' is a symptom. The defect can be corrected by means of surgery. (*See* PYLORUS.)

PYLOROSPASM means spasm of the pyloric portion of the stomach. This interferes with the passage of food in a normal, gentle fashion into the intestine, and causes distress from half an hour to 3 hours after feeding. It is associated with severe disorders of digestion.

PYLORUS is the name of the lower opening of the true stomach. Exit of food from the stomach is guarded by a strong ring of muscular tissue called the *sphincter of the pylorus*, which opens under nervous activity and allows escape of small amounts of partly digested food material into the small intestine. (*See* STOMACH; DIGESTION; and above.)

PYO- is a prefix attached to the names of various diseases to indicate the presence of pus or the formation of abscesses.

PYODERMA. A pustular condition of the skin. In dogs allergic skin disease is regarded as predisposing to infection by staphylococci.

PYOGENIC is a term applied to those bacteria which cause the formation of pus, and so lead to the production of abscesses.

PYOMETRA. A collection of pus in the uterus: a condition not uncommon in maiden bitches, and occurring in all species. (*See* UTERUS, DISEASES OF.)

PYORRHOEA. Inflammation of the gums, in which suppuration is produced and ultimately interference with the integrity of the teeth. It is a common condition in aged dogs and cats. (*See* TARTAR.)

PYOSALPINX. Distension of a Fallopian tube with pus.

PYOTHORAX. The presence of pus within the chest. It may be a sequel to pneumonia, or to a penetrating wound of the chest, perhaps a bite. This is a fairly common condition in the cat, which is likely to rest on its brisket, be disinclined to move, and to have laboured breathing. Cyanosis may be present. Tenderness of the chest is another symptom. The temperature may be 37°C. In many cases the condition develops very rapidly in the cat, death occurring before treatment has been obtained. Treatment involves aspiration of the pus, and the introduction of an antibiotic. In cats, however, the mortality despite treatment may be 50 per cent.

PYRAMIDAL DISEASE. An exostosis affecting the pyramidal process (extensor process) of the third phalanx of the horse's foot. It is usually found in association with low ringbone. (*See* RINGBONE.)

PYRETHROIDS. Synthetic equivalents of some of the active principles of pyrethrum flowers are useful and potent insecticides.

Commercial preparations: Outflank, Stomoxin. (*See* FLIES – Control.)

PYREXIA (*see* FEVER).

PYRIDINE is an alkaloidal substance derived from coal-tar, tobacco, etc. It is added to methylated spirit in order to render this unpleasant to drink.

PYRIDOXINE. Vitamin B_6.

PYRUVIC ACID. An organic acid which is an intermediate product in carbohydrate and protein metabolism. Excessive quantities accumulate in the blood-stream in cases of vitamin B_1 deficiency.

PYURIA. Pus in the urine produced by suppuration in some part of the urinary tract. (*See* URINE.)

Q

Q FEVER. A disease first recognised in Australia in 1935, and now known to have a world-wide distribution, Q fever is an infection of man, cattle, sheep, goats, fowls, and rodents. In Iran, serological evidence of Q fever has been found also in horses and camels.

CAUSE. A rickettsia, *Coxiella burneti*, which is resistant to heat and drying, and can be transmitted by ticks. Human infection can be acquired from these, from inhalation, and from drinking unpasteurised, infected milk; as well as from handling or coming into contact with the fetal membranes, faeces or urine of infected animals.

SIGNS. In farm animals, many Q fever infections may be present without obvious symptoms. However, the rickettsia is a cause of abortion, and less often of pneumonia.

INCIDENCE. In the UK a preliminary survey showed that 2581 farms in England, 553 in Wales, and 240 in Scotland were infected. It has been found possible to isolate the parasite from 3000-gallon milk tankers.

In a recent survey, sera from cattle and sheep in the north-east of Scotland were tested for antibodies to *Coxiella burnetii*. Approximately 1 per cent of 4880 cattle had antibodies to the organism. These potentially infected cattle were distributed throughout the area. Two flocks of sheep were tested; in one flock 30 per cent of sheep had antibodies, while the other was negative. The flock with the high prevalence of *C. burnetii* antibodies appeared to be associated with an outbreak of human Q fever on that farm.

TREATMENT. This is made difficult by the fact that antibiotics are rickettsiostatic rather than rickettsiocidal, and also because the organism can remain dormant for long periods *inside* cells.

Public health. Acute Q fever may involve the liver and heart (with resultant myocarditis). Mild cases may resemble food poisoning or influenza with headaches. Chronic Q fever occurs. Endocarditis was recorded in 11 per cent of human cases in England and Wales between 1975 and 1981.

Q fever in snakes. Many snakes imported into the USA are infested with ticks, which transmitted Q fever to dockside workers handling a shipment of Ball pythons.

Q fever from contaminated clothing. This was the presumed cause of sixteen out of 32 employees at a truck repair plant becoming ill with this disease. Serological tests on a cat were positive for *Coxiella burnetii*. The cat was fed at home by one of the workers at the plant.

QUADRICEPS means having four heads, and is the collective name applied to the powerful muscles situated above the stifle-joint. These are: medial and lateral *vasti*, and the *rectus femoris*; the fourth muscle (*vastus intermedius*) in the horse is so blended with the medial vastus that it has lost its autonomy.

QUADRIPLEGIA. Paralysis of all four limbs. (*See* PARALYSIS, TICK PARALYSIS, RACOON, CURARE.)

QUARANTINE implies governmental regulations for the prevention of the spread of infectious disease by which an animal or animals, which have come from infected countries or areas, are detained at the frontiers or ports of entrance, or at other official centres, for a period of isolation, before being allowed to mix with stock of the country.

The regulations dealing with quarantine of animals are altered from time to time, and so information on the matter is best obtained direct from the Government department that deals with live-stock in a particular country. (*See* RABIES, IMPORTING/EXPORTING ANIMALS, NOTIFIABLE DISEASES, PIGEONS.)

QUARTER HORSE (*see* AMERICAN QUARTER HORSE).

QUATERNARY AMMONIUM COMPOUNDS are used as antiseptics, and have found widespread application in dairy hygiene. Cetrimide – or cetyl trimethyl ammonium bromide – is an example. It is used in 0·1 per cent solution for washing cows' udders, teats, and milkers' hands, being effective against *Streptococcus agalactiae*. In higher concentrations it acts as a detergent. (*See also* CETRIMIDE, HIBITANE.)

QUEENSLAND ITCH. This is caused by sensitisation to bites of the midge – *Culicoides robertsi*. The lesions resemble those of mange or eczema, and are seen usually along the animal's back. Antihistamines are useful in treatment. The condition is regarded as an allergic dermatitis, and is similar to 'Sweet Itch'. (*See under* FLIES.)

QUEY. A heifer.

QUIDDING, or 'CUDDING', is the name given to that condition in horses, depending upon injuries to the mouth or diseases of the teeth, in which food is taken into the mouth, chewed repeatedly, and then expelled on the floor of the stall or into the manger. It may result from the teeth being too sharp, irregular in height, uneven in alignment, or from permanent teeth pushing the temporaries out from the gums; it may arise when the gums, cheeks, or tongue have been injured or are diseased; or it may arise in paralysis of the throat, or some other condition which causes inability to swallow. (*See* MOUTH, DISEASES OF; TEETH, DISEASES OF.)

QUININE is an alkaloid obtained from the bark of various species of cinchona trees in South America. It contains four alkaloids, of which *quinine* is the most active and important, the others being *quinidine, cinchonine,* and *cinchonidine.*

Quinine is usually used in the form of one of its salts, *i.e.* sulphate, hydrochloride, or hydro-bromate of quinine.

ACTION. Quinine causes a lowering of temperature in fevers. It stimulates the muscular wall of the uterus.

USES. These have dwindled. Before the advent of the sulpha drugs and antibiotics it was much used in influenza, distemper, and similar conditions. It is still sometimes used in the treatment of pyometra in the bitch. It is sometimes given as an intra-muscular injection. Owing to its very bitter taste it is seldom that it will be taken in the food.

TOXICITY. 'The dog is very susceptible to quinine and becomes blind at plasma concentrations readily tolerated by man.' (*Lancet*, Feb. 6, 1965.)

QUITTOR is a condition of the 'lateral' cartilages of the horse's foot, in which suppuration occurs, with pus escaping from an opening in the region of the coronet. This and the bulbs of the heels are swollen and painful. The cause is an injury to the cartilage or to infection, or both. There is usually some degree of lameness. Antibiotics are used in treatment.

QUIXALUD is an approved feed additive for pigs for use as a growth promoter. Based on Halquinol (a mixture of three chlorinated quinolines), it is effective against *E. coli* and several other organisms (but not those causing swine dysentery). (*See also under* ADDITIVES, GROWTH PROMOTERS.)

R

R FACTOR (*see* PLASMIDS).

RABBIT FUR MITE. This may cause itching in dogs and people. (*See Cheyletiella parasitivorax.*)

'RABBIT SYPHILIS' is caused by a spirochaete *Treponema cuniculi* (which does not affect humans). It is a venereal disease characterised by the appearance of nodules and superficial ulcers covered with thin, moist, scaly crusts and oedematous swellings of the surrounding tissues mainly in the region of the genitalia and also sometimes in the region of the nose.

RABBITS. Breeds of domesticated rabbits used for table purposes include: the New Zealand white, the California, and the Dutch rabbit. (*See also* PETS.)

Handling. When lifting a rabbit, a fold of skin over the shoulder and back should be grasped with one hand, while the other supports the rump. A rabbit should not be lifted by its ears. Struggling while being inexpertly handled can lead to fractures of limbs. A startled rabbit may leap and fracture the spine.

Diseases include APPENDICITIS, ATROPHIC RHINITIS, COCCIDIOSIS, HYDROMETRA (the accumulation of watery fluid in the uterus), IMPACTION of colon or stomach (often the result of insufficient hay being provided), LISTERIOSIS, MASTITIS, METRITIS, MYXOMATOSIS, PASTEURELLOSIS, PNEUMONIA, 'RABBIT SYPHILIS'/'vent disease', SALMONELLOSIS, SCHMORL'S DISEASE, TOXOPLASMOSIS, TUBERCULOSIS, TYZZER'S DISEASE, VIRAL HAEMORRHAGIC DISEASE, and YERSINIASIS.

Pasteurella multocida causes a pneumonia which may be acute and fatal in rabbits under twelve weeks old. It may cause also middle-ear disease with a loss of balance, circling, and head held to one side, epiphora, and also 'Snuffles' in which there is a discharge from eyes and nose and sneezing.

Rabbits act as hosts of the liver-fluke of sheep, and of the cystic stages of some tape-worms, *e.g. Taenia pisiformis, T. serialis.*

Rabbits have been used experimentally as incubators for sheep's eggs. (*See* TRANSPLANTATION OF MAMMALIAN OVA.)

A hermaphrodite rabbit served several females and sired more than 250 young of both sexes. In the next breeding season the rabbit, which was housed in isolation, became pregnant and delivered seven healthy young of both sexes.

Pregnancy diagnosis. An 'Ovucheck' ELISA test kit is available for this purpose. It can also differentiate between pseudo-pregnancy and pregnancy, and detect rabbits about to ovulate. (Dr J. M. Morrell, B.Vet Med, National Institute for Medical Research, London. *Veterinary Record* (1990) **127**, 521)

Anaesthesia. Premedication with atropine (1 to 3 mg per kg by hypodermic or intra-muscular injection) is advisable half an hour earlier. CT1341 (Saffan: Glaxo) is one of the recommended anaesthetics for surgery. Oxygen should be ready to hand.

Tranquillisers include Acepromazine.

For further information, see the following two papers: Caroline Wood, *Vet. Rec.* (1978) **102**, 304. J. Cowie-Whitney, *ibid.* (1977) **101**, 299.

RABIES (the Latin word for madness), is a specific inoculable contagious disease of virtually all mammals, including man; and occasionally it occurs in birds, e.g. domestic poultry and vultures. It is characterised by nervous derangement, often by a change in temperament, with paralysis occurring in the final – and sometimes in the intermediate – stages.

Foxes and cattle are both highly susceptible to infection.

Rabies occurs in all continents with the exception of Australasia and Antarctica. In Turkey dogs remain the principal vectors; in a few countries in Europe cats attack more people than do dogs. In Asia and South America dogs are still the most important vectors, but in many countries wild animals provide a reservoir of infection, and infect dogs and cats and farm animals – which in turn may infect man, who is an incidental host of the disease. (*See* Table of vectors.)

Rabies in wild animals – principal vectors in various regions	
Europe	FOXES, ROE-DEER, BADGERS, MARTENS
Asia	WOLVES, JACKALS, BATS MONGOOSES
North America	FOXES, SKUNKS, COYOTES, BATS
Central America	BATS
South America and Trinidad	VAMPIRE BATS

Public health. Rabies is virtually always fatal in the human being, and there is danger not only from being bitten by rabid animals, but also from contamination by their saliva of wounds, cut fingers, eyes, etc. Scratches may convey infection as well as bites.

People have died from rabies following attacks by rabid dogs, cats, foxes, wolves, badgers, skunks, racoons, mongooses, bats, rodents, etc.

Pet animals, such as rabbits, may be bitten by rabid animals and themselves become rabid; and it has sometimes happened that wild or exotic animals (originating in countries where rabies is endemic) were bought as pets while in the incubation stage of rabies, with unfortunate results.

In the UK as in most other countries rabies is a NOTIFIABLE DISEASE, and must be reported to the

Wild animal cycles   Domestic animal cycles

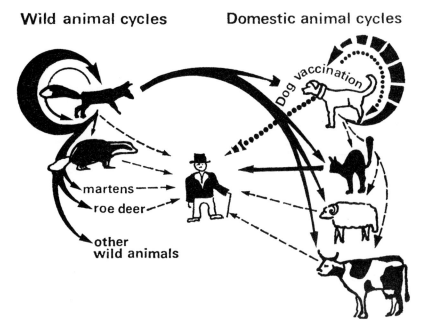

martens

roe deer

other
wild animals

Rabies in Europe.*

Ministry of Agriculture or to the police. Bitten persons should seek medical advice immediately.

CAUSE. A Lyssavirus (one of the Rhabdovirus group). When it is injected into the tissues, either naturally (from a bite) or artificially, the virus passes along the nerves and reaches the central nervous system. The time elapsing between infection and onset of symptoms varies greatly with the location of the bite, its severity, and – no doubt – the quantity of virus in the saliva. In the most rapidly developing cases the symptoms may be shown as early as the ninth day after being bitten, and at the other extreme cases have appeared several months after the incident. It is owing to this fact that the 6 months' period of quarantine insisted upon in Great Britain is something of a compromise. The average incubation periods in dogs, sheep, and swine are from 15 to 60 days, in horses and cattle from 30 to 80 days. In young animals the period of incubation is shorter than in adults.

SIGNS.

Dog. There are two distinct forms of rabies in the dog – the *furious* and the *dumb*; but these are in reality two stages only. It is customary to consider three stages of development of typical symptoms.
(1) *Melancholy.* The prodromal dull stage is often not noticed, or, if it is, only scant attention is paid to it. The habits of the dog change. It becomes morose and sulky, indifferent to authority, disregards its usual playthings or companions, shows a tendency to hide in dark corners, and may appear itchy or irritable as regards its skin. Noisy, boisterous animals become quiet and dull, while animals that are normally of a gentle, quiet disposition may become excitable. After 2 or 3 days of such behaviour the next stage is reached.

(2) *Excitement.* The symptoms described above become exaggerated, and there is a tendency towards violence. The dog pays no attention to either cajoling or threatening. It becomes easily excited and very uncertain in its behaviour. Food is either disregarded completely or eaten with haste. Vomiting is a not uncommon symptom. A fear of water is *not* a symptom to expect in the rabid dog, which will often drink or attempt to do so even when partly paralysed. After a time the appetite becomes deranged. The dog refuses its ordinary food, but eats straw, stones, wood, coal, carpet, pieces of sacking, etc., with great avidity. If the animal is shut up in a kennel, it persists continually in its efforts to escape. Should it be released or should it escape, it almost invariably runs away from home. It may wander for long distances. In its travels it bites and snaps at objects which it encounters, real or imaginary, animate or inanimate. Some rabid dogs bite several people. The tone of voice is altered.

The face has a vacant stare, and the eyes are fixed and expressionless, and the pupils are dilated. This stage lasts from 2 to 4 days, unless the dog's strength gives out sooner, and the next stage appears.
(3) *Paralysis.* The characteristics of the last stage in the train of symptoms of rabies are those of paralysis, especially of the lower jaw and the hindquarters. The dog begins to stagger in its gait, and finally falls. It may manage to regain its feet when stimulated, but soon falls again. The lower jaw drops, the tongue lolls out of the mouth, and there is great salivation. The muscles of the throat and larynx are soon involved in the progressive paralysis.

The *dumb* form of rabies consists of this paralytic stage; the stage of excitation having

*The diagram should really also have a horse and a pig on the right-hand side.

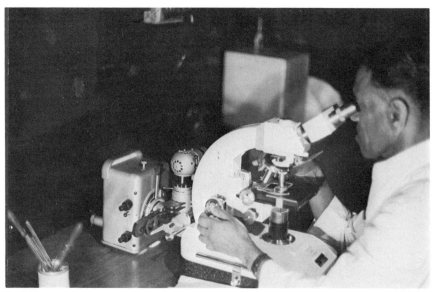

Diagnosis of rabies in an animal by means of the fluorescent antibody test. The microscope is equipped with a darkfield condenser and an ultra-violet light source. (World Health Organisation, taken at the Pasteur Institute, India.)

been omitted. The *dumb* form is the more common in the dog. Barking ceases – hence the name. Vomiting may suggest merely a digestive upset. Protrusion of the nictitating membrane partly across the eye, together with a dropped jaw, *i.e.* partly opened mouth which can be closed by gently raising the lower jaw by means of a stick, are highly suggestive of rabies.

In parts of Africa and Asia, the classical form of rabies in dogs (described above) is replaced by a form called in Africa OULU FATO (*see* separate entry for this).

Cat. In this animal the *furious* form is more common than in the dog. The aggressive stage is most marked, the cat attacking other animals and man with great vigour, and attempting to injure their faces with teeth or claws. Sometimes the rabid cat will at first show extra affection. The course of the disease is usually shorter than in the dog.

It is worth mentioning that occasionally dogs and cats die from rabies without any observed symptoms. They may be found dead or dying. It is not unknown for a cat to be found lying in a field or garden unable to walk but still able to bite.

Cattle. These animals are usually affected through having been bitten by a rabid fox or dog. The stage of excitement is short and the dumb stage is most evident. Affected cattle behave in an unusual manner; they may stamp or bellow, salivate from the mouth, break loose, and may do much damage. Rumination and milk production cease, muscular quiverings are seen, sexual excitement is noticed, and there is a great loss of condition. Exhaustion soon follows and paralysis sets in. Death occurs in from 2 to 6 days or more after the commencement of the condition.

Rabies may be mistaken for hypomagnesaemia,

milk fever, botulism, anaplasmosis, listeriosis, lead poisoning, choking, etc.

In the USA, in 1984, the number of confirmed cases of rabies in cattle totalled 154. In Central and South America, cattle are infected with rabies by vampire bats, and may show long streaks of blood on their shoulders, necks and backs.

Sheep, goats, and swine. The sheep and the goat are affected in a manner similar to cattle, but the stage of excitement is shorter or absent, and the dumb paralytic stage is more often noticed. Pigs become excitable, may squeal, show muscular spasms, before paralysis.

Horse. The *furious* form is common but the animal may appear calm between bouts of aggressiveness. Dumb forms also occur and may be mistaken for colic, paresis or encephalitis from other causes. Signs may include a facial twitch, biting of woodwork or self-mutilation, head-tossing, frequent whinnying, abnormal posture, apparent lameness, ataxia, paralysis of hindquarters. The horse may continue to eat and drink until shortly before death. The tone of voice may be altered.

DIAGNOSIS. The routine examination for Negri bodies has now in most countries been superseded by the fluorescent antibody test, with confirmation by mouse inoculation if necessary. (If a dog which bit someone is still alive after 10 days, it **cannot** be assumed that the dog is not rabid.)

DIFFERENTIATION between laboratory and street rabies virus, between rabies vaccine virus and street virus, and between rabies virus and rabies-like viruses (*e.g.* Mokola, Lagos bat, and Duvenhage viruses) is now possible by 'utilisation of selected panels of monoclonal antibodies (hybridomas).' (A. E. J. Okoh, The Wistar Institute, Philadelphia, USA.)

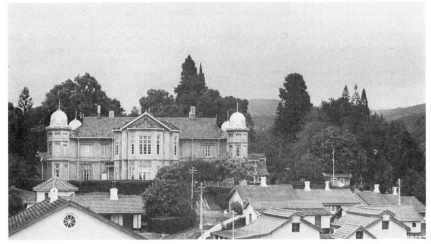

The Pasteur Institute of Coonoor, South India, is one of three World Health Organization International Reference Centres on Rabies – two others being in Paris and Philadelphia. A dog with subclinical rabies was studied here in the 1960s.

PREVENTION. Prevention of the disease in man and animals stems from the research of Louis Pasteur in the 1880s. He attenuated the ordinary 'street' virus by passage through rabbits, resulting in what he called a 'fixed' virus – one less virulent for dogs. Later he injected this 'fixed' virus into rabbits, and prepared the first anti-rabies vaccine following dessication of pieces of their spinal cords. His triumph came in 1885 when the vaccine saved the lives of two badly bitten boys.

In the intervening years many modifications have been made, and new techniques developed, to make rabies vaccines which would be safe and free from dangerous side-effects, and so could be used to immunise people and animals against rabies ('pre-exposure' vaccination), as well as provide 'post-exposure' treatment of those bitten by rabid animals.

The table shows examples of vaccines prepared from tissue culture cells. The last one, the Merieux, was developed by the Merieux Institute of France using a technique pioneered at the Wistar Institute of Philadelphia. Only 1 ml doses are required, and two injections (apart from any booster doses). (*See also* VERO CELLS.)

In the UK two vaccines approved by MAFF for use in dogs and cats are: (1) Rabiffa rabies vaccine (May & Baker) containing inactivated GS-57 Wistar virus strain; and (2) Delcavac-R (Mycofarm) containing cloned rabies virus strain RV675 in an inactivated form.

Mass vaccination of dogs is carried out in many countries as a control measure; and in Central and South America cattle on ranches are vaccinated against vampire-bat transmitted rabies. In France and other countries of Europe, hundreds of thousands of cattle are vaccinated against rabies (often a combined rabies/foot-and-mouth disease inoculation).

It must be remembered, however, that no vaccines are 100 per cent effective, that certificates of vaccination can be forged, and that consequently it is still essential to control the import of animals, whether vaccinated or not, and to enforce quarantine measures in countries where the disease is not endemic.

Control of rabies in Britain. From 1902 until 1918 no cases occurred in the British Isles, but in that year infected dogs were smuggled from the Continent, and the disease obtained a fresh hold for a period of little more than 3 years. Britain had been free since then, but in 1969 a dog released from quarantine 10 days earlier showed symptoms of rabies and bit two people at Camberley, Surrey; and a second case occurred in 1970. Several cases have also occurred in recent years *inside* British quarantine kennels, and in

Examples of vaccines prepared from tissue culture cells		
Live virus: ERA	Pig kidney	Cat, dog, cattle and other animals
HEP-Flury	Dog kidney	Cat, dog, and cattle
Inactivated: Fixed	Hamster kidney	Cat, dog, cattle, and other animals
(Merieux)	Hamster embryo	Cat, dog, horses, cattle and sheep

1965 there was a case in a recently imported leopard in quarantine at Edinburgh Zoo. In Britain, in 1969, the danger of allowing the importation of rabies-susceptible exotic animals, for sale as pets or for research, was officially recognised, and the quarantine regulations amended to include monkeys, mongooses, etc.

Following publication of the Waterhouse Report in 1971, it was decided that all dogs and cats must be vaccinated in quarantine – whether previously vaccinated or not. (This last measure was adopted partly in order to minimise the risk of rabies being spread within quarantine kennels.) (*See* IMPORT/EXPORT OF ANIMALS.) A dog died of rabies while in quarantine in 1983.

Other points to note: (1) The saliva is sometimes infective *before* symptoms of rabies appear – a hazard for a person licked; (2) Farmers have died through mistaking rabies for 'choking' and, with abraded fingers, examining their cow's mouths; (3) Non-typical cases of rabies are not uncommon; (4) A dog may bite a small child or household pet and promptly run away – rabies not being suspected, though running away is in itself a canine symptom; (5) The virus may be present in semen, as well as in milk, tears, faeces, and urine. (6) **Subclinical rabies,** and a **'carrier' state**, have long been recognised in Africa (*see* OULOU FATO) and in Asia. In 1983 Dr Makonnen Fekadu, of the Center for Disease Control, Atlanta, USA, referred to the experimental inducement of a carrier state. Young adult beagles were inoculated, either (1) intracerebrally or (2) intramuscularly, with a rabies strain from the saliva of an apparently healthy Ethiopian dog. All those in the first group died. Most of those in group 2 also died, but six recovered without supportive treatment. (Recovery was assessed on the basis of diminishing clinical signs and the development of high antibody titres in serum and cerebrospinal fluid. One of the six recovered dogs was studied for a year during which virus was isolated from its saliva on days 42, 169, and 305 after its complete recovery. These isolates of virus produced fatal rabies infection in inoculated mice. Other studies had shown, said Dr Fekadu, that rabid animals might secrete virus in their saliva and yet have no detectable amounts of virus in their salivary glands and brain at death. (Dr Fekadu's paper was presented at the 1983 WVA congress in Australia.)

Vaccination of Foxes. Success has been claimed in Switzerland and West Germany for the use of an attenuated vaccine put into chicken heads or chocolate drops and left for foxes to take them. Other countries had been reluctant to use an attenuated vaccine in this way.

RABIES ACT, THE. This extends the powers contained in the Disease of Animals Act 1950 in dealing with an outbreak of rabies outside quarantine premises. In a declared infected area, an order may be made for the destruction of foxes and other wild mammals, and for access to land for this purpose. Fences or other types of barrier may be erected to restrict movement of animals into or out of an area while such destruction is in progress.

Orders may be made for compulsory vaccination, confinement, and control of domestic animals, including strays. Anyone knowing or suspecting that an animal has rabies must notify his suspicion to the police. Deaths of animals in an infected area must also be notified, and the authorities can take over ownership of carcases and determine the means of their disposal. This is because it is essential to confirm a diagnosis of rabies, so that precautions can be taken concerning in-contact animals and human beings. The Act can override a dog-owner's reluctance or refusal to part with the body of a dead pet or working dog.

The Rabies (Importation of Mammals) Order 1971 stipulates which mammals (in addition to dogs and cats) must undergo 6 months' quarantine, and lists ports at which animals can be landed.

A 1984 amending order enabled licensing controls to be applied to animals returning from oil rigs outside British territorial waters.

RABIES-RELATED VIRUSES. These include **Duvenhage** virus, the cause in fruit-eating bats of a disease very similar to rabies; the **Mokola** virus, which has been isolated from shrews, and causes nervous symptoms in man; the **Lagos** bat virus, and the **Nigerian** horse virus.

RACEHORSES. Every year between 1400 and 1600 thoroughbred mares go to stud in the UK. About 67 per cent of them foal successfully, and for every thousand mares covered 270 or so of the resulting progeny finally appear on the racecourse. Temperament, unsoundness, or sale abroad account for the non-appearance of more here.

An epidemiological study of wastage among racehorses was conducted in 1982 and 1983 among six stables, five of which were in Newmarket. The basis of the survey was the inability of horses to take part in cantering exercise as a result of injury or disease. The greatest number of days lost to training was caused by lameness (67·6 per cent) and respiratory problems (20·5 per cent). Conditions of the foot (19 per cent), muscle (18 per cent), carpus (14 per cent), fetlock joints (14 per cent), tendons (10 per cent) and sore shins (9 per cent) were the major reasons for training days being lost in 198 cases in which a positive diagnosis of the site of lameness was made. (Rossdale, P. D. & others, *Veterinary Record* (1985) **116,** 66.)

Pulmonary haemorrhage. In horses which show blood at their nostrils after exercise such as racing, the blood does not come from the nasal cavity but from the lungs. Endoscopic examination showed an incidence of 42 per cent in a group of horses with only 15 per cent showing blood at the nostrils. Affected horses might appear distressed, with dilated pupils. (Pascoe, J. R., California University.)

Exercise-induced pulmonary haemorrhage was observed in 23 of 49 endoscopic examinations after high speed training, in nine of 37 examinations after cantering and in one of 17 after walking or trotting; it was not possible to predict its occurrence. Mucoid or mucopurulent exudate was observed in 60 of 118 examinations and the amount increased after exercise. (Burrell, M. H., *Equine Veterinary Journal* (1985) **17**, 99.)

Pulmonary haemorrhage was diagnosed by endoscopic examination in 255 two-year-old quarterhorses after racing. Only 9 (3·5 per cent) of the animals had visible epistaxis. (Hillidge, C. J. & Whitlock, T. W., *Research in Veterinary Science* (1986) **40**, 406.)

(*See* HORSES, BREEDS OF; HORSES; EXERCISING HORSES; etc.)

RACCOONS are, in Canada and the USA, among the wildlife creatures which sometimes transmit rabies.

A dog bitten by a (non-rabid) raccoon may become paralysed in all four limbs (*quadriplegia*).

RACHITIS (*see* RICKETS).

RADIAL PARALYSIS, or 'DROPPED ELBOW', is commonest in horses and dogs, though it may be seen in any animal.
CAUSES. Probably the majority of cases are due to a fracture of the 1st rib on the same side of the body, the broken ends of the rib lacerating the nerve-fibres as they pass the rib, or pressing against them. In other cases the origin of the paralysis seems to be situated in the end-plates of the nerve-fibres where they are distributed to the muscles, and in some cases a neuritis involving the radial nerve, or a tumour pressing upon it at some part of its course, is responsible for producing the condition.
SIGNS. In a typical case the horse stands with the elbow dropped lower than normally, and with the knee, elbow, and fetlock joints flexed. Little or no pain is felt, unless there is a fractured rib, or some inflammatory condition which has caused the paralysis. The limb is held in the position assumed at the commencement of a stride, but the animal is incapable of advancing it far in front of the sound limb. No weight is borne upon the leg, the muscles are flaccid and soft, and if the horse is made to move forward it either does so by hopping off and on to the sound fore-limb, or it may fall forwards. If the hand be forcibly pressed against the knee, so that the limb is restored to its natural upright position, the horse is able to bear weight upon it and may lift the other limb from the ground, but as soon as the pressure is released, the joints fall forward again. Sometimes the toe is rested upon the ground, but at other times the horse stands with the wall of the foot in contact with the ground. In cases that are not so severe, the flat of the foot may rest on the ground, and the limb can be advanced forwards to a considerable extent.
TREATMENT. The majority of such cases as these will recover in a few weeks. Patience on the part of the owner is essential.

RADIATION, EXPOSURE TO. The 1986 Chernobyl nuclear power-station disaster in the USSR led to controls being imposed by MAFF

on the movement and slaughter of sheep in parts of Scotland, Cumbria, and Wales, after between 1000 and 4000 Becquerels/kg of caesium-137 had been detected in lambs. Similar controls were applied in other countries affected by the fallout. The ban temporarily affected about 2 million sheep and lambs in some 500 flocks.

The Atomic Energy Authority stated that 10,000 Bq/kg represents a health risk.

However the contamination figures exceeded, in nine cases, the internationally recommended action levels for radiocaesium of 1000 Bq/kg. The highest figure was 4000.

'Although the physical half-life of radiocaesium is 30 years, its biological half-life is much shorter. In an adult animal, the half-life is estimated at between 30 and 100 days, but for lamb it would be between 25 and 50 days.' (MAFF).

After an earlier accident at Windscale, in the UK, radioactive iodine alone contaminated pasture in the area.

RADIOACTIVE IODINE ⎱ (*See below.*)
RADIOACTIVE STRONTIUM ⎰

Annual human exposure. Of the average UK citizen's annual exposure to radioactive discharges, only 0·1 per cent comes from the nuclear power industry, according to the Radiological Protection Board.

For radiation exposure associated with veterinary practice, *see* RADIOISOTOPES *and* X-RAYS.

Carbon-14 is 'among internal sources of natural radiation, and is present in the human body to the extent of about 2000 Bq.' (Dr B. Sansom, *Veterinary Record* (1986) **119**, 48, who defines a Becquerel as 'one radioactive disintegration per second.')

'RADIATION SICKNESS'. Dogs exposed to radiation following a nuclear explosion will vomit as a result of gastro-enteritis, become dull and lose their appetite. This may return after a day or two, but leucopenia develops, and may be followed by haemorrhage or septicaemia.

RADIOACTIVE CAESIUM. The explosion on April 26, 1986 at the Chernobyl nuclear power station contaminated the whole of western Europe with radioactive nuclides. Within 30 km of the reactor the authorities evacuated 135,000 people and 80,000 head of livestock. Later, so much caesium-137 was detected in sheep meat from some areas of Wales and Scotland, that the meat was declared unfit for human consumption; (Dr. K. L. Morgan, Vet MB, University of Bristol.)
ANTIDOTE: A ferric-cyano-ferrate (AFCF), in the form of a dark blue powder can bind radiocaesium both *in vitro* and in the gastro-intestinal tract of animals very effectively; so preventing the isotope from being absorbed and secreted into the milk or transferred to the meat of cows, etc. The addition of only 3 g AFCF per day to the diet of lactating cows reduced the radiocaesium content of their milk by between 80 and 90 per cent, and of their meat by 78 per cent.

The radiocaesium content of the meat from

sheep fed 1 g AFCF per day or of calves or pigs fed 2 g AFCF per day was reduced by approximately 90 per cent. The compound has been given official clearance as a feed additive against radio-caesium in West Germany. (Giese, W. W. *British Veterinary Journal* (1988) **144,** 363.)

RADIOACTIVE DISCHARGES. Of the average UK citizen's annual exposure, only 0.1 per cent comes from the nuclear power industry, according to the Radiological Protection Board.

Around 90 per cent comes from natural sources, principally Radon gas released from building materials.

For radiation associated with veterinary practice, *see* RADIOISOTOPES *and* X-RAYS.

RADIOACTIVE FALL-OUT, following the explosion of nuclear bombs, etc., or accidents at atomic plant, may be dangerous to farm livestock on account of the radioactive iodine and strontium released. After an accident at Windscale, radioactive iodine alone contaminated pasture in the area. (*See also below and above.*)

RADIOACTIVE IODINE. Cattle grazing pasture contaminated by fall-out pick up ten times as much radioactive iodine as do people in the same locality, according to American reports. Much is excreted in the milk, and much concentrated in the thyroid glands.

Feeding-stuffs or pasture contaminated by fall-out containing radioactive iodine and strontium may give rise to illness in cattle. Digestive organs may be damaged, changes in the blood occur, and deaths follow within a month or so, after a period of dullness and scouring. (*See below.*)

RADIOACTIVE STRONTIUM. Whereas the half-life of radioactive iodine is a matter of days, that of strontium is 30 years. Following the grazing of contaminated pasture or the eating of other contaminated feed, radioactive strontium is excreted in the milk, but much of it enters the bones and is liable to set up cancer many years afterwards.

The UK average ratio of strontium-90 to calcium in milk was 2·8 picocuries per gram of calcium in 1975, compared with 3·3 picocuries per gram in the previous year; this result is about one-tenth of the maximum reached in 1964. The average concentration of **caesium-137** (7 picocuries/litre) was about four-fifths of the value in 1974 and less than one-twentieth of the 1964 maximum (AFRC).

RADIO-FREQUENCY TREATMENT (*see under* CANCER, Treatment).

RADIOGRAPHY (*see under* X-RAYS).

RADIOIMMUNE ASSAY. A method of measuring antigen or antibody concentration by means of radioactively labelled reagents.

RADIOISOTOPES. Nuclear medicine involves the use of unsealed radioisotopes for diagnosis and therapy. For bone scanning, the most commonly used radiopharmaceutical is methylene diphosphonate, labelled with Technetium 99 mm (Tc-99). With a half-life of only six hours, high doses can be given for a low radiation burden, permitting high resolution pictures to be obtained. 'A point to stress is the extreme sensitivity in picking up lesions in bone, but the extreme non-specificity in pathological terms.' (Dr D. H. Keeling of the Department of Nuclear Medicine, Derriford Hospital, Plymouth, UK, 1985 BVA Congress paper.)

RADIO PILLS or telemetering capsules have been developed for research purposes. A radio transmitter, the size of an ordinary drug capsule, can give information concerning pressure, temperature or pH within an organ.

RADIUS is the inner of the two bones of the forelimb. In the horse and ox particularly, the radius forms the main bone of this part, the ulna being much smaller and not taking part in weight-bearing. (*See* BONE.)

RADON GAS (*see under* RADIO-ACTIVE).

RAGWORT POISONING causes losses among **cattle** and **sheep** in Great Britain, Canada, and New Zealand. It is the cause of the 'Pictou cattle disease' of Canada, and of 'Molteno cattle disease' in South Africa. The plant (*Senecio jacobaea*, or sp.) is very often fed off by sheep when it becomes too plentiful in grass land. In the UK fatal poisoning has followed the giving of hay contaminated with ragwort; death occurring many weeks after the last mouthful. The death of 28 head of cattle was caused 2 to 4 months after feeding ragwort-contaminated silage.

Ragwort contains PYRROLIZIDENE ALKALOIDS (which see).

Effect: Cirrhosis of the liver, inflammation of the fourth stomach, and other lesions.

Milk from a cow which has eaten ragwort may be dangerous to children, causing liver damage. SIGNS include loss of appetite and of condition, constipation, sometimes jaundice. Cattle may strain and later become excited and violent; horses may become drowsy, with a staggering gait.

In the UK after a mild, damp winter, when the plant grows earlier in the year than usual, and is sprouting among the grasses, horses may eat it.

Secondary gastric impaction and rupture in horses was reported by Dr E. M. Milne & others. *Veterinary Record* (1990) **126,** 502.
TREATMENT: There is no specific antidote, but methionine has been reported to be helpful.

Acute ragwort poisoning may also occur, causing death in 5 to 10 days with symptoms of dullness, abdominal pain, and sometimes jaundice. (*See* LIVER, DISEASES OF.)
DIAGNOSIS. S. W. Ricketts recommended a liver biopsy as being helpful in the diagnosis of chronic ragwort poisoning in horses 'probably the most common cause of chronic hepatic pathology in horses in the UK.'

'RAIN SCALD'. An old name for *Dermatophilus* infection in horses subjected to prolonged wetting. Lesions occur on withers, shoulders, and rump. For appearance of the lesions, see under 'GREASY HEEL', and DERMATOPHILUS.

RAINFALL may influence outbreaks of HYPO-MAGNESAEMIA, BLOAT, FOOT-AND-MOUTH DISEASE.

RALES, or MOIST SOUNDS, are sounds heard by auscultation of the chest during various diseases. They are divided into two main classes: (1) *Crepitant* or *vesicular râles*, which are heard in the first stages of pneumonia, and are sharp, fine, crackling noises noticed during inspiration only. (2) *Mucous râles* are heard during expiration as well as during inspiration and may be described as bubbling or gurgling sounds.

RAM EPIDIDYMITIS. This is a disease of economic importance in most of the sheep-farming areas of the world. The cause is *Brucella ovis.* Diagnosis by clinical means (palpation, mainly) is not very satisfactory, as epididymitis may be due to other infections, so that laboratory tests are necessary (see *Laboratory Techniques in Brucellosis,* 1975, World Health Organisation). Vaccination and culling are methods of control, but vaccination is not free from problems.

RANCIDITY of cod-liver oil or other fish oils, etc., can be extremely dangerous. Rancid mash may bring about deficiencies of vitamins A, D, and E, with acute digestive disorders and death in chicks. Growing and adult birds may also suffer losses from this cause; with osteomalacia, and decreased egg production. (*See also under* VITAMIN E.)

RANGOON BEANS (*see* JAVA BEAN POISONING).

RANULA is a swelling which sometimes appears below the free portion of the dog's tongue. It is caused by a collection of saliva in one of the small ducts that carry saliva from the glands below the tongue, or farther back, into the mouth, and when of some size a ranula may cause considerable interference with feeding. It is treated by incision or excision, and is usually not serious.

RAPE POISONING occurs in animals which are not given hay or other food in addition to rape. Poisoning can be extremely serious, especially in sheep. Symptoms include dullness, red-coloured urine, and blindness. In one outbreak reported by the Reading VI Centre, 36 out of 360 sheep died from rape poisoning.

A form of light sensitisation called 'Rape Scald' occurs in sheep on rape. Swelling of the head occurs, there is irritation leading to rubbing, the ears may suffer damage. Jaundice may occur.

RAPESEED OIL. This has been shown experimentally to be toxic to the hearts of rats. The degree of toxicity varies according to the erucic acid content of the oil, and perhaps to closely related mono-ethylenic acids (*e.g.* cetoleic and nervonic). It is apparently the breakdown of erucic acid in the myocardium and skeletal muscles which produces the damaging effects.

'With ten or more mammalian or avian species reacting to rapeseed oil in much the same way, the economic implications of its adverse effects when incorporated in animal feedstuffs have long been apparent' (*Lancet,* 1974). The use of the oil in margarine manufacture and as a substitute for more expensive olive oil has led to anxiety over the effects on the human heart.

Rapeseed meal fed to poultry may depress growth and egg yield, and cause hypertrophy of the thyroid gland, liver haemorrhage, abnormalities of the skeleton, and a fishy taint in the eggs. The liver haemorrhages closely resembled those associated with the 'fatty liver/haemorragic syndrome'. (Martland, M. F. & others, *Research in Veterinary Science* (1984) **36,** 298.)

RAPHE means a ridge or furrow between the halves of an organ.

RAREFACTION OF BONE. A decrease in the mineral content.

RAT-BITE FEVER. This is a disease recognised in man and caused, following the bite of a rat (or, sometimes, dog, cat, mouse, weasel, or squirrel), by infection with (1) *Spirillum minus,* (2) *Streptobacillus moniliformis.* In addition to fever there may be an extensive rash.

RAT and MOUSE POISONS (*see* RODENTICIDES).

RATS are important from a veterinary point of view as carriers of infection to cattle, pigs, dogs, etc. Examples of rat-borne diseases are: Aujeszky's, Leptospirosis, Salmonellosis, Ringworm, Trichinosis, and Foot-and-mouth. (*See also* PETS, RODENTS.)

RATIONS FOR LIVESTOCK
Dairy Cattle.
WINTER RATIONING. The home-grown foods available naturally vary from farm to farm. Farm-mixed rations often make good use of barley. Proprietary compound feeding-stuffs are well balanced and formulated to contain all necessary ingredients such as vitamins, trace elements, etc., and are nowadays extensively used. Proprietary barley balancers and straw balancers are also much used. (*See also under* WINTER DIET.)

Rations: Theoretical basis for calculation. It is customary to regard the ration as being composed of two parts: (*a*) the 'maintenance' part, which provides the material for all vital activities and makes good the normal wear and tear of the body without causing increase or decrease in liveweight; (*b*) the 'production' part, which supplies the materials used for increase in body size, fat production, growth of the fetus, and milk production.

A D A S Advisory Paper No. 11, *Nutrient Allowances and Composition of Feeding-stuffs for Ruminants* contains two valuable sets of information. Firstly, what different classes and weights of ruminant stock need for maintenance and production. Secondly, the analyses of a wide variety of feeds.

Maintenance and 1-gallon rations for cows of Friesian breed or similar:

(a) Hay	18
Brewer's grains	10
Dried sugar beet pulp	4
(b) Hay	18
Dried sugar beet pulp	4
Silage	50

with parlour-fed concentrates, 3½ lb per gallon, for both (a) and (b).

Maintenance plus 2:

Ryegrass/lucerne haylage	*ad lib.*
Brewer's grains plus minerals	15 lb

with 4 lb hammer-milled maize fed in parlour for every additional gallon.

A ration for dairy cows used at Boxworth Experimental Husbandry Farm for many years:

	cwt
Rolled barley	12
Sugar beet pulp	2½
Kibbled beans	4
Groundnut meal	1½
Minerals	½

This ration is fed at the rate of 4 lb per gallon to Friesian cows.

SUMMER RATIONING. Grass is the standard summer food for cattle. On a good, well-managed pasture – where over-stocking is avoided – young, leafy grass will supply enough protein for high yielders, but they will require additional carbohydrate. This may be supplied in the form of cereals, *e.g.* 4 lb for each gallon of milk over about 4 produced per day. If the pasture is less good, cereals will be required for each gallon over 3.

Kenneth Russell recommended that in April, cows grazing young, leafy grass 4 to 6 inches high for 4 hours daily, should receive 7 lb hay and cereals (plus a mineral mixture) at the rate of 4 lb for each gallon over 3. In May, with unrestricted grazing of grass 8 or 10 inches long at the pre-flowering stage, the hay is discontinued; the cereal ration remaining as before. In June and July, with grass at the flowering stage, the cows receive balanced concentrates for yields over 2½ gallons (June), then over 2. In August, grazing aftermath (or green fodder during a drought), the cows receive concentrates for each gallon over 1. In September, with young aftermath or maiden seeds, there is a hay ration of 7 lb (or 28 lb kale) plus concentrates for yields over 2 gallons per day.

Beef cattle (*see Table re suckler cows, and under* BEEF).

Calves. *See* CALF-REARING.

Pigs:

Creep Feed	Per cent
Barley meal	40
Flaked maize	30
White fish-meal	15
Wheatings	15

Breeders and Growers*	Per cent
Barley meal	70
White fish-meal	10
Wheatings	10
Ground maize	10

Fatteners*	Per cent
Barley meal	75
Soya bean-meal	5
Wheatings	20

*Plus mineral and vitamin supplements.

Rations for suckler cows						
	Autumn calvers			Spring calvers		
	Blue-Grey	Hereford × Friesian			Blue-Grey	Hereford × Friesian
	(kg per day)				(kg per day)	
Calving to mating			*Mid-pregnancy to calving*			
1. Grass silage			1. Grass silage			
(25% DM, 60D)	27	27			20	20
Mineralised barley	1¼	2	Mineralised barley		½	½
2. Hay (57D) 35%	8	10	2. Hay		6	7
protein concentrate	1¾	1¾	Protein concentrate		½	½
			3. Barley straw		7	7
			Protein concentrate		1½	1¾
Mating to turnout			*Calving to turnout*			
1. Grass silage	25	27	1. Grass silage		25	27
Mineralised barley	½	¾	Mineralised barley		1	1
2. Hay	7	8	2. Hay		8	8½
Protein concentrate	¾	¾	Protein concentrate		1	1
During this period cows can lose about 0·5 kg per day so that condition falls by about ½ score to turnout.			3. Barley straw		7	7
			Protein concentrate		2¾	3¼
Mid-pregnancy to calving						
	grazing	grazing			grazing	grazing

Sheep (*see under* SHEEP, *and* FLUSHING OF EWES).

Horses. (*See under* HORSES, FEEDING OF.)

Poultry:

Chicks to 12 weeks	*Per cent*
Maize meal	23
Ground barley	10
Ground oats	10
Ground wheat	20
Wheat bran	13
Grass meal	5
White fish-meal	10
Soya bean-meal	5
Dried yeast	1½
Ground limestone	1
Salt mixture	½
(10 parts of common salt, 1 of manganese sulphate)	
Vitamin pre-mix	1

Layers'/Growers' Mash (Balancer for grain)	*Per cent*
Ground wheat	30
Ground barley	25
Wheat middlings	8
Wheat bran	5
Grass meal	8
White fish-meal	3
Meat and bone-meal	3
Soya bean-meal	10
Ground limestone	3
Steamed bone-flour	2½
Salt mixture	½
Vitamin pre-mix	2

RAVC. The Royal Army Veterinary Corps, which has a long and honourable history. An Army Veterinary Service was established in 1796; this became the Army Veterinary Corps in 1906; the title of 'Royal' being bestowed in 1918.

A History of the RAVC 1796–1919 was compiled by Major-General Sir Frederick Smith, KCMG, CB, a former Director-General, Army Veterinary Services, and published by Baillière, Tindall & Cox. A second volume, by Brigadier J. Clabby, was published in 1963. (J. A. Allen & Co.)

RBV (*see* PROGENY TESTING).

RCVS. The Royal College of Veterinary Surgeons, 32 Belgrave Square, London. The governing body of the veterinary profession in the United Kingdom. (*See also* REGISTER.)

REAGINIC ANTIBODIES. These are immunoglobulins which become fixed to mast cells and, in the presence of antigen, cause the release of histamine (and other compounds) giving rise to allergic reaction. (*See* ALLERGY, ASTHMA.) They react with antigens produced by parasitic worms.

RECEPTORS. These are or contain antibody molecules, occur on the surface of lymphocytes, and enable specific antigens to be recognised. (*See under* IMMUNE RESPONSE, BLOOD.)

Physiological receptors include those for enzymes, and for hormones.

RECESSIVES (*see* GENETICS).

RECOVERY QUILTS for cats and dogs have been developed. Marketed as Flectabed, the quilts contain Flectalon, a special fibre developed for emergency blankets. It is stated that the product reflects back 95 per cent of the infrared heat lost by the body. Details from Flectabed, 17a Moor Street, Chepstow, Gwent BP6 5DB.

RECTUM commences on a level with the anterior opening of the pelvis and extends to the anus, passing through the upper part of the pelvic cavity. In most of the domesticated animals it possesses a dilatation, known as the 'ampulla', which serves to collect the faeces that are slowly passed into it from the colon, and holds them until time and circumstances are convenient for their evacuation to the outside. (*See* INTESTINE.)

RECTUM, DISEASES OF. With the exception of the dog the domestic animals are comparatively free from disease of this part of the alimentary system.

Impaction. This occurs mainly in dogs (and to a lesser extent in cats) when pieces of bone, string, and other foreign materials form with the faeces a hard mass. The affected animal attempts to pass faeces, but after considerable efforts fails to do so. If the impacted material contains spicules of bone or other hard material every effort at defaecation causes the animal to cry out with the pain.

Removal of the offending matter is effected by the administration of an enema of glycerine, oil, or soapy water, and the introduction of the lubricated finger. Hard masses are broken up and taken away in portions if too large to remove whole. A mild laxative should be given by the mouth after the impacted material has been cleared from the rectum, and the dog should receive a soft semi-fluid diet for some days afterwards.

Inflammation of the rectum may follow impaction, or it may commence as the result of an injury. The animal frequently strains, and the owner may surmise that it is constipated, but exploration reveals the absence of faeces.

Abscesses, tumours and ulcers may also affect the rectum, but they are not common. (*See also* ANAL GLANDS.)

Prolapse of the rectum may occur in any animal, but is especially common in the smaller animals. A portion of the gut is protruded from the anus to an extent of a few inches. It appears as a tumorous swelling of a bright-red appearance, cold to the touch, and usually covered with mucus or faecal material. There is usually some straining when the condition is of recent origin, but after a time the animal appears to become used to the protrusion of the piece of bowel, and only strains when it is handled or when attempts are made to return it. Anaesthesia or analgesia will be needed. It may be gently bathed with warm water containing common salt in solution (5 per cent) while awaiting assistance. An operation, in which the rectum is sutured to some part of the abdominal roof, is sometimes necessary to prevent its recurrence after replacement. Prolapsed rectum is not uncommon in the horse. Sometimes it may be easily returned by placing the neck of a quart bottle within the central depression that is always present, and pressing slowly and cautiously in a forward direction.

In some instances amputation of the protruded portion becomes necessary, especially if it has been outside for some considerable time and has become gangrenous.

RECUMBENCY. In a veterinary sense, this means not merely lying down but also a failure to get up. (*See* 'DOWNER COW' SYNDROME.) In animals in dorsal recumbency during anaesthesia, pressure of viscera on the posterior VENA CAVA may result in hypotension. It was suggested (Blakemore, W. F. and others, *Veterinary Record* (1984) **114,** 569) that a slightly oblique dorsal recumbency is advisable: and they reported a case in which hypotension was followed by spinal cord necrosis, leading to paralysis of a horse's hindlegs, necessitating euthanasia.

Anaesthetised horses, when positioned in left lateral recumbency, showed least muscle or nerve injuries when lying on a water mattress. Foam rubber was far from satisfactory.

RECURRENT LARYNGEAL NERVE is a branch of the vagus nerve which leaves the latter at different points on the right and left sides of the body. On the right side it leaves the parent nerve opposite the second rib, curves inwards round the subclavian or the costo-cervical artery, and runs up the neck on the lower surface of the trachea and below the carotid of the same side. In the case of the left, the branch leaves the vagus where that nerve crosses the arch of the aorta, winds inwards around the concavity of the aortic arch, and runs up the neck in a position similar to that of the right side. Both nerves supply the muscles of the larynx which are concerned in the production of voice and in maintaining the glottis open during ordinary and forced respiration.

RED SQUILL. Preparations of the dried ground bulbs of the sea onion, *Urginea maritima,* are used for poisoning rodents, baits being made up to contain 10 per cent Red Squill. Domestic animals refrain from eating such preparations owing to the smell and taste. Symptoms of poisoning include profuse vomiting in the pig but not in the cat, according to one report, excitement, muscular incoordination, and convulsions. Poisoning in rodents by Red Squill may be agonising and very prolonged. Its use in the UK is banned.

RED URINE. Causes of red discoloration of the urine include: Red water Fever, Leptospirosis, Post-parturient Haemoglobinuria. Azoturia, infection with *Clostridium haemolyticum,* kale and rape poisoning, dosing with phenothiazine, pyelonephritis, poisoning by turpentine, and the drinking of very large quantities of water.

RED-WATER FEVER (British Isles), BABESIOSIS or PIROPLASMOSIS, is a disease of cattle and sheep, due to the presence in the blood of a protozöon parasite which attacks the red blood cells, destroying their envelopes and liberating haemoglobin, which is excreted by the kidneys and colours the urine reddish or blackish. It occurs mainly in the south and west of England, in the north and west of Scotland, and practically all over Ireland, but it is also seen at times in districts that are not included in these areas. It is common in low-lying, rough-pastured, and moorland districts, where ticks, which harbour and transmit the parasite, can find abundant shelter and suitable breeding places. Cattle are exclusively attacked from the age of about 3 months upwards, but young calves are practically immune. One attack gives a degree of immunity, and cattle that have been bred upon infected farms, and from infected cattle, are more resistant than those brought from a clean district. It is more prevalent in the spring and autumn months, since the ticks are then at their maximum activity.

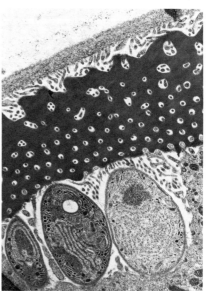

An electron microscope picture showing three profiles of *Babesia divergens* – the cause of redwater fever – inside the egg of a tick. (With acknowledgements to IRAD, Compton.)

CAUSE. *Babesia (Piroplasma) divergens.* This is transmitted by the common tick, *Ixodes ricinus,* and occasionally by *Haemophysalis punctata.* (*See under* BABESIA *and* TICKS; *also* MUSCLES, DISEASES OF; MYOGLOBINURIA.)

SIGNS. Two varieties of the disease are recognised: an acute and a mild form.

The *acute type* is sudden in its onset and frequently fatal. The animal becomes very dull and depressed, separates itself from the rest of the herd, moves slowly or not at all, grunts, groans, arches its back, salivates freely, grinds its teeth, and often staggers and falls. The coat becomes hard and staring, the skin is dry and often hidebound, and there is almost always a profuse, watery, violent diarrhoea. The temperature rises to as high as 105° to 107°F, the pulse is fast and weak (often 100 per minute), and the respirations are laboured, blowing, and rapid (80 to 100 per minute). The visible mucous membranes are pale. After a few days the animal's distress becomes less acute, and the most alarming symptoms subside. The signs of fever, however, are still evident, and the cow is still in a serious condition. The urine usually shows some degree of coloration, which varies from a clear reddish claret to a deep dark brown or black – almost like stout.

The duration of acute attacks varies, but it is seldom that the high temperature lasts for more than a week. Death may take place in from 3 to 5 days, or later on, when it is usually due to exhaustion.

In the *mild type* the urine is not usually highly coloured; there is only slight dullness and loss of appetite. The animals are ill for a week or 10 days, and the only marked sequel is anaemia.

There are *irregular forms* of red-water met with at times, in which the general symptoms are similar to these seen in the typical acute attack, but the urine does not become discoloured. Many of these cases end fatally.

TREATMENT. 'Imazol Injection' (Coopers Animal Health Ltd, Berkhamsted). For use under prescription only.

The main conditions of the licence are as follows:

— animals must not be slaughtered for human consumption during treatment;

— cattle may be slaughtered for human consumption only after at least a 90-day withdrawal period from the last treatment;

— milk for human consumption may be taken only from cattle after at least a 21-day withdrawal period from the last treatment; and

— the local ministry divisional veterinary officer is notified about each sale of Imizol Injection to a veterinary surgeon.

The conditions of granting the licence also include a requirement that veterinary surgeons who prescribe Imizol are advised that:

— full records of product administration to identifiable animals must be maintained and that it is the duty of the farmer to keep a careful record of all administration of the product, as required by the Animals and Fresh Meat (Examination for Residues) Regulations 1988;

— the local DVO must be notified of the address of the farm where treatment is to take place; and

— farmers should be informed that they must notify the local DVO when treated animals go for slaughter for human consumption or when milk from treated animals is intended for human consumption.

Any suspected adverse reactions, including evidence of lack of efficacy, should be reported to the Veterinary Medicines Directorate immediately. Dr J. M. Rutter, Veterinary Medicines Directorate, New Haw, Weybridge, Surrey. (*Veterinary Record*, July 28, 1990).

Ticks should be removed, either by hand-picking or by spraying with a suitable parasiticide. (*See* TICKS, CONTROL OF.)

The few piroplasms taken into the blood-stream, when young cattle are bitten by infected ticks, tend not to multiply but to give rise to a useful degree of immunity. This may wane if the piroplasms die, so that the animal becomes susceptible again. Immunity may likewise break down if the animal becomes ill from some other cause.

CONTROL. Measures involve tick control, and not mixing cattle from Redwater areas with susceptible cattle. Even then there are risks. Professor D. W. Brocklesby commented (1978):

'Recent work in Scotland has revealed that about 30% of the 100,000 cattle that are imported from Ireland through Glasgow each year are carriers of *B. divergens*. Similar cattle were responsible for 20 deaths when local cattle were placed on sea marsh land in Lincolnshire that had previously been used for fattening Irish steers. Cornish cattle brought to a farm in Sussex set up a focus of infection because infected ticks became established in the new habitat. Simmental, Charolais and other European breeds are imported into Britain with no screening for blood parasites: there is already a possibility that *Babesia bovis* may have been imported into Northern Ireland from France.'

RED-WATER (USA), also called Bacillary Hemoglobinuria, or ictero-haemoglobinuria, occurs in California, Colorado, Idaho, Louisiana, Montana, Nevada, Oregon, Texas, and Utah. *Clostridium haemolyticum* is the cause. (*See also* TEXAS FEVER, the American Red-water Fever.)

RED WORMS. The common name for Strongyles. These can cause severe anaemia, unthriftiness, and debility. (*See under* FOALS, DISEASES OF; *also under* VERMINOUS ARTERITIS; HORSES, WORMS IN.) Thiabendazole is a useful drug for the removal of red worms in horses. (*See also* ROUNDWORMS.)

'REDFOOT'. A condition seen in new-born lambs, in which the sensitive laminae of the feet become exposed owing to detachment of the overlying horn. The cause is unknown, no treatment effective, and the lambs soon die.

REDUPLICATION is a term applied to a duplication of the normal heart sounds as heard by auscultation. There are heard a first and a second sound in a normal heart-beat, and in the above condition one or both of these may be doubled. It is found in certain diseases of the heart, such as obstruction of the valve between the auricle and ventricle on the left side of the organ (the mitral valve).

REFLEX ACTION is one of the simplest forms of activity of the nervous system. For the mechanism *see* NERVES.

Superficial reflexes are well instanced in the sudden shivering movement that is seen when a fly or other insect settles upon the skin of a horse, particularly in the region of the back of the shoulder.

Visceral reflexes are those connected with various

organs, such as the narrowing of the pupil when the eye is exposed to a bright light. (*See* SPINAL CORD.)

REGIONAL ANAESTHESIA. This consists in the anaesthetisation of a region of the body by means of a local anaesthetic solution injected either into the connective tissue surrounding a sensory nerve trunk or into the spinal canal. (*See* EPIDURAL ANAESTHESIA, ANALGESICS.) The most common example of perineural injection is Plantar Block in the horse.

REGISTER OF VETERINARY SURGEONS, THE, lists members of the profession who qualified in the UK. It may be consulted in some public libraries or is obtainable from the Royal College of Veterinary Surgeons, 32 Belgrave Square, London. (*See also under* VETERINARY SURGEONS ACT, 1948.)

REHYDRATION. The restoration of the correct levels of water and electrolytes in animals suffering from DEHYDRATION (which see).

REINDEER. (*Rangifer tarandus.*) Parasites include the warble fly *Edoede magena tarandi*, and the nostril fly *Cephenomyia trampe.*

RELAPSE. A relapse occasionally occurs when antibiotic or sulpha drug treatment of an infectious disease is stopped – the infection having been suppressed but the animal's powers of resistance not having been stimulated to establish a sufficient degree of immunity. Some forms of lameness are particularly liable to relapses, especially those associated with sprains of tendons or ligaments.

RELATIVE BREEDING VALUE (*see* PROGENY TESTING).

'REMOTE INJECTION' METHOD (*see* PROJECTILE SYRINGES).

RENAL. Relating to the kidney.

RENIN. An enzyme, secreted by the kidneys, which may control the secretion of the hormone aldosterone by the adrenal glands.

REOVIRUS. The name derives from the words 'respiratory enteric orphan virus'. Reoviruses have double-stranded ribonucleic acid (RNA), and will replicate and produce changes in cells of cattle, pigs, dogs, cats, rabbits, monkeys, and man. (*See also* CALF PNEUMONIA.)

REPAIR of tissue after injury is described under WOUNDS, and for the repair of special tissues *see* under BONE, MUSCLE, NERVE, etc. (*See also* HOOF REPAIR.)

REPRODUCTION.

Ovulation. This is described under OVARIES.

At OVULATION (which see) the Graäfian follicle bursts, and the ovum is expelled by the rush of the escaping fluid. (*See* OVARY.) The cavity of the Graäfian follicle becomes filled with special cells to form the *corpus luteum*, and the ovum begins its career as an absolute entity. In normal circumstances the fimbriated and dilated funnel-shaped end of the Fallopian tube, or oviduct, is applied to the point at which a follicle will burst, so that upon escape of its ovum this latter may be caught and retained. The dilated end of the oviduct is usually known as the vestibule, and it is in this part that the sperm *usually* meets the ovum and fertilises it.

Coitus. The act of copulation. As mentioned under OESTRUS (which also see), service by the male is only allowed during the period of oestrus by the females of the majority of species of higher animals. At other times there is little or no desire exhibited by the male, and all attentions are resented by the female. Artificial methods of domestication have to some extent modified the frequency and duration of oestrus, so that the domestic animals sheltered under the protection of man, breed more frequently than do the majority of wild animals of similar species.

During one ejaculation of an adult vigorous stallion about 80,000,000 sperms are released. As soon as the sperms are free in the uterus or vagina, they travel towards wherever the ovum is situated. This they accomplish partly by a kind of wriggling movement of their tail, which drives them onwards always in one direction. They are attracted to the ovum by 'chemotaxis'.

Fertilisation. Somewhere in the oviduct, generally in its vestibule but not necessarily so, the spermatozoa arrive in the region of the waiting ovum. More than one sperm may *penetrate* the wall of the ovum, but except in rare instances (giving rise to PRIMARY MOSAICISM) only one sperm *fertilises* the ovum.

The sperm having penetrated the ovum, loses its tail, which is no longer required, and lies within the protoplasm of the ovum. The nucleus of the ovum and that of the head of the sperm now fuse, each contributing half the number of chromosomes that are to be found present in nearly all the cells of the future young animal. The fused body is known as the *segmentation nucleus*, and from it, when it begins to divide, all the body cells of the embryo are formed. The process of the formation of the young embryo is considered under EMBRYOLOGY, to which further reference should be made. (*See also* TESTIS, OVARY, OESTRUS, BREEDING OF ANIMALS, PREGNANCY, PARTURITION, PARTHENOGENESIS, etc.)

REPRODUCTIVE ORGANS (*see* diagrams following sections headed UTERUS and PENIS).

REPTILES. They tend to move to warmer places when they are ill. Accordingly, keepers often raise the temperature to help them recover; but sometimes this can worsen the disease and result in deaths. It is suggested that their housing should be divided up into areas having different temperatures (within the species' natural limits) so that the reptiles can choose which area suits them best at different stages of the disease. (Warwick, C. *Applied Animal Behaviour Science* (1991) **28,** 375). (*See also* PETS.)

RESECTION is an operation in which a part of some organ is removed, as, for example, the resection of a piece of dead bone, or resection of a part of the intestine which is diseased; resection of a rib in thoractomy; aural resection done to overcome chronic disease of a dog's ear.

RESERPINE. A tranquilliser, which lowers the blood pressure and has been used for this purpose in turkeys. (*See* AORTIC RUPTURE.) It is an alkaloid obtained from the roots of *Rauwolfia serpentina* and *R. vomitoria*, and has been used in the treatment of lathyrism; and it is an officially approved UK rodenticide.

RESISTANT STRAINS. This phrase is commonly used of bacteria which are not sensitive to antibiotics, or of insects which are not killed by, *e.g.* DDT.

RESISTANCE TRANSFERABILITY (*see under* PLASMIDS, ANTIBIOTIC RESISTANCE).

RESORPTION. Mummification. Resorption of the fetus occurs, *e.g.* in heifers receiving a high calcium and low phosphorus diet. It may occur in the sow with Aujeszky's disease, and is by no means a rare occurrence in the bitch and cat. (*See* MUMMIFICATION.)

RESPIRATION (*see* AIR PASSAGES, LUNGS).

Mechanism of respiration. For the structure of the respiratory apparatus *see* AIR PASSAGES, LUNGS, etc.

Inspiration is due to muscular effort which enlarges the chest in all three dimensions, so that the lungs have to expand in order to fill up the vacuum that would otherwise be left; and since, although the lungs are not fixed to the chest wall, surface tension between the pleura lining the chest and the pleura covering the lungs, has much the same effect.

In most vertebrates, except birds, the lungs are not normally attached to the walls of the chest, but are rather suspended in them from their 'roots', so that there is no direct pull upon the lungs when the chest cavity increases in size. The vertical diameter of the chest is increased during inspiration through the downward tilting of the sternum. This movement is best seen in the dog when it is out of breath; at other times, and in other animals, it is so slight that it escapes detection. The transverse dimension of the chest increases when any one of the ribs behind the first 2 or 3 are forcibly pulled forward by muscular action. Each rib only moves a small amount, but the mass effect of the series is very considerable. The muscles which bring about these changes in

ordinary inspiration are the diaphragm, the intercostal muscles which are situated in two layers between each rib and its two neighbours, and possibly the levators of the ribs, and the serratus muscles.

When the chest expands, the lungs expand too; but initially the quantity of air within them remains the same. Accordingly, the pressure falls, leading to an inflow of air.

Expiration is in ordinary circumstances merely an elastic recoil, the diaphragm moving forward and the ribs settling back into their original positions, partly through muscular action, and partly through the elasticity of their cartilages. It occupies a slightly longer period of time than does inspiration.

Nervous control. Respiration is usually an automatic act under the control of the *respiratory centre* in the medulla oblongata.

Although the respiratory centre is itself capable of carrying on respiration, it is in its turn liable to be controlled by the higher conscious centres. This is seen particularly well in human beings, where it is possible to 'hold the breath', or inhibit respiration for considerable periods, when diving underwater, for example.

Rate of respiration. The speed of the respirations varies with many internal and external factors. It is faster during fevers, after violent exercise, or even after mild exercise (though it soon returns to normal upon cessation); during powerful emotions, such as fear, anger, sexual excitement, etc.; during very cold or very hot weather; when the body condition is very fat, or when radiation is obstructed, through too thick a covering of wool, fur, etc., or too much clothing. (*See also* ANAEMIA.)

It is slower than normal during resting, either when merely lying or when sleeping; in cases of unconsciousness.

The normal rates in adult domesticated animals are as follows:

Horse	8–12 per minute
Ox	12–16 per minute
Sheep and goat	12–20 per minute
Pig	10–16 per minute
Dog	15–30 per minute

In each case the larger the particular animal the slower does it breathe, other things being equal; for instance, a Shetland pony respires about 12 times per minute, while a Shire stallion respires only 8 times; also, the young of any species breathe faster than do adults; and females breathe faster than males – especially during pregnancy.

	Inspired air	Expired air
	Per cent	Per cent
Nitrogen	79·04	79·04
Oxygen	20·93	16·02
Carbon dioxide	0·03	4·38

When this air is taken into the lungs its composition is altered, so that upon leaving the lungs its CO_2 content is about 4 per cent greater and its oxygen content about 4 per cent less.

Quantity of air. The lungs do not by any means completely empty themselves at each expiration and refill at each inspiration. What is left after maximum expiration is called the *residual volume.* The volume of air exchanged during normal breathing (*i.e.* passing in and out of the nose) is the *tidal volume* – about 5 litres in the horse. The volume of air in the airways leading to the alveoli of the lungs is the *anatomical dead space.* Air available for the supply of oxygen in the lungs is the tidal volume minus the anatomical dead space.

Irregular forms of respiration. Apart from mere changes in rate and force, the respiration is modified in various ways under certain conditions. *Coughing* is a series of violent expirations, during each of which the larynx is at first closed until the pressure of air in the lungs and lower passages is considerably raised, and then suddenly opened, so that the contained air is released under pressure and rushes to the outside; its object is to expel some irritating object from the air passages. *Sneezing* is a single sudden expiration, which differs from coughing in that the sudden rush of air is directed by the soft palate up into the nose in order to expel some source of irritation from the nasal chambers. It is particularly well exhibited by the dog.
Yawning is a deep slow inspiration followed by a short expiration, the air being taken in by the open mouth as well as by the nose. *Hiccough*, is due to a sudden spasmodic contraction of the diaphragm, along with a sudden closing of the larynx, producing a sound not unlike a very loud heart-beat. *Hyperpnoea* is a term applied to the slightly increased frequency and depth of respiration occurring during gentle exercise, or from some mild stimulus to the respiratory centre. *Dyspnoea* means that there is distinct distress in breathing,

due to a more powerful stimulus to the respiratory centre, and is usually characterised by convulsive movements of the chest and diaphragm. It is frequently the forerunner of asphyxia. *Apnoea* is seen when there is a hyperoxygenation of the tissues, and consequently no further immediate demands for oxygen. It consists of a complete cessation of the respiratory movements without the exhibition of any distress. It is artificially produced in human beings when a diver takes ten or twelve deep breaths before entering the water, where he must hold his breath. It is not commonly seen in the domestic animals; but the seal and other diving animals have developed the power of inducing apnoea to a very marked extent. (*See also under* ASTHMA, LARYNGEAL PARALYSIS, VOICE, TACHYPNOEA, etc.)

RESPIRATORY DIFFICULTY, FAILURE (*see under* BREATHLESSNESS, ANAEMIA, OEDEMA of the lungs, ASPHYXIA, BRONCHITIS, PNEUMONIA, FOG FEVER, ANAESTHETICS). Many poisons bring about respiratory failure; *e.g.* chloroform, hydrocyanic acid, paraquat.

RESPIRATORY DISEASE IN PIGS. A total of 65 pigs from 8 'problem' herds, in which clinical disease was present, and 44 pigs from 'control' herds, were bought and examined at the Central Veterinary Laboratory, Weybridge (Little, T. W. A., *Vet. Rec.* (1975) **96**, 540). It was found that 'a confused picture arises because there appears no clear-cut, one-way causal relationship between microbial agents and disease; indeed the same organisms appear in both diseased and healthy pigs'.

Although it was possible to find groups of pigs with rhinitis and groups with pneumonia, in most cases there was evidence of a combination of the two conditions of varying severity.

Inclusion-body rhinitis virus frequently infects very young pigs – even the fetus; and during the first 4 months of life the possible sequence of

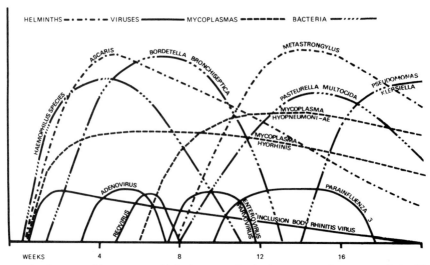

Diagram showing a possible sequence of infections occurring in the upper respiratory tract of pigs (Crown copyright. With acknowledgements also to Mr T. W. A. Little and the *Veterinary Record*.)

infections in the upper respiratory tract of pigs may be complex, with viruses, mycoplasmas, worms all perhaps involved (*see* diagram).

Enzootic pneumonia may depend in part for its cause on a synergism between a mycoplasma and an adenovirus. Then again, *Haemophilus* bacteria may be present in enzootic-pneumonia-like lesions, but replaced at some stage by *Pasteurella multocida.*

Not all the factors involved in respiratory disease are infections. Management factors play their part, too. Space allowance per pig, number of pigs per group, effects of mixing and crowding, temperature, humidity, nutrition, age and genetic status of the pigs all exert their effects. (*See also under* RHINITIS, ATROPHIC.)

RESPIRATORY STIMULANTS. These include niketamide (Coramine), Dopram-V (Willow Francis); Dalophylline Gel (Arnolds); Eatamiphylline camsylate, BP.

RESPIRATORY SYNCYTIAL VIRUS was first isolated from chimpanzees showing 'cold-like' signs; and since the mid-1950s it has been detected in clinical cases of respiratory disease in man, cattle, sheep, and goats, and horses. A cause of acute bronchiolitis and alveolitis.

RESTRAINT. In order to examine an animal thoroughly for signs of injury or disease; in order to carry out inoculations, or even to administer an anaesthetic, some form of restraint is often necessary.

The introduction of **Etorphine ('Immobilon')** facilitated the handling of horses and cattle, and also dogs (but *not* cats), and obviated the use of several means of restraint described below. (*See also* TRANQUILLISERS, XYLAZINE, ANALGESIA.)

The following methods should not be used indiscriminately upon any and every animal. A method that is sufficient to restrain one animal may prove aggravating to another; *e.g.* while the common twitch may serve for a heavy draught gelding, it is very likely to cause a thoroughbred stallion to be more restive than ever. A person who finds it necessary to employ some means of restraint should first of all consider the temperament, age, breed, and, if possible, the individual characteristics of the animal, as well as the purpose of the restraint, before deciding upon what methods will be employed. Firm gentleness, a kindly spoken word, and a hand-pat, with a little coaxing or urging, will very often allay an animal's fears, but there are those of a surly morose nature which will not respond to gentleness, and will only recognise mastery when they are cowed by a show of might; it is to such particularly that such methods as will be described here are applicable.

Horses. The usual halter, head-stall, or bridle is generally sufficient to control broken horses that are to be handled or examined without the infliction of pain. In some cases it may be necessary to tie the animal to a ring in the wall or manger, or to the heel-posts, but it is better in such cases to take a couple of turns round the ring and

have a man hold the end of the rope. For measures which involve handling of the hind parts of the body, it is usually advisable to have one of the fore-feet picked up and held (preferably that upon the same side of the body as the operator is to work).

For greater control a TWITCH (which see) may be applied. (*See also* TRANQUILLISERS, ANAESTHETICS.)

Cattle. A cattle crush, either of a commercial pattern or one constructed of timber by farm labour, is useful (*see* CRUSHES) for inoculations, etc. (*See also* VETERINARY FACILITIES ON THE FARM.)

In the case of comparatively quiet cattle, milk cows, etc., it will generally suffice if an assistant takes the animal by the nose. The thumb and middle finger of one hand are inserted into the respective nostrils, and the nasal septum is pinched between them. It is important that the stockman's fingers do not block up the airway.

The other hand may be placed under the jaw. In this position the majority of adult quiet cattle can be easily held. For bulls and those cattle that are more difficult to control it is usual to use a pair of *bull-holders, 'bull-dogs', 'bull-tongs',* or if the animal is already rung (with a copper or aluminium ring), to attach a rope or *bull-leader* to the ring in the nose. For drenching purposes it is necessary to keep the head and neck in as straight a line as possible to obviate the risk of choking. If an assistant is needed he should stand on the opposite side of the beast and take the horns in his hands so that he may tilt the head upwards and at the same time keep the head and neck straight out. A pair of bull-holders may be inserted into the nostrils, and have a rope attached to them which is passed over a beam and the head pulled up.

For lifting one hind-leg, a pole, broom handle, etc., may be placed in front of that hock and behind and above the other. Two men take hold of ends of the pole and pull the leg upwards and backwards, at the same time steadying the animal's balance by leaning against its thighs with their shoulders. For the fore-feet it is usual to pass a rope around the cannon or above the heels and over the back to the opposite side, where it is held by an assistant. (*See also* CATTLE CRUSH, VETERINARY FACILITIES ON FARMS, TRANQUILISERS.)

Sheep. For most purposes the sheep may be turned up into a position in which it sits upon its rump, by placing the left hand round under the neck from the near side, and the right hand over the back to seize the wool of the abdomen, lifting the animal's fore-end off the ground and twisting its hind-legs from under it. In this position its feet may be dressed, its fleece may be examined, etc. With in-lamb ewes it is not advisable to turn them owing to the possibility of doing them damage; they may be held against a wall or fence by an assistant while their feet, etc., are being dressed. Sheep stocks are sometimes used; or modern shearing tables.

Pigs. The adult pig is proverbially a difficult animal to handle and restrain, especially when the handling involves pain or discomfort, but piglets are easily held by the hind-legs with the hands, while the knees grip the dependent head. With large sows and boars it is wise to remember that they are apt to be vicious with strangers, and to use a shield of wood or a hurdle to prevent a rush by the angry animal.

A method of securing a large pig is to drive it into a corner and pen it there with a door, gate, or heavy hurdle carried by two men, and held so that the pig has no room to turn while a noose is dropped over its head and pulled tight round its jaws, and another is secured to a hind-leg above the hock. The ends of these ropes are then passed round a post or a rail in the fence and pulled tight when the pig is released from its corner.

Dogs and cats. These animals are usually more easily restrained than some of the larger animals because of their intimate association with man, but there are certain animals that present difficulty when angry or excited. A kind word and a caress will often be necessary to gain the animal's confidence before attempting to examine it, and, wherever possible, severe methods of restraint should be avoided except as a last resort. The human voice often exercises a degree of control over an excitable animal, and there are certain people who appear to possess the faculty of immediately gaining almost any dog's confidence and of being able to do anything with it.

However, it is always wise in any case of doubt to take no risks. The safest way of dealing with a dog is to muzzle it first.

A *tape muzzle* may be applied. This latter is simply a piece of tape or a bandage about 3 feet long whose middle is wound round the dog's nose, the ends being crossed under the jaw and tied round the neck or on to the collar. With bulldogs, and those with a short face and a pug nose, it is better to tie the tape round the jaws, finishing with the end above the nose, tying them together there, and then passing the ends back to the collar.

Cats can be rolled in a sack or towel. With cats it is important to prevent them from using their claws, which inflict injuries more often than do the teeth. (*See also under* TRANQUILLISER, ANAESTHETICS.)

RESUSCITATION. A simple method of pulmonary resuscitation with expired air, using a device portable and simple enough for emergency use by herdsmen and shepherds is in use on farms.

The device consists of a mouthpiece, non-return valve, flange, and mouth tube. (Weaver, B. M. Q. & Angell-James, J. *Veterinary Record* (1986) **119**, 86). (*See* ARTIFICIAL RESPIRATION, RESPIRATORY STIMULANTS, ACUPUNCTURE.)

RETENTION OF AFTERBIRTH (*see* PLACENTA, RETAINED).

RETICULOCYTES. The penultimate stage in the formation of red blood cells. Reticulocytes are numerous in the blood only in anaemic conditions and indicate an effort of the blood-forming tissues to restore the red-blood cell count to normal levels.

RETICULO-ENDOTHELIAL SYSTEM. This depends upon special cells present in the liver, spleen, lymph nodes and bone marrow. The system removes antigens from the body (*see under* ANTIBODY), and also red cells from the blood.

RETICULUM. The second stomach of ruminants. *See the diagram under* ABDOMEN.

RETINA. Detachment of, or haemorrhage into, is a cause of sudden blindness in dogs. It is often due to hypertension; the long-term effects of which may be hypertrophy of the left ventricle of the heart and kidney failure. (*See* EYE *and* EYE, INJURIES AND DISEASES OF).

RETINOBLASTOMA. A type of tumour which occurs on the retina.

RETRO- is a prefix signifying behind or turned backward.

RETROPHARYNGEAL ABSCESS is the name given to an abscess occurring at the back of the throat in the region behind the pharynx. Such abscesses generally make swallowing difficult or impossible until they burst, which they frequently do into the cavity of the pharynx, whence the pus is swallowed. (*See* STRANGLES.)

RETROVIRIDAE. The family of viruses which includes the LENTIVIRUSES (which see).

RETROVIRUS. Retroviruses are naturally occurring gene transfer organisms. When it infects a cell the virus is uncoated, the viral RNA is transcribed into DNA and this DNA integrates into one of the cell's chromosomes. This property could be used to produce disease resistant transgenic animals.

Certain viral groups appear to need the presence of a receptor on the cell membrane in order to gain access into the cell. Retroviruses carry a glycoprotein on their surface and a specific interaction with this glycoprotein and the cellular receptor are a prerequisite for infection. Blocking this receptor, said Mr Cameron, of the University of Glasgow, might prevent infection and he and his colleagues were currently producing cell lines and transgenic mice to test this hypothesis.

This group includes the Lentiviruses and Oncoviruses. (*See* VIRUSES table.)

(*See also* GENETIC ENGINEERING.)

RHABDOMYOLOSIS. A breakdown of skeletal muscle; in consequence of which the urine contains myoglobin. (*See* EQUINE MYOGLOBINURIA.)

RHABDOVIRUS. A group of bullet-shaped viruses which includes the rabies virus and that of vesicular stomatitis.

RHEUMATISM. A general term indicating diseases of muscles, tendons, joints, bones, or nerves, resulting in pain and disability.

Rheumatism is seen in dogs, pigs, and horses most commonly, but it affects all of the domesticated animals. Young animals are most often attacked by the acute type, especially young pigs and puppies, and adults by the muscular form and by chronic or articular rheumatism.

For the *muscular type see under* MUSCLES, DISEASES OF.

TREATMENT. There is no absolute specific, although certain drugs have enjoyed a great reputation in the alleviation of this disease, especially salicylates. Phenyl-butazone has been used with reported success. (*See also* CORTISONE.)

RHEUMATOID ARTHRITIS. This may occur in the dog from the age of about 2 years upwards, and in cats.

SIGNS are at first vague; the dog appearing depressed, often with a poor appetite and some degree of fever, but with no lameness. This appears later, sometimes involving several joints simultaneously, sometimes affecting one limb and then shifting to another. There may be crepitus when the limb is moved.

DIAGNOSIS depends for confirmation upon radiography and on laboratory tests.

(*See also* AUTOIMMUNE DISEASE.)

RHINITIS. Inflammation of the nose. (*See* NOSE.)

RHINITIS, ATROPHIC. This term cannot be precisely defined, but Done (1962) stated: 'Atrophic rhinitis (the macroscopic lesion) is the product of a severe persistent inflammatory reaction in the nasal mucosa of a growing, and therefore very young pig, and as such is non-specific with regard to aetiology.'

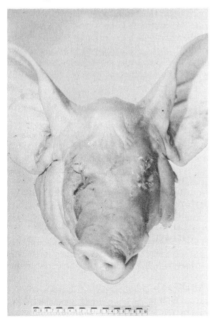

Distortion of the pig's snout as a result of atrophic rhinitis. (With acknowledgements to Professor R. H. C. Penny and the Royal Veterinary College.)

Although it has been suggested that this condition is hereditary or nutritional in origin these may be only predisposing or accessory factors. The generally accepted view is that in the first 2 or 3 months of life the rapidly growing nasal structures are extremely liable to attack by infectious agents but quite often recovery from these is complete. In herds with severe disease, however, the condition may progress to give rise to the marked displacement or atrophy of the turbinate bones and also to an associated pneumonia.

CAUSES. A paper 'Respiratory disease in pigs: a study' (Little, T. W. A., *Vet Rec.* (1975) **96**) stated that, in chronic rhinitis, inclusion-body rhinitis virus (IBR), *Bordetella bronchiseptica, Pasteurella multocida,* and *Pseudomonas aeruginosa,* 'all may have been dominant in the lesions at some stage'. The study – made by research staff of the Central Veterinary Laboratory and Veterinary Investigation Officers – showed respiratory disease in the pig to be a changing, developing process, with many agents and factors involved, and with rhinitis and pneumonia often-occurring together. (*See* diagram *under* RESPIRATORY DISEASE.)

From other sources it is known that *Bordetella bronchiseptica* secretes a substance which inhibits the deposition or transfer of calcium salts in the infected tissues. Accordingly the bones may fail to ossify properly or may become weak and liable to distortion.

ARC research suggested that the disease in a severe form may occur only when there is a double infection with *B. bronchiseptica* and *Pasteurella multocida.* In 1983 the ARC referred to evidence supporting 'the view that the lesions of severe progressive atrophic rhinitis are associated with infection by *toxigenic* strains of *P. multocida.*'

SIGNS. The acute form is to be found in piglets 2 or 3 weeks old, when there is no deformity of the snout to be seen and not always an overflow of tears. Sneezing is perhaps the most common symptom. The eye-lids may be puffy, and sometimes the piglet has a copious discharge from its nose and breathes through its mouth. The disease can be so mild that symptoms pass unnoticed, or so severe that death occurs within a week. In some outbreaks the mortality is 10 per cent or more, and survivors suffer a growth check from the disease which continues in the sub-acute form.

INCIDENCE. In a 1975 paper in the *Veterinary Record* Professor R. H. C. Penny and Dr P. A. Mullen concluded that the incidence of atrophic rhinitis 'could have increased markedly since the last survey in the UK was undertaken in 1956–57'.

Their own survey involved examination of the snouts from 2701 pork, bacon, and heavy pigs killed at five abattoirs in England and Scotland during March to July 1974. They found obvious atrophy of the turbinate bones in over 44 per cent and severe atrophy in over 17 per cent of the snouts examined.

PREVENTION. 'Conflicting but encouraging' trials with a *Bordetella bronchiseptica* vaccine were reported during 1980 by Dr R. Goodwin, University of Cambridge.

RHINOPNEUMONITIS (*see* EQUINE ditto).

RHINOSPORIDIOSIS. A chronic disease of the nasal mucous membrane, and associated with polyp-formation leading to difficulty in breathing, caused by a fungus *Rhinosporidia seberi.* The disease occurs in cattle and horses, in the USA, South America, Australia, and India.

RHINOTRACHEITIS, INFECTIOUS. A disease of cattle recognised in the USA in 1951. It is also called Infectious Bovine Rhinotracheitis, or IBR for short.

CAUSE: The bovine herpes virus 1, which can produce disease of the respiratory, reproductive, nervous and digestive systems.

SIGNS. In America the disease is usually severe in feedlot cattle, but mild in dairy/range cattle. In Britain outbreaks of severe IBR occurred in 1978–79, causing heavy losses on some farms, with reduced milk yield, loss of appetite, fever (up to 108°F), laboured breathing, a discharge from eyes and nose, and sometimes drooling of saliva. Reproductive disorders such as vulvo-vaginitis and orchitis have also occurred in Britain. In America abortion has followed natural infection or vaccination against IBR.

IBR is sometimes associated with a fatal pneumonia. The disease may closely resemble Mucosal Disease, with which at one time it was thought to be possibly identical, and also Malignant Catarrh.

At least one strain of the virus is neurotropic and has caused encephalitis in calves in Australia and elsewhere. (*See also under* FELINE.)

RHINOVIRUS. This genus of viruses have RNA as their nucleic acid and include equine rhinovirus.

RHODOCOCCUS (*see* CORYNEBACTERIUM).

RHODODENDRON POISONING is not common. There are about 20 varieties which have been recorded as causing poisoning in sheep, cattle, goats, and even man. The shrubs contain a glycoside called *Andromedotoxin.*

Poisoning may occur when sheep are brought in to graze former amenity land on an estate. In one outbreak, lambs were turned into a crop of rape bordered by rhododendrons, before having had time to adjust to the new diet. Fifty out of 300 lambs were found weak and salivating; two were attempting to vomit; six were recumbent; and three dead. (Hosie, B. D. & others, *Veterinary Record* (1986) **118**, 110.)

RHONCHI, or DRY SOUNDS, sometimes referred to as 'DRY RÂLES', are continuous sounds heard during breathing by auscultation of the chest, when there is some obstruction of the bronchi. (*See also* RÂLES.)

RIBOFLAVIN (*see* VITAMIN B₂).

RIBONUCLEIC ACID. A substance related to DNA, RNA includes the sugar ribose combined with nucleic acid. It appears to be concerned with protein synthesis within the cell. (*See* CELLS.) In some experiments it has been shown that RNA from malignant cells will cause normal cells *in vitro* to show characteristics of malignancy; and

the converse is possible. (*See* VIRUSES, CANCER, and GENETIC ENGINEERING.)

RIBOSOMES are granules containing RNA. (*See* CELLS.)

RIBS are the long bones which together form the cage of the thorax. Their numbers vary in the different animals, according to how many thoracic or dorsal vertebrae are present, as follows: horse, 18 pairs; ox, 13 pairs; pig, 14 or 15 pairs; dog, 13 pairs. In any of these animals an extra rib (often called a 'floating rib' because it possesses little or no cartilage to unite it to the costal arch) may be present on one or both sides of the body. The first 8 of these in the horse and ox, the first 7 in the pig, and the first 9 in the dog, have cartilages which are united to the sterum, and are called *sternal ribs,* while those farther back in the series in each case have cartilages which do not reach the sternum, but form an arch by overlapping each other, and are known as *asternal ribs.* (*See* STERNUM.)

Each rib possesses a 'head', by which it is joined to the anterior part of the vertebra to which it corresponds in number, and to the posterior part of that immediately in front, and this is succeeded by a 'neck', and a short distance farther down the shaft is a 'tubercle', which articulates with the transverse process of the vertebra to which it corresponds. The rest of the rib is composed of a long curved flat shaft, whose curve varies according to the position of the rib in the chest, being greatest about the middle of the series, and also according to the animal to which it belongs. Posterior to each runs the intercostal nerve and blood-vessels which are situated in a little groove along the borders of each rib. In life the ribs are attached to each other by the intercostal muscles to form the continuous wall of the chest. (*See* BONES.)

RICINE (*see* CASTOR).

RICKETS, or RACHITIS, is a deficiency disease of young animals characterised by a tendency towards the formation of enlarged extremities of the long bones, and a bending of their shafts. Dogs, pigs, lambs, foals, and calves are all affected, the first two more frequently than the other species of domesticated animals. It has also been met with in intensively managed poultry establishments where chicks are deprived of sunlight.

CAUSE. Rickets is an aphosphorosis essentially, which may be caused by a deficiency of either vitamin D or phosphorus, or in some cases both these.

Absence of sunlight is a contributory cause and animals kept in dark buildings, especially if inadequately fed, are prone to rickets.

Often a diet consisting largely of oatmeal or maize meal, such as is commonly the lot of sheepdogs, results in rickets. (*See* PHYTIN.)

SIGNS. The typical changes consist of the development of bony swellings upon the ends of the long bones of the limbs, where they meet other bones to form joints, and the production of swellings at the point where a rib joins its rib cartilage, *i.e.* along each side of the chest about two-thirds the way down from the spine. In puppies, there is also a tendency for the shafts of the long limb to bend in an outward direction under the influence of the weight of the body.

TREATMENT. A vitamin D supplement is recommended or fresh cod-liver oil. (*See* COD-LIVER OIL.) (*See also* OSTEOMALACIA.)

RICKETTSIA. The generic name for a group of minute micro-organisms which may be said to be intermediate between the smallest bacteria and the viruses. 'They have certain characteristics in common with Gram-negative bacteria; but their failure to grow in ordinary culture media, and their multiplication intracellularly, show that their metabolic requirements are more akin to those of the filterable viruses.' (Topley and Wilson, 1964.) They flourish in the alimentary canal of ticks, lice, etc. (*For rickettsial infections in cattle see* TICK-BORNE FEVER, Q. FEVER. *For tropical diseases caused by rickettsiae, see* BOVINE PETECHIAL FEVER, HEARTWATER, *and in dogs,* CANINE RICKETTSIOSIS *and* CANINE TROPICAL PANCYTOPANIA; *see also* ROCKY MOUNTAIN FEVER.)

RICKETTSIAL POX. A mild form of mite typhus transmitted to people by the mouse mite *Allodermanyosus sanguineus*, and caused by *Rickettsia akari.*

RIDA. A disease of sheep involving the nervous system, similar to SCRAPIE, in Iceland.

RIDEAL-WALKER COEFFICIENT. Expresses the comparative efficiency of antiseptics, as based on the R W Test, taking carbolic acid as unity. It does not take into account the influence of body fluids upon the efficiency or otherwise of the antiseptic.

RIFAMPICIN. This antibiotic, not available in the UK, has proved effective against some bacteria resistant to other antibiotics. It has been used to treat feline brain abscesses. It is not suitable for use in pregnant animals owing to the risk of neonatal haemorrhage. (A Hoffman-LaRoche product.)

RIDING ESTABLISHMENTS ACT, 1939. This empowers local authorities to authorise a veterinary surgeon to inspect premises and horses, and to prosecute in the event of unfit horses being used.

RIFT VALLEY FEVER, or ENZOOTIC HEPATITIS. A disease of sheep, cattle, buffaloes, goats, camels, horses, donkeys, and man, occurring in Africa. Until 1973 it had not been recorded in northern Africa, but in that year it reached the Sudan, and then Egypt, where major epizootics occurred in 1977–78. In 1982 WHO stated that this disease might be of greater concern outside Africa than in many of the countries where it is endemic; and expressed anxiety over its possible spread to Mediterranean and Middle East countries unprepared for it.

CAUSE: A bunyavirus, transmitted by mosquitoes. The virus causes necrosis of liver cells; also abortion.

SIGNS. The disease is seen at its most acute in young lambs, which die within a few hours. Fever, vomiting, ataxia, and death within a day or two may occur in older lambs, calves, and occasionally adult sheep. Mild or subclinical infections also occur in adult animals. Abortion accounts for much economic loss; also a temporary halt in lactation.

PREVENTION. A live vaccine made from the attenuated Smithburn strain of the virus was WHO approved in 1983.

Public health. The human illness is like an acute attack of influenza, and sometimes there is also an encephalitis lasting 5 to 15 days, which may prove fatal. Jaundice may occur in another fatal form of the disease. Impairment of vision may be permanent as a result of inflammation of the retina.

The 1977–78 outbreaks in Egypt involved over 200,000 human cases, with nearly 600 deaths, and about 800 cases of eye disease and encephalitis, respectively, in 1977.

A differential diagnosis has to include the possibility of rodenticide poisoning, such as occurred in Egypt in 1982, when an epidemic lasting three weeks was traced to the use of brodifacoum. (*See* RODENTICIDES.)

RIG, RIDGLING, or CRYPTORCHID. A male animal in which one or both testes do not descend into the scrotum from the abdomen at the usual time. (*See also under* CRYPTORCHID, MONORCHID GELDING.)

RIGOR MORTIS. Temporary stiffening of the muscles several hours after death (*e.g.* 4 to 8 hours in the pig carcase). It is associated with the breakdown in the muscles of adenosine triphosphate (ATP), which also occurs when muscles contract during life.

RIGORS. Shivering fits. When prolonged, rigors may be the warning sign of the approach of some disease or fever.

RIMA is a term, meaning a crack or fissure, applied to any narrow natural opening, *e.g.* rima glottidis, the space between the vocal cords.

RINDERPEST is an acute, specific, inoculable, and febrile disease of cattle, characterised by an ulcerative inflammation of mucous membranes, especially those of the alimentary tract.

This disease ravaged Europe intermittently for fifteen centuries. In the United Kingdom the 1865–6 outbreak alone involved over 324,000 cattle, but the disease was finally eradicated in 1877.

Vast areas of Asia and Africa are still subject to cattle plague, which remains one of the most serious threats to world food-supplies, and which – like foot-and-mouth disease – is caused by a virus, but one far more deadly. Indeed, when cattle plague strikes a herd, nine out of ten animals may die – a catastrophe which is not infrequently followed by famine – and the total loss of food and draught animals (cattle and buffaloes) from this cause is immense.

SUSCEPTIBILITY. Cattle are by far the most susceptible animals. Eland and bush pig are known to contract rinderpest, and ailing wild game may carry infection to healthy cattle. Sheep and goats occasionally become infected; and recent experience in Kenya led Drs P. B. Rossitter and D. M. Jessett to suggest, along with Dr W. P. Taylor of the Animal Virus Research Institute, England, that the disease may exist subclinically in sheep and goats for a time, with consequent risk of an outbreak among unvaccinated cattle. It is also possible that one or more strains of the virus may now be circulating independently of cattle, they suggested.

Most pigs show only a mild fever, with some depression and anorexia; they could, therefore, act as a very dangerous means of transfer of virus from contaminated meat to cattle. There is evidence that Asiatic pigs are more susceptible than those of European origin to infection with rinderpest virus, and they have long been known to be affected naturally in Indo-China. Horses are immune.

INCUBATIVE PERIOD. 3 to 9 days.

SIGNS include fever, dullness, and loss of appetite.

Soon the nasal mucosa becomes red and gives off a watery discharge which then becomes mucoid. The mouth is found to be pasty and inflamed.

Ulcers occur in front of the incisor teeth, on the gums, inside the cheeks, on the borders of the tongue, and in front of the dental pad. The epithelium comes off in bran-like scales, leaving a ragged surface. This feature of the ulcers is important as one of the distinguishing characters from the ulcers found in foot-and-mouth disease.

Constipation gives place to diarrhoea of a fetid nature, and much straining takes place. The diarrhoea is followed by dysentery. The anus becomes dilated and the mucous membrane of the rectum is exposed, appearing dark, or purple. The affected animal becomes very weak and emaciated.

In milking cows the milk falls off. Pregnant cows usually abort about the height of the disease. The lungs are affected only in chronic cases, as a rule.

COURSE AND DURATION. The disease is usually acute, lasting 4 to 10 days. Outbreaks of a more chronic type do occur in some countries. These produce a greater number of recoveries. In new outbreaks of cattle plague death may claim up to 90 per cent of the victims, while at other times the death-rate may be as low as 20 per cent.

PREVENTION. Several vaccines are available.

In continents other than Asia and Africa, quarantine measures are relied upon to exclude the disease from countries. In the event of an outbreak, immediate slaughter of all infected or in-contact cattle, sheep, goats, or other ruminants, must be carried out, and all movement of stock prohibited in a given area.

DURATION OF IMMUNITY. Cattle were immunised with a single dose of a rinderpest cell culture vaccine and maintained in a rinderpest-free environment for six to 11 years. They were then challenged by either parenteral or intra-nasal inoculation of virulent virus or by contact exposure to reacting cattle. None of the vaccinates reacted clinically and a rinderpest viraemia was never detected. (Plowright, W. (1984) *Journal of Hygiene* **92,** 285.)

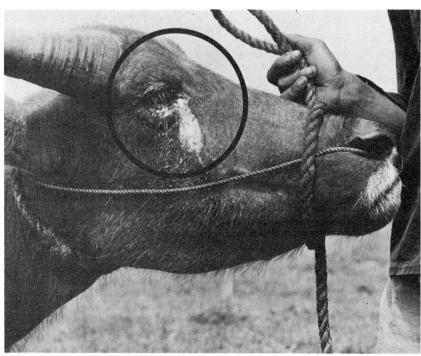

Rinderpest. This buffalo is showing what is usually the first symptom of the disease – a discharge from the eyes. (Unations picture)

CROSS-IMMUNITY. Infection of dogs with the rinderpest virus apparently confers immunity against distemper.

RING-BONES. A term used for any bony exostosis affecting the interphalangeal joints of the horse's foot, or indeed any bony enlargement in the same region: (1) *High ring-bone*, where the pastern joint (*i.e.* between the long and short pastern bones) is the seat of the disease; (2) *Low ring-bone*, where the deposit occurs round the coffin-joint, between the short pastern bone and the coffin-bone; and (3) *False ring-bone*, where the enlargement occurs upon the shaft of one of the bones and does not involve the edges of a joint surface (though it may do so later). From the point of view of etymology it would appear that the term 'ring-bone' should be restricted to conditions in which a partial or complete *ring of bone* is formed round one or other of the joints, and that all other bony enlargements affecting the surface of the shaft of the bones, but not involving the edges of the joint surfaces, should be called *exostoses*. Difficulty arises, however, when examining a horse's foot, in determining exactly whether the joint surfaces are affected, or are likely to become affected, in any particular given case.

CAUSES. Injury, inflammation of the periosteum or of the bone – sometimes following infection, possibly a vitamin D deficiency.

SIGNS. In the early stages nothing more than a fleeting lameness is seen. Eventually the horse will go lame all day if it is worked, or becomes too lame to take out of the stable. After a time one or other of the joints becomes enlarged, and the cause of the lameness becomes obvious. It must be understood that it is only in the case of high ring-bones (around the pastern joint) that the exostosis can be felt; when the lower (coffin) joint is affected there is at first no outward visible or palpable sign; but after a time the hoof alters in shape, becomes distinctly bulged or 'buttressed' at the coronet. This latter effect is due to the fact that in low ring-bone the extensor or pyramidal process of the coffin-bone is usually involved, and the deposit of bone upon it pushes the coronet, and the wall which grows from it, in an outward direction ('pyramidal disease'). At times the alteration in the outline of the hoof is not by any means regular; it may be bulged at any point from one heel to the other, denoting a deposit of bone wherever there is a bulge.

In 'true ring-bone' the joint that is affected almost always ends by becoming stiff (ankylosed), owing to fusion between its complementary bones and obliteration of the joint having occurred. In this state the horse may become fairly sound, because the pain occasioned by movement at the joint has disappeared, but the gait will always be stiff.

TREATMENT. Prolonged rest in a loose-box or, preferably, at grass is indicated. More harm than good results when blistering is carried out. Corticosteroids are used.

RING VACCINATION. This is carried out in the control of foot-and-mouth disease in a prescribed area around an outbreak. Vaccination is begun at the perimeter of the areas, progressing inwards towards the centre. For success, diagnosis, typing of virus and the vaccination itself must all be speedy.

RINGER'S SOLUTION consists of sodium chloride, 9 grams; calcium chloride 0·25 gm; potassium chloride, 0·42 gm per litre.

'RINGWOMB'. This is the colloquial name for a condition which sometimes complicates lambing, and is due to failure of the cervix to dilate. Usually, the *os uteri* will admit one or two fingers, which can feel what seems like a firm ring.

The shepherd may recognise the condition on seeing a small portion of fetal membrane protruding from the vulva. The ewe remains in good health (but does not lamb) until death and decomposition of the fetus occur.

Manual dilation of the cervix is practised by some veterinary surgeons. Should this prove impossible, Caesarean operation is the only alternative. (*See* UTERUS, *and* PARTURITION.)

RINGWORM. A contagious skin disease caused by the growth of certain fungi, which live either upon the surface of the skin or in the hairs of the areas affected. Ringworm may affect any of the domesticated animals, but it is probably commonest in young store cattle when they are enclosed in buildings during winter, and in pet cats and kittens. Dogs and horses are also frequently affected, but the disease is not often seen in the sheep and pig.

Ringworm and favus in the domesticated animals are caused by parasitic fungi which belong to the family GYMNOASCIDAE.

Lesions generally. Ringworm appears in the form of patches of dry, raised, crusty skin, from the surface of which the hairs have fallen and upon the surface of which there are scales or scabs. The patches are often more or less circular, but in bad cases large irregular areas may be produced, which result from the coalescence of adjacent areas. Favus is a type of ringworm in which the lesions have cup-shaped depressions which bear some similarity to a honeycomb, from which they get their name (*favus*, honeycomb). Favus affects the dog and cat, the mouse and rat, rabbits sometimes, and fowls occasionally.

Horses. Ringworm may be due either to parasites belonging to the class *Trichophyton* or to *Microsporum*. In cases due to the former, the first affected areas are usually confined to the head, neck, withers, and sometimes to the root of the tail. The hair becomes matted in patches about the size of a large coin and in the centre of each patch appears a bare area from which the hair has fallen off; this gradually extends until the whole area is denuded. The skin becomes raised and scurfy, and greyish-white crusts are formed; at times there may be grey or yellow scales adherent to begin with, but becoming detached later. There is usually little or no itchiness, except when due to *Trichophyton mentagrophytes*.

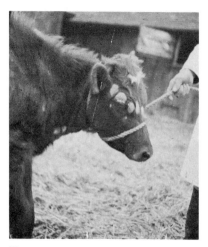

Ringworm.

When the horse is affected with ringworm due to *Microsporum* parasites practically any part of the body may be attacked.

Cattle. Ringworm is nearly always due to *T. verrucosum* infection. It is very common among young animals in autumn, winter, and early spring, especially if they are kept indoors. The head and neck are most often affected, especially the eye-lids, lips, ears, and above the jaws, but it may occur anywhere on the body. The lesion begins as a raised ring-like patch on which the hairs stand erect. In a day or so the hairs fall off, and the surface of the skin becomes covered with masses of scales heaped up into a greyish-white or greyish-yellow crust. The areas are usually very numerous and often become confluent, so that large areas become bare of hair and present roughened, crusty, hard, dry surfaces with a tendency towards pronounced wrinkling of the skin around and between them. Where calves are very extensively affected with ringworm there is always a good deal of loss of condition and itchiness.

Sheep. When they are affected the fleece becomes matted, and falls out in circular patches over the shoulders, neck, and chest. *Trichophyton verrucosum* is one cause.

Dogs. Ringworm may be one of four varieties: *Trichophyton, Microsporum, Oidmella,* or *Oospora,* the last named causing favus. The lesions produced by the first three of these are very similar in all respects to those seen in horses and cattle. In favus caused by *Oospora canina* the lesion appears as a raised circular patch upon whose surface there is a pale yellow crust with little depressions (honeycomb) scattered through it. The skin in such cases is often very much thickened.

Hedgehogs. Caused by *Trichophyton erinacei,* this infection may cause lesions on the face of dogs where the skin has been damaged by the hedgehog's spines.

Cats. Ringworm is of three kinds: due to *Trichophyton, Microsporum,* and *Achorion,* the latter producing favus. When due to the first two of these the symptoms and lesions are similar to those seen in other animals. (*See* ONYCHOMYCOSIS.)

Cats become infected from mice with mouse favus (*A. quickeanum* or *A. arlongi*), although it may also be due to *A. schoenleinii* – the favus of man. The lesions are chiefly confined to the fore-paws and the head and the neck, though they may spread to other parts of the body. Itchiness is usually absent. The areas affected vary in size from that of a pin's head up to a 5p piece or so, and are not always regular in outline. The skin is

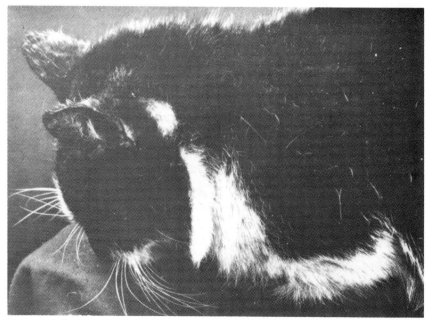

Ringworm in the cat: a whitish, scaly lesion can be seen to the right of the ear, above the white fur.

thickened and the edges are raised. When newly formed, the covering crust is yellow and soft to the touch, but when old it is grey and powdery. The characteristic cup-shaped depressions are seen in most cases, but when affecting the claws they may be absent.

Ringworm due to *Microsporum canis* Bodin is of considerable public health importance. It is often overlooked by owners; affected cats being a danger to children.

Cats, especially Persians and other longhairs, may be **'carriers' of ringworm** fungus. A survey carried out by M. Baxter involved 200 selected cats seen at a veterinary clinic, none of them showing any sign of ringworm. Fur samples taken with a brush showed that 39 per cent of the 200 were carrying spores of ringworm fungi. (In 72 samples the spores were those of *M. canis*.) A survey in England of fur samples taken at four cat shows revealed that, overall, 35 per cent of longhairs were carrying *M. canis* spores. (M. Baxter. *New Zealand Veterinary Journal* (1973) **21** 33; and R. A. Quaife & S. M. Womar. *Vet. Rec.* (1982) **110,** 333.)

Decontamination of households is important for human health after ringworm has been diagnosed. Hypochlorite, benzalkonium chloride,

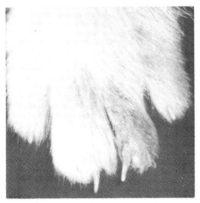

A bare, scaly patch on a kitten's toe due to ringworm – transmissible to humans.

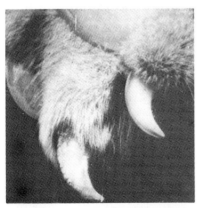

The roughened appearance of an infected claw. *Microsporum canis* Bodin was responsible in each case.

and glutaraldehyde-based compounds are recommended by the Mycology Unit, University of Glasgow.

Favus in the fowl, due to *Trichophyton gallinae*, affects the comb, wattles, and other parts of the fowl's head.

If the condition spreads down to feathered parts the feathers become dry, brittle, and break off at the surface of the skin, leaving large bare areas. There is always a most disagreeable odour from fowl favus, so much so that it is at times referred to as 'foul favus'.

TREATMENT. Oral administration of griseofulvin is by far the simplest method. Cattle and horses can be given a supplemented feed. This makes possible group treatment, and avoids handling of infected animals; thus reducing the risk of infection being transferred to man. However, it is inadvisable to use griseofulvin in pregnant animals. In a cat which could not tolerate griseofulvin, a THIABENDAZOLE dip was successfully used.

Another antibiotic, Natamycin, has been found to be effective when applied to infected cattle with a knapsack sprayer.

Another method is to use an aerosol spray, containing a fungicide and a dye; taking care to protect the animal's and the operator's eyes, and observing the manufacturer's instructions.

Otherwise, treatment consists, in the first place, of removing the hair from around the lesions, collecting it and burning it; soaking the scabs in hot soda and water, or caustic potash in water (a 10 per cent solution in either case), removing them with a spoon or piece of wood, and burning them; and, finally, painting the raw surfaces with some reliable dressing of which there are many. A choice may be made from the following: gentian violet solution; undecylenate ointment; isoquinolinium chloride lotion, which has given rapid and good results in the treatment of ringworm in cattle.

Dressing should be carried out twice a week for a fortnight for cattle and horses, and by then most of the fungus will be killed, but the cases should not be considered cured until there is a level crop of new hair over each of the areas. For the smaller animals it is better to use the dressing once every second day.

In all instances it is very important to remember that ringworm spreads from the centre outwards, and edges and margins of the areas should be especially well dressed.

Vaccination of calves against *Trichophyton verrucosum*, using a live Russian vaccine (L T F 130), has been practised in Norway. The first dose is given when the calf is four weeks old; a second dose 10 to 14 days later. Side-effects include a slight fever lasting a couple of days, and a noninfective lesion at the inoculation site. None of a batch of vaccinated calves had ringworm by day 90; whereas all the unvaccinated controls had lesions. However 'results vary'. In some herds calves do develop ringworm, mostly in the period between the two injections. (B. Naess & O. Sandvik. *Vet. Rec.* (1981) **109,** 199).

In the U S S R the vaccination of racehorses,

and other horses taking part in competitive events, is compulsory.

Public health. Ringworm is readily transmissible to human beings, so precautions such as hand-washing and disinfection after contact with known infected animals should not be neglected. Dettol is useful for these purposes.

DIAGNOSIS. Microscopic examination or culture methods. (*See also* WOOD'S LAMP.)

RNA (*see* RIBONUCLEIC ACID).

ROAD ACCIDENTS. Dogs and cats struck by cars may suffer chest injuries in addition to limb injuries. (*See* FRACTURES, ACCIDENTS, DIAPHRAGMATOCELE, HYDROTHORAX, PNEUMOTHORAX.)

ROAN (*see* COLOURS OF HORSES.)

'ROARING' IN HORSES. The abnormal sound is made when the horse breathes in, and the usual cause has for long been regarded as vibration of the slackened vocal folds on one or both sides of the larynx, due to paralysis of the muscles which move the arytenoid cartilages outwards. (For treatment and further details, *see* LARYNX, DISEASES OF – Laryngeal Paralysis.)

ROCK SALT (*see* SALT LICKS).

ROCKY MOUNTAIN FEVER, which is also called Rocky Mountain Spotted Fever, is a disease of man caused by *Rickettsia rickettsii*. Wild animals provide a reservoir of infection.

Rocky Mountain fever affects human beings usually between March and July. The onset of fever is sudden, and in 2 to 5 days a rash appears over the whole body, including the palms of the hands. The rash changes to a sort of mottling –

petechiae, scattered over the skin, which gives the condition its name of 'spotted fever'. The infection is transmitted by ticks, especially *Dermacentor andersoni* – the Rocky Mountain Wood Tick.

Dogs. The infection causes fever, abdominal pain, depression, loss of appetite, nystagmus, with sometimes conjunctivitis and petechial haemorrhages in the mouth. Oedema of a limb(s) is common, and the scrotum and prepuce may be similarly affected. Over 30 cases are confirmed serologically each year, with many more being diagnosed, in Long Island, New York.

Diagnosis is most reliably confirmed by the immunofluorescent test. Treatment is by antibiotics, e.g. tetracycline.

PRECAUTIONS: There is a risk to veterinarians taking a blood sample or carrying out a post-mortem examination, as the rickettsia is present in the blood during the acute phase (B. A. Lissman & J. L. Benach, *JAVMA* (1980) **176,** 994).

RODENT ULCER. In human medicine this term is reserved for carcinoma of the skin, but is sometimes misapplied by animal-owners to EOSINOPHILIC GRANULOMA or 'LICK GRANULOMA' (which see).

RODENTS. Rats and mice are important from a veterinary point of view on account of the diseases which they may transmit to domestic animals. For examples, see AUJESZKY'S DISEASE; SALMONELLOSIS; LEPTOSPIROSIS; RINGWORM, FOOT-AND-MOUTH DISEASE. In countries where the disease is present, rodents may transmit RABIES.

Zoonoses. *Muridae* (Old World rats and mice) can infect man with plague, tularaemia, listeriosis, pseudotuberculosis, erysipelas, leptospirosis, brucellosis, melioidosis, murine typhus, Q fever, scrub typhus and other

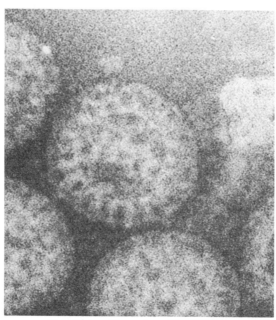

The rotavirus. (By courtesy of the AFRC.)

rickettsioses, histoplasmosis, lymphocytic choriomeningitis, Lassa fever, rabies and other viral infections, Asian schistosomiasis, Chagas' disease, rat-bite fever, and HANTAAN virus.

Rodenticides. In the UK brodifacoum was cleared by MAFF (for indoor use only) in 1984; and difenacoum had also been scrutinised under the Pesticides Safety Precautions Scheme. (No incidents linking barn owl deaths with these two rodenticides had been reported in the UK.)

A calciferol preparation, 'Rodin C' (Rentokil) – claimed to be effective against warfarin-resistant rats, had earlier received MAFF approval. (*See also* WARFARIN for information concerning that rodenticide.)

RESERPINE was officially approved for use against mice in 1975. Alpha-chloralose has been used for the same purpose.

A rodenticide containing vitamin D_3 caused the death of two dogs.

SIGNS: Weakness, anorexia, vomiting and passing blood. (Gunther, R. & others. *JAVMA* (1988) **193**, 211.)

Accidental poisoning of domestic animals has occurred from some of the above, and also from others banned in the UK; e.g. RED SQUILL. THALLIUM, ANTU. THIOUREA, PHOSPHORUS, FLUOROACETATE ('1080'), barium salts, zinc phosphide, strychnine.

ROMAGNOLA. An Italian breed of cattle, white in colour, and reared for beef. An importation of 200 Romagnolas into the UK was sanctioned in 1974.

ROMPUN (*see* XYLAZINE).

ROSE BENGAL PLATE TEST. A simple and quick screening test used in the diagnosis of brucellosis in cattle. Sera giving positive results may then be tested by means of the Serum Agglutination Test and Complement Fixation Test.

ROSTRAL TEETH are the incisors and canines.
Rostral. Towards the nose or front end of the body.

ROTAVIRUS. So-called because of its resemblance to a wheel. Research has demonstrated the importance of rotaviruses in the causation of diarrhoea in children, foals, calves and piglets. At the IRAD, Compton, it has been shown that, in piglets, only the pig and calf rotaviruses cause diarrhoea, although the human and foal rotaviruses can replicate in the pig. In IRAD experiments, rotaviruses from calves and piglets, given by mouth to gnotobiotic piglets, produced desquamation (stripping) of the epithelial cells lining the small intestine and severe stunting of the villi – small projections from the surface mucous membrane.

This rotavirus has also been isolated from scouring piglets, foals, lambs, monkeys and rabbits.

Research at the Moredun Institute led to a novel method of diagnosis – one based on the direct detection of the viral nucleic acid, which comprises 11 molecules of double stranded DNA. This method is 'rapid and as sensitive as ELISA'.

A vaccine was introduced in 1986, following research at Moredun, to protect calves against rotavirus (and also K99 *E. coli*). The vaccine, 'Rotavec K99' is a Coopers Animal Health product.

ROTENONE. The insecticidal principle of Derris root. Rotenone is highly poisonous to fish and is used deliberately for removing coarse fish from enclosed waters before establishing trout fisheries. (For details of this, and for the comparative toxicity of rotenone for different species of fish, see Meadows, B. S., *J. fish. Biol.* (1973) **5**, 155.)

ROTHERA TEST. A modified version of this test for ketones in milk or urine requires the following reagent: ammonium sulphate 100 grammes; anhydrous sodium carbonate, 50 grammes; sodium nitroprusside, 3 grammes.

If the bottom half inch of a test-tube is filled with this powder, and a little of the fluid to be tested run down the side of the tube, a red colour will develop after 3 or 4 minutes if ketones are present as with acetonaemia.

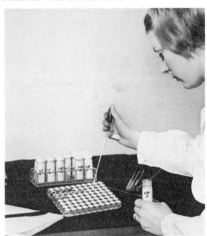

The Rothera Test for ketosis. The photograph shows milk samples being added to specially prepared Rothera powder. A colour reaction indicates a cow with ketosis and the test can be used very simply and cheaply to monitor dairy herds for the presence of the disease. (With acknowledgements to the AFRC.)

ROUGHAGE. By this is meant food of a bulky and fibrous nature, such as hay and straw. These have a low water-content, and are in a sense the opposite of succulents, *e.g.* kale, silage. (*See also* 'FIBRE' *under* DIET.)

ROULEAUX is the term applied to the columns into which red-blood cells collect as seen under the microscope. The appearance somewhat resembles a pile of stacked coins.

ROUND HEART DISEASE causes sudden death of turkeys in apparently good condition. The cause is inbreeding.

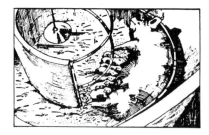

The New Zealand Pen: a drawing showing the position in which the sow voluntarily assumes, and, below, a plan for the pen's construction.

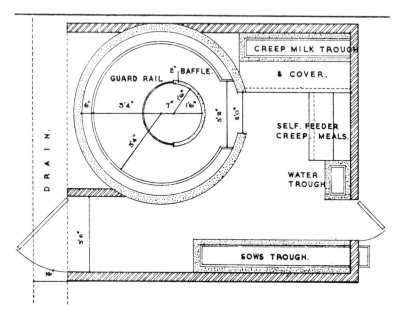

ROUNDHOUSE. A type of circular farrowing pen devised in New Zealand. A variant of the original described in *Agriculture*, consists of a circle of hardboard, about 8 feet in diameter and 4 feet high, bolted to a light iron framework and fitted with an internal creep rail. A smaller circle, about 3 feet in diameter, made partly of hardboard and partly of tubular rails, is fitted eccentrically within the larger one, and the whole is fastened with bolts to the concrete floor of the piggery. The smaller circle which is warmed by an infra-red lamp, acts as a creep for the piglets, while the sow is kept in the space between the two circles. Because of the shape of this space, the sow invariably lies in the same position, with her udder towards the piglet's creep. This gives the piglets the maximum degree of safety.

ROUNDWORMS. (Nematoda). Most nematodes lay eggs, but some produce living larvae. The life-history may be direct or indirect, *i.e.* an intermediate host may be necessary.

Nematodes can be the cause of anaemia, wasting, gastro-enteritis, bronchitis and pneumonia, aneurism, convulsions and blockage of the intestine. Some are of public health importance. (*See* TRICHINOSIS, TOXOCARA.)

Horse

I. Stomach. Two species of *Habronema* (*H. muscae* and *H. microstoma*), and *Drascheia megastoma*, inhabit the stomach of *equidae* in various parts of the world.

The worm larvae are passed in the horse's faeces, swallowed by maggots, and continue through the pupal and adult stages of the stablefly or house-fly; finally the larvae become located in the fly's proboscis. When the fly settles near a horse's mouth, the larvae enter it, and reach the stomach. However, if the horse has a wound, some of the larvae will be attracted to that, and give rise to the cutaneous or orbital form of *habronemiasis*, 'summer sores' or 'bursati'.

Habronemiasis is common in the tropics and subtropics, but has also been seen in the UK, for example.

Hard nodules or granulomas may form on the skin or at the inner canthus of the eye.

Drascheia megastoma forms nodules, in which it lives, in the stomach. *Habronema* worms may penetrate the gastric mucosa and become embedded; causing gastritis, thirst, colic and pica.

Trichostongylus axei, seldom more than 8 mm long, also causes gastritis. This worm also inhabits the duodenum.

II. Small intestine. Parascaris equorum. This is the common large roundworm of the horse. The female may be up to 50 cm long. Pica, colic, unthriftiness may result from heavy infections, which may also lead to partial blockage of the intestine.

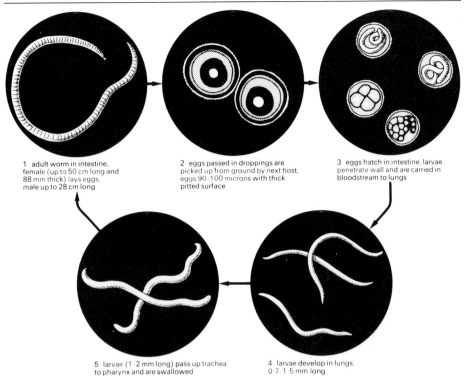

1 adult worm in intestine,
female (up to 50 cm long and
88 mm thick) lays eggs,
male up to 28 cm long

2 eggs passed in droppings are
picked up from ground by next host,
eggs 90-100 microns with thick
pitted surface

3 eggs hatch in intestine, larvae
penetrate wall and are carried in
bloodstream to lungs

5 larvae (1-2 mm long) pass up trachea
to pharynx and are swallowed

4 larvae develop in lungs,
0·7-1·5 mm long

Life cycle of the large roundworm of the horse, *Parascaris equorum*. Reproduced with permission from H. T. B. Hall, *Diseases and Parasites of Livestock in the Tropics*, Longman.

The larvae, which migrate to the lungs after hatching in the stomach, are capable of causing a catarrhal bronchitis or broncho-pneumonia; and possibly some damage to the liver also, during their migration through that organ.

Strongyloides westeri is another worm found in the duodenum, and a cause of diarrhoea in foals. This and other worms of this genus may also cause broncho-pneumonia.

III. Caecum and colon. *Strongylus.* Three species are important.

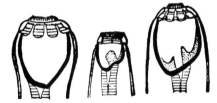

Strongylus (head). (Left to right) *S. edentatus, s. vulgaris, S. equinus.*

Strongylus (Delafontia) vulgaris is a cause of verminous arteritis, or thrombosis, affecting the cranial mesenteric artery. (*See* EQUINE VERMINOUS ARTERITIS.)

Strongylus (Alfortia) edentatus produces nodules in the peritoneum. If very numerous, the larvae may cause peritonitis, bleeding, and anaemia. After two or three months they return to the large intestine and become adult worms.

Strongylus equinus. The larvae of this large worm also produce nodules in the caecum and colon, and later migrate to the liver and pancreas.

Strongylus vulgaris was completely eliminated from three horses at pasture near Perth, Western Australia, by means of four oral doses of ivermectin (200 µg/kg bodyweight), at approximately monthly intervals, during the time of year when environmental conditions would be likely to eliminate all the non-parasitic stages of the parasite. *S. edentatus, Draschia megastoma* and *Habronema* species were also almost completely eliminated. (Dunsmore, J. D., *Equine Veterinary Journal* (1985) **17**, 191.)

Oxyuris equi. The female worm comes to the end of the rectum to deposit its eggs, which are ejected as yellowish or greenish mass surrounding the anus. Resulting pruritus can lead to emaciation in severe cases, and more usually to unsightly bare patches on the tail and hindquarters.

IV. Lungs. *Dictyocaulus arnfieldi* is the cause of a verminous bronchitis which may be recognised by a cough and, if the worms are numerous, by loss of appetite and emaciation.

'Demonstration of the presence of larvae in the faeces is sufficient to confirm the presence of infection in donkeys but even if respiratory symptoms are present, this finding should not be allowed to obscure the more likely possibility that other causal agents are involved. Diagnosis of infection in horses may be very difficult. Recovery of larvae from faeces will identify the 'silent carriers' but most horses have very low larval output and several examinations may be necessary. Most cases of clinical disease, in horses, are seen during the prepatent phase and larvae will not therefore be present in the faeces. Most infected horses, although showing respiratory signs, do not develop patent infections. It is therefore important not to exclude lungworm as a possibility just because it is not possible to recover larvae from the faeces. Naturally acquired infections are known in which larvae were not recovered from horses with clinical respiratory signs extending for more than a year. Complete recovery followed specific lungworm therapy. While an association with donkeys is added circumstantial evidence on which diagnosis can be based, infection may be transmitted from horse to horse in the absence of a donkey contact. This frequently occurs on thoroughbred studs.' (Round, M. C., *Veterinary Record* (1976) **99,** 393.)

The efficacy of orally administered ivermectin against induced *Dictyocaulus arnfieldi* infection was evaluated in a controlled study comprising 12 yearling ponies. Treatment with ivermectin paste, orally once, was 100 per cent effective against both adult and immature or inhibited stages of the horse lungworm. (Britt, D. P. and Preston J. M., *Veterinary Record* (1985) **116,** 343–345.)

V. Connective tissue. ONCHOCERCA. *O. reticulata* is found in the horse, especially in tendons. It is common near the suspensory ligament, but is also reported in the withers. They may cause no symptoms, or may induce hypertrophy of the tendon or may cause 'fistulous withers'. *O. cervicalis* occurs in the *ligamentum nuchae* of equines, and is often associated with poll-evil.

VI. Skin. Parafilaria multi-papillosa (Filaria haemorrhagica) is found in inter-muscular tissue or under the skin. The female worms penetrate the latter to lay their eggs on the surface, where hard nodules subsequently develop, and these open and bleed.

Haematobia flies in the USSR, and *Drosophila* in tropical regions, transmit the worm larvae.

VII. Nervous system. The larvae of *Setaria equina* invade the central nervous system of horses in Asia, causing epizootic cerebrospinal nematodiasis. This is characterised by paralysis, and the disease may prove fatal.

The adult worm, milky-white, lives in the peritoneal cavity. Transmission is by mosquitoes.

VIII. Eyes. Thelazia lachrymalis causes conjunctivis (and sometimes keratitis too). (*See* EYEWORMS.)

Cattle, sheep, goats and pigs

I. Oesophagus and stomach. Gongylonema. Two species occur in ruminants and one in pigs. They are found just below the epithelium in the thoracic third of the oesophagus. The intermediate hosts are various species of dung-beetles.

Haemonchus contortus. This is the large stomach worm or 'barber's pole' worm of ruminants, so called because of the female's spiral red and white stripes. The male is red. It is a trichostrongyle, with a length of about 30 mm and the thickness of a pin. It is a voracious blood sucker, and inhabits the abomasum.

It can cause serious anaemia and unthriftiness, especially in lambs.

H. placei is another of several species.

Ostertagia worms, which are of considerable economic importance, are peculiar in that while most infective larvae living in the abomasum moult twice to become adults, some – especially perhaps those ingested by the calf during late summer and autumn – moult only once and remain as fourth-stage larvae in a dormant state. These dormant larvae are unaffected by many anthelmintics but are usually, though not always, susceptible to fenbendazole and albendazole. Later they develop into adults causing a winter outbreak of gastro-enteritis. Calves should therefore be dosed in September and moved to 'clean' pasture.

Also known as the small brown stomach worm, Ostertagia cause severe irritation of the mucous membrane by the formation of nodules. Infested animals may lose weight, scour, and become anaemic.

II. Small intestine. Ascaris vitulorum. This large round worm of cattle is generally of little importance, but it may be a frequent and fatal parasite of calves in certain localities.

Nematodirus. This is a common trichostrongyle genus found in large numbers in the small intestine of sheep. It is a very slender form under an inch long. In recent years nematodirus infestation has caused severe losses.

The infestation is a 'lamb-to-lamb' one, and can be avoided – where practicable – by confining lambs to pasture which carried no lambs in the previous two seasons. Nematodirus species found in Britain are *N. filicollis, N. helvetianus, N. spathiges,* and *N. battus. N. helvetianus* and *N. battus* are parasites of calves. (*See* PASTURE, CONTAMINATION.)

Cooperia species are important. They are usually present in association with other species of worms, *e.g.* Ostertagia, trichostrongylus. They seldom cause anaemia, but are responsible for weight loss and scouring.

Similar symptoms are produced by Trichostrongylus species. These are very small (only 2–7 mm long) and inhabit the abomasum and duodenum.

Bunestomum (Hookworms) live in the small intestine. The larvae may either enter their host via the mouth or penetrate the skin. They suck blood and accordingly cause anaemia and sometimes oedema under the throat. (*See* HOOKWORMS.)

Oesophagostomum. This is a genus of strongyle worms related to the horse forms, and found in

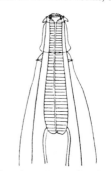

Oesophagostomum (head-end).

ruminants and pigs. They are about an inch or so long. They are the cause of nodular disease of the intestine ('pimply gut'). If present in small numbers, the only result is to render the intestine unfit for sausage skins. If in large numbers, the symptoms are anaemia, emaciation, diarrhoea, and oedema. The disease in this case often has a fatal termination.

Trichuris. This genus of whip-worms occurs in the caecum of various animals, but is usually of little importance. The worms have very slender necks with stoutish bodies. The necks are threaded through the mucous membrane of their host.

They may cause inflammation at the point of insertion of the head and may admit bacteria.

Strongyloides worms are found in the small intestine, often deep in the mucosa. Scouring is caused in heavy infestations. The worm larvae can enter the body via the skin.

III. Lungs. *Dictyocaulus.* Three species are known in cattle, but only one is important. *Dictyocaulus viviparus* which causes a form of bronchitis. The male is about 4 cm long and the female is about 7 cm. Eggs hatch in the lung, and the larvae climbing up the trachea are swallowed, and pass to the exterior with the faeces. After moulting twice, they reach the resistant infective stage, and can live thus on pasture through the winter. When swallowed, they continue their development.

The signs and treatment are described under PARASITIC BRONCHITIS.

PARASITIC BRONCHITIS ('HUSK')
Several species of roundworm occur in sheep and goats.

Dictyocaulus filaria is the largest and most common species. The male is about 5 cm long and the female 8 cm. The infective stage is reached in about 10 days. Apparently lambs can be infected prenatally. This worm is cosmopolitan in its distribution. Its life-history is direct.

The symptoms are those of a verminous bronchitis, sometimes complicated by bacterial infection, but otherwise similar to those in cattle.

Protostrongylus (*Synthetocaulus*) *rufescens* is a red and much smaller form. The male is about 2 cm and the female 3 cm long. It is found mainly in Europe. These worms live in the bronchioles and in the pulmonary parenchyma, and cause a verminous lobular pneumonia. The eggs cause a diffuse nodular pneumonia. Cough is less prominent than in the above form, but breathing is difficult.

IV. Connective tissues. *Onchocerca.* Several species occur in cattle in various parts of the world. They are the cause of 'worm nodules'.

The nodules are found mainly in the brisket, but also occur in the flank and forequarters. They appear to cause little harm to their host, but as the capsule is a product of inflammation, beef containing worm nodules is condemned, and in Australia they have caused considerable loss in the export trade.

Dracunculus. Only one species of this worm is found in the domestic animals, *D. medinensis*, the 'guinea worm'. It is found in India, Africa, and South America. The female is of considerable length, but is generally recovered from the host in small pieces. It is milky white in colour, smooth and without markings. Nearly the whole of the worm is occupied by the uterus, packed with coiled-up embryos. The worm occupies a subcuticular site, as a rule in the extremities, with the head-end projecting to the exterior. The larvae are released by a prolapse of the uterus through the cuticle of the worm. They escape into the water, are swallowed by a cyclops in which they develop. The cyclops is in due course swallowed in the drinking water by a suitable host – practically any of the domestic animals will do – and larvae are released by the digestive juices and proceed to their adult habitats. The worm may give rise to local abscesses, and sometimes affects the feet of dogs.

V. Eye. *Thelazia.* (*See* EYE WORMS.).

Pigs

I. Stomach. The most important worm here is *Hyostrongylus rubidus.* Its life cycle is direct. (*See also* 'THIN SOW SYNDROME'.) The latter may sometimes be due to various species of Oesophagostomum worms. (*See* OESOPHAGOSTOMIASIS.)

II. Small intestine. *Ascaris suum.* This worm is a very common parasite of pigs in all countries. The eggs have a remarkable vitality, and have been kept alive for as long as five years. The egg, in a few weeks after passing to the ground, develops an embryo, but this does not hatch until the egg is swallowed. When this happens, the larva, which is about $\frac{1}{100}$ in long, bores through the intestine, reaches the bloodstream, and is carried through the liver and heart to the lungs. Here it remains for some days, but it finally climbs up the trachea and is swallowed. The larva which leaves the lung has grown to about $\frac{1}{10}$ in in length. In the intestine it continues its development, taking about two and a half months to do so.

In passing through the lungs a certain amount of bleeding is caused, and if the larvae are numerous, pneumonia results. During this period the animal shows the symptoms known as 'thumps'. If it survives the lung symptoms, it often fails to grow properly and remains small and stunted.

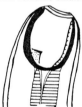

Globocephalus (head). A bloodsucking worm found in the intestines of pigs.

Macrocantorhynchus hirudinaceus is found in the small intestine of pigs. It is a whitish worm, the male being 5 to 10 cm long, while the female is 20 to 35 cm long. The neck is thin and the posterior region stout. The intermediate stages are found in beetles.

The parasite may cause a catarrhal enteritis or even actual perforation with peritonitis.

Trichuris suis, the pig whip-worm, causes mainly subclinical disease in temperate climates, but in the tropics it may cause dysentery, anaemia, and even death. In the Americas up to 85 per cent of pigs may be infested; in some areas of the UK, from 75 per cent. *Trichuris* occurs in the caecum.

Treatment in the pig can be undertaken with 'Shell Atgard' resin pellets containing dichlorvos.

III. Lungs. In pigs two species are common, both belonging to the genus *Metastrongylus*. They are about the same size, 2 cm in the male and 4 cm in the female. Both species are common in Europe and America, and may occur in the same pig. They cause a verminous bronchitis and sometimes pneumonia. Young animals are more susceptible and may die from it. Both species are carried by earthworms. (*See also diagram under* WORMS, FARM TREATMENT AGAINST.)

IV. Muscles. Trichinella spiralis. This is a small worm found in the intestine. The female produces living larvae (0·1 to 0·16 mm long) which migrate through the mucosa, reach the blood-stream, and are carried to various muscles. Here they pass into a cystic stage (the cyst being formed by the host), in which they remain until they are swallowed by some flesh-eating host or until they calcify and degenerate. In the intestine of the new host they reach sexual maturity and produce a new lot of larvae, which in turn migrate to the muscles.

The normal hosts are carnivores (dogs and cats). Rodents may be infected, and rats can be a source of infection to pigs. Man may be infected from the pig. (*See under* TRICHINOSIS.)

V. Kidney. Stephanurus dentatus is a thickish worm of fair size, the male being nearly 3 cm long and the female a little larger. It is found as a rule in the kidney fat of pigs, but also occurs in the liver and other locations in these animals and in ruminants. It is found in America and Australia, and is responsible for considerable damage. Its life-cycle is similar to that of the hookworms. Thiabendazole has proved effective in controlling this parasite.

Dogs and cats

I. Oesophagus. Spirocerca lupi is found in nodules in the oesophagus and, less frequently, the stomach of the dog, in all hot countries and in Europe.

It is a reddish worm. The male is 3 to 5 cm long. The intermediate hosts are various beetles and cockroaches.

The disease is often undiagnosed during life, but in countries where it is common the presence of the worm may be suspected from a frequent cough followed by repeated vomiting. They may result in death from exhaustion.

Damage to the carotid artery by *Spirocerca lupi* worms (3 in each of two nodules attached to the oesophagus) led to the death in the UK of an alsation from internal haemorrhage. (Bannor, T. T., *Vet. Rec.* (1976) **98**.) This parasite appears also to be closely associated with sarcoma of the oseophagus.

II. Stomach

A microscopic gastric nematode of cats, *Ollulanus tricuspis*, has been found in the Americas, Australasia, and Europe. The worm causes unthriftiness and vomiting in kittens. (*JAVMA*, **178**, 468.)

III. Small intestine

ASCARIDS include several species that occur in dogs and cats. In cats the species seem to be *A. tubaeforme* and *A. braziliense.*

HOOKWORMS IN DOGS. Two species of hookworm are found in dogs: *Ancylostoma caninum* and *Uncinaria stenocephala*. The latter is found in Britain. These are smallish worms, about ¾ in long, found in the small intestine.

Eggs are passed to the exterior in the faeces and hatch in the soil or water. After several moults, the resulting larva become infective. This larva is able to gain access to the host either in the food or by penetrating the unbroken skin. It enters the blood-stream and is carried to the lungs. It then passes up the trachea and is swallowed. It completes its development in the small intestine, where it becomes mature.

IV. Caecum. The whip-worm *Trichuris vulpis* occurs in the UK, and gives rise to diarrhoea/dysentery, loss of condition and a harsh, staring coat.

V. Heart. Dirofilaria. There are two species occurring in dogs and cats. *D. immitis* occurs in the heart of the dog and occasionally the cat. The female may reach a length of 30 cm, but the male is little more than half this size. It is found in Asia and, of recent years, in Britain. The embryos are hatched in the body of the female, and the young larvae, passed into the blood-stream, are sucked up by a mosquito in which they develop. After a certain period they escape from the fly, when it attacks another dog, and entering the blood are carried to the heart, where they complete their development.

The worms interfere to a greater or lesser extent with the circulation. No symptoms may be shown; or the dog may suddenly die. Other symptoms include anaemia, respiratory troubles, ascites, and so on. Various complications may be due to emboli, such as cough, dyspnoea, etc. Diagnosis is by demonstration of the microfilaria in the blood.

Another heart worm of the dog is *Angiostrongylus vasorum*, which has as intermediate hosts, slugs and snails. This worm, which has caused an outbreak of infestation in kennels in Ireland, lives in the pulmonary artery and the right ventricle of the heart. Symptoms include malaise, stiffness on running, and subcutaneous swellings (due to suppression of normal blood clotting by the parasites). Some lung damage may be caused; likewise anaemia.

(*See also under* HEARTWORMS.)

VI. Kidney. Dioctophyme renale. The kidney worm of dogs and wild carnivores is very large, reaching 1 m in length, and is a blood-red colour. It is found in Europe and USA. It occurs in the pelvis of the kidney, and occasionally destroys the kidney tissue, to leave only the wall as a cyst filled with a purulent fluid. The other kidney usually shows a compensatory hypertrophy. It is occasionally found in the bladder. Infestation follows the eating of raw fish.

The worm's eggs are barrel-shaped and maybe seen in the urine, under the microscope.

VII. Bladder. In the UK the bladder-worm *Capillaria plica* is rare, and seldom gives rise to obvious symptoms. A severe infestation can lead to inflammation of the bladder and a mucoid discharge from vagina or prepuce. In cats cystitis may rarely be caused by *C. feliscati*.

VIII. Trachea. Oslerus (Filaroides) osleri occurs in the UK and gives rise to a sporadic but persistent cough, especially on exercise or if the dog is excited. Retching may be caused. Severe infestation can give rise to emaciation despite a fair appetite, laboured breathing, sleeping standing, and death in young dogs. For control, Thiabendazole has given promising results.

Another tracheal worm *Capillaria aerophilia* seldom gives rise to obvious symptoms.

IX. Lungs. A minute worm lives in the lungs of cats in Britain and elsewhere in Europe and America. It may cause a fatal form of parasitic pneumonia. The parasite (*Aelurostrongylus abstrusus*) is transmitted to cats by mice. In Africa, *Bronchostrongylus subcrenatus* is found.

Lung lesions found at the autopsy of 5 out of a batch of 20 beagles were due to *Filaroides* species, 'probably *F. milksi* rather than *F. hirthi.*' The lungs had the appearance of being peppered with black spots. Signs of larval migration were seen microscopically in the liver, mesenteric lymph nodes, and gastro-intestinal tract. (J. Plumb, Beechan Pharmaceuticals. *Vet. Record* (1981) **109**, 267.)

Public health aspects (*see under* TOXOCARA).

ROUS SARCOMA of chickens. This is produced by a virus. (*See under* CANCER.)

-RRHAPHY is a suffix meaning an operation in which some opening or tear is closed by stitches.

RUBARTH'S DISEASE (*Hepatitis contagiosa canis*). This is named after the Swedish scientist Rubarth who, in 1947, described for the first time a disease in dogs which he called, on account of its contagious nature and the damage caused to the liver, *Hepatitis contagiosa canis*. This is now commonly known as CANINE VIRUS HEPATITIS (which see). He regarded this disease, on the basis of the microscopical findings, as identical with Fox Encephalitis which had been known in America for some seventeen years previously.

RUBBER BANDS. These sometimes get, or are put, on to the legs of cats (and possibly dogs), where they may remain unnoticed until the continual pressure has destroyed the skin beneath the band and caused damage to the underlying structures. Gangrene or loss of use of the limb results.

A successful prosecution has followed the application of rubber bands to cows' teats in the UK.

Rubber rings have been used for castration of lambs and calves, and for the docking of lambs. (*See* ELASTRATOR, etc.)

'RUBBER JAW'. A condition seen in the dog in some cases of chronic nephritis. It may be associated with enlargement of the parathyroid glands. Softening of the bones of the skull, particularly the jaw, occurs, and in a severely affected part the bone can be cut with a scalpel. There is resorption of bone and its replacement by vascular fibrous tissue. 'Rubber jaw' is not of course, seen in all cases of chronic nephritis, though some changes may be detected microscopically.

RUMEN is the first stomach of ruminants. It lies on the left side of the body, occupying the whole of the left side of the abdomen and even stretching across the median plane of the body to the right side. It is a capacious sac which is subdivided into an upper or *dorsal sac* and a lower or *ventral sac*, each of which has a *blind sac*, at its posterior extremity. These divisions are defined by the presence of grooves on the outside of the organ and by pillars or ridges internally. The whole organ is lined by mucous membrane which possesses a papillated, stratified, squamous epithelium containing no digestive glands, but mucus-secreting glands are present in large numbers. Its entrance is through the oesophagus, and its exit is into the reticulum or second stomach through the *rumeno-reticular orifice*.

Coarse, partially-chewed food is stored and churned in the rumen until such time as the animal finds circumstances convenient for rumination. When this occurs, little balls of food are regurgitated through the oesophagus into the mouth, and are subjected to a second more thorough mastication. Each bolus is chewed from 30 to 60 times and mixed with copious amounts of saliva, to be swallowed and pass onwards into other parts of the compound stomach.

In rare instances, the rumen is situated on the right-hand side. (*See* D. H. Ellicott and A. Jones, *Vet. Rec.* (1976) **99**, 318.)

RUMEN FLUKES. Belonging to the genus *Paramphistomum*, these are found both in the tropics and North America.

Conical in shape, round in cross-section, they inhabit not only the rumen but also the reticulum, and – when immature – the duodenum. They are also found occasionally in the bile ducts and urinary bladder.

Little damage is caused to the rumen, but in young animals a severe enteritis is the important aspect of the disease; resulting in diarrhoea, unthriftiness, anaemia, and sometimes death.

Paramphistomum flukes have a life-history similar to that of the common liver fluke *Fasciola hepatica*; several species of snails being the intermediate hosts.

RUMEN, ULCERATION OF. In calves ulcers in the rumen may be associated with lesions of the liver caused by *Bacteroides* (*Fusiformis necrophorus*). (*See also* STOMACH, DISEASES OF.)

RUMINAL DIGESTION. In the rumen, bacteria break down the cellulose (which forms the structural materials of plants), and starch by means of enzymes, and convert them into fatty acids. The bacteria fall a prey to the protozoa which, besides digesting starch, thus perform the useful task of converting plant protein into animal protein. This becomes available to the cow when the protozoa are, in their turn, destroyed further down the digestive tract and themselves digested.

A sample taken from the rumen, at the Hannah Research Institute, contained 100 million protozoa and 5 million bacteria (giving some idea of the proportion of the two). Examples of protozoa included *Entodiniomorph* species, which feed on plant material, bacteria, and each other; and *Holotrich* species, which ferment soluble sugars from plants and feed on bacteria. (*See also under* FIBRE in the section on DIET, *and under* LACTIC ACID.)

RUMINAL TYMPANY (*see* BLOAT).

RUMINATION, or 'CUDDING', is the process whereby food taken into the stomachs of ruminants is returned to the mouth, subjected to a second more thorough chewing, and is again swallowed.

The act occurs at intervals of from 6 to 8 hours, and occupies a longer or shorter time according to the nature of the food and the amount taken at the last meal. It usually commences about half an hour after feeding ceases, and probably continues until all the coarser constituents have been re-chewed, or at least until the animal is disturbed. This fact is of considerable importance practically; cattle and sheep should be allowed at least 2 hours' rest after feeding before they are subjected to any severe exertion. Disregard of this is a fruitful contributory cause of stomach disorders in both cattle and sheep. (*See also under* RUMEN.)

The act of regurgitation appears to be in reality a complex one, but it may be briefly summarised as follows:

(1) The tension of the oesophagus relaxes, partly by dilatation, and partly through an inspiratory movement of the diaphragm (the glottis being temporarily closed) which reduces pressure in the thorax.

(2) The rumen and the reticulum powerfully contract and squeeze upon their contents.

(3) The abdominal muscles contract and raise the intra-abdominal pressure.

The direct result is that ingested foodstuffs are forced from the area of high pressure (*i.e.* the rumen and reticulum) through the open oesophagus into an area of lower pressure (*i.e.* into the thoracic portion of the oesophagus). When a small quantity, sufficient to form a bolus or 'cud', has entered the oesophagus, the lips of the oesophageal groove and the muscles in the vicinity close the terminal part of the oesophagus, and there commences an antiperistaltic movement which conveys the 'cud' upwards past the closed glottis, underneath the soft palate, and so into the mouth. Excess fluid is immediately squeezed from the mass and swallowed, and chewing movements commence at once. Each bolus is chewed from 30 to 60 times according to its consistency, size, and to the nature of its constituents; coarse straw or hay fodder requiring the longest time.

The chewing occupies from ½ to 1¼ minutes, and then the bolus is rolled up by the dorsum of the tongue and again swallowed. In from 3 to 6 seconds another bolus has reached the mouth, and so the process is continued.

'RUN-BACK'. This must be avoided by means of back fences. (*See under* STRIP-GRAZING.)

RUNCH (*see* CHARLOCK POISONING).

'RUNNERS'. This is an old, popular term for hounds unable to gallop properly. 'Runners' are usually recognised as such when they return to hunt kennels at about 7 months old after being walked; and they are then often culled from the pack. Technically, the condition is known as osteochondrosis of the spine. Symptoms include: poor muscular development in the spinal region, poor bodily condition, an unnatural gait, and often inability to jump a fence successfully negotiated by the rest of the pack. Some curvature and rigidity of the spine may also be observed. It seems that this is, in part at least, an inherited defect of foxhounds.

RUNT PIGS. Many of these can be reared with the help of antibiotic supplements. (*See* ADDITIVES.)

RUPTURE is a popular name for hernia. (*See* HERNIA.) The term is also applied to the tearing across of a muscle, tendon, ligament, artery, nerve, etc. Rupture of the aorta is a cause of death in male turkeys 5–22 weeks old.

RUSSIAN GAD-FLY. *Rhinoestrus purpureus.* This attacks horses in Europe and North Africa.

RUSSIAN SPRING-SUMMER VIRUS causes an encephalitis of man and goat, caused by a virus and transmitted by the tick *Ixodes ricinus* in Russia, Poland, and Czechoslovakia.

RYE-GRASS poisoning has caused the death of cattle and horses restricted to grazing rye-grass pasture. (*Lolium perenne.*) In New Zealand and Australia, a fungus present on the rye-grass may cause facial eczema. A staggering gait – and convulsions – may occur in cattle and sheep on rye-grass pasture giving rise to the colloquial name 'Rye-grass staggers'. In a UK outbreak in sheep, they had 'a rocking-horse gait, and when chased fell down and trembled violently'. (Veterinary Investigation Service report, 1976.) Fungal toxins are now regarded as the most likely cause of 'Rye-grass staggers' both in the UK and New Zealand. (*See also* CEREBROCORTICAL NECROSIS.)

RYZAMIN-B. A proprietary syrup made from rice-polishings, used in vitamin B therapy.

S

SABULOUS. Gritty, sandy.

SACKS may be a means of passing infection from one farm to another, for when empty they are put to many uses. Poisoning has occurred through contamination of feeding-stuffs by sacks previously used for sheep-dip. For these reasons, non-returnable paper sacks have advantages over jute sacks.

SACRUM is the part of the spinal column lying between the lumbar region and the tail. It consists of 5 vertebrae in the horse and ox, 4 in the sheep and pig, and 3 in the dog and cat, fused together in each case. It is roughly triangular in shape in all animals, and forms the roof of the pelvic cavity, lying midway between the two 'points of the hip' or 'haunch bones'.

SADDLE-SORES are formed through uneven pressure upon the back by some part of the saddle. They may be found in the middle line, immediately over the upper ends of the spinous processes; they may occur on either side of the middle line where the fore arch of the saddle-tree presses; or they may be found just behind the elbow, when they are caused by badly fastened girths, and are often called 'girth-galls'.

The injuries consist of raw areas from which the hair has been rubbed or chafed off and, later, ulcers. Or, alternatively, patches of the skin, varying in size from an inch in diameter to almost 3 inches, may become hard and leathery, pus being formed underneath. These are known as 'sitfasts'.

TREATMENT. Attention must first of all be paid to the saddles. They should fit evenly all over the back, and the stuffing or padding should be adequate to protect the skin from pressure by the rigid framework of the saddle-tree. The hollow of the arch of the saddle should never press upon the middle line of the back, and the girth should never be fastened with the skin folded under it. Rest from work will be necessary. (*See* ULCERS, WOUND TREATMENT.)

SAGITTAL. A structure or section running transversely across the trunk or a limb.

SAINFOIN. (*Onobrychis sativa*). A forage crop with great potential in the UK. Being a legume it fixes its own nitrogen; it contains tannins, so its rumen protein degradability is low (this means that the protein is used more efficiently); and it does not cause bloat. Voluntary intake by animals is high – trials at GRI have shown intakes of sainfoin can be 25 per cent higher than ryegrass. Furthermore, it is drought-resistant.

Unfortunately, sainfoin does not grow as well as bred strains of grasses, clovers and lucerne; a figure of 30 per cent less yield than lucerne is quoted. Work is in progress at GRI and else-where to try to overcome this. (*Grassland Research Institute*—1986)

ST JOHN'S WORT. This plant, *Hypericum perforatum*, which may be present in hay, does not lose its poisonous character when dried. It causes LIGHT SENSITISATION (which see) in cattle, sheep, and pigs, especially in Australia.

ST LOUIS ENCEPHALITIS. Transmitted by mosquitos, and caused by a flavivirus, this disease occurs in North and South America, affecting wild birds, bats, horses and man (in which it may cause encephalitis and death in the elderly, although only fever in other people).

SALICYLIC ACID and the **SALICYLATES** are prepared either synthetically, or, when a pure compound is wanted, from oil of wintergreen or oil of sweet birch. *Aspirin*, which is acetyl-salicylic acid, largely replaced the other salicylates as pain relievers (*see* ANALGESICS), and has been given in fevers (*but see* ASPIRIN).

Salicylate **poisoning** has occurred in young animals following overdosage. Symptoms include depression, loss of appetite and vomiting. Treatment involves the use of an emetic or gastric lavage and respiratory stimulants.

It has been found in human medicine that repeated administration of salicylates may give rise to anaemia following slight internal haemorrhages. In the cat, gr. 5 daily may prove fatal within 12 days.

SALINE (*see under* NORMAL SALINE).

SALINOMYCIN. An IONOPHORE (which see) used as a coccidiostat in chickens, and also (overseas) as a growth-promoting feed additive for pigs.
Salinomycin poisoning. Four hundred point-of-lay turkeys died within a week after the introduction of a diet containing 50 ppm salinomycin.

In horses the signs of poisoning were eyelid swelling, anorexia, colic, weakness, ataxia. (Rollinson, J. *Veterinary Record* (1987) **121** 126).

SALIVA is the fluid which, normally, is always present in the mouth, and is secreted from the salivary glands, especially copiously immediately before and during feeding. Saliva contains much mucus and, in the domestic animals, very little ptyalin – an enzyme which acts on starches (changing starch into maltose), and in samples taken from the mouth there are always large numbers of the usual bacterial inhabitants. In domestic animals, the chief action appears to be one of lubrication, rather than one of digestion of the starch in the food. This is particularly the case in dogs, which bolt their food before time has been allowed for enzyme action to take place, and in cattle swallowing their food for the first time; in them, however, it appears probable that during rumination the ptyalin (if present) acts upon the starch in a more efficient manner, although, even at the best, the action is never so thorough as in man.

An excessive flow of saliva is referred to under SALIVATION and in some types of poisoning. (*See also under* MOUTH.)

SALIVARY GLANDS include the *parotid gland*, lying in the space below the ear and behind the border of the lower jaw; the *submaxillary gland*, lying just within the angle of the lower jaw, under the lower part of the parotid; and the *sublingual gland*, which lies at the side of the root of the tongue. Each of these glands is paired, so that actually there are six glands, not all of which function at the same time.

SALIVARY GLANDS, DISEASES OF. As with all tissues, local inflammation and infection may occur. Calculi and tumours may occur. In rabies the salivary glands must become infected before transmission of the virus to another host can occur through a bite. (*See also* MUMPS.) A foreign body, such as a grass seed, may cause an obstruction to one of the ducts, particularly in the dog.

Salivary gland tumours in dogs and cats are rare. The majority of 138 tumours in dogs (81) and cats (57) involved animals of 10 years of age or more, were malignant and of epithelial origin (84 per cent). Local recurrence after excision occurs frequently and metastasis to regional lymph nodes and beyond is common (Carbeny, C. A. and others (1988) *Journal of the American Animal Hospital Association* **24**, 561).

SALIVATION. 'Foaming at the mouth', to use a colloquial but apt expression, is seen in the dog, *e.g.* in an epileptic or other fit. (*See* FITS.) 'Drooling of saliva' is seen in the dog with a bone wedged across the roof of its mouth, or in a cat

with a needle embedded in its tongue – or in cases of RABIES in all species.

Salivation is a symptom of CHOKING, of almost any painful condition of the mouth or tongue, and of poisoning (*e.g.* by benzoic acid in the cat; arsenic, lead, phosphorus and organophosphorus compounds; and *see* TOAD.

Salivation is also an important symptom of FOOT-AND-MOUTH DISEASE, and of other diseases and conditions mentioned under MOUTH.

'SALMON POISONING' in dogs occurs on the Pacific coast of the USA, and is the result of eating salmon or trout infested with the fluke *Troglotrema salmincola*, containing a rickettsia. The latter, *Neorickettsia helminthoeca*, produces a haemorrhagic gastro-enteritis which is usually fatal unless antibiotics are used in time.

SALMONELLOSIS. Infection with organisms of the *Salmonella* group is of importance from two distinct aspects: (1) food poisoning in man, and (2) disease in domestic animals.

Salmonella poisoning – routes of infection (*see diagram*).

In cattle and calves. Salmonellosis and brucellosis have four points in common – both are important from the public health point of view, both can lead to abortion in cattle, to a carrier state likely to perpetuate infection on the farm, and to considerable financial loss to the farmer.

While the salmonella group of bacteria includes over 1000 different serotypes, the two of most importance to the dairy farmer are *Salmonella dublin* and *Salmonella typhimurium*. Either can produce acute or subacute illness in adult cattle and in calves.

S. typhimurium infection is of greater public health importance, and is a notorious cause of outbreaks of food poisoning in man. In 1944, in

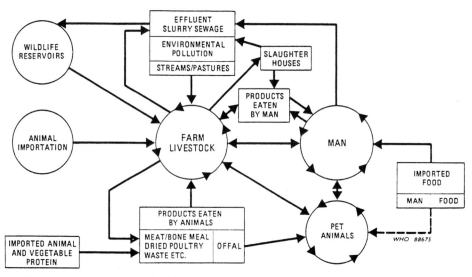

(With acknowledgement to the World Health Organisation's *Technical Report* no. 774, 1988.)

the West Riding of Yorkshire, no less than 79 households, involving 162 people, suffered from food poisoning as a result of this organism being excreted by an apparently healthy cow.

An outbreak of this same infection involved over 200 cows on a single farm, and led to the death or slaughter of 29 of them.

S. dublin infection may be associated with abortion, sometimes without any other symptoms being observed. Animals which recover may excrete the organisms for years. Besides this carrier state, which may keep infection on the farm, there is also a latent carrier state in which the organism remains dormant within the animal until it is subjected to some stress or superimposed disease, and then excretion of the organism occurs and fellow members of the herd become infected.

SIGNS. The two infections are usually very similar and can be distinguished only by laboratory means. In the acute form of the disease, the cow becomes dull, feverish, goes off her food, and the milk yield suddenly drops. Scouring is usually severe, and the animal may pass blood and even shreds of mucous membrane from the intestine. Death may occur within a week. If treatment is delayed, mortality may rise to 70 per cent or so; whereas early treatment can bring the death rate down to 10 per cent. In animals which recover, scouring may persist for a fortnight, and it may be several weeks before the cow is fit again.

The sub-acute form in adult cattle runs a milder course and, indeed, the infection may exist without any symptoms being shown. A latent infection may become an overt one following stress of any kind or when another disease becomes superimposed – sometimes masking the symptoms of salmonellosis itself. A liver-fluke infestation may be a precipitating factor.

Salmonellosis may run through eight calves out of a batch of 10, and kill four of them. Some calves collapse and die without ever scouring; others become very emaciated as a result of persistent scouring. Pneumonia, arthritis, and jaundice may be among the complications; and occasionally the brain is involved, giving rise to nervous symptoms.

S. typhimurium infection seldom persists from one season to another on any particular farm because there are fewer 'carrier' animals than there are with *S. dublin*; it is often brought on to the farm by calves bought in from markets and suffering from the effects of stress, rough travelling conditions, lack of food or a change of diet. The infection occurs in many species of animal including, as the name suggests, mice.

S. dublin infection arises mostly from other cattle. It can be spread from farm to farm via slurry and streams. The Ministry's veterinary service has pointed out that infection may enter even a closed herd if it is grazing flooded pasture land.

Lack of shelter, overcrowding, dirty surroundings, and faulty feeding were all implicated in outbreaks investigated by M A F F during the last six months of 1980. In adult cattle, the fortnight after calving is regarded as a danger period, especially where the calving has been a difficult one.

It was shown in 1969 that *S. dublin* could survive in slurry for at least 12 weeks.

It is also known that salmonella organisms can survive for 6 months or so in dung and litter, and *S. dublin* can survive for up to 307 days, if not longer, on dung splashes on a wall, so that

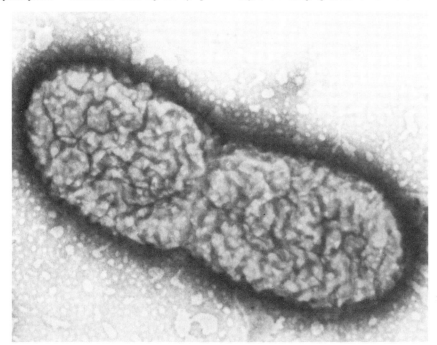

An electron-micrograph of *Salmonella dublin*. (Magnification ×50,000.) Reproduced by courtesy of Dr J. R. Walton, Department of Veterinary Preventive Medicine, The University of Liverpool.

thorough cleaning and disinfection of buildings are necessary, and reliance must not be placed on a simple 'resting period' between batches of calves.

Salmonella organisms may be present in domestic sewage, and river pollution from this source has led to an outbreak of salmonellosis in cattle.

There is not much which the farmer can do about feeds and fertilisers, but preventive measures which can be taken include keeping rats and mice off feed, avoiding pig and poultry effluent for organic irrigation, having piped drinking water for cattle, and not buying in through markets or dealers but rather from farms with a known health record. The earlier housing of cattle in the autumn may help, and it is important not to neglect liver fluke infestation which can sometimes act as a 'trigger' to outbreaks of salmonellosis in which the infection was hitherto latent.

With salmonellosis in mind, MAFF introduced the Diseases of Animals (Protein Processing) Order 1981 and the Importation of Processed Animal Protein Order 1981.

TREATMENT. Drugs used include furazolidone, chloramphenicol, and ampicillin.

Calf vaccination is recommended.

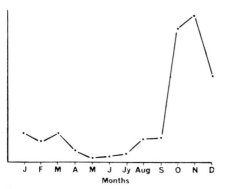

Seasonal incidence of salmonellosis (with acknowledgements to the *British Veterinary Journal*).

In sheep. *S. typhimurium* has caused diarrhoea and abortion. *S. agona* has caused abortion, death of ewes from septicaemia, death of lambs within a week of birth, and *sometimes* diarrhoea. *S. dublin* is likewise a cause of abortion and diarrhoea.

One outbreak in an upland sheep flock was characterised by rapid spread and heavy mortality in ewes and young lambs. Clinical signs included diarrhoea and abortion. Abomasitis was the most striking and consistent post mortem lesion. Vaccination was the only control method that was apparently successful. Infection also occurred in the cattle, farm personnel, and a dog.

(*See also under* ABORTION – Ewe.)

In pigs. The term 'salmonellosis' is now usually reserved for a severe septicaemia. *Salmonella cholerae suis* causes this; symptoms including fever, huddling together, purple discoloration of ears, unsteady gait, *sometimes* scouring. The same organism may give rise to a chronic infection with scouring. The organism can infect man.

A live vaccine is available for prevention on farms where this infection is a recurrent problem.

Infection with *Salmonella dublin* sometimes occurs in pigs, and may give rise to dysentery.

More common is infection with *S. typhimurium*. This causes fever, scouring, vomiting, unsteady gait, usually in younger pigs than the first-named organism. Sulphamezathine has proved useful in treatment.

In horses. *S. typhimurium* has caused serious outbreaks of illness in young horses. Horses may also be symptomless carriers of this infection. In 1976 an outbreak of *S. newport* infection caused the death of many horses in the UK. (*See also* FOALS, DISEASES OF.) Overseas *S. abortus equi* is a cause of abortion in mares.

Stress, associated with the hospitalisation of horses, is said to have led to acute enteritis, often from *S. senftenberg*.

In dogs. Illness may be mild, with fever and malaise; or there may be severe gastro-enteritis and death. Many *Salmonella* serotypes infect dogs. It is possible for a dog to become a symptomless carrier of *S. typhimurium* and to infect man. Pneumonia and convulsions may occur, as well as diarrhoea and vomiting. Of rectal swabs from 672 dogs (472 household pets, 181 kennel dogs, and 19 strays) in Teheran, 7·7 per cent yielded Salmonellae of 20 different serotypes. (A. Shimi *et al.*, *Vet. Rec.* (1976) **98**, 110.

Feeding raw offal to dogs had been suspected as an important source of salmonellosis in West Berlin. Accordingly, 408 samples of edible offal (liver, lungs, heart, bovine rumen, and porcine oesophagus) were examined bacteriologically. It was found that 231 samples (57 per cent) were infected with salmonella. *S. typhimurium* was the most prevalent of 24 serotypes. (Sinell, H. J. & others., *Journal of Food Protection* (1984) **47**, 481.)

In cats. Infection with *Salmonella enteritidis* and *S. typhimurium* may be set up following the catching of infected rats and mice. For this reason cats should not be allowed to lie on uncovered foodstuffs. Cats may also become infected through contaminated meat sold at some pet shops.

In poultry. Over 50 members of the *Salmonella* group have now been isolated from poultry in this country, and several have caused outbreaks of disease in broiler plants. (*See* PULLORUM DISEASE, FOWL TYPHOID.)

Arthritis, due to a variant strain of *Salmonella pullorum*, gives rise to a mortality of 5 per cent or so, as a rule, but in one outbreak 200 deaths occurred in a 1000-bird unit. Apart from lameness and swelling of the foot and hock joints, symptoms include poor feathering and under-development. Deaths can be expected between the ages of 10 days and 5 weeks.

It was found that survivors did not react to a blood test carried out with standard *S. pullorum* antigen, but reacted strongly to antigen prepared from the variant strain. This probably accounts for carrier birds having remained undetected in the past.

During a 5-year period birds in 144 flocks in Sweden were given cultures of caecal contents as a means of controlling salmonella infection by the competitive exclusion technique. In all 2·86 million birds were treated and it was concluded that this treatment was associated with a reduction in salmonella infections. No adverse effects were reported. (Wierup, M., and others (1988) *Poultry Science* **67**, 1026).

Salmonellas will remain alive for periods of up to 6 months or more in dung and litter. Therefore such material should be stacked so that heating occurs; no animals should have access to the heap.

In ducks. Salmonella species sometimes cause a high mortality in ducklings. Fatal cases of human food poisoning have occurred as a result of infected ducks' eggs.

Public health. As already mentioned, salmonellosis is an important cause of 'food-poisoning' in man, often leading to serious illness. In a 1967 survey in the Portsmouth region, a link was established between isolates of *S. seftenberg* from human beings and a poultry processing plant. *S. kiambu* and *S. enteritidis* were isolated from frozen turkeys from the same batch which caused 64 cases of illness in people. *S. panama* and *S. brandenburg* were similarly isolated from abattoirs/processing plants and human beings.

A vet suffered an unusual salmonella infection following a difficult calving/abortion of a cow subsequently found to be infected with *Salmonella dublin*. Protective gloves were worn as a precaution but they split during the procedure.

In 1969 and 1970, stated the *Lancet* (September 1, 1973), *Salmonella agona* emerged as a public-health problem in the USA, the UK, Netherlands, and Israel. In each country an initial isolation from Peruvian fish-meal was followed by recovery of *S. agona* from domestic animals and subsequently from man. By 1972, *S. agona* was the eighth most commonly isolated serotype in the USA, accounting for more than 500 cases in man, and the second most common serotype in the UK, causing approximately 700 cases. An investigation of an outbreak in Paragould, Arkansas, traced the source of infection from a restaurant back to a Mississippi poultry farm using Peruvian fish-meal. 'This outbreak illustrates the complexity of the chain of transmission of salmonellosis and emphasises the importance of animal feeds in salmonellosis in man.' (*See* ZOONOSES ORDER.)

Unpasteurised milk is another source of human salmonellosis. A 65-year-old woman was infected in this way, and was ill with diarrhoea and meningitis. After her death a brain abscess was found. Both the latter and meningitis are 'rare complications of salmonellosis in man'. Seventeen other people were ill with salmonellosis from drinking the unpasteurised milk. (M. E. Ellis and others, *British Medical Journal* (1981) **283**, 273.)

Viable salmonellas were found in the meat fraction of domestic refuse from 120 houses. This 'could provide a reservoir of infection accessible to wild animals'. Tipping should be carefully controlled, and refuse covered immediately.

(D. S. Durrant and S. H. Beatson, *Journal of Hygiene* (1981) **86**, 259.

The protective gloves, worn by a veterinary surgeon while calving a cow, unfortunately burst. 'Within 48 hours numerous *non-pruritic papules* had appeared over both my arms, especially the upper arm, where the gown cuffs had chafed the skin. The papules developed into pustules which burst and resolved in approximately 10 days without treatment. No other symptoms were observed.

'A pustule was swabbed and a pure growth of *Salmonella* species was recovered, (unfortunately, not typed.)'

(*See also under* SAUSAGE.)

SALOLITHS. These are CALCULI, found mainly in STENSON'S DUCT of horses.

SALPINGITIS is inflammation in the Fallopian tubes or oviducts, sometimes the cause of sterility in cattle. (*See* INFERTILITY.)

SALT, A. A chemical substance in which a metal is substituted for the hydrogen of an acid.

Sodium chloride (common salt) is an essential ingredient of body fluids. Sodium depletion results, ultimately, in circulatory collapse. (Michel, A. R. *Veterinary Record* (1985) **116**, 653.)

Salt is an appetiser, and commonly incorporated in animal feeds in carefully measured proportions.

Dr Michel pointed out that ruminants, like people, avidly consume salt in quantities greatly exceeding their physiological requirements; and that sodium deficiency, other than in high-yielding dairy cows, or those with diarrhoea, is seldom encountered in ruminants.

His advice is: be liberal with salt; any excess is harmlessly excreted in the urine and faeces. **Salt licks.** Previously other authorities had suggested that a 10-cwt cow needs ¾ oz salt a day for maintenance and a further ⅛ oz for every gallon of milk produced. Therefore, a 700-gallon cow requires about 30 lb of salt yearly.

On some pastures or under some systems of management they may not obtain sufficient. To obviate this danger, salt licks are commonly provided. In some salt licks traces of iodine are incorporated and sometimes also other 'trace elements' such as copper, manganese, cobalt, magnesium. (*See* LICKING SYNDROME.)

SALT POISONING has been reported in both pigs and poultry. It is essential that pigs are not kept short of water, or given too salt food.

An outbreak, reported from Scotland, involved piglets aged 6 weeks brought indoors from field arks at weaning. A proprietary meal was fed dry. The water bowls in the house were not very accessible, and some of the piglets were not strong enough to depress the levers. Two days after being housed, 23 out of the 32 piglets were showing symptoms of salt poisoning, and some died.

SIGNS. Often a number of pigs are found dead without symptoms having been observed, the remainder being weak and very thirsty. Vomiting and diarrhoea may occur. (For other symptoms, *see under* MENINGOENCEPHALITIS.)

In poultry, adult birds show excessive thirst and diarrhoea, with sometimes cyanosis of the wattles, somnolence, and sudden death. In young birds gasping and ascites may occur. (*See* BRINE *also*.)

SAND COLIC is a form of colic due to the collection in the caecum and colon of quantities of sand. It may be caused through feeding horses with food contaminated with sand; horses grazing on the seashore or along tidal mud flats learn that the sand contains salt, and may lick up large quantities of it in their endeavour to get the salt. The symptoms set up are chiefly those of colic with impaction. (*See* COLIC.)

Cattle feeding on the seashore take in with their food quantities of sand, which in some cases may be so great as to hinder the movements of the rumen (where the sand always collects), and, by upsetting digestion, may cause unthriftiness and even emaciation.

SANDCRACK is a pathological condition affecting horses' feet, in which a deep fissure or crack forms at some part of the wall of the hoof, extending downwards from the coronet, and usually involving the whole of the thickness of the wall.
CAUSES. Anything which interferes with the proper nutrition of the horn at the coronet predisposes to sandcrack, the actual splitting of the horn occurring as the result of the strains put upon the foot. Treads on the inside of the coronet, occasioned by hurried turning when at work, are frequent causes in the fore-feet, and continual pressure on the coronary matrix by the second phalanx, especially when the toes have been allowed to grow too long, appears to be the commonest cause in the hind-feet. A predisposition to sandcrack may be inherited.

With all cases it is advisable to place the animal under veterinary care. (*See* HOOF REPAIR.)

'SANDFLIES' (*see* FLIES).

SAND TAMPAN, *Ornithodorus savignyi.* (*See* TICKS – Family Argasidae.)

SANGUINEOUS means containing blood.

SANTA GERTRUDI. This breed of cattle are ⅝ Shorthorn and ⅜ Brahman in origin.

SAPO is the Latin name for soap.

SAPONINS. These are natural detergents, present in some plants such as Corn cockle and Soapwort. Saponins contain a sugar and a steroid-like compound, and with water form a lather. Poisoning by them results in gastro-enteritis. The central nervous system may also be affected, with consequent paralysis. Saponins break down red blood cells. In the USA the leaves and nuts of the Tung tree, grown for the sake of its oil, can cause fatal poisoning.

SARCO- is a prefix signifying flesh or fleshy.
Sarcolemma. The membrane covering each voluntary (striated) muscle fibre.

SARCOCYSTIS. A genus of protozoal, coccidian parasites having a two-host life-cycle. Carnivorous animals such as dogs, cats and foxes ingest the cysts when eating infected flesh of cattle, sheep, pigs and horses. Human infection also occurs, and sarcocystis is a ZOONOSIS.

While the cysts in the intermediate host's muscles may not have any serious effect upon health, the second-generation schizonts are certainly harmful; damaging the endothelium of blood vessels, and causing serious illness in many cases.
SIGNS. Cattle showed loss of appetite, fever, anaemia, and wasting, after feeding them sporocysts from canine faeces, and some cattle died within 33 days. Sarcocystosis has also killed sheep. In horses signs of central nervous system damage may be seen, as well as signs of muscle inflammation, resulting in lameness.
PREVALENCE. In Europe between 61 and 99 per cent of slaughtered cattle have been found to be infected. In West Germany a prevalence rate of 5 per cent in pigs has been recorded.

Human sarcocystosis may give rise to abdominal pain, diarrhoea, fever, tachycardia, and an increased respiratory rate.

'SARCOID'. A tumour which resembles histologically a sarcoma, but which is regressive in character, disappearing within a matter of months. It has the appearance of a reddish button, raised about an eighth of an inch above the surrounding skin. It affects the **dog**.

A fibroma-like sarcoid is perhaps the most common tumour of **horses,** especially older ones, occurring on limbs or head. Believed to be caused by a virus, the equine sarcoid commonly ulcerates and recurs following surgery. Cryosurgery may be tried, or a BCG vaccine. A guarded prognosis should be given.

Bovine papillomavirus is involved in the process by which sarcoids develop from equine fibrous tissue. (Wood, A. L. & Spradbrow, P. B. *Research in Veterinary Science* (1985) **38,** 241.)

SARCOMA (*see* CANCER).

SARCOPTES are members of a class of parasitic acari, which cause mange in animals and man.

Sarcoptic mange occurs in cattle, horses, sheep, pigs, and dogs – also in man, when it is called Scabies – and is caused by the parasitic mite *Sarcoptes scabei.* (*See* MITES.) Cats are only very rarely infected.

SARCOSPORIDIA, SARCOSPORIDIOSIS (*see* SARCOCYSTIS).

SAUSAGE. Discarded portions of sausage, or sausage-skin, can be a source of infection when fed, unboiled, to pigs, etc. Foot-and-mouth disease has been transmitted in this way. African

Swine Fever and Swine Fever could similarly be spread by this means. (*See* SWILL.)

The incidence of salmonella contamination of pork and beef and pork sausages taken from a large factory during the course of production was 65 per cent and 55 per cent respectively. The salmonella serotypes isolated (in descending order of incidence) included *Salmonella derby, S. dublin, S. newport, S. stanley, S. typhimurium, S. heidelberg, S. infantis* and *S. agona.* (Banks, J. G. and Board, R. G. (1983) *Journal of Hygiene,* **90,** 213.)

SAVAGING OF LITTERS by sows. – Various causes of this have been suggested, including: an inherited tendency; absence of any straw for nesting purposes; a painful udder; insufficient time to have become used to her farrowing quarters; and fright resulting from the use of a farrowing crate. (*See* PIGS, SEDATION OF.)

SAWDUST (*see under* BEDDING *and* MASTITIS).

SAWFLIES. Four-winged insects which have a saw-like ovipositor. The larvae can cause poisoning if swallowed.

Sawfly poisoning. This affects both sheep and goats.
CAUSE: The larvae of the birch sawfly (*Arge pullata*).
SIGNS: Depression, anorexia, muscular incoordination with a difficulty in rising to their feet.
AUTOPSY FINDINGS: Liver necrosis petechial haemorrhages, and sometimes degeneration of the kidney tubules. (S. M. Thamsborg, *et al. Veterinary Record* (1987) **121**, 253.)

SCABIES (*see* MITES – Sarcoptic mange).

'SCAD'. A colloquial name for a transitory lameness, in sheep, which may follow frost. (*See* 'SCALD'.)

'SCALD'. Inflammation between the digits of young sheep, causing acute lameness. Its onset is said to be associated with frosts and moisture. Recovery may occur spontaneously under dry conditions. The term is vague, however, and has been used to include the non-progressive form of foot-rot. It has to be differentiated from foot-and-mouth disease. (*See also* 'SCAD' *and* OVINE INTERDIGITAL DERMATITIS.)

SCALDS (*see* BURNS).

'SCALY LEG' (*see* MITES, mange in the fowl).

SCANNER, BODY. The EMI-Scanner is briefly described under X-rays.

Scanning. (*See also* RADIOISOTOPES.)

SCAPHOID. A small bone present in the carpus and tarsus. In the racing greyhound, fracture of the right hind scaphoid is a common accident. Treatment has included the removal of bone fragments and the successful insertion of a plastic 'scaphoid'.

SCAPULA is the shoulder blade, the large, triangular, flat bone that lies on the outside of the front of the chest, to which are attached many of the muscles that unite the fore-limb to the trunk.

SCHEDULED DISEASES (*see under* NOTIFIABLE DISEASES).

SCHISTOSOMIASIS. Infestation with *Schistosoma* worms or flukes, which are also known as **bilharzia** worms. They inhabit the portal and mesenteric veins mostly; one species preferring veins of the urinary bladder, and another the veins of the nose. Cattle and sheep and virtually all domestic animals, and man, may become infested.

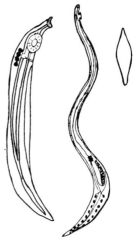

Schistosoma, ♂, ♀, and egg.

Several species have been reported from mammals in India, Africa, and Europe. *S. bovis* may cause anaemia, emaciation and death of cattle in Africa, or the infestation may be sub-clinical. In India *S. nasalis* may produce a nasal discharge and difficulty in breathing, with sometimes the formation of a granuloma. In the Far East, *S. japonicum* occurs in water-buffalo and infests man, in which the disease is very serious.

The life-cycle differs from the typical case, in that the free cercaria may pierce the skin of its host instead of being swallowed.

The sexes are separate, and are usually found with the female lying in a groove formed by the incurved edges of the male.

SCHMORL'S DISEASE is a disease of rabbits, involving areas of necrosis of skin or mucous membrane, and caused by *Bacteroides necrophorus* (often after the animal's resistance has been lowered by some other pathogen).

SCHRADAN. An organo-phosphorus insecticide used in agriculture and a potential danger to farm live-stock. (*See also* PARATHION.) Symptoms of poisoning may include vomiting, lachrymation, salivation, straining, twitching, distressed breathing, and coma.

SCIATICA means pain connected with the sciatic nerve which runs down the thigh.

SCINTIGRAPHY. The application of nuclear medicine to the diagnosis of bone pathology and lameness. It has applications for dogs and horses. (*See* NUCLEAR MEDICINE.)

SCIRRHOUS CORD is a condition in which there is a chronic fibrous enlargement of the cut end of the spermatic cord following castration. In most cases the castration wound does not completely heal, but a small sinus discharging a thick white pus persists. The discharge may cease later, but the swelling of the cord goes on increasing slowly in size, until eventually it may be nearly as large as a man's head. In extreme cases the swelling extends upwards through the inguinal canal and into the abdomen and a mass weighing as much as 100 lb has occasionally been encountered in the horse on *post-mortem* examination. The treatment is entirely surgical.

SCIRRHUS is a term applied to a growth or to other hard fibrous conditions of various organs.

SCLERA, or SCLEROTIC COAT is the outermost hard fibrous coat of the eye. (*See* EYE.)

SCLERITIS means inflammation of the sclerotic coat of the eye. (**Sclerotitis.**)

SCLERODERMA (*see* CHANCRE).

SCLEROSIS means hardening of tissues.

SCOLIOSIS. Lateral curvature of the spine.

SCOMBIOTOXIC poisoning is a chemical intoxication which occurs as a result of eating food, almost always fish, that contains large amounts of histamine. The histamine is produced by bacterial degradation of histadine when the fish, particularly tuna, bonito and mackerel, and also sardines, pilchards and herrings, are stored for prolonged periods at elevated temperatures. Between 1976 and 1986, 258 incidents of suspected scombiotoxic fish poisoning were reported in human patients in Britain. The symptoms most consistently reported were rash, diarrhoea, flushing and headache. (Bartholomes, B. A. & others (1987) *Epidemiology and Infection* **99**, 775.)

SCORPION VENOM. This affects the nervous system, causing pain, salivation, erection of hair, dilated pupils, increased blood pressure, and muscular spasm.

'SCOTTIE CRAMP'. A condition apparently confined to the Scottish Terrier, and occurring usually for the first time at 4 to 8 months of age. There is cramp following exercise. In mild cases the animal may be seen to be in difficulties when negotiating steps; in severe cases a hundred yards' brisk trot will cause the animal to double up and collapse, and in a few instances excitement without exertion will give rise to cramp. Mild attacks often become worse, reaching a maximum severity at 12 or 15 months of age. At 2 or 2½ years of age the dog may have outgrown 'Scottie Cramp'. The cause is unknown. Intravenous injections of calcium borogluconate, or parathyroid extract administration, have been recommended. The condition could be eliminated by breeders.

'SCOURS, SCOURING' (*see* DIARRHOEA).

SCRAPIE is a disease of sheep mainly confined to the district of the English and Scottish Borders, to Spain, France, and Germany. Sheep imported into Australia, New Zealand, Canada, and the USA have brought the disease with them.

Australia and New Zealand are believed to have quickly eradicated the disease.

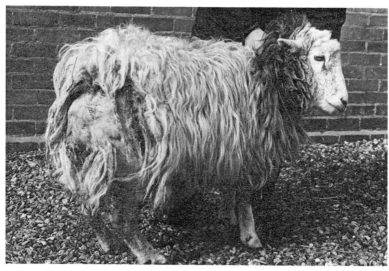

Scrapie.

Scrapie, BSE and other 'prion' diseases. It is possible that scrapie has a relationship with the human diseases kuru, Creutzfeld-Jakob disease and Gerstmann-Straussler-Scheinker syndrome. (Prusiner, S. B. & others (1991) *Cornell Veterinarian* **81**, 85.)

DIAGNOSIS. One method is to detect scrapie-associated fibrillar protein (PrP) by means of a rabbit-anti-sheep PrP polyclonal antibody by Western blot analysis; but consistent results have not, it seems, been obtained.

Experimentally, scrapie has been transmitted to goats, mice, rats, and hamsters.

CAUSE. An infective agent, possibly a prion.

At the 1985 BVA Congress Dr R. H. Kimberlin, of the joint AFRC and MRC Neuropathogenesis Unit, Edinburgh, said that examination of crude extracts of scrapie-infected brain had revealed accumulations of material known as scrapie-associated fibrils (SAF), which were also found in scrapie-like diseases.

Conventional selection of scrapie-resistant animals is protracted and costly but in 1989 the AFRC/MRC Neuropathogenesis Unit developed a blood test which can identify resistant animals within days.

A major component of SAF was a glycoprotein, and there was a close correlation between the amount of this and infectivity.

SIGNS. The most striking and easily seen symptom of scrapie is the torn, ruffled, and untidy appearance of the fleece, and when very severe, the bruised or scratched condition of the skin. In many cases, especially those occurring during the late spring, the fleece may be almost entirely rubbed off against fences, posts, trees or may be greatly removed by the mouth. In addition, the condition of the sheep is noteworthy; whereas the remainder of the flock may be in fair bodily condition, the scrapie sheep are thin, gaunt, and apt to become weak on their legs, lagging behind when going uphill, and losing their foothold when descending. Muscular tremors are often seen, and later there is evidence of intense itching.

Occasionally, when startled, as for instance, when being moved by dogs, or when a gun is fired near the unwary scrapie sheep, convulsive seizures are seen, usually lasting from 3 to 5 minutes, and leaving the animal temporarily dazed.

SCREW-WORM FLIES. These include *Chrysomyia bezziana* in Australia, *Cochliomyia hominivorax, C. Americana.*

The screw-worm (*Cochliomyia hominivorax*), a significant parasite of both humans and animals, had not been recorded outside the New World until its accidental introduction into Libya, probably in 1988–89. Hundreds of cases of wound myiasis including many fatalities were recorded in various species of domestic animals during 1989 and 1990.

An international campaign to eradicate the American screw-worm fly from North Africa appears to be succeeding, according to a bulletin from the organisers.

The campaign involved the release of sterile male flies imported from Mexico. The flies are dispersed by air at densities of 500 to 1200 per km² over an area of 40,000 km². Since the releases began in December 1990, 745 million flies have been used and currently 40 million a week are being dispersed, stated Dr Patrick Cunningham, director of the eradication programme. (*See* FLIES, MYIASIS *and* 'STRIKE'.)

SCROTAL. Relating to the scrotum.

SCROTUM, the pouch of skin in which the testicles are lodged, consists of a purse-like fold of skin that is generally hairless, within which each organ has an investment of muscle-fibres, several layers of fibrous tissue, and a serous membrane called the 'tunica vaginalis'.

SCRUB TYPHUS. (Japanese River Fever). A disease caused by *Rickettsia tsutsugamushi*, and transmitted by mites.

SCUR. A loose, horny growth, not attached to the skull, at the site normally occupied by a horn in a horned breed of cattle.

A bull calf with a scur, or with a bony protuberance beneath the skin at the horn site, is not a pure polled animal. Without these, a bull can be expected to breed true as regards the poll character; this can be checked by a progeny test of the bull mated to horned cows – the result should be polled heifer calves or bull calves with scurs or bony protuberances, but no calves with horns.

SEALIONS (*see* VESICULAR EXANTHEMA).

SEALS. Deaths of these around the UK and Dutch coasts have been attributed to a morbillivirus, possibly the canine distemper virus. Bordetella was found, by the Inverness V.I. Centre, to have killed seals in the Liverpool Bay area, UK.

SEASON (*see* OESTRUS).

SEAT-WORM is another name for the threadworm or oxyuris.

SEAWEED. A source of agar and a food grazed by sheep on the seashore and sometimes given to horses and cattle. A source of iodine and other trace elements and (in the case of brown seaweeds) of vitamins A, B_1, B_2, C, and D. Animals do not take readily to seaweed as a rule, nor are they able to digest it well at first, but after a few days it usually proves an acceptable supplement to the ration.

It was found at the Institute of Physiology, Babraham, England, that the ruminal microflora of sheep feeding almost entirely on seaweed were devoid of cellulolytic bacteria and anaerobic bacteria which are so numerous in sheep grazing pasture.

SEBACEOUS GLANDS are found in the skin (*see diagram under* SKIN), and secrete the oily sebum which prevents excessive dryness of hair and skin. The glands are liable to become invaded during some parasitic diseases; and sometimes a blocked duct leads to a retention cyst.
Seborrhoea is an excessively oily skin due to over-production by the sebaceous glands.

SECRETIN. A hormone secreted by the mucous membrane near the beginning of the small intestine when food comes into contact with the latter. On reaching the pancreas via the bloodstream, the hormone stimulates the flow of pancreatic juice.

SECRETORY IgA. It has been shown that in some infections, especially those of the respiratory and digestive tracts, immunity is conferred by antibody found in the local secretions – and not by the antibody circulating in the bloodstream. For example, the IgA found in secretions is quite different from that found in serum. Secretory IgA is relatively resistant to breakdown by digestive enzymes and has an affinity for mucus. (*See* IMMUNE RESPONSE, IgA.)

-SECTOMY. Words ending in this way mean surgical removal of.

SEED CORN, dressed with a mercury dressing, has been fed to pigs with fatal results.
Dieldrin seed dressings lead to poisoning in wild birds and, indirectly, have killed dogs, cats, and foxes which have eaten poisoned birds. (*See also under* GAME BIRDS.)

SEEDY TOE. A condition affecting the hoof of the horse, in which there is a separation of the wall from the laminar matrix below, and the formation in the space so produced of a dry, crumbly, friable variety of horn, which bears some resemblance to pumice-stone. It may occur at any part of the wall of the foot.
SIGNS. In most cases the condition is generally first noticed by the blacksmith when paring down the wall prior to fitting a new shoe. Lameness is only seen when the extent of the separation is large, or when foreign matter becomes forced up into the space, and causes pressure upon the sensitive matrix.
When struck with a hammer the affected part of the foot gives out a hollow resonating note, and the margins of the separated area can usually be fairly well determined by this means.
TREATMENT. All the soft friable horn should be cleared away and an antibiotic applied within. A suitable shoe should be fitted to cover the base of the cavity. (*See* HOOF REPAIR.)

SEITZ FILTER. An asbestos composition disc used in bacteriological work.

SELENIUM. Sodium selenate is used by horticulturists as an insecticide, and accordingly there is a possibility of toxic effect occurring in animals. Sterility results, and also loss of hair. These symptoms are also observed in parts of the USA and Eire where the soil contains an excess of selenium. In the acute form of poisoning, animals may be found wandering aimlessly or in circles. Paralysis precedes death. A horse weighing approximately 450 kg received 25 mg selenium as sodium selenate daily for five consecutive days. The horse became lethargic, walked stiffly and was unwilling to undertake pace work. The main signs were loss of hair from the mane and tail, disintegration of the skin of the lips, anus, prepuce and scrotum, and separation of the hooves from the coronary corium. There were strong correlations between the selenium concentrations in blood, hair and hoof parings. (Dewes, H. F. & Lowe, M. D. (1987) *New Zealand Veterinary Journal* **35**, 53.)
Selenium is a **trace element**. In some parts of Britain home-grown animal feeds may not contain enough selenium, and unless concentrates are fed as well, nutritional muscular dystrophy may result.
In other areas the soil may contain an excess of selenium.
However, as with other micronutrients (TRACE ELEMENTS), if selenium is provided in excess, toxicity may result, as noted above. Dr B. C. Cooke has pointed out that the normal level in animal feeds would be around 0·2 ppm; and that the maximum level of selenium allowed in pig diets without a veterinary prescription is 0·5 mg/kg; this level being specified under the Feedingstuffs Regulations 1982.
Supplements of the selenium can be given not only in the feed, but also in drinking water, by subcutaneous injection, by BOLUS, and (for **lambs**) by an oral dose.
Externally, selenium sulphide is used in wet shampoos for dogs and cats infested with fleas, harvest mites, or cheyletiella mites. (*See also* VITAMIN E, LATHYRISM; MUSCLES, DISEASES OF; IONOPHORES; *and* TRACE ELEMENTS.)
Retention of placentas in a dairy herd in the north of England was associated with a selenium deficiency.

SELLA TURCICA is the name applied to the deep hollow on the upper surface of the sphenoid bone in which the pituitary gland rests.

SEMEN, or seminal fluid, consists of the secretions of the accessory sex glands with, present among those secretions, the mature spermatozoa (or sperms) from the epididymis. A single ejaculation by a bull may produce semen containing millions of sperms.
The secretions of the accessory sex glands act as a vehicle for the sperms, probably as a nutrient, and neutralise any acidity in the female genital passages.
The accessory glands are the prostate; the ampullae of the *vasa deferens* (absent in the boar); the seminal vesicles; and (except in the dog) the bulbo-urethral (Cowper's) glands situated on

either side of the urethra. (*See also under* SPERMATOZOA, ARTIFICIAL INSEMINATION.)
IMPORTS of semen in Britain are subject to MAFF's 1984 regulations.

SEMINAL VESICLES (*see under* TESTICLE, ACTINOBACILLOSIS).

SENDAI VIRUS. This causes respiratory disease in the mouse but is most noteworthy for its use in experimental cell fusion work.

SENKOBO. Cutaneous Streptothricosis, caused by *Dermatophilius congolensis*, occurring in tropical Africa in cattle, sheep, goats, and horses. The hair stands erect and matted on small patches along the back. Moist, raw areas are left, then crusts form, and eventually a 'crocodile-skin' effect is produced. The disease occurs in association with tick infestation, and can therefore be controlled by means of a BHC dip (banned in the UK) (*see* DERMATOPHILUS).

SENNA. A standardised preparation of this household laxative has been recommended in treating or preventing constipation in pigs - especially in pregnant sows. A sub-laxative dose of 3 g is recommended during the farrowing period.

SENSITISATION (*see* ALLERGY).

SEPSIS (*see* SUPPURATION, ANTISEPTICS).

SEPTICAEMIA. A condition of the bloodstream when bacteria are circulating in it. It is very serious because the organisms and the products of their activity (toxins) become widely distributed throughout the tissues, and practically every organ is affected by them. In most cases, septicaemia terminates in death. Examples are ANTHRAX, HAEMORRHAGIC SEPTICAEMIA.
SIGNS. In many cases, especially when the animal is in a weakened state, sudden death, preceded by a very high temperature, may be the only sign of the presence of septicaemia.
TREATMENT. Antibiotics and/or the sulphonamides, and antisera (where appropriate) are given.

SEPTUM. A thin wall dividing two cavities or masses of tissue.

SEQUELAE. Symptoms or effects which may follow disease or injury. Thus pneumonia may follow a simple influenza, and chorea may follow distemper.

SEQUESTRUM. A fragment of bone which, in the process of necrosis, has been cast off from the living bone and has died, but still remains in the tissues.

SEROCONVERSION. The appearance in the blood serum of antibodies following vaccination, (or natural exposure to some infective agent).

SEROSAL PATCH. Perforated and leaking hollow viscera were successfully treated in 8 dogs by suturing the surface of a loop of healthy bowel over the leaking areas to form a serosal patch. The technique was used also in 3 dogs and 1 cat to reinforce areas of potential leakage. Experimentally, it was found that healthy bowel serosa could be used to repair perforations in even grossly infected visceral wounds. (Crow, D. T. *Veterinary Surgery* (1984) **13**, 29.)

SEROUS MEMBRANES are smooth, glistening, transparent membranes that line certain of the large cavities of the body and cover the organs that are contained in them. The chief of the serous membranes are: (1) the peritoneum, lining the cavity of the abdomen; (2) the pleurae, one of which lines each side of the chest and surrounds the corresponding lung; (3) the pericardium, in which the heart lies; (4) the tunica vaginalis, one on each side, enclosing a testicle; and (5) the mesentery supporting the small intestine.

SERTOLI CELLS. The function of these is believed to be the nourishment of spermatids. (*See diagram under* SPERMATOZOA.)

SERTOLI-CELL TUMOUR. This may be associated in the dog with feminisation, urethral bleeding, and urinary obstruction. (*See also* SPERMATIC CORD, TORSION OF.)

SERUM is the fluid which separates from blood, when the process of clotting takes place. It is, in effect, defibrinated plasma without the red cells, platelets or white cells. (For a description of plasma, *see* BLOOD.) (*See also* ANTISERUM.)

SERUM GONADOTROPHIN (*see* HORMONES).

SERUM SICKNESS. In human medicine this term is applied to the fever, glandular enlargements, oedema, pain in the joints, which may occur 8 to 12 days after the injection of a 'foreign' serum. Immediate reaction, denoting sensitisation by a previous injection of the same kind of serum, is regarded as anaphylactic shock. (*See* HYPERSENSITIVITY.)

SERUM THERAPY (*see* ANTISERUM).

SERVICE PERIOD. An 85-day service period would appear to be the optimum number of days between calving and successful service. If the trend of heat periods after calving is detected at about 6 weeks, checked again around 9 weeks, the cowman can, with a fair degree of accuracy, be on the look-out for bulling at or about the twelfth week (or 84–85 days).
Very early service *may* produce prolonged infertility.

SETAE. Stiff hairs. (*See* CATERPILLARS, SPIDERS.)

SEWAGE. Human excreta should not be used for manuring pasture, as the eggs of the tapeworm *Taenia saginata* can survive for weeks and give rise to cysticercosis in cattle. (The eggs are not destroyed or filtered off in *all* sewage plants.) (*See also* SALMONELLOSIS, SLURRY, COPPER POISONING in sheep.)

SEX DIFFERENTIATION in the fetus is briefly described under EMBRYOLOGY. (*See also under* GENETICS, CYTOGENETICS, FREEMARTIN.)

SEX-HORMONES (*see* HORMONES).

SEX-INVERSION. Animals which at birth, and for a variable period afterwards, are of normal sexual structure and function, but which later in life acquire properties of the opposite sex, are said to undergo sex-inversion. This has been seen in Ayrshire cows permanently kept indoors. (*See also* FEMINISATION in the dog.)

SEX PILUS (*see* PLASMIDS).

SEXUAL CYCLE (*see* OESTRUS).

SHAVINGS (*see under* BEDDING).

SHEARING. In Britain, the usual time for shearing is May in the southern counties, early June on upland semi-arable farms, and during July in mountain flocks.

The newly-shorn sheep is very sensitive to cold. This is particularly so with machine shearing 'which in the most professional of hands leaves a fleece of about 6 mm depth compared with about 12 mm' after hand shearing (Dr K. L. Blaxter). In Australia, late winter and early spring shearing of ewes has led to a high mortality, so that the practice is being abandoned or the usual shears replaced by 'snow combs' which leave a longer fleece. 'In Britain, losses of weight or poor gains in lambs shorn during the summer can largely be attributed to an effect of cold.'

In the USA trials have been carried out with a drug, cyclophosphamide, (or cytoxan, to use another name for it) which causes the wool to loosen so that it can easily be plucked. The sheep is left naked and unprotected against cold.

Chemical shearing is likely to become the most economical way of defleecing sheep in the long-term, according to the New Zealand Wool Board. At the Commonwealth Scientific and Industrial Research Organisation in Sydney three drugs have been found – cyclophosphamide, mimozone and PAP – that remove wool from live sheep. (*NZ Journal of Agriculture*, January 1977.)

SHEEP, ABORTION and infertility in (*see* ABORTION).

SHEEP BREEDING AND MANAGEMENT. The use of hybrids, referred to under SHEEP, BREEDS OF (British) is a relatively new trend. Another is the in-wintering of sheep – one aspect of intensive live-stock production.

Other developments. Sheep management has undergone change due to other economic factors. For example, a full-time shepherd is now expected to look after 1000 rather than only 400 ewes. Average flock size in Britain in 1978, according to the MLC, was 179 breeding ewes (hill flocks averaging about 210, lowland flocks about 130 ewes). Some flocks had over 10,000 breeding ewes.

Then again, in the UK the market for mutton, except for processing, has disappeared, and virtually the sole requirement is lamb. Lightweight carcases of under 40 lb are in demand. Fat is not wanted.

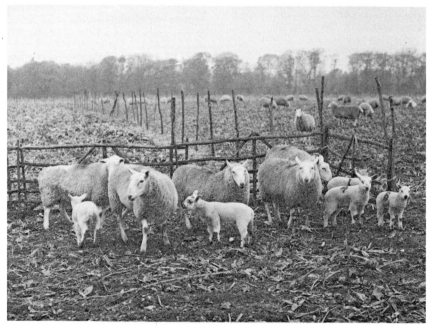

October lambs: a second crop in the year obtained by means of hormone injections. (*An Esso photograph*.)

It may prove possible to reduce the present high costs of zero-grazing and then use this to prevent the high wastage (up to 40 per cent) of grass trampled underfoot.

Greater use may be made of the various forms of creep-grazing in order to obtain higher stocking rates. (*See also under* STRESS.)

A plan put forward by the Grassland Research Institute, Hurley, involves rearing lambs artificially from day-old, keeping ewes on high/marginal land leaving lusher lowlands for growing stock.

Research at the GRI. Professor C. R. W. Spedding listed ways by which productivity can be raised: (a) by growing more herbage (or other sheep foods) per acre; (b) by ensuring that more of what is grown is eaten by the sheep; and (c) by improving the efficiency with which the sheep convert their food into meat and wool. The last really means improving the sheep.

'With bred varieties of grasses and legumes, and liberal use of fertilisers, very high levels of herbage production can be achieved. Sheep performance – especially that of lambs – has been better on legumes than on grasses. Sainfoin and lucerne have proved most effective but, on balance, a ryegrass/white clover mixture will generally give the greatest total production with sheep.

'The main disease hazard is excessive worm-infestation, especially in lambs that receive less milk than they could readily use. Ensuring good milk output from the ewe is therefore important, but this may not be enough for twins and triplets. The problem remains greatest where high stocking rates and high lambing percentages are combined. Possible solutions include better use of modern, efficient anthelmintic drugs, the use of grazing management and supplementary feeding of the lambs. Weaned lambs do best when they have plenty of herbage, provided that its quality is also high, especially in terms of digestibility.

'Since food costs may amount to 60 per cent of the total costs of sheep production, the efficiency with which food is converted is bound to be important. In a lowland ewe flock, most of the food is consumed by the ewes – the lambs eat about 10 per cent of the total, if they are singles, and up to 25 per cent if they are twins. In other words, the proportion of the total food that goes towards meat production depends chiefly on the number of lambs per ewe.

'A ewe requires so much food for the year, whether she produces any lambs or not; for a little more food she can produce 30–40 lb of lamb carcase, and for a little more again, nearly twice as much meat. Wool production is still important – and will remain so whilst sheep production is not very profitable and whilst the wool can be sold – but it is on meat production that the British sheep industry of the future will surely rest.

'The most important factor at present appears to be the number of lambs per ewe per year. What we want, it seems, is a small ewe (thus reducing the food bill – cheaper still if the food comes from cheap by-products), crossed with a large ram to produce a lot of lambs that will achieve heavy carcase weights.

'Experimentally, we have been producing large litters (up to 6) by hormone injections and breeding more than once a year (in some animals) by hormones and by light treatments.

'It is *unlikely*, nevertheless, that ewes will be bred that are capable of rearing all the lambs they can produce.

'For this reason, and to ensure that loss of young lambs is minimised, a great deal of work has been done to develop methods of artificial rearing for lambs. We are now at the stage where large-scale rearing, housed or in the field (weather permitting), either fully-automated or managed by simple methods, can be visualised in practice.'

In-wintering. In Scotland the in-wintering of sheep denotes a revival rather than an innovation, for it was, of course, the usual practice on many hill farms until a change was made to transferring the sheep to a lowland farm for the worst of the winter. Now that such an arrangement has become too expensive or otherwise proved impracticable, the ewes are being housed again on hill farms. It is, however, on mixed farms in England that in-wintering is chiefly gaining popularity, and it is here a part of the general process of intensification affecting live-stock production. A flockmaster of some 30 years standing has commented: 'If more live lambs are reared because of closer supervision and the avoidance of bad weather hazards, then there is every justification for the use of permanent buildings for flocks which lamb in the December to April period.'

Professor M. McG. Cooper stated that the biggest single cost in fat lamb production is flock depreciation. With winter housing, it is possible to retain ewes to a greater age, as a result of their being spared the stress arising from exposure in severe weather, and of their having their food provided for them. He has also commented, with reference to the lowlands: 'The case for in-wintering only really arises with high-intensity stocking on land subject to poaching.'

Mr L. J. Williams has commented: 'Portable feeding racks or boxes have two main advantages: they can be easily removed to give an unobstructed floor area should this be necessary, and they can be used to divide the flock into sizeable units – generally about 70 upland sheep or 50 lowland.

'There are two types in general use. The first, which is more often used for upland sheep, consists of a hay rack with a small concentrate trough below. The rack should not be too flat otherwise hay seeds will get into the eyes of the sheep and cause serious trouble. The other feeder is of the box type where a metal grille or wooden ladder can be used to prevent the hay being wasted.

'These box troughs have the advantage in that they can be used by the shepherd to walk down to feed the flock – a real advantage where large heavy sheep are involved. As to trough lengths a space of 9 in to 10 in is adequate for mountain lambs while 12 in to 14 in is necessary for heavy lowland breeds.

'Sheep will only drink water which is absolutely clean, fresh and, above all, cold. Water that is only slightly fouled or warm will be rejected even to the point of death. The ideal is a supply running through a trough in the shed but this can seldom be achieved. The alternative is to have a trough continually being fed from a very slow running tap with a good overflow to an outside area. The trough should be so positioned as to cause the sheep to step up to drink as this helps to prevent fouling. A trough 1 ft long is adequate for about 40 sheep.'

It is essential that sheep houses are very well ventilated, and ample use of Yorkshire boarding helps in this direction.

Where slatted floors are used, Mr Williams recommends that the slats are laid parallel to the door openings. (*See also under* HOUSING OF ANIMALS.)

Lamb survival research. Every winter in Britain over a million sheep are lost – many of them through exposure – and cold kills many thousands of lambs soon after birth.

Almost all newborn lambs are subject to cold stress. This, Dr J. Slee explained in the A B R O report for 1977, 'is because the environment is colder than the critical temperature below which the lamb must increase its metabolic rate in order to maintain body temperature. Critical temperatures during the first few hours after birth range from about 32°C for heavy lambs to about 37°C for light lambs'.

A lamb born outdoors is 'transferred suddenly from a temperature of about 39°C in the mother's uterus to an environmental temperature which may vary from about 15°C down to 0°C; or effectively even below −10°C if the cooling effects of wind and rain are taken into consideration'. A wind speed of 12 mph can effectively reduce an environmental temperature, in terms of its cooling power, by 15–20°C; and heavy rain may cause a similar, additional amount of cooling.

Even if a lamb survives the first few hours after its birth, exposure to cold remains harmful by causing the lamb to raise its heat production and so deplete its reserves of energy, which are mainly in the form of fat. In severe conditions, with ambient temperatures near or below zero and accompanied by wind and rain, lambs will require peak metabolic rates to maintain body temperature. Survival time would then be limited to between five and 17 hours.

While a lamb will normally begin to replenish its store of energy within an hour of birth by sucking, work in Australia has shown that the urge to do so is reduced if its body temperature falls below 37°C. In some breeds of sheep such temperatures occur in weather not unusually severe for March and April in Scotland. So cold not only increases the demand for energy, but may prevent that demand being met.

Starvation, on the other hand, exaggerates the effect of cold by reducing heat production capability, so increasing the risk of death from hypothermia.

'The provision of shelter, and extra food to give more warmth, is costly and not always feasible, so a genetic approach to the problem could provide a useful alternative method of helping sheep to survive under harsh conditions,' commented Dr Slee, of the A F R C's Animal Breeding Research Organisation in Scotland.

Experiments there suggest that it may indeed be possible to breed for greater resistance to cold. Results have shown that there are significant differences between breeds in their tolerance of body cooling; and within breeds, some individual sheep have a cold-resistance several times greater than that of other individuals, and preliminary trials have indicated that this character is moderately well inherited.

Lambs, stated Dr D. J. Mellor and L. Murray, require between 180 and 210 ml of colostrum per kg body-weight during the first 18 hours after birth, in order to provide sufficient fuel for heat production; and usually enough immunoglobulins for protection aginst infections.

Ewes which are well fed during late pregnancy produce more colostrum than their lambs need; those with singletons having enough for a second lamb. By contrast, most underfed ewes do not produce enough colostrum.

Colostrum can be readily obtained and stored for subsequent use. Yields are markedly increased when hand milking is preceded by an oxytocin injection. There is little practical benefit in milking ewes more than three times during the first 18 hours after lambing. The ewes should *not* be up-ended during milking. (Mellor, D. J. & Murray, L., *Veterinary Record* (1986) **118,** 351.)

Life-saving techniques on the farm. The following recommendations were made by the Moredun Institute, Edinburgh, in 1982. Two danger periods should be recognised: (1) from birth to five hours afterwards; (2) 10 hours to three days after birth.

During the first period, moderate hypothermia (a body temperature of 37° to 39°C) usually responds to drying the lamb, feeding it colostrum by stomach tube, and moving it to shelter along with the ewe. Serious hypothermia (below 37°C) requires in addition that the lamb be warmed in air at 37° to 40°C until its body temperature has reached 37°C. When removed from the Moredun-type bale-warmer (heated by a domestic blower-heater), the lamb is then given colostrum and, if strong enough to suck vigorously, can be reunited with the ewe. If not strong enough, the lamb must be housed for a day or two in its own cardboard box in an intensive care unit. There colostrum is given three times daily, and warmth provided by an overhead infra-red lamp.

During the second danger period, when serious hypothermia is then usually due to depressed heat production as a result of starvation, and often complicated by low glucose levels in the blood, treatment consists of drying the lamb, the injection of glucose, and warming – in that order.

Further details of bale warmers, lamb warming boxes, the Moredun lamb thermometer (which indicates by flashing, coloured lights, whether a lamb has hypothermia, and if so how badly), and techniques can be obtained from the Institute at 408 Gilmerton Road, Edinburgh EH17 7JH.

Worm control. Most sheep at pasture are

infected with roundworms. These, if numerous, can cause outbreaks of scouring and obvious unthriftiness. Subclinical infestations of the stomach or intestine can, research at the Moredun Research Institute has shown, reduce the weight gain of growing lambs by 20–50 per cent. (*See* WORMS, FARM TREATMENT AGAINST.)

Winter feeding. Work at the Hannah Dairy Research Institute has indicated the wisdom of hand feeding with starchy concentrates (rather than high protein or high roughage rations) to obviate the hill ewe burning up her own tissues in order to keep warm and alive during very cold weather. (*See under* ABORTION, FEED BLOCKS.)

For other aspects of sheep husbandry, and related health and disease problems, *see under the following headings:* ABORTION, BARLEY-POISONING, BRACKEN, 'BROKEN MOUTH', CASTRATION, CLOTHING, COBALT, COLOSTRUM, 'CONTROLLED BREEDING', COPPER, COPPER POISONING, DIET, DIPS and DIPPING, DOCKING, 'DRENCHING', EXPOSURE, FEED BLOCKS, FLEECE, FLUSHING OF EWES, GENETICS, HOUSING, INFECTION, INFERTILITY, ISOLATION, LIGHTNING, 'LUMPY WOOL', NOTIFIABLE DISEASES, OESTRUS, PARASITES; PARTURITION, DRUG-INDUCED; PASTURE CONTAMINATION, PASTURE MANAGEMENT, POISONING; SEAWEED, SHEARING, SHEEP, DISEASES OF; SHEEPDOGS, SOIL-CONTAMINATED HERBAGE, STELL, STOCKING RATES, STRESS, TRACE ELEMENTS, TRANSPLANTATION OF MAMMALIAN OVA (Embryo transfer), TROPICS, VAGINA (for rupture of), VITAMINS, WATER, WEANING, WOOL BALLS; WORMS, FARM TREATMENT AGAINST.

Clipping (*see* SHEARING *and* CLOTHING FOR ANIMALS, and 'WOOL SLIP'.).

SHEEP, BREEDS OF

Introduction. Sheep are maintained, generally speaking, with the object of producing both wool and meat. In some countries ewe's milk is valued for cheese-making. In the UK the importance of the fleece tends to be disregarded (*see* FLEECE).

Hardiness, prolificacy, milking capacity of the females, activity, are all important. What will constitute the most profitable type must be carefully considered in relation to local conditions.

British breeds of sheep. British breeds offer a wide choice of types, adapted to almost every conceivable set of conditions under which sheep are maintained in the country, from the highest mountain grazings in Scotland and Wales to the richest lowland pastures, or the dry arable farms of the Wolds.

At the 1965 Oxford Farming Conference, Mr N. R. Woods of New Zealand House, London, gave a friendly but frank appraisal of the British sheep industry, and his criticisms could be summed up as 'too much tradition'. This applied to our 40 breeds of sheep and the size of our flocks. He pointed out that a reduction (possibly by amalgamation) in the number of breeds would give immeasurably greater opportunities for breeding, culling, and selecting according to defined performance standards. In New Zealand they manage with two breeds and a cross – Merino, Romney, and Merino Romney – which

between them thrive from sea-level to an altitude of 5000 feet, and in areas with a rainfall varying from 12 to 200 inches.

In New Zealand the farmer himself will commonly look after a flock of up to 1000 or 1200 ewes, and will hand-feed them as a matter of course during the winter months. Mr Woods referred to the reluctance of hill farmers here to feed their sheep even in the face of a more severe winter. In the name of 'hardiness – whatever that might be' – prolificacy, lamb performance, and wool were sacrificed.

There was already, before this Conference, a move towards the development of new breeds of sheep in Britain. For example, Mr Oscar Colburn had produced his COLBRED (which see), and Mr J. Brian Cadzow had been working in Scotland. He started with the Finnish Landrace, a prolific breed, crossed with the Dorset Horn to give out of season lambing. The Ile-de-France was used because of its fame as a mutton producer to bring in the live-weight gain factor, and the Westfalen brought in for its great milking capacity.

The aim of the first development is to produce a ewe which will live long and average two lambings a year; giving four to five lambs a year or more.

In the USA the Morlam has achieved six lambs in two years.

Cambridge. This new breed was developed at the University of Cambridge by Prof. John Owen in collaboration with Alun Davies. The breed is now regarded as one of the most prolific in the world with litter sizes of 1.7, 2.5 and 2.9 for one, two and three year old females respectively. Both sexes are polled, ewes weighing 70 kg and rams 90 kg. (*See also* TEXEL, COOPWORTH.)

The British breeds are commonly classified as Longwools, Downs, other Shortwools, and Mountain breeds.

LONGWOOL breeds include: Leicester, Border Leicester, Lincoln, Wensleydale, Kent or Romney Marsh, Devon Longwool, South Devon, and Roscommon.

DOWNS breeds include: Southdown, Suffolk, Hampshire, Dorset Down, Shropshire, and Oxford.

OTHER SHORTWOOL breeds include: Dorset Horn, Wiltshire Horn, Ryeland, Devon closewool, Kerry Hill.

MOUNTAIN breeds include: Scottish Blackface, Cheviot, Swaledale, Hetdwick, Lonk, Welsh Mountain, Exmoor, and Dartmoor.

UK sheep survey. In 1988 the Meat & Livestock Commission carried out the first survey for 17 years of the composition of the UK's sheep; and they stated that 70 pure breeds were being maintained. However, crossbred ewes were becoming increasingly popular, and numbered about half of the UK total.

The UK's National Sheep Breeders' Association has listed 40 affiliated Breed Societies; plus ten in the Half-bred section; and 7 in the Rare Breeds section.

SHEEP DIPPING (*see* DIPS AND DIPPING).

SHEEP, DISEASES OF (*see under* ABORTION; ACTINOBACILLOSIS; ANTHRAX; ARTHRITIS; BALANITIS; BLACK DISEASE; BLACK-QUARTER; BLINDNESS (*under* EYE, DISEASES OF); BLOUWILDEBEESOOG; BLUE TONGUE; BORDER DISEASE; BRAXY; 'CAPPIE'; CASEOUS LYMPHADENITIS; ENTEQUE SECO; FOOT-AND-MOUTH DISEASE; FOOT ROT; GAS GANGRENE; HYPOMAGNESAEMIA; JAAGSIEKTE; JOHNE'S DISEASE; JOINT-ILL; LAMB DYSENTERY; LIVER FLUKE; LOUPING-ILL; MILK FEVER; MOREL'S DISEASE; OVINE EPIDIDIMYTIS; OVINE INTERDIGITAL DERMATITIS; NEMATODIRUS; PARASITES; 'PINING'; PNEUMONIA IN SHEEP; PREGNANCY TOXAEMIA; PULPY KIDNEY; 'REDFOOT'; 'RINGWOMB'; SCALD; SCRAPIE; SWAYBACK; TICKS; TOXOPLASMOSIS; UDDER, DISEASES OF; 'WATERY MOUTH'; WESSELSBRON DISEASE; 'YELLOWSES'). (*See also* ARIZONA infection; ENZOOTIC OVINE ABORTION; HAEMORRHAGIC SEPTICAEMIA, MAEDI/VISNA, 'MILKSPOT LIVER', PULMONARY ADENOMATOSIS, RIFT VALLEY FEVER, ULCERATIVE DERMATOSIS and *under* RAM.)

SHEEP KED (*Melophagus ovinus*) is a wingless blood-sucking parasite. (*See* KED.)

SHEEP: Names given according to age, sex, etc. There are probably more names for any given class of sheep than is the case among any of the other domesticated animals, and it is almost impossible to give a list that will include all the various designations that are used, but the table gives a list of commoner terms.

SHEEP POX (*see* POX).

SHEEP SCAB. This is the popular name for psoroptic mange, a Notifiable Disease in the UK. Sheep scab was eradicated from the UK in 1952 but re-appeared in 1973. There were numerous outbreaks in 1980 to 1984, with compulsory dipping in England and Wales. (*See* MITES.)

SHEEP, WINTER COATS FOR (*see* CLOTHING OF ANIMALS).

SHEEPDOGS. Sheepdogs are popularly regarded as exceptionally healthy, but a 1953 survey in Scotland showed that at least 11 per cent were suffering from Black Tongue (which see) as a result of an inadequate diet. On average, this consisted basically of ½ lb oatmeal, ½ lb maize, and (by no means always) ½ pint of milk; the first two ingredients being made into a brose or mash by pouring on boiling water. The occasional

NAMES OF SHEEP GIVEN ACCORDING TO AGE, SEX, ETC.

Periods	Male		Female	Remarks
	Uncastrated	Castrated		
Birth to weaning	Tup lamb Ram lamb Pur lamb Heeder	Hogg lamb	Ewe lamb Gimmer lamb	A sheep until weaning is a lamb
Weaning to shearing	Hogg (also used for the female) Hogget (also used for the female) Haggerel or Hoggerel Tup teg Ram hogg Tup hogg	Wether hogg Wedder hogg He teg	Gimmer hogg Ewe hogg Sheeder ewe Ewe teg	Hogget wool is wool of the first shearing
First to second shearing	Shearing, or Shearling, or Shear hogg Diamond ram Dinmont ram tup One-shear tup	Shearing wether Shear hogg Wether hogg Wedder hogg Two-toothed wether	Shearing ewe Shearling gimmer Theave Double-toothed ewe Double-toothed gimmer Gimmer	'Ewe', if in-lamb or with lamb; if not a 'barren gimmer'; if not put to a ram is a 'yield gimmer' (Scotland)
Second to third shearing	Two-shear ram Two-shear tup	Four-toothed wether Two-shear	Two-shear ewe	A ewe which has ceased to give milk is a 'yeld ewe'; taken from the breeding flock she is a 'draft ewe' or a 'draft gimmer'
Third to fourth shearing	Three-shear ram Three-shear tup	Six-toothed wether Three-shear wether	Three-shear ewe Winter ewe (Scotland)	
Afterwards	Aged tup or ram	Full-mouthed, full-marked or aged wether or wedder	Ewe Ewe	After fourth shearing 'aged' or 'three-winter'

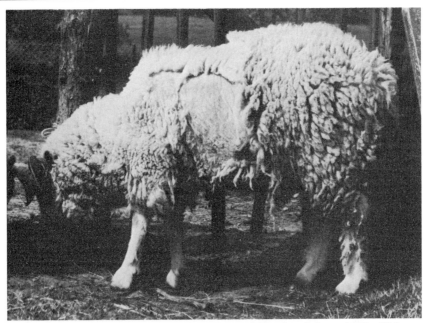

An advanced case of sheep scab, showing loss of wool. (With acknowledgement to the Wellcome Foundation Ltd.)

rabbit, or piece of boiled mutton from a dead sheep, or – at lambing time – the afterbirths, were not sufficient to prevent Black Tongue.

Sheepdogs may walk or run 90 miles per day at lambing time and must have meat if stamina and health are to be maintained. Even fishmeal is of service – also dried blood – if meat or fish are unobtainable. (*See under* GID, RICKETS, *and* BLACK TONGUE.)

Sheepdogs may become infected with brucellosis as a result of eating infected cattle afterbirths; and through eating dead sheep they may become infested with the tapeworm causing HYDATID disease. Regular worming is essential (*see also* GID, ORF, ANTHRAX, BOTULISM).

SHELTERS, NEED FOR (*see under* EXPOSURE, TROPICS; *also* STELL).

SHEPHERDS. Occupational hazards include the following diseases: CAMPYLOBACTER infections, CHLAMYDIA, HYDATID DISEASE, LISTERIOSIS, LOUPING ILL, ORF, PASTEURELLOSIS, Q-FEVER, SALMONELLOSIS *and* TOXOPLASMOSIS. (*See under* these headings and ZOONOSES.)

Shepherdesses, if pregnant, are at risk when helping with lambing. (*See* CHLAMYDIA.)

SHIGELLOSIS. Infection by one of the Gramnegative Shigella bacteria. (*See* 'SLEEPY FOAL' *under* FOALS, DISEASES OF .)

'SHIPPING FEVER'. A disease of cattle caused by a virus and/or *Pasteurella multocida, Pasteurella haemolytica.* 'Shipping fever' is very common in American feedlots, among cattle 6 months to 2 years old, and often follows the stress of transport, castration, de-horning, winter weather,

change of food, etc. In the USA the term 'Bovine respiratory disease complex' is a synonym. (*See* PASTEURELLA.)

SIGNS include fever, loss of appetite, weakness, followed by nasal discharge, a discharge from the eyes, distressed breathing, coughing, and signs indicating bronchopneumonia. Mortality is usually 1 to 2 per cent, but may exceed this if cases are neglected.

TREATMENT AND PREVENTION. Antibiotics and sulfa drugs are used. Immunisation has been tried using myxovirus parainfluenza-3 and *P. septica*, for example.

'SHIVERING'. A nervous disease of horses. It runs a slowly progressive course, and constitutes an unsoundness.

CAUSE. This is unknown, though it seems that there may be a hereditary predisposition to it.

SIGNS. In a well-marked case, the muscles of the hindquarters are seen to quiver or tremble. At the same time, the tail is usually elevated and also shows the quivering movements. In advanced cases it may be difficult or impossible to pick up either of the hind-feet, and shoeing is only accomplished with difficulty. When the hind-limb is raised from the ground during backing, in many cases it also quivers, or 'shivers', and in some instances one or both of the fore-limbs, or the muscles of the fore-quarter, exhibit the same feature.

Shivering in the dog may occur, especially in fox-terriers, for no apparent reason and may be unconnected either with cold or fear. At the prospect of a walk the dog may suddenly cease trembling.

SHOCK is an abrupt fall in blood pressure (acute hypotension).

SIGNS include weakness, pale and cold mucous membranes, subnormal temperature but no shivering; a weak and rapid pulse; shallow breathing at an increased rate; cold extremities.

CAUSE. Shock may follow severe trauma, haemorrhage, surgical operations, a sudden decrease in the heart's pumping capacity, burns and scalds, toxaemia. (*See also* ELECTRIC SHOCK, ANAPHYLACTIC SHOCK.) Pain, fright, and any airway obstruction may exacerbate the condition.

TREATMENT. Although corticosteroids are often used, it has been stated that there is little or no evidence that they are effective. A blood transfusion, adrenalin, and lactated Ringer's solution given intravenously, may each have a place in treatment, as appropriate.

The patient must be kept warm.

SHOEING OF CATTLE. This may be undertaken to reduce weight bearing on an injured claw, especially where there is a fracture of a phalanx.

SHOTGUN INJURIES (*see* GUNSHOT).

SHOULDER, the joint formed between the scapula and the upper end of the humerus. (*See* DISLOCATIONS.)

SHOULDER-BLADE (*see* SCAPULA).

SHOVEL BEAK. A disease occurring in intensively reared chicks fed dry mash. It affects usually birds of 2 to 8 weeks old. The upper or lower beak (or both) may be deformed, with ulceration or necrosis. Infection with *Fusiformis necrophorus*, *Staphylococcus aureus*, or *Clostridium welchii* may follow.

SHYING (*see* 'VICES').

SI UNITS. The Système International d'Unités was adopted by the Conférence Générale des Poids et Mesures in 1960. Based on seven units – metre, kilogram, second, ampere, degree kelvin, candela, and mole – it admits only one unit for any one physical quantity. Derived units in any science or technology can be made up from the seven basic units by division or multiplication without numerical factors being involved. The SI unit joules replaces calories. The seven basic SI units and their symbols are as follows: –

(length)	metre	m
(mass)	kilogram	kg
(time)	second	s
(electric current)	ampere	A
(thermodynamic temperature)	degree Kelvin	°K
(luminous intensity)	candela	cd
(amount of substance)	mole	mol

(*See under* METABOLISABLE ENERGY.)

SIALOCOELES. Cyst-like swellings, usually lined by granulation tissue rather than epithelium, containing saliva. (P. J. Brown & others. *Vet. Record* (1989) **125**, 256.)

SIALOGOGUES are substances which produce a copious flow of saliva, *e.g.* pilocarpine and arecoline.

SICKNESS (*see* VOMITING).

SIDEBONES. Ossification of the lateral cartilages of the horse's foot. (*See* LATERAL CARTILAGES.) When this occurs in a young animal it is looked upon as an unsoundness. In old horses, all cartilages, not only in the foot, tend to become ossified as an almost natural course of events, and sidebones are accordingly not looked upon as so serious.

CAUSES. Heredity is considered as a predisposing cause, but in many instances no such relationship can be shown. It has been suggested that a vitamin D deficiency in foalhood may be partly responsible.

SIGNS. Ordinarily, the upper part of each cartilage can be felt at the coronet as a flexible ridge or edge, lying immediately below the skin, but when the cartilage has ossified, this ridge is no longer flexible, and is more or less thickened as well. In some instances the ossified cartilage can be easily seen when the feet are viewed from the front. The condition is more common by far in the fore-limbs, and may occur on the outside or inside, or in both places, on one or both of the fore-feet.

When sidebones have formed, there is no lameness, pain, heat, or other signs of inflammation, but when forming, there may be pain over the quarters involved, and lameness – characterised by the taking of a shorter step by the affected foot, and the tendency to do this may result in a peculiar short and long step.

TREATMENT. As a rule, in horses with wide open feet and well-developed frogs, no treatment is required. The sidebone does not interfere with slow work of a regular nature. (*See also* RINGBONES.)

SIDE-EFFECTS. The side-effects of a drug are those produced in addition to that for which purpose the drug is given. Examples: deafness in humans following the administration of streptomycin, moniliasis after the use of chlortetracycline, aplastic anaemia after the use of chloramphenicol. (*See also* IATROGENIC DISEASE.)

SILAGE, or ensilage, is a succulent food.

Dr H. Ian Moore classified it as follows: Grade I containing 15 per cent and over crude protein, and made from young grasses – none in flower; clover, lucerne, or sainfoin in bud stage. Grade II containing 12 to 14·9 per cent crude protein, and made from grasses in their flowering stage, late autumn grass, clover passed full flower, marrow stem kale, pea pods, cereal-legume crops cut when cereal is 'milky'. Grade III containing less than 12 per cent crude protein, and made from seeding grasses, stemmy clover, maize, pea haulm and pods, sugar-beet tops, potatoes.

Grade I makes a substitute for cake, whereas Grade III is good enough only as a substitute for roots, straw, or low-grade hay.

Ensilage involves fermentation. Lactic, acetic and butyric acids are produced. In good silage, lactic acid predominates. Silage with a high butyric-acid content must be fed with caution, and may be recognised by its unpleasant smell and lighter colour – yellowish-green instead of dark brown.

The Dorset Wedge system of silage-making has enabled better quality to be achieved.

ADAS comment: 'Most farmers still make silage at the wrong time.' This criticism is levelled from many directions, and refers, of course, to not cutting at the optimum stage of growth but tending to delay until there is more to cut. Wilting, judicious choice of harvester, type of silo, sealing, consolidation, and use of additives are all being applied by the more progressive farmers.

As with hay, there are extremes of quality in silage. At the Rowett Research Institute cows have maintained a yield of up to 5 gallons daily for 2 months while receiving no other feed. With the average quality silage it would, however, be unrealistic to expect to be able to dispense with supplements.

Acetonaemia is often seen in cattle receiving large quantities of silage of low quality. Hay should be made available as well; also 2 oz per head of bone flour with salt added.

When self-feeding of silage is practised care must be taken that conditions underfoot do not become dirty and slushy to an extent where softening of the horn of the hoof occurs and foot troubles develop.

Silage must be free of ragwort. (*See under* RAGWORT POISONING; *also* HAEMORRHAGIC SYNDROME in dairy cows.)

Listeria in silage. Listeriosis in ruminants has often been associated with silage feeding. In a survey carried out in Scotland *Listeria monocytogenes* was isolated from 2·5 and 5·9 per cent of samples of clamp silage obtained in 1983 asnd 1984, respectively. In samples of big bale silage the incidence was 22 per cent and when mouldy samples were selected, 4 per cent. (Fenlon, D. R., *Journal of Applied Bacteriology* (1985) **59**, 537.) (*see* LISTERIOSIS).

SILAGE EFFLUENT has been described as one of the strongest of all agricultural wastes and pollutants. Some 3500 gallons of clean water are needed to dilute 1 gallon of silage effluent to bring it to the recommended level for treated ('safe') effluents.

In a wet season a 400-ton silage clamp with grass at 10–15 per cent dry matter at ensiling may produce 40,000 gallons of effluent, most of which discharges in the first month. It takes only a little of this effluent to kill fish and other forms of aquatic life if it reaches a stream.

'SILENT HEAT' (*see under* OESTRUS DETECTION *and* INFERTILITY).

SILICA CONTAMINATION can be a problem with sugar-beet tops and other arable residues. Crops windrowed and then picked up may contain up to 30 per cent silica. Direct loading might keep the figure down to 10 per cent. (*See also* SOIL-CONTAMINATED HERBAGE, SAND COLIC.) Silica is silicon dioxide, present in sand.

SILICON. A non-metallic element. In the form of silicic acid or its derivatives, silicon is essential for growth, and is found mainly in connective tissue. It has been suggested that lack of sufficient silicon may be a factor in the cause of atherosclerosis in man. (K. Scwartz, *Lancet* for Feb. 26, 1977). (*See also above.*)

Silicone implant repair. A year-old Arabian filly had a depression over its right frontal sinus as the result of an injury sustained six months earlier when it ran into a steel pipe and the frontal bone had been broken. A heat-vulcanised silicone implant was used to repair the deformity and the normal facial contour was restored by suturing the sculpted implant to the periosteum over the defect. One year after the surgery the cosmetic results were excellent. (Bohanon, T. C. & Gabel, A. A. (1991) *Journal of the American Veterinary Medical Association* **198**, 1957.)

SILICONE SOLUTION. An anticoagulation solution used in connection with blood transfusion apparatus and syringes to prevent clotting.

SIMIAN HAEMORRHAGIC FEVER (*see* MONKEYS, DISEASES OF, *and* EBOLA VIRUS).

SIMMENTAL. A dual-purpose breed of Swiss cattle, now to be found throughout Europe and in the USA. In Germany the Simmental has been developed with emphasis on beef production.

SIMULIUM (*see under* FLIES). In the UK the gnat, *S. ornatum*, which breeds in running water and is difficult to control, sometimes causes eye lesions in cattle.

SINUS is a term applied to narrow hollow cavities (especially in bones) occurring naturally in the body, or produced as the consequence of disease. (*See* SINUSES OF THE SKULL.) (*See also* FISTULA.)

In pathology, 'sinus' refers to a blind infected tract, leading from a site of suppuration to the surface of the skin or of a mucous membrane.

SINUSES, DISEASES OF THE. The sinuses of the head are lined with a membrane which is continuous with that of the nasal cavities, and which acts as a periosteal covering for the bone.

CAUSES. Sinusitis may arise as a result of a spread of inflammation from that affecting the nasal mucous membrane. It may follow strangles in the horse; occasionally the cause is a diseased tooth, the root of which has suppurated and the pus burrowed through the thin plate of bone that separates the tooth socket from the sinus cavity. In other cases, the cause is a penetrating injury from the outside, such as is occasioned by a blow on the forehead which fractures the external plate of bone and allows the ingress of infection. Gunshot wounds are also a cause of pus in the sinuses. Animals living near the seashore or in sandy and windy localities are sometimes afflicted with collections of fine sand in the sinuses. In sheep, and sometimes in the horse, sheep nostril fly larvae of the *Oestrus* family may be found in the sinuses, and are generally associated with pus formation. In dogs especially, but also in other animals, tumour formation is often accompanied by the presence of pus in the sinuses, and the condition may be complicated by a fungal infection (*see* FUNGAL). In the dog, a foreign body such as a grass seed may give rise to the discharge from one nostril which is characteristic. Either cancer, or a fungal infection which may follow, can lead to distortion of the dog's or cat's face. (*See also* LINGUATULA, LEECHES.)

SIGNS. The most prominent sign of the presence of any amount of pus in the sinuses is the usually slight, but continual, dribbling of discharge from **one** or both nostrils. This discharge is usually more marked when the animal lowers its head.

TREATMENT. This consists of opening, under anaesthesia, the diseased sinus by trephining the bone over the surface, and irrigation and evacuation of the cavity. When a tooth has been the primary cause of the condition it is extracted, and its cavity temporarily plugged with gauze until healthy tissue fills up the space between the tooth socket and the sinus. Parasitic inhabitants are removed, either by the injection of fluids that will kill them, or by picking each out separately with forceps. Chloroforming the animal will often kill such parasites.

SINUSES OF THE SKULL, also called the PARANASAL SINUSES, are directly or indirectly connected with the nose. There are four pairs: (1) maxillary; (2) frontal; (3) spheno-palatine, or sphenoid; (4) ethmoidal.

SINUSITIS. Inflammation of the sinuses.

SINUSITIS, INFECTIOUS. This is common in turkeys, and also in game birds. In turkeys it is sometimes a sequel to de-beaking. The cause is a mycoplasma. Symptoms: a swelling below the eyes, and sneezing. Treatment may consist of surgically draining the infra-orbital sinus and using antibiotics. Birds which recover often remain 'carriers' for a time.

Infectious Sinusitis in pheasants and partridges may be confused with 'Gapes', Fowl-Pox, Newcastle Disease, nutritional roup caused by vitamin A deficiency, aspergillosis, and perhaps with pasteurellosis. In artificially reared poults, the disease occurs mainly between 2 and 8 weeks of age. Mortality may be as high as 90 per cent.

SIRE IDENTIFICATION (*see* DNA 'FINGERPRINTING').

SITFASTS (*see* SADDLE-SORES).

SKIM MILK. This is a valuable food, retaining, as it does, the solids-not-fat after most of the fat has been removed. These solids include the valuable milk-protein, the sugar lactose, valuable minerals, and vitamins of the B group. It is poor in the fat-soluble vitamins A and D; and also in vitamin E; and if given along with cod-liver oil to beef stores, may lead to cod-liver oil poisoning or MUSCULAR DYSTROPHY (which see).

Skim milk is a useful food for pigs, but is not suitable on its own. It can be fed *ad lib.* to suckling pigs; weaners may receive 5 pints per day; fatteners from 14 weeks to slaughter, about 6 pints.

Skim milk is, if from infected cattle, a source of tuberculosis in pigs, and pasteurisation may be desirable in many countries.

For sows and piglets, skim milk should be fresh or completely sour; 0·1 per cent formalin is sometimes added to skim milk for fattening pigs.

SKIN, the protective covering of the body, is continuous at the natural openings with the mucous membranes. It consists of two main layers, which differ in structure and origin.

The epidermis. This is a cellular layer of non-vascular, stratified epithelium of varying thickness, covering the outer surface of the body, which presents the openings of the cutaneous glands and of the hair follicles. In animals it is divisible into two layers, the outer, hard, dry *stratum corneum*, and the deeper, softer, moist *stratum germinativum*. The cells of the latter are pigmented, and by their growth compensate for the loss by exfoliation or shedding of the surface cells from the stratum corneum, which forms the scurfy deposit upon an ungroomed horse. This inner layer consists of the part of the skin which is living, and is formed by several layers of cells set upon the corium and nourished by it. The cells continually multiply, and are slowly pushed upwards to replace the constant wear and tear which occurs on the cells at the surface. There are no blood-vessels in the epidermis, but there is a ramification of the surface sensory nerves which supply the skin with its delicate sense of perception. A *blister* is a collection of fluid separating the stratum corneum from the stratum germinativum.

The dermis (corium) consists of a felt-work of fibrous tissue and elastic fibres. It is very vascular, contains the hair follicles, the sudoriferous (or sweat) glands, and the sebaceous glands, as well as a certain amount of involuntary muscle. The most superficial part is known as the *corpus papillare*, on account of the presence of numbers of tiny papillae, which are received into corresponding depressions in the epidermis. These papillae contain loops of blood-vessels, which nourish the epidermal cells, and numerous sensory nerves, which act as tactile organs, affording sensations of touch, pain, temperature, etc.

The sweat glands glands are situated partly in the deeper parts of the corium, known as the *tunica propria*, and partly below it in the layer of subcutaneous fibro-fatty tissue. In this deepest layer, which forms the bulk of the skin, or lying in the deeper part of the corium, there are certain tactile bodies, known as *Pacinian corpuscles*. The fibrous tissue of the skin consists of interlacing bundles of white fibrous tissue which form a dense felt-work. Here and there elastic fibres are mixed with them, and these serve to give the skin its pliability, and at the same time keep it in place and stretched reasonably tightly.

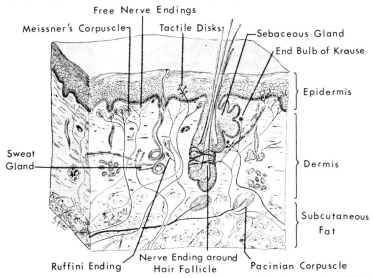

Free Nerve Endings

Meissner's Corpuscle — Tactile Disks — Sebaceous Gland

End Bulb of Krause

Epidermis

Sweat Gland

Dermis

Subcutaneous Fat

Ruffini Ending   Nerve Ending around Hair Follicle   Pacinian Corpuscle

The nerve supply to the skin. (In Miller, Christensen and Evans, *Anatomy of the Dog*, courtesy of W. B. Saunders Co.)

Hair. Practically the whole of the body of each domesticated animal is covered by hair, except in the pig. Portions of the skin which appear to be bare are found on close inspection to be covered with very fine hair of delicate texture. The hairs are constantly being shed and replaced by others, while at certain periods of the year in the horse, and to a less extent in the other animals, they are cast off in great numbers, and constitute the 'shedding' or 'casting of the coat'. This normally occurs twice a year, once in the autumn, when it is more marked, and again in the spring with the first warm weather of the year.

Hairs are of several kinds: in the first place there are the ordinary hairs which, on account of the small amount of pigment that each carries, give the coat its characteristic colour; and there are different kinds of special hairs. Among these ordinary hairs scattered over almost the whole body are: *tactile hairs* of the lips, nostrils, and eyes; *cilia*, or *eyelashes*, growing from the free rim of the eyelids; *tragi*, in the external ear; and *vibrissae*, round the nostrils. In addition to the ordinary and tactile hairs, certain regions carry specially long and coarse hairs, such as the mane (*juba*), the forelock or foretop (*cirrus capitis*), the tail, where the hairs (*cirrus caudae*) are very large and long, and the 'feather' of the fetlocks and cannons (*cirrus pedis*), which gave the name of this region (fetlock = feet-lock – a lock of hair on the foot).

Each hair has a shaft, the part above the surface, and a root, embedded in the hair follicle. Below this is a little fibrous papilla possessing blood-vessels, which is capped by the expanded end of the hair root, and known as the hair bulb. The follicles are set somewhat obliquely in the corium and at varying depths; the long tactile hairs reaching down to the underlying muscle. Most of the follicles have little bands of plain muscle attached to one side, known as the *arrectores pilorum*; these serve to erect the hairs during anger, fear, or extreme cold, and also to express

from the sebaceous gland a small portion of sebaceous secretion.

Glands of the skin are of two kinds: sweat and sebaceous. The former are scattered over the body in nearly all animals, being most numerous in the horse, and least in the dog (which is essentially a non-sweating animal), where the largest are found only on the pads of the feet. Each sweat or sudoriferous gland consists of a long tube, usually greatly coiled in its inner part, which has a duct leading up to the surface of the skin. (*See* PERSPIRATION.)

The sebaceous glands, except in certain places, open into the follicles of the hairs a little way below the surface. Each consists of a little bunch of small sacs, within which fatty or oily material is produced. This secretion is forced from the sacs by the contractions of the arrectores pilorum muscles, and during exercise it also escapes on to the shafts of the hairs. Its function is to keep these pliable and lubricated and prevent them from becoming brittle through drying. A copious secretion from the sebaceous glands results in a sleek shining coat, such as is associated with a well-fed and well-groomed horse.

Appendages of the skin. In addition to hair, the skin possesses certain appendages, which in reality are modified hair only. Thus, horns, hoofs, claws, nails, ergots, chestnuts, and other horny structures, are closely packed epidermal cells which have undergone keratinisation or cornification. Spurs of poultry are horny epidermal sheaths covering a centre of bony outgrowth from the metatarsal in the case of poultry. Feathers are highly specialised scales. The down feathers of the chicken are simple, and consists of a brush of hair-like 'barbs' springing from a basal quill or 'calamus'. From the whole length of each barb a series of smaller 'barbules' comes off not unlike the branches of a shrub. The adult or 'contour feathers' are formed at the bottom of the same follicles that lodged the down feathers, which by the growth of the adult feather become pushed out of place. At first they are nothing more than enlarged down feathers, but soon one of the barbs grows enormously, and forms a main shaft or 'rachis' to which the other barbs are attached on either side. From the sides of the barbs grow the barbules, just as in the down feathers, and these, in the case of the large wing feathers ('remiges') and the tail feathers ('retrices'), are connected by minute hooks so that the feather 'vane' has a more resistant surface for flight than in the case of the breast feathers, for instance. Moulting in birds occurs periodically, and the bird casts off the old feathers and gets a complete new set.

Functions of the skin. The main use of the skin is a *protective* one. It covers the underlying muscles, protects them from injury, and in virtue of its padding of fat prevents them from extremes of temperature. The hair, fur, wool, or feathers assist this heat-regulating mechanism more still, and usually the growth of the coat is determined by the temperature of the surroundings; for example, when horses are kept out of doors during winter they grow long thick coats, while when kept in warm stables and covered with rugs they assume a close sleek coat, and the same applies to other animals.

Heat regulation is one of the most important functions of the skin. When cold air, water, or other cooling substances come into contact with a large area of the skin, the numerous blood-vessels of the skin immediately contract, reducing the amount of blood circulating in them, and therefore reducing the amount which will be exposed to the cooling action from outside. On the other hand, when the surrounding medium is at a higher temperature than the normal – *i.e.* when it is approaching body heat, or rises above it – the blood-vessels of the skin dilate, more blood is brought to the surface, and this stimulates sweating, or excretion, and when the perspiration evaporates, especially when the surrounding atmosphere is dry, considerable cooling of the skin surface occurs. (*See* TEMPERATURE, TROPICS, HYPOTHALAMUS.)

SKIN, DISEASES OF. The majority of the commoner diseases of the skin in animals are due either to parasitic invasion, or to conditions of an allergic origin, *e.g.* eczema. These are treated under separate headings – *e.g.* mange, of all varieties, is dealt with under MITES; ECZEMA; URTICARIA; RINGWORM; ACNE, CONTAGIOUS, etc.; *see also* TUMOURS, NECROSIS (BACILLARY), IMPETIGO, POX, BRIDLE INJURIES, SPOROTRICHOSIS, SWINE ERYSIPELAS, LIGHT SENSITISATION, DERMATOPHILUS, GRANULOMA, ABSCESS, HYPERKERATOSIS, LUPUS, AUTO-IMMUNE DISEASE, CUTANEOUS ASTHENIA.

Cats may suffer from cancer of the sweat glands.

SKIN GRAFTING TRANSPLANTATION. The pedicle technique, in which the transplant is attached at one end to adjacent skin, has been applied in cats and dogs. A broad flap of skin is formed by incision to cover the denuded area,

with a narrow strip to form the pedicle or bridge to carry the blood supply to the broad flap or graft. The edges of the pedicle are sutured; and the flap is sutured to adjacent skin. (For further details *see Vet. Rec.* (1976), **98,** 52.)

In horses, skin grafting has also been carried out, using free, whole-thickness grafts of skin taken from other sites in the same animal. Such grafts will give rise to normal hair growth. (*Vet. Rec.* (1976), **98,** 105.)

In a cat a badly damaged tail was used as a source of skin for a graft before tail amputation; extensive skin loss having resulted from a fan-belt accident.

SKIN, POISONING THROUGH (*see under* POISONING, HYPERKERATOSIS).

'SKIN TUBERCULOSIS'. This is characterised by the appearance of swellings, varying in size from that of a pea to that of a tangerine, on the limbs and occasionally on the trunk of cattle. Lesions are often multiple and in the form of a chain. They are unsightly but appear to cause the cow no discomfort, and their economic importance lies only in the fact that they apparently sensitise the animal to mammalian and/or avian tuberculin, thus complicating the interpretation of the tuberculin test. This, indeed, may give rise to anxiety on the part of the owners of attested herds. A re-test after an interval of 30 to 60 days will, however, in the absence of tuberculosis, usually give a reaction justifying retention of the animal within the herd.

Microscopically, the lesions of 'skin tuberculosis' closely resemble those of tuberculosis, and acid-fast bacilli resembling *M. tuberculosis* are present in them.

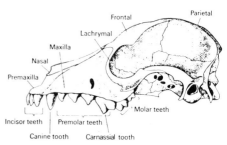

The dog's skull, and teeth of the upper jaw.

SKULL. Excavated in it there are large irregular spaces known as 'sinuses'. (*See* SINUSES OF SKULL.)

General arrangement of the skull. The skull is divided into two parts: (1) the *cranium*, and (2) the *face*. The former consists of the posterior part, which encloses the brain.

Most of the bones of the skull are flat bones developed from a structure which is partly cartilage and partly fibrous membrane. Centres of ossification appear in these during early life, and soon after birth the greater part of each bone has assumed its eventual outline, but is separated from its neighbours by an intimately dovetailed joint. These joints, none of which is movable, allow growth until the animal is adult, when bony fusion usually occurs, and the joints become obliterated. Many of these joints – 'sutures', as they are called – can be felt in the skull of a newly born animal, particularly over the dome of the head in a foal or puppy, and for a time constitute especially vulnerable parts of the skull.

Bones of cranium. The bones which enclose the brain and its membranes are ten in number – four single and three paired. They are occipital, sphenoid, ethmoid, interparietal (single), and parietals, frontals, and temporals (paired). The occipital lies at the posterior lower aspect of the skull, and forms the hinder wall of the brain cavity. Through it passes the spinal cord, which emerges by the 'foramen magnum', and to a roughened prominence above this foramen is attached the very powerful 'ligamentum nuchae', which supports the head. On either side of the foramen are the 'occipital condyles' which articulate with the atlas – the first of the cervical vertebrae. The lower part of the occipital – the 'basilar part' – runs forward along the base of the brain to meet the body of the sphenoid bone. The inner surface is adapted to the cerebellum – the most posterior upper part of the brain, while above the basilar portion lies the medulla which is continued backwards into the spinal cord. It has the form of a body with two pairs of wings and one pair of projections. It is supposed to resemble a bird with two pairs of wings in flight trailing its legs behind it. The body is continuous with the basilar part of the occipital, and helps to form the base of the brain.

SKUNKS and foxes are now the two most important wildlife hosts of the rabies virus in the USA.

SLAG (*see* BASIC SLAG).

SLATTED FLOORS. These were tried in England in the last century and described in the *RASE Journal* of 1860, and had been used for many years in Norway, before being re-introduced in Britain as a means of saving money on straw. The current practice is sometimes to sprinkle sawdust on the slats (of wood or concrete), but to use no straw. The use of slatted floors can hardly be regarded as anything but a retrograde step from the animal husbandry point of view, however attractive commercially. The animals obviously cannot rest as comfortably as on straw, and if strict precautions are not taken (as in Norway) they may be subjected to severe draughts with resultant ill-health and poor food conversion ratios. Teat and leg injuries, and injuries or abnormalities of the feet, may also develop in animals on slats. (*See also* EPIPHYSITIS.)

The space between the slats is critical, and there must be no sharp edges on the concrete. (*See* LAMENESS.)

A slatted dunging area and a bedded area are satisfactory. (*See also under* SOW STALLS *and* SLURRY.)

SLAUGHTER (*see under* EUTHANASIA, STUNNING). Specified intervals between cessation of treatment of food animals with certain drugs are required before slaughter. (*See* IVERMECTIN.)

SLEEP. The rest obtained by horses sleeping in an erect position is, actually, not sufficient for their needs. They require complete relaxation of their muscles, and this can only be furnished in the recumbent position. When from fear, ankylosis of vertebrae, or other cause a horse does not lie down, it should be placed in slings, or given some form of support, such as a rope between the heel posts upon which the hindquarters may bear, so that it may obtain the requisite rest.

On board ship, and for surgical or other reasons, horses may be kept standing without harm for considerable periods, but they should be exercised for a short while two or three times daily, in order that the muscles may be prevented from becoming stiff. Horses are liable to fall while standing asleep, and may, in rare cases, actually come to the ground through the relaxation of their extensor muscles; what happens more frequently is that they knuckle over on to their fetlocks, recovering themselves almost at once, but not before a slight injury has been inflicted to the skin over the joint. The fall always occurs in front, not behind, probably because of the extra weight carried by the fore-legs.

'SLEEPER' SYNDROME. This takes the form of a septicaemia, is caused by *Haemophilus somnus*, and occurs in cattle in feedlots in the USA. The syndrome is associated with an encephalomyelitis though, as well as brain and spinal cord, many other tissues may be involved. It has also been seen in the UK.

SLEEPING SICKNESS. Human trypanosomiasis transmitted by tsetse flies and caused by *T. gambiense* and *T. rhodesiensis*. (*See* TRYPANOSOMES, TROPICS, FLIES.) Sleeping sickness caused by *T. rhodesiensis* can also be transmitted from person to person.

'SLEEPY FOAL DISEASE' (*see under* FOALS, DISEASES OF).

SLINGS. A device whereby a large animal may be kept in the standing position for long periods without becoming completely exhausted. The apparatus consists essentially of a broad strong sheet which passes under the animal's chest and abdomen, supported by a block-and-tackle or other means to a beam overhead. Connected with this there are two strong straps, one passing round the front of the chest, and the other passing round the buttocks. These latter serve to hold the sling in position, and prevent the animals from struggling free. The whole is adjustable so that it may fit animals of different sizes. The sling is often made with a metal or wooden bar along each end of the sheet; these bars serve to distribute the weight of the animal along the whole width of the sheet, and afford a rigid means of attachment to the cross-beam of the slings, to which the chain or rope of the block-and-tackle is attached.

In addition to the above use, slings are one of the means of lifting a horse that has either fallen or lain down in a stable and is unable to rise. The horse is placed so that the slings may be pulled under it, or is rolled on to them, and after the chest and breeching straps are arranged the horse is lifted by the block-and-tackle high enough to be able to use his feet. It sometimes happens that if the horse has lain for a considerable time it refuses to support its weight on its feet, but hangs 'like a herring' in the slings. In such cases it may be necessary to startle the horse, when it will generally make a plunge and 'find its feet'.

Slings are employed in a variety of conditions: e.g. fractures.

When slings are applied to an animal, they should not be fixed up so tightly that the animal is unable to walk a step or so in each direction. They are only required as a means of support for the animal when it so desires, and not as a suspensory apparatus which is always in use. The animal soon learns to lean on the slings and rest its feet. The hand should be able to be passed under the sling webbing when the animal is standing immediately under the centre of the block-and-tackle, and neither the chest strap nor the breeching should be buckled up tightly. It is generally necessary to secure the head of the animal by a halter to restrict its movements, and to supply a suitable manger or other receptacle from which it may feed easily.

(*See also* 'DOWNER COW' SYNDROME for a means of lifting a cow.)

SLINK CALVES. Immature or unborn calves improperly used for human food. The flesh of slink calves is often called *slink veal*.

'SLIPPED'. A colloquial expression meaning aborted; also dislocated (*see below*).

'SLIPPED SHOULDER' (*see* DISLOCATIONS *and* SUPRASCAPULAR PARALYSIS).

SLIPPED STIFLE is the popular term for dislocation of the patella. It may be partial, when the patella slides in and out of the trochlear depression on the femur with each step; or it may be complete, when the patella becomes fixed above the outer lip of the pulley-like trochlear surface, causing all the joints of the affected leg to become straightened, and the limb to be held pointing behind. Dislocation of the patella is a common condition in the dog.

'SLIPPED TENDON'. A condition seen in chickens, turkey poults, and ducklings, in which there is displacement of tendons and an inability for the leg to support the bird's weight. It is due to a manganese deficiency, and may arise from feeding lime to excess.

SLOPE CULTURE. A method of growing micro-organisms on solid media (*e.g.* agar) in tubes which are usually arranged in racks at the correct angle for the agar to solidify on cooling.

SLOUGH means a dead part separated by natural processes from the rest of the living body. The

slough may be only a small part such as a piece of skin that has been burnt by heat or chemicals, or it may be a whole foot. (*See* GANGRENE.)

SLOW-MILKING COWS (*see under* MILKING MACHINES).

SLUGS. The common field slug, *Agriolimax meticulatus*, is of veterinary interest as intermediate host of the sheep lungworm *Cystocaulus ocreatus*. (For the danger of **slug poisons**, *see* METALDEHYDE.)

SLURRY is the liquid mixture of urine and faeces, together very often with washing-down water and rain-water, which has to be disposed of from pig, beef and dairy units. Deaths of pigs have been reported following agitation of slurry during the emptying of tanks or pits under the piggery slats. It is recommended that slurry should never be allowed to come within 18 inches of the slats, and that especially in hot weather emptying should be carried out at least every 3 or 4 weeks. Methane, hydrogen sulphide, ammonia, and carbon dioxide may all be given off as the result of bacterial action on slurry; giving rise to a mixture both lethal and explosive.

Cows, too, have been overcome by slurry gas.

For methods of slurry disposal *see* DAIRY HERD MANAGEMENT. (*See also under* SALMONELLOSIS, PASTURE CONTAMINATION, 'MILK-SPOT LIVER', SILAGE.)

SMEAR PREPARATIONS. A film of blood, pus, etc., smeared on to a slide, fixed – and if necessary stained – for microscopical examination.

'SMEDI' VIRUSES were obtained from pig herds, in the USA, having stillbirths (S), mummified fetuses (M), embryonic death (ED), and infertility (I). The viruses were serologically of two groups: (a) swine picorna viruses, (b) related to Ontario polio-encephalitis and oedema disease viruses.

SMEGMA. Sebum with a distinctive odour found in the region of the clitoris and penis. For a test using smegma, *see* EQUINE CONTAGIOUS METRITIS.

SMELL. The sense of smell is situated in the nasal mucous membrane, and in the nerve centres of the brain which are connected with the nasal mucosa by the olfactory nerves. The power to appreciate smell depends upon the stimulation of tufts of hair-like processes found in certain cells in the nasal mucous membrane, by particles of matter given off by an odoriferous substance. These particles, either gaseous or solid, are dissolved in the secretion present, and so far as present knowledge goes, appear to act chemically on the nerve tufts. The act of 'sniffing', familiar in the case of the dog especially, simply ensures that the particles are rapidly and forcibly drawn upwards into the nose. There are certain substances which act more quickly than others in particular animals: thus the smell of fish, blood, and offal has a remarkably stimulating effect upon the carnivorous animals, while grass, grain, and vegetable substances stimulate the sense organs of herbivorous creatures particularly. The odour of flesh, blood, etc., is repulsive to the herbivora, and may cause great nervousness and fright. Most of the wild grass-eating animals have remarkably well-developed powers of smell, and are able to locate their enemies at great distances: thus deer and antelope can detect a carnivorous animal which has recently made a kill at a distance of two miles if the wind is favourable. It is through the sense of smell that the male is attracted to the female during the season or oestrus of the latter; the odour at this period is most persistent, and can be appreciated at great distances. Females recognise their offspring by their sense of smell, and dams whose young have died can often be deceived and persuaded into accepting other young animals by clothing these in the skins of the dead ones. This fact is made use of in the case of ewes which have lost their lambs. (*See* JACOBSON'S ORGAN, PHEROMONE.)

SMELLS AS EVIDENCE OF DISEASE. In certain cases the presence of a smell connected with an animal is almost a diagnostic feature of disease. Thus in decay of the teeth or decomposition of bone there is a characteristic smell which, when once it is appreciated, can never be forgotten, although it is difficult to describe. The breath, urine, and the milk of a cow suffering from acetonaemia have a characteristic sweetish sickly smell. Poisoning by certain drugs, *e.g.* carbolic acid, can be diagnosed to some extent by the smell of the drug that is left in the mouth or on the skin. The urine of the horse has the smell of violets after the administration of turpentine in large quantities.

It has been suggested that dogs might be trained to recognise certain smells associated with human diseases, and so aid diagnosis at an early stage.

SMOG. This is the popular name for fog containing a dangerously high proportion of sulphur dioxide and other harmful gases derived from coal fires and factory chimneys. (*See also* OZONE for a further description of smog.)

SNAILS. One or two species are of veterinary interest in connection with LIVER-FLUKES and tapeworms.

The giant African snail (*Achatina fulica*) is commonly kept in UK schools to show to biology class pupils; but it is a potential human health risk. Third-stage larvae of *Angiostrongylus cantonensis*, passed out in rats' faeces, are infective for mammals, and in the Far East have caused meningitis in people; though the majority of cases have occurred through eating uncooked snails. (Mr J. E. Cooper BVSc, DTVM & Mr A. R. Mews BVM&S, MSc. *Veterinary Record*.)

SNAKES. Many snakes imported into the USA from West Africa arrive infested with ticks. An outbreak of Q fever occurred among men handling a shipment of pythons.

A fungal disease of pythons, caused by *Geotri-*

chum, is believed to occur only when the reptile's resistance has been lowered by some other disease.

Types of snake. With most snakes, the venom is, of course, introduced by their fangs, which have either a groove on the surface, as in cobras, or a canal down its centre, as in adders.

The African Ring-hals, however, squirts its venom with uncanny accuracy for a distance of about 6 feet into the eyes of its victim; the snake rising and opening its mouth wide; its head thrown back.

The rattlesnake venom contains five or so compounds containing zinc, plus an enzyme which causes destruction of muscle tissue, stated Dr Anthony Tu, a biochemist at Colorado State University, in the May 1984 issue of *Science Digest*.

The Russel's Viper in Burma disrupt pituitary gland function. Five people (out of many) who died had haemorrhage from the gland.

Hong Kong snakes. Over a 4-year period, at the Prince of Wales Hospital, 242 patients were treated for snake-bite. Five different species of snake were involved, including cobras, kraits, and adders. One in ten of the patients developed 'disturbances of blood-clotting and three died.' (*Journal of Tropical Medicine & Hygiene* (1990' **93** 79.)

Animals susceptible. Dogs are most frequently killed by snake bites, both at home and abroad, and sporting dogs suffer more than others. Sheep, cattle, and horses come next in frequency, whilst cats and pigs are only very rarely killed. The reasons for this appear to be that hunting dogs most often disturb snakes, and that grazing herbivorous animals, moving only slowly over a tract of country, disturb snakes less; while the cat is not often attacked because of its greater caution when hunting, and because of its superior agility. Pigs apparently are least often killed because of the protection they possess in a hard tough skin, with a padding of fat immediately below it.

Identification of snakes. Broadly speaking, those which have *two rows* of small solid, equal-sized teeth on either side of the upper jaw are non-venomous; while those with *one row* of small teeth on either side of the upper jaw, and two or more large, curved, hollow or grooved fangs on the outside of the smaller teeth, should be considered venomous.

SIGNS. Two kinds of symptoms are produced, depending upon the kind of venomous snake involved. In those of the cobra type there is a period of excitement immediately after the bite, lasting only for a few minutes and followed by a period of normality. Then nervous excitement appears, convulsive seizures follow, and death takes place from asphyxia. If death does not occur at once, dullness and depression are seen and death or recovery takes place some hours later. There is usually but little pain at the site of injury, and practically no local reaction in rapidly fatal cases.

The symptoms of bite by the adder (*Vipera berus*) are similar, except that there is local pain and considerable swelling. The skin becomes a livid colour, tumefied, and if in a limb there may be severe lameness. The dog often appears to be frightened.

In Australia snake bite was diagnosed at the University of Melbourne in 41 cats over a six-year period; the Tiger Snake having been positively identified in seven of these cases. Symptoms included weakness, dilated pupils and absence of normal reaction to light by the pupils, with vomiting and laboured breathing in some instances. Paralysis and a subnormal temperature suggest a fatal outcome. A high rate of recovery followed the use of 3000 units of Tiger Snake antivenin. (F. W. G. Hill & T. Campbell, *Austr. Vet. J.* (1978) **54**, 437.)

TREATMENT. Injection of antivenin as soon as possible.

SNEEZING is a sudden expulsion of air through the nostrils, designed to expel irritating materials from the upper air passages; the vocal cords being kept shut till the pressure in the lungs is high, and then suddenly released, so that the contained air is driven through the throat into the nose. Entrance to the mouth is prevented by the soft palate closing the exit from the mouth.

Sneezing is induced by the presence in the nose of particles of irritating substances, such as pungent odours, smoke, dust, spores of certain species of fungi, pollen from some grasses, etc. It is also the forerunner of chills, colds, influenza, etc., when it is usually accompanied by a running at the nostrils, and it is a sign of the presence of certain parasites, such as *Oestrus* larvae in sheep and horses, and rarely *Linguatula* in dogs. In pigs, sneezing is an important sign of atrophic rhinitis and Aujeszky's disease.

S-N-F (see SOLIDS-NOT-FAT).

SNOOD. The long fleshy appendage extending from the front of a turkey's head over its upper beak.

'SNOW BLINDNESS' IN SHEEP (see under KERATITIS under EYE, DISEASES OF).

SOAPWORT POISONING is possible when the soapwort plant (*Saponaria officinalis*) grows abundantly in pasture. The plant contains a poisonous glycosidal substance called *saponin*, which causes frothiness when stirred in water. When saponin is introduced into the body it causes solution of the red blood-cells, stupefaction, paralysis, vomiting, and purging with the passage of large amounts of frothy faeces, which are mixed with blood.

SOCIAL BEHAVIOUR (see BUNT ORDER).

SODIUM. A metal the salts of which are white, crystalline, and very soluble in water. Common salt, or sodium chloride, is contained in the fluids of the body under natural circumstances, and therefore the salts of sodium, when used as drugs, act not through their metallic base but according

to the acid radicle with which the sodium is combined. Generally speaking, the salts of sodium act in a manner very like corresponding salts of potassium (see POTASSIUM) but are better tolerated.

SODIUM CARBONATE, commonly called 'washing soda', is an irritant internally, and is therefore never given by the mouth except, in an emergency, as an emetic for the dog.

The citrate, acetate, sulphate, and hydroxide of sodium are used in a similar manner to those of potassium. (See POTASSIUM.) SODIUM IODIDE has many uses and a solution of it can, if necessary, be given intravenously whereas an effective concentration of potassium iodide may prove fatal by this route.

SODIUM DEFICIENCY. This may occur in dairy cattle in the UK in July. (See also SALT, SALT LICKS, METABOLIC PROFILE TESTS, LICKING SYNDROME.)

SODIUM METABOLISM. Sodium is important in maintaining osmotic pressure in the body fluid outside cells, and so controlling body fluid volume. (See also KIDNEYS, Function, and ALDOSTERONE.)

SODIUM MONOFLUOROACETATE. Also known as '1080', this is a rodenticide. In the dog symptoms of poisoning with '1080' include yelping, sometimes vomiting, and convulsions. This compound was sometimes used in wild-life rabies control operations against foxes, etc.

SODIUM NITRITE (see under NITRITE POISONING).

SODIUM PROPIONATE (see under PROPIONATE).

SOFT PALATE. For a condition of this causing distressed breathing in the race-horse, see under PALATE; likewise for Prolonged Soft Palate in the dog.

SOIL-CONTAMINATED HERBAGE. Experiments in Australia and New Zealand with intensively grazed sheep were undertaken to investigate tooth wear in ewes and wethers at various stocking densities. It was found that 'tooth wear was low when soil content of faeces was low and they rose to a peak simultaneously'. Moreover, in the majority of cases, soil content of the faeces was highest where stocking rates were high; when stocked at nine adult sheep to the acre, the daily intake of soil per head could be as much as 13 oz in the rainy season.

In Britain, a NAAS officer suggested, July thunderstorms over first-year leys may – by a combination of splashing by rain and poaching by feet – produce a herbage that is seriously contaminated with soil. This could well irritate the sensitive lining of the gut in young lambs with consequent scouring, which is often seen among lambs believed reasonably free from parasitic worms. (See also SAND COLIC, SILICA CONTAMINATION.)

SOLIDS-NOT-FAT. These include the protein casein, milk-sugar, and minerals.

Deficiencies of solids-not-fat lead to difficulties in processing the milk and render it unsuitable for manufacture into high-class products. Milk produced by a cow affected with mastitis, or by one approaching the end of a lactation, is particularly undesirable.

Maintaining the S-N-F percentage at a satisfactory level is a more difficult problem for the milk producer than rectifying variations in the butterfat percentage. The causes of S-N-F deficiency are not always apparent, and attempts at remedying them may have no rapid effect.

Factors involved include: breed of cow, her inherited capacity, age, stage of lactation, the season of the year, feeding, management, and attacks of mastitis.

The diet should contain adequate fibre as well as protein. There is some evidence suggesting that an all-silage diet may lower S-N-F, unless the silage is of the highest quality. Hay, as well, is desirable. (*See* WINTER RATIONS.)

The percentage of solids-not-fat is relatively high in October and November, after which time it begins to decline and falls to a minimum in February and March. It then starts an upward trend, reaches a high level in May, and may drop again in July and August.

Milk from cows of the Jersey and Guernsey breeds is relatively high in solids-not-fat. British Friesians, as a rule, give milk low in S-N-F. Inherited capacity is important.

The percentage of solids-not-fat in milk varies according to the stage in the lactation. It is high at the beginning, but falls rapidly to a low level in from 6 to 8 weeks after calving. Thereafter, it rises gradually if the cow is pregnant, while it tends to decline further if she is not again in calf. Towards the end of the lactation, when the cow is drying off, it may fall very low.

SOMATIC means all the cells belonging to the body except the germ cells in the gonads.

SOMATIC NERVES. Sensory or motor nerves of the somatic division of the central nervous system; they deal with awareness of sensation and with voluntary control of muscles. (*See* CENTRAL NERVOUS SYSTEM.)

SOMATOSTATIN. A peptide hormone, produced by the hypothalamus at the base of the brain, which acts as a brake on growth by regulating release of growth hormone directly responsible for tissue growth. Animals immunised against somatostatin are not subject to this 'braking' effect, and research at the A R C's Meat Research Institute suggests that this new technique may be more effective than conventional steroid growth promoters used in meat production.

Dr Stuart Spencer and colleagues found that immunisation of lambs in this way resulted in their putting on weight almost twice as fast as their un-immunised twins used as controls. The treated animals also grew taller (a result not obtained with growth-promoting steroids), an advantage so far as lean-meat production is concerned. It is (1983) expected that cattle and pigs can be similarly immunised.

SOMATOTROPHIN. The growth hormone, produced by the pituitary gland, stimulates growth of all body tissues, and influences mammary gland development. Like insulin, somatotrophin maintains correct glucose levels in the blood.

In the 1930s the National Institute for Research in Dairying found that the hormone could increase the milk of dairy cows. In 1983 research was being directed towards production of growth hormone by genetic engineering techniques, with the aim of producing a commercial product which could increase milk yields. (*See* SOMATOSTATIN, PITUITARY GLAND.)

SORES (*see* ULCERS).

SORE THROAT is a popular term for laryngitis or pharyngitis, which is often present during catarrh, strangles, influenza, etc. (*See* THROAT, DISEASES OF.) A cowman with a sore throat may pass his infection to a cow's udder, setting up mastitis.

SORGHUM. Poisoning in horses has been recorded in horses grazing pasture containing sorghum species. Hindquarter weakness and paralysis of the bladder may result.

SORREL POISONING (*see* DOCKS, POISONING BY, *and* SOURSOB).

SOUND is a metal rod, either curved or straight, which is used for passing along a natural channel or duct of the body. They are generally used to discover whether there are any hard or solid foreign bodies present.

SOUNDS are made both normally and abnormally by some of the organs of the body. For example, during the heart-beat there can be distinguished two definite sounds normally. The first of these, known as the 'first heart sound', is a long booming noise, similar to the syllable *lūb*, which is heard when the ventricles are contracting and the atrio-ventricular valves are closing, and which is produced by these processes. The 'second heart sound' is a short, sharp, sudden sound, similar to the syllable *dŭp*, and is heard at the end of the contracting period of the ventricles, when the semilunar valves at the bases of the pulmonary artery and the aorta are closing.

Respiratory sounds are also present normally. The sound made by the air entering the alveoli is generally called the *respiratory*, or *vesicular murmur*. It is a soft, low, quiet blowing sound, which can be imitated by the gentle blowing of air from a pair of bellows. In addition to the friction of the air in the alveoli there is also a sound produced by the air in its course down the trachea and along the greater bronchi, but as this is quite indistinguishable from the former the two are classed together.

The stomach and the intestines produce audible sounds, always of a very varied character, during the process of digestion.

During disease there are unusual sounds produced, especially by the organs in the chest: for these *see* RALES; RONCHI; HEART, DISEASES OF; LUNGS, DISEASES OF; etc.

SOURSOB. The Australian name for *Oxalis cernua*, a member of the sorrel family, found in Australia, South Africa, the continent of Europe, and now the West of England. It has caused fatal poisoning in sheep.

SOW'S MILK. The production of colostrum lasts for about 5 days during which time the milk composition changes rapidly to 'normal'. In reality, however, there is no such thing as 'normal' milk because its composition changes continually throughout lactation. 'The protein and mineral contents rise steadily, while lactose and fat contents fall.

'Sow's milk is particularly rich in fat having, on average, some 8·5 per cent, or 45 per cent of the dry matter. The fat percentage, although very erratic, tends to reach a peak around the third week of lactation and has been reported as high as 17·2. This sudden, very high fat level in the diet ... may be of considerable significance in the incidence of piglet scours which frequently occurs at about 3 weeks of age.

'The diet of the sow, both quantitatively and qualitatively, affects the fat content of the milk. Weight loss during lactation, associated with high pregnancy and low lactation feed allowances, results in a reduced yield of milk but of higher fat content. It appears that milk of high fat content, and so of higher than usual energy value, has a depressing effect on the growth rate of the pigs.

'Apart from its inadequate iron level, sow's milk appears to be an ideal feed for young pigs, allowing as it does an efficiency of feed conversion on a dry matter basis of some 0·8 lb feed per lb of gain. Its failure is quantitative rather than qualitative; thus, an average yield is about 100 lb milk per piglet suckled, or 20 lb dry matter in 8 weeks which, at an efficiency of conversion of 0·8, is sufficient to allow a weight gain of 25 lb. With an average birth-weight of 3 lb this would allow the production of 28 lb weaners at 8 weeks, so a 40-lb pig at this age must have consumed some 24 lb creep-feed at an efficiency of feed conversion of about 2:1.

'Sow's milk has a crude protein content increasing from about 25 to 33 per cent of the dry matter as lactation advances; the major requirement, therefore, is for energy. This fact seems frequently to be overlooked in the compounding of creep-feeds which tend to have needlessly high protein levels. While an early-weaning diet requires to have a high protein content, which will vary with the age of pig to which it is given, this is not so for a creep-feed which is merely an energy supplement to milk – already higher than it need be on its percentage of protein.' (Dr G. A. Lodge.)

SOW'S MILK, ABSENCE OF, following farrowing, may be due to prior feeding with excessive quantities of fodder beet, or to inflammation of the uterus (metritis). Another cause is an endocrine failure. Post-parturient fever is an important cause. Wet, cold floors and cold, draughty premises appear to predispose sows to mastitis and agalactia.

In herds where agalactia is common, administration of prostaglandin (PG) $F_{2\alpha}$ to induce parturition reduces the number of cases of lactation failure. (Peter, A. T., Huether, P., Doble, E. & Liptrap, R. M. *Research in Veterinary Science* (1985) **39,** 222.)

In parts of Africa heavy losses of piglets have resulted from this failure of the sows' milk supply, and the cause was traced to the fungus ergot, parasitic on bulrush millet ('Munga'). (*See* PREDNISOLONE, POSTPARTURIENT FEVER *and* ERGOT OF MUNGA.)

SOW STALLS have been now widely used for dry and pregnant sows, and ensure that each animal obtains her fair share of food. However, in partly slatted stalls high culling rates have sometimes resulted from defective slats causing foot and leg injuries, leading in some instances to partial or complete paralysis of the hind-quarters. Also the sow is cramped, and cannot move out of draughts; so the use of these stalls can lead to stress. (*See* 'THIN SOW'.)

SOYA BEANS are rich in protein and fat. Soya flour contains about 40% protein and 20% fat, and is a good source of thiamine, riboflavin, vitamin A, and lysine.

SPANISH FLY (*see* CANTHARIDES).

SPARGANOSIS. Infestation with Spirometra larvae of muscles and subcutaneous tissue. The adult worms infest dogs, cats, and wild carnivores in Australia, the Far East, and North and South America.

Sparganosis is a ZOONOSIS, as people can become infested through eating pork or drinking water containing the larvae at one stage in their development.

SPASM. Means an involuntary and, in severe cases, a painful contraction of a muscle, or of a hollow organ with a muscular wall. Further information is given under ASTHMA; COLIC; CHOREA; CONVULSIONS; CRAMP; EPILEPSY; MUSCLES, DISEASES OF; SPINAL CORD, DISEASES OF; STRYCHNINE; TETANUS; TETANY; RABIES; HYPOMAGNESAEMIA, etc.

SPASTIC is a term applied to any condition showing a tendency to spasm, such as 'spastic gait'.

In British Friesian cattle, an inherited spastic form of lameness may appear when the calf is 6 or 8 weeks old, but sometimes not until it is 6 months old. Before long, the toe may not touch the ground as the calf walks, and the affected hindleg is held backwards. Later, the leg becomes shortened and useless. If, however, the case is treated early enough, a simple operation will correct the deformity and prevent these unfortunate sequels. But of course, that calf, grown to maturity, can transmit the deformity to a proportion of his offspring. The condition has also been seen in Shorthorns and Aberdeen-Angus crosses. (*See* TENOTOMY.)

SPAVIN (*see* BONE SPAVIN, BOG SPAVIN).

SPAYING. Surgical removal of the ovaries, and usually of the uterus also, carried out mainly in cats and bitches. (*See* OVARIO-HYSTERECTOMY for reasons for the operation.)

Also, mares to be used in cavalry regiments, or polo pony mares, as well as certain thoroughbred racing mares, where the occurrence of oestrus and its associated phenomena would interfere with the proper performance of work, and mares which are suffering from some definitely hereditary disease, are subjected to the operation.

In 'nymphomania', ovariotomy, when performed before the symptoms have been in existence for long, usually results in a complete cessation of the kicking, squealing, and fractiousness which generally render the mare unfit for work.

In the past it was common practice to spay both cows and sows; the former giving a continuous milk supply for 18 months or even much longer.

Cats are spayed to prevent the birth of unwanted kittens, adding to the problems of stray and feral cats. The operation is almost invariably satisfactory, and involves few if any disadvantages.

Bitches are spayed to a less extent than cats. The operation may be requested by the owner on account of domestic difficulties or convenience, or it may be advised as a means of preventing pyometra. It is desirable after fracture of the pelvis or in the treatment of 'sexual alopecia'. Bitch puppies can be spayed as early as 8–10 weeks of age; kittens also, though probably most are spayed between 3 and 4 months of age.

Ovariohysterectomy is performed usually through a flank incision.

SPECTACLES, so-called, of plastic material are sometimes used to prevent poultry from resorting to cannibalism, etc. 'Spectacles' for horses in mines are really eye-shields. (*See also* 'LENS', CONTACT.)

SPECULUM is an instrument designed to aid the examination of the various openings of the body surface. Many are provided with small electric lamps which illuminate the cavity under examination.

SPEEDS OF ANIMALS.
Racing camel. In Australia the record is ¼ mile in 27 seconds.

Cheetahs. 63 mph.

Greyhounds. The record is 41 mph.

Ostriches can achieve a speed of 45 mph over short distances.

Pigeons can fly at 46 mph.

Porpoises can swim at 40 mph.

Racehorses have reached 43 mph.

Killer whale. 30 knots.

(with acknowledgements to *The Guinness Book of Records*.)

SPEEDY-CUT is the name given to the injury that results from a horse striking the inside of carpus or metacarpus with some part of the inside of the shoe of the opposite foot. (*See* BRUSHING AND CUTTING.)

SPERMATIC. Blood-vessels, nerves, and other structures that are associated with the testicle.

SPERMATIC CORD (*see* INGUINAL CANAL and the illustration, Genitalia of the Bull, adjacent to PENIS).

SPERMATIC CORD, TORSION OF. This has been reported, as a rare condition, in the dog. In a review of 13 cases Pearson and colleagues (Pearson, H. and Kelly, D. F., *Vet. Rec.* (1975) **97**, 200) found the testicle involved was intra-abdominal in 11 dogs, and inguinal and scrotal in two others. In most cases the torsion appeared to result from enlargement of the testis due to tumours. Two of the dogs died – one of uraemia due to retention of urine, the other from shock – and a third after surgery. However, 10 dogs recovered completely after castration.

SPERMATOZOA, or sperms, are the motile male sex cells which, having matured in the Epididymis, are ejaculated at orgasm and are normally capable of fertilising the ovum or egg. The sperms are derived from non-motile cells in the seminiferous tubules of the testicle. The first-stage cells, *Spermatogonia*, divide to form the *Primary Spermatocytes*. When these latter in turn divide, the chromosomes become paired, one from each pair being found in the resulting *Secondary Spermatocytes*, which accordingly have half the number of chromosomes found in all the somatic cells. The *Spermatid* is a further stage of development which includes acquisition of the flagellum or tail which provides the sperm with its motility. For their journey to the Fallopian tubes, it appears that the sperms are not wholly dependent upon their own motive powers; the muscles of the female genital organs apparently assist onward movements of the semen.

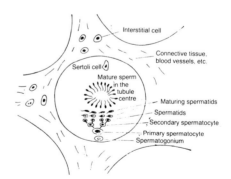

Sperm formation in the testis. (From Dr D. F. Horrobin's *Medical Physiology and Biochemistry*, courtesy of the author and Edward Arnold, 1968.)

Each spermatozoon has three main parts: the head, containing the cell's nucleus; a middle portion; and the tail. (*See also* SEMEN, REPRODUCTION, *and* ARTIFICIAL INSEMINATION.)

'It takes about 50 days from the time a sperm begins to be formed in the testicle to the time it appears in a bull's semen.' (Dr Gareth Williams.)

All normal semen contains some genetically deleterious diploid spermatozoa, distinguishable by their large size. The number of these can be reduced by differential centrifugation.

Fever may result in increased numbers of abnormal spermatozoa. For example, in Australia many abnormalities have been found in the middle portions of sperms from bulls suffering from bovine ephemeral fever.

SPERMIOPHAGES are macrophages which engulf sperms, thereby causing infertility. They have been found in both human and canine semen. (For a case history, see W. E. Allen, *Veterinary Record* (1981) **109**, 296.)

SPF. Specific Pathogen-free. In Britain as in the USA, SPF pigs are available for repopulating farms where disease has become a problem. SPF piglets are removed from the uterus by surgery in a sterile manner, reared in elaborate isolation premises, and immunised and prepared for a normal farm environment. (*See also* 'DISEASE-FREE' ANIMALS.)

SPHENOID is a bone lying along the base of the skull in front of the occipital bone, and immediately above and slightly behind the throat.

SPHINCTER. A circular muscle which surrounds the opening from an organ, and by maintaining constantly a state of moderate contraction prevents the escape of the contents of the organ. The muscle fibres forming the sphincter relax under nervous influence when the contents of the organ are due to be discharged to the outside past the sphincter. Sphincters close the outlet from the stomach, bladder, rectum, and regulate the escape of the contents from these organs. Under certain conditions the nervous mechanism which keeps these sphincters shut is liable to become upset, so that faeces and urine, for instance, can escape freely. This incontinence is one of the important symptoms seen in fracture of the spinal column, and in some forms of paralysis.

SPHYGMOGRAPH is an instrument used for recording the pulse.

SPICA BANDAGE (*see* BANDAGES).

'SPIDER SYNDROME'. A name given by Minnesota sheep breeders to a crippling congenital disease seen mostly in black-faced lambs. The forelimbs may be bent, spines 'twisted', rump angled steeply from *tuber sacrale* to *tuber ischii*. In 1986 the disease was said to be on the increase in the USA (Vanek, J. & others. *Veterinary Medicine* (1986) July 663.)

SPIDERS. In the USA and South America dogs are often bitten by the Black Widow spider (*Latrodectus mactans*), which tends to lurk among piles of logs or in dark outhouses. The bite is extremely painful, and may be followed by vomiting, laboured breathing, weakness, and paralysis. Death follows within hours or days, unless the antivenin is administered.

In the USA bites by the spiders of the suborder Labido are fairly common in horses and dogs; the bites being mostly on the head. Cats are mostly bitten on the face or forepaws. Two puncture marks provide a clue aiding diagnosis. Within minutes or hours, signs of neurotoxicity appear and may last for several days. Myalgia, abdominal rigidity, vomiting, panting, disturbance of vision, and shock occur.

Another spider, the Brown Recluse (*Loxoceles reclusa*) causes an erythematous lesion, from which a central blister emerges; the skin there turning purple or black. Convulsions followed by death are not uncommon; the preliminary signs being those caused by the Labido spider. (Northwood, R. B., *Veterinary Medicine* (1985) **80**, 38.)

Several of the larger 'bird-eating' spiders have setae, which they brush off their abdomens with their hind-legs. These setae (described under CATERPILLARS) can give rise to dermatitis, pharyngitis, and eye inflammation.

Such spiders are becoming popular as pets, and veterinary advice is increasingly sought on their care. The management of spiders and methods for their restraint was described in 1987. (Cooper, J. E. *Journal of Small Animal Medicine* **28**, 229.)

The Sydney funnel-web spider (*Atrax robustus*) is poisonous to a degree which varies with its sex. Seventy-five per cent of mice, and 95% of guinea pigs died after being bitten by male spiders; but only 20% or so after bites by females. (Tibbals, J. & others. *Australian Veterinary Journal* (1987) **64**, 63.)

SPINA BIFIDA. A congenital abnormality of the vertebral column, involving a defect in closure of the arch formed by the dorsal laminae of one or more vertebrae. The worst lesions prove lethal. Symptoms of less serious lesions includes paresis or paralysis and incontinence. The condition has been found in dogs.

SPINAL ANAESTHESIA (*see under* EPIDURAL).

SPINAL COLUMN, the chain of bones reaching from the base of the skull along the neck and back to the tip of the tail, is composed of the vertebrae, and forms the central axis of the skeleton. Through the spinal canal, formed by the arches of adjacent vertebrae, runs the spinal cord, which gives off the spinal nerves running to various parts of the body. (*See* BONES, NERVES, SPINAL CORD.)

SPINAL CORD is the posterior part of the central nervous system and is situated within the spinal canal of the spinal column. It forms the direct continuation of the medulla of the brain, being usually arbitrarily held to commence at the *foramen magnum*, the large opening in the occipital bone at the back of the skull. Posteriorly, it ends about the middle of the sacrum, although in this region the cord has lost its original form, and consists of a bundle of nerves, the actual termination being at about the level of the joint between fifth and sixth lumbar vertebrae, the continuation of bundles behind this being known as the *cauda equina*, owing to its supposed likeness to a horse's tail. The spinal cord is thus considerably shorter than the spinal column which houses it. During its course in the horse it gives off 42 pairs of spinal nerves, each of which takes origin by means of a dorsal and ventral root, which join each other, before emerging from the spinal canal. These spinal nerves, according to their position, are known as *cervical* (8), *thoracic* (18), *lumbar* (6), *sacral* (5), and *coccygeal* (5). The cord itself is divided into cervical, thoracic, lumbar, and sacral parts. Like the brain the cord is surrounded by three membranes, the *dura mater, arachnoid*, and *pia mater*, from without inwards. In the spaces of the arachnoid is a quantity of cerebro-spinal fluid, and between the outside of the dura and the inside of the bony canal is a padding of fat and blood-vessels, which together prevent injury to the spinal cord itself during the movements of the spinal column.

On section the spinal cord is found to be composed partly of grey, but mainly of white matter. It differs from the arrangement in the brain in that while in the brain the grey matter is on the outside of the white mass, in the cord the white matter is superficial. The arrangement of grey matter, as seen in section transversely across the cord, resembles the capital letter H 'horn', and the masses at each side are joined by a wide bridge of grey matter known as the 'grey commissure'. In the middle of this commissure lies the 'central canal' of the cord, which communicates with the ventricles of the brain.

Microscopic structure. The *grey matter* consists greatly of 'neuroglia' cells, the supporting scaffolding fibrous-tissue cells of nerve regions, and in the meshes formed by these cells lie the large multipolar motor nerve cells, and the fibres which spring from them and unite one cell to another, or pass out of the cord to form the fibres of the nerve trunks. The *white matter* is composed almost entirely of bundles of nerve fibres, most of which possess a myelinated sheath, the white colour being due to the appearance of these sheaths in the mass. (*See* NERVES.) There is also in the white matter a certain amount of supporting tissue. Blood-vessels are found in both white and grey matter.

Functions. The spinal cord conveys nerve impulses to and from the brain, but it also deals with *spinal reflex* actions. For example, sensation of pain in a dog's paw will cause the animal to snatch the paw away from the source of pain, *e.g.* a hot cinder. Such protective action is a spinal reflex, involving sensory and motor nerves, taken without reference to the brain. (*See also* CENTRAL NERVOUS SYSTEM and BRAIN.)

SPINE AND SPINAL CORD, DISEASES AND INJURIES OF. These will be considered together, because the chief danger of injury or disease in the spine is that the spinal cord and its nerves may be simultaneously injured or diseased.

FRACTURE of the spinal column is probably the commonest severe injury that affects this part. It may be met with in any animal, but is probably commonest in the horse and dog. It usually occurs from external violence, such as falls, falling timber, running into stationary objects

and other run-away accidents, in the larger animals, and in the smaller animals it is often occasioned by run-over accidents, kicks or blows from large animals, falls from great heights, etc. It may occur from powerful muscular contractions when a horse is cast, or falls in a loose-box, and cannot easily regain its feet; while suddenly pulling up during a gallop in a hilly field occasionally causes it in saddle-horses. Paralysis of the hindquarters, with loss of sensation, and often local sweating behind the injury, are symptoms of fracture, in addition to severe shock, occasioned by the laceration of the cord. (*See also* PARAPLEGIA *and* PARALYSIS.)

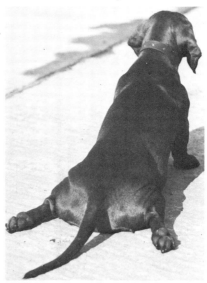

Paralysis due to a ruptured inter-vertebral disc.

CONCUSSION of the cord, occasioned by factors similar to but milder than those which cause fracture, is also common. Generally speaking, if the onset of the symptoms of paralysis occurs a day or two after the accident, instead of at the time, concussion, with or without haemorrhage, should be suspected, and hope of recovery can usually be entertained so long as there is not much systemic disturbance. (*See also* HORSES, BACK TROUBLES IN.)

INTERVERTEBRAL DISC PROTRUSION. Each intervertebral disc, which has a soft, pulpy centre and a fibrous or gristly outer ring, acts as a shock-absorber between the vertebrae, and supports the spinal cord between them. The nature of the usual disc injury is one of partial or complete rupture, with compression of the spinal cord to a lesser or greater extent. The injury is most common in Pekingese, Dachshunds, Sealyhams, and Spaniels. It also occurs in cats.

The cause would appear to be a gradual wear of the disc with age, and perhaps the extra strain on the spine which may be imposed upon the short-legged breeds. In some cases there is no history of violence; in others, a sudden muscular effort, *e.g.* in jumping to catch a ball.

Symptoms consist of pain and weakness or paralysis of the hindquarters, and may appear

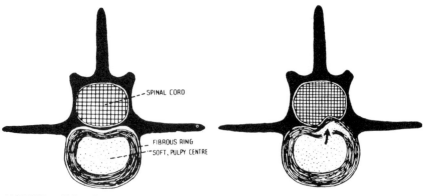

NORMAL : This diagram shows a cross-section through the vertebral column, with the spinal cord above and the disc below.

PARTIAL RUPTURE of the inter-vertebral disc, with pressure being exerted upon the spinal cord.

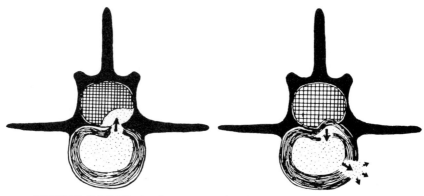

COMPLETE RUPTURE of a disc, with severe compression of the spinal cord.

" FENESTRATION " OPERATION sometimes performed to relieve pressure on the spinal cord by making a counter opening.

Intervertebral disc lesions.

shortly after the dog has been observed to jump, slip, or fall, or they may appear in cases where the owner has not observed any violent movement whatever. For example, a dog apparently normal at night may be found paralysed in the morning.

The muscles which control the passage of urine and faeces may become paralysed.

In many cases natural recovery takes place within a fortnight, and this applies even to dogs with paralysis. Where this persists, the outlook becomes progressively less hopeful; though a complete recovery after twelve months is not unknown.

A 'fenestration' operation is occasionally performed to relieve pain by relieving pressure upon the spinal cord, but it is not of much use for paralysis. Other measures are for the treatment of paralysis generally. (See also NANDROLONE.)

CERVICAL SPONDULOPATHY ('wobbler' syndrome) in the dog is most commonly seen in the Great Dane but also occurs in other breeds, especially the Doberman. It is usually first seen between 8 and 12 months and the clinical signs include hind limb inco-ordination, abduction of the limbs, a prancing gait, and dragging of the feet causing wearing of the toe nails. Diagnosis of cervical spondylopathy is confirmed by radiography. Lesions include stenosis of the vertebral canal,

exostosis of the articular facets, and subluxation. (*J. Amer. anim. hosp. Ass.* (1975), **11**, 175.)

HEMIVERTEBRA ('wedge-shaped' vertebra). In many cases this condition in dogs gives rise to no obvious symptoms, but in others the condition is characterised clinically by progressive hind-leg weakness, spinal pain, abnormalities of the nervous system, and evidence of muscle atrophy or other abnormalities of conformation. Confirmation of the clinical diagnosis is by radiography. It is suggested that the condition is congenital in origin. Breed incidences are reported. The occurrence of the disorder in certain families of dogs suggests also that it may be hereditary. (Done, S. H., *et al.*, *Vet. Rec.* (1975), **96**, 313.)

ANKYLOSIS of the vertebrae is not rare in horses. It originates from diffuse inflammation of the spinal column, frequently due to rheumatic causes, and one after another of the vertebrae becomes fused to its neighbour in front or behind. In severe cases practically the whole of the thoracic and lumbar regions of the horse may fuse into a rigid bar. Such horses usually can perform straightforward work for some time, but are unable to carry any weight, to back heavy loads, or to lie down or rise with ease. They may develop into 'shiverers', but so long as the spinal cord is not compressed they may live for years.

PACHYMENINGITIS, or inflammation of the membranes of the cord, sometimes occurs in old dogs. It is called 'ossifying pachymeningitis' in these animals, because of the tendency for bone to be deposited in the dura mater. Like most conditions of the spinal column it cannot be treated.

ABSCESS in the cord, or in one of the vertebrae, may be discovered only at a knackery or at autopsy; or it may lead to symptoms of paresis/paralysis. (*See also* SPINA BIFIDA.)

SPIRILLUM. A bacterium with a wavy shape. (*See* RAT-BITE FEVER.)

SPIRIT (*see* ALCOHOL *and* SURGICAL SPIRIT).

SPIROCERCA. Worms which are found in nodules on the oesophagus. In the dog they may sometimes give rise to cancer (sarcoma) of the oesophagus; and also to fatal haemorrhage. (*See* ROUNDWORMS.)

SPIROCHAETE is one of the names applied to bacteria possessing a more or less spiral or wavy outline. Another term applied to this group is 'spirillum'. There are three genera which are important causal agents of disease: *Borrelia*, *Treponema*, and *Leptospira*. The first has large wavy spirals and is flexible; the second has regular rigid spirals, while the last has small spirals and one hook-like end.

Many spirochaetes produce disease in man and animals, the best known among which is: *Treponema pallida*, the cause of syphilis in man. *Treponema cuniculi* in rabbits causes 'rabbit syphilis', in Britain, on the Continent, and in America. *Borrelia galinarum* is responsible for a form of spirochaetosis affecting fowls in the tropics and sub-tropics, and is transmitted by the fowl tick. *Leptospira canicola* causes nephritis in dogs and canicola fever in man; *L. icterohaemorrhagiae* causes Weil's disease in man and jaundice in dogs. Leptospirosis also occurs in cattle and pigs, and there are many serotypes. (*See* LEPTOSPIROSIS and, for infection with *Treponema* in pigs, SWINE DYSENTERY.)

SPIROCHAETOSIS OF FOWLS is met with in Africa, Asia, West Indies, South America, Australia, and in Europe. It occurs in fowls, ducks, geese, and turkeys. Canaries and other birds are susceptible to artificial infection.

Transmission. The disease is transmitted from diseased to healthy fowls by the fowl tick, *Argas persicus* one of the most important parasites of poultry. The ticks are very active at night, and may travel long distances to reach a host. They remain hidden during the day in crevices and underneath the bark of trees. Myriads of these ticks may attack fowls on the roost, a large quantity of blood being sucked, the affected birds becoming weak and unthrifty and having ragged plumage.

If, however, the ticks have fed on a bird affected with Spirochaetosis, they become carriers of this disease and may transmit the infection through the egg to the next generation of ticks.

SIGNS. Affected fowls show diarrhoea, loss of appetite, loss of power of the head, and may die in convulsions. A more chronic course is also described, birds becoming paralysed and emaciated, and dying in about a fortnight.

TREATMENT. Penicillin is very effective.

PREVENTIVE TREATMENT. This consists in ridding the premises of ticks.

SPIROCHAETOSIS OF PIGS (*see under* PORCINE ULCERATIVE SPIROCHAETOSIS *and* SWINE DYSENTERY).

SPLANCHNIC means anything belonging to the internal organs of the body as distinguished from its framework.

SPLAYLEG, CONGENITAL of piglets may involve either the fore-legs or all four. Recovery from this defect can be expected if the piglet can manage to keep out of the sow's way. (*See* VITAMIN E.)

SPLEEN. A soft, highly vascular, plum-coloured organ, possessing a smooth surface formed by a dense fibrous capsule over which the peritoneum is closely applied.

STRUCTURE. Beneath the outermost covering of peritoneum lies the dense fibrous tissue coat, from the inner surface of which numerous strands or 'trabeculae' run into the organ. The fibrous coat and the trabeculae possess elastic fibres and a fair number of plain muscular fibres. The trabeculae branch and rebranch throughout the substance of the organ, and in the meshes so formed lies the spleen-pulp. This consists of delicate connective-tissue fibres passing between the trabeculae, and numbers of leucocytes and red blood corpuscles. Blood-vessels run through the trabeculae and end in areas where the blood cells appear to be highly concentrated; these concentrations are known as 'Malpighian corpuscles' or 'bodies'. The blood escapes into the pulp of the spleen instead of travelling through capillaries everywhere as in other organs.

FUNCTIONS. The spleen destroys old red blood cells, acts as a blood store, and appears to play some part in the formation of lymphocytes.

An animal is able to survive after removal of the spleen. There is a compensatory increase in the lymph nodes all over the body, and, after a period of adjustment, life continues.

The spleen is apparently concerned with bodily defence, and resistance to liver fluke infestation is reduced after removal of a sheep's spleen. (*See* RETICULO-ENDOTHELIAL SYSTEM.)

(A person who has had his spleen removed and works with cattle may become ill with BABESIOSIS.)

SPLEEN, DISEASES OF. It is often only at post-mortem examination that spleen diseases are revealed in the large animals. In anthrax it becomes greatly enlarged, and also in babesiosis, for example. In the dog, splenectomy is occasionally performed in cases of tumour formation or injury. Rupture of the spleen, with resultant internal haemorrhage, occurs in small animals which have fallen from a height or have been involved in a road accident.

SPLENECTOMY. Surgical removal of the spleen.

SPLINTING MATERIALS. For the immobilisation of limbs to achieve external fixation of fractured bone, or to provide additional support for internal fixation, plaster of Paris and resin-impregnated materials are used.

For large-animal use, plaster of Paris has several disadvantages: 'it does not achieve its maximum strength for up to 24 hours after application, and is liable to break. The cast is often heavy and cumbersome, and will soften in contact with moisture'.

'Fibreglass casts are light, waterproof, and very strong,' but are difficult to apply, and need a primary cast of plaster of Paris; they also need special plaster saws for removal.

A new thermoplastic material (Hexcelite) was found to be quickly and easily applied, and 'all the casts ... withstood the stresses to which they were subjected when the animal regained its feet on recovery from anaesthesia.' It is, however, a costly material. (G. B. Edwards and D. G. Clayton Jones, *Vet. Rec.* (1978), **102**, 397.)

Another splinting material is Baycast (Bayer), a polyester cotton bandage impregnated with a water-actived prepolymer resin. It has been successfully used for both large and small animals. Cast removal is not necessary for radiography. (J. E. F. Houlton, *Veterinary Record* (1981), **109**, 10.)

Scotchcast consists of polyurethane resin on a fibreglass bandage.

SPLINTS IN HORSES . After a painful osteoperiostitis, involving the small metacarpal and metatarsal bones, splint formation usually starts in the periosteum or ligament. The amount of new bone formed depends on the extent and duration of the inflammation. The lameness disappears as the inflammation subsides.

The causes include an inherited defect.

SIGNS. Usually, lameness appears before any bony enlargement can be seen or felt, although pressure over the region of splints causes pain. This lameness usually increases with exercise. The horse may walk sound, but trots lame to a surprising extent, considering the apparently 'sound' walk. Later on, a soft putty-like swelling can be felt, and this becomes harder with time, until it can be finally recognised as bone. In knee-splint the leg is carried to the outside, and appears stiff. As a rule splints are not serious, since with rest and treatment the bony fusion becomes complete, and the horse goes sound. When they are placed high up, however, there is a danger that the new bone formation may involve the knee-joint, and when they are situated far back, so as to interfere with the tendons, they may produce permanent lameness and injury to the tendon. In a horse under six years old they should be looked upon as liable to cause future trouble, but in a horse over six years old they can be disregarded unless lameness is present.

TREATMENT. Most mild cases require nothing further in the way of treatment than a rest from work, and later a run at grass for a fortnight or so. Fomentations may help to relieve pain during the acute stage.

SPONDYLITIS. Inflammation of a vertebra, due to trauma or an infection.
Spondylosis. A degenerative condition of the spine which can lead to ANKYLOSIS.

SPONDYLOPATHY. Disease of the vertebrae such as may cause compression of the spinal cord, disc degeneration, and narrowing of the intervertebral space.

SPONGES. In modern stables it is recognised that if a contagious disease breaks out, the sponge used for a number of horses is an important factor in the spread of the disease, and consequently a piece of flannel or other material which can be boiled is generally used instead for 'quartering' (*see* GROOMING). A sponge used at the end of a hosepipe for udder-washing of cattle led to an outbreak of mastitis due to *Pseudomonas aeruginosa.*

SPONGIFORM ENCEPHALOPATHY (*see under* BOVINE *and* FELINE ditto).
Human spongiform encephalopathy. The human spongiform encephalopathies – Creutz-feldt-Jakob disease (CJD), Gerstmann-Straussler-Scheinker syndrome (GSS) and kuru – are pathologically very similar to scrapie in sheep and to bovine spongiform encephalopathy (BSE). Like them too they are transmissible, although there is very little evidence of person to person transmission, except in a very few iatrogenic cases, such as the grafting of corneal or dura mater tissues from donors subsequently shown to have had CJD, and the use of human growth hormone prepared from the pituitary glands of patients dying with CJD. (Baker, H. (1990) *State Veterinary Journal* **44**, 19).

SPORADIC DISEASE is a disease occurring in single cases here and there, as distinct from disease occurring as an enzootic, throughout a district, or epizootic, through a country or large tract of land.

SPORES. Reproductive cells of protozoa, bacteria, and fungi, etc., usually able to withstand an adverse environment.

SPORIDESMIN. A poisonous substance, isolated from the fungus *Pithomyces chartarum*, which causes Facial Eczema and liver damage in sheep and cattle in New Zealand and Australia.

SPOROTRICHOSIS. A fungal disease of horses, cattle, dogs, cats, and man, caused by *Sporothrix schenckii*. This gives rise to nodules under the skin, and thickening of the lymphatics with ulceration. In the dog, liver, lungs and bone may show lesions. Of 19 people reported to have acquired this infection from cats, 14 had no history of traumatic injury at the site; and 12 were veterinarians or assistants/nurses. All had a localised cutaneous lymph node infection; lesions resolving in 1 to 10 months after potassium iodide treatment. One patient had a deep ulcer on a finger. Although rare, infection through inhalation has been recorded in people. (Dunstan, R. W. and others. *J A V M A* (1986) **189**, 880.)

SPOROZOA. This is a group of Protozoa which are all parasitic and produce spores at some stage of their life-cycle. It is divided into a number of orders, of which only two are important. These are the HAEMOSPORIDIA which are parasites of the red blood-cells, and the COCCIDIA which are parasites of epithelia.

SPOTTED FEVER (*see* ROCKY MOUNTAIN FEVER).

SPOTTED HORSE (*see under* APPALOOSA).

SPRAINED TENDONS is an extremely common condition both in the heavy and light draught horse. The flexors, superficial and deep, are mostly affected.
CAUSES. The superficial flexor tendon is sprained during maximum weight-bearing by the limb, and the deep flexor becomes sprained at the period of thrust.
SIGNS. There are the usual signs of inflammation – heat, pain, swelling. A horse with a badly sprained deep flexor may walk almost sound, but goes pronouncedly lame when made to trot. A localised sprain of the check ligament and its insertion into the deep flexor tendon often produces acute lameness, but the condition is not so serious as a sprain of the tendons lower down. From an owner's point of view, however, differential diagnosis between the various forms and situations of sprain is not important.
TREATMENT. Antiphlogistine, spread with cotton-wool, and applied hot, being bandaged with an elastic bandage, fairly firmly, gives good results. The horse must be kept at rest.
Generally a horse with a badly sprained tendon is not fit for work for from a month to 6 weeks, although it may be apparently sound before this time.
Chronic sprained tendons are often incurable, but good results have sometimes been obtained with diathermy. (*See* DIATHERMY.)

SPRAINS involve the wrenching of a joint, often with the simultaneous tearing of a ligament. The term is also applied to an inflammation of a tendon, generally the result of an excessive stretching of its fibres. (*See* SPRAINED TENDONS, SYNOVITIS.)

SPRAY 'DRIFT'. By this is meant droplets of spray liquid carried by the wind to fields adjacent to that which is being intentionally sprayed with some farm chemical for purposes of weed control, pest control, haulm destruction. It is a potential cause of poisoning in grazing animals. (*See* SPRAYS USED ON CROPS.)

SPRAY RACE. A race which can be used for spraying sheep or cattle. Nozzles are arranged at intervals and fed with suitable parasiticide liquid by means of a pump.

SPRAYS USED ON CROPS include weedkillers such as D N O C, insecticides such as Parathion, and potato haulm destroyer such as arsenites. Such substances constitute a hazard to livestock which gain entry into fields. (*See* POISONING, INSECTICIDES, WEEDKILLERS, etc.)

'SPREADING FACTOR' (*see* HYALURONIDASE).

SPURGES, POISONING BY. The various species of spurges (*Euphorbia* sp.) are, apparently, mostly poisonous, though not to the same extent. Animals are not very likely to eat them because of the acrid milky juice. Species which have been blamed for causing poisoning are as follows: Caper spurge, *Euphorbia lathyris*, Irish spurge, *E. hibernica*; Petty spurge, *E. peplus*; and the Sun spurge, *E. helioscopia*; and of these the first seems to be the most dangerous.
SIGNS. Inflammation and swelling of the mucous membranes of the mouth and tongue, pains in the abdomen, coldness of the extremities of the body, dizziness, fainting, leading to unconsciousness and death in 2 or 3 days. In one of the South African spurges, *E. genistoides*, the typical symptom, in addition to these mentioned here, is an acute inflammation of the urethra, accompanied by frequent and painful attempts at urination. Symptoms of acute enteritis may also be seen.
TREATMENT. Veterinary advice should be sought at once, and since the milk of affected cows may cause illness to people drinking it, it should not be used either for human or animal consumption.

SPUR VEINS. The veins liable to damage by the horseman's spurs.

'STABLE COUGH' (*see* EQUINE INFLUENZA).

STABLE FLY is a serious pest to horses and other animals, and transmits diseases such as surra and anthrax in the tropics. (*See* FLIES, FLY CONTROL, 'SUMMER SORES'.)

STABLES FOR RACEHORSES. A survey of 96 racehorse stables in the south west of England showed that a 'typical' racehorse is kept in a loose box with a floor area of 12 m^2 and is bedded on straw; it shares its airspace of 39 m^3 with seven other horses. In calm conditions, with the top door of the stable open, natural convection would provide 6·6 air changes/hour, but with the door closed, only 2·2 changes. The top door should rarely, if ever, be closed. It is concluded that present day stables are based on designs which are worse than the best available in the 19th century. (Jones, R. D. & others (1987) *Equine Veterinary Journal* **19**, 454.) (*See also* BEDDING.)

STABLE VICES AND TRICKS (*see* 'VICES' *and* VICIOUSNESS).

STAG. An ox or pig castrated late in life, or a turkey cock (over one year old).

'STAGGERS WEED'. A poisonous South African plant. (*See* 'PUSHING DISEASE'.)

STAINING for differentiation of bacteria. (*See* ACID-FAST, GRAM-NEGATIVE.)

STALLION. An adult male horse, uncastrated, over 4 years old.

STANDARD INTERNATIONAL UNITS (*see* SI UNITS).

STAPHYLOCOCCUS (*see* BACTERIA).

STARCH (*see* CARBOHYDRATES, DIETETICS, *and* DIGESTION).

STARCH EQUIVALENT. This term is no longer used. METOLISABLE ENERGY replaces it.

The starch equivalent in the UK was replaced in 1975 by units of METABOLISABLE ENERGY (which see) as part of the introduction of metric and SI units.

STARCH GEL ELECTROPHORESIS. This is one of the commonest techniques for studying the genetic variation in serum proteins, and could well become important in the future for selecting superior stock. (*See* ELECTROPHORESIS.)

STARING COAT, A. In the dog there are several causes of this, but one is lack of suitable fat in the diet. As a first-aid measure, offer bread and butter or dripping (but not margarine) for a few days as an 'extra'. (*See also under* WORMS.)

STASIS is a term applied to stoppage of the flow of blood in the vessels or of the food materials in the intestinal canal.

'STEAMING UP'. A term used by dairy farmers to describe the practice of feeding a concentrates ration 4–5 weeks before calving in order to provide for growth of the fetus and provide reserves against the onset of lactation. For detailed advice on 'steaming up', *see under* ACETONAEMIA – prevention.

Excessive steaming-up is regarded as one cause of LAMINITIS (which see) and lameness.

STEATITIS. A yellow discoloration of fat occurring in cats, mink and pigs fed mainly on fish scraps or tinned fish. Listlessness, tenderness over the back and abdomen, and a reluctance to move are observed. Treatment: administer vitamin E; also the B complex.

In cats steatitis may follow prolonged and continuous feeding not only with red tuna or pilchards, but also with white fish such as coley. The symptoms include stiffness and pain. Treatment includes a change of diet and a vitamin E supplement.

Steatitis in horses has also been reported. Pathological changes in the fat taken from the abdominal wall was found in 44 of 173 horses and ponies examined *post-mortem* at the Institute of Veterinary Pathology, Utrecht, over a 2-year period. Steatitis was found in fetuses from normal mares, and in adult horses. Sub-clinical steatitis was the most common type, but a few deaths were attributed to this cause. Lesions varied from the presence of macrophages in the fat, to some fibrosis in addition, and to necrosis. (Wensvoort, P., *Tijdschr. Diergeneesk.* (1974), **99.**)

STEATORRHEA. Fatty faeces.

STELL. A circular stone or corrugated metal shelter for sheep or cattle, built on moorland or hill, and affording good protection against snow drifts. Stells were in use in the early nineteenth

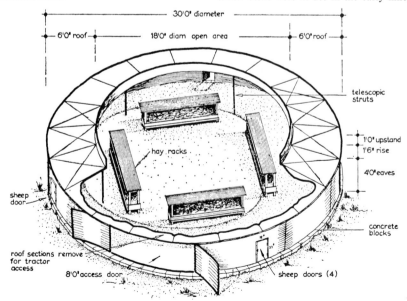

Of metal construction, on a base of concrete blocks, this modified Stell at the Rowett Research Institute, Aberdeenshire, was designed by Dr E. Cresswell. Sheep doors and an 8 ft doorway for tractor access are shown.

century, if not earlier, but metal ones have now come on to the market.

STENOSIS is any unnatural narrowing of a passage or orifice of the body. It is specially reserved for application to the heart valves, and to the opening through the larynx – the glottis – but is applied to any of the large arteries, as well as to the parotid ducts. (*See* HEART DISEASES, LARYNX, PAROTID DUCT, PYLORIC STENOSIS.)

STENSON'S DUCT is the duct which carries saliva from the parotid gland into the mouth. (*See* PAROTID GLAND.)

STENT. This is woven in the form of a tubular mesh from surgical-grade stainless steel, and is self-expanding when released from a small-diameter delivery catheter.

Stents were developed originally for endovascular use, but are now a new treatment for urethral stricture, in human patients. When the latter were seen at 'follow-up' 6 to twelve months later, all had a good-calibre urethra. Urethroscopy showed complete epithelial covering of the implant. (Milroy, E. J. G. & others. *Lancet* July 25th 1991, 1424.)

Stents obviously have a potential for use in veterinary surgery.

STEPHANOFILARIASIS. A chronic skin disease occurring in cattle in parts of the USA, and caused by the nematode worm *Stephanofilaria stilesi*. The intermediate host is the horn fly.

STERILISATION (*see* CASTRATION; *also* SPAYING for sterilisation in the sexual sense).

With reference to sterilisation in its other sense, *see* DISINFECTION, ANTISEPTICS, ASEPSIS, *and* WOUNDS. For most general purposes the best sterilising agent is boiling water. Boiling should be continuous and should last for at least 10 minutes in order to kill vegetative bacteria, viruses, and most other types of micro-organisms.

STERNUM. This forms the floor of the chest, provides attachment for the pectoral muscles, and for the costal cartilages of the sternal (true) ribs. (The asternal (false) ribs are not directly connected to the sternum.) The sternum comprises *sternebrae* – segments which fuse together with advancing age. The horse and dog each have eight of these; the cow seven; pig and sheep six.

STEROIDS. Chemical substances closely related to the sterols. Examples: the sex hormones, hormones of the adrenal cortex, bile acids. (*See also* CORTICOSTEROIDS *and* DIABETES.)

Prescribing steroid hormone products (where allowed). Steroid hormone growth promoters are substances with an androgenic, oestrogenic or gestagenic action. In general they must not be administered to farm animals. 'Farm animals' includes cattle, sheep, pigs, goats, horses, poultry, the wild animals of these species and any ruminants raised on a holding.

The prohibition does not apply to:
(a) the administration for therapeutic treatment by a veterinarian in the form of an injection of oestradiol-17-beta, progesterone or testosterone or derivatives of these substances which readily yield the parent compound on hydrolysis after absorption at the site of application;
(b) the administration of a steroid hormone product for the termination of unwanted gestation or the improvement of fertility;
(c) the administration of a steroid hormone product by, or under the direct responsibility of, a veterinarian for the synchronisation of oestrus or the preparation of donors or recipients for the implantation of embryos.

For the purposes of the controlling regulation the term 'injection' does not include implantation and the term 'therapeutic treatment' has a very restricted meaning, ie, the treatment of a fertility problem diagnosed by a veterinarian in an animal not intended for fattening.

A small range of products is licensed in the UK for the purposes listed above. In the course of time there will be a list of such products authorised by the European Community.

STEROLS. Solid alcohols, waxy substances derived from animal (and plant) tissues. Examples: cholesterol, ergosterol.

STERTOR. Noisy breathing resembling snoring.

STIFF LAMB DISEASE. This is a mild disease occurring in East Anglia due to infection with *Erysipelothrix rhusiopathiae*, the cause of swine erysipelas. The same name is also applied to Muscular Dystrophy, a condition similar to that occurring in cattle as a result of vitamin E deficiency.

'STIFF-LIMBED LAMBS'. This is a hereditary condition affecting newly born lambs, to which the name *Myodystrophia fetalis deformans* has been given. It is commoner among Welsh Mountain sheep than among other breeds. The condition is an arrest of the development of muscular tissue during fetal life, and a replacement by fibrous tissue. This contracts and pulls the limb into an unnatural, stiff attitude, and gives rise to difficulty in parturition.

The condition is a Mendelian recessive lethal.

The condition has also been reported from Britain and America affecting cattle, but is not at all common in them.

STIFF SICKNESS (*see* THREE-DAY SICKNESS *and* STYFZIEKTE).

STIFLE, THE. The joint corresponding to the human knee. (*See* BONES *and* JOINTS.) In horses, stifle lameness is often the result of OSTEOCHONDROSIS DISSECANS or of subchondral bone cysts.

In 42 cases of stifle lameness in cattle, the diagnoses included subchondral bone cysts (18 cases), joint instability (15), degenerative joint disease (12), cranial cruciate ligament injury (9), sepsis (9), collateral ligament injury (3), femorotibial luxation (2) and intra-articular fracture (2). The prognosis for animals with bone cysts was good, irrespective of treatment (75 per cent recovered), while it was much poorer for animals with sepsis (22 per cent) or joint instability (27 per cent). (Ducharme, N. G. & others., *Canadian Veterinary Journal* **26**, 212.)

STILBENES. Substances consisting wholly or partly of stilboestrol, hexoestrol, dienoestrol, or benzestrol. (*See* HORMONES IN MEAT.)

In accordance with an EC Directive, the sale of stilbenes for use in veterinary medicines, veterinary products or animal feeds containing these products, was banned in 1982 in the UK.

The ban deprived veterinary surgeons of the use of stilboestrol for treating enlarged prostate glands, adenoma, misalliance in the bitch, and urinary incontinence in spayed bitches.

STILBOESTROL. An oestrogen formerly used both therapeutically and as a growth promoter in food animals. (*See* HORMONES, HORMONE THERAPY, HORMONES IN MEAT PRODUCTION, STILBENES.)

STILLBORN PIGS. Breeding stock should, of course, have access to pasture, but if for any reason this golden rule is going to be broken, then rations should be supplemented in summer as well as in winter, with vitamin A. In a group of 20 gilts which were suddenly switched from succulent feeding to dry, fibrous grazing late in pregnancy, severe constipation resulted, and there were dead piglets in 19 of the litters.

A survey carried out by the Veterinary Investigation Service in England and Wales showed a 4·8 per cent incidence of stillbirths out of a total of 4394 piglets born in 371 litters. The incidence varied widely from herd to herd, as would be expected; ranging from 0·4 to 12·9 per cent. Constipation appears to be a cause of stillbirths, and SENNA may be used.

There are several infections which give rise to abortion and stillbirths. (*See* AUJESZKY'S DISEASE, ABORTION, MUMMIFICATION, INFERTILITY, CARBON MONOXIDE.)

STIMULANTS. Heart stimulants include caffeine, digitalis, coramine, etc. (*See also* RESPIRATORY STIMULANTS.)

STINGS (*see* BITES AND STINGS).

STIRK. A young female bovine of 6 to 12 months old, sometimes a male of the same age, in Scotland.

STITCHING, or SUTURING (*see* WOUNDS).

STOCKING RATES. During the peak of grass growth from early April to mid-June, 8 to 10 ewes and their lambs can be carried per acre. But this is a maximum figure for this period only. For cattle, continuous grazing, the figure is perhaps 1 to 3 acres.

In Britain, 'most grass is greatly understocked during the grazing season, chiefly due to the lack of capacity to carry more stock over winter.

'Good farmers, using intensive grass-farming methods, require 1½ acres or more per cow, even when winter feeding is supplemented considerably with concentrates.

'Estimates in New Zealand have suggested that dairy cows at 1·2 per acre may consume as little as 30 per cent of the available herbage.' (Director, Grassland Research Institute, Hurley.)

The most skilful dairy farmers were soon achieving 0·9 to 1·0 acre per cow without purchasing more than 10–15 per cent of their winter feed requirements other than production concentrates.

STOCKMEN/WOMEN. For health hazards *see under* COWMEN, PIGMEN, SHEPHERDS, MEAT-HANDLERS, and ZOONOSES.

STOMACH.
Functions of the stomach (*see* RUMEN, RUMINAL DIGESTION, RETICULUM, OMASUM, ABOMASUM). Broadly speaking, the function of the stomach is to store, warm, soften, and prepare food materials, and then to pass them on in regulated amounts into the intestine, where the more important digestive processes and absorption occur.

STOMACH, DISEASES OF. In all animals bacterial diseases, such as SALMONELLOSIS, may be involved in diseases of the stomach; likewise parasitic worms.

Horse. In view of the comparatively simple arrangement of the stomach, and the natural fastidiousness of the horse in the matter of food, stomach disease is not so common as in some other animals.
GASTRITIS, or INFLAMMATION OF THE STOMACH, is usually brought about by the ingestion of irritant, poisonous, or otherwise harmful substances, or by the presence of bots, or spread of disease from other parts of the body. (*See also* SALMONELLOSIS, BOTS, ROUNDWORMS.)

Signs. Attacks of violent abdominal pain, occurring shortly after feeding or even before feeding is completed, indicate that the stomach is affected. Dullness and depression are noticed; patchy sweating may break out; food is refused; the temperature rises slightly in mild cases, and to as high as 106°F in severe instances. Usually in from 2 to 3 hours after taking food the acute pain ceases, but the horse remains dull, and gives the impression that it is affected with a dull ache rather than with acute pain. Vomiting does not usually occur unless the stomach is ruptured or the oesophagus is dilated.
IMPACTION OF THE STOMACH is a condition in which engorgement of the stomach with food takes place. It may be due to lack of vitality (atony) in the muscular walls, to impaired gastric secretion.

Signs. Signs of impaction may occur, suddenly or gradually. There is depression, uneasiness, and perhaps colic, in those cases where a horse over-eats. (*See* COLIC.)

Sometimes a horse obtains relief by vomiting through the nostrils a quantity of the impacted material, which reduces the amount in the stomach so that the remainder can be dealt with in the usual way.

Prevention. It is easier to prevent impaction of the stomach than it is to cure it.

Whole beans, peas, wheat, or barley should not be used for horses. Horses should always be allowed as much water as they desire to drink, and should be watered before feeding in all cases. Diseased or rough and irregular teeth should be treated.

TYMPANY OF THE STOMACH. When vegetable food ferments from any cause, gas is produced. Certain foods, especially when unsound, undergo fermentation in the stomach instead of digestion, and the gas so formed is liable to collect in that organ often under pressure producing great distension. Foods which ferment easily are: succulent green crops, clovers, lucerne, potatoes eaten in quantity.

Signs. There is no remission of pain, such as is usually seen when the intestines are tympanitic. Horses may roll, plunge, and paw the ground during the earlier part of the attack. Respirations increase in rate, and become laboured. The abdomen becomes tense and often swollen, and in many instances horses assume a crouching attitude with their hindquarters, not unlike the way in which a dog sits. When the tympany is severe, unless relief is afforded by the passage of the stomach-tube, rupture of the stomach may occur, and death follows. (*See* COLIC.)

RUPTURE OF THE STOMACH may also occur when a horse falls violently to the ground soon after a big feed, *i.e.* when the stomach is full.

Signs. The distress characteristic of engorgement and tympany suddenly cease when the stomach ruptures, and for a short time the horse appears so much better that the owner imagines recovery will result. After a short time, however, the more serious symptoms of peritonitis and shock occur. Profuse perspiration usually breaks out; the pulse changes to what is called a 'running down pulse', *i.e.* there are a few strong beats which gradually become weaker until they are almost imperceptible, and then a succession of strong beats return; this is repeated rhythmically. Ears and feet become cold and clammy to the touch; respiration is blowing; and the expression on the face of the horse is one of anxiety. Vomiting is said to characterise rupture of the stomach, but it is probable that in most cases the vomiting occurs *before* the rupture takes place; the food material escapes into the abdominal cavity after rupture has occurred rather than up into the pharynx and nostrils. (*See also* COLIC.)

Treatment is useless; euthanasia advisable.

Cattle. ACUTE INDIGESTION with acidosis and, sometimes impaction of the rumen, may follow over-eating of grain or green foods. (*See* ACIDOSIS.)

TYMPANY OF THE RUMEN, 'bloat', consists of a collection of gas in the rumen. (*See under* BLOAT for symptoms, prevention and treatment.)

INFLAMMATION OF THE RUMEN (*see also* RUMEN ULCERATION) may be due to ingestion of irritant poisons, either of chemical or vegetable origin, to penetrating foreign bodies, or to the spread of inflammatory conditions from other parts in specific diseases.

FOREIGN BODIES IN RETICULUM are of great importance in both young and adult cattle, because of the close proximity of this organ to the pericardium and heart. In the reticulum two things may happen to them; they may fall to the lowermost part of the sac and remain there for an indefinite period, or they may slowly penetrate its wall and wander forwards through the diaphragm. Their subsequent course has been described under the section on HEART DISEASES, Sub-heading: *Traumatic pericarditis of cattle*, to which reference should be made. (*See also* HAIR BALLS, WOOL BALLS.)

INFLAMMATION OF THE ABOMASUM, abomastitis, or gastritis, is probably most commonly due to parasitic round worms.

(For the causes, symptoms, and treatment of parasitic gastritis in cattle and sheep, *see* PARASITIC GASTRO-ENTERITIS.)

DISPLACEMENT OF ABOMASUM may be associated with stenosis of the sigmoid curve of the duodenum in cattle. The abomasum is then found to be distended with fluid and gas, and displayed to the right. (M. A. van der Delden, *Vet. Record* (1983) **112**, 452.)

Symptoms include a distended abdomen, loss of appetite, loss of weight, and depression of milk yield, may sometimes be successfully treated by casting the cow and, with her lying on her back, rotating or rocking her through an angle of 45° from the vertical each way. Surgical treatment may be necessary. (*See* TYMPANITIC RESONANCE.)

ULCERATION is a condition by no means rare in cattle. It is sometimes associated with displacement of the abomasum, and may give rise to symptoms a few days after calving. Death follows perforation. Symptoms are similar to those given above. Ulceration is not uncommon in calves after weaning, giving rise to capricious appetite and sometimes evidence of abdominal pain. *Fusiformis necrophorus*, *Corynybacterium pyogenes*, and *Pasteurelle* organisms in other parts of the body may be associated.

Sheep. The diseases of the stomachs of the sheep resemble in general those of the same organs in cattle.

BRAXY is characterised by a patch of acute inflammation in the wall of the abomasum, usually about the size of the palm of the hand, where the mucous membrane is to a large extent destroyed.

Another form of gastritis is due to parasitic worms in the young lambs. (*See* WORMS.)

Pigs.

GASTRITIS. Irritating or poisonous substances, specific disease, or parasites, are among the causes. Salt poisoning is a cause of gastritis, as are also poisonings by arsenic, copper, saltpetre, sheep dips, etc. During the course of swine fever, swine erysipelas, foot-and-mouth disease, and even tuberculosis, the wall of the stomach may become involved, and inflammation may result. (*See under* GASTRIC ULCERS.) Parasites may also cause this condition. (*See* WORMS, TREATMENT AGAINST, MUCORMYCOSIS.)

Signs. Vomiting is the first and most important symptom of stomach disturbance. Thirst, depression, and sometimes skin discoloration are other symptoms. Convulsions and twitching of the limbs may be seen in young pigs.

Treatment. All solid foods must be withheld, and soft light foods given instead. Whole milk is one of the best. Where it is believed to be due to poisonous substances the appropriate antidotes must be given. (*See* ANTIDOTES.)

Dog. Gastritis may be bacterial in origin, caused by parasitic worms, irritating substances which include poisons, or be associated with foreign bodies. It is probably less common than enteritis or nephritis, both of which may give rise to vomiting.

Causes. Gastritis/gastro-enteritis may be a complication of distemper, canine virus hepatitis; or may arise during Salmonellosis and other bacterial disease; or follow the eating of infected or decomposing food.

Ulceration of the stomach in dog and cat may be associated with gastritis – sometimes with tuberculosis, malignant growths, and actino-bacillosis. Ulcers similar to peptic ulcers in human beings, and leading to perforation occur occasionally.

Signs. As a rule, a severe attack of vomiting immediately after a feed, and refusal to touch food subsequently. Thirst is nearly always excessive, and if gratified, vomiting usually follows.

If capillary haemorrhage occurs into the stomach, perhaps as the result of retching, the blood which slowly oozes from its walls, collects in the cavity of the stomach, undergoes partial digestion, and becomes changed into a brownish granular material, strongly resembling moist coffee grounds. This always has a most foul and objectionable odour. The dog itself becomes extremely miserable, dragging itself slowly from place to place, and showing preference for cold places where it may lie stretched out with its hind-legs straight behind it, so that the lower wall of the abdomen is in close contact with the cold surface, *e.g.* a stone step, or linoleum in a passage. Constipation usually occurs unless the intestines become involved, when diarrhoea is noticed. Pressure on the abdomen causes pain, and sometimes a dog lifted by the hand under the abdomen cries out. The temperature is raised at first.

Treatment. Hot packs applied to the abdomen soothe pain. Dogs affected with gastritis should be under the charge of a veterinary surgeon, who will vary the treatment according to the circumstances.

At first food is better withheld. (*See* PYLORIC, GLUCOSE, SALINE, HYDROLISED PROTEIN, etc.)

FOREIGN BODIES IN THE STOMACH may include: pieces of carpet, or other fabric, the rubber from a golf ball, the covers of tennis balls, bones, pieces of wood, etc. A depraved appetite may be due to hunger, a mineral or vitamin deficiency, rabies, or to bad habits – such as picking up and swallowing pebbles (often misguidedly thrown by the owner).

Signs. Ineffectual attempts to vomit, accompanied by painful retching, an arched back, salivation from the mouth, and signs of discomfort. Sharp-pointed bodies may cause perforation

of the stomach walls, peritonitis, and death. (*See* PERITONITIS.)

In small toy dogs it is quite usual for symptoms of acute nervous excitement to be shown.

With chronic gastritis due to swallowed pebbles, symptoms are those of occasional vomiting, discomfort, and even a rattling sound as the dog walks.

First-aid. An emetic (e.g. a crystal of washing soda and water).

Treatment. Apomorphine given by hypodermic injection, will rid the stomach of the greater part of fibrous or soft ingesta, but where sharp-pointed foreign bodies have been swallowed, obviously it is unsafe to give emetics. To remove these and large rounded objects which cannot be easily vomited, surgery will be necessary.

TORSION OF THE STOMACH. Except in the giant breeds of dogs, torsion or twisting of the stomach is rare. The abdomen becomes painful to the touch, swelling may be apparent, and vomiting likely to occur. The dog is soon in a very distressed condition, and needs emergency treatment or death will result.

PYLORIC STENOSIS and PYLOROSPASM (see under these separate heads for disease affecting the pylorus of the stomach).

STOMACH-TUBE is a rubber tube from 9 to 10 ft long for horses and cattle, and about ½ to ⅝ths of an inch in diameter. It is used for introducing into the stomach (either through the mouth or more often through the inferior meatus of the nostril on one side), with a view to relieving tympany, or introducing medicines in the treatment of disease. A larger-sized tube which possesses two channels is sometimes used to attempt to remove from the stomach portions of poisonous plants which may have been eaten. Water is pumped down through one channel, and when the stomach is full it runs from the other carrying with it small pieces of the harmful material. It is not possible to empty completely the stomach by the double stomach-tube, but considerable amounts of the harmful material may be removed.

The stomach-tube is extremely useful in those cases of colic which depend upon disturbances in the stomach, and if warm water is introduced by it in impaction of the large colon, peristalsis can often be stimulated. (*But see* DEHYDRATION.)

Its use demands care and a knowledge of the structure of the nasal passage, pharynx, gullet, and stomach.

STOMATITIS. Inflammation of the mouth. (*See* BOVINE PAPULAR STOMATITIS; FOOT-AND-MOUTH DISEASE; VESICULAR STOMATITIS; SWINE VESICULAR DISEASE; MOUTH, DISEASES OF, FELINE STOMATITIS.)

-STOMY is a suffix signifying formation of an opening in an organ by operation, *e.g.* gastro-stomy and colostomy.

STONES (*see* CALCULI *and* FOREIGN BODIES).

STORING FEEDS (for safe storage periods *see under* DIET).

STOT. A steer.

STRAIGHTS. Single, feeding-stuffs of animal or vegetable origin, which may or may not have undergone some form of processing before purchase; *e.g.* flaked maize, soya bean meal, fish meal, barley.

STRAIN. The over-stretching of muscle fibres, often a few of these are ruptured. A painful condition requiring rest. The same is true of over-stressed tendons. (Compare a SPRAIN which involves ligaments of a joint).

STRAMONIUM is the leaf of *Datura stramonium*, which is popularly known as the thorn apple or the Jamestown weed. It contains an alkaloid called *daturine*, which is almost identical in its actions with atropine.

The plant has caused fatal poisoning in pigs in Britain. However, 'Thornapple seems far less likely to cause poisoning in housed pigs than is generally believed. The fatalities which have been reported appear to be the result of ingestion of large quantities of the plant in a situation of alternative starvation'. (T. R. Worthington *et al.*, *Veterinary Record* (1981) **108**, 208).

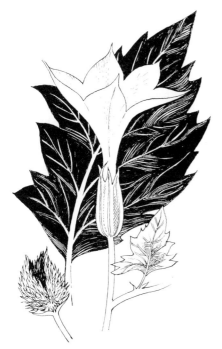

Thorn apple (*Datura stramonium*), which is also known as Jamestown, or 'Jimson' weed. The flower may be white or purple. On the left is a fruit capsule. Well developed plants may be 5 ft high.

STRANGLES is an acute contagious fever of horses, donkeys, and mules.
CAUSE. *Streptococcus equi.*

Strangles is commonest and most serious in horses under 6 years of age. Mature horses living in a stable where an outbreak has occurred are frequently unaffected.

SIGNS. *Typical attacks* being with dullness, lack of appetite, rise in temperature to between 103°F and 105°F, and congestion of the visible mucous membranes, especially of the nose and eyes. Nasal discharge is at first thin and watery, but soon becomes thicker, and profuse. There is often a cough. One or both of the submaxillary nodes, or perhaps one of the pharyngeal nodes, becomes enlarged, hot, tense, and painful to the touch; until a soft spot, usually over a most prominent part of the swelling can be detected. This indicates the 'pointing' of the abscess. Following its resolution the horse improves greatly; temperature falls, appetite returns, and the animal becomes much brighter.

Complications. Occasionally a suppurative pneumonia occurs. There may also be abscess formation in the liver or other abdominal organs.

TREATMENT. The owner should call in a veterinary surgeon. Immediate isolation of affected horses is necessary. (The box or stall where they stood must be disinfected as carefully and thoroughly as possible, and should be left vacant for 3 to 4 weeks afterwards.) The sick horse should be clothed and made comfortable. Soft foods, such as mashes, are indicated as swallowing may be painful. (*See* NURSING OF SICK ANIMALS.) Antibiotics and/or sulpha drugs are used.

PREVENTION. An efficient vaccine can be produced only if encapsulated *Streptococcus equi* is used (*i.e.* from very young cultures) and the capsule not destroyed by formalin and excessive heat. In older cultures, the capsule is lost and the organism no longer invasive.

HUMAN INFECTION by *Streptococcus equi* has been recorded.

STRANGULATION is an occasional cause of death in cattle in Africa, and has been reported from quarantine camps. A ligature is usually employed for the purpose. Unless human malice is suspected, deaths may be attributed to other causes.

Strangulated hernia. The term strangulation is also applied to a loop of intestine becoming trapped in a hernia, so that the blood supply to that section of it is cut off. (*See* HERNIA, 'GUT TIE', VOLVULUS, INTESTINES, DISEASES OF.)

STRANGURY. Difficulty and pain in passing more than a few drops of urine at a time. It is a sign of an inflammatory condition situated in the kidneys, bladder, or urethra.

STRAW. Reference to this will be found under BEDDING, DAIRY HERD MANAGEMENT, DEEP LITTER.

Straw feeding of cattle. The system originally was a strictly maintenance diet of 4 lb each of barley and a low protein-mineral-vitamin concentrate with some 10–12 lb barley straw.

Experimental work was carried out by Professor Lamming and his colleagues at Nottingham University on the use of pulverised straw. Using Feedmobile mobile milling and mixing plants, up to 30 per cent of ground straw has been conveniently incorporated into beef rations, along with 10–20 per cent molasses, 45 per cent cereals, and 5 per cent total minerals, vitamins and urea to provide a complete ration. Fed *ad lib* this is claimed to have consistently given daily live-weight gains in excess of 2·8 lb with Friesian steers in commercial trials.

Hitherto the main snag with ground straw had been its tendency to produce frothy bloat (with loss of appetite and loss of weight in subclinical cases). This has been overcome, it is claimed, by inclusion in feeds of an anti-bloat preparation (Poloxalene).

(*See also* MOULDY STRAW, NITRITE POISONING.)

'STRAWBERRY FOOT-ROT'. The colloquial name applied to a condition caused by the fungus *Dermatophilus pedis* or *D. congolensis*.

'STRAY VOLTAGE' (*see under* ELECTRIC SHOCK).

STREAMS. As a source of drinking water for cattle these should always be suspect, since they often carry infection from one farm to another, *e.g.* COCCIDIOSIS, JOHNE'S DISEASE, SALMONELLOSIS.

'STREET' VIRUS. This term refers to the naturally occurring rabies virus, such as may be isolated from a rabid dog, as opposed to 'fixed virus' which is passaged through a series of animals, increasing in virulence for that species and giving rise to a shorter incubation period.

STREPTOCOCCAL MENINGITIS (*see under* PORCINE).

STREPTOCOCCUS. A micro-organism which under the microscope has much the appearance of string beads. It is responsible for strangles, mastitis, acute abscess formation, etc. (*See* BACTERIA.)

STREPTODORNASE, STREPTOKINASE. Enzymes used to dissolve pus, fibrin, and blood-clot in infected wounds. They have also been used in the treatment of mastitis.

STREPTOMYCIN. An antibiotic obtained from *Streptomyces griseus*. Active almost entirely against Gram-negative organisms, streptomycin has given good results against infection with *C. pyogenes, Staph. pyogenes, C. renale, E. coli,* and *Past. septica.*

It has been used in cases of calf pneumonia and calf scours, some types of bovine mastitis, and complications of virus diseases in the dog, and in septic conditions in the cat. (In medical practice, streptomycin is regarded as one of the most toxic of the antibiotics in common use. It may cause deafness and vestibular disturance in dogs and cats.) Resistance to this antibiotic develops readily and is usually multiple. For these two reasons, other antibiotics are to be preferred.

STREPTOTHRICOSIS. Infection with streptothrix organisms.

In Britain, the name is applied to the disease in cattle equivalent to 'Lumpy Wool' or 'Wool Rot', caused by *Dermatophilus dermatonomus*. A scurfy, scaly condition of the skin is produced, and scabs come away with a bunch of hairs attached if plucked. The *Dermatophilus* parasite responsible for this condition is hardy in the sense that it can probably survive on a large scale in the vicinity of an infected animal. Anything which lowers the resistance of a hitherto healthy animal facilitates infection; and prolonged wetting, insect bites, thistle pricks, and other tiny breaks in the skin may all predispose to infection.

In the tropics, the name is applied to infection with *Dermatophilus congolensis.*

The onset of the rains brings an increase in the incidence and severity of the disease, which is of great economic importance in central and west Africa. Flies, ticks, and thorn bushes appear to play some part in the production and spread of the disease. Zebu cattle, as exotic cattle, appear highly susceptible; while N'dama and Muturu humpless cattle are resistant. It seems that infection does not give rise to later immunity.

Treatment with antibiotics or sulphonamides offers most chance of success, but is impracticable in many areas. Local applications of sulphur in groundnut oil are less effective. (*See* DERMATOPHILUS.)

STREPTOTHRIX (*see above*, and SENKOBO).

STRESS. In human medicine it is now recognised that mental stress, anxiety, and frustration can exert a profound effect for the worse upon bodily health, and that many people who are now ill would become well again if only they could, before too long, recapture peace of mind. The minds and thoughts and emotions of domestic animals are undoubtedly far dimmer and simpler than our own, but certainly not non-existent. Undoubtedly there is some equivalent of our peace of mind – call it a familiarity with surroundings, an absence of fear, or an absence of frustration.

Dr Joseph Edwards has referred to a farm in New Zealand where theoretical considerations were all against high milk yields, yet where the yields were, in fact extremely high. After a detailed investigation it was concluded that the reason could only be sympathetic handling at milking time by the owners – father, son, and daughter – who were strikingly 'in harmony' with their cattle.

By contrast, on another New Zealand farm where everything – staff, milking machines, and herd management – remained the same, the strangeness of a new milking shed was apparently the sole cause of a 15 per cent reduction in milk yield (*see also* CALF HOUSING.)

Stress is recognised as a predisposing cause of diseases in pigs, following the mixing of litters, castration, etc.; and in all species following parturition.

Subjection of animals to noise in intensive livestock production, or in the course of transport, can be a source of stress. Reduction of noise could have considerable economic benefits. (*See* Marschang, F., *Deutsche tierärztliche Wochenschrift* (1978) **85**, 28.) (*See* TRANSPORT STRESS.)

Sheep. Problems arise in paddock grazing. The grassland breeds, said Stephen Williams, 'need a greater space, if they are to remain happy, than those of the Down breeds. The open flocking types of sheep reveal indications of stress and unhappiness under compression. They are the hedge-breakers and fence-testers. They "work away" at weak places with a will to escape. The answer is clearly strong, reliable fences.

'There is much disappointment in the practice of intensive sheep management where a very large number of sheep are dealt with in one unit. It is especially desirable, in our experience, to break up the flock of grass sheep into units of 80 ewes during the intensive management period at grass. To have more grass ewes in a unit is to magnify the psychological problems.' Stress can result in a subclinical infection turning into overt illness. (*See also* BUNT ORDER, INTENSIVE LIVESTOCK PRODUCTION, INFECTION.)

Dogs. Stress may result from being left tied up for long periods, or alone in an otherwise empty house; sometimes from ill-treatment by one member of a family. Dog fights are another cause, or merely the presence of a large dog in the vicinity, known to be a fighter. Being lost or abandoned, placed in boarding kennels, change of ownership, etc. can all cause stress. Diarrhoea, sometimes vomiting, and 'compulsive' polydipsia may result.

Cats. The presence of a particularly aggressive tom (perhaps newly arrived in the district); the addition of another cat or dog to the household, or a mother paying less attention to the cat after the birth of a baby; or too many cats in the same house or confinement in a boarding cattery – these are all potential causes of stress.

During times of stress, a cat may develop a transient hyperglycaemia. This could lead to a mistaken diagnosis of diabetes.

STRICTURE. An abnormal narrowing of one of the natural passages of the body, such as the gullet, bowel, or urethra.

'STRIKE'. Blowfly myiasis, the condition resulting from infestation of the living skin of sheep by the larvae of blow-flies which, in certain circumstances, lay their eggs in the wool. The flies are, apparently, attracted by putrefactive odours, and strike accordingly most often occurs in the region of the hindquarters in sheep which have been scouring. Some cases of strike begin, however, in the clean wool covering the shoulders and loins; and other parts may be affected.

Where there is sufficient moisture the eggs hatch in about 12 hours and the resulting larvae attack the skin with their mouths and secretions, causing raw areas. The consequent moisture favours the larvae, and their excreta attracts further blowflies which give rise to further generations of larvae.

SIGNS. A characteristic twitching of the tail is seen when the hindquarters are affected. Tufts of white wool, discoloured wool, and the odour are indications of strike in other parts of the body. Death may occur within a week, and the mortality may be high among hill sheep especially, as the trouble may in them go undetected.

TREATMENT consists in the use of a dressing which will kill the larvae and facilitate healing of the wounds.

PREVENTION (*see* DIPS, INSECTICIDES).

STRING as a foreign body. It might reasonably be thought that string would be the least dangerous of foreign bodies, but such as not the case. Gravy-soaked string may inadvertently be included in a dog's or cat's meal of chicken scraps or leftovers from a joint of beef. Occasionally string will form a loop around the base of the tongue, but more often it will pass into the stomach, causing local inflammation and sometimes obstruction. In the intestine swallowed string is apt to lead to an accordion-pleated appearance of the bowel wall, which may perforate. One dachshund had no less than 15 such perforations, each of which had to be sutured during the course of a life-saving operation.

STRINGHALT is the sudden snatching up of one or both hind-legs of the horse when walking or, less often, when trotting.

All classes and ages of horses may be affected, although it is perhaps commonest in older horses. It often appears about the time when maturity is reached – *i.e.* 5 to 6 years or a little sooner.

CAUSES. The cause of stringhalt is unknown.

An Australian form of stringhalt is seasonal in incidence, and possibly associated with plant poisoning. Several horses in a locality may be affected. Recovery occurs after weeks or months, but not in all cases.

Neither pain nor lameness is associated with stringhalt, but the condition constitutes an unsoundness, and is incurable.

STRIP-CUP (*see* MASTITIS).

STRIP-GRAZING of cattle behind an electric fence tends to give greater production per acre, but it carries with it a risk of worm infestation under lush condition unless a back-fence is brought up at 5-day periods, and 'resting pastures' avoided. The use of an electric fence for strip-grazing on 'early-bite' is valuable. It induces the cattle to eat the whole plant instead of nibbling off the most succulent leaf-tips – which predisposes to Bloat. (*See* illustration on page 560.)

'STROKE' (*see* APOPLEXY).

STROMA. Tissue which supports a gland's secreting part but does not itself secrete.

STRONGYLES. These can cause anaemia, unthriftiness, debility, intermittent colic. (*See* FOALS, DISEASES OF; VERMINOUS ARTERITIS; *and under* ROUNDWORMS.)

STRONTIUM (*see under* RADIOACTIVE STRONTIUM).

STRUVITE (*see* FELINE UROLOGICAL SYNDROME).

STRYCHNINE is one of the two chief alkaloids of the seed of *Strychnos nux vomica*, an East Indian tree, the other being *brucine*, which is less

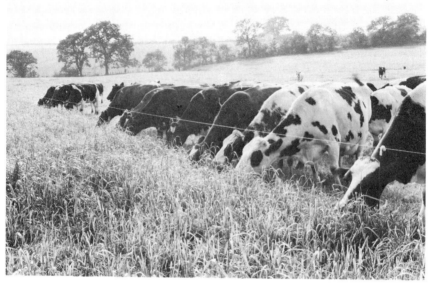

Controlled grazing, showing use of an electric fence. (*Farmers Weekly.*)

powerful and not used medicinally, although its actions are similar to those of strychnine. Strychnine itself is a white crystalline substance, possessing an intensely bitter taste. Strychnine (or nux vomica) was at one time much used as a tonic, especially during convalescence from debilitating illnesses, in pneumonia, and in atony of the bowels.

STRYCHNINE POISONING occurs mostly in the small animals, and particularly in the dog, which may be poisoned by relatively small doses. It may arise from overdosage (*see* EASTON'S), from malicious use of poisons for trespassing dogs, from indiscriminate use of rat-poisons containing the drug, and from its cumulative effects when used in small doses for a long period. This latter effect must always be kept in mind, for the drug is excreted very slowly from the system, and it may still be found in the urine as long as a week after administration has ceased.

SIGNS. In the larger animals the symptoms consist of convulsive seizures, characterised by a pronounced spasmodic contraction of the muscles of the limbs and trunk, and by a drawing back of the head and hollowing of the back (opisthotonus). In the horse, the eye-balls roll and the eye-lids are seen quivering and often becoming drawn back, exposing the white of the eye. In the smaller animals the same symptoms are seen, but the seizures are of a more violent nature, and the periods of relaxation are shorter.

FIRST-AID. If a large dose has been taken, an emetic should be given to the smaller animals at once, preferably apomorphine given hypodermically; the larger animals should have their stomachs emptied as far as possible by the use of the stomach-tube. Tannic acid or strong tea is indicated for immediate first-aid.

TREATMENT. Expert advice should be sought without loss of time. The patient should be anaesthetised.

'STUD TAIL'. An over-production of sebum by the modified sebaceous glands on the dorsal aspect of a cat's tail. The fur tends to become matted, and bare patches may occur. The precise cause is unknown, but it has been suggested that close confinement, and a consequent failure of the cat to groom itself, leads to 'stud tail'. Prolonged treatment may be necessary, on the line of that for acne.

STUNNING, ELECTRIC, OF CATTLE. This is practised in Sweden and the Netherlands by means of the Elther apparatus (prior to Jewish ritualistic slaughter or otherwise). It is used also for calves, sheep, and goats.

STUNNING, ELECTRIC, OF PIGS. This has been practised extensively since the 1930s, and involves the use of brine-soaked electrodes, applied on each side of the pig's face, by means of which the electric current is passed. A voltage of not less than 75 is recommended by Dr Phyllis G. Croft, and a current of not less than 250 millampères, assuming 50 cycles-per-second alternating current. An electroplectic fit is caused, with anaesthesia lasting for about 60 seconds, *when conditions are satisfactory*. After 60 seconds, there may be a half-minute period of paralysis during which sensation is present. Therefore, the pigs must be stuck *during the first 60 seconds.* If care is not taken and the apparatus be faulty or unsuitable, paralysis only, and not anaesthesia, may result; the pig being conscious when stuck.

High-voltage stunning. The tend towards the use of 180 to 600 volts has been impeded by the commonly held belief that it might adversely affect 'bleed out'. However, the A R C's Meat Research Institute has shown that this need not be so.

'STUNTING'. This syndrome in chickens was first recognised by Kouwenhoven and others in

1978, and has since been found to occur world-wide. (Kouwenhoven, B., Vertommen, M. & Van Eck, J. H. H., *Veterinary Science Communications* (1978) **2**, 253.)

The cause is believed to be a virus.

STURDY (*see* COENURIASIS).

STYE (*see* EYE).

STYFZIEKTE is a name meaning 'stiff sickness', which is used to describe either the symptoms associated with chronic aphosphorosis, which is the forerunner of lamziekte in South Africa, or those associated with a mineral deficiency in certain parts of Northern Nigeria.

SUB-CLINICAL. A disease is said to be sub-clinical when the symptoms are so slight as to escape the notice of the animal owner. Examples: sub-clinical mastitis, which by lowering the milk yield of a herd of cows may be of considerable economic importance; similarly, a sub-clinical infestation with parasitic worms. (*See* STRESS.)

SUBCUTANEOUS means anything pertaining to the loose connective tissue lying under the skin, such as a subcutaneous injection, where the injected fluid is introduced below the skin. (*See* HYPODERMIC INJECTIONS.)

SUBLUXATION A partial dislocation. Atlanto-axial subluxation is a cause of neck pain and muscle dysfunction in some toy breeds of dogs. TREATMENT: In 13 cases the atlas and axis were stabilised with a wire suture; in 10 cases lag screws were used for fixation of the ventral articular facets. Nine of them recovered within two months.

SUCKING or INTERSUCKING. This habit or 'vice' occurs among dairy calves. The M M B has commented: 'If allowed to go unchecked, the practice may become habitual, involving a risk to the health of the calves, and, if persisting into adulthood, the welfare of the herd in general may be affected.' A particularly severe case was encountered in a herd of 50 Friesian cows where the habit grew so pronounced that the herd became uneconomic and had to be dispersed. Cattle of all ages were involved and milk loss was considerable. Purchased calves acquired the same habits after a short while. Intersucking is a problem in only a small proportion of herds, usually those of above average size, where the calves are bucket fed, or where they are grouped at or shortly after birth.

The most effective remedy is to separate the calves after feeding, but if this is not practicable, mechanical devices or the provision of dry food are good alternatives. It seems that a useful preventive measure is to delay grouping calves until they are more than four weeks of age.

SUCKLING (*see* NURSE COWS, CALF REARING).

SUDDEN DEATH (*see under* DEATH).

SUDORIFICS are drugs and other agents which produce a copious flow of perspiration. (*See* DIAPHORETICS.)

SUFFOCATION (*see* ASPHYXIA and CHOKING).

SUGAR is a substance containing the elements carbon, hydrogen, and oxygen, and belonging therefore to the chemical group of carbohydrates. This group includes three main subdivisions as follows:

Monosaccharides, or glucoses
(1) monosaccharides, or glucoses
   ($C_6H_{12}O_6$):
   e.g. Dextrose or grape-sugar,
      Levulose.
(2) Disaccharides, or sucroses
   ($C_{12}H_{22}O_{11}$):
   e.g. Cane-sugar,
      Lactose or milk-sugar,
      Maltose or malt-sugar.
(3) Polysaccharides, or amyloses
   ($C_6H_{10}O_5$)n:
   e.g. Starch,
      Glycogen (animal starch),
      Dextrin and other gums.

Glucose is the form of sugar present in the blood, and reserves are stored in the liver in the form of glycogen.

Starch is mentioned under a separate heading, and its use as a food-stuff is described under DIET AND DIETING.

SULPHA DRUGS (*see* SULPHONAMIDES).

SULPHADIMIDINE (*see* 'Sulphamezathine' *under* SULPHONAMIDE DRUGS).

SULPHAQUINOXALINE. A yellow powder given to poultry, mixed in their food or in their drinking water, for the control of coccidiosis.

SULPHASALAZINE. (*See* 'DRY-EYE' *under* EYE, DISEASES OF (in dogs); *also* PROCTOCOLITIS.)

SULPHONAMIDE DRUGS are, to susceptible organisms (*e.g. streptococci*) bacteriostatic rather than bactericidal; that is to say, they prevent the multiplication of bacteria rather than killing them. Sulphonamide drugs are all synthetic and closely related to π-aminobenzoic acid, which is believed to be essential to bacteria, and which is absorbed by them; and it is believed that the sulphonamides are absorbed by the bacteria similarly, with the result mentioned above. Individual sulpha drugs do not have specific action against specific bacteria; their differences lie in the differing concentration or level which can safely be obtained in the animal's blood-stream, and their excretion route.

USES. Sulphonamide drugs are extensively employed in veterinary medicine for dressing wounds, for the prevention of post-operative sepsis, and in the treatment of pneumonia, metritis, enteritis, 'joint-ill', foul-in-the-foot of cattle, and arthritis in young pigs, etc. They must be used in full dosage, or resistant strains of bacteria may be set up.

TOXICITY. Sulphonamides may have an adverse effect upon the host's cells as well as upon the invading organisms. For this reason (and to avoid giving rise to resistant strains) sulphonamides should be used only under veterinary advice and not indiscriminately. Fortunately, however, domestic mammals, with the exception of the goat, show few signs of intolerance. Sulphanilamide is, however, highly toxic to birds.

NAMES OF INDIVIDUAL COMPOUNDS. The list of these is being continually extended, but mention may be made here of:

SULPHANILAMIDE. Of value as a dry dusting powder for wounds, teat sores, etc. It may be combined with 1 per cent neutral proflavine sulphate.

SULPHAPYRIDINE ('M. & B. 693'). Gained a great reputation in human medicine in the treatment of lobar pneumonia. Has been used in calf pneumonia. More toxic than several other sulphonamides.

SULPHATHIAZOLE. Has been used in the treatment of calf pneumonia.

SULPHADIAZINE. Has been used in the treatment of calf pneumonia, etc.

SULPHAMERAZINE. Has been used in the treatment of calf pneumonia, etc.

SULPHAGUANIDINE. Used in the treatment of White Scour of calves, necrotic enteritis in pigs, and enteritis in other animals. Readily taken in the food.

SULPHAQUINOXALINE. Used in the control and treatment of coccidiosis in chickens and turkeys.

'SULPHAMEZATHINE' (Sulphadimidine). Of value in 'Foul-in-the-foot' in cattle, pneumonia, enteritis. Is readily accepted in the food by all animals.

SULPHUR is a non-metallic element which is procurable in several different allotropic forms, *e.g.* 'flowers of sulphur'. As a parasiticide sulphur has been largely replaced by derris, etc., although proprietary *organic* preparations of sulphur are still used in the treatment of mange.

Internally, sulphur was at one time a popular laxative and mild tonic, and no doubt still enjoys a vogue among some animal-owners.

Poisoning. Overdosage must be avoided – 3 oz of flowers of sulphur has killed cattle. Dosing by guesswork on the part of a shepherd killed 140 ewes in a single flock.

Accidental poisoning occurred in 14 horses, two of which died.

SULPHUR DIOXIDE. A poisonous gas which is a constituent of Diesel engine exhaust fumes. (*See* SMOG.)

'SUMMER MASTITIS'. Recent studies have implicated both the Headfly and *Peptococcus indolicus* in the aetiology of this disease. (*See* MASTITIS, FLIES.)

'SUMMER SORES' in horses are caused by infective *Habronema* larvae deposited in wounds by stable- or house-flies. They are very itchy. Eyelids may be affected. The infestation results in the formation of fibrous nodules which may later ulcerate. Summer sores are uncommon in Britain.

SUNBURN. (*See* LIGHT SENSITISATION, *and cancer under* EYE, DISEASES OF.)

Small animals may be similarly affected; also fish in clear water with no shade available.

SUNLIGHT (*see under* RICKETS, INFERTILITY, LIGHT SENSITISATION, TROPICS).

SUNSTROKE (*see* HEATSTROKE).

SUPERFETATION. The presence in the uterus of fetuses of different ages, due to successive services.

For example, a cow is got in calf at one service, comes on heat again, and settles to a further service; in due course producing a calf as the result of the first mating, but more often than not having little or no milk. She later calves again, as the result of the second mating, and this time lactation begins. Calves born in this way are not, of course, twins. Although contemporaries within the dam, they are of different ages, and can have different sires!

An elderly cow which had always had single calves, was 'put to A I again and subsequently on three occasions at normal intervals, after which she appeared to hold'.

Presuming that she had held to the last service, her owners were very surprised to find her one morning two months before she was expected to calve, licking a full-term heifer calf which was 'quite obviously hers'. The milk yield was poor, and so the cow was left at grass to suckle her calf. Two months later she 'suddenly bagged up well and calved a live, full-term bull calf in circumstances that left no doubt it was hers also'.

Subsequent blood-tests, carried out in Copenhagen, showed that the first calf was not by the A I Centre's bull as stated. The second was.

The remarkable features of this example of 'double pregnancy' are that artificial insemination did not disturb a 2-month embryo; and the stress and exertion of calving did not affect a 7-month fetus, either.

SUPERINVOLUTION is the contraction of the uterus after parturition when the shrinkage proceeds beyond the normal, and the organ is less in size than before conception. It may proceed to such an extent that the dam is subsequently unable to breed, or it may result in a reduction in size of the organ which is not very important.

SUPEROVULATION. The production of extra (mammal's) eggs. It can be induced by means of hormones. (*See* TRANSPLANTATION OF OVA, TWINNING.)

SUPERPURGATION is excessive purgation which continues for some considerable time, and may end fatally. It is most serious in the horse, where it may follow the administration of aloes. It may also arise through the ingestion of foodstuffs which are unwholesome, such as sprouted potatoes, decomposed mouldy oats; and it may result from horses breaking out from a stable and getting into a field of clover or lucerne. (*See* PURGATIVES, LAXATIVES, COLIC.)

SUPPLEMENTARY FEEDING (*see* FLUSHING OF EWES, FEED BLOCKS, UREA, SUPPLEMENTS, CREEP FEED).

SUPPLEMENTARY VETERINARY REGISTER (*see under* VETERINARY SURGEONS ACT).

SUPPLEMENTS. Technical products for use at less than 5 per cent of the total ration, in which they are included, and designed to supply planned proportions of vitamins, trace minerals, one or more non-nutrient additives and other special ingredients.

SUPPOSITORY is a small conical mass made of glycerine, and containing drugs intended for introduction into the rectum.

SUPPURATION. For further information *see under* ABSCESS; CELLULITIS; FISTULA; INFLAMMATION; PHAGOCYTOSIS; WOUNDS.

SUPRARENAL BODIES (*see* ADRENAL GLANDS).

SUPRASCAPULAR PARALYSIS occurs as a result of injury to the suprascapular nerve. The term 'slipped shoulder' is applied to the symptoms which are shown in a typical case. The supraspinous and infraspinous muscles act as ligaments of the shoulder-joint, and when they are paralysed the shoulder slips outward each time the foot is placed upon the ground and when weight is put upon it. After the paralysis has been in existence for some few days two distinct hollows appear over the shoulder, due to atrophy of the muscles, and the spine of the scapula stands out prominently between these hollows. When viewed from in front the animal appears to have lost the symmetry of the two shoulder regions. In typical cases there is difficulty in bringing the limb forward, and often the leg appears to swing outwards with a circular movement. When a horse stands quietly, the affected limb is usually brought well under the body, and may even take up a position across the middle line of the body. The paralysis may disappear in 6 weeks; but in more severe cases, 18 months may elapse before the horse is fit for work. First-aid: fomentations, soap liniment may be helpful until the acute symptoms subside; thereafter a run at grass generally results in improvement.

In the dog there may be permanent paralysis, sometimes requiring amputation of the leg or other surgery.

SURAMIN. A drug used against trypanosomes.

SURFACTANTS. Surface active agents used in America and elsewhere to increase growth rate of poultry. They are less effective than antibiotics. The fluid lining the alveoli of the lungs is an example of a natural, physiological surfactant.

SURGICAL SPIRIT. This commonly contains half a fluid ounce of castor oil per pint of industrial methylated spirit, together with a little methyl salicylate and brucine.

SURRA is a disease of most economic importance in camels and horses, but it can affect all the domestic animals. The disease occurs in Africa (north of the tsetse fly belt), Asia, Central and South America. In the latter, *T. equinum* is responsible; elsewhere it is caused by *T. evansi.*

The infection is spread by blood-sucking flies, such as Tabanids and stable flies. Vampire bats are believed to transmit the infection also. Animals which eat the meat from carcases infected with trypanosomes may themselves become infected in the case of surra.

In the Sudan surra affects mainly camels, which die within weeks or a few months, after showing symptoms of fever, anaemia, progressive emaciation, oedema, and paralysis. In Asia, surra in camels is often a chronic disease which may persist for years.

In horses, symptoms are similar, but the dropsical swellings (oedema) are especially noteworthy, affecting several parts of the body (as they do also in the dog). Mortality is high, and occurs in horses after a matter of weeks or months. Loss of power in the hind limbs, and exaggerated heart sounds may precede death.

In Central America the names 'murrina' and 'derrengadera' have been used for vampire-bat and fly-transmitted infection with *T. equinum.*
TREATMENT involves use of drugs such as 'Antrycide' and 'Suramin' which have specific action on trypanosomes. Fly control is also important in reducing the incidence of the disease.

SUSPECTED ADVERSE REACTION SURVEILLANCE SCHEME (SARSS). During 1990, a total of 317 field reports of suspected adverse reactions to veterinary medicines were received; 277 were from veterinary surgeons and 40 from companies. In 29 cases (9 per cent) the product was used outside the licence indications and there were 17 reports (5 per cent) involving the use of unlicensed products or human medicines. To aid assessment, an additional 321 product reports were requested from companies during the year. (Alastair Gray B.Vet. Med., MRCVS, Medicines Unit, Central Veterinary Laboratory, Weybridge. *Veterinary Record* July 27th 1991.)

SUTURE is the name given either to the close union between two adjacent flat bones of the skull at their edges, or to a series of stitches by which a wound is closed. (*See* WOUNDS.)

SWABS. Swabs are used for sampling mucus, etc., for diagnostic purposes; the material subsequently being cultured so that pathogenic organisms, if present, may be identified. For swabbing as a guide to infertility in the thoroughbred mare *see under* EQUINE GENITAL INFECTIONS.

SWALLOWING. As soon as food ready for swallowing enters the pharynx it touches areas of mucous membrane supplied with nerves which automatically inhibit breathing, in order to prevent food 'going the wrong way'; close the larynx, which is pulled forwards and upwards, while the base of the tongue folds the epiglottis over the opening of the larynx. The pharynx is shortened and its muscles force the food into the oesophagus, where peristalsis takes the food to the stomach.

Swallowing is one-third voluntary and two-thirds reflex. The voluntary part is placing the food on the upper surface of the tongue which is raised, tip first, against the hard palate towards the rear. At the same time the soft palate is raised, closing the gateway to the nose. The base of the tongue forces food into the pharynx. The next two stages of swallowing are involuntary, reflex actions. (For difficulty in swallowing, *see* DYSPHAGIA.)

'SWAMP CANCER'. A condition affecting horses in Australia. The lesion is, in fact, a fungal granuloma caused by *Hyphomyces destruens*.

SWAMP FEVER (*see* EQUINE INFECTIOUS ANAEMIA).

SWAYBACK is a disease of new-born and young lambs, characterised by progressive cerebral demyelination, which results in paralysis and often death. It occurs in many parts of the United Kingdom. Knowledge as to its cause is still incomplete, but prevention can be effected by the provision of mineral licks containing 1 per cent of copper.

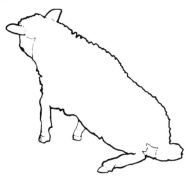

Swayback – a characteristic posture.

SIGNS. A staggering gait or inability to walk. Severely affected cases all die. New-born lambs cannot rise and suckle.
TREATMENT. None.
PREVENTION. Allow the pregnant ewes access to copper licks or injections of a suitable copper poisoning.

SWEAT or PERSPIRATION. There are parts of the horse's skin which sweat more readily than others, *e.g.* the bases of the ears, under the forearm, and around the dock, and generally speaking, fore parts of the trunk sweat more quickly than do the hinder parts. Mules and donkeys do not sweat readily, and when they do it is generally confined to the bases of the ears. In cattle, sweating occurs chiefly at the neck and over the chest. In Brahman cattle the hump is an important sweating site. Panting (and loss of water vapour from the lungs) is the chief means of heat loss in sheep, but they do sweat. The dog, cat, and pig are, for all practical purposes non-

sweating animals, though sweating may occur from the pads of the feet of dogs and cats; dogs rely mainly on panting. (*See also* ANHIDROSIS, HYPERTHERMIA, HYPOTHALAMUS, TROPICS.)

SWEAT GLANDS (*see* SKIN). Like all other tissue, the sweat glands can become the site of cancer. For example, ten cases were diagnosed in cats at the New York State College of Veterinary Medicine during 1985–1987. Head, neck, pinna of the ear and base of the tail were affected in cats aged 6 to 17 years.

'SWEATING SICKNESS'. This is a tick-borne disease of cattle in Southern Africa, affecting mainly calves. (Sheep can also become naturally infected.)
SIGNS. Fever, eczema. (*See also* TICKS.)

SWEDISH RED AND WHITE CATTLE. This is the main breed of Sweden. The herdbook dates from 1928, when the Swedish Ayrshire and the Swedish Red-white breeds – similar in origin and characteristics – were amalgamated. Each was the result of breeding from old Swedish stock to which had been introduced some Dairy Shorthorn and Ayrshire blood.

It is a long-lived breed, with an overall milk yield average in excess of 950 gallons at 4·1 per cent butter fat. The dams of all bulls sold at the 1958 Breed Society sales had averaged in all their recorded years (5·8 per cow) over 1196 gallons.

There is very little white in the coat-colour; and some animals are entirely red.

'SWEET ITCH'. A seasonal inflammation of the skin of horses, caused by hypersensitivity to the bites of Culicoides midges.

Fly repellents are effective for such short periods as to be worthless for control, probably best achieved by stabling at around 6 p.m. (a Vapona strip being hung in the stable to kill any midges entering). Treatment is by means of a calamine and antihistamine cream. (P. S. Mellor and J. McCaig. *Vet. Rec.* (1974) **95**, 411.)

'Sweet-itch often affects obese ponies at grass which are suffering from subclinical laminitis. I have seen cases of pedal bone prolapse in all four feet within 48 hours of corticosteroid administration to such animals. Eighty-two per cent of the acute laminitis cases with severe pedal bone rotation or prolapse cases referred to this centre during the last 14 months had received corticosteroids.

'The risk of steroid induced or potentiated laminitis is real and in my opinion this class of drugs should not be used to treat sweet-itch or laminitis.' (R. A. Eustace, Department of Veterinary Clinical Science, University of Liverpool.)

SWEET VERNAL GRASS (*Anthoxanthum odoratum*). Hay containing this has caused poisoning owing to its DICOUMAROL content (*see* HAEMORRHAGIC SYNDROME IN CATTLE). The dicoumarol content of the grass varies, but may increase in hay which has become overheated or mouldy.

SWILL. The feeding of unboiled swill – a practice which is illegal – is a frequent source of swine fever, swine vesicular disease, and foot-and-mouth disease infections. (*See also* BAKERY WASTE.) Scouring and deaths occurred among swill-fed pigs on premises where it was the practice to use daily only 500 gallons out of a total of 2000 gallons of steam-sterilised swill, the remainder being stored. There was no further trouble after the tank was emptied and the swill fed as soon as possible after processing.

'SWIMMERS'. The colloquial name for puppies showing the juvenile femoral rotation syndrome. They are unable to rise on to their hind legs at the usual age, due to the head and neck of the femur being wrongly positioned on the shaft. Sometimes the name 'Flat Pup' Syndrome is applied.

SWINE DYSENTERY. An important disease, characterised by haemorrhagic enteritis, and dependent for its cause upon synergism between the spirochaete *Treponema hyodysenteriae* and *Bacteroides vulgatus* and 'other, as yet unknown' bacteria. This was stated by the I R A D, Compton, in 1978; research there having confirmed that Treponema will cause swine dysentery in 80 per cent of ordinary pigs but will not do so in gnotobiotic pigs.

About 1 in 3 pigs in a herd become ill, and the mortality rate is 10 to 60 per cent. Chronic scouring, without dysentery, may persist. The faeces are greyish. Treatment with arsenicals is effective; but the treatment of choice is dimetridazole.

Swine dysentery and chickens. Retarded growth rate and delayed onset of egg production in pullets have, as one of the causes, infection with *Treponema hyodysenteriae*. Pullets reared on deep litter with 'indirect contact with pigs' became infected.

SWINE ERYSIPELAS is an infectious disease of pigs and characterised by high fever, reddish or purplish spots on the skin, and haemorrhages on to the surfaces of certain of the internal organs in acute cases; and by general debility, lameness, and difficulty in breathing in chronic cases. In these latter there are usually found characteristic cauliflower-like masses on the valves of the heart.

The disease may occur in man; also in chickens, turkeys, ducks, pheasants and grouse. According to American research, dogs are susceptible to one strain of the organism, which gives rise to bacterial endocarditis.

INCIDENCE. In Europe it is usually prevalent both in the acute form and in the chronic, and at times it assumes the nature of an epizootic, sweeping throughout large territories, and leaving a high percentage of death in its wake. In Britain the chronic form is usually met with in small outbreaks in different parts of the country, but from time to time in certain areas, especially in East Anglia, and during hot dry summer weather, it breaks out in a more menacing form, and large numbers of pigs become affected with the acute form, and considerable numbers die.
CAUSE. *Erysipelothrix rhusiopathiae*, which

may also infect sheep at shearing or dipping time through small wounds or abrasions.
SIGNS. There are three recognised forms of swine erysipelas: the subacute, the acute, and the chronic.

Mild or *subacute* attacks come on suddenly; there is high fever, loss of appetite, dullness, a tendency to lie buried in the litter, and when moved to do so reluctantly, and the skin over the chest, neck, back, and over the thighs, becomes flushed at first, and soon changes to a red or purple colour. The outlines of the areas affected are often square, or they may be the shape of the playing-card diamond, from which the diseases gets one of its names – 'diamond disease'. The areas are usually raised above the level of the surrounding skin, are painful to the touch at first, but not so later, and, appearing about the second or third day of the attack, last for 4 days, and then disappear. Recovery may be followed by the chronic form. In some cases, pigs may show painful swellings of the knees and hocks, but this is not invariable. Young pigs between 3 and 5 or 6 months old are most commonly attacked; it is rare before 3 months, but may occur in older animals.

Acute type, or *Septicaemic type*, often results in sudden death.

Chronic type, is the most insidious, and pigs affected with it are probably responsible for causing most of the outbreaks of the previous types, since, being bad thrivers, they are often disposed of through the open market and bought by owners of clean herds. They feed, but do not always finish their food; they have a normal temperature, but are easily distressed when made to take exercise. Breathing becomes shallow, and a cough generally develops. The pulse becomes thready, and if the heart be listened to, a flowing murmur can be heard over the left side of the chest. This is due to the vegetative (or verrucose) endocarditis, which is almost *the* characteristic feature of post-mortem examination of pigs dead from chronic swine erysipelas. The chronic form may last for several weeks, or even for 2 or 3 months, especially in strong robust young breeding gilts, but towards the end emaciation and prostration become very obvious.

Infertility, involving abortion, stillbirths, and mummified fetuses, commonly results from erysipelas.
TREATMENT consists in the administration of antiserum as soon as possible. Penicillin is also very effective.
PREVENTION consists in avoiding any pigs in the open market which appear to be thin and not thriving, especially sows and boars, or older pigs. Any showing wrinkling of the skin of the ears, or patches or flushing on the skin, those which have swollen joints, or those which have diarrhoea, should not be bought. Pigs showing extreme breathlessness upon mild exertion should be likewise avoided. Protective inoculation gives good results but is somewhat costly. This confers a strong degree of immunity, which, if not life-long, is at least long enough to protect fattening pigs. It is of most use in a district where there are enzootic outbreaks of the mild or acute types.

Arthritis and heart disease may be a result of

pigs becoming hypersensitised to the bacteria, and not the result of attack by the bacteria themselves. This must be borne in mind when prescribing the vaccine.

Public health. Stockmen exposed to infection must be careful to wash their hands.

SWINE FEVER, hog cholera, pig typhoid, is a highly infectious and contagious disease of pigs.

Cause. The cause of swine fever is a Pestivirus (a member of the Togavirus family). Secondary bacterial invaders include: *Salmonella suipestifer*, or *B. cholera suis*; *Pasteurella suiseptica*. None of these secondary organisms is, however, necessary for the production of swine fever.

It inevitably happens that pigs harbouring the virus of swine fever, but not yet showing symptoms of the disease, are slaughtered for human food. Under such circumstances, the virus can survive in the skin and muscle for 17 days. In frozen pork the survival time has been quoted as over four years; in bacon 27 days. No wonder that unboiled swill is responsible for so many outbreaks.

At public markets, the urine of infected pigs so often drains into adjoining pens and alleyways. The urine may, too, get splashed on to men's clothing, boots, etc., and droplets of it find their way into lorries and on to farms. In 1953 about 30 outbreaks, spread over 10 counties, arose from the sale of a single infected pen at a large market.

It seems probable that the virus may be carried by rats and mice for short distances at least. Horse-flies can carry the virus, which – according to an American report – can be harboured by larvae of the pig lungworm. These larvae are, in turn, harboured by earthworms.

The use of antibiotics contained in feeding-stuffs has had the effect of masking the classical symptoms of swine fever, and is sometimes said to have extended the incubation period.

Signs. In young pigs the disease is often acute or peracute, while in older pigs it tends to assume a chronic form, although they also may be affected with the severe rapidly fatal form.

ACUTE TYPE. After an incubation period of 5 to 10 days, signs of the disease include thirst, sometimes vomiting, shivering, loss of appetite. There is a tendency to lie with backs arched and tails uncurled. If forced to move, they are seen to be unsteady on their legs. If their temperature is taken, it is found to be high. Initial constipation is usually followed by diarrhoea, with a foul odour. There is often a discharge from the eyelids. The skin becomes reddened or purplish. Some pigs may cough or show laboured breathing. Convulsions may precede death. The mortality rate can be as high as 90 per cent or so.

Pneumonia is a common *post-mortem* finding and 'button ulcers' may be present in the intestines.

CHRONIC TYPE. The pigs are dull and unthrifty, lose weight, have a variable appetite; coughing and/or diarrhoea may be other signs. The temperature may be only slightly raised or as high as 106°F. A partial recovery may be followed by relapse and death.

SUBCLINICAL. Swine fever may exist in a herd in a subclinical form; pregnant sows showing no obvious signs (though fever may be present), and the disease remaining unsuspected until the finding of a few dead piglets, or of others showing muscular tremors.

Death of the fetus may occur (*see* MUMMIFICATION) or weak or deformed piglets may be born. If infected late in pregnancy, piglets may die without signs of swine fever. Meanwhile, being viraemic, they may have infected others.

Infection of a pregnant sow can be followed by the presence of virus in her piglets, either stillborn or living. The sow is not a 'carrier' in the usually accepted sense, since after the birth of her piglets the virus – having crossed the placental barrier – no longer remains within her body. A period of 56 days may elapse between the last deaths on a farm and a recrudescence of the disease.

Diagnosis. The fluorescent antibody test.

Treatment. The best results are derived from hyperimmune serum. Sulpha drugs and antibiotics are not effective against the virus but combat the secondary invaders.

Prevention. Ensure that swill is boiled, for pieces of infected pig meat may otherwise give rise to an outbreak of the disease. Pigs introduced into a herd should be from premises shown to be free from the disease. Visits by pig-dealers should be discouraged.

Control. In Britain swine fever is NOTIFIABLE (which see).

A swine fever eradication programme, with compulsory slaughter, and compensation, was introduced in Britain in 1963. The disease was eradicated in 1966, but re-appeared briefly in Yorkshire in 1971; and a single outbreak occurred in 1986.

SWINE FEVER, AFRICAN. This disease, formerly restricted to the African continent, appeared in Spain and Portugal during 1960. Including animals compulsorily slaughtered, Spain lost 120,000 pigs and Portugal 16,000.

During 1978 there were outbreaks in both Sardinia and Malta, and – with the aeroplane (and passengers' food) as its main vector – the risk of introduction of the disease into Britain is a serious one. In 1985 there were five outbreaks in Belgium.

The disease is also known as Wart-Hog disease, as these animals besides bush-pigs are affected. In some parts of Africa, pig-raising has had to be abandoned on account of the disease, which is highly contagious, nearly always fatal, and gives rise to 'carriers' – those few that survive often transmitting the infection to other pigs for a year or more.

CAUSE. A pestivirus, resistant to heat, drying, and putrefaction, and which can survive in smoked or partly cooked sausage and other pork products. The virus attacks blood-vessel cells and the disease is accordingly characterised by haemorrhages.

SIGNS. After an incubation period of 5 to 15 days, there is fever; the pig running a temperature of 105° or so. There may be no other symptoms for about 5 days. Then the fever subsides, and there are more obvious signs of illness – followed by death within a day or two. Clinically, the disease is indistinguishable from acute classical swine fever.

CONTROL. Live vaccine has been used in Portugal and Spain, but has given rise to 'carriers'.

At the beginning of 1978 there were approximately 80,000 pigs in the islands of Malta and Gozo, supplying the inhabitants with all their requirements of fresh pork and bacon. By the end of January 1979 there were no pigs at all.

It was the first time that any country had slaughtered all the surviving members of a species in order to eliminate a disease – in this instance African Swine Fever. The decision to slaughter all survivors was taken when the pig population had fallen to 13,975. The cost of the outbreak was estimated at £5 million. Swill feeding and the movement of weaners to fattening premises helped to spread the disease. (P. J. Wilkinson *et al.*, *Vet. Record* (1980) **106,** 94.) (*See map.*)

SWINE INFLUENZA. An H1N1 virus was causing the disease in Europe in 1986, and was isolated from an outbreak involving a 400-sow unit in the UK. Morbidity was nearly 100 per cent, but all recovered. H3N2 virus is also present in the UK. (Dr D. H. Roberts & others. *Veterinary Record* (1987) **121,** 53.)

In many outbreaks, several deaths are to be expected. (*See also under* INFLUENZA.) (*See also* ENZOOTIC PNEUMONIA.)

CAUSE. An orthomyxovirus; important secondary invaders include: *Haemophilus influenzae suis, Pasteurella suiseptica, Brucella bronchiseptica,* and *streptococci.*

SIGNS. Coughing, fever, anorexia, laboured breathing. (*See also under* INFLUENZA.)

SWINE PLAGUE is the term applied to what in Britain is considered to be the pneumonic form of swine fever, but what in America and the continent of Europe has been regarded as a separate disease. (*See* SWINE FEVER.)

SWINE POX (*see* POX).

SWINE VESICULAR DISEASE first appeared in the UK in 1972. In the Staffordshire outbreak of that year it was at first mistaken for foot-and-mouth disease, from which it cannot be differentiated on clinical grounds alone. However, within 3½ days of receipt of material from the lesions, it was shown at the Animal Virus Research Institute, Pirbright, that the virus was not that of foot-and-mouth disease but related to an enterovirus which had caused outbreaks in Italy and Hong Kong.

All cases in the UK had (up to late 1973) been linked either to swill feeding of pigs or to the movement of pigs from infected to clean

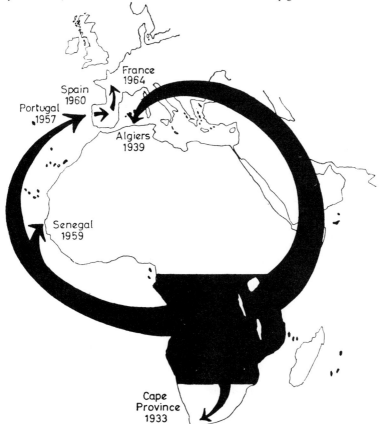

The spread of African swine fever.

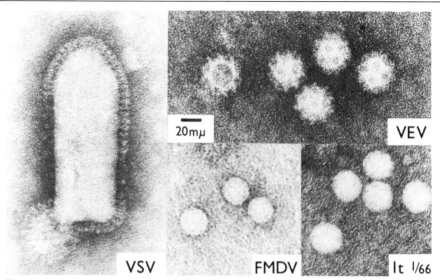

The virus causing swine vesicular disease is shown bottom right, labelled It 1/66. Extreme left is the bullet-shaped virus of Vesicular Stomatitis (VSV), and top right is the virus of Vesicular Exanthema (VEV). Centre bottom picture shows foot-and-mouth disease virus. All these viruses affect pigs and have to be differentiated. (The scale shows 20mu = 0·00002 mm. Photographs by electron microscope, with acknowledgements to Mr C. J. Smale and the Animal Virus Research Institute, Pirbright.)

premises. The disease appears to be spread rapidly through contact, with an incubation period of perhaps 4–8 days. Airborne infection appears less likely than with foot-and-mouth disease.

A similar disease has been reported in Austria among pigs imported from Poland, and also in France.

SVD virus is very closely related to Coxsackie B5 virus, which causes not only influenza-like symptoms in man but also sometimes heart disease and meningitis. It is thought possible that SVD arose as a result of pigs becoming infected by people ill because of Coxsackie B5 virus, which locally then became adapted to pigs or underwent mutation.

SVD has been transmitted to laboratory workers; so precautions must be taken.

CONTROL. Experience has shown that the incidence of the disease has been quickly reduced by the imposition of Controlled Area measures, and this fact led to the Movement and Sale of Pigs Order, 1975, designed to slow down the movement of pigs so that infection can show up and be dealt with before it spreads further.

Licences, issued by local authorities, are required for all movement of pigs except for those going direct to slaughterhouse or to a slaughter market from premises where no waste food is used. Swill-fed pigs can move only to a slaughterhouse. All pigs consigned to a slaughter market or to a slaughterhouse must be marked with a red cross of specified dimensions.

SVD reappeared in the UK in 1979 and persisted during 1980–81. Sixty outbreaks occurred during 1980. In 1982–83 there were none. The infection can be subclinical.

MODE OF INFECTION. Although the SVD virus belongs to the enterovirus group, it has been difficult to obtain evidence for infection by mouth. Many experiments, in which precautions were taken to prevent entry of virus by other routes, have failed to produce the disease. In contrast, infection by rubbing or scarification of the skin regularly produces infection, and it seems that the most likely route of infection in the field is through damaged skin.

SWINGE COAT. An abnormality in which the hair is short, sparse and curly.

SWOLLEN HEAD SYNDROME in chickens.
CAUSE: The TURKEY RHINOTRACHEITIS VIRUS (of the genus Pneumovirus.)
SIGNS: Opisthotonus. If picked up the birds became incoordinated, rolled over, and had difficulty in regaining a normal posture; swelling around the eyes and on top of the head; diarrhoea. (Pattison, M. & others. *Veterinary Record* (1989) **125**, 229.)

SYMBIOSIS means an obligatory association between two different species for their mutual benefit.

SYMPATHETIC NERVOUS SYSTEM (*see* CENTRAL NERVOUS SYSTEM, AUTONOMIC NERVOUS SYSTEM).

SYMPHYSIS. A joint, in which bones are united by a flattened disc of fibro-cartilage.

SYN- is a prefix signifying union.

SYNAPSE (*See* NERVES.)

SYNCHRONISATION OF OESTRUS (*see* 'CONTROLLED BREEDING').

SYNCOPE (fainting) is generally due to cerebral anaemia occurring through weakened pulsation of the heart, sudden shock, or severe injury.

It is common in dogs and cats, especially when old; but cases have been seen in all animals.

'SYNCRO-MATE' (*see* PROGESTAGENS).

SYNCYTIAL VIRUSES (*see* RESPIRATORY SYNCYTIAL VIRUS).

SYNCYTIUM. Tissue composed of a mass of nucleated protoplasm without cell boundaries, such as the outer layer of the trophoblast of a placenta; or a mass of cells united by protoplasmic bridges.

SYNDROME. A group of symptoms.

SYNECHIA (*see* IRITIS *under* EYE, DISEASES OF).

SYNERGISM is the opposite of antagonism. Synergism between drugs, *e.g.* penicillin and sulphathiazole, may be of practical value, for with the two it may be possible to obtain the required effect with a dosage of one which, if used alone, would be insufficient, but which cannot be increased because larger amounts would cause side-effects. Another advantage of using two drugs is the possibility that this would tend to prevent the multiplication of mutants resistant to one of the compounds.

The word 'synergism' is also used to describe an interaction between a virus and bacteria in their combined invasion of, for example, the lungs; implying that the result of the 'combined forces', as it were, is greater than the sum of the effects produced by the agents individually. Synergism occurs in calf pneumonia between *Mycoplasma bovis* and *Pasteurella bovis*. (For another example, *see* SWINE DYSENTERY.)

SYNOSTOSIS is the term applied to a union by bony material of adjacent bones usually separate. It may occur in the spinal column in old animals. (*See also* HORSES, BACK TROUBLES IN.)

SYNOTIA. The (virtual) absence of head in a stillborn animal.

SYNOVIAL MEMBRANE forms the lining covering the surfaces of the opposed articular cartilages, which enter into the formation of a joint. (*See* JOINTS.)

SYNOVITIS. Inflammation of the membrane lining a joint. It is usually accompanied by effusion of fluid within the synovial sac of the joint. It is found in various injuries and inflammation of joints.

SYNOVITIS, INFECTIOUS. This is a disease of chicks, of about 2 to 10 weeks old, and of turkeys; first diagnosed in Britain in 1959.
CAUSE: *Mycoplasma synoviae*.
SIGNS: Reluctance to move, lameness, swelling of joints, anorexia.

The confined conditions under which broilers are raised appear to render them particularly susceptible to this disease. Mortality is low, but a third of the survivors may be down-graded, so that severe financial loss may be caused. Control depends upon hygiene, and being careful about the breeding stock.

SYRINGE (*see* INJECTIONS, *and* DETERGENT RESIDUE; *also* PROJECTILE SYRINGES).

SYSTOLE means the contraction of the heart as opposed to the resting phase, which is called 'diastole', and which alternates with the former contracting period. In the cardiac cycle systole takes about one-third, and diatole about two-thirds, of the whole period of the heart-beat. (*See* HEART.)

T

T. CELLS. These are lymphocytes from the thymus gland concerned with cell-mediated immunity. (*See* IMMUNE RESPONSE, *and* LYMPHOCYTES.)

T$_2$ TOXIN. This may poison cattle or poultry eating stored corn containing the fungus *Fusarium tricinctum*. In cattle, the toxin may cause multiple haemorrhages and sometimes death; in poultry, there may be mouth lesions.

TACHYCARDIA is a disturbance of the heart's action which produces great acceleration of the pulse.

TACHYPNOEA. An increase in the rate of breathing due to some pathological condition. (*See* BREATHLESSNESS *and* PARAQUAT POISONING.)

TAENIA (*see* TAPEWORMS).

TAIL, AMPUTATION OF (*see under* DOCKING, WELFARE CODES).

TAIL-BITING. In pigs this 'vice' can be of great economic importance.

Tail sores in pigs. These may follow tail-biting by one or two pigs out of a large batch, and if untreated can lead to pyaemia.

In 6 months, out of 135 pig carcases condemned in an Oslo abattoir, 56 were affected with pyaemia – and of these 43 had tail-sores.

Feeding only concentrates is regarded as a contributory factor in tail-biting. Boredom, absence of bedding, and floor space of less than 5 square feet per pig, are also regarded as conducive to tail-biting. High temperature and humidity are possible causes. Bitten tails require amputation or dressing if pyaemia is to be prevented.

TALFAN DISEASE. This is a disease of pigs, and its cause is a virus. Experimentally, the incubation period is stated to be 12 days. Piglets 3 weeks old and upwards are affected. The disease has also been seen in pigs aged 8 months, but this is rare. By no means all piglets in a litter or on a farm become ill and the mortality is usually low. The main symptom is weakness or paralysis of the hindlegs. There is little or no fever or loss of appetite. Recovery occurs in a proportion of animals which are hand fed. The disease is present in Britain to a small extent, and apparently may be associated with abortion. (*See also under* PORCINE ENCEPHALOMYELITIS.)

TAMPAN. A soft TICK of the family Argasidae. (*See* TICKS.)

TAMPONADE, CARDIAC. A rapid accumulation of blood or other fluid in the pericardial sac, compressing the heart and sometimes suddenly arresting its function.

TANNIN, or TANNIC ACID, is a non-crystallisable white or pale-yellowish powder, which is very soluble in water and glycerine. It is prepared from oak-galls. Tannin is also found in strong tea or coffee. When brought into contact with a mucous surface, tannin causes constriction of the blood-vessels. When brought into contact with many poisonous alkaloids it renders them temporarily inert by forming the insoluble tannate, and so is a valuable antidote.
USES. Tannic acid has been used in diarrhoea and dysentery in young animals, more often as catechu or kino, two vegetable drugs which contain a large amount of tannin. It is often administered as the first step in the antidotal treatment of poisoning by ALKALOIDS.

Tannic acid jelly is a valuable burn dressing, and tubes of this should be included in every first-aid kit. It lessens the absorption of breakdown products from the burned area and hence diminishes the secondary effects of a serious burn. It is not suitable for large areas owing to the danger of liver damage if large quantities are absorbed.

TAPEWORMS. Their life-cycle requires two hosts, sometimes three. The presence of the adult worm may give rise to few if any symptoms or, on the other hand, to anaemia, indigestion, and nervous symptoms – or even to blockage of the intestine. The cystic stage of tapeworms may involve the brain. Tapeworms are of considerable public health importance.

A typical tapeworm has a head or *scolex*, provided with suckers and, in some species, with hooks also.

Behind the *scolex* follows a neck, and behind that are the segments; each being called a *proglottis*. The segments nearest to the head are the smallest, and are immature. Next follow mature segments, and lastly the gravid, segments containing eggs. These older segments fall off and are passed out of the host's body in the faeces.
TAENIA. This is the common genus of worms found in dogs and cats, and include:
T. pisiformis (*T. serrata*) is one of the commonest. Its cystic stage, *Cysticercus pisiformis*, is found in rabbits and hares.
T. hydatigena (*T. marginata*) is the largest form, with mature segments wider than long. It may reach a length of over 16 feet. Its cystic stage, *Cysticercus tenuicollis*, occurs in the viscera of various animals, especially sheep, cattle and pigs.
T. ovis is frequently mistaken for the last form, from which it can be distinguished only by microscopical examination. Its cysticercus, *C. ovis*, is found in the muscles and organs of sheep and goats. It is a small form, easily overlooked.
T. multiceps (*T. coernurus*) is a more delicate form than the others, semi-translucent. The intermediate stage is a coenurus, found in the nervous system of sheep and other ruminants and man.
T. serialis is a more robust form, its coenurus

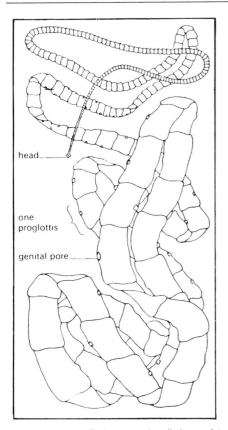

A typical tapeworm. Each segment is called a proglottis. (From H. T. B. Hall's *Diseases and Parasites of Livestock in the Tropics*, Longman.)

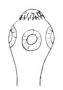

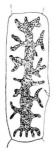

Taenia. Head, mature and gravid segments.

being found in rabbits and hares. Only one species is common in the cat, *T. Taeniaeformis* (*T. crassicollis*). The cystic stage, *Cysticercus fasciolaris*, is found in the liver of rats and mice.

DIPHYLLOBOTHRIUM. *D. latum* is the broad tapeworm of man, the dog, and the cat. It is rare in Britain, but has a wide distribution. Several species are found, but this is the commonest. The life-history is interesting. The ciliated larva liberated from the egg is swallowed by a crustacean. *Cyclops strenuus* or *Diaptonius* spp., in which it becomes an elongated form with a terminal sphere containing three pairs of hooklets, called a 'procercoid larva'. The crustaceans are swallowed by a fish, when the larva, migrating to the muscles, becomes an elongated infective larva called a 'plerocercoid'. The fish is eaten by a suitable host, and the adults develop. In man, the tapeworm may attain a length of 60 feet, and it may cause a grave form of anaemia (bothriocephalus anaemia) associated with gastric and nervous symptoms.

D. mansoni is also widely distributed and has a similar life-history, but the infective stage is found in many hosts, including man, pig, and carnivores. It is common in frogs in Japan. The adult worm is found in carnivores.

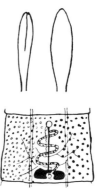

Diphyllobothrium. Head and segment.

Treatment of dogs infested with tapeworms is very important, not so much from the point of view of the dog; but because some of the species in their intermediate stages are dangerous to food animals. Farm dogs should never be allowed to harbour tape-worms. Routine use of anthelmintics is essential. All material passed should be destroyed.

Dipylidium caninum infests cats also; and may be transmitted by swallowing a flea.

In pigs, cattle, and sheep cysts of the tapeworm *Taenia hydatigena* (which infests the dog and may occasionally attain a length of 16 feet) may be so numerous in the liver that the latter ruptures, causing death.

Tapeworms in horses. Three species occur in horses, all belonging to the genus ANOPLOCEPHALA. *A perfoliata* and *A. mammillana* are not uncommon in Britain, while *A. magna* is also sometimes encountered.

A. perfoliata, a stoutish worm with large head and

no hooks, is a cause not only of unthriftiness but occasionally also of ileal and caecal obstruction, and/or intussusception, where numerous *A. perfoliata* are present; so the infection may be more serious than is generally supposed.

The intermediate host is a mite.

Tapeworms in ruminants. All the tapeworms of ruminants have four suckers and no hooks. In Moniezia the intermediate host is a free-living mite.

MONIEZIA. This is the only genus found in Britain; but it is world-wide in its distribution. The segments of these worms are much broader than long. The worms may attain a length of several yards, with a minute head little larger than a pin-head. Over 1000 worms have been recorded from a single host. Numerous species have been recorded. *H. giardi* is found in Europe, Australia, and Africa. Is from 1 to 2 metres long.

A closely related form, *Thysanosoma actinoides*, is found in North America. It is about 30 cm long, and is found in the liver. The sheep show general symptoms of malnutrition.

Bovine cystercercosis in Denmark. Studies were conducted on 14 farms with a history of this disease. On six of the farms the source of infection was sludge from septic tanks applied to pasture or crops. In two herds the cattle grazed pasture near a sewage plant; while on three farms people defaecating on pasture was a possible source. (Ilsoe, B. & others. *Acta Veterinaria Scandinavica* (1990) **31**, 159.)

Tapeworms in poultry. A number of tapeworms have been found in poultry, of which the commonest are *Davainea proglottina*, which has a larval stage in slugs and snails and is widely distributed, several species of *Raillietina*, with the larvae in house-flies, dung beetles and ants; these are also common in many countries, *Amoebotoenia*, with larvae in earthworms, and *Hymenolepis* of various species, some of which may be very numerous in individual birds.

The worms are only likely to cause serious loss when present in very large numbers, and often they are only identified at post-mortem examination.

'Measles' in beef due to the presence of the cyst stage (*Cysticercus bovis*) of the tapeworm *Taenia saginata*, which is a parasite of man. Cattle swallow the eggs of the adult tapeworm, and these hatch in the intestines, liberating young embryos, which burrow until they settle in muscle fibre or connective tissues. Here they appear as small oval cysts, containing fluid, and each possessing the head of a potential tapeworm. The disease causes no symptoms in cattle, but it is of great importance from the meat inspection point of view, since if the meat is not well cooked, a person eating it becomes infested with tapeworms.

'Measles' in pork is due to the presence of the cyst stage (*Cysticercus cellulosae*) of the tapeworm of man *Taenia solium*. It is extremely common among pigs in eastern lands, which have access to garbage and human faeces; from whence they pick up the eggs passed through the human intestines. The eggs undergo a development similar to those of the beef measles tapeworm. Man may also himself harbour the cystic stage.

Cysticercosis in man. Very high sporadic infection rates have been found in Africa with *Taenia saginata* and *T. solium*, the two tapeworms of major importance in man. Where *T. solium* is present, serious human infections with the cysticercus stage may be observed, as well as mild infections with the adult tapeworm. When it occurs in beef cattle, the cysticercus of *T. saginata* is a major economic problem and a serious obstacle to the export of meat.

A single human carrier of *T. saginata* led to an outbreak of cysticercosis among cattle on a large farm in the USA. (*WHO Chronicle.*)

Coenuriasis ('Gid' or 'Sturdy') in sheep. This disease is caused by the pressure of cysts of the tapeworm *Taenia multiceps* on cells of the brain (or spinal cord).

Sheep become infested by swallowing the unhatched eggs, excreted in a dog's faeces, while grazing. In the digestive tract the eggs hatch, and pass via the bloodstream to various parts of the body; only those reaching the central nervous system developing. Here they form small cysts, each containing one tapeworm head. This larval stage is known as *Coenurus cerebralis.* Over a period of months, each cyst increases in size, and more heads are budded from the lining membrane of the translucent cyst wall. Eventually a single *coenurus* may contain 50 or 100 or more tapeworm heads (*scolices*) projecting inwards.

The life-cycle is completed if a dog eats the head of an infested sheep.

SIGNS. These include impairment of vision, a staggering or high-stepping gait, circling, standing with head lowered, raised, or pressed against an object. Backwards somersaults have been recorded. Recumbency and opisthotonus may occur. A softening of the bone of the skull, due to internal pressure of the cysts, is found in a proportion of cases.

DIAGNOSIS. Skerritt and Stallbaumer found in 62 cases of coenuriasis that 58 per cent did *not* have any palpable skull softening. In the absence of this, their paper states, 'the proper interpretation of the neurological signs is the only guide for surgery.' First they recommend careful observation of the sheep's spontaneous behaviour, then the application of various tests to show the animal's reactions. Accurate localisation of cysts was then possible in 68 per cent of cases.

An intradermal 'gid' test was used in 34 cases (of which 29 proved to be gid); 0·1 ml of cyst fluid being injected into a shaved area of skin, with a similar quantity of sterile water being injected at a similar site. Any skin thickening within 24 hours was regarded as positive.

Seven of the sheep had a cyst in the cerebellum, and became recumbent after showing a high-stepping gait. Only six of the sheep with cerebral cysts became recumbent.

TREATMENT. The authors anaesthetised the sheep with a single injection of pentobarbitone sodium, after intravenous injections of sodium benzylpenicillin and dexamethasone. In the absence of any skull softening, a trephine was used to remove a disc of bone 1·5 cm in diameter. Draining the fluid from the cyst before its removal obviated the need to enlarge the hole. The cyst was removed completely. (If this is not done, the remaining cyst wall is apparently capable of replacing the fluid.)

The surgical technique, fully described in their paper (Skerritt, C. G. and Stallbaumer, M. F., *Veterinary Record* (1984) **115,** 399), gave a success rate of 74 per cent of the 42 cases selected for surgery.

Hydatid disease is caused by the cystic larval stage of the tapeworm *Echinococcus granulosus*, of which the **dog** and **fox** are the usual hosts. Eggs released from tapeworm segments passed in the faeces by these animals are later swallowed by grazing cattle, sheep and horses, which may become infested also through drinking water contaminated by wind-blown eggs.

People become infested through swallowing eggs attached to inadequately washed vegetables, and possibly eggs may be inhaled in dust or carried by flies to uncovered food. The handling of infested dogs is an important source. In Beirut the risk is put at 21 times greater for dog-owners than others, by the World Health Organisation, who state also that in California nomadic sheep rearers are 1000 times more likely to have hydatid disease than other inhabitants of the state. (WHO Technical Report 637, 1970).

There have been successful campaigns to control human hydatid disease in both Cyprus and Iceland; by compulsory treatment and/or banning of dogs.

Swallowed eggs hatch in the intestines and are carried via the portal vein to the liver. Some remain there, developing into hydatid cysts; others may form cysts in the lungs or occasionally elsewhere, *e.g.* spleen, kidney, bone marrow cavity, or brain. Inside the cysts brood capsules, containing the infective stage of the tapeworm develop, and after 5 or 6 months can infest dog or fox.

In Wales, where the incidence of hydatid disease is relatively high, farm dogs and foxhounds are important in its spread.

Only some seven people are known to die from this disease in England and Wales each year – a figure which would probably be higher were diagnosis less difficult. Condemnation of sheep and cattle offal from this cause runs into hundreds of thousands of pounds annually. Routine worming of dogs is essential for control.

Echinococcus granulosus is far from being a typical tapeworm, as it has only three or four segments and a total length of a mere 3–9 mm, so that the dog-owner will not notice the voided segments.

A problem of diagnosis also arises, in that this worm's eggs are indistinguishable from those of *Taenia* tapeworms. Previously, Professor M. J. Clarkson has pointed out, one could dose dogs with arecoline hydrochloride and examine the faeces for the presence of the intact tapeworm, but in Britain this anthelmintic is no longer obtainable, having been replaced by more modern drugs which destroy the tapeworm but leave it unrecog-

nisable. (M. J. Clarkson. *In Practice.*) (For effective anthelmintic treatment of dogs, *see* DRONCIT.)

Equine hydatidosis in Britain is caused by a strain of *E. granulosus* which has become specifically adapted to the horse as its intermediate host, and is often referred to now as *E. granulosus equinus.* This apparently is of low pathenogenicity for man.

In a survey covering 1388 horses and ponies examined at two abattoirs in the north of England, 8·7 per cent were infected. Prevalence of infection was closely related to age; rising from zero in animals up to two years old to over 20 per cent of those over eight years old.

Sixty-six per cent of the infected animals had viable cysts. Prevalence appears to be greatest in central and north-west England. (G. T. Edwards, *Veterinary Record* (1982) **110,** 511.)

Treatment of human patients. 'Hydatid disease is one of the rare parasitic conditions that can be treated only by surgery ... However, the result is often incomplete, with frequent local recurrences or accidents of secondary dissemination. Repeated interventions are often mutilating and do not guarantee a definite cure.' (A. Bekhti and others., *British Medical Journal* (1977) **2,** 1047). They used mebendazole successfully in four patients, but WHO points out that while success has been obtained in some, others have died despite it.

TAPPING (*see* ASPIRATION).

TAR is the thick, oily, strong-smelling, black liquid which is obtained by distillation from shale, coal, and wood. Tar from the road is a common cause of irritation between a dog's toes, causing the animal to lick or bite the part. The tar must be removed with a bland fat or oil. Crude tar, *e.g.* from a gasworks, should never be used on an animal's skin.

Wood-tar, which is also known as 'pix liquida', is obtained by the destructive distillation of various species of pine tree. Wood-tar ('Stockholm tar') is slightly soluble in water, and more readily in alcohol, oils, and strong alkaline solutions. **Uses.** Externally, Stockholm tar is used as a preservative for horn and hoof. (*See also* PITCH POISONING.)

TARSORRAPHY. An operation for producing union of upper and lower eyelids. It is performed as a permanent measure after enucleation of an eyeball; and sometimes as a temporary expedient to give protection to an ulcerated or perforated cornea (but *see* 'LENS', CONTACT.)

TARSUS. The hock. (*See under* BONES; EYELIDS.)

TARTAR is the concretion that often forms upon the crowns and upon the necks of the teeth, as well as upon exposed portions of the roots. The material is of a brownish, yellowish, or greyish colour, and consists chiefly of phosphate of lime which has been deposited from the saliva, with which are mixed numerous food particles and bacteria of a harmful nature. Tartar is most often seen in the mouths of dogs and cats, although the herbivorous animals may also be affected.

It is important that accumulated tartar be removed from time to time, for if it is allowed to collect for an indefinite period the gums shrink before the advancing deposit, the root becomes exposed and ultimately affected, and the tooth loosens and falls out. In addition to this, there are generally signs of systemic disturbance, such as a bad smell from the breath, indigestion from inability to feed properly, and in bad cases, great irritability and loss of condition. (*See* PERIODONTAL DISEASE.)

TASMANIAN GREY. An Australian breed of beef cattle, similar to the Murray Grey but developed from Aberdeen Angus and white Shorthorns.

TASTE. This special sense is dependent upon the taste buds, located in the crevices of the papillae. The taste buds have minute projections – the endings of nerve fibres. It is necessary for the purpose of taste that the substance should be dissolved in a fluid, and it seems that this is one of the functions of the saliva. The sense of taste is closely associated with the sense of smell. (*See* TONGUE, SMELL, *and* JACOBSON'S ORGAN.)

TATTOOING. This is done, by means of a special pair of forceps, etc., for the purpose of identifying farm live-stock. On black skins, tattooing is not an effective method, and the use of NOSE PRINTS has been tried for cattle. The tattooing of dogs is widely practised in France (where it is compulsory for the Kennel Club's register of pedigree dogs), and in Canada and the USA.

Tattooing is not entirely free from the risk of introducing infection, *e.g.* blackquarter, tetanus; and has been largely replaced by FREEZE-BRANDING (which see). (*See also* DANGEROUS DOGS ACT 1991.)

TAURINE. An amino-acid. In the USA feeding of cats on canned dog foods is reported to have led to a taurine deficiency, resulting in degeneration of the cat's retina. (C. D. Aguirre. *JAVMA* (1978) **172**, 791.)

However, a level of taurine in the cat's diet sufficient to prevent degeneration of the retina may be insufficient to prevent the heart disease DILATED CARDIOMYOPATHY (DCM). (Pion, P. & others, *Science* (1987) **237**, 764).

TAXIS is the method of pushing back into the abdominal cavity a loop of bowel which has passed through the wall as the result of a rupture or hernia.

TEAR-STAINING of the face in the dog may be due to atopic disease or to blockage of a lacrimal duct.

TEARS (*see* EYE. For 'soapy' tears *see* ALGAE POISONING; *see also* NAPHTHALENE POISONING).

'TEART PASTURES, SOILS' (*see under* MOLYBDENUM).

'TEASER', A (*see under* VASECTOMISED).

TEAT CANAL, as a first defence against pathogens. (*See* last but one paragraph of MASTITIS IN THE COW; *and also* ORIFICES, IMMUNITY AT.)

TEAT DIPPING. First practised by a veterinary surgeon in 1916, this has proved a most useful measure for the control of mastitis in cattle. The liquid chiefly used for the purpose is an iodophor; but good results can be obtained with hypochlorite teat dips containing 1 per cent available chlorine. (*See under* MASTITIS IN THE COW.)

TEATS, DISEASES OF (*see* BOVINE HERPES MAMMILITIS, TEAT NECROSIS, VIRUS INFECTIONS OF COW'S TEATS).

TEAT NECROSIS. This is seen in piglets under intensive conditions of rearing, and is sometimes accompanied by skin necrosis affecting the limbs. Inadequate bedding and abrasive concrete may be contributory factors. (*See also* NECROSIS, BACILLARY.)

TEATS, COW'S (*see under* MAMMARY GLAND; *also* VIRUS INFECTIONS OF COW'S TEATS, MASTITIS).

TEETH are developed in connection with the mucous membrane of the mouth, being actually calcified papillae. They are implanted in sockets or 'alveoli' in the upper and lower jaws, being only separated from actual contact with the bone by a layer of 'alveolar periosteum'.

The *incisors* are implanted in the incisive bones of the upper jaw, and in the anterior part of the mandible; they are situated in the front of the mouth, and purely prehensile in all animals, and are absent from the upper jaw of cattle, sheep, and goats, as well as other ruminating animals.

The *canines* are situated behind the incisors, and are used mainly for fighting purposes, being most developed in carnivores and omnivores. They are useless to the domesticated herbivorous animals, and in them are usually of small size. They are not present in the upper jaws of ruminants, and in the lower jaws have the shape and function of incisors.

The *molars* are the remaining teeth, situated farther back in the mouth. They are used for chewing mainly, and specially adapted for this purpose by having broad strong irregular tables or grinding surfaces. The term 'cheek teeth' is often applied to these teeth, since, strictly speaking, they are composed of 'pre-molars', which are represented in the milk dentition, and 'molars' which are not so represented. (*See* DENTITION.)

Each tooth has a portion covered with enamel, the 'crown'; a portion covered with cement, the 'root'; and a line of union between these two parts known as the 'neck'. A constriction occurs at the neck in the temporary incisors of the horse, in the incisors of the ruminants, and in incisors and molars of the dog and cat; in the remaining teeth there is no such constriction.

Structure. Teeth consist of four tissues. In the

middle of the tooth is the 'pulp', occupying the 'pulp cavity'. It is soft and gelatinous, well supplied with blood-vessels and nerves, and is large in the young tooth. It nourishes the remaining tissues, and forms dentine for so long as the pulp cavity is open. In later life it is small or absent, the pulp cavity having filled with dentine formed from the pulp. The 'dentine' forms the greater part of the tooth. It is hard, yellowish, or yellowish-white in colour, and is surrounded in the crown by enamel, and in the root by cement. The 'enamel' consists of a comparatively thin layer of a brilliant white colour and extremely dense and brittle, which forms a cap to the dentine, or is arranged in layers through it. The 'cement' is always the outermost layer of a tooth, being formed on the outside of the dentine in the root, and filling up the irregular spaces and hollows of the crown. The implanted part of a tooth is fixed into the socket by a layer of vascular fibrous tissue, which serves as the periosteum both of the tooth root and of the lining of the alveolus. It is known as the 'alveolar periosteum'.

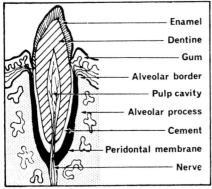

Enamel

Dentine

Gum

Alveolar border

Pulp cavity

Alveolar process

Cement

Peridontal membrane

Nerve

Tooth structure. (From de Coursey's *The Human Organism*, McGraw-Hill.)

Enamel is the hardest tissue in the body, and consists mainly of phosphate of lime. It is composed of prisms placed side by side, with one end resting on the dentine and the other end towards the free surface in a simple tooth, such as the canine of a dog. Cement is practically of the same structure as bone, without possessing Haversian canals.

Arrangement and form (*see* DENTITION).
(For times of cutting of the various teeth, *see* DENTITION.)

TEETH, DISEASES OF. Most diseases or disorders affecting the teeth are associated with pain or discomfort, which results in absence of appetite, capriciousness in feeding, or other disturbances.

Irregularities. In certain cases, the incisor or molar teeth develop out of their normal positions in the jaw, with the result that perfect apposition between the upper and lower teeth is not possible, and the rate of wear is not uniformly distributed over the tables of the teeth. In other instances, extra or 'supernumerary' teeth are formed; in the incisor region these are usually placed behind the

arch of normal teeth, while extra molars may be found as projections from the gums on the inside or the outside of the line of normal teeth.

When the temporary teeth are shed, it sometimes happens that the permanent teeth erupt irregularly to one side or behind the temporaries, and are distorted accordingly. This frequently happens in puppies, and to a less extent in the herbivora. In the former, trouble is likely to be experienced between 3½ and 5 or 6 months, and in young horses at 2½ and 3½ years of age. In such cases it is necessary to extract any temporaries which persist, so that the permanent teeth can arrive in their proper places in the mouth.

In dogs frequently, in sheep sometimes, and in other animals less commonly, there may be a discrepancy in length between the upper and lower jaws. When the upper jaw is too long, the condition is known as an 'overshot jaw', and when the lower jaw projects too far forward, it is popularly spoken of as an 'undershot jaw'. In bulldogs, pugs, and other breeds of dogs with very short upper jaws the undershot condition is practically normal, while in certain breeds with extremely long upper jaws, such as the greyhound and show collie, overshot jaws are very common.

Abnormal wear, which is due to malformations of the jaws, to excessive softness of the teeth, or to the direction of the teeth, is another mechanical cause of tooth disorder. (*See* SOIL-CONTAMINATED HERBAGE *with references to sheep.*)

Abnormal wear varies in different cases, and is productive of some well-known conditions, as follows: (1) *shear mouth*, in which the molar teeth of the upper and lower jaws wear so that in time they appear like the blades of a pair of sheep-shears, the upper row being worn away on its inner border, and the lower one along its outer border; (2) *step mouth*, where the cheek teeth, instead of being all at the same level, are arranged with some higher than others, somewhat like steps, a high tooth in the lower jaw being opposite a short one in the corresponding upper jaw; (3) *overhanging* upper jaw, which is where the first upper cheek tooth on either side is placed too far forward in the mouth, and does not come into accurate apposition with the tooth immediately below it, causing the formation of a hook. At the same time the last lower cheek tooth is situated too far back and also forms a hook; (4) *curved tables*, where the line of cheek teeth in the upper jaw shows a convexity in its centre, and a corresponding concavity exists in the lower row.

SIGNS. In most of these instances the animal affected (almost always a member of the horse tribe), instead of chewing its food and swallowing it in the usual way, rolls it round and round in the mouth until it collects into a sodden mass, often about the size of a couple of fingers, and puts it out of the mouth instead of swallowing it. (*See* QUIDDING.) Pain may be shown when the hand is passed along the outside of the cheek, especially when pressure is put upon the line of teeth.

TREATMENT. Rasping the teeth by means of a special tooth-rasp will reduce smaller irregularities, and bring the teeth back into their proper function.

Caries is *not* synonymous with tooth decay, although the term – borrowed from human dentistry – is often used in veterinary practice to include all tooth decay.

In man, the superficial appearance of caries comprises 'margins of the cavity lined by partially de-mineralised tissue which can be penetrated by a sharp probe, and in which the latter "sticks".' The essential lesion, in dentine, is a destructive invasion by bacteria. (G. W. Schneck and J. W. Osborn. *Vet. Rec.* (1976) **99**, 100.)

True caries has been confirmed in dogs but not in cats, and the above authors refer to its 'comparative rarity in animals'.

Neck lesions in cats' teeth. The above authors referred to a 'frequent and clearly painful condition affecting middle-aged to elderly cats, and characterised by cavitation of the necks of teeth, making extraction difficult because of breakage of crowns. These lesions did not show the bacterial invasion and destruction of the dentine ahead of the margins of the cavity – which is typical of human cases of caries'.

TREATMENT consists of the removal of the diseased tooth or teeth by extraction.

Inflammations of the periosteum lining the root cavity of a tooth are common. They may be due to small particles of food getting forced down into the socket of the tooth, to fractures or fissures of the teeth, to caries, tumour formation, depositions of tartar, and to certain specific diseases, such as actinomycosis, etc.

SIGNS. These vary from a slight redness of the gum around the root of the tooth, which is painful when pressed by the finger, to a large suppurating tract running alongside the root of the tooth down into its socket, and perhaps through the skin to the outside or into one or other of the sinuses. Abscess formation in the tooth socket may take place, and the abscess may burst into the mouth, to the outside through the skin, or up into a sinus. In many cases there is a distinct bulge of the surface above the diseased tooth, which may give to the face a one-sided appearance.

TREATMENT. The affected tooth or teeth must be extracted, and the areas of suppuration cleansed and curetted if necessary. The cavity usually has to be packed with antiseptic gauze afterwards for a few days until it begins to fill by healthy granulation tissue.

Periodontal disease is a name for chronic infection of the periodontal membrane. It is one form of inflammation of the periosteum, or alveolar periostitis. It causes loosening and shedding of the teeth, pain, failure to masticate, and loss of weight.

Odontomata are tumours formed in connection with the root of one tooth, or they may be found in the jaw, sinuses, or even involving part of the nasal passage, and be composite or compound, when multitudes of small rudimentary teeth are present. They cause swelling and bulging of the surface of the face, and can only be treated surgically.

Porphyria gives rise to a pink or brown discoloration of teeth. (*See under* BONE, DISEASES OF.)

Toothache is most spectacular in the dog, which rubs its mouth along the ground, paws at its nose or mouth, works its jaws, salivates, and may whine or moan.

A veterinary surgeon will offer a diagnosis and initiate the necessary treatment.

'Broken mouth' is important in hill sheep. (*See under this heading.*)

Fractures of the canine teeth in dogs are not uncommon. If the pulp is exposed, subsequent infection can lead to a painful abscess. Extraction of the remainder of the tooth obviates this but, for show dogs or guard dogs, is undesirable. Metal crowns have been applied to dogs' teeth, but are liable to be dislodged.

Tooth transplantation has accordingly been used in veterinary practice but unfortunately the results are seldom lasting, due to root resorption and bone replacement. Fracture of the transplanted tooth is likely after a couple of years or so. One technique involves fixing the transplanted tooth in position by means of stainless steel wiring and an acrylic splint.

TEETH, EWE's, 'TRIMMING'. 'Between 60 and 70 per cent of culling of ewes is on account of their teeth.' (Hindson, J. C., *Veterinary Record* (1986) **118**, 706.) 'A small percentage will involve loss of molars or incisor wear, but the vast majority will be incisor loss.'

Ewes have been treated for 'bite correction' by means of an electric grinder, and in 1986 this practice by laymen attracted the attention of the Farm Animal Welfare Council, who called for a temporary ban pending further research. The Council called for a permanent ban on the grinding down of teeth to the gum, as practised in Australia.

(*See also* 'BROKEN MOUTH'.)

TEETH SCALING. The use of ultrasonic dental scalers has now become widely accepted in veterinary dentistry.

During the scaling, an aerosol of water droplets is formed, with a variable amount of peridontal debris spattered from the patient's mouth. In the debris there are likely to be viruses and/or bacteria – a danger for operator, assistant, or subsequent patient. An aerosol of mouth flora can remain airborne for up to 30 minutes following scaling.

The BVA has accordingly recommended that (1) the working area should be well ventilated; preferably with forced air extraction. (2) Masks should be worn at all times by anyone in the working area. (3) A 0·2 per cent chlorhexidine solution should be used as the coolant supplied to the scaling equipment.

TELOGEN. The resting phase in the cycle of hair growth.

TEM. Triethylenemelemine, a gametocide which, in America, has been used in field trials for the control of birds. The chemical is mixed with corn, and has the effect of making the male bird infertile. The birds continue to defend their territories and nest, but do not produce any young.

TEMPERAMENT, CHANGE IN. This may follow a brain tumour or infection, giving rise to aggressiveness – as occurs in RABIES, for example. A horse may become bad-tempered as the result of a VERMINOUS ARTERITIS. Poisoning may cause frenzy or aggressiveness; e.g. BENZOIC ACID poisoning in the cat. (*See also* BRAIN DISEASES, STRESS, FUCOSIDOSIS.)

TEMPERATURE, AIR (*see under* HOUSING OF ANIMALS, HEAT EXHAUSTION, TROPICS.)

TEMPERATURE, BODY, is controlled by the heat-regulating centre in the brain – the hypothalamus, which also influences blood circulation, secretion of urine, and appetite: all three of which have a bearing on body temperature.

Heat is produced by the muscles and by the digestive organs, and during very cold weather or exercise, heat from the former increases, while that from the liver and other digestive organs decreases. The animal may also absorb heat from the sun's rays.

Heat is lost by evaporation of water, and by SENSIBLE HEAT LOSS (which see). Water loss is achieved via the lungs and the skin: *e.g.* by panting and sweating. (The dog is, for all practical purposes, a non-sweating animal apart from the pads of its feet, and has to rely mainly on panting.)

Diurnal variations in body temperature are normal; in the early hours of the morning it is usually at its lowest, and at its highest in the late afternoon.

For ordinary practical purposes the usual average temperatures of animals are given as follows:

Horses	100·5°F (38·0°C)
Cattle	102·0°F (38·9°C)
Sheep, Goats	104·0°F (40·0°C)
Pigs	103·5°F (39·7°C)
Dogs	101·0°F (38·3°C)
Cats	102·0°F (38·6°C)
Rabbits	100·8°F (38·2°C)
Fowls	106·9°F (41·6°C)
Small birds	108·6°F (42·5°C)
Elephants	97·6°F (36·4°C)
Camels	99·5°F (37·5°C)

Temperature-taking. The most satisfactory place is within the rectum. In females the thermometer may also be inserted into the external part of the genital canal; as a rule, the vaginal temperature is about half a degree higher than the rectal temperature, so than when a series of temperatures is to be taken, one site or the other should be selected.

With dogs and cats, one person should hold the animal, preferably on a table, while another inserts and holds the thermometer. In each animal, after the bulb of the thermometer has been lubricated with a little soap or Vaseline, etc., the tail is raised vertically by the left hand, and the thermometer is inserted through the anal ring and into the rectum, by a screwing movement if any resistance is encountered. It is held in position for

½, or 1 minute, according to the make of the thermometer, and is then withdrawn. With a piece of cotton-wool any adherent faeces are wiped away, and the temperature is read off. Subsequently, the thermometer should be washed in cold water, and a *cold solution* of disinfectant should be used to disinfect it.

For purposes of temperature stress research, American scientists use a special ear thermometer in cattle. As in similar medical research, this tympanic thermometer is more reliable than the rectal thermometer, and can sense changes as small as $\frac{1}{50}$°F

Temperature in disease. A high temperature is one of the classic symptoms of fever, and in greater or less measure accompanies practically all acute cases of disease. A comparatively steady rise in temperature is as a rule succeeded by a correspondingly steady fall, and is to be looked upon as a more favourable sign of the natural course of a disease than when the temperature rises and falls with greater suddenness. The reduction of temperature in simple fevers is in almost all cases much slower than the rise. A wavering temperature, which shows little tendency to come down to normal, generally indicates that there is some active focus of disease, such as an abscess, which the body cannot overcome. Sudden rise in temperature in an animal which has shown a steady fall previously is an indication of a relapse or recurrence of the disease. (*See also* FEVER, HYPERTHERMIA, HEATSTROKE, TROPICS).

Fall of temperature may be occasioned by great loss of blood, starvation, collapse, or coma; it is characteristic of certain forms of kidney disease. Certain chronic diseases in which emaciation is marked are also associated with a subnormal temperature. (*See also* HYPOTHERMIA.)

Temperature, near calving time. A healthy cow – even though showing the familiar signs – is unlikely to calve during the next 12 hours if her temperature is 102°F. This is a useful guide to herdsmen. (*See also under* FEVER, HOUSING, etc.)

TEMPERATURE CONTROL in animal housing (*see* CONTROLLED ENVIRONMENT HOUSING).

TEMPERATURE-SENSITIVE (ts) VIRUSES (*see* VACCINES).

TENDERNESS is pain that is felt only when a diseased part is handled.

TENDON is the dense, fibrous, slightly elastic cord that attaches the end of a muscle to the bone or other structure upon which the muscle acts when it contracts. Tendons are composed of bundles of fibrous tissue, white in colour, and arranged in a very dense manner, so as to be capable of withstanding great strains. Some are rounded; some are flattened into ribbons; others are arranged in the form of sheets; while those of a fourth variety are very short, the muscle fibres being attached almost directly on to the bone or cartilage which they actuate. Most tendons are surrounded by sheaths lined with membrane similar to that found in joint cavities, *i.e.* synovial membrane. In this sheath the tendon glides smoothly over surrounding parts. The fibres of a tendon pass into the fibres of the periosteum covering a bone, and blend with them. One of the largest tendons in the animal body is the '*tendo Achilles*', which runs from the large muscles at the back of the stifle down to the point of the hock; it is often called the 'hamstring', and is the structure that is injured in the condition known as 'hamstrung'.

TENDONS, DISEASES AND INJURIES OF
(*see also under* MUSCLES, SPRAINED TENDONS).

In most cases the injuries to which tendons are liable are in the nature of minute lesions in which fibres have been torn across through over-extension of the tendon as a whole. Accompanying these there are often slight haemorrhages or extravasations of blood into the substance of the tendon, and the tendon itself is thickened at the injured part or, when severe, practically over the whole of its length. At the same time, a certain amount of damage has usually been sustained by the tendon sheath, or by its lining, and an unusually large amount of the lubricating synovial fluid is thrown out, which fills the tendon sheath to the point of dilatation, causing it to stand out on the surface of the limb.

When recovery occurs, the swelling subsides, fluid is absorbed, and the broken ends of the fibres become attached by strands of fibrous tissue to other intact fibres near by, pain disappears, and the animal becomes sound. Sometimes, however, permanent thickening results. (*See also* KNUCKLING.)

Certain of the tendons of the horse's limb are liable to become ruptured when subjected to great or sudden strains. Suture of the ruptured ends of the tendon has given good results when performed early, and when a sufficient amount of support can be provided by splints or other means. (*See* CARBON FIBRE.)

Severing of tendons in dogs' legs has been successfully treated. (*See also* TENOSYNOVITIS.)

TENESMUS. Straining to pass urine or faeces with little or no result.

TENOSYNOVITIS affects the legs of broiler chickens and is caused by a virus. Tendons may enlarge and cease to function. (*See also* SYNOVITIS.)

TENOTOMY. The surgical severing of a tendon.

TEPP. Tetra-ethyl pyrophosphate, used in agriculture as a pesticide, is a potential danger to live-stock. A Texas rancher diluted 1 gallon of TEPP with water to make 120 gallons, and sprayed 20 head of cattle. All were dead within three-quarters of an hour. Symptoms of poisoning in a puppy comprised drowsiness, muscular in-coordination, and vomiting. The antidote is atropine sulphate.

TERATOGENIC agents, called Teratogens, are those known to cause congenital defects. Such agents include drugs (*e.g.* thalidomide, griseoful-vin) and viruses. (*See also* HEMLOCK.)

TERATOMA is a developmental irregularity in which the embryo, instead of growing normally in the uterus, develops structural defects or, in extreme cases, develops into a monster. The latter are comparatively common in cattle, and give rise to difficulty at parturition. 'Teratology' is the study of monstrosities. (*See also under* TUMOURS.)

TERMITES. Whitish, ant-like insects of the tropics. Some species feed on wood; damaging buildings.
CONTROL: Heptachlor and chlordane.
POTENTIAL HEALTH HAZARDS: 'Widespread use of these compounds in the past ensures that their metabolites will be detected in humans for years to come,' commented Dr M. R. Zavon (*Lancet* (1991) **337**, 306). He added: 'Despite extensive research, no harmful effects have been found.'

TERRAPIN. A web-footed reptile. Mr Trevor Farrell BVSc was brought one which had torn a claw. When this had been treated, the reptile's owners mentioned that the creature had a swimming problem. He had damaged his shell when quite tiny, and ever since had swum in circles at an angle of 45°. A radiograph showed Mr Farrell that one lung was much smaller than the other – probably it had been compressed at the time of the shell damage – and that was affecting the terrapin's buoyancy. So he made a plaster of Paris mould of the compression, and then a poly-styrene float. The patient no longer has a list to port, and can now swim in a straight line.

TESCHEN DISEASE. A virus disease of pigs, first recognised in Czechoslovakia, and now known to occur in Germany, Switzerland, Yugo-slavia, and France. In the UK (where it had not so far been reported), Teschen disease was made Notifiable in 1974.
SIGNS. Fever, excitement, paralysis, jerky movements of the eye. Death occurs in about 50 per cent of cases. In the others recovery is often incomplete, paralysis persisting.
TREATMENT. None. (*See also under* PORCINE ENCEPHALOMYELITIS.)

TESTICLE, or TESTIS, is the essential male generative gland or gonad, which, along with the epididymis and its associated structures, lies in the scrotum in each of the domesticated animals.

Normally, in the fetus or soon after birth, the testicle, guided by the fibrous cord known as the gubernaculum, moves down from a position close to the kidney to a 'cooler climate' in the scrotum. Into this it is pulled by the guber-naculum, which either fails to lengthen or actu-ally shortens.

In some animals e.g. foals, one or both testicles may go up again through the inguinal canal. This occurs occasionally in pigs, in which a returning testicle has been known to become a mere vestige by the age of six months.

In certain of the wild animals, such as the rat,

and in many tropical animals, *e.g.* the elephant, the testes are found in the abdominal cavity, either permanently or temporarily between periods of sexual activity. In the foal the testes appear in the scrotum usually very soon after birth, but they are subsequently drawn up into the abdomen, and do not reappear until between 5 or 6 months and 10 to 12 months. In a certain proportion of cases the testes are retained in the abdomen until 2 years of age, and then descend into the scrotum; in a number of cases they do not descend at all. The name 'rig', or 'cryptorchid', is applied to such animals, and the condition is known as 'cryptorchidism'. (*See* CRYPTORCHID.)

The testes consist of a dense fibrous coat, the 'tunica albuginea'. Blood-vessels run throughout the fibrous tissue, and nourish microscopic tubules, lined by layers of specialised cells which form the spermatozoa. The tubules, known as 'Seminiferous tubules', are connected with each other near the centre of the testes, and communicate with the coiled tubes of the epididymis, from which springs the 'vas deferens' connecting with the urethra at the opposite end. In the epididymis the sperms mature. The 'spermatic cord', which consists of the vas deferens, spermatic artery, veins, and nerves, enclosed in the layer of serous membrane (tunica vaginalis), passes upwards through the inguinal canal and enters the abdomen, whence it runs back to the region of the neck of the urinary bladder, opening finally into the urethra. Along its (i.e. urethra's) course are the openings of the ducts from the secondary sexual glands – seminal vesicles, prostate, and bulbo-urethral glands – which pour out a secretion which mixes with, nourishes, and protects the masses of spermatozoa coming from the testes.

Externally, the testicle is covered by a layer of serous membrane, lying immediately outside the tunica albuginea, and known as the 'tunica vaginalis propria', which also covers the epididymis. On the outside of this tunic is the 'tunica vaginalis communis', or the parietal layer. Outside this is a fairly thick layer of scrotal fascia, in which is deposited the 'cod-fat' of the bullock and wedder. A strong reddish, fibro-elastic 'tunica dartos' forms the next outermost layer, and provides the septum between the right and left pouches of the scrotum. Finally, on the outside, there is the practically hairless, thin, elastic, oily-feeling skin of the scrotum.

Functions. The essential function of the testis is to produce sperms. (*See under* SPERMATOZOA.) Between 60 and 80 million sperms are discharged at each copulatory act by the stallion at the beginning of the breeding season. Since a stallion may serve more than 100 mares during the season, many of them upon two separate occasions, it will readily be understood that the testes are extremely active organs, and make a considerable demand upon the vitality of the body generally. The necessity for a recuperative period in breeding males will also be obvious.

The other function of the testis is that associated with elaboration of the male sex-hormones, resulting in the production of the secondary

sexual characteristics, such as the arched neck and great body size of the stallion, the broad forehead, massive development of horns, and deep voice of the bull, the horns of the ram, and the tusks of the boar, etc., as well as the instinctive desire for sexual intercourse. The chief hormone is *Testosterone. (See also* REPRODUCTION, ENDOCRINE GLANDS, STERILITY, ARTIFICIAL INSEMINATION.)

TESTICLE, DISEASES OF. During service, an irritable mare may kick a stallion and rupture one of the testes, or seriously injure it. Damage may also be occasioned to these organs by the bites of dogs when fighting, by gores from cattle, or by injuries from the tusks of boars, gunshots, etc. However, infection is probably the most common cause.

Orchitis, or inflammation of the testis, may be the result of infection (*e.g.* by *Actinobacillus seminis, Brucella abortus, Brucella suis, Corynebacterium pseudotuberculosis, Tuberculosis*) or of trauma which – if the skin is broken – may itself lead to infection. A virus infection of bulls – Infectious Orchitis – has been reported in Czechoslovakia. Necrotic orchitis in the bull has been caused in Britain by actinobacillosis. The testis, being enclosed in a fibrous, comparatively non-elastic capsule, is not able to swell to any great extent, although the loose tissues of the scrotum often swell to an great extent. The scrotum becomes reddened in animals which have unpigmented skin in the inguinal region, and the whole area is very painful to the touch.
TREATMENT. Antibiotics or other therapy may be needed to deal with an infection.

Epididimytis (*see under* this heading and also under RAM).

Hydrocele is a local oedema affecting usually one tunica vaginalis, and distending that side of the scrotum with fluid. It is met with in the dog mostly although it may affect other animals.

Hypoplasia (*see under* INFERTILITY).

Tumours affecting the testicle and/or scrotum include CARCINOMA, SARCOMA, FIBROMA, PAPILLOMA, SEMINOMA, *and* SERTOLI-CELL TUMOUR.

Torsion (*see under* SPERMATIC CORD, TORSION OF).

TESTOSTERONE. The hormone, secreted by the testicle, which controls development of the secondary sex organs, sex characteristics and libido. (*See* ENDOCRINE GLANDS, HORMONES.)

TESTS (*see* LABORATORY TESTS).

TETANUS ('LOCKJAW') is a specific disease of the domesticated animals and man, caused by *Clostridium tetani*, which obtains access to the tissues through a wound. Horses are most commonly affected. The organism is present in most cultivated soils, especially such as receive heavy dressings of farmyard manure.

In certain districts tetanus is so common that it is usual to take precautions by inoculating horses with antitoxin whenever they receive even comparatively slight wounds, and always before

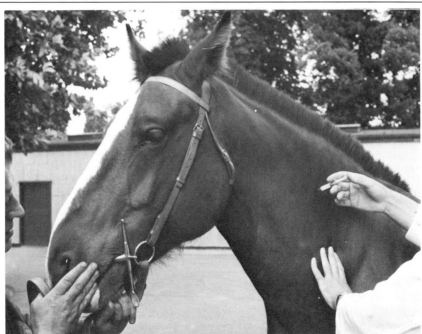

A tetanus vaccine introduced in 1971 by Burroughs Wellcome is claimed to overcome the disadvantage previously experienced in active immunisation of horses against the disease – it does not give rise to a painful swelling at the site of inoculation.

castration or major operations. Lambs are lost each year after docking and castration, or before the umbilicus (navel) has closed after birth, from tetanus.

Cl. tetani is an anaerobe, *i.e.* it thrives only in an absence of oxygen.

Its serious effects are produced by the elaboration of a toxin, which is absorbed into the general circulation, and exerts its effects upon the nervous system of the brain and spinal cord. This toxin is one of the most powerful known.

Deeply punctured wounds, from which oxygen is excluded, are much more serious than even large superficial wounds, the surfaces of which are exposed to the action of sunlight and fresh air. Picked-up nail wounds, cracked heels, injuries from the prongs of stable-forks, etc., are examples of wounds which often become contaminated with *Cl. tetani*. Tetanus may occur in an animal which has had a slight wound which appeared to heal without any complication. It may follow tattooing. Cases are met with where no wound can be found on the surface of the body, nor is there any history of an accident; such cases are probably the sequel to injuries inflicted by worms in the intestinal wall, or to slight scratches from unusually hard or rough herbage.

Intramuscular injections are a potential route of infection. (They led to tetanus in 48 out of 216 human patients admitted to a Spanish hospital between 1970–1982. (Garces-Bruses, J. & Nolla-Salas, M., *Journal of Infectious Diseases* (1984) **149,** 659.)

SIGNS.

Horses become stiff and disinclined to move. There is difficulty in turning the head round to the side, and the fore-legs are splayed outwards as though to enable the unfortunate animal better to retain its balance.

The ears may be turned in towards each other.

If the head be lifted sharply up, by placing the hand under the chin, the 'haw' or third eyelid (nictitating membrane), is seen to flicker across the eye to an extent much greater than usual.

Fixity of the jaws, or 'trismus', which has been responsible for the popular name given to tetanus (*i.e.* 'lock-jaw'), is not always in evidence in the early stages of an attack.

The tail may be held out quivering, and OPISTHOTONOS (which see) may be evident.

During the course of an attack, faeces and urine are usually withheld, and digestive disturbances may occur, sometimes resulting in fatal collections of gas in the large intestines.

(*See* HYPERAESTHESIA, another sign.)

Cattle. The symptoms are very similar to those in horses, trismus and protrusion of the haw being well-marked. Muscular stiffness is usually severe; flatulence and tympany are noted, and the tail may be outstretched. Tetanus in cattle is not, however, at all common.

Sheep. Standing is generally impossible; the affected animals lie on their sides, rapidly become tympanitic, and die after a very short illness. In lambs after castration or docking, the disease is very rapid in its effects, and several are affected at the same time.

Pigs. Tetanus is not common.

Dogs. The owner may notice 'something peculiar about the eyes and mouth', and either stiffness or recent lameness. Later, the limbs are usually stretched out as far from each other as possible, in a sawhorse position. Squinting and grinning are common, but closure of the jaws is not always in evidence. When it is present it is complete, and death practically always follows. Hyperaesthesia is also very marked. The ears may be bent inwards (as in the horse).

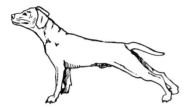

Diagram of attitude assumed by a dog affected with tetanus. The hind-limbs are kept well out behind the body, the tail is held rigidly or quivering, and the muscles of the face are drawn into a sardonic grin – the 'risus sardonicus' of ancient authors.

TREATMENT. Farm animals should be placed in a darkened loose-box, away from noise, and with food and water placed at a new level which they can reach despite their stiffness.

If nursed at home, a dog should be in a room where there are no bright lights, noise, television, or family activity.

Tetanus antiserum, penicillin, and muscle relaxants (such as acepromazine, which can obviate exhaustion and save life) are all needed. Treatment must also include glucose saline injections, e.g. in a dog which cannot drink or eat; and large animals similarly. (See DEHYDRATION, NORMAL SALINE.)

PREVENTION: On land where tetanus is rife, the most susceptible animals should be immunised.

Lambs are given antitoxin on the day of docking or castration. Toxoid can be injected at a different site on the same occasion.

Horses. The usual practice is to give two injections at an interval of 4 to 6 weeks; with a booster dose 6 or 12 months later. Further booster doses may be required. It is practicable to vaccinate pregnant mares so that later their new-born foals will be protected against tetanus infection via the navel. (See last paragraph under IMMUNITY.)

PROGNOSIS. In the absence of first-class nursing and intensive care, not many animals (other than cattle) recover from tetanus.

If an animal regains the ability to drink, that can be regarded as a favourable sign.

TETANY is a condition in which localised spasmodic contraction of muscles takes place. There may be twitching or convulsions. Tetany occurs when the level of blood calcium falls below normal. (*See also under* PARATHYROID, HYPOMAGNESAEMIA, TRANSIT, MILK FEVER, RABIES.)

TETHERING. The Horses, Ponies and Donkeys (No. 2) Bill to protect these animals against cruel tethering was passed in the UK in 1988.

TETRACYCLINES are bacteriostatic antibiotics with a wide range of activity which includes Gram-positive and Gram-negative bacteria, certain protozoa, rickettsia, and mycoplasma. Tetracyclines are absorbed from the gut, but oral

administration may upset the gut flora. They are irritant when injected.

Tetracyclines cause fluorescence in bone and teeth. In late pregnancy or in young growing animals, high dosage can result in teeth discoloration and can interfere with the formation of enamel.

Horses treated with tetracyclines while suffering from stress may become affected with diarrhoea and die. (*See* DIARRHOEA in horses.)

In cats tetracyclines occasionally cause severe loss of hair.

TETRAIODOPHENOLPHTHALEIN is used in radiography of the gall-bladder and bile ducts for diagnostic purposes.

TEXAS FEVER is a tick-borne disease. (*See* BABESIOSIS.)

SIGNS. Stained urine (redwater), high temperature, no appetite, and constipation followed by diarrhoea. Cerebral symptoms may be evident. The animal dies within 3 to 10 days. On post-mortem examination the blood is bright red and abnormally fluid, while the tissues are paler. The spleen is enlarged from 2 to 4 times its normal size and is reddish-brown ('anthrax spleen'). The liver is swollen and pale and the gall-bladder is distended with thick, viscid, dark-coloured bile. The muscles are normal.

The chronic form is similar but milder, and occurs in late autumn. Recovery is frequent, but convalescence is long (although it is stated to be very short in Argentine cattle).

TREATMENT is now fairly effective. Several proprietary preparations have replaced the 'trypan blue' formerly used.

TRANSMISSION is by the following ticks:

Boophilus (*Margaropus*) *annulatus* (N. America)
B. microplus (S. America)
B. australis (many countries)
B. argentinus (S. America)
B. calcaratus (Asia)
B. decoloratus (S. Africa)
Rhipicephalus appendiculatus (S. Africa)
R. evertsi (S. Africa)
R. bursa (N. Africa)
Haemaphysalis punctata (Europe)

TEXEL. A Dutch breed of sheep, and the most common breed in Europe. Noted for its milk production, it has good growth rate and meat potential.

TGE. Transmissible gastro-enteritis of pigs.

THALAMUS. (*See* diagram and accompanying text under BRAIN.)

THALLIUM. Thallium sulphate is used in poison baits to destroy rats, ants, and other pests, and accidental poisoning in domestic animals may occur. Thallium poisoning in dogs gives rise to gastro-enteritis, profuse vomiting, and severe pain. If death does not immediately follow, there may be a brick-red discoloration of lips, skin of groin or axilla. Hair begins to fall out. In human medicine, thallium poisoning has been successfully treated with prussian-blue.

THEAVE (*see under* SHEEP).

THEILERIOSIS. Infection with tick-borne parasites of the *Theileridae.* (*See* EAST COAST FEVER, TZANEEN DISEASE, CORRIDOR DISEASE.)

They vary in shape, some being spherical, others ovoid, pear-shaped, or elongated rod-like. Division by binary fission within the blood corpuscle may occur. Sexual multiplication occurs within the tick which transmits the parasite when it bites a new host.

There are several species in cattle and in sheep, including:

T. parva — East Coast fever in tropical Africa.
T. mutans — Benign bovine theileriosis.
T. lawrencei, causing Corridor disease.
T. annulata, causing Mediterranean fever, (*see separate entry* MEDITERRANEAN FEVER).

THEINE is the alkaloid which gives its stimulant properties to tea. It is the equivalent of caffeine. (*See* CAFFEINE.)

THELAZIA (*see* EYE WORMS).

THEOBROMINE is the alkaloid upon which the stimulant action of cocoa and chocolate depends.

THERAPEUTIC SUBSTANCES ACT (*see* ADDITIVES).

THERMOGRAPHY. The mapping of temperature over surfaces. Infra-red thermography, using a camera, has been tested in the diagnosis of orthopaedic lesions in horses.

THERMOLABILE. Subject to the loss of characteristic properties caused by heat.

THIABENDAZOLE (*see* ANTHELMINTICS).

THIALBARBITONE SODIUM. This barbiturate is used as a short-acting anaesthetic, mainly for dogs, cats, and sheep.

THIAMIN, THIAMINE. Thiamine hydrochloride, or vitamin B_1. A secondary deficiency occurs in bracken poisoning and horse-tails poisoning in horses, and in pigs due to the enzyme *thiaminase.* Thiaminase-producing bacteria have been isolated from sheep dying from polio-encephalomalacia (cerebro-cortical necrosis). (*See also* CHASTEK PAPALYSIS.)

Thiaminase is present to a varying degree in raw fish. Accordingly, fish should be cooked before feeding it to cats, etc.

SIGNS of this deficiency include loss of appetite, a staggering gait, and muscular spasms.

'THIN SOW' SYNDROME. Groups of sows or gilts lose weight, usually in the middle or later stages of pregnancy, and remain emaciated for perhaps 6 months or more. Prolonged underfeeding may eventually result in some sows being unable to cope with adverse conditions encountered at times of stress, *e.g.* weaning. It has also been suggested that infestation with the stomach worm *Hyostrongylus* or with the nodular worm *Oesophagostomum* may be a cause. The use of sow stalls, in which animals cannot move away to escape draughts, is another possible cause.

THIOURACIL. An antithyroid agent which lowers the rate of metabolism.

THIOUREA. This is naphythyl antu, a rat poison which causes oedema of the lungs. It is dangerous to domestic animals and birds.

THIRST (*see* WATER, DIABETES, SALT POISONING, COMPULSIVE POLYDIPSIA).

THOGOTO virus was first isolated from a tick, *Rhipicephalus appendiculatus,* near Thogoto in Kenya, and has caused widespread abortions in ewes. In one flock of some 600 Dorper ewes, more than 200 aborted over a two-month period. (Davies, F. G. & others, *Vet. Record* (1984) **115,** 654.)

THORACIC DUCT is the large lymph vessel which collects the contents of the lymphatics proceeding from the abdomen, hind-limbs, part of the thorax, etc., and which discharges its contents into the left innominate vein. (*See* LYMPHATICS.)

THORACOCENTESIS. Tapping of the fluid found in certain diseases of the chest. (*See* ASPIRATION.)

THORACOTOMY. A surgical operation involving opening of the chest cavity.

THORAX (*see* CHEST).

THORN-APPLE (*see* STRAMOMIUM).

THOROUGH-PIN, is a distension of the sheath of the deep flexor tendon where it passes over the arch of the tarsus (hock). It is characterised by swellings one on either side of the hock, about the level of the 'point of the hock' (summit of the tuber calcis), and lying in front of the strong Achilles' tendon.

THREAD-WORM is a popular term for *oxyuris* worms. (*See* ROUNDWORMS.)

THREONINE. One of the essential amino acids.

THROAT (*see* PHARYNX). Information will also be found under LARYNX, NOSE AND NASAL PASSAGES, MOUTH.

Throat diseases. Most of these will be found under separate headings such as CHOKING; LARYNX, DISEASES OF; TONSILLITIS. For 'sore throat', *see* PHARYNGITIS.

THROMBASTHENIA. This is a rare, congenital disorder of the blood, occurring in man and dogs, in both sexes (compare HAEMOPHILIA). It arises from a defect of the platelets, and gives rise to prolonged bleeding resulting in anaemia. It has been described in foxhounds, otterhounds, etc.

THROMBOCYTOPENIA. A condition of the blood in which the number of platelets is below normal. Causes include viral infections, poisoning, auto-immune disease. The signs *may* include petechial haemorrhages and fever.

This syndrome is being increasingly recognised in veal calves in the USA.

THROMBOSIS. The blocking of a blood vessel by a blood clot. It may follow atheroma, or some injury to the vessel. In cats, thrombosis of the femoral arteries is by no means rare, and causes paralysis of the hind legs and often pain. There is complete absence of pulse in the arteries. In dogs, thrombosis of the iliac and femoral arteries occurs occasionally. Euthanasia is nearly always necessary. (*See also* PARAPLEGIA.)

Aortic-iliac thrombosis is seen in the horse; the worm *Strongylus vulgaris* sometimes being a cause.

Thrombosis of a blood vessel in the brain is a cause of apoplexy (a 'Stroke' in human medicine). (For thrombosis of the vena cava in cattle, *see under* VENA CAVA.) (*See also under* ANTI-COAGULANTS.)

THROMBUS. A blood clot in a blood vessel or the heart.

'THUMPS' is the colloquial name for respiratory symptoms in the pig caused by the migrating larvae of Ascaris worms.

THYMUS GLAND, situated in the anterior part of the chest cavity, attains its largest size during early life and thereafter gradually dwindles. The thymus has a role in immunity. (*See* T. CELLS, which are thymus derived.) (*See* LEUKAEMIA.)

THYROID CARTILAGE is the largest cartilage of the larynx, and forms a well-marked prominence at the upper end of the trachea. It gives attachment to one end of each of the vocal folds, which are concerned in the production of voice. (*See* LARYNX.)

THYROID GLAND. This is a very highly vascular ENDOCRINE GLAND, situated near the thyroid cartilage of the larynx. The gland usually consists of two lobes, one on either side of the larynx, joined by an isthmus in some species and individuals.

Located within or near the thyroid gland are the PARATHYROID GLANDS.

Minute structure. Each lobe is enveloped in a thin capsule of fibrous tissue, strands from which pass into the organ, dividing it into lobules.

Function. The most important hormone secreted by the thyroid gland is an iodine-containing compound called *thyroxin.* This increases the rate of metabolism, and is released when an animal is exposed to cold, for example. In hot weather, thyroid activity is reduced. Thyroxin is essential for growth and reproduction, and influences lactation.

Secretion of the hormone is controlled wholly or in part by a hormone from the anterior lobe of the pituitary gland. (*See also* PARATHYROID GLANDS.)

THYROID GLAND, DISEASES OF. Enlargement of the thyroid gland is known as GOITRE (which see). Goitre may occur when there is either too little or too much of the thyroid hormone, thyroxin, produced.

Dwarfism in young animals ('cretinism') can result from failure of the gland to produce sufficient thyroxin.

Hypothyroidism. An insufficiency of thyroxin is known as *hypothyroidism,* and may be associated with insufficiency of iodine in the diet (*see* GOITRE). The rate of metabolism is slowed, there is an increase in body weight, loss of hair, and lethargy.

One form of hypothyroidism, MYXOEDEMA, affects the skin, causing its deterioration.
TREATMENT includes the use of thyroid extract; and iodides if appropriate.

Hyperthyroidism, or excess thyroxin in the blood, is characterised by loss of weight, sometimes an increase in appetite, polyurea, thirst, increased rate of metabolism and heart beat. Enlargement of the gland may be detected on palpation. The animal may become restless or irritable. Protrusion of the eyeballs ('exophthalmic goitre' may occur).

Hyperthyroidism is seen in elderly cats. They are mostly thin, and it is this loss of weight which causes the owner to seek veterinary advice in many instances. In addition to the symptoms mentioned above, diarrhoea may occur.
TREATMENT is surgical: removal of one gland, or ligation of the anterior arteries; or the use of drugs such as sodium fluoride or methylthiouracil.

Tumours of the gland include ADENOMA, SARCOMA, CARCINOMA, and EPITHELIOMA.

THYROXIN. A hormone secreted by the THYROID gland.

TIAMULIN. A semi-synthetic antibiotic with pronounced *in vitro* activity against *Treponema hyodysenteriae*, various Gram-positive organisms, and *Mycoplasma hyosinoviae* (a cause of arthritis in pigs). (*See also* SALINOMYCIN.)

TIBIA is the larger of the two bones which lie between the stifle and the hock. In animals which possess less than five digits in their hind-limbs the tibia has become modified so that it sustains the greater part of the weight borne by the limb, the fibula, its complementary bone, having become reduced in size and importance. The tibia lies just below the skin on the inside of the limb, in such a position that it is liable to be injured by kicks, blows, etc., and in this connection is of more importance than those bones that are surrounded by massive muscles which afford some protection. It is not uncommon for the tibia to become fractured, but the parts remain held together by the very dense periosteum that covers the bone. In the smaller animals the setting of the fractured bone is a routine. (*See* BONES, FRACTURES.)

Tibial dyschondroplasia. A crippling

deformity occurring in certain strains of chickens, ducks, and turkeys selected for high growth rates. It is due to a cartilage abnormality. (AFRC News, 1989.)

TICKS. These are among the most serious parasites of domestic animals. In the tropics they transmit bacterial, protozoal and viral diseases; in the UK, tick-borne fever, Redwater fever and louping ill.

Some cause illness by means of a toxin, while all feed on the host's blood – which can result in a serious anaemia. Large numbers of ticks also 'worry' the host, and cause unthriftiness. Suppurating wounds may also result.

Life-cycles. On this basis, ticks can be divided into three groups:

1-host ticks, such as *Boophilus*, which spend all three stages of their life-cycle on the same animal. Larvae having attached themselves to the host, they feed on it, moult, feed again on it as nymphs, moult, and the adult ticks also feed on it; the mated females subsequently dropping to the ground to lay their eggs.

2-host ticks. These, such as some *Hyalomma* species, feed both as larvae and nymphs on the same host, but then moult on the ground; emerging adults then finding and feeding on a second house.

3-host ticks. Larva, nymph, and adult each feeds on a different host, with moulting taking place on the ground between each stage in the life-cycle. *Ixodes* and *Dermacentor* species are included in this group.

Family ixodidae, HARD TICKS. In this family the dorsum of the body is more or less protected by a hard shield of chitin, and in some species the male has ventral plates also.

The principal species attacking the domestic animals are dealt with below. (*See also* **dog ticks** for those occurring in Britain.)

IXODES. There are over fifty species in this genus, including the following:

(*a*) *Ixodes ricinus* attacks all the domesticated animals and is found in most parts of the world. It is known locally as the 'castor-bean tick', or 'European sheep tick'. A 'three-host' tick, it leaves its host before each moult, and then seeks a new host. In this way three animals are attacked by the same tick: one as a larva, one as a nymph,

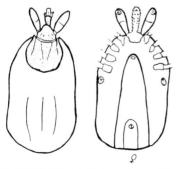

Ixodes. (Dorsal and ventral views of a small female. × 8.) In this and subsequent drawings of ticks only the fore parts of the legs are shown in diagrams of the ventral surface.

and one as an adult. The animals attacked need not be of the same species. This tick transmits 'tick-borne fever' in sheep, louping-ill, and causes 'tick paralysis' in sheep and cattle. It can also transmit *Babesia*, the cause of 'red-water'.

(*b*) *Ixodes hexagonus* attacks especially the dog, but is found on other hosts, notably sheep. It occurs in Europe, North Africa, and America; and is common on hunting dogs in France. In addition it is a transmitter of babesiosis.

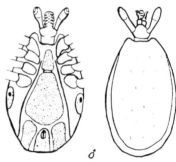

Ixodes. (Ventral and dorsal views of male. × 12.)

(*c*) *Ixodes canisuga* is the common species found on the dog in Britain. It occurs also in Western Europe and North America. Like the last species only females are found on the host. It is known popularly as the British dog tick.

(*d*) *Ixodes pilosus* attacks all the domestic mammals in South Africa. It is a reddish-brown tick, with the body larger behind than in front. It is known locally as 'the russet tick', and is a causal agent of 'tick paralysis'.

(*e*) *Ixodes rubicundus*, another South African tick, which is found only on sheep, also causes 'tick paralysis'.

(*f*) *Ixodes holocyclus*, in Australia and India, is found on ruminants, dogs, and pigs. It is the cause of Australian 'tick paralysis', symptoms of which may appear within an hour of attachment. It transmits Q-fever.

HAEMAPHYSALIS.

The following species are important:

(*a*) *Haemaphysalis punctata* (*H. cinnabarina* var. *punctata*) is a common tick in Europe, North America, and North Africa on all the domestic animals. The life-history is identical with that of *H. leachii*. It transmits *Babesia bovis* in Britain.

(*b*) *H. leachii* is a 3-host African species which has been found in Western Asia and Australia. It attacks carnivores, but is sometimes found on ruminants. In East Africa it is called the yellow dog tick. It is also known as the South African dog tick. It transmits canine babesiosis, Q-fever, and tick-bite fever.

DERMACENTOR.

The following species are important:

(*a*) *D. reticulatus* is common in Europe, but also occurs in North Asia. It attacks ruminants, and also the dog and the horse. It is occasionally found in Western England. It transmits equine and canine babesiosis.

(*b*) *D. variabilis* (*D. electus*) is found on dogs in North America. It also occurs on cattle and horses. It is known as the American dog tick.

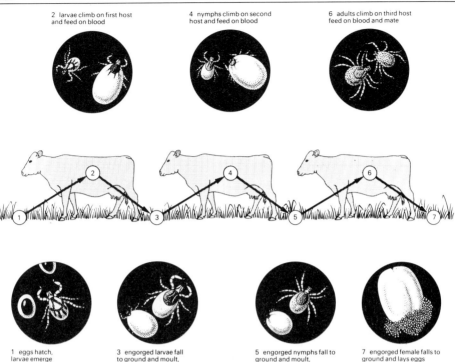

Life cycle of a 3-host tick, *Ixodes ricinus*. Reproduced with permission from H. T. B. Hall, *Diseases and Parasites of Livestock in the Tropics*, Longman.

(*c*) *D. occidentalis* occurs in Western North America on various domestic mammals. It is considered by some authorities to be *D. reticulatus* or *D. venestus*. It is called the Pacific Coast tick.

(*d*) *D. venestus* is found in the Rocky Mountain District of North America. Adults are found on various mammals, including man. It is the transmitter of 'Rocky Mountain spotted fever' in man, and of canine babesiosis. It is the cause of American 'tick paralysis'. It is a 3-host tick.

RHIPICEPHALUS. The following species are important:

(*a*) *R. sanguineus* is found in all parts of the world on dogs and ruminants. It is brown in colour. It is known as the 'European brown tick' and also as the 'European dog tick' – a name shared with *Ixodes hexagonus*.

(*b*) *R. appendiculatus* is found in Africa, where it attacks cattle, sheep, goats. It is called the 'brown tick', and is a 3-host tick.

This species transmits: East Coast Fever, Corridor disease, mild gall sickness, red-water, Nairobi sheep disease.

(*c*) *R. bursa* is found in North Africa and South Europe on all animals. It is a two-host tick. It transmits ovine babesiosis in Europe.

(*d*) *R. capensis* is found in South Africa on cattle, horses and dogs. It is called the 'Cape brown tick'. The life-cycle is similar to the second species. It can transmit *Theileria parva*.

(*e*) *R. simus* is found in Africa on dogs and herbivores. It is called the 'dark pitted tick'. Its life-cycle is similar to the second species. It can transmit: *Theileria parva, Anaplasma marginale, Theileria mutans.*

(*f*) *R. evertsi* in Africa may be found on all the domestic mammals except pigs. It has orange-red legs with round convex distinct eyes. The scutum is black and densely pitted. The under side of the male is red. The females are brown or reddish brown. It is called the red tick or the red-legged tick. This 2-host species transmits: *Nuttallia equi, Theileria parva:* causing East Coast Fever, babesiosis; spirochaetosis.

BOOPHILUS.

(*a*) *B. decoloratus* is found on cattle and other animals in Africa. It is a 1-host tick, called the 'blue tick'.

This tick, which may be a variety of *B. annulatus*, transmits: *Babesia bigemina; Anaplasma marginale;* and *Spirochaeta theileri.*

(*b*) *B. australis* is found in Australia, India, Africa, and Tropical America. It is called the 'Australian blue tick'. It also is probably a variety.

(*c*) *B. annulatus* is the Texas fever tick, and is found in southern North America.

The tick remains on the host for 3 to 9 weeks. It transmits *B. bigemina.*

HYALOMMA. This genus has an oval body with longish pedipalps and distinct eyes.

H. aegyptium is found on all the domestic animals in Africa, Southern Europe, and Asia. It has a brown scutum. Only adults are found on the domestic animals, the younger stages being found on small mammals. It is called the 'striped-leg tick', or the 'bont-leg tick'.

The tick produces ulcerating sores in cattle, and is frequently the cause of lameness in sheep and goats owing to its attachment between the

COMMON TICKS IN EAST AFRICA*

Tick species	Number of hosts	Preferred site of attachment	Animal affected	Parasite	Disease transmitted
Brown-ear tick (*Rhipicephalus appendiculatus*)	3	Ears, base of horns, around eyes, tail brush, and heels	Cattle	*Theileria parva*	East Coast Fever
			Cattle	*Theileria lawrencei*	Corridor disease
			Cattle	*Theileria mutans*	Mild gall-sickness
			Cattle	*Babesta bigemina*	Red-water
			Sheep and goats	Virus	Nairobi sheep disease
			Sheep, cattle, and goats		Louping-ill
			Man	*Rickettsia*	Tick-bite fever
Red-legged tick (*Rhipicephalus evertsi*)	2	Larvae and nymphae in ears. Adults perineal region	Cattle	*Babesia bigemina*	Red-water
			Cattle	*Theileria parva*	East Coast Fever
			Cattle	*Theileria mutans*	Mild gall-sickness
			Horses	*Babesia nuttali* / *Babesia caballi*	Biliary fever
			Cattle, horses sheep, and goats	*Spirochaeta theileri*	Spirochaetosis
			Lambs	?*Tick toxin*	?Paralysis
Yellow dog tick (*Haemaphysalis leachi*)	3	Whole body	Dogs	*Babesia canis*	Biliary fever
			Man and animals	Virus	'Q' fever
			Man	*Rickettsia*	Tick-bite fever
Blue tick (*Boophilus decoloratus*)	1	Face, neck, dewlap, and sides of the body	Cattle	*Babesia bigemina*	Red-water
			Cattle	*Anaplasma marginale*	Gall-sickness
			Man	*Rickettsia*	Tick-bite fever
			Horses, cattle, goats, and sheep	*Spirochaeta theileri*	
Bont tick (*Amblyomma* spp.)	3	Larvae and nymphae on head and ears Nymphae and adults on perineum, udder, scrotum, and tail	Cattle/Sheep/ Goats	*Rickettsia ruminantium*	Heartwater
			Sheep	Virus	Nairobi sheep disease
			Man and animals	Virus	'Q' Fever
			Man	*Rickettsia*	Tick-bite fever
Bont-legged tick (*Hyalomma* spp.)	2 or 3	Adults on perineum, udder, scrotum, and tail brush	Cattle, sheep, goats, and pigs	*Tick toxin*	Sweating sickness
			Man and animals	Virus	'Q' fever
			Man	*Tick toxin*	Tick paralysis
			Man	*Rickettsia*	Tick-bite fever

*Reproduced by courtesy of Cooper, McDougall, & Robertson (East Africa) Ltd.

claws. It is believed to transmit both species of *Theileria*, and equine and bovine babesiosis.

H. truncatum, the African bont-legged tick, is usually a 2-host, occasionally a 3-host parasite. Cattle and goats are the main hosts. It transmits Sweating Sickness and Q fever. A toxin is thought to be produced by this species capable of causing necrosis of skin and mucous membrane at the site of bites as well as some degree of paralysis. A case in a terrier bitch was reported by E. W. Burr (*Veterinary Record* (1983) **113**, 260) in which the necrosis extended from vulva to umbilicus, with exposure of the urethra and much sloughing.

AMBLYOMMA. In this genus the body is broadly oval.

(*a*) *A. hebraeum* is an African tick attacking all the domestic mammals. It has a conspicuously marked scutum, yellowish with a red and blue tinge, and brown or black markings. The eyes are flat and flush with the body. It is called the 'bont tick'.

This species causes ulcerating sores at the points for attachment, and is a frequent cause of sore teats. It conveys heart-water to ruminants.

(*b*) *A. variegatum* is an African species attacking herbivores. It has distinct convex eyes. The scutum is reddish yellow bordered with green with black markings. It is called the 'variegated

tick'. Its life-history is as above. It also transmits heart-water, Nairobi sheep disease, and Q-fever.

A. lepidum, an African 3-host bont tick, apparently transmits no diseases but gives rise to unpleasant sores.

A. gemma, an African 3-host bont tick which infests cattle, camels, and other domestic animals. It can transmit both heartwater and Nairobi sheep disease.

(*c*) *A. cayannense* in South and Central America attacks all the domestic mammals. It is a most vicious biter, and transmits equine nuttalliosis.

(*d*) *A. americanum* is similar to the last species, but the scutum has a silvery white spot, giving it its popular name of the 'lone star tick'.

An American species of Amblyomma transmits *Anaplasma argentinum*.

Family argasidae. SOFT TICKS. This family is distinguished from the hard ticks by the absence of a scutum and by the fact that the males and females are almost indistinguishable. Looked at from above the capitulum is invisible in the adult, whereas in the *Ixodidae* the head is always visible.

Only two genera exist in this family, *Argas* and *Ornithodorus*. The adults do not permanently attach themselves to one host, like the hard ticks, but resemble the bed-bug in habits. The female also generally lays more than one batch of eggs.

Some ticks in this family are carriers of spirochaetal diseases to man and birds.

ARGAS. (a) *Argas persicus* (*A. miniatus*) is the well-known 'Fowl tick', or 'blue bug', or 'tampan'. It is practically cosmopolitan in its distribution.

It is essentially a bird tick; but will bite man and other mammals (horses and cattle) on occasion. It particularly attacks chickens. A large number on a fowl will suck so much blood that the bird will die from anaemia. It is the carrier of fowl spirochaetosis, and fowl piroplasmosis.

The tick normally feeds at night, spending the day in crevices, and accordingly is seldom seen – as is the case with bed-bugs, which also attack chickens. It is easily distinguished from this pest by the presence of eight legs – the bed-bug being an insect, and in consequence having only six legs. The larval tick (seed tick) remains several days on the host, and is more frequently seen. The adults can live for two years without food.

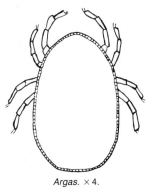

Argas. × 4.

(b) *Argas reflexus*, a closely related species, is found mainly on pigeons, but also attacks poultry and man. It is found in Europe, Africa, and America.

ORNITHODORUS.

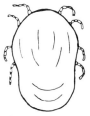

Ornithodorus. × 3.

(a) *Ornithodorus savignyi*, the Sand Tampan, is a soft tick of great economic importance in Africa, Asia, and the Near East. The tick lives below the surface of the sand; emerging to feed on the blood of cattle, other domesticated stock, wild animals, and man. The tick's saliva contains a potent toxin and this, together with massive blood loss, readily kills young or debilitated animals. In field trials, ivermectin has proved a successful means of control. (M. D. Soll *et al.*, *Veterinary Record* (1984) **114**, 70.)

(b) *O. megninii* is the spinose ear tick of America and S. Africa. The larvae creep into the ear of some mammalian host, and in a few days moult. The nymphs, which are covered with minute spines, may live for 1 to 7 months in the ear, increasing in size from ⅛ in to ⅔ in. They finally drop to the ground, moult, mate, lay their eggs, and die. The adult is not parasitic. The eggs hatch in about 10 days. As many as eighty ticks have been found in one ear. The irritation is considerable and heavy losses may result. A modern treatment is IVERMECTIN.

(c) *O. coriaceus* (*pajaroello*) is a venomous species (found in North America) which causes a very painful bite.

Transmission of disease. When an infected tick feeds upon a calf, it transmits the parasites – or causal organisms – of the tick-borne disease in question. The calf soon becomes ill, and either dies or recovers. As a rule, recovery is associated with immunity. However, relapses may occur in animals thought to be immune to Redwater, for example:

Except with ticks of the *Boophilus* species, larvae hatching from a tick's eggs will not immediately be infective because these larvae have not yet fed on any host; but as soon as they start feeding they may ingest the causal organisms of a tick-borne disease. When they moult and become nymphs, they may then be capable of transmitting disease. Similarly, when the nymph, on moulting, becomes an adult tick, it will be infective if there were already parasites in its blood.

Not all tick vectors will transmit all causal organisms; and, of course, not all species of host are susceptible to the same causal organisms.

An infective three-host tick feeding on a non-susceptible host 'cleans' itself of infection and will not transmit disease in the next stage of its life cycle. This fact provides a useful control measure.

The specific parasites transmitted by the ticks are not passed on mechanically, but must undergo a special development in the tick. This is easily understood when it is realised that any one stage in the life-history of a hard tick bites only one animal. Accordingly, a tick infected in one stage must be capable of producing the disease in some succeeding stage, which depends on the tick.

Control of ticks. In many tropical countries energetic measures for the regular and frequent **dipping** of cattle and sheep are necessary. In order to achieve adequate control of the tick-borne diseases, it is important that 'hand-dressing' of certain parts of the body should be carried out in addition to the dipping or spraying. This applies to inside the ears, around the base of the horns, around the eyes, anus, etc.

The acaricides, or tick-killing chemicals, have comprised (1) arsenical compounds, (2) chlorinated hydrocarbon compounds (3) the organo-phosphorus compounds and (4) ivermectin.

Dipwashes containing arsenic are unsuitable for spraying because of the danger of pasture contamination. Although cheap, stable, and soluble, arsenic compounds are very poisonous.

Another disadvantage is that some species of ticks acquire a resistance to arsenic preparations. Accordingly, a change to chlorinated hydrocarbons followed. Of these, BHC and toxaphene have been widely used. Unfortunately, ticks can become resistant to these too; (*and see* BHC.)

Organo-phosphorus compounds tend to be expensive, and are used mostly against ticks resistant to other acaricides. DELNAV may be combined with chlorfenviphos. Coumaphos compounds (e.g. 'Asuntol') and trichlorphon compounds (e.g. 'Neguvon') are all effective acaricides, but must be used with care to avoid poisoning.

For tick control in temperate regions, *see also* DIPS and DIPPING and DOG TICKS.

SYSTEMIC ACARICIDES could have considerable application in cattle raising areas that lack dipping or spraying facilities, or in areas where there is widespread resistance to conventional acaricides. (Pagram, R. G. & Lemche, J., *Veterinary Record* (1985) **117,** 551.)

They carried out field trials in Zambia to assess the efficacy of multiple subcutaneous injections of ivermectin in the control of naturally occurring tick infestations on traditionally managed Tonga-Ila (Sanga type) calves and yearlings. In the first trial *Boophilus decoloratus* infestations were decreased following treatments at monthly intervals. In the second trial, with weekly and two weekly treatment intervals, infestations of *Rhipicephalus appendiculatus* were controlled less effectively than infestations of *Amblyomma variegatum* or *Hyalomma truncatum*. However, no engorging females of any of the tick species were found on treated animals. In treated cattle, significantly greater liveweight gain occurred than can be attributed to the control of tick infestations alone.

In Australia and elsewhere ivermectin has been formulated for use in a slow-release BOLUS for tick control.

TICKS IN BUILDINGS, such as quarantine premises, kennels in the tropics, private houses, etc., can be eradicated by placing a block of 'dry ice' on the floor and closing all doors and windows. Adults, nymphs, and larval ticks will be found, after a time, clustering around this source of CO_2 and can then be easily collected and destroyed. (Captain B. J. Thompson, RAVC, 1969.)

TICK-BITE FEVER of man in Africa.
CAUSE: A RICKETTSIA. Local reactions, swelling of lymph nodes, occur in some individuals. So far as is known, tick-bite fever is not fatal.

The bont tick, bont-legged, blue tick, yellow dog tick, and the brown tick – all common in East Africa – transmit this disease. It can be transmitted to the guinea-pig by inoculation of blood.

TICK-BORNE ENCEPHALITIS (TBE). A dog in Switzerland was suspected of having rabies; but laboratory tests showed that its brain infection was caused by another virus – that causing tick-borne encephalitis (TBE). This occurs in 19 countries in Europe; being especially prevalent in mountainous areas with mainly conifer forest. The virus is transmitted by the sheep/cattle tick *Ixodes ricinus*. The ticks become infected by field mice, voles, shrews, and occasionally moles.

The human illness resembles influenza in its symptoms, with a high fever. This may be followed by meningitis. Mortality is about 1 per cent. The incidence of TBE in Austria has been greatly reduced among forestry workers and farmers by means of a vaccine, the World Health Organisation stated.

In differential diagnosis, the flavivirus causing TBE has to be distinguished from louping ill virus.

TICK-BORNE FEVER OF CATTLE is caused by *Cytoectes* (*Erlichia*) *phagocytophila*, transmitted by the common sheep tick, *Ixodes ricinus*. Symptoms of this infection are high but transient fever, and a considerable reduction in milk yield. Abortion may also occur. Oxytetracycline is used in treatment. (Redwater, caused by *Babesia divergens*, often occurs simultaneously.)

TICK-BORNE FEVER OF SHEEP is a disease transmitted by the tick *Ixodes ricinus*.

Tick-borne fever is a mild febrile disease of sheep in which the essential symptom is a rise in temperature occurring after an incubation period of 4 to 8 days, and lasting about 10 days, when it subsides. During this period (which may be prolonged) there is dullness and listlessness, and a considerable loss of weight may occur. Death occurs in only a small percentage of cases; most sheep recover unless some other complicating condition such as louping-ill supervenes. Abortion is an important result of infection in many instances, and may affect 50 per cent of breeding stock introduced from tick-free areas.

Rickettsiae can be demonstrated in the polymorphonuclear white cells of the blood.

The importance of tick-borne fever is that it is capable of rendering the vasculo-meningeal barrier of the central nervous system vulnerable to the virus of louping-ill, while without its presence, though the louping-ill virus may be introduced into the blood-stream (by the bite of a tick) it cannot pass this barrier to attack the nerve cells and so produce the typical nervous symptoms. It has been shown that both infective agents – that of tick-borne fever and of louping-ill – frequently exist together in ticks found on animals on farms where louping-ill is common, and it is probable that under natural conditions the great majority of adult sheep on such farms have been infected with tick-borne fever infection and have recovered.

Tick-borne fever increases the susceptibility of lambs to **tick pyaemia**, often caused by infection with *Staphylococcus aureus* following tick bites. Abscesses occur in the joints and elsewhere, causing lameness, unthriftiness, and death.

TICK PARALYSIS affects man, cattle, sheep, horses, pigs, dogs, cats, and poultry.

It occurs in Africa, Australia, and Canada. It is caused by the presence on the animal of various species of *Ixodes* (especially the dog tick) in South Africa and Australia, and *Dermacentor* in America. In East Africa, the bont-legged tick

(*Hyalomma spp.*) and possibly the Red tick (*Rhipicephalus evertsi*) cause paralysis.

The paralysis is caused by toxin(s) present in the saliva of ticks.

In human beings, 3 or 4 days after the ticks attach themselves, paralysis of the legs occurs, then paralysis of the arms takes place, later the chest and neck become involved, and ultimately the heart and respiratory centres are attacked. In the sheep, the parts are affected in the same general sequence.

This form of paralysis is peculiar in that symptoms disappear in from 2 to 6 days after the ticks are removed, and recovery takes place subsequently. Individual lambs, for example, can be reinfected and recover more than once, if the ticks are removed by hand. They are usually not easily seen unless a deliberate search is made in the wool over the vertebral column from the base of the skull back to the tail.

In the dog, they may cause QUADRIPLEGIA.

TICK PYAEMIA (*see under* TICK-BORNE FEVER OF SHEEP).

TIMBER (*see* WOOD PRESERVATIVES, BEDDING – pigs, dogs and cats).

TINCTURE is an alcoholic solution, *e.g.* tincture of iodine.

TINEA (*see* RINGWORM).

TISSUE CULTURE VACCINES (*see* VACCINES).

TISSUES OF THE BODY include five groups:

(1) *Epithelial tissues*, including the cells covering the skin, those lining the alimentary canal, those forming the glands, etc. (*See* EPITHELIUM.)

(2) *Connective tissues*, including fibrous tissue, fat, bone, and cartilage. (*See* these headings.)

(3) *Muscular tissues* (*see* MUSCLES).

(4) *Nervous tissues* (*see* NERVES).

(5) *Fluid tissues*. (*See* BLOOD, LYMPH.)

TITRE. The extent to which an antibody-containing biological substance can be diluted before losing its power of reacting with a specific antigen. 'High titres' indicate, in practical terms, that a patient's blood serum contains high levels of antibody, *e.g.* to the rabies virus.

TOADFISH (Puffer Fish), if eaten, can cause paralysis in cats. (*See* Atwell, R. B. and Stutchbury, G. B. *Austr. Vet. J1* (1978), **54**, 308.)

TOADS have a defensive venom which is secreted by skin-glands and by the parotid salivary gland. The principal toxic substance is BUFOTALIN (which see). Symptoms of poisoning in the dog are profuse vomiting followed by the emission of ropy saliva and by loss of consciousness, which may persist for a couple of hours. Adrenalin has been used in treatment.

The Central American toad, *Eufo marinas*, is very large, and has a powerful venom which can cause prostration, convulsions, and death within 15 minutes.

TOADSTOOLS. A MAFF V.I. Centre found that the death of a cairn terrier was due to the eating of *Nolanea sericeum* toadstools growing on a lawn. Death occurred within three hours.

SIGNS of poisoning by this fungus are severe vomiting and abdominal pain.

TOBACCO (*see* NICOTINE). Stalks of tobacco plants fed to pigs have resulted in piglets born with limb deformities.

TOCOPHEROL. Vitamin E.

TOES, CURLY ('CURLY TOE DISEASE', 'CURLED TOE PARALYSIS') is a condition arising in chicks from a deficiency of riboflavin. The toes curl underneath the feet. (*See* VITAMINS.)

TOES, TWISTED ('CROOKED TOES'). A condition also seen in chicks; one or more toes twisting inwards or outwards. There is, at least, a hereditary disposition to this abnormality, but it may occur in *temporary* and *reversible* form where infra-red brooders are in use.

TOGAVIRUSES. Formerly known as Arboviruses, this group includes ALPHAVIRUSES, BUNYAVIRUSES, FLAVIVIRUSES, ORBIVIRUSES, and PESTIVIRUSES. (*See* VIRUSES table.)

TOMOGRAPHY. Body section radiography. (*See* EMI SCANNER.)

-TOMY is a suffix indicating an operation by cutting.

TONGUE (*see also* MOUTH) is a muscular and fibrous organ, richly supplied with blood-vessels and nerves, and covered with a highly specialised mucous membrane. Its shape varies in the different animals, but in all it consists of a free part or 'tip', a middle part, the 'body', and a hinder part, the 'root'. In the horse the tongue is long and spatulate, with a blunt tip, freely movable, and there is a definite narrowing just behind the tip. In the ox the tip is short, and pointed or conical; mobility and pliability are not so great; and on the upper surface is a hump-like eminence or 'dorsum', divided from the tip by a distinct, deep, transverse groove. The dorsum is of the greatest use in swallowing, and in bringing the small balls of cud from the back of the mouth forward for chewing by the cheek teeth.

TONGUE, DISEASES OF (*see under* MOUTH, DISEASES OF; SALIVATION; RANULA; 'CURLED TONGUE' in turkey poults).

Condition of the tongue. The tongue of any animal in health should be of a pink glistening appearance, soft and moist to the touch in the horse, sheep, pig, and dog; rough in the cow and cat. (There are a few breeds of dogs, such as the chow, in which the tongue is normally black or bluish.) When handled the tongue should possess a considerable power of retraction; a weak flabby tongue usually indicates general muscular weakness. When at rest the tongue should touch the inner edges of all the lower teeth. When it becomes greatly swollen it presses against the teeth and these leave indentations around its margin. In cattle there is a raised part or 'dorsum', behind the free tip, which is instrumental in forming the food into boli for swallowing.

Inflammation of the tongue (*Glossitis*) is usually accompanied by SALIVATION, and may result from injuries, irritant or corrosive poisons, infections, and vitamin deficiencies.

Glossitis may be accompanied by the formation of vesicles which burst, leaving ulcerated areas. (*See* FOOT-AND-MOUTH DISEASE, SWINE VESICULAR DISEASE.) Ulcers are also a symptom of CATTLE PLAGUE, MUCOSAL DISEASE, ORF in sheep. FELINE CALICIVIRUS and FELINE RHINOTRACHEITIS VIRUS may cause tongue ulcers in the cat; likewise FELINE ENTERITIS.

Raised irregular swellings or abscesses on the tongues of cattle suggest ACTINOBACILLOSIS.

Ulcers along the free edges of the tongue may be produced by diseased teeth.

In the disease called 'calf diphtheria', the tongue may be the seat of raised areas of false membrane which will also be seen in other parts of the mouth.

The tongue may be injured or wounded from too severe a bit in the horse, or from carelessness in breaking in a young colt. In such cases there is usually a distinct mark across the tongue's upper surface, behind which the organ appears normal, and in front of which it is reddened and swollen.

Foreign bodies, such as fish-hooks, needles, wire, splinters of bone, etc., may become fixed in the tongue, and lead to protrusion of the organ, difficulty in swallowing, salivation, and a disinclination on the part of the animal to allow of the mouth being handled or examined.

In canine LEPTOSPIROSIS/kidney failure there are often areas of necrosis around the tip (which may slough off) and a foul odour.

A brown discoloration may be present in the above condition. (*See also* BROWN MOUTH.) A soapy-white appearance of the tongue, again accompanied by an unpleasant odour, often indicates some digestive disorder. (*See also* 'BLACK TONGUE', BLUETONGUE (a specific disease of sheep and cattle), MYOTONIA *under* MUSCLES, DISEASES OF; *and* ASPHYXIA.)

'TONGUE WORM' is the colloquial name for *Linguatula serrata*, a parasite of the nose of the dog and other animals. (*See* MITES.)

TONIC means, in one sense, a continuous muscular spasm, as compared with CLONIC. (*See also* TONICS.)

TONICS. Generally tonics are most useful when given during the convalescent stages of debilitating diseases, fevers, and during recovery from starvation, exhaustion, overwork, haemorrhage, etc.

Vitamin supplements are most valuable (though overdosage can be extremely harmful).

Various bitters such as ginger, gentian, and malt, stimulate appetite.

Liver extracts, iron compounds, and certain phosphates are used as tonics in anaemia and debility. Turning out to grass is in itself a tonic to animals which have been confined indoors. (*See also under* HEART TONICS, PROTEIN, HYDROLISED; VITAMINS.)

TONSILS are collections of lymphoid tissue, situated between the anterior and posterior pillars of the soft palate at the back of the throat. In the horse there is not a compact tonsil, as in man, the dog, etc., but a diffuse collection of lymphoid tissue, mucous glands, etc., causing elevations on the surface, in which are seen the numerous depressions or crypts which characterise the tonsil and differentiate it from other lymphoid tissue. In the sheep the tonsil is bean-shaped and does not project into the throat, as in most other animals. In health, the dog's tonsils are not conspicuous, being situated in a depression; but when inflamed they appear as two bright red lumps.

TONSILLITIS. Inflammation of the tonsils, a symptom of, *e.g.* canine virus hepatitis. The dog may retch or cough, and be slightly feverish.

TOOTHACHE (*see* TEETH, DISEASES OF).

TOPICAL APPLICATIONS of a drug are those made locally to the outside of the body.

TOPPING OF PASTURES. This practice is beneficial from a veterinary point of view in that it is unfavourable to the survival of parasitic worm larvae.

TORSION, or twisting, occasionally involves the intestine (*see* VOLVULUS); the pedicle of the spleen; the stomach; uterus; and spermatic cords.

TORTICOLLIS. A lateral deviation of the neck.

TORTOISES. In Britain an amendment to the Endangered Species Act, in 1982, required that every buyer of tortoises must sign an undertaking to provide them with appropriate care, attention, and living quarters necessary for their survival. Failure to comply can result in a fine of up to £400 for an offending supplier, pet trader, or private individual. This little piece of legislation may help to mitigate the extremely high mortality of tortoises imported into this country, often due to their being crammed into unsuitable containers for their journey here and badly looked after subsequently.

It has been suggested that outbreaks of viral disease are present among tortoises (*Testudo* species) in the Mediterranean region.

Imported tortoises should be carefully examined for the presence of exotic ticks.

Tortoises and turtles have been known to infect dogs, cats, and people with salmonellosis. (*See also* AMERICAN BOX TORTOISES, PETS.)

For euthanasia, an injection into the abdomen of pentobarbitone sodium is recommended.

TORTOISESHELL CATS, MALE. Although nearly all tortoiseshell cats are female, males do occasionally occur. It appears that the most common chromosome complements are 39XXY, 38XY/38XX, 38XY/39XXY and 38XY/38XY. A 38XY is needed for the cat to be fertile. (S. E. Long & others. *Research in Veterinary Science* (1981) **30**, 274).

TOUCH. This sense depends upon receptors at the end of nerves, or upon the nerve endings themselves.

Touch sense proper, by which touches or strokes are perceived, such as the lightest sensation caused by a fly settling on the skin; the size and shapes of bodies in contact with the skin which are not seen is also appreciated by this sense. *Pressure sense*, by which the weight of heavy objects and their hardness can be determined.

Heat sense, by which the heat of the surrounding atmosphere, or of bodies in contact with the skin, is appreciated as being above that of body temperature. (Receptors for warmth in the human body number about 16,000 as compared with 150,000 for detecting cold.)

Cold sense.

Pain sense.

Muscle sense, by which the weight of an object can be tested, and the amount of energy necessary for an effort can be gauged.

Sense of position, by which, without using the powers of vision, the attitude and position of any part of the body is known.

The distribution of the sense organs which are concerned with the reception of these sensations is very widespread. There is no part of the surface of the body, except the horns, hoofs and claws, which can be cut without giving evidence of pain, and there is no part, including horny structures, which is insensible to touch.

Pain is detected, it seems, by free nerve endings in the layers of the skin, connective tissue, and cornea. The sense of touch is apparently dependent upon Meissner's corpuscles, situated under the epidermis; upon Merkel's discs in tongue, lips, muzzle. Tactile hairs on muzzle, etc., function through free nerve endings surrounding the hair follicle. Pacinian corpuscles in connective tissue, penis, clitoris, etc., react to pressure and contact. Receptors for heat and cold are named Ruffini's corpuscles and Krause endbulbs, respectively. (*See also* SKIN, HYPERAESTHESIA, PARALYSIS.)

TOURNIQUET is an appliance for the temporary stoppage of the circulation in a limb or appendage of the body, for use only in very severe haemorrhage. Application of a tourniquet is a risky procedure, best not undertaken by the animal-owner unless raising the limb and application of a pressure pad has failed to control the haemorrhage, which appears to be endangering the animal's life; and to be avoided on cats.

In emergencies, a handkerchief may be tied round the part, the knot being arranged above the principal artery, and a rigid object, piece of wood, pencil, etc., used to twist the loose part up tightly.

A tourniquet must not be left in position round a limb for longer than 20 minutes, or gangrene of the lower part will result. Occasionally, a circular bruise may occur under a tourniquet, especially in the limbs of horses; this, after healing, leaving a ring of white hair marking the place where the tourniquet was applied. Such a circular mark is due to a destruction of the pigmentary apparatus of the hair follicles. (*See also* BLEEDING, ARREST OF.)

TOXAEMIA. The presence of toxins in the bloodstream.

TOXAPHENE. An insecticide which remains active for a long time on the hair of cattle, and of value against ticks also.

TOXASCARIS (*see under* TOXOCARA).

'TOXIC FAT SYNDROME' of broiler chickens, mainly between 3 and 10 weeks old, has occurred in the USA and Britain. It is associated with oedema of the pericardium and abdomen, a waddling gait, squawking, laboured breathing, and sudden death. Mortality may reach 95 per cent. Recently it has been seen in chicks only a few days old.

This condition has to be differentiated from Roundheart disease, which usually occurs sporadically among older birds and is not associated with the feeding of fat-supplemented rations.

TOXICOLOGY (*see* POISONS).

TOXINS are poisons produced in animal tissues, by some bacteria, ticks, and fungi. Waste products, not removed from the body during liver or kidney failure, are also sometimes referrred to as toxins. (*See* TETANUS, BOTULISM, TICKS, MYCOTOXICOSIS, VENOM, TOXOID, MOULDY FOOD.)

TOXOCARA. A genus of roundworms which includes *Toxocara canis*, a parasite of dog and fox, *T. cati*, and *T. vitulorum* of cattle (the last-named not present in the UK). Infection with these worms is known as **Toxocariasis.** This is important not only from the veterinary aspect but also as regards public health, since Toxocara worm larvae cause *visceral larva migrans* in man.

In dogs *T. canis* is primarily a parasite of the young puppy, which commonly becomes infected before birth by larvae crossing the bitch's placenta. Post-natal infection may occur through the milk. During the first few weeks of the puppy's life, the life-cycle of Toxocara is completed; adult worms being found in the intestine. (In severe infestations, complete impaction of the bowel has been known to occur in puppies as young as seven weeks.)

Larvae acquired prenatally from the bitch arrive in the puppy's intestine within three days of birth, and mature at about the ninth day. Egg production begins when the puppy is about two months old. The number of worm eggs excreted by the puppy may be as many as 15,000 per g of faeces.

As the puppy becomes older, the degree of infestation diminishes. It seems that larvae from ingested eggs migrate within the tissues but are unable to complete the life-cycle. Some of these larvae must remain viable, or prenatal infection could not occur in succeeding generations. However, Dr Dennis Jacobs has stated that 'mature male dogs are more likely to carry patent infection than adult bitches.' The lactating bitch apparently experiences a hormonal suppression of immunity, resulting in a brief patent infection of *T. canis* from larvae formerly arrested in somatic tissues. Dr R. A. W. Girdwood found that of 740 unwanted Glasgow dogs examined after euthanasia, just under 21 per cent carried *T. canis*.

CONTROL. This is, unfortunately, dependent upon what action dog-owners take or fail to take. Several anthelmintics are effective against the adult worm; notably piperazine. Dr R. Herd has advised: 'Start treating pups at two weeks old, before eggs are passed in the faeces, and at 3, 6, and 8 weeks.' Many owners do not seek professional advice, and either use no anthelmintic at all or an unsuitable one. Some rely on grated carrot or garlic!

The BSAVA recommends that the nursing bitch should be dosed when the puppies are two, four, six and eight weeks old. Adult dogs should be wormed every two to three months. A 'recently introduced worming preparation' is safe to use in the bitch from day 40 of pregnancy and for the first three weeks of nursing, as well as the above recommended ages.

In Kittens, kidney damage, sometimes severe, may affect the glomeruli of the kidneys, as a result of larvae of *T. cati*.

Public health. Toxocara eggs are sticky and readily adhere to children's hands, blankets, dog baskets, etc., but fortunately the eggs are not immediately infective when excreted in canine faeces but require a period of weeks to become so. Research in America has shown that two larval moults occur before hatching of the egg, so the infective stage is the *third*-stage larva. (Dr R. Herd. *JAVMA* (1979) **174**, 180.)

The danger of transmission lies in the fact that the eggs are very resistant and can survive for long periods in the soil. Garden soil, and that of parks, playing fields, and grass verges, is an important source of eggs and larvae. One survey showed that (in Great Britain) 24·4 per cent of soil samples from public parks contained Toxocara eggs. (O. A. Borg & A. W. Woodruff. *Brit Med. J.* (1973) **4**, 470.) That figure is far higher than indicated by other surveys, in which soil sampling in parks and playing-fields have given a figure of about 7 per cent for viable Toxocara eggs.

Children can easily become infected through not washing their hands after contamination by such eggs – many of which will have undergone development rendering them infective. The World Health Organisation (WHO) has stated: 'Many patients with proven toxocariasis have not owned or had close contact with a dog or cat,' but have become infected from eggs in soil. Moreover, 'even though Toxocara eggs are unlikely to mature on an animal's coat, infective eggs from the soil may adhere to the hair so that contact with it can lead to infection.' (WHO Technical Report 637, *Parasitic Zoonoses*, 1979.)

PREVALENCE IN MAN. Human toxocariasis is encountered throughout the world. Surveys have demonstrated that about 2 per cent of people over 10 years old in London, and over 30 per cent in various African cities, showed a positive reaction to a Toxocara skin test.

A medical/veterinary team compared the results of blood tests made on 102 dog-breeder volunteers, at the 1977 Windsor championship dog show, with samples from 922 non-dog-breeders. Antibodies to *T. canis* were found in over 15 per cent of the dog-breeders' samples, as compared with only 2·6 per cent of the controls.

Visceral larva migrans affects, states WHO, mainly children between 18 months and three years of age. Tumours – eosinophilic granulomata – are formed in organs such as the liver, lungs, eye, and occasionally the brain. In some patients blindness is caused; in others the symptoms may resemble those of asthma or epilepsy. Debility and occasionally partial paralysis may occur. Eosinophilia is usually present.

About 50 cases of ocular toxocariasis are reported each year in England and Wales.

A young woman, who had kept dogs and rabbits for many years, presented with blurred vision in one eye in April 1977. This condition was treated with corticosteroids. In the November she developed a transient swelling and stiffness of the right elbow and the left ankle and wrist. Between January 1978 and January 1979 she suffered repeated episodes of choroiditis in the left eye and arthralgia. A toxocaral fluorescent antibody test was positive and after treatment with diethylcarbamazine citrate her symptoms subsided. (Williams, D. & Roy, S., *British Medical Journal* (1981) **283**, 192.)

Apart from the skin test already mentioned, an indirect immuno-fluorescent test or the ELISA test may be used in human medicine for diagnosis. Diagnosis of Toxocara affecting the eye may be difficult. In a case described by Professor Norman Ashton FRS, fragments of a larva were not found until the 186th section of an eye had been made.

TOXOID. A toxin which has been rendered non-toxic by physical or chemical means, while retaining its antigenic properties. An example is TETANUS toxoid for immunisation.

TOXOPLASMA EYE INFECTION IN HORSES. The first UK case of this was reported in 1991. SIGNS: Inflammation and degeneration of the retina and of the sclera ('white of the eyeball'). (Turner, C. B. & Dr Sava, D (University of Reading.) *Veterinary Record* (1991).)

TOXOPLASMOSIS. This is a disease of man and of most warm-blooded animals. CAUSE. A coccidian (*see* COCCIDIOSIS) parasite, *Toxoplasma gondii*, closely related to the genus *Isospora*. The reproductive cells (gametes) form in the intestine of cats (and probably of other members of the cat family).

Cats (and other carnivores) can become infected through the ingestion of the cystozoites within cysts in the muscles of their prey; or they can – like other animals and man – become

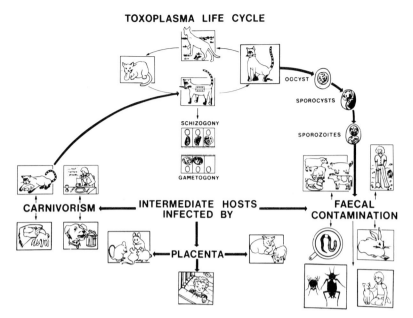

TOXOPLASMA LIFE CYCLE

OOCYST

SPOROCYSTS

SPOROZOITES

SCHIZOGONY

GAMETOGONY

CARNIVORISM ← INTERMEDIATE HOSTS → FAECAL
                    INFECTED BY   CONTAMINATION

← PLACENTA →

infected by oocysts present in feline faeces. (The oocysts can survive outside the body for 17 months). Dr W. M. Hutchison, University of Strathclyde, has commented: 'There seems to be little doubt that the ingestion of oocysts constitutes the major source of human urban toxoplasmosis in the United Kingdom.'

Toxoplasma gondii has been isolated from the milk of bitches, cows, ewes, and sows, and it has been shown that the young of these may be born already infected. The parasite can live in ticks and lice, so that the spread of toxoplasmosis by these is not unlikely. The parasite has been recovered from the semen of rams.

For diagnosis, laboratory techniques are essential e.g. using Sabin-Feldman dye, latex agglutination tests.

Sheep. After ingestion of feed or water contaminated with *Toxoplasma* oocysts, susceptible (seronegative) sheep become, and remain, infected for life. Infection of the ovine placenta and conceptus occurs only when the initial infection establishes in susceptible pregnant sheep, following ingestion of oocysts. The oocysts excyst in the digestive tract and the released sporozoites penetrate the cells lining the gut so that tachyzoites eventually reach and infect the placenta and fetus.

Infection in very early pregnancy causes fetal resorption and the ewes subsequently appear to be barren, while infection between about 50 and 120 days gestation presents the clinical picture typical of the disease, with the premature birth of stillborn and weakly lambs, outwardly of quite normal appearance, often accompanied by a mummified fetus.

Goats. Toxoplasmosis causes abortion and perinatal mortality similar to that seen in sheep. Goats also appear to stay infected for life, but experiments carried out in the USA suggest that, unlike sheep, they may, in subsequent pregnancies, pass infection on to their kids in utero and

may even abort with overt toxoplasmosis more than once. Infection can spread also via semen and milk but the relative importance of these two routes within a herd is uncertain, as is the risk to humans ingesting milk from infected goats.

SIGNS. Toxoplasmosis may be sub-clinical – no symptoms being shown, but a degree of immunity being acquired; or the infection may give rise to very varied symptoms which, in different cases, have included coughing, distressed breathing, mastitis, abortion, still-births, diarrhoea, and encephalitis.

A report in the *Australian Veterinary Journal* stated that 7 out of 48 penned **ewes** aborted because of infection with *Toxoplasma gondii.* They had been eating grain contaminated by faeces from cats which lived in the feed shed.

In a Canadian farm outbreak only 12 out of 50 chicken, reared indoors, survived three months after being turned out into the farmyard for the summer. Antibodies to Toxoplasma were found in the chickens, in 23 out of 24 of the cows, in all the farm cats, a mare, the farmer, his wife and daughter, but not their son. The source of infection in this outbreak was considered to be wild birds, many of which had been found dead around the farmyard.

Cats. The infection is often subclinical. Acute feline toxoplasmosis may prove fatal, a few days after symptoms such as a high fever, lethargy, loss of appetite, and dyspnoea. Chronic toxoplasmosis is often a relapsing disease, with loss of appetite, anaemia, nervous symptoms, abortion or sterility. Heart disease and liver disease may be found. The fever does not respond to antibiotics. Dyspnoea may be seen in the terminal stages. (Margaret Petrak & others. *JAVMA* (1965) **146,** 728).

Public health. Probably all practising veterinary surgeons, and many cat-owners, have had antibodies to Toxoplasma in their blood serum;

yet of these people probably only a small percentage were ever *ill* as a result of the infection though a proportion may have suffered malaise.

The World Health Organisation (WHO) has stated that the only real danger to human health appears to be (1) acute, generalised toxoplasmosis, especially in patients undergoing immunosuppressive therapy: and (2) congenital infection which can lead to miscarriage, stillbirth, or abnormality in the baby.

Dr D. Reid commented at the 1979 environmental health conference held at the University of Dundee: 'My impression is that the small number of clinical cases which are reported in man are only the tip of the iceberg. Although second to rubella as a cause of human embryopathy, congenital toxoplasmosis occurs in only one infant in 2500. In these it causes a 12-per-cent case-fatality rate,' and leaves many survivors with severe eye or brain disability. (*Veterinary Record* (1979) **104**, 331.)

In the USA 3000 of the 3 million babies born each year are reckoned to have congenital toxoplasmosis, but many of the babies are well or only mildly affected.

Medical opinion is that pregnant women should be advised against eating or handling raw or undercooked meat, and should not themselves empty cat litter trays. (*Lancet* (1980) **1**, 578.)

There is danger for the baby only if the mother becomes infected *during* pregnancy; if infected previously there is no such danger.

The immunosuppression occurring in AIDS has resulted in some deaths from toxoplasmosis. (*See* AIDS.)

A family outbreak of Toxoplasmosis, attributed to the eating of lamb served rare, was described by Henry Masur et al. (*American Journal of Medicine* (1978) **64**, 396.) The husband suffered fatigue, malaise, muscle pains, headache and fever. After 11 days in hospital, he was discharged; the cause of his illness undetermined. Some weeks later toxoplasmosis was diagnosed, following an immuno-fluorescent test. A complement fixation test and a Sabin-Feldman dye test were also positive. Three months later an eye lesion affecting the retina was discovered. Treatment involved the use of prednisone, sulfadiazine, and pyrimethamine, but while the lesion decreased in size, vision was not restored to normal. The wife's illness left her tired and lethargic for nearly 10 weeks, with weakness, fever and a rash. Neck swelling, with lymph node enlargement, was a feature of illness in two boys. The family had no pet animals.

TRABECULA. A band of fibrous tissue.

TRACE ELEMENTS are those of which minute quantities are essential for the maintenance of health in animals (or plants). They include: iron, manganese, iodine, cobalt, copper, magnesium, zinc, selenium. (*See under* HYPOMAGNESAEMIA, PIGLET ANAEMIA, PINING, IODINE, HYPOCUPRAEMIA, PEROSIS, ZINC, SALT LICKS.) Calcium and phosphorus are also needed, but in much larger quantities than is the case with trace elements. (*See also* VITAMIN E.)

TRACHEA is another name for the windpipe. (*See* AIR PASSAGES.)

Foreign bodies have included a spanner in a dog's trachea; a chip of stone in a cat; a snail; and – not strictly 'foreign' – a cat's own tooth. An incision into the trachea, to admit an endoscope from the outside, was necessary in this last case.

TRACHEA, DISEASES OF. These include hypoplasia, with a narrow lumen – a congenital defect in several breeds of dogs.

SIGNS: A chronic moist cough, wheezing, dyspnoea, aversion to exercise. (Van Pelt, R. W. *Veterinary Medicine* (1988) March 266)

TRACHEAL WORMS. In the dog, infestation with the worm *Filaroides osleri* gives rise to a persistent cough, and sometimes to retching. The cough may be like that in 'Kennel Cough', and hoarse. This disease occurs in Britain. Diagnosis depends on use of an endoscope (which can reveal the characteristic pink nodules), or of X-rays. Treatment can be successful, using an appropriate anthelmintic, *e.g.* oxfendazole.

Another tracheal worm, which seldom gives rise to symptoms, is *Capillaria aerophilia*. (*See also under* COUGH.)

TRACHEITIS. Inflammation of the trachea. The trachea may be severely damaged as the result of a dog fight, involving bites of the neck. (*See also above.*)

TRACHEOSTOMY refers to an artificial opening into the trachea, and is usually taken to include the insertion of a tracheostomy tube to overcome nerve dysfunction. **Tracheotomy** is the surgical procedure of creating a tracheostomy, although some authors use these words interchangeably.

Severe upper respiratory obstruction presents as an anxious, sweating horse with possibly stridulous breathing noises at rest, flared nostrils, extended neck, increased costo-abdominal respiratory effort, cyanosis and functioning accessory muscles of respiration. Particularly if the last two signs are present, a **temporary tracheostomy** is imperative.

Permanent tracheostomy. A tracheostomy tube is used to by-pass a permanent upper airway obstruction. A permanent tracheostomy is most commonly used in performance animals to by-pass performance limiting, less severe respiratory obstruction eg, cases of laryngeal paralysis non responsive to conventional surgery. The term permanent tracheostomy is not absolute because for ease of management many owners request the removal of 'permanent' tracheostomy tubes at the end of each working season, with its replacement at the beginning of the following season.

Thirty-four cases of permanent tracheostomy involving eleven dogs and 23 cats were reviewed. The pet-owners assessed the results as good in 16, and fair in 6, cases. The most common post-operative problem was occlusion of the trachea by a fold of skin. (Medlund, C. S. & others. *JAVMA* (1989) **24**, 585.)

A surgical accident. Abscesses due to *Strep-*

tococcus equi caused upper airway obstruction in a 2-month-old Standardbred foal. Unfortunately, while attempting surgical relief, four mid-cervical tracheal rings were completely severed. This led to dyspnoea and a loud respiratory noise even with mild exercise; and an endoscopic examination showed that the lumen of the trachea was now key-shaped for a distance of 6 cm.

When six months old, the foal was referred to the Ohio State University veterinary hospital, where it was found that the severed ends of the four tracheal rings had not healed but were connected solely by fibrous tissue.

In order to effect repair, a prosthesis was made by cutting in half longitudinally a 60-ml syringe, and then cutting segments 2 to 5 cm in length, with 2-mm holes drilled to take sutures.

Two ¾-thickness incisions were made transversely at 1-cm intervals in each ring on both sides of the defect, and sutures placed, avoiding penetration of the tracheal mucosa.

Nine days after surgery, endoscopy showed the tracheal lumen to be nearly normal and the mucous membrane free from inflammation. Ten months later the surgical site was normal. As a 2-year-old the colt was raced successfully, a tribute to the technique of Drs James Robertson and G. H. Spurlock of the Ohio State University.

TRACHEOTOMY is indicated when some foreign body has gained entrance into the trachea or larynx and hinders the flow of air; it relieves breathing when an abscess develops at the back of the throat in strangles in horses, and threatens to occlude the passages; it is also undertaken in oedema of the glottis; in roaring; and in other conditions.

An incision is made into the trachea, through the skin and muscles, usually in the middle line (in cattle sometimes at the side), and a tracheotomy tube is inserted and fixed in place.

The air in the stable must be kept as clean and free from dust as possible, and during foddering or bedding operations a plug should be put into the tube to prevent pieces of chaff, hay seeds, etc., from getting drawn in by the inspired air.

TRACHOMA (*see* EYE, DISEASES OF).

TRACK LEG. A condition seen in the racing greyhound. There is a swelling of the triceps muscle or the semitendinosus muscle – due to sprain. Prolonged rest is necessary.

TRAINING (*see* MUSCLES, EXERCISE).

TRANQUILLISERS. This term usually implies drugs which reduce anxiety without inducing sleep or drowsiness. They include phenothiazine derivatives ('Pacatal' and 'Nutinal' are proprietary examples) and are used in veterinary practice to calm or restrain vicious or nervous animals; to obviate travel sickness; and to facilitate the induction of anaesthesia. Their use is not permitted at Kennel Club shows.

(For horses, *see* DETOMIDINE.)

In human medicine, some tranquillisers which were stated to be safe have been proved dangerous in practice, *e.g.* methylpentynol and meprobomate, thalidomide.

Tranquillisers have been administered to cattle, zoo and wild animals, by firing a hypodermic syringe from a cross-bow, gun, or blow-pipe. (*See* DART GUNS; *see also* SEDATION OF PIGS, ROMPUN, AVICALM.)

Natural tranquillisers. At the Institute of Animal Physiology, during investigation of the hormones contained in extracts of ovarian tissue, several steroids have been found which exert a strong sedative effect on the central nervous system. Variations in secretion rates of these steroids during the reproductive cycle may be partly responsible for cyclic variations in behaviour, states the AFRC. Slight tranquility could occur when the blood concentration of the steroids is relatively high; restlessness or even aggressiveness might result from a low concentration.

TRANSFERABLE RESISTANCE (*see under* ANTIBIOTIC RESISTANCE, PLASMIDS).

TRANSFERRIN. A β-globulin present in blood plasma and acting as a carrier of iron. Transferrin is an ideal protein for blood typing. (*See also* IRON, EQUINE BLOOD TYPES, BLOOD TYPING.)

TRANSFUSION OF BLOOD (*see under* BLOOD TRANSFUSION).

TRANSGENIC ANIMALS. Those bred by 'genetic engineering' methods involving the isolation of genes from one animal, modification of them in the laboratory, and introduction of them into animals of the same or different species. (AFRC). (*See also* RETROVIRUSES.)

TRANSIT OF ANIMALS (Road and Rail) ORDER, 1975, lays down certain rules concerning the humane treatment of farm animals and horses and the standard of vehicles used.

TRANSIT TETANY is the result of HYPOCALCAEMIA. It is mostly seen in lactating mares, about 10 days after foaling or a day or two after weaning. It can also occur, it has been said, in fillies and colts, though rarely; so alternative names such as lactation tetany or eclampsia may not be entirely appropriate. It is no longer common.

CAUSE. The stress of transport over long distances is regarded as the precipitating cause.

SIGNS. These vary according to the extent to which the blood calcium level is reduced. A slight reduction causes the mare to be excitable; but a further fall produces muscular incoordination and staggering, and the animal appears obviously distressed. Sweating may occur; rapid and noisy breathing and flared nostrils are other signs. The mare walks stiffly, the tail may be raised, and spasms similar to those of tetanus occur.

Another similarity is that eating and drinking may become impossible, Recumbency, coma, and death follow within a couple of days.

While mild cases recover, the mortality is high in untreated animals showing the more severe signs.

TREATMENT. Measures should be taken to remove the horse from all sources of excitement or fear. It should be housed in a loose-box and made comfortable. The injection subcutaneously of 50–80 cc of calcium gluconate solution (5 per cent) repeated in an hour usually serves to terminate an attack. If untreated, the horse usually falls to the floor of the horse-box and injures itself – often seriously – in its endeavours to regain its feet. It may pass into a state of coma and die.

TRANSLOCATION. In cytogenetics, this means transfer of a broken-off fragment of one chromosome to another. (*See* CYTOGENETICS.) A cause of some congenital diseases.

TRANSMISSIBLE GASTRO-ENTERITIS OF PIGS (TGE). This viral disease was first recognised in the USA, and in Britain has caused a great many deaths of piglets 3 weeks old or under. The stomach becomes severely inflamed, sometimes with ulceration and bleeding.

In the first East Anglian outbreak of 1957–8, many pregnant sows became ill at farrowing – with resultant agalactia and also with the piglets being involved, too. Severe diarrhoea was the principal symptom – faeces of piglets being greenish. Some piglets vomited. Mortality was 90 per cent during the first week of life. Fattening pigs survived but their growth rate was greatly reduced during the scouring. The disease is periodically of considerable economic importance. For example, in 1973 persistent TGE caused the loss of 1000 piglets in a single herd.

In the USA a live and virulent transmissible gastro-enteritis virus has been given by mouth 3 weeks before sows farrow. This provides passive immunity for the piglets during their first few weeks of life, but the method is not without risk. For example, the infection may become established and spread to other herds.

In Canada dogs have been shown to have antibodies to a TGE-associated virus, and rectal swabs from dogs have led, when fed to pigs, to the latter's death from TGE. An identical or associated coronavirus has been isolated also from cats and foxes. (*See also* 'EPIDEMIC DIARRHOEA'.)

TRANSMISSIBLE MINK ENCEPHALO-PATHY. A scrapie-like disease, the cause of which has not yet been fully elucidated.

TRANSPLANTS. (*See* EMBRYO TRANSFER *and* SKIN GRAFTING. For skeletal muscle transplants, *see* CANINE HEART REPAIR.)

TRANSPORT STRESS. When farm animals are transported, meat quality may deteriorate and some animals may even die. A method has been developed for measuring the adverse nature of the noise and vibration components of transport, using operant conditioning. The equipment is a modification of a machine originally developed for testing tractors and consists of a pen which is tilted up and down in all directions and generates a noise of 80 decibels. It was found that pigs soon learn to press a panel with their snouts in order to obtain a 30 seconds' respite from vibration and keep the machine immobile for 70–80% of the time. The animals switch the machine off more frequently when the speed of vibration is increased and also when they have eaten a large meal just before the test. During a one hour session the frequency with which the machine was switched off tended to increase showing that aversion to the conditions does not diminish with time. Pigs which have experienced the machine will press the switch when exposed to a recording of the noise even when there is no movement. In contrast, naïve animals do not learn to operate the switch when exposed to the noise alone. The advantage of this technique is that specifications for improved methods of transport can be based on the animal's own preferences. (AFRC.)

TRANSTRACHEAL ASPIRATION. This, it has been claimed, is a quick and simple technique to perform in the field; innocuous to calves; and providing ready access to pathogens of the lower respiratory tract. 'Furthermore, by entering this rather than using the nasopharyngeal route, the risk of contamination from the upper respiratory tract is avoided.' (Espinasse, J & others. *Veterinary Record* (1991) **129**, 339.)

TRAUMATIC PERICARDITIS (*see* HEART DISEASE).

TRAVEL SICKNESS is observed in dogs and cats – some individuals being particularly susceptible – and may be relieved by the administration of a suitable tranquilliser prior to the journey. Fitting a chain to a car so as to act as an 'earth' has been recommended, but may be less effective than periodic stops and adequate ventilation. (*See also* TRANSIT TETANY.)

TREADS are injuries inflicted at the coronet of the horse's foot, either by the shoe of the opposite foot, or, when horses are worked in pairs, by the adjacent horse. When situated in the posterior half of the foot the upper free edge of the lateral cartilage may be damaged and a quittor result.

TREFOIL is a cause of Light Sensitisation in Australia.

TREMATODE. An unsegmented flat worm or fluke. (*See* LIVER FLUKES, LUNG FLUKES, RUMEN FLUKES, *and* SCHISTOSOMIASIS.)

TREMBLING IN DOGS (*see under* SHIVERING).

'TREMBLINGS' IN EWES (*see* 'MOSS ILL').

TREMORS. Very fine jerky contractions of a muscle or of some of the fibres of a muscle. They are often seen in nervous animals when frightened, and they are one of the signs of viciousness in a horse when seen on the quarters, especially when the horse is 'watching out of the corner of his eye'. They are, however, met with in certain nervous affections, such as shivering in horses and chorea in dogs. (*See also* 'CRAZY CHICK' DISEASE.) HYPOMAGNESAEMIA in cattle, and RABIES in many species, also give rise to tremors.

(For tremors in **pigs**, *see* SWINE FEVER.)

TREPHINING is an operation in which a small disc of bone is removed from the cranium to permit of the elevation of a depressed portion, or to allow access into the brain cavity. In certain purulent conditions of the air sinuses of the horse's head trephining may be required to give drainage for the pus.

TREPONEMA. A genus of spiral organisms of the family Treponemaceae, which includes also *Borrelia* and *Leptospira*. (*See also* SWINE DYSENTERY.)

TRIATOMID BUGS are the most important vectors of human trypanosomiasis in South and Central America.

TRICHIASIS (*see* EYE, DISEASES OF).

TRICHINOSIS is an infestation of the muscles of the pig, man, dog, etc., with the larvae of *Trichinella spiralis*, a small roundworm. Pigs become infected by eating infected rats or raw swill or garbage containing pieces of infected pork. Trichinosis constitutes a serious problem among sledge-dogs in the Arctic and may follow the eating of walrus, bear, seal, or fox-meat. In 1941 an outbreak of trichinosis occurred among human beings at Wolverhampton, where 500 cases were reported. There have been several smaller outbreaks in Britain since the Wolverhampton one. A temperature of $-15°C$ for 20 days is needed to kill the larvae. (*See* ROUNDWORMS.)

Infection in man occurs through the eating of raw or undercooked meat. Human symptoms include pain in muscles. Myocarditis, meningitis, encephalitis, and rarely death have occurred.

An outbreak of trichinosis in Paris, involving 300 proven cases, followed the eating of horsemeat either raw or served rare. All this meat had come from two shops, and originated from a single horse imported from the USA.

The main symptoms in this outbreak were fever, muscle pain, swollen face and eyelids, a rash, and digestive system upsets. (Ancelle, T. & others, *Lancet* (1985) **2,** 660.)

TRICHOCEPHALUS or WHIP-WORM, is the name of a worm that infests the caeca of various animals. (*See* ROUNDWORMS.)

TRICHOGLYPHS (*see* WHORLS).

TRICHOMONAS. The flagellates of the genus *Trichomonas* are usually pear-shaped, with 3 to 5 anterior flagella, and undulating membrane and, in some species, one free flagellum directed backwards. Species of this genus very commonly occur in the intestinal canal of many different species of mammals and birds.

Trichomoniasis. *T. fetus* causes abortions, pyometra, and sometimes sterility in cattle. The cow becomes infected by the bull at coitus, or *vice versa.*

CAUSES. *Trichomonas suis.* This, it has been shown experimentally, can give rise to infertility and other symptoms in cattle similar to those caused by *T. fetus.* The two organisms, which cannot be differentiated by the mucus agglutination test, may well be identical. The unwise disposal of pig manure on a dairy farm might lead to an outbreak of trichomoniasis.

T. rumentium inhabits the rumen and appears not to be pathogenic.

In budgerigars, trichomoniasis affecting the oesophagus and/or crop is a common cause of retching and vomiting. (Baker, J. R., *Veterinary Record* (1986) **118,** 447.)

SIGNS. A transient vaginitis, which is often overlooked. If conception has not occurred, a chronic form of endometritis follows. If the cow is pregnant, the fetus dies and is either aborted 1 to 4 months later or is retained in the uterus where it becomes macerated and a pyometra develops.

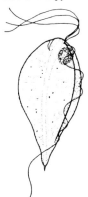

Trichomonas fetus.

CONTROL of the disease includes the disposal of infected bulls, withholding all breeding operations on infected cows for at least 3 months, and the serving of non-infected cows and virgin heifers by a 'clean' bull. Freezing bull semen to $-79°C$, in the presence of 10 per cent glycerol, kills *Trichomonas fetus* but allows the spermatozoa to survive. This method of deep-freeze commonly practised at AI centres, is one way of getting rid of the infection from semen.

TRICHOPHYTON (*see* RINGWORM).

TRICHOTHECENES are found in animal feeds and human foods. Examples are deoxynivalenol and nivalenol. The most potent toxin is T_2 TOXIN (which see).

Throat irritation and digestive disorders are caused in people. Baking does not destroy the toxin.

TRICUSPID VALVE is the valve lying in the heart between the right atrium and the right ventricle, which possesses three cusps or flaps. (*See* HEART.)

TRIGEMINAL NERVE is the fifth of the cranial nerves. (*See* NERVES.)

TRIMETHOPRIM. A drug which inhibits the growth of many bacteria and some protozoa through reducing their synthesis of folinic acid (necessary for synthesis of nucleic acids). Effective against many Gram-positive and Gram-negative bacteria. Trimethoprim is combined with Sulphadiazine, which is synergistic, in Wellcome's 'Tribrissen'.

TRIORCHIDISM. A condition in which three testicles are present. This was found in a cock; all three being functional, and structurally independent. A case in which there was duplication of the right testicle was seen in a calf. (In man, triorchidism is not extremely rare, and even five testes in a scrotum have been recorded.)

TRIPLET CALVES. In the U K in 1985 a Friesian cow had triplets. The first was delivered with veterinary aid, but breathing was unsatisfactory until Dopram-V was given intravenously. The two other calves ceased breathing but this was restarted after similar treatment; and all three survived and were described as 'fine, strong calves.' **Quintuplets** have been recorded.

TRIPLOID. An animal having one and a half times as many chromosomes in its cells as a normal (*i.e.* diploid) animal. (*See* COLCHICINE.)

'Triploidy accounts for up to 13 per cent of embryonic loss in animals, and for 20 per cent of all chromosomally-caused spontaneous human abortion' (*ARC Annual Report*, 1974–5). (*See* CHROMOSOMES, CYTOGENETICS.)

TRISMUS. The locking of the jaws, which is characteristic of tetanus.

TRISOMY. The presence in triplicate of a particular chromosome. In the cow, such a condition would be denoted as 61,XXX.

X-Trisomy was associated with nymphomania and infertility in a 30-months-old cow.

A 7-year-old Spanish-bred horse was considered to be a mare, though it looked masculine, was aggressive towards males, and attempted to copulate with females. It had a very large clitoris. (Moreno-Millan, M. Faculty of Veterinary Studies, University of Cordoba, Spain. *Veterinary Record* (1989) **124,** 969).

'TRIVETRIN'. An antibacterial drug containing trimethoprim and sulfadoxine intended for use where antibiotics are contra-indicated or ineffective, and stated to be efficacious in treating calf diphtheria, salmonellosis, *E. coli* infection.

TRIXYLPHOSPHATE. A substance used in the manufacture of plastics. Poisoning of cattle has occurred through contamination of molasses with this substance. Symptoms included diarrhoea, coughing, unsteady gait, partial paralysis.

TROCHANTER. One of the protuberances on the femur which serve as attachment sites for hindquarter muscles.

TROMBICULOSIS. Infestation with *Trombicula autumnalis,* the harvest mite.

TROPHIC. The influence that nerves exert upon the tissues to which they are distributed, for health and nourishment.

TROPHINS. Gland-regulating hormones.

TROPHOBLAST. The outer layer of BLASTOCYSTS which make contact with the wall of the uterus, and through which nutrients and waste products are exchanged between fetal and maternal circulations. (*See also* SYNCYTIUM.)

TROPICS, LIVESTOCK PRODUCTION IN THE. Livestock farming in the tropics, and even in some sub-tropical developing countries, is beset with difficulties not experienced to anything like the same degree in developed countries having a temperate climate.

In developing countries there is often the additional problem of limited financial resources. Money may not be available for measures to counter or ameliorate adverse conditions for animals; to provide adequate supplies of safe drinking water, good-quality feeds, vaccines, prophylactic drugs, or to support disease eradication programmes on a large scale. Veterinarians are usually few in number in relation to the large areas in which they are needed (*see* VETERINARY PROFESSION), and faced with great distances to cover and an absence of local laboratory services.

Heat. Animals can *survive* in temperatures of up to 60°C. Temperatures above that are lethal. Cattle in Death Valley, California, and in Queensland, Australia, for example, exist at temperatures of 52 to 58°C. Such heat, however, is far above the *comfort zone* – air temperature at between 21 and 26°C. (E. S. E. Hafez); 'about 13 to 18°C for adult cattle' (J. I. Richards).

High temperatures impose stress upon the animal's physiological processes and productive capacity.

Records for over 12,000 inseminations over a two-year period in a Florida herd indicated a sharp decline in conception rates of cows when a maximum air temperature the day after artificial insemination exceeds 86°F. (95°F for heifers.)

Besides air temperature, radiation, air movement, and humidity all influence the animal's immediate environment. Body temperature is controlled by the heat-regulating mechanism (*see* HYPOTHALAMUS), and affected not only by environmental heat but also by the heat generated in the tissues (*see* METABOLISM). The more the animal eats, the more heat its body will produce. Water intake also plays a part in the physiological reactions; as does sweating, but in this respect cattle are less efficient than people. In great environmental heat, the point may be reached where normal body temperature cannot be maintained, and it rises – a state of HYPERTHERMIA. Death may result.

Even at non-lethal levels, tropical heat is a limiting factor so far as fertility and yields of milk, meat, and eggs are concerned. Poor feed, and water deprivation, can further depress growth rates, fertility, and yields. Humidity can increase heat stress.

SIGNS. Heat stress may cause the body temperature to rise to 42 to 43°C (110°F) in cattle. The earlier symptom of rapid breathing progresses to panting. The mouth may be kept open, tongue lolling out, and frothy saliva may be in evidence. Appetite is lost. Cattle may remain standing, huddling together (J. I. Richards).

PREVENTIVE MEASURES. If heat stress is to be avoided or minimised, livestock must have shade (from trees or shelters) to protect them from the sun's rays. Cooled drinking water is beneficial to all livestock in tropical heat. Pigs need to be able to wallow – their normal, instinctive method of cooling themselves. Cool water sprays can help dairy cattle to withstand high temperatures. Grazing should take place at night rather than during the day. **Zero-grazing** (*which see*) may be practicable in some places and beneficial too. Poultry in the tropics grow larger combs and wattles than do similar birds in temperate climates, as a physiological means of body cooling. At very high temperatures they dip combs and wattles into water, for an extra cooling effect. It has been suggested (Marsden and Morris) that the design of drinkers in intensive poultry units should be such as to make possible this beneficial practice.

Antibiotics and poultry. Throughout the developing countries in the tropics, Dr A. A. Ojeniyi stated, the widespread, uncritical, and uncontrolled use of antibiotics – especially the tetracyclines – in modern battery poultry units encourages the proliferation of drug-resistant bacteria. Where such reckless use is coupled with poor sanitation and low personal hygiene, the situation may constitute a danger to public health.

The policy in these countries is based on a tacit assumption that success in poultry rearing achieved in Europe and the USA was largely attributable to regular prophylactic use of antibiotics.

All 1248 strains of *E. coli* from battery hens at the University of Ibadan, Nigeria, and 2196 strains from a commercial poultry farm, were resistant to tetracycline, streptomycin, (and also sulphonamides). By contrast, all strains isolated from free-range town and village poultry were sensitive to these drugs. (Ojeniyi, A. A., *Veterinary Record* (1985) **117**, 11.)

Altitude. In some regions, altitude mitigates the effect of heat. The uplands of Jordan are regarded as suitable for intensive poultry production; and Iran's uplands, with their dry climate, make dairy farming practicable despite very high summer temperatures of 43°C upwards, and very cold ones in winter (W. J. Jordan). When temperature falls during night-time hours, cattle may withstand a higher day-time temperature than they otherwise could.

Very high altitudes, *e.g.* in the mountains of Peru, can themselves be an obstacle to livestock production. (*See* ALTITUDE, MOUNTAIN SICKNESS).

Stock improvement. When high-yield stock are imported into tropical regions from countries having a temperate climate, disappointment often follows. At first yields – whether of beef, milk, pork, or eggs – are better than those of the indigenous stock, as expected; but before long, in many instances, the initial gains are offset by a high mortality rate. The exotic animals may not be able to tolerate the heat, may not produce so well when fed on local feeds of lower quality, and will have no resistance to many local diseases and parasites, especially ticks. (For cattle resistant to heat and ticks, *see* DROUGHTMASTER, ZEBU, SANTA GERTRUDI, AFRICANDER.)

In many situations it is often preferable to improve indigenous stock first, before introducing new blood from overseas, by selective breeding and better management; ensuring that they are better fed and not deprived of adequate quantities of drinking water. After improvement has been obtained by these means, but not before, crossbreeding with exotic high-performance stock may be begun, preferably on a small-scale trial basis to start with. Use may be made of AI.

Desert dairies. It could be said that a new concept of livestock production in the tropics is illustrated by Saudi Arabia's dairy farm at Al-Kharj in the desert. With no balance of payments problem in this oil-rich state, 60,000,000 dollars were spent in establishing the farm in 1980. By March the following year there were 4,000 cows on the 60 sq km farm, and it was claimed that after 9 months' milk production most of the problems had been solved. Expansion continued, with a target of 18,000 cows there by 1985. Water is pumped from wells 150 m deep in the Al-Kharj oasis, and some of this water is used for pivot irrigation sprinklers, which make crop growing possible. The cows there in early 1981 were Friesians from the Netherlands, but it was planned to start importing Holsteins from the USA and Canada. Management was in the hands of Alfa-Laval of Sweden; the owners of the farm being the Saudi Arabian Agriculture and Dairy Company (Saadco). (Source: *International Agricultural Development*, March 1981 issue).

Animal power in India. Dr. N. S. Ramaswamy, director of the Indian Institute of Management, commented that in view of the importance of animal power to India's economy, there is an urgent need to expand its veterinary services. He estimated that work animals provide as much energy as the entire electrical system of the country. The government, he stated, had invested the equivalent of over 37 billion US dollars in building up electricity generating capacity, but only a third of that figure in work animals – 70 million bullocks, 8 million buffaloes, 1 million horses, and 1 million camels. (*See* WATER BUFFALOES.)

Dr Ramaswamy emphasised that animal power usage is not a mere passing phase in India's social and economic development, as many policy-makers appear to believe. He pointed out that half India's farms are too small for tractors ever to be used on them; that only half the villages have roads suitable for trucks; and that animal power is the only energy source within reach of the rural poor. (Ramaswamy, N. S. *World Health Forum* (1982) **3**, 352.)

His comments will undoubtedly have relevance for many other countries in the tropics.

Animal feeds. In poorer countries the cost of importing cereal grains or high-quality protein feeds may be prohibitive, and local stock will then be dependent on feeds which may restrict their yields; though obviously this is not always the case.

Imported feeds sometimes deteriorate to some extent during long sea voyages and subsequent storage in a hot and often humid climate. There may, for example, be a serious loss of vitamin E, so that a supplement is required if ENCEPHALOMALACIA is to be avoided. (*See* also VITAMINS.)

Local crops such as groundnuts, cotton seed,

sorghum and sunflower seed may be contaminated by AFLATOXINS, so that precautions are needed. Groundnuts may be affected in this way through being left too long in the ground before harvesting, or during subsequent storage.

Minerals. In many parts of the tropics milling and processing facilities are lacking, at any rate in the more remote areas, and this fact makes feed supplementation more difficult. Mineral and trace element supplements are necessary for avoidance of deficiencies. In South Africa many years ago, Sir Arnold Theiler showed that the need of cattle for phosphorus drove them to eat the bones of dead animals, and many cattle became infected with botulism in that way and died. (*See* LAMZIEKTE.) In several parts of the world a deficiency of copper in the herbage has impeded livestock production, and appropriate dressings of the land have brought great benefit. (*See* TRACE ELEMENTS).

Some tropical crops. Apart from the crops mentioned above, many others – or their by-products – are used. For example, cattle may have the leaves of shade trees, or sugar-cane; pigs may be given dried leaf meal, banana waste, coca pod husks, or sweet potatoes; poultry may receive millet (if any can be spared from human food requirements) or sago.

(*See* GOSSYPOL POISONING, CASTOR SEED POISONING, COCOA POISONING).

Tropical diseases. In some tropical regions the presence of animal parasites and their vectors makes livestock production difficult, costly, or even impracticable. This is true of the African tsetse-fly belt, extending roughly from latitude 15°N to 30°S. Here control of trypanosomiasis (*see* TRYPANOSOMES) is dependent on drugs for prevention, drugs for treatment, and use of insecticides against flies. Aerial spraying, bush clearance, and attempts to eradicate reservoirs of infection among wild animals will, if undertaken, obviously add to the cost, which in some territories may be beyond local resources. For many years control of tsetse flies had been successfully achieved by aerial spraying with insecticides, but the ever-rising cost of these, and of aviation fuel, has led to the abandonment of many such government schemes. Fly traps have had to be used instead. The Manitoba trap designed specially for Tabanids is reported to be very successful. Another widely used trap is the Laveissire. In other territories long-term, government-controlled campaigns have prove successful in maintaining and extending production.

Humpless cattle, such as the N'Dama, in West Africa had long been regarded as historic relics, and their reduced susceptibility to trypanosomiasis as a biological oddity. A survey had shown, however, that despite their relatively small size, N'Dama cattle could survive and be productive in endemic trypanosomiasis areas where Zebu cattle died. (Murray, M. & others, *Veterinary Record* (1981) **109**, 503.)

Comparative studies on two types of large East African zebu (*Bos indicus*) Boran cattle, on a beef ranch in Kenya, indicated that a Boran type bred by the Orma tribe has a superior response to tsetse

fly challenge. The Orma Boran when compared with an improved Boran was found to have lower trypanosome infection rates and, when untreated, better control of anaemia and decreased mortality. (Njogu, A. R. & others *Veterinary Record* (1985) **117**, 632.)

In a paper given at the 1986 BVA Congress, Professor Murray commented that some well established drugs can be surprisingly helpful if used correctly. This had been shown on a 47,000 hectare ranch in Tanzania over 10 years.

Seventy to 80 per cent of the 4800 breeding females were Boran cattle and the area was one in which cattle succumbed to trypanosomiasis if left untreated. The strategic use of isometamidium chloride (Samorin; May & Baker) every 80 days and diminazene aceturate (Berenil; Hoechst) every 520 days allowed cattle to survive without the development of drug resistance or other side effects. Not only did the cattle survive but their productivity compared quite well with Boran ranches in tsetse-free areas of Kenya – 80 per cent – and they were 35 per cent more productive than N'dama herds in West Africa.

Trypanosomes cause disease also in Asia and Central and South America.

Ticks are of great importance in the tropics, transmitting numerous protozoal parasites, viruses, and rickettsias. (*See under* TICKS.)

Among the major diseases caused by viruses are cattle plague (rinderpest), African swine fever, foot-and-mouth disease, and various types of encephalitis. Bacterial diseases include anthrax, botulism, haemorrhagic septicaemia (pasteurellosis), and salmonellosis. A notable mycoplasmal disease is contagious bovine pleuropneumonia; another is contagious agalactia of sheep and goats. (*See also under* TROPICAL DISEASES, above.)

Vaccine storage/transport. One of the problems of veterinary medicine in the tropics is the storage of vaccines at a low enough temperature (below 8°C.) With the high cost and scarcity of kerosene or liquid propane gas in many rural areas, and the fact that electricity supply is often unreliable or non-existent, there is scope for solar refrigerators. Under a WHO scheme these have been tried in 13 countries. Photovoltaic panels exposed to the sun supply electricity direct to an ordinary commercial refrigerator. The latter can also be used for making 1 or 2 kg of ice every 24 hours.

Sterilisation. In the tropics the sun's rays can be used for sterilisation purposes. Research at the American University of Beirut showed that oral rehydration solution, for treating dehydration, can be sterilised in plastic bags or transparent plastic or glass vessels by exposure to sunlight. In an experiment such a solution, contaminated with fresh sewage, proved to have a zero coliform count after one hour. It appears that the sterilising effect is not heat, since the temperature of the solution rises by less than 5°C after 2 hours, but solar radiation in the near ultra-violet range.

Another application is the 'Solomon solar sterilizer' which uses only solar energy to boil water and sterilise needles and syringes. The prototype consisted of a metal-lined plywood box topped with a truncated pyramid of glass. The steriliser, in use in the Solomon Islands, is easily constructed, has no moving parts, and requires no fuel; but it does need orienting to the sun every half hour. (Source: World Health Organisation.)

Carcase disposal, following post-mortem examinations, may present problems in recently established laboratories or research centres still lacking much in the way of buildings or equipment. An Australian veterinarian working at an Indian sheep project found the answer. If unsuitable for boiling as dog food, and yet not likely to spread infection, the carcase is dragged out into the open, He timed events on one occasion. At 2.46 p.m. post-mortem examination completed; no vultures to be seen in a clear sky. At 2.50 the first arrived; at 2.53 there were approximately 40 vultures around the carcase; at 2.58 carcase stripped to bones and sinew – vultures leaving.
References:
E. S. E. Hafez, *Adaptation of Domestic Animals*, Lea & Febiger, 1968.
J. I. Richards, A. Marsden, T. R. Morris, and W. J. Jordan, *Intensive Animal Production in Developing Countries*, Brit. Soc. Anim. Production (1981).

TRYPANOCIDE. A drug which will kill trypanosomes within the host's body.

TRYPANOSOMES are small single-celled parasites that are found in the blood-stream in certain diseases that are classed together as the 'trypanosomiases'.

The trypanosome is of an elongated shape with a single flagellum and an undulating membrane. There are two nuclei – a large nucleus (macronucleus or trophonucleus) near the centre of the body, and a small kinetoplast (micronucleus) at the posterior end remote from the flagellum. In some forms there is no free flagellum.

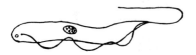

Diagram of Trypanosome.

Transmission is generally by the bite of an insect (except in the case of Dourine). The transmission may be mechanical, *i.e.* carried directly from an infected animal to an uninfected one by the bite of a blood-sucking fly, or cyclical, when the insect host is not infective for a definite time after ingestion of the parasite. In this case the parasite passes a definite part of its life-cycle in the fly. In many cases transmission may be both mechanical and cyclical. Thus, the tsetse fly may have two infective periods, one immediately after biting a sick animal and the second some time later (about 20 days) after the trypanosome has progressed to its infective stage along normal lines.
LIFE HISTORIES OF TRYPANOSOMES. In the blood of the mammalian host the trypanosomes reproduce by splitting lengthwise (longitudinal fission). A quantity of blood is sucked up by the tsetse fly, a species of *Glossina*, and in that host the flagellates undergo a developmental cycle. The location

chosen by the parasite for its development varies with the species. Thus some will develop only in the salivary glands, others in the gut, and still others in the proboscis. After some time they assume the infective form, and are ready to be passed with the salivary fluids into the bloodstream of a suitable vertebrate host.

African trypanosomiasis. Tsetse-borne trypanosomiasis renders approximately 10 million square km of prime African land unsuitable for cattle production. It has been estimated that if this disease could be controlled, the infested area would increase its cattle holding capacity from 20 million head to 140 million head generating an additional yearly income of US$75 million at 1974 prices. (Njogu, A. R. & others. *Veterinary Record* (1985) **117,** 632.)

The disease is of greatest importance in **cattle**, which are hosts of the following trypanosomes: *T. congolense, T. vivax, T. uniforme,* and *T. evansi.*

Usually a chronic disease, acute cases also occur, and the mortality may be high. (*See also* PREMUNITION; *and,* for resistant breeds, TROPICS.)
SIGNS. These include intermittent fever, anaemia, anorexia or pica, a progressive loss of condition, and increasing weakness. (*See under* CHANCRE for the hard swelling which is often the first pointer to trypanosomiasis.) Lymph nodes are enlarged in many cases, the coat harsh, and abortion may occur.

Some cattle recover, but in others apparent recovery is followed later by a relapse and death. In acute cases, death may occur within a fortnight.
Horses. Additional signs include oedema of the limbs and abdomen, and corneal opacity. Species of trypanosome infecting horses are *T. brucei, T. vivax, T. evansi;* (*See also* DOURINE, caused by *T. equiperdum,* transmitted at coitus, and occurring also in Asia.)
Dogs. The eyes may be affected, as in horses. Canine trypanosomiasis is caused by *T. brucei, T. congolense,* and *T. evansi.*
Pigs often suffer from acute and fatal trypanosomiasis caused by either *T. simiae* or *T. evansi.*
CONTROL. This is difficult, on account of trypanosomiasis existing in wild animals in the vicinity of cattle herds, and the fact that vaccination has not been practicable.

In well-managed herds in areas where tsetse fly numbers are relatively low, drugs are used for preventive purposes against the trypanosomes; but as the latter develop drug resistance, it is usually necessary to change drugs.

In other areas, reliance is placed on drugs for treatment rather than prophylaxis; and they can achieve survival of cattle where untreated animals die.

(*See also under* TSETSE FLY for another aid to control of the disease, and under TROPICS for breeds resistant to trypanosomiasis, and for drugs in current use.)

Diseases caused by trypanosomes are separately described under NAGANA, DOURINE, SURRA and (for human trypanosomiasis) SLEEPING SICKNESS and CHAGAS' DISEASE. The latter also affects domestic animals and is described below, under the subheading American trypanosomiasis.

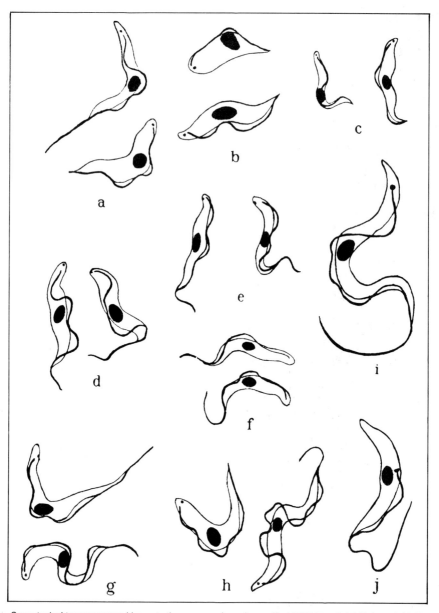

Some typical trypanosomes (drawn to the same scale and magnified 2000 times): (a) *T. brucei*; (b) *T. montgomery*; (c) *T. congolense*; (d) *T. vivax*; (e) *T. simiae*; (f) *T. equiunum*; (g) *T. equiperdum*; (h) *T. evans*; (i) and (j) *T. theileri*.

(For one symptom of trypanosome infections, *see* CHANCRE.)

American trypanosomiasis (Chagas' disease). Caused by *T. cruzi*, this occurs in South and Central America, and also in the southern states of the USA. WHO estimates that at least 7 million people are infected with *T. cruzi*.

The infection can be carried from both wild and domestic animals to people by blood-sucking triatomid bugs; and the latter also cause people-to-people infections. Blood transfusions, and infection of the human fetus *in utero*, have also to be borne in mind.

Dogs, cats, and guinea-pigs are among domestic animals which are hosts; and pigs and rabbits also have the disease. Rats, mice, foxes, ferrets, and vampire bats are other vectors.

SIGNS. Fever, anaemia, emaciation, ascites, with death from heart failure following myocarditis in children.

TRYPSIN is a proteolytic enzyme of the pancreatic secretion. It changes proteins into peptones. It is often helpful in cases of non-specific diarrhoea in dogs.

TRYPTOPHAN. One of the essential AMINO ACIDS.

TSETSE FLY is the insect vector which is of such importance in the transmission of African TRYPANOSOMES. (*See also* FLIES, Glossina; TROPICS.)

Destruction of tsetse flies in the fly-belts – tracts of bush country in which only cattle which have acquired some degree of immunity to trypanosomiasis can survive – has proved an almost insuperable problem. One method is the sterilisation of tsetse flies by the chemicals tepa or metepa, or by gamma radiation, and the release of sterile males. This can be complementary to the use of insecticides. A difficulty at present is the rearing of tsetse flies in sufficient quantities.

Wide use is also made of fly traps, to which tsetse flies may be attracted by means of PHEROMONES or other chemical compounds such as CO_2, acetone, or octenol. (*See also under* TRYPANOSOMES.)

TUBERCLE is a term used in two quite distinct senses. As a descriptive term in anatomy a *tubercle* means a small elevation or roughness upon the surface of a bone, such as the tubercles of the ribs. In a pathological sense a *tubercle* is a small mass, barely visible to the naked eye, formed in some organ as the starting-point of the disease which has been called after the tubercle, viz. *Tuberculosis.*

TUBERCULIN TEST. We owe the tuberculin test, the original form of which came into use in 1890, to Koch, who grew his tubercle bacilli on broth. Today a special Purified Protein Derivative ('PPD') is used for culturing the bacilli: a feature which adds to the reliability of the test. Tuberculin is prepared by killing and filtering off the bacilli from the culture medium. To the liquid which remains trichloracetic acid is added. This precipitates tuberculo-protein, which is poured into cylinders to form a sediment, is centrifuged, diluted to a standard strength, and bottled.

Tuberculin has in the past been used by instillation beneath the lower eyelid of one eye (the ophthalmic test); by subcutaneous injection (the subcutaneous tuberculin test); and by injection with a special syringe into the thickness of the skin of a defined area (the intradermal test). Today, in this country, the test used is the intradermal Comparative Test. Two different tuberculins are used – one bovine and one avian. (Bovine tuberculin replaced human tuberculin for this purpose in 1975.)

A fold of skin is measured with special calipers before the injection, and again 70 hours later. Interpretation of the test is based upon the resultant swelling of each infection site.

Bovine tuberculosis is not the only disease which can bring about this sensitisation. Human tuberculosis and tuberculosis of birds will also do it; so will so-called skin tuberculosis and Johne's disease. Hence the advantage of the Comparative Test which helps the veterinary surgeon to distinguish between these various possible causes of a positive reaction.

So-called 'skin tuberculosis' (see under this heading) may also cause confusion. A re-test after an interval of 30 to 60 days will, however, in the absence of tuberculosis, generally give a reaction justifying retention of the animal within the herd. (*See also* JOHNE'S DISEASE *vaccine.*)

If cattle are running on the same land as poultry, and some of these happen to be infected with

tuberculosis, the cattle may react when tested with the avian tuberculin. There will not be a significant reaction at the site where the mammalian tuberculin was injected, however; hence the value of the Comparative Test. Avian tubercle bacilli are not virulent for cattle, which usually cease to react within a few months of the infected birds being removed. Reaction to avian tuberculin may also occur in an animal suffering from Johne's disease.

TUBERCULOSIS. A contagious disease of man, all the domesticated animals, many wild animals in captivity, birds, fishes, and reptiles. It is caused by *Mycobacterium tuberculosis* (bovine, human, or avian strains).

The disease is usually a chronic one; though the *miliary* form is acute. It is characterised by the formation of nodules or tubercles in almost any or all of the organs or tissues of the body. (*See also* 'SKIN TUBERCULOSIS'.)

Occurrence. The prevalence of tuberculosis in animals bears a direct ratio to the intensity of the methods of agriculture in an area. Cattle closely confined, and housed to a great extent in buildings, are much more often affected than are those living a free open-air life. The cattle in the prairies of North America, on the tablelands of Central Africa, and in the steppes of Eastern Europe, are almost entirely free from its ravages, while it is unknown in many islands (Iceland, Sicily, etc.).

Bovine tuberculosis eradication campaigns have succeeded in several countries.

Animals affected. Among the ordinary domesticated animals, cattle and pigs are much more commonly affected than are other species. Cats and dogs are not uncommonly affected. Horses, sheep, and goats appear to be more resistant. Donkeys and mules are only very seldom attacked.

Age is an important factor. The following table illustrates incidence according to age. Of 9046 cattle examined and found to be diseased the ages were as follows:

Age	Numbers	Age	Numbers
3–4 weeks	3	3 years	81
5 months	1	4 years	118
7–9 months	4	5 years	326
1 year	12	6 years	1223
2 years	39	7 and over	7239

Methods of infection. Cattle are infected in two chief ways: (1) by the respiratory system, and (2) by the digestive tract. They are susceptible to infection from humans suffering from bovine tuberculosis and serious 'breakdowns' in attested herds have been traced to cowmen suffering from the disease. Cattle are also susceptible, to a lesser degree, to infection of the human type. (*See also under* COMPARATIVE TEST *re* avian tuberculosis.)

Sometimes tuberculosis may be contracted through a wound (*e.g.* after de-horning) or by direct introduction into the tissues of a penetrating instrument, and an infection of the udder may easily occur through the teat canal.

An aerosol infection commmonly results from coughing cows, and infected sputum may contaminate feed or be swallowed; spreading infection to the intestines.

Within the body infection may spread via the lymphatic system or the bloodstream.

Tuberculosis of the vagina occurs in cows, and the disease may be spread from them to healthy cows through the medium of the bull. Infected dung can be a source of infection.

Nature of the lesions. A typical lesion is a *tubercle* – a small nodular swelling whose centre contains either pus or dry yellowish cheesy material. The peritoneum, liver, lymph nodes, lungs, etc., may be affected. Sometimes the disease remains localised to the area of its first infection and does not spread. In other cases the defensive forces of the body overcome and destroy the focus of infection.

Tuberculosis may affect bones and one or more joints, causing arthritis.

Superficial, as well as deep, lymph nodes may become enlarged.

A subclinical infection may occur, and result in overt illness only when stress, under-feeding, exposure or some other infection lowers the animal's resistance.

1. Cattle. As a rule a considerable period of time elapses between infection and the appearance of the first symptoms.

Tuberculosis of the lungs – the commonest type – gives rise to a hard, dry, short cough in the early stages. Later, coughing becomes more frequent and DYSPNOEA is evident.

Appetite is variable. Sometimes a difficulty in swallowing is noticed. Loss of condition follows, with pale mucous membranes, and a 'staring' coat. There may be diarrhoea.

Superficial lymph nodes may become enlarged. Those at the back of the throat or at the corner of the lower jaw, or the glands of the neck, shoulder, or stifle, may be swollen.

Tuberculosis of the udder – which is all-important from the milk standpoint – begins insidiously. The gland slowly becomes diffusely thickened, and more solid to the touch than normally. After milking, it does not feel quite so elastic as it should, and in some cases distinct hard nodules can be felt.

(**Tuberculoid** mastitis. Over 700 cases of this, due to rapidly growing acid-fast organisms other than *M. tuberculosis*, occur in the UK annually – mainly due to not cleaning the teats before introducing antibiotics).

Tuberculosis sometimes involves the brain or spinal cord, giving rise to symptoms described under MENINGITIS.

Tuberculosis of the bones and joints is not uncommon.

In the skin there occasionally develop hard tumours, about the size of a hazelnut (*see also* 'SKIN TUBERCULOSIS'), which, if they be opened, are found to contain cheesy or mortar-like masses in their centres. Later, ulcers may develop.

Miliary tuberculosis is an acute form (which may follow the chronic) with the formation of multiple small abscesses in any or all of the organs. The abscesses are millet-seed sized (hence 'miliary'). This form of tuberculosis is rapidly fatal.

2. Sheep and Goats. A distressing painful cough, always present, but most noticeable upon exertion, a gradual, but quite definite, loss of condition, with progressing weakness, are the main symptoms observed in these animals. Sheep are very rarely affected, but milking goats kept in the vicinity of infected cattle not uncommonly develop tuberculosis. There is nearly always a marked anaemia, pneumonia, sometimes diarrhoea, and occasionally an infection of the udder corresponding to that found in cattle.

3. Horses. Tuberculosis in the horse is not very common, but there are certain symptoms which should always lead one to suspect its presence; a gradual emaciation in spite of good food and without any other established possible cause; a slight fluctuating increase in the temperature; an occasional moist weak cough; a tucked-up appearance of the abdomen, or in some cases (where ascites exists) a heavy pendulous condition, 'Pot-bellied'.

Cases in which the abdominal organs are affected sometimes terminate by lung complications – *i.e.* miliary tuberculosis sets in – the animal becomes feverish, distressed in its breathing, refuses all food, and generally dies in a few days. Tuberculosis may also become localised in the skin, lymph nodes, brain, or udder, but these are not common. It is comparatively often found that sooner or later some part of the skeleton (the bones of the neck being a very usual situation) becomes infected.

Occasionally, tuberculosis in the horse may be caused by the human or avian type of the tubercle bacillus.

4. Pigs. When tuberculosis affects the pig it may be due to feeding with infected whey from cheese-making establishments and creameries, or with infected and unboiled swill from sanatoria. (*See* AVIAN TUBERCULOSIS.) Tubercular poultry, or wild birds such as wood-pigeons, are a not uncommon source of infection.

A diagnosis may be established by means of the tuberculin test.

Symptoms are as in the horse. Scouring and emaciation may occur. Anaemia is common. As in horses, the bones are especially vulnerable to attack.

Lesions which, to the naked eye, appear identical with tuberculosis, may be caused by infection with *Corynebacterium equi*. Even the use of a microscope sometimes fails to differentiate between the two infections.

5. Dogs and cats. Owing to their close relationship with man these animals are liable to become infected with tuberculosis, either as the result of receiving tubercle-containing milk, or as the result of infection from sputum or discharges from a human case. Not only may dogs and cats contract the disease from man, but may occasionally be sources of infection to healthy human beings, and especially to children.

As in other animals, the symptoms are somewhat vague until the disease is well established. The first signs may be no more than a capricious appetite, slight loss of condition, general weakness, and exhaustion when at exercise. Pulmonary tuberculosis usually begins with a short dry cough. It is less common in these animals than the abdominal form, (but see PLEURISY). (*See also* BREAKDOWNS.)

Tuberculosis of the abdominal organs is indicated by impaired nutrition and anaemia, attacks of diarrhoea and constipation alternating with each other. There may be vomiting; also *ascites*. Body temperature is very variable.

Joints and sinuses may be sites of infection in the cat. Occasionally skin tuberculosis is seen in dogs and cats, and may take the form of raised plaques with a tendency to ulcerate. **In both these animals tuberculosis is much less common in the UK than it was in the 1930s and earlier.**

TREATMENT. The treatment of tuberculosis in the domesticated animals is not attempted, for four reasons: (1) because of the nature of the disease; (2) because of the ever-increasing danger to human beings who have to attend affected animals; (3) economic reasons; and (4) humanitarian ones. In zoological gardens animals are sometimes treated. (*See* PAS *and* INH.)

PREVENTION. Good hygiene, good feeding and good ventilation all help.

History of control in Britain. It was not until 1928 that measures to control bovine tuberculosis was introduced by the Government. In that year the Tuberculosis Order, enacted in 1915, came into force, and the attempt to control the disease by the detection and elimination of 'open' cases began. In 1935 the Attested Herds Scheme carried control measures a stage further.

Area Eradication, which began in 1950, and meant, at first, an extension of the Attested Herds Scheme on a voluntary basis, and then the compulsory slaughter of reactors within the prescribed areas, followed.

In October 1960, the whole of the UK was declared one Attested Area; bovine tuberculosis being virtually eradicated from all herds of cattle.

In 1962, the incidence of bovine tuberculosis in herds in England and Wales was 0·14 per cent. The number of reactors slaughtered was 8846.

During 1968, 5,854,915 cattle were tested in 108,452 herds and as a result 2170 reactors (including 2 'affected' animals) and 202 contacts in 1040 herds were slaughtered.

The Tuberculosis Orders, 1964, provide for the notification and slaughter of cattle found to be affected with certain forms of tuberculosis – *i.e.*, tuberculosis of the udder; giving tuberculous milk; tuberculous emaciation; chronic cough accompanied by clinical signs of tuberculosis; or found to be excreting or discharging tuberculous material. Two animals were slaughtered in 1968 as being 'affected' as defined in these Orders. In 1973 just over 70,000 herds were tested, and reactors found in 647 of them. The number of reactors was 1574 – an incidence of 0·032 per cent.

In 1990 16 cattle were found positive for TB in UK slaughterhouses..

INTERVAL BETWEEN TESTS. In Denmark, where herds were freed of bovine tuberculosis in 1952, testing was at first done at two-year intervals, but is now done at three-year intervals.

INSURANCE. Lloyd's Underwriters offer a TB Reactor Insurance Scheme.

The relationship of tuberculosis in animals and man; Bovine Tuberculosis. This is not a pedantic way of saying 'tuberculosis in cattle', but indicates that one is referring to disease set up by the bovine strain of tubercle bacillus as opposed to the human strain or the avian strain. Man may become infected by any one of the three strains. The bovine strain of the tubercle bacillus is particularly pathogenic for children under 16 years of age.

In considering statistics dealing with incidence of bovine tuberculosis in humans, it must be borne in mind that bovine tuberculosis can be spread from one person to another, just as it can be from animal to man.

Human infection with tuberculosis may also arise from eating infected meat, but this risk, is, in civilised countries, not great owing to (*a*) meat inspection services, (*b*) cooking of the meat. But in 1949 the British Veterinary Association issued a warning to the public against buying uncooked meat at 'pet food stores'. Some of this meat may have been condemned as unfit for human consumption on account of its being affected with tuberculosis or other disease. There is an obvious danger of dogs and cats becoming ill from this cause unless the meat is thoroughly cooked, but there is also a danger to animal owners handling such meat before it is cooked, and so contaminating their hands and kitchens.

As previously mentioned, tuberculosis in human beings may arise from infected dogs, cats, poultry and other birds; and from drinking unpasteurised milk. (*See* BREAKDOWNS, BADGERS.)

TUBERCULOSIS (AMENDMENT) ORDER 1973, made under the Diseases of Animals Act 1950, requires anyone who suspects a carcase to be affected with tuberculosis to notify a veterinary inspector and to retain the carcase (or parts of it) for him to examine. The purpose of the Order is to enable the herd of origin to be traced. Isolation of suspected tubercular cattle is also empowered.

TUBERCULOSIS, AVIAN (*see* AVIAN TUBERCULOSIS).

TULARAEMIA is a disease of hares (*see* HARES), ground squirrels, rabbits, and rats, caused by the *Francisella tularensis*, and spread mechanically either by flies or ticks, or by direct inoculation; for example, into the hands of a person engaged in skinning rabbits. In man, the disease takes the form of a slow fever, lasting several weeks, with much malaise and depression, followed by considerable emaciation. It was first described in the district of Tulare in California, but is found widely spread in North America, also in parts of Europe and Japan. Sheep and pigs are attacked and many die. Streptomycin may prove effective in treatment.

Dogs are susceptible, too.

TUMBU FLY (*see under* SCREW-WORM FLIES).

TUMOUR. This word is nowadays reserved for solid swellings resulting from abnormal growth, such as benign tumours or malignant tumours (cancer); or hollow swellings containing fluid such as cysts.

Malignant tumours are those which tend to grow and spread rapidly, destroying neighbouring tissues and infiltrating the healthy structures near by. They are liable to ulcerate through the skin when superficial, are non-encapsulated, and may spread to distant parts of the body by the blood- or lymph-stream, giving rise to secondary tumours there. (Further information upon malignant tumours appears under the heading CANCER.)

Benign tumours grow slowly at one place, press neighbouring parts aside, but neither invade nor destroy them, only seldom ulcerate through the skin or mucous membrane, have usually a capsule of fibrous tissue surrounding them, and when once completely removed by surgical excision or other means, do not recur.

While this classification serves in a measure to differentiate typical varieties into two classes, it is by no means absolutely satisfactory. There are certain kinds of normally benign tumours which may remain comparatively small and circum-scribed for a number of years, and then suddenly become malignant.

Benign or simple tumours include ANGIOMA, CHONDROMA, FIBROMA, GLIOMA, LIPOMA, MYOMA, MYXOMA, NEUROMA, ODONTOMA, PAPILLOMA. The last-named may be benign in the beginning but become malignant later; also MELANOMA and ADENOMA. (*See under those headings, also* CYSTS, WARTS, CANCER.) While normally all tumours tend to increase in size – either slowly or rapidly – some grow to a certain size, remain stationary, then decrease in size, and a few may even disappear completely.

Two of the most common tumours of the dog are mammary carcinoma and anal adenoma (usually benign). (*See also* EOSINOPHILIC GRANULOMA.)

TUMOUR ANGIOGENESIS FACTOR (TAF).

This has been isolated from human and animal tumours. It stimulates mitosis in endothelial cells and rapid formation of new capillaries for tumour nourishment. (Unlike a skin-graft, which sends out capillary shoots to join the capillaries of the recipient tissue, a tumour has to rely entirely on the host, and makes use of TAF for this purpose.)

TUNGIASIS. Infestation with *Tunga penetrans*, the jigger flea. (*See under* FLEAS.)

TUP (*see under* SHEEP).

TURBINATE BONES (*see under* NOSE *and* RHINITIS).

TURKEY CORYZA. A disease caused by Gram-negative motile bacteria named (1980) *Al-caligenes faecalis.*

TURKEY VIRAL HEPATITIS. This occurs in Europe, the USA, and Canada; and in 1982 isolation of a picorna-like virus causing hepatitis

and disease of the pancreas was isolated from an outbreak in Scotland. The infection is often, if not usually, subclinical, but may take an acute form, and prove fatal.

TURKEYS. Diseases include: Arizona Disease, Blackhead, Coccidiosis, Erysipelas, Fowl Pest, Hexamitiasis, Haemorrhagic enteritis, Mon-iliasis, Oregon disease, Ornithosis, Leukosis, Mycoplasmosis, Pullorum Disease, Rupture of the Aorta, Sinusitis, Synovitis (and *see also* above, *and* GROUNDNUT MEAL; *also* MANIOC).

Turkey meningo-encephalitis occurs in Israel. Influenza viruses cause disease in North American domestic turkeys.

Turkey rhinotracheitis has been seen in several countries, and appeared in the UK in 1985, causing severe financial losses due to deaths, carcase rejections, and lowered egg production. The first sign is sneezing.

TURNIPS. Like kale, these contain a goitre-producing factor, and if fed in large amounts to pregnant ewes are liable to cause abortion – unless iodine licks are provided. (*See* VAGINA, RUPTURE OF.)

TURPENTINE, MEDICINAL OIL OF. Turpen-tine is the oleo-resin which exudes from various members of the pine family, especially the *Pinus Australis, Pinus taeda,* and *Pinus sylvestris.* The oil distilled from this oleo-resin is known as oil of turpentine. The natural turpentine is not used in medicine, as it is highly irritating and when the word *turpentine* is employed the oil of turpentine is indicated.

In collections of gas in the abdominal organs medicinal turpentine has been used, *e.g.* tympany in horses and cattle. Large doses are liable to irritate the stomach and kidneys.

Turpentine should *never be given* when an animal is suffering from congestion of the kidneys, nephritis, inflammations of the bladder, stomach, or bowels, as its active irritant action only in-creases the already existing inflammation. (*See under* SMELLS.)

Externally, oil of turpentine is used as a consti-tuent of liniments.

TURTLES (*see* AMERICAN BOX TURTLE).

Threat to public health from pet turtles. Six of 28 lots of embryonated eggs of the red-eared turtle (*Pseudemys scripta elegans*) imported into Canada from Louisiana were found to harbour salmonellae. *Salmonella poona* and *S. arizonae* were often isolated from the eggs and the pack-aging moss, and the turtles hatched from the con-taminated eggs continued to shed salmonellae into the tank water for up to 11 months. Of the 37 strains of salmonellae isolated, 30 were resistant to gentamicin, probably because of the wide-spread use of the antibiotic to try to produce sal-monella-free eggs for export. Such high levels of antibiotic-resistant salmonellae in turtle eggs could pose a serious risk to human health. (D'Aoust, J.-Y., & others. (1990) *American Jour-nal of Epidemiology* **132,** 233.)

'TWIN LAMB' DISEASE. A colloquial name for PREGNANCY TOXAEMIA.

TWINNING, ARTIFICIAL. In the interests of increased beef production, attempts were begun in 1959 to exploit commercially an experimental technique for the production of twin calves. A suitable dose of pregnant mare's serum (PMS), injected subcutaneously at a suitable time, *e.g.* 4 days before oestrus, will on average give twins; but there will be some triplets and singles. The follicle-stimulating hormone (*see* FSH) contained in the serum causes an extra follicle to mature and shed an extra egg with resultant twinning. Over-dosage, however, leads to undesired quadruplets, etc.; or to numerous eggs which pass quickly down the Fallopian tubes without being fertilised; result – no calf at all. There is a risk of stillbirths and of strain on the dam. (*See also* TRANSPLANTATION).

TWINS (CALVES). Twins tend to run in families. For example, one cow had three pairs of twins, her daughter four pairs, and a granddaughter two pairs. That might be called twinning at its best. Of course, there is sometimes trouble. Perhaps the condition of the dam is pulled down; or perhaps the 'cleansing' is retained, becomes infected, and infertility follows.

Predicting twins. The concentration of oestrone sulphate, a hormone produced by a cow carrying a viable fetus and present in blood plasma or milk, can be used to confirm pregnancy.

The concentration was higher in cows carrying twins, but the difference did not become significant until about the 220th day of gestation. However, even at this late stage, the prediction of twins could be used as a guide to increase the feed allowance of cows carrying more than one fetus. (Worsfold, A. L. & others. *British Veterinary Journal* (1989) **145**, 46.)

In strains not noted for twins, twinning may occur on farms where there is a herd infertility problem.

Identical twins – always of the same sex – result from the division of the fertilised egg into two; whereas ordinary twins are produced as the result of the fertilisation of two eggs.

These two eggs may come from the same ovary, when the two fetuses may develop in the same horn of the uterus. Sometimes they result in a FREEMARTIN.

Dr Joseph Edwards once quoted a Swedish research worker who found that there is evidently, with cattle, a close affinity between identical twins – as their undoubtedly is with human beings. **Six pairs of twins were split at birth and reared separately, for fifteen months. At this age they were all put into a field together. Within a few days each twin had found and paired off with its sister.** (*See* ERYTHROCYTE MOSAICISM; *also* GENETICS, SUPERFETATION *and* TWINNING *above*; *also* TRIPLET CALVES.)

TWINS (FOALS). In the mare, the presence of twins in the uterus is a common cause of abortion. About 3 per cent of pregnant mares conceive twin fetuses, but the birth of healthy twins is exceedingly rare – about 0·01 per cent.

TWINS, MONOZYGOUS. Identical twins, from the same ovum.

TWITCH. This consists of a loop of soft rope threaded through a hole near the end of a stout piece of wood. The twitch is applied to the horse's upper lip, where it compresses the sensitive nerves. It used to be thought that the twitch merely diverted the horse's attention away from other parts of the body, but this view was disputed by Lagerweij and others, who consider that pain perception or awareness are diminished through the activation of ENDORPHINS (which see). They demonstrated that the twitching significantly increased plasma levels of β-endorphin, which returned to normal 30 minutes or so after the twitch was removed. Twitching could therefore be said to be analogous to ACUPUNCTURE. (Lagerweij & others, *Science* (1984) **225**, 1172.)

'TYING-UP SYNDROME'. Also known as setfast, this condition in racehorses appears to be identical with azoturia. Symptoms include stiffness, a rolling gait, blowing and sweating and, if exercise continues, the adoption of a crouching attitude. Pain is evident. The animal may lie down and be unable to rise. (*See* AZOTURIA.)

'TYLAN' (*see below*).

TYLOSIN. An antibiotic. (*See* ADDITIVES.)

TYMPANITES the drum-like condition of the abdomen, which results from distension of the stomach or bowels with gas, as the result of fermentation, constipation, or of simple obstruction. (*See under* STOMACH, DISEASES OF; INTESTINES, DISEASES OF; BLOAT; TYMPANITIC.)

TYMPANITIC RESONANCE IN CATTLE. Right side tympanitic resonance (ping) caused by gas distention of intra-abdominal structures was diagnosed in 366 adult cattle. The source of the ping was identified as the abomasum in 137 animals, various segments of the intestinal tract in 157 and peritoneal gas in two. The source of the noise was not identified in 70. The principal final diagnoses were: left displacement of the abomasum (116), right displacement of abomasum (77), abomasal (and omasal) volvulus (60). other gastrointestinal conditions (73) and non gastrointestinal conditions (40). Smith, D. F and others (1982) *Cornell Veterinarium* **72**, 180.

TYMPANY is distension of a hollow organ with gas. (*See* TYMPANITES, BLOAT.)

TYPHILITIS. Inflammation of the caecum or first part of the large intestine, into which the termination of the small intestine opens.

TYPHUS OF RATS & MICE, caused by *Rickettsia mooseri*, may kill about 5 per cent of people infected by it.

TYZZER'S DISEASE. This was first described in mice in 1917, and has since been reported in horses, cats, and laboratory animals including rats, rabbits, gerbils, and Rhesus monkeys.

CAUSE. The spore-forming, Gram-negative, motile *Bacillus piliformis.*

SIGNS. The disease is characterised as a rule by severe diarrhoea, debility, and death; though sudden death in foals without preliminary symptoms has been reported in the USA. Jaundice, slight or marked, was a *post-mortem* finding, together with some liver necrosis and enteritis.

In the cat, the infection gives rise to symptoms of loss of appetite, depression, diarrhoea, collapse and death. Necrosis of the ileum and hepatitis are among *post-mortem* findings.

TZANEEN DISEASE. This is a tick-borne infection with *Theileria mutans* in cattle, the African buffalo, and the Indian water buffalo, and often occurs simultaneously with other infections. There may be only a mild fever or, less commonly, serious illness, and death. Antimalarial drugs are of use.

U

UDDER (*see* MAMMARY GLAND).

UITPEULOOG ('Bulging Eye Disease'). A recently described oculo-vascular myiasis of domestic animals in South Africa.

ULCER. A breach on the surface of the skin, or of any mucous membrane of a cavity of the body, which does not tend to heal. The process by which an ulcer spreads, which involves necrosis (death) of minute portions of the healthy tissues around its edges, is known as 'ulceration'. Most ulcers are suppurative; bacteria preventing healing and often extending the lesion.

An ulcer consists of a 'floor' or surface which, in consequence of the loss or destruction of tissue, is usually depressed below the level of the surrounding healthy structures, and an 'edge' around it where the healthy tissues end.

Callous ulcer is a type of chronic ulcer often met with in horses and dogs, when there is any pressure or irritation that interferes with the blood-supply but does not necessarily cause immediate destruction of the skin. In most cases it is covered by a hard leathery piece of dead skin from under which escapes a purulent fluid. Bedsores in all animals may be of this nature.

'Rodent ulcer' is a term reserved in human medicine for an ulcerating carcinoma of the skin, but it is often colloquially used by dog- and cat-owners for an EOSINOPHILIC GRANULOMA. Skin cancer occurs in domestic animals, and such malignant tumours *may* ulcerate.

Tubercular ulcers may occur in dogs' and cats' skin in the form of raised plaques which ulcerate.

Internal ulcers may occur in the mouth (*see* MOUTH, DISEASES OF), in the stomach (*see* GASTRIC ULCERS), in the bowels (*see* INTESTINES, DISEASES OF), and in other parts.

Glanders ulcers, which are typically met with in the mucous membrane of the nostrils, and have a 'punched-out' appearance.

Lip-and-leg ulcers, which occur in sheep affected with the condition known as 'orf'.

CAUSES. Any condition that lowers the general vitality of the animal, such as old age, chronic disease, malnutrition, defective circulation, will act as a predisposing cause. Among direct causes may be bacteria gaining access to wounds. Irritation from badly fitting harness, pressure of bony prominences upon hard floors insufficiently provided with bedding (*see* BEDSORES), and application of too strong antiseptics to wounds.

TREATMENT. In the smaller animals a vitamin supplement may be indicated. An antibiotic or one of the sulpha drugs may be used.

Local treatment aims at converting the ulcer into what virtually becomes an ordinary open wound. The surface is treated with some suitable antiseptic, such as gentian violet, 'TCP', acriflavine, etc. If one or two days of such treatment does not result in a clean, bright-red, odourless wound, or where there are shreds of dead tissue adherent to the surface, it may be necessary to curette the surface so that the dead cells may be separated from the healthy below them.

Animal-owners should note that after the surface of the ulcer has been rendered as healthy as possible, use of strong antiseptics or (worse still) disinfectants, should cease, as these retard healing by the destruction of surface tissues. The use of what are often referred to as 'heroic measures' is in itself a possible cause of ulceration.

Corneal ulcers are referred to under EYE, DISEASES OF – Keratitis. (*See also* CRYOSURGERY.)

ULCERATIVE DERMATOSIS of sheep. A viral infection, which has to be differentiated from ORF, and is characterised by ulcers on face, feet, legs, and external genitalia. It is also called INFECTIOUS BALANOPOSTHITIS (which see), and occurs in Europe and Africa.

ULCERATIVE LYMPHANGITIS, also called ULCERATIVE CELLULITIS, is a contagious chronic disease of horses characterised by inflammation of the lymph vessels and a tendency towards ulceration of the skin over the parts affected.
CAUSE. Is usually *Corynebacterium ovis.* It gains access through abrasions. Infection may be carried by grooming tools, harness, utensils, etc., from one horse to another.
SIGNS. The commonest seat of the disease is the fetlock of a hindleg. This part becomes swollen and slightly painful. Small abscesses appear, ulcers follows. The condition gradually spreads up the leg.
TREATMENT. Encouraging results have followed antibiotic treatment.

ULCERATIVE SPIROCHAETOSIS OF PIGS. This has been reported in the UK, Australia, New Zealand, South Africa, USA. It may give rise to footrot in pigs, ulceration of the skin, and scirrhous cord.

ULNA is the inner of the two bones of the forearm. The shaft has gradually become less and less in size in ratio as the number of digits has decreased, so that while the ulna is a perfect bone in the dog and cat, in the horse its shaft has almost completely disappeared and the bone is only represented by the olecranon process which forms the 'point of the elbow'. The shaft of the ulna is liable to become fractured from violence to the fore-limb, but the commonest seat of an ulnar fracture is the olecranon process. This occurs from a fall in which the fore-limbs slip out in front of the animal, and the weight of the body comes down suddenly on to the point of the elbow. (*See* FRACTURES.)

ULTRA HIGH TEMPERATURE TREATMENT
of milk involves heating it to between 275° and
300°F for a few seconds. Suggested in 1913, this
process is used to produce 'Long-keeping' milk,
on sale in Britain from 1965 onwards. This process does not affect the calcium nor the casein, but
destroys some vitamins and probably some serum
proteins (immune globulins). Calves grow less
well on it than on raw or pasteurised milk.

ULTRASONIC (*see below, and also* PREGNANCY
DIAGNOSIS). ☞

ULTRASOUND. Sound at a frequency above
20,000 cycles per second. Propagated by applying
an electric current to one side of a piezoelectric
crystal, which deforms and produces a sound
wave. (R. E. Carter *et al. JAVMA* (1980) **176 (5)**
426.)
   Ultrasound is generally defined as an auditory
frequency beyond that perceived by the human
ear. Most humans hear and emit sound in the
frequency range 2 to 20 kHz, while in some
animals ranges are much greater. Bats, dolphins,
many rodents and some insects have ranges that
extend as high as 120 kHz, well beyond the limit
of human detection. (Kock, K., *Veterinary Record*
(1986) **118**, 588.) (*See also* PREGNANCY DIAGNOSIS.)
   In human medicine, ultrasound has been
shown to be beneficial for wound healing, both in
the treatment of pressure sores and in the preparation of trophic ulcers for skin grafting. Studies
have shown that it influences the activity of
fibroblasts. (Callam, M. J. and others. *Lancet*
(1987) **87**, 204.)

ULTRA-VIOLET RAYS are used in the treatment
of various skin diseases, etc., and in the diagnosis
of ringworm and porphyria and also in the
fluorescent-antibody test for various infections
including rabies.
Ultra-violet rays and eye cancer. Analysis of
data from 14 veterinary colleges in the USA
where 147 cases of eye cancer in horses were
studied, led to the conclusion that ultra-violet
radiation may be of primary importance. (Dugan,
S. J. & others. *JAVMA* (1991) **198**, 251.)

UMBILICAL CORD, CUTTING THE (*see under*
PARTURITION).

UMBILICUS is another name for the navel.

UNCINARIASIS. Infection with *Uncinaria
stenocephala*, one of the hookworms of the dog.

UNCONSCIOUSNESS (*see under* COMA, FITS,
SYNCOPE, EPILEPSY, NARCOLEPSY).

UNDECYLENATE OINTMENT. A fungicide,
used in the treatment of ringworm, etc.

UNDULANT FEVER IN MAN is caused by
Brucella melitensis; Brucella abortus suis; or
Brucella abortus. The latter organism is responsible for 'contagious abortion' (brucellosis) of
cattle, and it is probable that most cases of
undulant fever in man caused by *B. abortus* arise

through handling infected cows or from drinking
their milk. Infection can readily occur through
the skin. Numerous cases have occurred in veterinarians, following mishaps with Strain 19 vaccine; *e.g.* accidental spraying into the eyes or injection into the hand. In America, *Brucella
abortus suis* is an important cause of undulant
fever in man; *B. canis* likewise.
SYMPTOMS are vague and simulate those of
influenza except that undulant fever lasts for a
much longer time, even many months. Temperature is generally raised but fluctuates greatly;
there are muscle pains, headache, tiredness and
inability to concentrate. One or more joints may
swell. There may be constipation. The organisms
are present in the blood-stream and in the spleen.
   The disease is serious, not so much because of
its mortality (1 to 2 per cent), but because of in-
capacity occasioned by its long duration. (*See*
BRUCELLOSIS *and* CHEESE.)
PREVENTION. Anyone handling aborting
cows, or their fetal membranes, or even calving
an apparently normal cow, should wear protective gloves or sleeves (which nevertheless sometimes tear), and wash arms and hands in a disinfectant solution afterwards. Avoid drinking any
cold milk that has not been pasteurised.

UNSATURATED FATTY ACIDS (*see under*
LIPIDS, VITAMIN E).

UNSTABLE   SUBSTANCES (*see   under*
INJECTIONS).

URAEMIA results when the waste materials that
should be excreted into the urine are retained in
the body, through some disease of the kidneys,
and are circulated in the blood-stream. Blood-
urea is in excess. The condition is very serious and
nearly always fatal. Death may be preceded by
convulsions and unconsciousness. In the slower
types there is usually a strong urinous odour from
all the body secretions. In acute cases the administration of glucose saline subcutaneously may
help; likewise withdrawal of a quantity of blood
(provided saline is given). (*See* URINE, ABNORMAL
CONDITIONS *and* LEPTOSPIROSIS, KIDNEY, DISEASES
OF.)

URATES (*see* URIC ACID).

UREA, or CARBAMIDE, is a crystalline substance
of the chemical formula $CO(NH_2)_2$, which is very
soluble in water and alcohol. It is the chief waste
product discharged from the body in the urine,
being formed in the liver and carried by the blood
to the kidneys. The amount excreted varies with
the nature and the amount of the food taken,
being greater in the carnivora, and when large
amounts of protein are present in the food. It is
also increased in quantity during the course of
fevers.
   Urea is rapidly changed into ammonium
carbonate after excretion and when in contact
with the air, owing to the action of certain
microorganisms.
   Determination of the blood urea level is an
important aid to the diagnosis of kidney failure.

UREA AS A RUMINANT FEED. As long ago as the beginning of the century it was known that some of the micro-organisms which inhabit the rumen could synthesise protein from urea, and it was accordingly suggested that urea might be substituted for protein in concentrates fed to cattle. This has since been referred to as the protein-sparing effect of urea.

In recent times, the emphasis has shifted more, perhaps, to the value of urea in increasing the intake and aiding the digestion of low-quality roughages, and it has been widely used as a dietary supplement for cattle and sheep on poor pasture in many parts of the world. **Where extra energy, in the form of readily digestible carbohydrate, is provided in addition to the urea,** both roughage digestibility and feed intake improve. In these circumstances the urea stimulates multiplication of cellulose-digesting organisms, so that the urea-fed animal may be able to make more effective use of roughage than the one receiving no urea.

In the ruminant animal any injudicious feeding of urea will give rise to poisoning by ammonia, since it is this which the rumen bacteria convert urea into. An excess of ammonia in the rumen can cause death. It is essential, therefore, that urea is taken in small quantities over a period, and not fed a large amount at a time. 'Ideally,' Dr E. C. Owen, of the Hannah Research Institute, emphasised, 'urea must be intimately mixed with the carbohydrates or fibrous part (or both) of the ration,' and for this reason he would strongly deprecate the direct sale of pure urea (as opposed to a commercial mix) to farmers. On the other hand, farmers who use a proprietary preparation of urea in the way advocated by Dr M. H. Briggs should have no fears about poisoning.

Dr R. C. Campling, of the National Institute for Research in Dairying, comments: 'When the crude protein content of the diet is about 10 per cent or over, the addition of urea would not be expected to be beneficial.' Dr Owen agrees: 'If the ration is already adequate in protein equivalent, there will be little response.'

The crux of the matter, therefore, seems to be whether farmers can get good enough results from a ration containing urea but under 10 per cent crude protein. At the present time, many farmers seem convinced that they can, and in addition to its use in beef and sheep rations, urea is also being used as a supplement for dairy cows on a high barley diet.

There are several proprietary preparations of urea on the market; for example, Promax, Rumevite, Mozine molasses meal. Dr M. H. Briggs stated:

'Promax is a solution of urea in mineralised molasses. It is fed in special inexpensive ball-valve feeders which allow single licks but prevent its being drunk to excess. By this method the animals receive the urea in small amounts over a long period; and it is just these conditions that allow the maximum use to be made of the urea by the animal. Tests have shown that cows can be fed large amounts of urea in this manner with no ill effects.

'Under practical farming conditions, where optimum animal production is the aim, only 15 to 30 per cent of the dietary protein is replaced by urea.

'Urea is not merely a protein-replacer for ruminants. It also stimulates the production of cellulose-digesting organisms in the rumen, with the result that the animal can eat and efficiently digest much more cheap roughages than a protein-fed animal.' (*See also* STRAW FEEDING.)

Professor M. McG. Cooper and Dr M. B. Willis stated in their book *Profitable Beef Production* that 'a survey of the evidence leaves no doubt that urea substitution of protein will lead to reduced gain (about 6 per cent) and reduced feed efficiency (about 5 per cent), in beef cattle. Nevertheless, they agree that these disadvantages may, in economic terms, be more than offset by a saving in feed costs, so that the use of urea becomes financially advantageous to the farmer.

Dr A. Eden, of MAFF, has stated: 'Urea can be toxic if used too freely or if it is not uniformly incorporated throughout the ration. A 1 per cent usage (22 lb/ton) has not only been shown to be quite safe and, together with a cwt of barley, can replace a cwt of ground nut meal in a ton diet, but also will sustain yields and milk compositional quality equal to those on more conventional feeding. Such usage may also reduce the cost of a dairy production ration, depending on the make-up of the latter and the extent to which purchased foods are being used. There appears, as yet, little evidence to show whether urea-containing diets are as fully satisfactory with really high-yielding cows.

'There is no doubt that urea has higher potentialities in the diets of fattening cattle fed virtually *ad lib.*, because this scheme of feeding lessens the risk of suddenly flushing the rumen with urea (and hence leading to ammonia poisoning) than is likely to occur in the dairy cow given large quantities of concentrates twice daily at milking times. Moreover, the protein needs of fattening cattle are less than those of the dairy cow and in the finishing diets of such cattle the level of urea can be raised to 3 per cent (67 lb/ton).'

Some guide-lines for urea feeding

1. Introduce urea feeding gradually, *i.e.* at a slowly increasing level over a period of 3–4 weeks, with adequate minerals and vitamins provided.

2. Avoid starting newly calved cows* on it, or giving it to calves under 3 months of age.

3. Ensure that urea is fed with adequate readily digestible carbohydrate, as is contained in cereals, molasses, sugar-beet pulp, maize silage, etc.

4. Do not exceed levels of urea recommended above.

5. Ensure that urea is fed little and often, and not irregularly or at long intervals.

Urea poisoning. Symptoms include salivation, excitement, running and staggering, jerking of the eye-balls, and scouring.

---

*But urea may be included in the steaming-up ration.

Acute urea poisoning killed 17 beef cows in a group of 29 in the south of Scotland during 1990, according to the Scottish Veterinary Investigation Service. The animals died over an eight-hour period as a result of drinking water which had been carried to a trough in a tanker previously used for transporting urea fertiliser. It was calculated that as little as 10 litres of the water would have provided a fatal dose of urea to a 500 kg cow.

UREAPLASMAS. Formerly known as T-mycoplasmas, these have been isolated from the lungs, and also the uro-genital tract of several species of animals. They are a likely cause of pneumonia and infertility.

URETER is the tube which carries the urine excreted by a kidney down to the urinary bladder. Each ureter begins at the pelvis of the corresponding kidney, passes backwards and downwards along the roof and walls of the pelvis, and finally ends by opening into the neck of the bladder. The wall of the ureter is composed of a fibrous coat on the outside, a muscular coat in the middle, and this is lined by a mucous membrane consisting of cubical epithelium.

URETHRA is the tube which leads from the neck of the bladder to the outside, opening at the extremity of the penis in the male, and into the posterior part of the urino-genital passage in the female, and serves to conduct the urine from the bladder to the outside; and also the semen.

URETHRA, DISEASES OF. Owing to its extreme shortness in the female the urethra is not subject to the same diseased conditions as in the male, where the tube is considerably longer. In fact, disease of the urethra in the female hardly ever arises except as a complication of either disease of the bladder, on the one hand, or the vagina on the other.

Urethritis. Inflammation of the urethra is usually associated with cystitis, and may be the result of an infection, or of some irritant poison (such as CANTHARIDES) present in the urine. The lining mucous membrane may also be inflamed by crystalline deposits. (*See* FELINE UROLOGICAL SYNDROME, UROLITHIASIS, URETHRAL OBSTRUCTION.)

In most cases of urethritis there are signs of pain and distress whenever urine is passed or when the parts are handled. A little blood may be seen.

Stricture is an abrupt narrowing of the calibre of the tube at one or more places. In almost all cases of true stricture there has been some injury to the urethra or penis, resulting in the formation of scar tissue, which eventually contracts and decreases the lumen of the tube. A few cases, however, are caused by a rapidly growing tumour.

Injuries to the urethra may follow a severe crush or blow which causes fracture of the pelvis or of the os penis in the dog. They are usually obvious when the injury has involved the surface of the body, and may be suspected if there is an inability to pass urine, or if the urine contains blood or pus following upon a severe injury to the hindquarters of the body. A complication of urethral injuries is abscess formation around the urethra and consequent stricture at a later period.

URETHRAL OBSTRUCTION. In **sheep,** the injudicious use of hormones to increase live-weight gain, has killed lambs, apparently as the result of urethral obstruction. In one outbreak in the USA, 200 out of 9000 lambs died after receiving 12 mg stilboestrol by injection. In the UK an increased incidence of urethral obstruction in male calves and lambs was noted during 1981. The common cause was too high a level of magnesium in the concentrates fed, and analysis of the calculi or 'stones' causing the obstruction showed them to be crystals of magnesium ammonium phosphate, Dr.E. R. Orskov and Mr J. J. Robinson stated (*Vet. Record* (1981) **109**, 107). Since reducing the level of magnesium supplementation over 10 years ago to 200 mg MgO per tonne of feed, they had not had a single case of urolithiasis in intensively fattened male lambs offered a cereal-based diet *ad lib.* (*See also under* BLADDER, DISEASES OF – Urinary calculi.)

Five outbreaks in male **calves** of various ages investigated by Mr. D. A. Rice and Dr. C. H. McMurray, of the Veterinary Research Laboratory, Stormont, showed a magnesium content of the concentrates (fed from the first week of life) to range from 4·9 to 9·2 g/kg dry matter. (The ARC recommendation is not more than 1·4 g/kg dry matter.) (*Vet. Record* (1981) **109**, 88.)

Cattle, sheep, cats and camels are stated to be more susceptible to urethral CALCULI during cold weather. (Koch, R. A., *Veterinary Record* (1985) **117**, 494.)

Obstruction of the male urethra is a common condition in **cats**, and fairly common in the **dog**. (*See* FELINE UROLOGICAL SYNDROME.)

Unless relieved, urethral obstruction can lead to rupture of the bladder and death.

URETHROSTOMY. Perineal urethrostomy is a surgical operation for the treatment of urethral obstruction; and consists of making a permanent opening in the urethra, the lining mucous membrane and the skin being joined by sutures. (Urethrostomy differs in this respect from **urethrotomy**, in which the urethra is incised—to remove a wedged calculus, for example—but immediately closed.)

Urethrostomy is performed mainly in cats suffering from the feline urological syndrome (FUS). It is not in itself a cure for this, but rather for the often associated urethral obstruction. The operation is an alternative to euthanasia when the cat cannot be catheterised, or has already been subjected to this on two or more occasions, when repetition could be regarded as inhumane.

Urethrostomy, skilfully performed, can be successful, both in the short term and the long term.

Complications can arise, however, after both urethrotomies and urethrostomies, and include extravasation of urine into surrounding tissues; haemorrhage; and stricture, as the result of scar formation. Should the latter occur, it leaves the cat in the same state as it was before the operation; so that nothing has been gained.

Urethrostomy makes the male cat anatomically similar to the female, so that ascending infections may occur.

Some veterinary surgeons remove the penis; others leave it.

(For the surgical technique, the reader is referred to the article by G. P. Wilson on pages 237–243 of *Current Techniques in Small Animal Surgery I*, published by Lea & Febiger, Philadelphia.)

URIC ACID is a crystalline substance, very slightly soluble in water, white in the pure state, and found in the urine of flesh-eating animals in normal conditions. It is also found in some kidney stones and urinary calculi, and may be present in joints affected with GOUT.

URINARY ANTISEPTICS include hexylresorcinol, mandelic acid, hexamine (for acid urine; not effective in alkaline urine), buchu.

URINARY BLADDER. In some animals the bladder is situated in the pelvis, but in the dog and cat it is placed farther forward in the abdomen, while in the pig and ox it may be almost entirely abdominal when distended. The size of the organ varies with the breed and sex of the animal, and its capacity depends upon the individual. Two small tubes – called *ureters* – lead into the bladder, one from each kidney, and the larger, thicker *urethra* conveys urine from it to the exterior. The constricted portion from which the urethra takes origin is called the *neck* of the bladder, and is guarded by a ring of muscular tissue – the *sphincter*.

Structure. The wall of the bladder is somewhat similar to that of the intestine, and consists of a mucous lining on the inside, possessing flat, pavement-like epithelial cells, a loose submucous layer of fibrous tissue very rich in blood-vessels, a strong complicated muscular coat in which the fibres are arranged in many directions, and on the surface an incomplete peritoneal coat covers the organ. In places this peritoneal covering is folded across to parts of the abdominal or pelvic wall in the form of ligaments which retain the bladder in its position.

In young animals the bladder is elongated and narrow and reaches much farther forward than it does in the adult. In the unborn fetus its forward extremity communicates with the outside of the body until just before birth, when the passage becomes closed at the umbilicus, or navel, and the bladder shrinks backwards.

URINARY BLADDER, DISEASES OF.

Cystitis. Inflammation of the bladder is often infective in origin, with micro-organisms coming either from the kidneys via the ureters, or, in the female, in the reverse direction, *i.e.* via the urethra from an infected vagina.

Leptospirosis is a common cause of nephritis and cystitis in farm animals and in dogs. *E. coli* is another common pathogen in dogs; and *Corynebacterium suis* in pigs.

In dogs cystitis is occasionally found to be due to the bladder worm *Capillaria plica*; and in cats to *C. feliscati*. The parasites' eggs may be found in the urinary sediment. Levamisole may be used for treatment.

Some poisons cause cystitis; for example, cantharides, turpentine.

Inflammation of the bladder may be caused by the abrasive action of a sand-like crystalline deposit as in the FELINE UROLOGICAL SYNDROME (FUS) or, to a lesser extent, by sizeable urinary calculi.

SIGNS. In acute cystitis small quantities of urine may be passed frequently, with signs of pain and/or straining on each occasion. Blood may be seen in the urine. The larger animals may walk with their hindlegs slightly abducted, and the back is often arched in all animals.

TREATMENT. This will naturally vary according to the cause. An appropriate antibiotic may be used to overcome infection, along perhaps with a urinary antiseptic. Pain relievers may be needed.

Urinary calculi. These, associated with high grain rations, and the use of oestrogen produce heavy losses among fattening cattle and sheep in the feed-lots of the United States and Canada. 'However, this condition does not seem to present the same problem in the barley beef units in this country, although outbreaks do occur in sheep fed high grain rations. Udall found that the inclusion of 4 per cent NaCl in the diet decreased the incidence of urinary calculi.' – H. C. Wilson.

In male calves and lambs, crystalline deposits of magnesium ammonium phosphate cause urethral obstruction if the animals are receiving too high a level of magnesium supplement in their concentrate feed. (*See* URETHRAL OBSTRUCTION.)

Urinary calculi may occur in an individual animal irrespective of its diet, or of hormone implants. There may be one large calculus present in the bladder, or several small ones, or the crystalline sand-like deposit already mentioned. In such cases, although hyaluronidase might be tried, treatment usually has to be surgical; *i.e.* cystotomy.

Rupture of the bladder. This condition is usually quickly fatal, and is brought about by a painful over-distension of the bladder due to urethral obstruction.

Tumours. These may cause difficulty in passing urine, and sometimes the presence of blood in the urine.

Of 70 cases in the dog, A. G. Burnie and A. D. Weaver (*Journal of Small Animal Practice* (1983) **24,** 129) found no urinary signs in 9. In the other 61, signs included haematuria, dysuria, tenesmus, incontinence, and polyuria. Sixty-two dogs had primary tumours; 44 of these being carcinomas. Several papillomas were found during cystotomy for urinary calculi.

URINARY CALCULI (*see above, and under* URINARY BLADDER, DISEASES OF).

URINARY INCONTINENCE in dogs and cats. (*See* INCONTINENCE.)

URINARY ORGANS (*see* KIDNEYS, URETERS, BLADDER, URETHRA).

URINE. A brief outline of the formation of urine is given under KIDNEYS – Function. (*See also* HOMEOSTASIS.)

Not only are waste products removed from the bloodstream by the kidneys; most poisons taken into the body are eliminated from the system by way of the urine; thus, quinine, morphine, chloroform, carbolic acid, iodides, and strychnine can be recognised in the urine by means of appropriate tests, while there is abundant evidence to show that during bacterial diseases the kidneys eliminate toxins.

Specific gravity. The specific gravity of the urine of animal varies between wide limits; for average purposes the following figures are given.

	Lowest	Average	Highest
Horse	1014	1036	1050
Cow	1006	1020	1030
Sheep	1006	1010	1015
Pig	1003	1015	1025
Dog and cat	1016	—	1060

Reaction. The urine of the herbivorous animals is usually alkaline, and that of the flesh-eating animals is acid. The alkalinity in herbivores is due to the salts of the organic acids that are taken in with the vegetable diet, such as malic, citric, tartaric, and succinic; these acids are converted into carbonates in the body, and these latter are excreted in solution. In the case of some foods, such as hay and oats, an acid urine may be produced when they are fed to the horse. In the carnivorous animals the acidity is due to sodium acid phosphate. The pig's urine may be acid or alkaline according to the nature of its food.

Amount. The quantities of urine excreted depend upon many factors, among which may be noted: season, diet, amount of water consumed, condition of the animal, secretion of milk, pregnancy, age, and size of the animal. (*See* PREGNANCY DIAGNOSIS TESTS.)

The following are average figures of the amounts excreted during 24 hours:
Horse: 5 to 20 pints, average 9 pints.
Cow: 10 to 40 pints, average 22 pints.
Sheep: 0·5 to 1·5 pints, average 1 pint.
Pig: 2·5 to 14 pints, average 8 pints.
Dog: 0·75 pints to 1·75 pints, average 1·25 pints.

Abnormal constituents of urine. *Albumin* may be excreted when there is some disease of the kidneys. *Sugar* is found in diabetes and it is also found in smaller amounts after an animal has been fed on a diet that is too rich in sugar. In this latter case – known as 'glycosuria' – the sugar disappears when the feeding is corrected. *Pus* and *tube-casts* are the signs of inflammation or ulceration in some part of the urinary system. *Bile* in the urine is a sign that there is some obstruction to the outflow of bile into the intestines, and that the bile is being reabsorbed into the blood-stream and excreted by the kidneys.

URINE-DRINKING, or licking, by cattle may be a symptom of sodium deficiency. (*See* LICKING SYNDROME.)

URINE-SPRAYING by cats. This is the normal method used by the male cat to mark out his territory. Under natural conditions this may be some five acres or so in extent (Dr W. R. Kirk). The territory-marking serves as a warning to other males to keep out, and perhaps also as an invitation to females in oestrus to enter.

Urine-spraying is not confined to the entire male, but may also be indulged in by the entire female, and even by neuters of either sex. It may also be an expression of sexual excitement.

Spraying indoors is often the result of stress, caused by neglect of the cat following the arrival of a baby, or by the addition of another cat (or dog) to the household, or by being left alone for long periods, or the presence locally of an aggressive tom. A move to a new home may initiate urine-spraying indoors. Spraying is common in households where several cats are kept.

Tranquillisers during short stress periods may be prescribed, or anabolic steroids similarly. Food can be put down in places usually sprayed, or foil can be used to cover the target areas in the hope that the noise will disconcert the animal.

URINOMETER is an instrument designed for the estimation of the specific gravity of urine.

UROLITHIASIS. The formation of calculi ('stones'), or of a crystalline sand-like deposit, in the urinary system. A bacterial or viral infection may precede or follow the condition. (*See* URETHRAL OBSTRUCTION; URINARY BLADDER, DISEASES OF; FELINE URINARY SYNDROME, *and* URETHRA, DISEASES OF.)

UROLITHS. The mineral composition of 2700 of these were studied, after their removal from dogs. Their composition was struvite in nearly 60 per cent of those tested. In cats the prevalence of struvite uroliths declined between 1984–1989; corresponding with the introduction of Prescription Diets. In horses the most common mineral was calcium carbonate. (Osborne, C. A. & others. *Veterinary Medicine* (1989) **84,** 750.)

UROTROPINE (*see* HEXAMINE).

URTICARIA, or 'NETTLE RASH', is a disease of the skin in which small areas of the surface become raised in weals of varying sizes. It occurs in horses, cattle (when it is often called 'blaines'), pigs, and dogs.
CAUSES. The condition is not necessarily specific. It may follow exposure to the leaves of the stinging nettle (hence one of its names); insect bites may produce it; it may be associated with diet; it may occur during the course of certain specific conditions, such as purpura, dourine, influenza, etc. Urticaria is usually, if not always, of an allergic nature.

Factitious urticaria, common in the dog but not recorded in the cat, is a term for an abnormal tendency for the skin to weal when rubbed or scratched.

SIGNS. As a rule there is little to be seen beyond the local swellings of the skin. These may vary in size from a pea to a walnut, and are generally more or less almond-shaped. They are painless to the touch, show no oozing discharge, are scattered irregularly over the whole body, and sometimes involve the skin of the eye-lids, nostrils, and perineum. In cattle especially they may attain a great size in the throat region and produce difficulty in breathing.

TREATMENT. Consists in the use of ANTIHISTAMINES (which see), a laxative, a light diet, and calamine lotion. An antibiotic may be used to prevent infection occurring.

UTERINE INFECTIONS. These are discussed under UTERUS, DISEASES OF and under INFERTILITY. A list of the principal organisms which infect the uterus in the various species is given under ABORTION; but for the **mare**, *see* EQUINE GENITAL INFECTIONS.

UTERUS, is a Y-shaped organ consisting of a body and two horns or 'cornua', and is lined by an elaborate mucous membrane which presents special features in different species of animals. The uterus lies in the abdomen below the rectum and at a higher level than the bladder. It becomes continuous with the vagina posteriorly. Its most posterior portion, known as the 'cervix', usually lies partly in the pelvis. From the tip of each horn to the ovary on the corresponding side runs the fallopian tube or oviduct, which conducts the ova from the ovary into the uterus.

In the human female the body is large, and horns for practical purposes do not exist. In rabbits the two horns open into the vagina separately. The uteri of domesticated animals are intermediate between these types. (*See later*.)

The walls consist of three coats – a peritoneal covering on the outside continuous with the rest of the peritoneum; a thick muscular wall arranged in two layers, the fibres on the outside being longitudinal and those on the inside circular; the innermost coat is mucous membrane. This latter is very important, since it is by its agency that the ovum and the sperms are nourished before they fuse, and it is through the mucous membrane that nutrients and oxygen are conveyed from dam to fetus, and that much of the waste products leave the fetal circulation to pass into the maternal blood-stream. It consists of epithelial cells, amongst which lie the uterine glands which secrete the so-called 'uterine milk' which serves to nourish the newly fertilised ovum.

The most posterior extremity of the uterus is called the 'os uteri', and this forms the opening into the 'cervix uteri', which is a thick-walled canal guarding entrance into the cavity of the body of the uterus. Normally this is almost or completely shut, but during oestrus it slackens, and during parturition it becomes fully opened to allow exit of the fetus. The uterus is held in position by means of a fold of peritoneum attached to the roof of the abdomen, which carries blood-vessels, nerves, etc. This is known as the 'broad ligament'; it is capable of a considerable amount of stretching.

The mare. The shape of the uterus of the mare most nearly approaches that of the human being. It possesses a large body and comparatively small horns. During pregnancy the fetus generally lies in horn and body. The mucous membrane is corrugated into folds.

The cow. The body is less in size than the

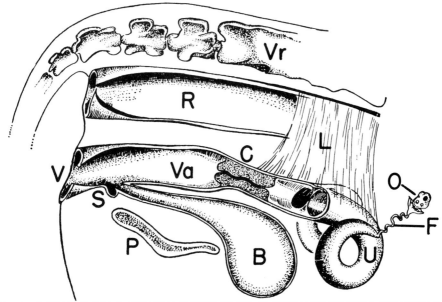

The reproductive tract of the cow (side view). *B*, Urinary bladder; *C*, cervix; *F*, fallopian tube; *L*, broad ligament; *O*, ovary; *R*, rectum; *P*, pelvic bone (*os coxae*); *S*, suburethral diverticulum; *U*, uterine horn; *Va*, vagina; *V*, vestibule; *Vr*, vertebral column. (Hafez, *Reproduction in Farm Animals*, Lea & Febiger as reproduced in R. D. Frandson: *Anatomy and Physiology of Farm Animals*, Baillière, Tindall & Cassell.)

horns, which are long, tapering, and curved downwards, outwards, backwards, and upwards to end within the pelvis at about the level of the cervix. The fetus lies in the body and one horn in single pregnancy, and when twins are present each usually occupies one horn and a part of the body. The mucous membrane presents upon its inner surface a large number (100 upwards) of mushroom-shaped projections – 'cotyledons'. The fetal membranes are attached to the dome-like free surface of the cotyledons, in which are a large number of crypts, which receive projections called 'villi' from the outer surface of the chorion.

The ewe's uterus is similar to that of the cow except that it is smaller and that the cotyledons are cup-shaped.

The sow has a small uterine body and a pair of long convoluted horns that resemble pieces of intestine. The mucous membrane is ridged but has no cotyledons. The young lie in the horns only.

The bitch and cat have uteri with comparatively short bodies and long straight divergent horns that run towards the kidneys of the corresponding sides.

(*See* PREGNANCY, PARTURITION.)

UTERUS, DISEASES OF. Inflammation of the uterus (*metritis*) may be acute or chronic, localised (*e.g.* confined to the cervix) or involving more than one uterine tissue.

A list of uterine infections giving rise to infertility and abortion in the various species will be found under ABORTION, but for the mare, *see under* EQUINE GENITAL INFECTIONS.

The mare.
ACUTE METRITIS. This may occur either before or after foaling. When it takes place prior to the act it is usually associated with the death of the foal and its subsequent abortion, with or without discharge of the whole or a part of the membranes. In such cases the inflammatory condition may persist in an acute form and cause the death of the mare, or it may assume a chronic form after the abortion and render the mare incapable of further breeding; other cases are followed by recovery. Acute metritis occurring after normal foaling may arise through the conveyance of infection into the uterus by the arms or hands of the attendants, or by the ropes, instruments, or other appliances that are used to assist the birth of the foal, or it may be the direct result of retained membranes that undergo bacterial decomposition. (This may happen after a large part, but not all, of the fetal membranes have come away.)

Signs. Acute metritis is a severe and often fatal condition. Within 24 to 48 hours, the mare becomes greatly distressed and loses all interest in the foal. She lies most of the time and refuses food; her temperature is usually high. Greyish blood-flecked discharge escapes from the vagina and soils the tail and hindquarters. The mare may become tucked up in her abdomen and stands with her back arched.

Laminitis may develop. (*See* LAMINITIS.)

Prevention. During foaling and after the act the greatest attention should be paid to the cleanliness of everything that is to come into contact with the genital tract of the mare. The attendant's finger nails should be trimmed short, and his hands and arms should be well scrubbed with soap and water containing some antiseptic, such as Dettol. Finally the hand and arm should be lubricated with a suitable preparation marketed for this purpose. All appliances that are to be used should be boiled and kept in a pail of hot water when not actually in use.

One other factor is of the greatest importance. After a mare foals the fetal membranes should be given attention. Normally they are discharged by means of a few comparatively mild labour pains within an hour of the birth of the foal. If they are retained for longer than this period the person in attendance should suspect that something may be wrong and give continual attention to the mare.

In other cases a series of violent pains may commence, when the bulk of the membranes are passed to the outside, where they hang suspended. Should this happen a sack or sheet should be placed under the dependent mass, and held so as to support the weight and relieve the tension on that portion that is still retained in the uterus. This is necessary lest the weight of the external membranes causes a tearing away from the non-separated part. *Gentle traction* should now be exerted upon the imprisoned portion, and as a rule it will gradually detach itself and come to the outside. If no progress is made, veterinary assistance should be sought promptly.

Injections of PITUITRIN (which see) may obviate manual removal of the fetal membranes. A synthetic oestrogen may be preferred. (*See* HORMONE THERAPY.)

Regarding complete retention of the fetal membranes – when only a very small portion is seen hanging from the vagina – professional help should be obtained if there is no sign of any attempt at expulsion within from 4 to 6 hours after foaling.

Generally speaking, membranes that have remained in position for 8 to 12 hours are commencing to decompose, and decomposition means bacterial infection of the uterus (*i.e.* metritis) in almost every case.

Treatment. The case must be considered most serious. The use of antibiotics or one of the sulpha drugs is indicated. (*See also under* NURSING.) Any retained fetal membrane must be removed from the uterus by hand and as much discharge as possible cleared out. A solution of acriflavine, proflavine, or brilliant green, 1 part in 1000 of boiled water, or some other suitable non-irritant antiseptic solution at blood heat, is douched into the cavity of the uterus by a length of rubber tubing, and, after allowing it to act for 2 to 5 minutes, is syphoned off. A special two-way tube is sometimes used for this purpose – the solution entering by one channel and leaving by the other. When all the fluid has been removed an antiseptic pessary may be inserted. When complications such as laminitis or pneumonia co-exist, they must receive separate attention. (*See* LAMINITIS, PNEUMONIA, etc.)

CHRONIC METRITIS. This may originate as a sequel to an acute attack in some cases, but more commonly it is directly due to an injury or infection which is not sufficiently severe to produce an acute attack.

Signs. There may be a general unthriftiness following upon foaling. The mare's appetite is capricious, but her thirst is unimpaired. The temperature fluctuates a degree or two above normal. There may or may not be a dirty, sticky, grey, or pus-like discharge from the vagina, which causes irritation and frequent erections of the clitoris. The mare resents handling of the genital organs, but if the lips of the vulva are gently separated the mucous membrane is seen to be inflamed and swollen.

In other cases the pus collects in the cavity of the uterus and is retained there through closure of the os. (*See* PYOMETRA.) It sometimes happens that after the pus has collected for a certain period the os suddenly opens and a gallon or more of pus is discharged. The os then closes once more. Intervals between these evacuations may vary from a few days to 3 or 4 weeks. The mare's general condition shows an improvement immediately following a sudden discharge of pus, but as it reaccumulates she relapses into her former chronic state. Chronic metritis may get gradually worse, and the mare dies. Cases taken in time usually recover with treatment, but further breeding is often impossible.

Treatment. An early opportunity should be taken to evacuate the pus from the uterus, by douching and syphonage, or by irrigation as already described under acute metritis.

Sulpha drugs or antibiotics may be used.

It should be emphasised that expert advice should be sought at the earliest opportunity.

The cow. In the following brief account much of what has been said in relation to the mare must be understood to apply to the cow as well, and only the main differences will be stated.

ACUTE METRITIS. In some cases where birth of the calf has taken place easily and naturally, metritis supervenes in the course of the first week or 10 days after calving, but in the majority of cases there has been some injury or infection at, or shortly after, parturition. Retention of the fetal membranes, which is so much more common in the cow than in other animals, is very often the contributory factor to an attack of acute metritis. The conveyance of infection by the hands and arms of the cowman, in his capacity of accoucheur, (or insemination of a cow not in oestrus), are other causes.

Signs. The cow generally becomes obviously affected between the second and eighth day after calving. The vulval lips swell and are painful when touched, the lining membrane of the vagina is intensely reddened and swollen. There are frequent and painful attempts at the passage of urine, the temperature rises to 107°F or 108°F, the appetite is lost and there is a gritting of the teeth, rumination is suppressed, the pulse is hard and fast, the milk secretion falls off or stops altogether. A discharge appears at the vulva.

Treatment. Acute metritis in the cow should be looked upon as a contagious disease and precautions taken to prevent infection being conveyed to other cows that are soon due to calve.

Actual treatment is similar to that as applied to the mare.

CHRONIC METRITIS very often follows an acute attack in the cow. The animal partially recovers, the more acute symptoms subside, and there is apparently little or no pain. The general health, however, remains indifferent. Milk secretion does not continue, flesh is lost, there is either a constant or an intermittent discharge from the vulva, which soils the tail and hindquarters, and has in many cases a putrid smell.

Chronic metritis may be due to *Brucella abortus* (*see* BRUCELLOSIS), *Trichomonas fetus*, *Corynebacterium pyogenes*, or *Campylobacter fetus*, among other organisms.

Another form of chronic metritis that attacks cattle is seen in virgin heifers that have never bred.

Pyometra (a collection of pus in the uterus) may result from infection introduced during natural service, insemination, or at or after calving. Treatment with cloprestonol may be helpful.

Treatment of chronic metritis in the cow is much the same as that in the mare, but *see also under* HORMONE THERAPY.

The ewe, sow, and goat. What has been said in respect to the larger animals applies to these animals to a great extent. It should be remembered that flesh from an animal that is suffering from a severe inflammatory condition, such as metritis, is not suited for human food. (*See also* SOW'S MILK, ABSENCE OF.)

The bitch and cat. In these carnivores, owing to the diffused placenta, and to the consequent sudden stripping bare of protective covering of a large surface, inflammation of the uterus is very prone to follow protracted or difficult parturition, especially when manual assistance from unskilled persons has been undertaken. As in other animals, an acute and a chronic form are recognised.

ACUTE METRITIS. May follow difficult whelpings, and retention of one or more fetal membranes. The membrane most commonly retained is that which belonged to the fetus that was born last and occupied the extremity of one of the horns of the uterus.

Signs. The onset of inflammation of the uterus generally occurs within a week after whelping, but some cases are delayed a little longer than this, especially in cats. A rise in temperature, increased pulse and respiration rates, dullness, disinclination for movement, and an absence of appetite occur.

Cats and dogs seem to get ease from the pain by sitting crouched in an upright position on their hocks and elbows, and this posture is almost continually assumed. A discharge appears at the vulva. Vomiting may occur. The secretion of milk ceases and the puppies or kittens become clamorous for food. The sides of the abdomen are held tense and rigid, and any attempt at handling these parts is resisted. The animal may groan or grunt if the flanks are firmly pressed between the hands.

Treatment. The use of antibiotics or sulpho-namides is important. The uterus is syringed out with non-irritant antiseptics such as acriflavine solution; and pituitrin, ergometrine or dinoprost is given. (*See* QUININE.) Antiseptic pessaries may be introduced into the uterus. (*See* NURSING, NORMAL SALINE, ANTIBIOTICS.) The puppies or kittens should be removed from their mother, and may be reared either by hand or through the agency of a foster-mother.

CHRONIC METRITIS is very common in the smaller animals, and is sometimes the sequel of an acute attack that has never completely cleared up. The cervix remains closed in most cases, so that the uterus becomes filled with pus (PYOMETRA) and the abdomen consequently enlarges. It is this increase in size that first draws attention to the condition, as a rule.

Treatment. In cases of pyometra where some pus is coming away a course of pituitrin injections may be useful and it may be tried even where the cervix is closed. (*See* PITUITRIN.) Stilboestrol is no longer an alternative in EC countries. A two-way catheter may be used to wash out the pus. Penicillin or acriflavine may be used for irrigation of the uterus, and antibiotics or sulphonamides systemically. Success has been reported following the use of quinine by mouth. Ovario-hysterectomy is indicated in a number of cases but should not be postponed until toxaemia is far advanced or the animal too weak to stand the operation. Shock is severe.

Stricture of the cervix is one of the results of an inflammatory condition of this part. When inflammation has been severe a certain amount of fibrous tissue is laid down around the canal, contracts and causes a narrowing of the passage.

Treatment is described under 'RINGWOMB' – a term used only for stricture in ewes, in which it is most often seen.

Tumours. Benign tumours include: lipoma, fibroma, papilloma, myoma, and haemangioma (rare). Malignant tumours include lymphosarcoma, adenocarcinoma, squamous cell carcinoma.

Prolapse. A partial or complete turning-inside-out of the organ, in which the inside comes to the outside through the lips of the vulva and hangs down, sometimes as far as the hocks. When the displacement is only slight nothing may be seen at the outside – as *e.g.* when one horn only is inverted into the body of the uterus. It is most common in ruminants, less frequent in the mare.

Signs. With an incomplete inversion, the uterine horn that carried the fetus becomes turned in upon itself like the finger of a glove, but it remains inside the passages, and nothing is seen to the outside. The animal is distressed for a time, paws the ground, stamps, lies and rises from the ground frequently, and a series of mild or violent labour pains occurs. She may settle down in a short while, but in a few hours she generally has a repeated attack, when the bulk of the uterus will be expelled to the outside of the body. In the early stages of such a case the real nature of the condition is seldom suspected. On the other hand, a large pear-shaped mass may be seen hanging from the vulva.

The state of the mucous membrane lining of the uterus, which in the prolapse is of course on the outside of the mass, serves as a rough guide to the length of time that has elapsed since the accident occurred. For the first two or three hours the mucous membrane appears moist and of a reddish or brownish colour over the whole surface in the mare and sow. In the cow, sheep, and goat, the general surface is red or pink, but the cotyledons show as deep-red mushroom-like eminences scattered over the outside of the tumour. In the bitch and cat there is a wide dark-brown zone. Later, the surface becomes dry – owing to its exposure to the air – and becomes deep reddish, violet, or purple, according to the amount of congestion and strangulation.

In the cow the whole of the outer upper surface may be covered with the faeces that are passed as the result of the severe straining. In all animals – but especially in ruminants – parts of the fetal membranes may be adherent to the outer surface of the mass, and can be easily recognised.

The surface is not sensitive to the touch, but any manipulation of the mass is provocative of further straining.

Various complications may occur. The vagina is always displaced when the prolapse is complete; this obstructs the urethra, and dams back the urine.

Treatment. Prolapse of the uterus is always an extremely serious condition in any animal, and in the mare and sow very often proves fatal. A good percentage of cows and ewes recover, when the prolapse is replaced *without loss of time,* and when there are *no complications.*

When treating a case – in whatever animal – it is absolutely necessary to comply with certain essentials as follows:

(1) *The prolapsed uterus must be protected from further damage.* To ensure this the animal must be secured at once, and a large sheet or blanket – which has been previously dipped in mild antiseptic solution – must be placed under the mass, and held by two men so that the tension is relieved from the neck, and so that it cannot be further contaminated or injured.

(2) *The surface of the organ must be carefully cleansed.* For this purpose a clean pail containing a warm solution of potassium permanganate and common salt (one teaspoonful of the former and ¼ lb of the latter to the gallon of water) or diluted Dettol may be used. All the larger particles of straw, debris, etc., are picked off, and the smaller pieces removed by gentle washing. Care must be taken not to make the surface bleed.

(3) *The prolapsed portion must be replaced.* To effect this the larger animals may require epidural or general anaesthesia to prevent the powerful expulsive pains that otherwise accompany the process, and make return difficult. When the animal has been anaesthetised the hindquarters are raised as high as possible by building up the floor with straw bales, by hoisting the hind legs, or by other means. When the protruded mass is very large and has a distinct neck, the main bulk is raised to a slightly higher level than the

external passage, and a process of 'tucking in' is begun near the vulva. This is carried out by the two hands – one at either side – using the hands half closed, so that the middle joints of the fingers come into contact with the uterus. The finger tips should not be employed owing to the danger of laceration or even puncture of the walls. The resistance is gradually overcome and the mass eased along the passages back into the pelvis – a labour that often makes great demands upon the strength and endurance of the operator, and frequently takes an hour or more to effect. Moreover, when once the organ has been returned, unless it is straightened out into its normal position, it may be reinverted a second time.

(4) *Measures must be taken to retain the uterus in position:* the animal may be given an analgesic or a tranquilliser to lessen the chance of subsequent straining; and sutures may be inserted.

Bedding etc. is arranged so that the animal is compelled both to stand and lie with the hindquarters raised above the level of the forequarters. This throws the abdominal contents forwards, and helps to maintain the uterus in place. It is, of course, mainly applicable to mares and cows. Bandages may prove helpful.

Amputation of the prolapsed uterus becomes necessary when all attempts at its reduction are futile, when the organ has received so much injury or has become so much decomposed and gangrenous that it would be certainly fatal to return it to the abdomen, or when prolapse occurs time after time in spite of its repeated re-position, and in spite of all attempts at retention.

Hydrops amnii. A condition in which the quantity of amniotic (*see* AMNION) fluid is greatly in excess of normal. It is often associated with a similar condition of the ALLANTOIS, which is sometimes erroneously called *hydrops amnii.*

Occurring mainly in cattle, and only rarely in other farm/domestic animals, *Hydrops amnii* is often associated with 'bulldog' calves and monsters. Sometimes a recessive gene is responsible. It may also occur when crossing an American bison on a cow, *i.e.* when producing hybrids.

Where oedema of the allantois alone occurs, the cause may be disease of the uterus, especially of the caruncles.

Sometimes oedema of both the fetal membranes and the fetus occurs. In mild cases the condition may not be suspected until calving, when an unusually large amount of fluid will be expelled. Retention of fetal membranes and subsequent metritis may follow.

In severe cases, the cow may lose appetite, appear distressed, be constipated, with rumination adversely affected or depressed. Abdominal swelling may suggest bloat. In extreme cases, the cow may be unable to get to her feet, and Professor Stephen J. Roberts, of the New York State Veterinary College, has had cases of dislocation of the hips or backward extension of the hind legs in cases of combined fetal and fetal membrane oedema involving amnion and allantois, and uterus (*hydrops uteri*).

Rupture, involving the uterine wall, may occur before or during parturition in any animal, during the reduction of a torsion or prolapse, or, in the bitch or cat, as the result of a car accident. (*See* ECTOPIC PREGNANCY.)

Torsion, or TWISTING, of the uterus is commonest in the cow and other ruminants, and rare in other domestic animals. This accident consists of a partial or complete rotation of the uterus around its long axis, and usually involves the neck of the organ.

Signs. As a rule there is no indication of the presence of the displacement until parturition is due to commence. The animal is then seen to prepare herself in the usual way, but the preliminary labour pains are exceptionally feeble and separated by long intervals. After the lapse of some hours – when the 'waterbag' and other signs of the approaching act should have become evident in an ordinary case – nothing happens. The animal is slightly disturbed, shows an occasional pain, walks round aimlessly, may feed spasmodically, but does not appear to be greatly distressed. This condition may persist for as long as 48 hours. In other cases the animal is very much upset. It has spasms of violent and painful uterine contraction.

Treatment. In the small animals laparotomy is performed, and the twisted organ untwisted. In the cow, it may be possible to rectify the twist by rolling the animal.

Congenital defects (see the diagram under INFERTILITY.) (*See also* HYDROMETRA.)

UVEITIS. Inflammation of the uvea (iris, ciliary body and choroid coat of the eyeball).

UVULA is the small downward projection that is found on the free edge of the soft palate of the pig. It is not present in the other domesticated animals.

V

VACCINATION. A method of producing active immunity against a specific infection by means of inoculation with a vaccine, *i.e.* a preparation of the necessary antigen(s). (*See* IMMUNITY, IMMUNISATION, IMMUNE RESPONSE, and below.)

Mass vaccination of poultry has been successfully carried out against Newcastle Disease by dispersing finely divided particles of vaccine over the heads of the birds with simple dust pumps. Vaccines prepared from temperature-sensitive viruses, which will replicate in the nose but not in the lungs, have been used in cattle. (*See* illustration.)

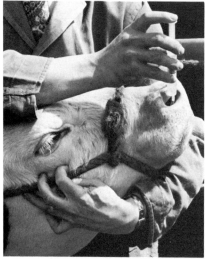

Painless vaccination by nasal spray is possible where temperature-sensitive virus vaccines are being used. (*Picture by Smith Kline Animal Health Products.*)

Multiple vaccines are available against a number of diseases. For example, sheep can be simultaneously immunised against Pulpy Kidney disease, Lamb Dysentery, Braxy, Blackleg, Black disease, Struck, Clostridium oedematiens infection and Tetanus by a single 8-in-1 vaccine.

(In connection with foot-and-mouth disease, *see also* RING VACCINATION.)

VACCINE. When an animal is inoculated with a vaccine as protection against a specific disease, *e.g.* blackleg, this is carried out with the object of stimulating production of 'antibodies' in its system, which will confer active immunity against blackleg organisms.

Vaccines are sometimes used for treatment as well as for prevention of a particular disease.

A vaccine may consist of live but attenuated viruses or bacteria, or dead (inactivated) viruses or bacteria; or parts of them. Some vaccines may also contain toxoids. Occasionally the live viruses used are related but non-pathogenic strains, useful because they will stimulate antibody pro-

duction but will not produce the disease. In most instances the virulence of the micro-organisms is reduced (*attenuated*) by *passage* through a series of animals other than the normal host species; *e.g.* cattle plague vaccine used to be prepared from the virus *passaged* through goats, but is now grown in chick embryos.

Live viruses may be inactivated by phenol or ultra-violet rays, for example; or they may be modified in some way, such as by artificially induced mutation, *e.g.* to produce a temperature-sensitive (*ts*) virus which will replicate in the nose but not in the lungs. Such a virus vaccine can be administered by nasal spray.

Tissue culture vaccines have been used in the prevention of canine distemper, rabies, etc., and in treatment of benign skin papillomata (warts) of cattle.

X-irradiated worm larvae vaccine is used in the prevention of PARASITIC BRONCHITIS. A similar vaccine has been used against *Haemonchus contortus* in sheep in recent experiments carried out at the University of Glasgow Veterinary School. Similar vaccines have been prepared for use against gape-worms in birds and hook-worms in dogs; and against the tapeworm *Jaenia saginata*.

It is important that, in the commercial production of live vaccines involving the use of chicken embryos (or of tissue cultures derived from them), contaminant viruses are eliminated. For example, the avian leukosis virus has contaminated distemper vaccine and would represent a risk to vaccinated poultry if contaminating vaccines for them. Scrapie was accidentally spread by an early louping-ill virus contaminated by the scrapie agent.

It is essential that vaccines are stored under suitable conditions of temperature, etc.; that they are not used after the expiry date shown on the package; that where two doses are stated to be necessary both are given – and at the correct interval. Failure to observe these rules can mean that the vaccinated animal does not become an immunised animal; it has led to dogs presumed properly vaccinated against rabies becoming rabid after exposure to a natural infection. (*See also* INJECTIONS, GENETIC ENGINEERING.)

Vaccine development. In 1985 Dr Nathan Zygraich referred to two techniques of great importance: (1) recombinant DNA production of protein and polypeptide antigens. This could eliminate many of the imperfections of present vaccines by creating subunit vaccines free from infectious material; (2) the hybridoma production of monoclonal antibodies, would allow the selection of microbial agents of direct relevance to immunity.

VACCINIA VIRUS. This term may refer to the virus of naturally occurring cow-pox, or to a strain which has undergone mutation and was used for vaccination against smallpox. (*See* POX.)

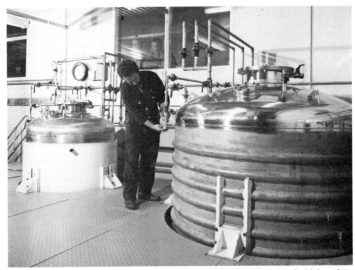

Vaccine production. The finishing touches being put to a blending vessel which makes possible batches of foot-and-mouth disease vaccine of up to 1½ million doses in the 1973 extension to the Wellcome foot-and-mouth disease vaccine laboratory at Pirbright, Surrey.

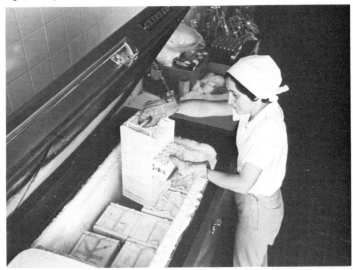

Vaccine production. Stocks of foot-and-mouth seed virus (140 different strains) are kept in a refrigeration plant ready for use at the Wellcome foot-and-mouth disease vaccine laboratory at Pirbright. To combat the intense cold, assistants use asbestos gloves when handling containers.

VACUOLE. A cavity within a cell.

VAGINA, extends from the cervix of the uterus to the vulva.

Vaginal mucus is altered in character during pregnancy, a fact which is made use of in pregnancy diagnosis. (For inflammation of the vagina, *see* VAGINITIS.)

Vaginal prolapse in ewes. This may precede lambing by up to 55 days, but most cases occur within the last 21 days of pregnancy.

Rupture of the vagina, with protrusion of the intestine and rapid death, occurs not uncommonly in ewes of a large breed, of mature age,

carrying a twin – a week or two before lambing is due. Bulky foods – swedes, turnips, kale – are often involved. An artificial vagina is used at A I centres for the collection of semen.

Vaginoureteral fistula. This has been recorded in dogs and cats, as a complication of ovariohysterectomy or a caesarean operation, and leads to urinary incontinence. It has been suggested that the fistula may occur following accidental ligation of the ureter during surgery, or because the ureter becomes involved in an inflammatory adhesion originating in the vaginal stump. (De Baerdemaecker, *Veterinary Record* (1984) **115,** 62.)

Intermittent haemorrhage occasionally occurs

in mares having very prominent varicose veins at the dorsal aspect of the vulva-vaginal area; but does not appear to affect health or fertility. Persistent vulval haemorrhage from varicose veins of the dorsal wall of the vagina has also been described. It yields to local haemostatic treatment. (White, R. A. S. & others, *Veterinary Record* (1984) **115**, 263.)

VAGINITIS. Inflammation of the vagina. (*See under* INFERTILITY – Diseases of the Genital Organs in Female; *also* 'WHITES', 'EPIVAG', VULVOVAGINITIS, PROLAPSE.)

VAGOTOMY. Severing of the vagus nerve. (*See* HYPERTROPHIC OSTEOPATHY.)

VAGUS (Pneumogastric Nerve) is the tenth cranial nerve. This nerve is remarkable for its great length, and for the attachments which it forms with other nerves and with the sympathetic trunks. It arises from the side of the medulla, passes out of the skull, runs down to the jugular furrow of the neck, where, along with the sympathetic, it accompanies the carotid artery to the entrance to the chest. From this point the right and left vagi differ from each other in their course. They both pass through the chest cavity, giving branches to the pharynx (which run up the neck again), to the heart, bronchi, oesophagus, etc. Each nerve then splits into two parts and the two upper branches fuse with each other to form the dorsal trunk, the lower branches behaving similarly to form the ventral trunk. These two branches now pass through the diaphragm, with the oesophagus, into the abdominal cavity, and end by giving branches to the stomach, duodenum, liver, and various ganglia near by. (*See* Parasympathetic system *under* CENTRAL NERVOUS SYSTEM, *also* BRAIN.) (*See* GUTTURAL POUCH DIPHTHERIA).

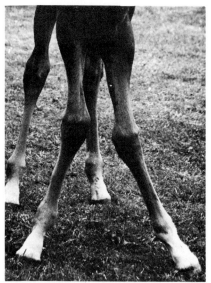

One-month-old foal with bilateral carpal valgus. (With acknowledgements to Professor L. C. Vaughan and the Royal Veterinary College.)

VALGUS. A bone growth-plate defect. (*See under* BONE, DISEASES OF.)

VALINE. One of the essential amino acids.

VALVES are found in the heart, veins, lymph-vessels, etc., and serve the purpose of ensuring that the fluids will only circulate in one direction. (*See* HEART, VEINS, ILEOCAECAL.)

VALVULAR DISEASE (*see* HEART DISEASES).

VAMPIRE-BATS are important transmitters of rabies in parts of South and Central America, the West Indies, etc. The bat laps blood from the wounds inflicted with its upper incisor teeth on cattle, horses, etc. In Mexico infected vampires have made necessary the preventive inoculation of 800,000 cattle a year. Trypanosomiasis can also be transmitted by vampire bats.

VARIED DIET, NEED FOR (*see* DIET, AMINO ACIDS, CAT FOODS, DOGS' DIET).

VARIOCELE is a condition in which the veins of one or both testicles are greatly distended.

VARICOSE VEINS (*see under* VEINS).

VARIOLA, or POX, is the inclusive term for fevers of animals and man, in which a skin eruption takes the form of a 'pock', caused by a pox virus (*see* POX).

VAS DEFERENS (*see under* TESTICLE).

VASCULAR. Consisting of, or containing a high proportion of, blood-vessels.
Vasculitis. Inflammation of a blood-vessel.

VASECTOMISED. A male animal in which the *vas deferens* has been cut. Such an animal is sterile though it retains its libido and may be used for the detection of oestrus (*e.g.* in cattle). In breeding catteries one or two toms are sometimes vasectomised for the sake of peace, quiet and contentment of queens not being bred from until a later oestrus.

Sterility does not immediately follow vasectomy (or castration), as some sperms will be in the seminal vesicles and can lead to conception after mating. It may be three weeks or more before the animal is sterile.

VASODILATOR. Anything which causes dilation of blood vessels. A drug used for this purpose is Isoxuprine hydrochloride. (*See* NAVICULAR DISEASE.)

VASOMOTOR NERVES are the small nerve fibres that lie in or upon the walls of the blood-vessels and connect the muscle fibres of the middle coat with the nervous system. By the continuous action of the nerves the muscular walls of the vessels are maintained in a moderate state of contraction. Any continuous and generalised increase in this action results in a raising of the blood-pressure of the body, while a diminution produces a lowering of the pressure. Such vasomotor nerves are called vaso-constrictors, but there are vaso-dilators as well. These latter are able to dilate the vessels, and cause either a general or a local fall in the blood-pressure, along with an increased supply of blood to the part.

VASOPRESSIN. A hormone secreted by the posterior lobe of the pituitary gland. (*See* PITUITARY.)

VEINS are the vessels which carry the blood back to the heart after its circulation in the tissues of the body. With one or two exceptions the veins lie alongside or near to the corresponding arteries – thus the renal vein brings back blood that has been carried to the kidney by the renal artery and lies alongside it. The veins are, however, more numerous and more irregular in their courses than are the arteries, especially on the surface of the body. In regions, such as the cheeks, brain meninges, and in the abdomen and thorax, there are veins arranged quite irrespective of the distribution of the arteries.

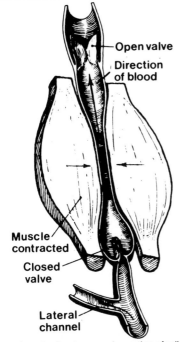

Valves of a vein showing pumping action of adjacent muscles. (Grollman: *The Human Body*, The Macmillan Co.; as used in Frandson: *Anatomy and Physiology of Farm Animals*, Baillière, Tindall).

Structure. A vein is a thin-walled tube which possesses a structure similar to that of an artery, and consists of three coats, viz. an outer fibrous, a middle composed of muscular and elastic fibres, and an inner coat composed of an elastic membrane and flattened epithelial cells. If an ordinary vein be split open along its length there are seen to be a number of flap-like valves attached to its inner surface. These are like little pockets, and are so arranged that they offer no resistance to the blood when it is flowing in the right direction, but

they prevent any back-flow. These valves are most numerous in the veins of the limbs, where gravity would naturally tend to produce a back-flow, and least numerous in the veins of the internal organs.

Chief veins. The arrangement and relations of the veins are very different in animals of varying species, and even in different individuals, so that only a general description can be given here.

Pulmonary veins–as many as 8 or 9 in the horse and fewer in other animals – return the oxygenated blood from the lungs to the left auricle of the heart. They possess no valves. Opening into the right auricle are four veins; these are: (1) coronary sinus; (2) anterior, and (3) posterior vena cava; and (4) the azygos vein. The *coronary sinus* is a short thick trunk that discharges the blood used by the heart walls back into the general circulation. The *anterior vena cava* drains the blood from the head, neck, two fore-limbs, and much of the chest wall. It is formed by the confluence of the *jugulars* and the *brachial veins*, and receives other branches from the neck, vertebral region, and the chest wall. The *posterior vena cava* drains all the remainder of the body except the region of the diaphragm, the posterior intercostal areas, the oesophagus, and the bronchial tubes; the blood from these parts being collected into the *azygos vein* which joins the right auricle separately in most animals. The posterior vena cava is formed under the lumbar region by the union of the right and left *common iliac veins*, which drain the blood from the pelvis and hind legs, and which are distributed in a more or less similar manner to the corresponding arteries of these parts. From here it passes forward below the lumbar muscles in company with the abdominal aorta, until at the level of the last thoracic vertebra it passes downwards and forwards, past the pancreas, and reaches the liver. Its further course is partly embedded in the liver substance until it arrives at a special opening in the diaphragm, called the *foramen venae cavae*, by which it gains the thoracic cavity. From here it passes along in a groove in the right lung to reach the right auricle. Its main tributaries are as follows: (1) *lumbar veins*, which empty blood from the lumbar muscles, etc.; (2) *internal spermatics* in the male, and *utero-ovarian veins* in the female, from the generative organs in either sex; (3) *two renal veins*, one from each kidney, satellites of the corresponding arteries; (4) several large *hepatic veins*, which return not only blood carried to the liver by the hepatic arteries, but also that which comes from the digestive organs by the *portal vein* to undergo a second capillary circulation in the liver (*see* PORTAL VEIN); and (5) the *phrenic veins* returning blood from the diaphragm.

In the venous system, even more so than in the arterial system, there is an intricate arrangement of anastomoses by which, when one vein becomes damaged or diseased, lateral branches from it may enlarge and carry away the excess blood into other veins so that no great hindrance to the return flow of the blood to the heart may be occasioned. If this were not so, the circulation might be easily upset from quite minor causes.

The following labels appear on the figure:
Open valve
Direction of blood
Muscle contracted
Closed valve
Lateral channel

VEINS, DISEASES OF. Those lying near to the surface are frequently injured along with other tissues when contusions or lacerations have been sustained, but so extensive is their communication with neighbouring veins that it is usually possible for these latter to enlarge and undertake the functions of the damaged vessels, and thereby prevent serious consequences. The deeper veins are protected from all but the most severe, and usually fatal, injuries.

Inflammation of a vein, or PHLEBITIS, may follow the collection of blood samples when unclean instruments have been used, or when the resulting skin wound has not received attention. In other cases it follows thrombosis and infection. (*See also under* THROMBOSIS.)

Varicose veins are those which have become stretched or dilated to an extent not justified by the blood flow. (*See* VARIOCELE *and under* VAGINA.)

VELD SICKNESS (*see* HEART-WATER).

VENA CAVA. Each of the two large veins that open direct into the right auricle of the heart. (For further details *see under* VEINS.)

Thrombosis of the posterior vena cava, which may follow abscess formation in the liver or elsewhere, is in cattle not infrequently followed by the presence of clots in the pulmonary vessels, abscess formation and sometimes erosion of the pulmonary artery wall – giving rise to a fatal haemorrhage. Symptoms may include dullness, rapid breathing, a cough, chest pain, the presence of blood in material coughed up, anaemia, and widespread rhonchi. (*See* RECUMBENCY.)

VENEREAL DISEASES. Animals, with the exception of the monkey, are not subject to infection by the two great human venereal diseases – syphilis and gonorrhoea, but there are several important contagious diseases that can be transmitted from animal to animal by coitus. These include brucellosis, trichomoniasis, *Campylobacter fetus* infection, and infectious vaginitis of cattle, venereal granulomata or venereal tumours of dogs, and dourine or 'Mal du coit' of horses. (*See* PROTOZOA, EPIDIDYMITIS, 'EPIVAG', VULVO-VAGINITIS, CONTAGIOUS EQUINE METRITIS.)

VENEREAL TUMOURS, or INFECTIVE GRANULOMATA, characterise a contagious disease of dogs.
SIGNS. In the female the original tumour is a warty excrescence which soon grows and becomes cauliflower-like. In advanced stages there is a large mass of pinkish or greyish-red tissue, which easily bleeds when touched, occupying the greater part of the vaginal passage and often causing a bulging and swelling of the perineal region. A dirty sticky blood-stained discharge accompanies the condition, and the animal's general health suffers. In the male the watery growths usually have a distinct stalk, and are attached to the skin or mucous membrane of the prepuce, or to the penis. (*See also under* WARTS.)

VENEZUELAN EQUINE ENCEPHALO-MYELITIS. A strain recognised in the 1930s. A severe outbreak occurred in Venezuela and Colombia in 1962–4, when thousands of horses died and about 30,000 people were infected. A later outbreak spread to Mexico in 1970 where 6000 or more horses died, and then to Texas, USA. (*See also* EQUINE ENCEPHALITIS.)

VENOM (*see* SNAKE BITE; TOAD, *and* BUFOTALIN; TOADFISH, SPIDERS, SCORPION).

VENT GLEET. This condition in poultry is an inflammation of the cloaca, with which is associated a thin yellowish watery discharge which has a characteristic and particularly unpleasant odour. The cloaca and adjacent skin appear swollen and congested, and the bird exhibits signs of irritation. Other birds attracted by the reddening of the region may peck at vent; this leads on to cannibalism.

Egg production drops, and in some cases egg binding and impaction of the oviduct result. Culling is advisable.
TREATMENT. Cases of severe infection of the eyes of poultry-keepers treating this condition are not uncommon.

VENTILATION may be summed up as 'the measures necessary to rectify the pollution of the air in a building – without the production of a draught'. Whenever animals are enclosed in a confined building they gradually use up the oxygen and discharge into the air quantities of carbon dioxide, water vapour, until, if no fresh air be supplied, the percentage of oxygen decreases below the amount required.

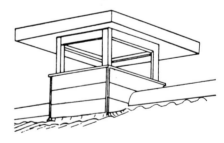

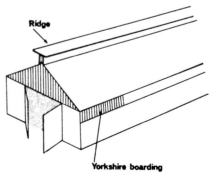

Ventilation methods for cattle houses: A, Chimney; B, Continuous ridge outlet. (With acknowledgements to *UFAW Handbook on Care & Management of Farm Animals*, Churchill Livingstone (Longman Group).)

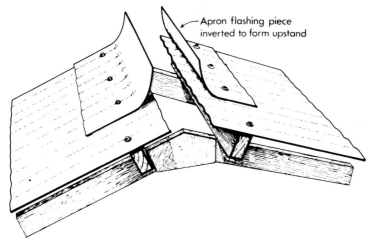

Open ridge

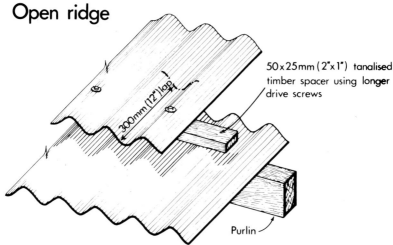

Breathing roof

(With acknowledgements to the Scottish Farm Buildings Investigation Unit.)

One of the problems in livestock buildings is condensation, which can lead to bronchitis and pneumonia. For buildings used for cattle and sheep, provision of Yorkshire boarding is one of the best and least expensive methods of avoiding or curing condensation.

Necessary air space in cubic feet.

Cow, Horse (Byre or stable)	200
(Loose-box or Yard)	600–1200
Bacon pig	60
Poultry	
(layers on slats)	6
(layers on deep litter)	12

The required amount of air for each animal must be continuously brought in from the outside, and an exit must be provided for an equal amount. This is arranged for by the provision of *inlet* and *outlet* ventilators.

Inlets. These include windows, direct inlet pipes,

perforated bricks and gratings, Yorkshire boarding, and electric fans.

Windows, of which the Sheringham Valve type is the most common and useful, serve the dual purpose of lighting and ventilation. Those on the lee side of a building serve as outlets when the wind is strong. In the Sheringham Valve windows the incoming air is deflected upwards by the hopper-like flap that falls inwards, so that it is spread over a greater area than is the case with other openings. Inlet pipes are used, often in conjunction with windows, to ensure a supply of fresh air in the region of the animals' heads.

Ventilation rates – (maximum)

	Changes of air per hour	Cubic feet per hour
Bacon pig	20	200–1200
Broiler chicken	40	240
Laying birds	30	360

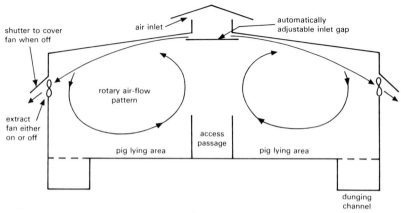

Outlets. These include an open ridge, louvre-board ventilators, outlet shafts, open eaves, exhaust fans, and other devices. The most satisfactory outlet is undoubtedly an open ridge along the whole length of the building. The heated impure air rises and is drawn through the open space by the suction of the wind. The disadvantages of this system are that the open space will allow entrance to a certain amount of rain or snow in bad weather, and that the system is inapplicable to buildings possessing lofts.

Extraction area.

(Necessary with natural ventilation.)

	Outlet: sq. ins per beast
Cowhouse	144
Farrowing house	15
Fattening house	10
Calf house	10
Poultry (adult) house	2

Mechanical ventilators may be either of the *plenum* or in-forcing type, or of the *vacuum*, exhaust, or out-forcing variety. In the former a larger power-driven fan is enclosed in a chamber with communication to the outside of the building, and is connected by ducts or shafts with all parts that are to be ventilated. In the exhaust variety one or more electric fans are enclosed in turrets placed along the ridge of the roof.

The temperature in a livestock building is a result of the heat released from the stock (for example, a dairy cow gives off heat equivalent to ½ kW; and with a heavy milker the figure may be 1 kW) and the varying quantity of ventilating air drawn from outside. 'Because heating and refrigeration are only economic for young stock, the properties of the air entering the building are those of the outside air and vary considerably, depending on the weather. In hot weather a large amount of air is used, but in cold weather only a small amount is required and in many traditional systems this gives rise to different patterns of internal air flow. By studying the relevance of airflow patterns to the conditions near the stock and to the response of the ventilation system the Environment Department, N I A E, has designed a ventilation system which provides near uniform internal conditions as the outside temperature changes. The system ensures a desired airflow pattern by automatically adjusting the inlet gap to maintain an air speed of about 5 m/s. Calculations and experiments have shown that this system will maintain the required airflow pattern for outside temperatures down to 0°C.

'Another shortcoming of traditional systems is the influence of wind on ventilation rates, particularly in cold weather when fans are running slowly. For this reason the N I A E have discarded the method of varying fan speed to control rate of ventilation and recommends switching the fans on or off. When fans are off they are covered by simple backdraught shutters and when on they are at full speed and so are least affected by wind. The fans are switched on or off in predetermined steps and the inlet gap is adjusted automatically to match the steps in ventilation rate.

'The diagram [above] shows the essence of the system which has proved effective in fattening piggeries, broiler houses and turkey buildings and is fully described in the N I A E Report No. 28.' (*See also* HOUSING, CARBON MONOXIDE POISONING.)

Fan failure. (For this and the resulting mortality, *see under* CONTROLLED ENVIRONMENT.)

VENTRAL in Anatomy indicates that a particular organ or structure is situated towards the abdominal surface of the body, as distinct from the spinal or dorsal aspect.

VENTRICLE (*see* HEART, BRAIN).

VENTRICULUS (*see* GIZZARD *and diagram for* PROVENTRICULUS).

'VERMINOUS ANEURYSM' is a misnomer for EQUINE VERMINOUS ARTERITIS.

VERMINOUS BRONCHITIS (*see* PARASITIC BRONCHITIS *and* 'GAPES').

VERMINOUS DERMATITIS (*see* STEPHANOFILARIASIS, 'SUMMER SORES').

VERMINOUS OPHTHALMIA (*see under* EYE, DISEASES OF).

VERO CELLS. A continuous heteroploid cell line derived from African green monkey (*Cercopithecus aethiops*) kidney tissue. These cells are approved as a substrate for the production of virus vaccines, including rabies. They are much easier to grow than human diploid cells, and provide a better yield; so that manufacturers are keen to use them for vaccine production. Latent virus in these cells is a potential danger.

VEROTOXIN. A total of 1012 milk filters were collected from 498 diary farms in south-west Ontario. The supernatants of 20 (2 per cent) of the milk filter cultures had verocytotoxic activity. Seven verotoxin producing *Escherichia coli* strains were isolated; two of which had been previously associated with disease in humans. (Clarke, R. C. & others. (1989) *Epidemiology and Infection* **102,** 253.)

VERRUCA (*see* PAPILLOMA).

VERRUCOSE. Covered with warts or vegetative growths. In pigs a verrucose endocarditis is recognised, the growth being found on the heart valves. The condition may be associated with swine erysipelas or be caused by staphylococci or streptococci.

VERSION, or TURNING, means the changing of a presentation at parturition so that some other part of the fetus than that which was presented originally comes through the pelvic opening first.

VERTEBRA (*see* SPINAL COLUMN).

VESICLE, or small blister, is a collection of fluid in the surface layers of the skin or of a mucous membrane. Vesicles are present in a number of diseases, and according to their location, some assistance is afforded for diagnostic purposes. For example, in foot-and-mouth disease the vesicles are present in the mouth and on the feet, in cow-pox they are found on the teats, udder, and other parts.

VESICLES, SEMINAL. These secondary sex glands, like the prostate, have openings into the urethra and are situated close to the neck of the urinary bladder. (*See also under* SEMEN.)

At a bull-rearing unit four yearlings appeared fit and well. Their appetite was good and they showed no signs of pain or discomfort. When, however, samples of their semen were taken, clots of pus were noticed. This finding led to a careful examination of the bulls being made, and it was then discovered that each had a hard, painful swelling of one of their seminal vesicles. Inflammation was found to be due to infection with *Actinobacillus actinoides.* Other organisms sometimes involved include: tubercle bacilli; *Brucella abortus; streptococci; C. pyogenes.*

VESICULAR DISEASE of pigs is described under SWINE VESICULAR DISEASE. (*See also* VESICULAR STOMATITIS below.)

VESICULAR EXANTHEMA. A virus disease of pigs (and rarely of horses but not of cattle) which has to be distinguished from foot-and-mouth disease. It was eradicated from the USA in 1959 and has never been recorded elsewhere. It is thought that the vesicular exanthema virus may have been a 'land variant' of the San Miguel sea-lion virus, isolated from sea-lions off the coast of California.

VESICULAR STOMATITIS of horses resembles in some respects foot-and-mouth disease but is caused by a rhabdovirus. The disease may also affect cattle and pigs. In Canada in 1951, foot-and-mouth disease was mistaken for vesicular stomatitis with serious consequences. It has become important in cattle and pigs, and occasionally affects sheep. It is a disease of the summer, and mainly of the Western Hemisphere, especially in the Caribbean area. An insect vector is likely, and the virus has been isolated from mosquitoes.

In man the disease is influenza-like, with fever, sore throat, and several days' malaise.

Two strains of the virus are recognised – the New Jersey and the Indiana. Experimentally, numerous mammalian species can be infected – likewise ducks.

VESICULAR VAGINITIS (*see* VULVOVAGINITIS, GRANULAR).

VESICULITIS (*see* VESICLES, SEMINAL, *above*).

VETERINARY DEGREES are obtainable in the UK at the universities of Cambridge, London, Liverpool, Bristol, Edinburgh, and Glasgow, and lead to membership of the Royal College of Veterinary Surgeons. Higher degrees – MSc, PhD and DSc or equivalent – are obtainable after postgraduate study.

VETERINARY FACILITIES ON THE FARM. Every breeding cow and heifer in Britain has to be caught, ear-tag read, restrained and a blood sample taken from neck or tail vein. 'This will take place at least 2 or 3 times, quite apart from any herd or individual handlings necessary for clinical reasons or breeding management. Taking a blood sample can take as little as 30–45 seconds given efficient holding facilities; 200 cattle could be sampled in a morning's work. On most farms there is a lack of cattle handling facilities of the right type, so that the catching of a single animal can and does take all the farm staff about 20 minutes with the very real possibility of broken gates, and fences and varying degrees of personal injury even before blood sampling is attempted.'

P. Davidson continues: Experience in the design and erection of over 30 cattle handling units for dairy and beef cattle has shown the main points to be as follows:

The essential elements:

Collecting pens should be large enough to hold all stock to be handled, or all the stock in units as they are housed, *e.g.* 50s or 100s. A post-and-rail pen 9 × 18 m (30 × 60 ft) or 12 × 13·5 m (40 × 45 ft) will hold 100 cows with calves at foot. A pen of 9 × 12 m (30 × 40 ft) will hold 60 adult cattle or 80 young cattle.

The forcing pen leads from the collecting pen to the race or chute, and should be funnel-shaped. It should hold not less than 12 cows plus calves or 15 adult cattle – enough to provide a group for handling without having repetitive stops while two or threes are run into the cow-race. The

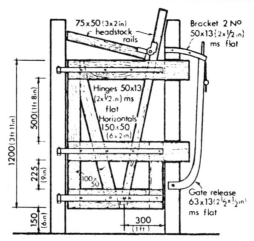

optimum dimensions are as shown and should not be made larger for large units. The dimensions are those within which cattle cannot evade pressure to go into the race by adopting a 'whirlpool' movement.

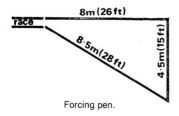

Forcing pen.

Race. An 18 m (60 ft) long race 680 mm (2 ft 3 in) wide internally and 1·680 m (5 ft 6 in) to the top rail will hold 10–12 cattle. It should be made up of verticals (sleepers) 2 m (6 ft 6 in) between centres sunk 900 mm (3 ft) into ground, the bottom concreted with a brushed surface. There should be four horizontal rails. Height above ground of the second and third rails is specific in that it accommodates the large, fat or pregnant animal.

Catwalk and working space. Catwalks should be provided on both sides of the cow race 760 mm (2 ft 6 in) above ground level and not less than 300 mm (12 in) wide, in wood. Space should always be provided for two catwalks, even when building in close proximity to an existing wall, *i.e.* the face should be stood off from the wall, however tempting it may be to use an existing wall for one side. Cattle can then be run in either direction for procedures on either flank (vaccinations, branding, testing, etc.).

Crush and veterinary gates. The crush should be stood-off 1·079 m (3 ft 6 in) from the end of the cow race with same internal width of 680 mm (2 ft 3 in), and suitable gates to hold animal No. 1 firmly, stop animal No. 1 from backing out of crush before being held and prevent animal No. 2 from pushing up. The materials and sizes are the same as for the race.

Yoke or headstock. The headstock is of bolted timber throughout to the detailed design and specifications illustrated. It has a quick-release frame to free any animal that goes down in the crush. The design of the bars restraining the head gives no opportunity for the head and neck to flail up and down and helps to raise pressure in jugular veins for blood sampling. Any movement of the animal locks the restraining bars even more tightly. This type of headstock is silent in use, due to its timber construction and the absence of any ratchets or springs.

The horizontal rails of the crush on the animal's left side should be checked into the inside face of that vertical post against which the head-stock closes. 'This presents a smooth surface for different thicknesses of neck.'

Three-way cattle shedder. If fat cattle are weighed, cows examined for breeding function or large stores sexed, then this at once dictates grouping by weight, pregnancy or other findings. A three-way shedder immediately after the crush renders this separation an easy task.

Dispersal and recirculation. Having dispersed any large group of cattle to their appropriate categories of in-calf, empty, etc., there should be a series of gates in the far end of all holding pens, allowing cattle to be recirculated, retained or individually extracted.

Suckler cows and calves. 'Suckler cows are usually handled for clinical reasons (vaccinations, treatment, blood-sampling) or to find out breeding status at that time (in-calf, ovulating, empty). This usually means that calves are at foot. To simplify handling, calves can go with their dams right into the forcing pen without any attempted separation. If a calf race is then sited to run from near the mouth of the cow race, with a shedder gate, then calves of 1–7 months can be run off separately. This allows S.19 vaccination, castration, dehorning or weighing to be done very quickly with no time and energy dissipated on catching each calf individually. Critical dimensions for the calf race are 410 mm (1 ft 4 in) internal width and 1·040 m (3 ft 6 in) to top rail. The shedder gate should be close-boarded to prevent visual contact between calves and cows in cow race. Calves will run into the calf race quickly if the shedder is operated from an overhead platform but they tend to flinch at an operator working through the rails at head or shoulder level.'

In addition to the cattle handling facilities which Mr Davidson has described above, it is useful to have a footbath suitable for cattle (*See* FOOTBATHS), and loose-boxes for calving or isolation purposes. With a very large herd of, say, 500 cows, 15 loose-boxes would not be too many.

VETERINARY INVESTIGATION CENTRES.
There were 23 of these in England and Wales in 1980, operating as part of the Ministry of Agriculture. They provide laboratory facilities and a consultative service for veterinary surgeons in private practice, assisting with the diagnosis of disease and herd problems. Their work includes autopsies, serological tests, biochemistry and parasitology. VIC staff carry out research into disease problems of local importance, and also provide a surveillance function for the Ministry in warning of local disease which might become important nationally. In Scotland similar VICs operate but are affiliated to the Scottish agricultural colleges.

VETERINARY NURSES.
People wishing to train as veterinary nurses must first find employment for not less than 35 hours per week in a veterinary practice or other veterinary centre approved by the Royal College of Veterinary Surgeons. The greater part of the training is given 'on the job', to quote the handbook published by the RCVS.

The practical training is supplemented by formal tuition to provide the necessary background knowledge. Residential courses are available.

All pre-enrolment queries about training are now being dealt with by the British Veterinary Nursing Association, The Seedbed Centre, Coldharbour Road, Harlow, Essex CM19 5AF.

There are over 80 training centres, approved by the RCVS, where student nurses can study for the two qualifying examinations.

A diploma in Advanced Veterinary Nursing can also be obtained.

VETERINARY PRACTITIONER.
Someone on the Supplementary Veterinary Register; *not* a MRCVS (*see below*).

VETERINARY PRODUCTS COMMITTEE (VPC).
This, under the Medicines Act 1968 advises the Medicines Commission, and ultimately, the Licensing Authority, on the marketing of medicines for animals. Its approval is needed before an animal medicine may be licensed for sale. It has to consider the safety of the treated animal, the safety of consumers of produce derived from treated animals, and the safety of farmer, pet-owner, and the environment.

In 1989 the membership comprised eight veterinary surgeons including a FRS) and two medical doctors.

(*See also* the SUSPECTED ADVERSE REACTION SURVEILLANCE SCHEME (SARSS).)

VETERINARY PROFESSION.
This comprises those engaged in private practice, in the Animal Health Division of the Ministry of Agriculture, the Royal Army Veterinary Corps, the overseas veterinary services, in research and teaching at the universities, and also at ARC research establishments, and those of the Ministry of Agriculture, etc., in food inspection and other municipal services, in AI Centres, in research and advisory appointments with, *e.g.* FAO, and commercial undertakings.

In Britain, the veterinary profession continues to grow. At the beginning of 1966, the register of the Royal College of Veterinary Surgeons contained a little under 7500 names – about twice as many as there were in 1935. Allowing for 1500 overseas, this left about 4800 veterinary surgeons in the UK. Of these, 3000 or so were in general practice; a little over 1000 in research, advisory, teaching, and other posts. In 1981 the total rose to over 10500.

Figures for 1975 from the SWANN REPORT showed that out of some 5570 active veterinarians in the UK about 70 per cent were in private practice, 13 per cent in government service and 6 per cent in teaching; the remaining 11 per cent being in commerce and industry, in research institutes or with animal welfare societies, or postgraduate students. About half the time of those in private practice was given to small animals (dogs, cats and other domestic pets), about 42 per cent to farm animals and about 8 per cent to horses.

'In Great Britain, there is one veterinarian to every 30 sq. miles, in the United States, one to every 270 sq. miles. In South Africa, there is one to every 1700 sq. miles and in Canada, one to every 1900 sq. miles, while in an under-developed region, such as East Africa, there is only one veterinarian to every 5000 sq. miles.' – Dr K. L. Kesteven, Director of FAO's Animal Production and Health Division, 1960.

In the USA in 1980 there were 35,489 veterinarians; of whom nearly 17,000 were engaged in small animal practice, and about 6000 were concerned with large animals.

VETERINARY SURGEONS ACT, THE, 1966.
This relates to veterinary education, the management of the profession and the registration and professional conduct of veterinary surgeons and practitioners. The practice of veterinary surgery continues to be limited to veterinary surgeons and practitioners whose names appear on the registers maintained by the Royal College of Veterinary Surgeons. Unregistered persons may carry out only the very limited treatments, tests, or operations specified in section 19 of the Act, any exemption orders made thereunder, or Schedule 3.

The Supplementary Veterinary Register was established under the 1948 Act.

VIAL (*see* AMPOULE, GLASS EMBOLISM).

VIBICES are long tapering markings that sometimes occur on visible mucous membranes during certain diseases, such as purpura haemorrhagica and pernicious anaemia of horses.

VIBRIO is a bacterium of curved shape.
Vibrio fetus (*see* CAMPYLOBACTER FETUS).
'Vibrionic Scours' in pigs. (*See* SWINE DYSENTERY.)

VIBRISSAE. The thick, stiff hairs or whiskers which project from the faces of cats, dogs, and other animals. They are minor sense organs. (*See* SKIN.)

'VICES' and VICIOUSNESS. A definition comprehensive enough to include 'bad habits'. *See* TAIL-BITING (in pigs), SUCKING (in calves), *and* FEATHER-PICKING, CANNIBALISM (in poultry). What follows here concerns the horse.

'Bad habits', mild vices, or whims. Horses which are shut in stables without exercise or work frequently learn vices and tricks which not only may be harmful to the animals themselves, but may be dangerous to persons who attend them. Perhaps the most objectionable is the habit of kicking when being approached. (*See under* KICKING.)

Eating the bedding may be merely an endeavour on the part of the horse to acquire a sufficiency of coarse bulky food when the ration is too concentrated, or it may be a bad habit. It can be prevented by supplying sawdust instead of straw, or peat moss litter.

Chewing the head ropes, which is a bad habit often acquired by mules, can usually be stopped by soaking the rope in a mixture of spirits of tar and aloes for 12 hours, and then hanging it out to dry in the air. The objectionable taste of aloes and the smell of the tar combine to make the animal stop the habit. The use of a chain instead of a rope will prevent the animal from breaking loose, when the above measures fail.

Refusing to lie is often due to fear, nervousness, or physical inability, such as ankylosis of the spinal column. Horses may lie when housed in a loose-box instead of a stall, or a stout rope from one heel post across to the other may allow the horse to obtain some amount of rest. (*See* SLEEP, etc.). Gnawing the walls is usually a sign of the presence of worms, bots, a mineral or other deficiency, or indigestion, and appropriate measures should be taken to determine which condition is present, and to treat it accordingly.

Pawing in the stable may be a sign of impatience or loneliness; then it is not important, but sometimes it develops into a vice of such persistency that it entails great wear of the shoes, and may result in the production of holes in the stable floor. It should be remembered that pawing is sometimes a sign of abdominal pain (colic).

More serious vices (*see* CRIB-BITING *and* WINDSUCKING; WEAVING).

Aggressiveness may be due to pain (*see* HORSES, BACK TROUBLES); and, in countries where the disease is present, to RABIES. (*See also* BRAIN, DISEASES.)

When an animal shows an ungovernable temper under the pressure of sexual disturbances, it is unfair to consider it vicious. Cruel treatment in the past may also be an underlying factor (*and see* too the effect of 'EQUINE VERMINOUS ARTERITIS).

Kicking. (*a*) *Rearing and striking with the fore-feet* is a dangerous vice that is more common among the light horses than among the heavy draught. Sometimes the animal merely rears from a desire to get started with his work; sometimes he will not allow himself to be held by the head when in harness, but rears and strikes out at anyone approaching him; at other times he may strike out without rearing. A saddle horse, when rearing, may with his head strike the face or chest of his rider and unseat him and may so lose his balance that he falls over backwards and perhaps crush the rider.

(*b*) *Kicking with the hind-feet.* 'With a kicking horse, pass in front', is a proverb that it is well to remember when dealing with the horse that uses his hind-feet for kicking. The hind-feet can be used to strike an object within a radius of from 4 to 6 feet *all around them.* It is a well-known fact that a mule can deliver a kick with his hind-feet to a person standing at its shoulder, and there are many horses able to do likewise. Two methods of kicking with the hind-limbs are commonly employed; in the first, which is the horse's natural method of defence and offence, the head is lowered, the body is lifted from the withers backwards, and both the hind-limbs are suddenly extended as far backwards as possible with tremendous force; in the second, the horse lifts one hind-foot and deals a short vicious backward or side-way kick without always fully extending the limb.

In addition to these there are 'cow kickers', which project one hind-limb forwards, outwards, and backwards, so that they may reach a person standing as far forward as the shoulder. These are especially dangerous.

(*c*) *Biting* is commonest among stallions, and the remarks at the beginning of this section on *Serious Vices* should be noted. It is well to take precautionary measures, such as muzzling while grooming, tying up short, using double head ropes, one to either side of the stall, etc.

Shying. In many cases where horses suddenly stop, plunge to one side, snort, tremble, attempt to turn in the opposite direction and run away, when confronted by some unusual sight, sound, or smell, the same causes as occasion bolting are operative. The horse does not trust his eyesight, is unable to interpret an unusual sound or smell, and consequently loses his head. Among the many objects at which horses are liable to shy may be mentioned the following: pools of water shining in the sun-light, fluttering pieces of paper, clothes hung out to dry, dogs, cats, fowls, and other small animals darting into the roadway. The odour of wild beasts, and the smell of blood and offal, that an animal perceives when passing a menagerie or a knackery or abattoir, are also likely to frighten it and cause it to shy.

Aversion to special objects. Occasionally a horse is encountered which has an absolute horror of some special, usually quite harmless, common object; for example, pieces of white or coloured paper or rag, cock turkeys, pigs, goats, donkeys, small white inanimate objects of any nature, etc. Grey horses have been known to attack bay horses, and a brown-bay horse, light grey horses.

VILLUS is the name given to one of the millions of minute processes which are present on the inner surface of the small intestine. These are structures concerned in the taking up of fat. (*See* DIGESTION, INTESTINE.)

VIRAL. Relating to viruses.

VIRAL HAEMORRHAGIC DISEASE of rabbits. This is encountered in the Far East and Europe, including the UK.
SIGNS: fever, quickly followed by death in as many as 95 per cent of the infected rabbits.
AUTOPSY FINDINGS: congestion of respiratory tract, and haemorrhages in various organs. (AFRC).

VIRAL HEPATITIS in dogs. (*See* CANINE VIRUS HEPATITIS.)

VIRGINIAMYCIN. An antibiotic which may be included in live-stock rations.

VIRINO. A low-molecular-weight nucleic acid and a host-derived protein. (Morgan, K. L. *Veterinary Record* (1988) **122** 445). (*See* SCRAPIE for a possible example.)

VIRION. A mature virus; the ultimate phase in viral development.

VIROLOGY. The study of viruses.

VIRUS DIARRHOEA OF CATTLE (*see* BOVINE VIRUS DIARRHOEA).

VIRUS HEPATITIS OF DUCKLINGS. This is a Scheduled disease which attacks ducklings under 3 weeks old. Death occurs suddenly, and on *post-mortem* examination the liver is seen to be enlarged, with haemorrhages. The Virus Hepatitis Order, 1954, refers.

VIRUS INFECTIONS OF COW'S TEATS. These include *cow-pox.* Nowadays, true cow-pox is (in the UK) considered to be a rare disease. Another infection common to man and cattle is **pseudo-cow-pox** or **milkers' nodules.** The skin disease in cowmen is indistinguishable from that in shepherds who have been handling sheep suffering from orf. It is now thought that the milkers' nodules virus very closely resembles the orf virus, but that they are two distinct entities.
In 1965 two medical men in Dorset, had seven patients with milkers' nodules and with the aid of a veterinary colleague they found that the six dairy herds in which the men worked all had some cows with pseudo-cow-pox (or milkers' nodules) lesions on the teats. There are two types of this infection: one is described as benign or chronic, this lasts for months, it is painless throughout, and starts with a mild redness of the teats, followed by the formation of many scabs which get rubbed off at milking. The second, or acute, form involves pain before scabbing begins, but not afterwards. First there is reddening, then blisters which burst, then very large scabs form. So-called proud flesh is formed beneath the scabs. When these drop off, a characteristic horse-

shoe-shaped ring of minute scabs at the circumference is left. All this takes 7 to 10 days. What looks like a wart remains for several months.
This pseudo-cow-pox differs from true cow-pox in that the latter infection is associated with more pain, fewer scabs, quicker development of them and recovery within 3 weeks.
The virus which causes pseudo-cow-pox or milkers' nodules may be identical with, or closely related to, that of **bovine papular stomatitis** (BPS). According to research workers at Pirbright, this may well be a common disease in southern England. A disease clinically indistinguishable from BPS has been seen in Devon steers used at the Animal Virus Research Institute. In June, 1964, 14 typical cases were observed in a group of 64 animals.
Raised, roughened, brownish plaques were seen on the muzzle, and there were lesions on the lips and inside the mouth.
An ulcerative infection of the teats of dairy cows has recently been described in Scotland, and given the name **bovine ulcerative mammillitis.** It is caused by a herpes virus, and was seen in eighteen herds. In these, 50 per cent of the milking stock showed symptoms, and of these 22 per cent developed mastitis.
The disease has been seen only in early winter, and lasts for up to 15 weeks. In severe cases it was of sudden onset, often appearing between milkings; the whole teat being swollen and painful. Blue discoloration was common. 'The resultant ulcer covered most, if not all, the teat.' In a less severe form (and six forms were described) vivid red discoloration was noted.
On account of the impossibility of milking cows with badly ulcerated teats, and because mastitis often followed, several animals had to be slaughtered.
The same disease has been the subject of another report from south-west England where the onset 'appeared to follow a prolonged period of wet weather. If the virus is of the herpes type it may be that it is endemic in the cattle population and produces lesions only under conditions which result in devitalising of the tissues.' Another possibility is that biting flies transmit the infection. (*See also under* FOOT-AND-MOUTH DISEASE.)

VIRUS PNEUMONIA OF CATTLE (*see* infections listed under CALF PNEUMONIA).

VIRUSES. These are minute entities which carry their genetic information in one type of nucleic acid. They use the energy system of the host cell for their own biosynthetic needs and can be differentiated from bacteria by their size and by their inability to multiply except in living cells.
Most viruses produce disease in man, animals and plants. They can be transmitted from one animal to another and stimulate the production of antibodies in infected animals.
Viruses are mostly invisible under the light microscope although some of the larger examples (*e.g.* the pox viruses) can be seen readily under the light microscope. Most viruses can only be visualised in the electron microscope. There is

Some viruses of veterinary importance

Group	Diseases caused	Animals affected
ADENOVIRUSES	Canine viral hepatitis	Dogs
	Fox encephalitis	Foxes
	(See also KENNEL COUGH.)	
ALPHAVIRUSES	Equine encephalitis	Horses, birds, man
APHTHOVIRUSES	Foot-and-mouth disease	Cattle, sheep, goats, pigs, deer, hedgehogs, and (very rarely) man
ARBOVIRUSES	(See TOGAVIRUSES below.)	
ARENAVIRUSES	Lymphocytic choriomeningitis	Mice, hamsters, man
	(See also LASSA FEVER.)	(Man)
BUNYAVIRUSES	Rift Valley Fever	Sheep, cattle, goats, buffaloes, camels, man
	Nairobi sheep disease	Sheep and goats
	Gumboro disease	Poultry
CALICIVIRUSES	Feline calicivirus disease	Cats
	Vesicular exanthema	Pigs; horses (rarely)
CORONAVIRUSES	Transmissible gastro-enteritis	Pigs
	Feline infectious peritonitis	Cats
	Infectious bronchitis	Chickens
	Enteritis	Calves, foals, dogs, cats
ENTEROVIRUSES	Swine vesicular disease	Pigs; rarely man
	Teschen/Talfan disease	Pigs
	Duck virus hepatitis	Ducklings
	Avian encephalomyelitis	Chickens
FLAVIVIRUSES	Louping ill	Sheep, cattle, deer, dog, man
	Wesselbron disease	Sheep, man
	Japanese B encephalitis	Horses, man, pigs, birds
	Tick-borne encephalitis	Rodents, goats, cattle, man
	Kyasanur forest disease	Monkeys, rodents, man
	Omsk haemorrhagic fever	Rodents, man
	Murray Valley encephalitis	Wild birds, children
	St. Louis encephalitis	Wild birds, bats, horses, man
HERPESVIRUSES	(See table on page 285.)	Horses, cattle, pigs, dogs, cats, man
IRIDOVIRUSES	African swine fever	Pigs, African warthog
LENTIVIRUSES	Maedi-Visna	Sheep
	Caprine arthritis-encephalitis	Goats
MORBILLIVIRUSES	Canine distemper	Dogs, ferrets, mink
	Cattle plague (Rinderpest)	Cattle, sheep, goats
ONCOVIRUSES	Leukaemia, leukosis, cancer	Mammals and birds
ORBIVIRUSES	Bluetongue	Cattle, sheep
	African horse sickness	Horses (but not donkeys)
ORTHOMYXOVIRUSES	Influenza	Horses, pigs, birds
ORTHOPOXVIRUSES	Cowpox	Cattle, man
PAPILLOMAVIRUSES	Warts/papillomas/cancer/sarcoids	Cattle, horses, dogs, man
PARAMYXOVIRUSES	Newcastle disease	Poultry, pigeons
	Parainfluenza	Cattle, dogs (see KENNEL COUGH)
PARAPOXVIRUSES	Pseudocowpox	Cattle, man
	Orf	Sheep, cattle, goats, dogs
	Bovine papular stomatitis	Calves
PESTIVIRUSES	Bovine virus diarrhoea	Cattle
	Border disease	Sheep
	Swine fever	Pigs
	Equine viral arteritis	Horses
PICORNAVIRUSES	(This group includes Enteroviruses, Rhinoviruses, and Aphthovirus – which see)	
POXVIRUSES	(See ORTHOPOXVIRUSES and PARAPOXVIRUSES above.)	
REOVIRUSES	Respiratory disease, enteritis	Calves, pigs, dogs, cats, rabbits, man
RETROVIRUSES	(See LENTIVIRUSES and ONCOVIRUSES above.)	
RHABDOVIRUSES	Rabies (See LYSSA VIRUS, DUVENHAGE, MOKOLA, LAGOS BAT, and NIGERIAN HORSE VIRUS.)	
	Vesicular stomatitis	Horses
TOGAVIRUSES	(See ALPHAVIRUSES, FLAVIVIRUSES and PESTIVIRUSES above.)	

considerable variation in size. Foot-and-mouth disease virus is about 25 nm in diameter, whereas African swine fever virus is about 10 times that size. (*See* NANOMETRE.)

Many pathogenic viruses are capable of altering their antigenic structure, or their pathogenicity, or both, in response to pressures put upon them by, for example, vaccination.

The classical example is provided by influenza viruses, which are able to change from harmless to extremely virulent forms very quickly within the same species. (*AFRC News* 1985)

The nomenclature and classification of viruses has in recent years undergone many changes, and further changes are likely as new viruses are discovered and new information on the properties of viruses accrues. (See the table opposite.)

Anti-virus agents. Since virus infections are not controllable by antibiotics, there has been a long search for other compounds which might achieve anti-viral activity. Much hope was pinned on INTERFERON (which see), but at present its use is very limited, and research has switched to attempts to stimulate natural production of interferon, or to find drugs effective against viruses.

Two drugs which showed significant *in vitro* activity against bovine herpes mammillitis virus, when tested at MAFF's Central Veterinary Laboratory, were: (E)-5-(2-bromovinyl)-2′-deoxyuridine (BVDU) (G. D. Searle & Co.) and phosphonoacetic acid (PAA) from Sigma Chemical Co. (Harkness, J. W. & others, *Veterinary Record* (1986) **118**, 282.)

(*See also* ROTAVIRUS, ASTROVIRUS, ONCOGENIC VIRUSES, DNA, RNA, CANCER.)

VISCERA is the name given to the larger organs lying within the chest and abdominal cavities. The term 'viscus' is applied to each of these individually.

'VISCERAL GOUT'. A condition, of unknown cause, in which chalky white deposits occur on the liver, spleen and heart of chickens. It is sometimes associated with PULLET DISEASE.

VISCERAL LARVA MIGRANS. A syndrome produced in Man by the larvae of *Toxocara canis*. Occasionally it is the cause of death. (*See* TOXOCARA.)

VISION (*see also* EYE). Rays of light pass, in the first place, through the cornea, then through the aqueous humour that fills the anterior chamber of the eye. The light then enters the hinder part of the eye, through the pupil, a round, slit-like, or elliptical hole in the iris, which can be automatically narrowed according to the strength of the light rays that are passing through it. Immediately behind the iris lies the crystalline lens, a clear structure arranged in layers somewhat like an onion, which also by automatic alterations in its curves, brings the rays to a focus upon the retina after they pass through a second clear jelly-like humour – the vitreous humour. The retina is the innermost of the three coats of the eye-ball, and consists of the specialised terminations of the fibres of the optic nerve. (*See* EYE.)

Monocular and binocular vision. In animals whose eyes are laterally placed in the head it is impossible for both eyes to look at an object directly in front of them. One eye can be focused upon an object at any one time, while the other eye sees a completely different picture. This is called 'monocular vision'. When the eyes are placed towards the front of the head so that they can both be concentrated upon an object, as in man, horse, and dog, each eye sees a slightly different picture, but the two ranges of vision overlap. This is called 'binocular vision'. It is partly owing to the fact that in binocular vision each eye sees slightly 'round the corner' of the object, that a sense of depth and distance is conveyed to the higher brain centres. The two pictures are not quite superimposed, and the previous experience of the animal enables it to judge distance by this difference in superimposition. This is technically known as 'stereoscopic vision'.

A striking point in connection with the eyesight of animals is that, although many of them have their visual powers obviously very highly developed, they seldom *trust* their eyes in matters of emergency. The visual images alone do not convey to the mind the reality of the external world. It becomes necessary that the animal shall verify his visual impression by tactile or olfactory impressions. In practically every case the fear of a harmless object may be immediately or shortly dispelled by allowing the animal to smell and examine it by touching it with the nose.

VISNA. A disease of sheep. (*See* MAEDI.)

VITAMINS are substances present in natural foods, essential for health, and which exercise an influence in nutrition out of all proportion to the amounts consumed. Several vitamins are synthesised in the animal body, some being thus available independent of the diet, but it is important to note that a vitamin synthesised in the *lower* part of the alimentary canal may be available to an animal only if it eats its own droppings. (Nocturnal coprophagy is a regular practice with rabbits.)

Vitamin supplements now form an essential part of farm live-stock feeding.

Animals, when feeding under natural conditions, with a free choice from a wide range of food-stuffs, consume, as a rule, all the vitamins they require. But under the influence of domestication, and especially of intensive rearing, animals often have no choice in the matter and suffer from vitamin deficiencies (which see) either because their artificial diet is too restricted, or because vitamins naturally present have been destroyed in the preparation of the food.

Vitamin A is formed from yellow *carotene* found in carrots, green vegetables, egg-yolk, fish roe, liver, cod-liver oil, kidney and milk.

This vitamin is necessary for the growth and general well-being of the young animal in particular. Vitamin A is also necessary for healthy skin and teeth.

Too little or too much vitamin A can both be harmful; and in 1991 MAFF announced a 20-per cent reduction in the level of supplementation for fattening animals. 'For certain ruminant rations it has been possible to exclude this vitamin altogether.' (1991)

Vitamin B complex, water-soluble, includes: riboflavin, nicotinic acid, pantothenic acid, choline, biotin, thiamin. (*See also* CHOLINE, FOLIC ACID.) Most of these are present in yeast and liver. (For nicotinic acid, *see* NIACIN.)

Vitamin B$_1$ (Thiamin, aneurine) is present in the husks of cereal grains, yolk of egg, yeast, liver. A deficiency can be caused by overheating the food of pet animals, or by the enzyme present in some fish. Horse and cattle which eat bracken are affected by the thiaminase in that plant. (*See* BRACKEN POISONING.)

Vitamin B$_2$ (Riboflavin) is present in milk (and is not destroyed by pasteurisation), as well as in foods mentioned under B$_1$.

Riboflavin is a constituent of the flavoproteins – hydrogen transporting enzymes, concerned with the animal's energy metabolism.

Biotin, formerly known as vitamin H, is another of the B group of vitamins. It is necessary for the health of skin and hoof. It is referred to below under Vitamin Deficiencies.

Vitamin B$_3$ (Pantothenic acid). Necessary for skin health, and growth.

Vitamin B$_6$ (Pyridoxine), present in liver, yeast and cereals, is important for growth and protein metabolism.

Vitamin B$_{12}$ is the anti-pernicious anaemia factor of importance in human medicine, and contains cobalt and is also known as Cobalamin.

Vitamin C. This is ascorbic acid; it is found in the juices of most fruits and vegetables, and its absence causes scurvy.

Vitamin D. This was identified as radiostol or irradiated ergosterol. It is the anti-rachitic principle found in cod-liver oil, meat juice, cow's milk, and egg-yolk. The absence of this vitamin causes rickets. There is an intimate association between the presence of this vitamin, the action of sunlight or the artificial irradiation by ultraviolet rays, and the mineral balance in the body.

With its help salts of calcium and phosphorus, instead of being eliminated from the intestinal canal, are absorbed into the system and made use of in the calcification of bone. (*See* COD-LIVER OIL.) *Too much* D is harmful. (*See* RODENTICIDES.)

Vitamin E (tocopherol) (fat-soluble). This vitamin is found in red meat, oil of seeds, milk, egg-yolk. It is necessary for fertility, and its absence from a diet has been shown to cause sterility in rats, by inducing firstly the death, and later the absorption, of the embryos.

Vitamin K complex, mostly fat-soluble. Concerned with the formation of PROTHROMBIN (which see), and hence might be regarded as 'the anti-internal-haemorrhage factor'. Present in alfalfa. Synthetic preparations available for therapy.

Vitamin excess (*hypervitaminosis*) may result in serious disease. (For an example, see under CAT FOODS – chronic hypervitaminosis A occurs in cats fed almost exclusively on liver.)

An excess of yeast, fed to pigs as a vitamin B supplement, has resulted in severe rickets.

Vitamin deficiencies. These may occur as the result of a vitamin-deficient diet, or a failure – in some instances – to synthesise a particular vitamin within the body. 'Secondary' or 'conditioned' deficiencies may also arise from any disease which impairs absorption from the alimentary tract, injuries to the liver, infections (which increase the consumption of vitamins), metallic poisoning, and as the result of some enzyme which destroys or inactivates a vitamin. (For examples of the last-mentioned cause, *see* CHASTEK PARALYSIS.)

Biotin-producing bacteria live in intestines and contribute a variable amount. But biotin deficiency is not rare – except in adult ruminants. Signs of deficiency are: dermatitis on ears, neck, shoulder and tail of the pig, together with cracking of the walls and sole of the hoof; retarded growth and brittle feathering, foot dermatitis, swollen eyelids, eruptions on mouth and beak, perosis, leg weakness, poor hatchability and embryonic malformations in birds.

Stress in domestic animals increases their need for vitamin C.

A report from Finland stated that bleeding from the navel, which was a serious problem in a breeding herd of 85 Finnish Landrace and 85 Large White sows, could be successfully controlled by vitamin C (not vitamin K as might have been expected). An ascorbic acid supplement was given to the sows for from 8 to 2 days before farrowing. Piglets from the treated sows were also 5·5 per cent heavier than those from untreated controls at three weeks of age. (M. Sandholm *et al.*, *Vet. Rec.* (1979) **104,** 337.)

Vitamin E could with advantage be added to all compound feeds as a precautionary measure; and at higher levels if the feed contains polyunsaturated fatty acids. Less vitamin E is absorbed from the intestine if the latter are present. Some feeds contain vitamin-E antagonists – present in lucerne and beans. The activity of vitamin E may be reduced by a high nitrate content in feed or drinking water. Animals which do not receive an adequate supply of the trace element selenium need extra vitamin E, because selenium has a vitamin-E sparing effect. Application of fertilisers rich in sulphates inhibits the absorption of selenium by plants from the soil, and in these circumstances grazing animals will require extra vitamin E.

Vitamin E contents of feeds/crops may be reduced to a dangerous level on storage. (*See also* MUSCULAR DYSTROPHY.) Anti-vitamin E factor may be present in barley as well as fats of animal origin.

Despite a current tendency to increase vitamin levels in animal feeds, cases of vitamin E deficiency appear to be becoming more prevalent in all classes of farm livestock: resulting in mulberry heart in pigs, muscular dystrophy in calves, and 'crazy chick disease' in poultry. Perhaps this has something to do with the faster growth rates expected of animals nowadays. Certainly the low vitamin E content of some cereals is important. This is especially the case with some samples of barley grown on selenium-deficient soil but fed on a farm where selenium is no problem and where the possibility of such a deficiency might well be overlooked.

It is generally accepted that 30–35 international units of vitamin E are required by the animal, on average, and on the basis that cereals will provide, say, 20 of those units, another 10 units are added by the feed manufacturer or by the farmer doing his own mixing, and using a conventional mineral and vitamin supplement. However, some samples of barley and other cereals contain little or no vitamin E; in which case the added 10 units would clearly be insufficient.

It has also been shown that moist grain storage can result in serious losses of vitamin E. Farmers using this technique should therefore be watchful for symptoms and, better still, ensure as far as they can that vitamin supplements are never omitted or used at levels below those recommended.

Vitamin E deficiency leads to MUSCULAR DYSTROPHY (which see); and a supplement of this vitamin has been shown to reduce the incidence of retained placenta, metritis, and cysts of the ovaries when given with SELENIUM. (Harrison, J. H. & Others, *Journal of Dairy Science* (1984) **67**, 123.)

(*See also under* Vitamin E on the previous page.)

A vitamin E supplement may also help in reducing the incidence of clinical mastitis.

Horses. Vitamin A deficiency is unlikely to occur except in town horses denied adequate green food. Deficiency symptoms are stated to include night-blindness, hoof lesions, corneal lesions, respiratory symptoms, and reproductive difficulties. Some of the B vitamins are synthesised by adult horses, but backward foals may benefit from vitamin supplements. Infertility in the mare may sometimes be associated with a Vitamin C deficiency. It has been suggested that splints, sidebones, ringbones, spavins may be associated with a Vitamin D deficiency.

Cattle. Vitamin A deficiency leads, in cattle denied adequate green food, to abortion or the birth of weak, blind calves, or of those suffering from diarrhoea which die within a few days. Corneal lesions and blindness may also result in growing cattle. For example, Hereford bulls on a diet of beet-pulp nuts, high-protein nuts, and barley straw went blind owing to a lack of vitamin A. (1977 MAFF report.) (*See also* HYPERKERATOSIS.) Vitamins of the B complex are mostly synthesised in the rumen, but in the new-born calf a deficiency may occur.* Vitamin C is apparently synthesised by adult cattle, but some cases of infertility may, it is believed, be due to a deficiency, and some cases of 'navel-ill' benefit, it is said, from Vitamin C treatment. In some parts of this country pasture or fodder crops contain too little Vitamin D, while sunlight during the winter months is insufficient to enable the shortage to be made good within the animal's body; the result is rickets. Vitamin E deficiency is associated with muscular dystrophy.

Pigs. Vitamin A deficiency results in failure to grow in piglets and infertility in adult pigs, paralysis of the hindquarters. A nicotinic acid deficiency gives rise to a condition simulating necrotic enteritis and poor growth. Yeast supplements will correct deficiencies of the B complex, but excess may result in rickets.

A vitamin E deficiency in new-born piglets can result in their sudden death after being given iron injections to prevent anaemia. It is advisable to delay the injection until the piglet is a week old, when it is more tolerant of iron. Gilts' rations low in vitamin E or high in fatty acid predispose to this condition in the offspring.

Biotin deficiency in pigs gives rise to symptoms which include dermatitis. Lameness can affect a whole herd where there is a biotin deficiency causing cracks in the sole or wall of the hooves.

Dog and cat. Vitamin A has been used with success in the treatment of diarrhoea in kittens. Corneal lesions, even blindness in extreme cases, and sometimes deafness, have also been attributed to a Vitamin A deficiency. Vitamin B (thiamin) deficiency results in fatigue and loss of appetite, and may be associated with cramp. Yeast may prove effective in cases of 'depraved appetite' and chorea. 'Black-tongue' in the dog and an ulcerative stomatitis in the dog are seen in the USA in naturally occurring cases of nicotinic acid deficiency. Lack of riboflavin is associated with eye lesions and skin disease. Rickets results from lack of vitamin D, especially in the larger breeds, but overdosage is harmful and can lead to deposits of calcium salts in or between muscles. (*See* 'SCURVY RICKETS'.)

Poultry. Vitamin A deficiency will occur only in birds deprived of adequate green food. Maize and cod-liver oil (which must not be rancid) are alternative sources of this vitamin. Lack of it leads, in chickens, to drowsiness, weakness, staggering, stunted growth, and often a discharge from the eyes. Adult birds become dishevelled looking, weak and emaciated, and show a watery or cheesy discharge from eyes and nostrils. Deficiency of riboflavin (Vitamin B_2) in the diet is not uncommon, particularly in wire-floor battery brooders, in which the chicks have no access to droppings. (On solid floors chicks may correct the deficiency by eating their droppings, which contain riboflavin synthesised by organisms in the lower part of the gut, but not otherwise available to the body.) Symptoms are leg weakness and a curling inwards of the toes in chicks; decreased egg production and poor hatchability. (*See also* BIOTIN *under* vitamin B above.) Thin shells, reduced hatchability, and sometimes a temporary paralysis after laying, are indications of a Vitamin D deficiency. Chicks are unthrifty, walk with difficulty, and later show typical symptoms of rickets. Bone deformity and softening of the beak occur in adult birds. Sunlight, green food, and the judicious use in winter of cod-liver oil overcome this deficiency. Vitamin E, necessary for hatchability, is present in whole grain and, to a lesser extent, in greenstuff. The latter also contains ample Vitamin K, a deficiency of which leads to anaemia as a result of internal haemorrhage.

VOICE is the sound produced as the result of the vibration of a column of air forced through the larynx by contraction of the respiratory muscles.

*See THIAMIN.

The means by which this is produced are analogous to those by which sound is produced in a reed instrument, except that in the living animal the pitch of the voice can be altered at will. This is accomplished by the amount of tension exerted by muscular action upon the vocal cords; the more tense these are the higher is the pitch of the voice. In the majority of mammals the vibrations are produced when a blast of air is expelled from the chest, but in the donkey the higher notes of the bray result from inspiration of air, and the lower notes from expiration.

The character of the voice can be altered to some extent by changes in the resonating chambers of the nose, mouth, pharynx, etc.; thus, the false nostrils of the horse are used to produce the 'snort' of fear or excitement, the nasal cavities transmit the whinny and neigh of pleasure, and the mouth and pharynx furnish the character of the neigh of impatience, loneliness, and sometimes the challenge of anger of the jealous stallion.

Neighing or *whinnying* in the horse is an expiratory act produced partly through the mouth and partly through the nose; the *bray* of the ass is expiratory for the low notes and inspiratory for the high; *bellowing* in the ox, *bleating* in the sheep, *barking* in the dog, and the *mew* of the cat, are all produced by expiratory efforts.

Animals use their voices upon widely different occasions. It seems probable that they make the greatest use of this faculty for the purposes of enabling the young to recognise their dams from a distance, and to maintain cohesion of herds or flocks. Stragglers getting left behind, or separated from their special companions, can be heard calling for long distances. Male animals of many species will give a warning upon the approach of newcomers or danger. Females may produce little cries or screams when attended by males during periods of oestrus, or when making acquaintance with their newly-born progeny. Almost all the domestic animals emit cries when suffering pain. In the horse tribe the sounds are often merely grunts or groans, especially when the pain is abdominal. In other cases horses will scream when they are suddenly subjected to acute pain, or to very great fright. Cattle and sheep in agony behave similarly to horses; they usually groan, but cows, ewes, and heifers may issue a long drawn-out bellow or bleat during difficult parturition. The pig has a range of notes from the satisfied grunt of suckling a sow, to the frightened squeals and screams of those that are being handled by man. The dog has a note for all occasions; he generally expresses all the emotions of which he is capable by differences in his bark. (*See also* LARYNX *and* MUTING.)

In rabies the character of the voice may be changed. In the 'dumb' form, barking is suppressed.

VOLAR. At the back of the fore-limb.

VOLVULUS. An intestinal obstruction is produced by the twisting of a loop of bowel round itself. It is usually due to some spasmodic contraction of the muscular coat, or to the presence

of gas, and is very dangerous owing to the great risk of strangulation of the blood-supply and consequent necrosis. Excessive gas formation in the caecum and colon of whey-fed pigs may lead to volvulus. (*See* HAEMORRHAGIC GASTRO-ENTERITIS *and see* INTESTINE, DISEASES OF.)

VOMICA. A cavity in the lung tissue produced by disease. Vomicae are most commonly met with in cattle suffering from either tuberculosis or contagious pleuro-pneumonia.

VOMITING involves not merely a contraction of the stomach walls and a dilatation of the gullet, but it is a complex act in which the abdominal muscles, the diaphragm, the muscles of the chest and larynx, and those of the lower part of the neck all play a part.

Before the act there is usually a profuse secretion of watery saliva which serves to lubricate the passage of the stomach contents. The animal appears uneasy, and will usually seek a secluded spot. Soon rhythmic contractions of the abdominal muscles commence and culminate in the ejection of a quantity of frothy material. The diaphragm is generally fixed, and there is a powerful closing of the glottis to prevent any fluids from gaining access into the trachea.

The dog and cat vomit with relative ease. They are able to induce vomiting by eating portions of the green shoots of couch grass (*Triticum repens*), ingestion of which brings on vomiting in from 5 to 10 minutes. In the pig the process is more exacting than in the carnivores. Cattle and sheep may vomit occasionally, but the act is an unusual one, and generally points to serious stomach trouble. Vomiting in the horse is rare, and often is associated with a rupture of the stomach, and when it occurs it should be considered a very grave symptom indeed. The material always escapes through the nostrils in the horse.

CAUSES. It will be sufficient to deal with vomiting under the headings as follows:

Travel sickness (which see).

Stress (which see).

Simple indigestion. When the stomach has received either a quality or a quantity of foodstuff with which it is unable to deal the process of digestion does not proceed, or only proceeds up to a point. The material brought up is recognisable as food, but it is mixed with quantities of frothy mucus, water, and perhaps may be stained brownish from bile. It has a faintly sour smell which is greater the longer the process of digestion has been enabled to proceed. The ejecta is generally easily brought up, and the animal soon settles down and becomes normal.

Indigestion from foreign bodies. (*See* 'CHOKING', IMPACTION, FOREIGN BODIES.)

Gastritis. The walls of the stomach are inflamed and thickened, the mucous membrane is swollen and painful, and the nervous system is in an irritable state. Whenever food or water enters the organ vomiting immediately takes place. The vomit consists of the solid material swallowed, coated on the outside with mucus and froth. If liquids have been taken they are returned almost unchanged. When the inflammatory condition is very severe there are quantities of blood that have undergone partial digestion and have an appearance not unlike coffee-grounds, seen in the vomit. In such animals there will be a very offensive smell both from the ejecta and from the mouth of the patient.

Pyloric stenosis, which may be congenital, is said to give rise to 'projectile' vomiting.

Enteritis is associated with vomiting but there is diarrhoea as well.

Impaction of the rectum, whether from particles of undigested bone, or hair, hard faeces, etc., generally induces vomiting in which not only does the stomach expel its contents, but there are masses of bowel content as well.

Acute nephritis is an extremely common cause of thirst and vomiting in the dog.

Pyometra in the bitch, cat, sow is frequently accompanied by vomiting.

Accidents. The shock of a severe burn or accident will cause vomiting, although the injuries have not been inflicted upon the stomach itself. In other cases, where the head has been injured, the area in the case of the brain which control the act of vomiting becomes disturbed and the animal evacuates its stomach.

Poisons. Very many irritant substances will produce vomiting. Of the commonest may be mentioned – tartar emetic, mustard, salt, carbolic acid, areca-nut, castor oil, etc.; and of substances less common, but more drastic, the following are examples – strychnine, arsenic, phosphorus, apomorphine, croton oil, zinc and copper sulphates, and many of the metallic salts. Some of these have special characteristics; *e.g.* phosphorus vomit is luminous in the dark.

Diseases. The symptom of vomiting is common to many other diseases – meningitis, peritonitis, nephritis, leptospirosis, rabies, 'vomiting and wasting' syndrome in pigs, etc.

TREATMENT. In the dog and cat the use of normal saline or glucose saline by injection is frequently indicated as an alternative to giving food (liquid or otherwise) by mouth during an illness (such as nephritis, uraemia, enteritis) in which vomiting is persistent.

'VOMITING AND WASTING' SYNDROME.

This occurs in piglets five days old and upwards, and is characterised by vomiting, depression, loss of appetite, constipation, emaciation, and a hairy appearance. It is probably caused by a virus. (*See also* 'ONTARIO ENCEPHALITIS'.)

VON WILLEBRAND'S DISEASE.

An inherited bleeding disorder which has been found in some 25 breeds of dogs, and is associated with an autosomal trait causing a high morbidity but a low mortality. Signs may include: epistaxis, haematuria, lameness, bleeding from genital mucosa, and prolonged bleeding from cut nails, etc.

VULTURES (*see* TROPICS, CARCASE DISPOSAL).

VULVA. It has in domesticated animals only simple, single labia or lips.

Diseases of the vulva. In Kenya squamous cell carcinoma of the vulva is common in cattle of the Ayrshire breed. Cryosurgery has given good results when treatment has not been delayed until the tumour becomes too large. In 62 cases, 55 were successfully treated. (Omara-Opyene & Others, *Veterinary Record* (1985) **117**, 518.)

Persistent bleeding from the vulva. (*See* VAGINA.)

In the tropics, especially, a thick purulent discharge from the vagina may be a sign of tuberculosis involving the uterus/vagina.

VULVOVAGINITIS (*see under* RHINOTRACHEITIS *and below*).

VULVOVAGINITIS, GRANULAR. A venereal disease of cattle caused by *Mycoplasma bovigenitalium*, affecting vulva and vagina or seminal vesicles and skin of the penis. The lesions are nodules.

W

'WALKABOUT DISEASE' (*see* KIMBERLEY HORSE DISEASE).

WALLABIES. Smaller than kangaroos, these marsupials are a source of human HYDATID DISEASE in the southern tablelands of New South Wales.

Despite a reduction of the disease in domestic dogs and sheep, eleven out of eighteen wild dogs which were trapped proved to be infected with *Echinococcus granulosus*.

WALL-EYES (Leukoma) in horses are met with when the greater part of the face, or that portion around the eyes, is white. The condition consists of an absence of colouring matter in the iris. The pupil of the eye appears to be encircled by a ring of bluish or greyish white, and the expression of the horse's face is consequently unusual. It is not a serious defect except in tropical countries.

WARBLE FLY ORDER came into force in 1989, and requires treatment where a blood test indicates an infestation. In order to wipe out whole fly populations, both the affected herd and any herd within 3 km will have to be treated.

WARBLES are swellings about the size of a marble or small walnut occurring upon the backs of cattle in spring and early summer caused by the presence in them of the larvae of one of the warble flies – *Hypoderma bovis* or *Hypoderma lineata*. These are of very great economic importance. The adults – especially *Hypoderma bovis* – cause great annoyance to stock during the period when eggs are being laid. Not only does this result in injuries, animals rushing around ('gadding') to avoid the 'attacks', but the milk yield is reduced, sometimes by as much as 25 per cent, and condition is impaired.

H. lineatum in its migration through the body irritates the gullet; and both species may injure the spinal cord. The warbles on the back are really so many small abscesses which not only reduce condition very considerably but may, when many are present, result in the death of

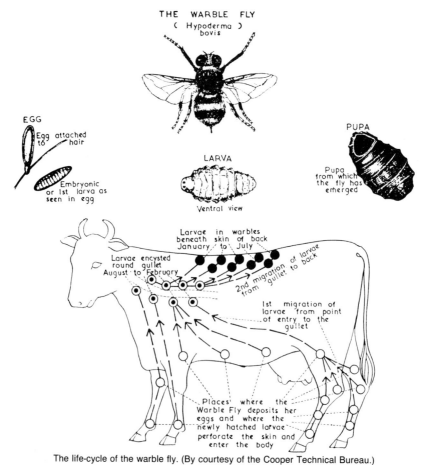

The life-cycle of the warble fly. (By courtesy of the Cooper Technical Bureau.)

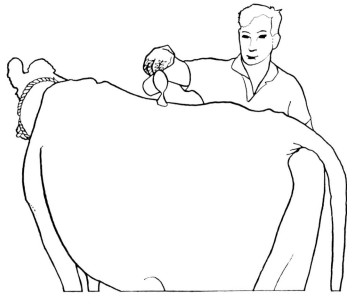

Dressing against warbles.

young animals. The accidental crushing of a number of the larvae in these cavities may cause the death of the animal from anaphylactic shock.

In the carcases there is considerable destruction of valuable meat around the warbles; 'Butchers' Jelly' or 'Licked Beef' is an oedematous, straw-coloured, jelly-like substance, which infiltrates the tissue near the larvae. The holes which the larvae produce in the hides reduce their value; heavily infected hides are often useless for leather.

Warbles are most frequent in young animals, in which loss of condition is most serious; but they have been found in small numbers in animals up to 15 years old. They are sometimes found in young horses. The larvae occasionally enter the spinal canal and produce very serious lesions. Horses are attacked mostly by *Hypoderma bovis* larvae, which affect the area of the saddle chiefly; but brain involvement has been reported in the horse. In deer larvae of the warble fly *Hypoderma diana* are often found.

Methods of control. Satisfactory control depends on artificial interference with the life cycle. (*See* IVERMECTIN.)

A systemic insecticide, on the other hand, will kill a high percentage of larvae *before* they complete their migration and penetrate the back.

Another **eradication programme** was announced for Britain in 1978, when MAFF stated that 40 per cent of cattle in England and Wales, and 20 per cent in Scotland, were affected with warbles. The new Order to control warble fly applied between March 15 and July 31 each year. It provides that during this period:

(a) owners of infested cattle must treat them;

(b) warbled cattle may not be moved even to a

Organophosphorus pour-on warblecide compounds which have been used in Great Britain

Standard name	Registered name	Trade name	Supplier
Famphur	Famphur (Cyanamid of Great Britain)	Cyanamid Systemic Warble Fly Dressing	Cyanamid of Great Britain Ltd
Fenthion	Tiguvon (Bayer Agrochem)	Tiguvon	Bayer Agrochem Ltd Ciba-Geigy Agro-chemicals
Phosmet	Prolate (Stauffer Chemical Co)	Orbisect	Beecham Animal Health
		Dermol	Crown Chemical Co
		Young's Poron Systemic Warble and Lice Fluids for Cattle	Robert Young & Co Ltd
		Rycovet Warblecide Pour-on	Rycovet Ltd

slaughterhouse without having been treated and they must be accompanied by a statutory declaration by the owner that they have been treated;

(c) untreated cattle being moved may be sent compulsorily for slaughter or to a specified place for treatment. In these circumstances veterinary inspection of the herd of origin and treatment under veterinary supervision of warbled animals may be required at the owner's expense. Similar measures may be applied to untreated warbled cattle found on any farm. (*See* FLY CONTROL.)

An amending Order 1981 enabled the Agriculture Departments to require treatment in the *autumn* of cattle aged 12 weeks and over on farms where there had been warbled cattle in the preceding spring. (Autumn is the more effective time for treatment, even though infestation cannot be detected then, and all cattle owners are advised to treat their herds in the autumn voluntarily.)

Reindeer. In Canada they are attacked by the warble fly *Edoede magena tarandi.* Ivermectin has been used for control.

Goats. Ivermectin has been used also against the goat warble *Przhevalskiana silenus.*

Warble fly infestation was reduced from 360 herds in 1989 to only about 100 in 1990. (MAFF survey).

The Tropical Warble fly of Central America is *Dermatobia hominis,* which lays its eggs on an intermediary vector – fly or mosquito – which it catches for the purpose. (*See also under* FLIES, and **Ivermectin**.)

WARFARIN. An organic rat poison approved by the Ministry of Agriculture and internationally known. It is an anticoagulant, its use leading to death of rats and mice from internal haemorrhage. In the strengths used, 0·005 per cent and 0·025 per cent, it is considered that properly prepared baits will not prove dangerous to livestock if used with ordinary care. Cases of accidental poisoning have occurred, however, in domestic animals; and food contaminated by rodents' urine may be dangerous where Warfarin is used.

Treatment of Warfarin poisoning:
Vitamin K_1 (phytomenadione – Konakion, Roche) by intra-muscular injection. Blood transfusion may be necessary. (See Dr Morag G. Kerr. *Veterinary Record* (1986) **119**, 435.)

Once symptoms have appeared, use of glucose saline, or blood transfusion, is indicated. The poisoned animal must be handled very gently, or further internal bleeding may occur. (*See also* NAVICULAR DISEASE.)

WARTS (*Papillomas*) are small growths which appear on skin or mucous membrane, and occur in all farm and domestic animals. Papillomas are benign, but an individual wart can become malignant. (*See* PAPILLOMAS.)

Around the mouth they may interfere with feeding, and when occurring about the nostrils they may obstruct the breathing. Soft warts in the oesophagus sometimes make swallowing difficult, and upon the penis or in the urethra they may hinder the passage of urine. (*See also* EYE.)

Horses. The commonest situations are the skin of the udder or sheath, the lips and nostrils, the eye lids, outer and inner skin of the ears, the region of the breast, the insides of the limbs.

Cattle. The commonest seats of warts are the teats of cows. Young cows in winter are often affected about the skin of the eyelids and along the lower line of the abdomen, but the growths often drop off spontaneously from these positions when the young animals are turned out to grass in the early spring. Otherwise warty growths are found as in the horse. (*See* VIRAL PAPILLOMATOSIS.)

Dogs and cats. In the dog especially, less so in the cat, warts are common. Single small warts with a cauliflower-like extremity or with a rounded top, are commonly found about the eyelids, lips, ears, paws, etc., as well as upon the general surface of the body. They usually grow very slowly and may be present for years without causing any pain or inconvenience. In other cases warts appear in connection with the gums, tongue, and insides of the cheeks; in these positions they arise in clusters and grow very rapidly. Cases such as these are usually accompanied by a great amount of salivation and a fetid discharge from the mouth.

REMOVAL OF WARTS. Multiple warts in cattle have been successfully banished by means of intramuscular injections of Anthiomaline (lithium antimony thiomalate). After a few injections the globular type of warts can then be 'shelled out' easily. Autogenous and other vaccines have also been used against multiple warts.

WASHING OF ANIMALS (*see* BATHS).

WASP STINGS (*see under* BITES).

WASTE FOOD (*see* BAKERY WASTE, SWILL, CHOCOLATE POISONING).

WASTING (*see* ATROPHY).

WATER AND WATERING OF ANIMALS.

Amounts required. The quantity of water needed per day by the various domestic animals depends upon the nature of the food, the climate, the temperature, and the size and the activity of the animals themselves. When very dry food is given, such as hay, bran, oats, etc., more water is required than when roots or growing grass is eaten.

Drinking water should be freely available to animals, so that they can drink as and when they choose. (*See below under* **Water supply.**) Stress may occur in an animal deprived of the chance to drink sufficient water, and actual dehydration (which can lead to death) may be caused. Production of milk, etc., will obviously be adversely affected.

With an *ad lib.* water supply, the amount of water required by various animals under various conditions is of mainly theoretical interest, apart from practical aspects of planning adequate supplies of piped water, trough space, etc. Water requirement figures can be taken only as approximate guidelines, and authorities differ to some extent.

Cattle. Dry cows of the larger breeds require between 36·5 and 45 litres (about 8 to 10 gallons) per day. Those in milk 'need in addition about five times as much water as the volume of milk produced,' Professor J. O. L. King has stated*, while 'for the last four months of pregnancy, the daily consumption may rise to about 70 litres (approximately 15 gallons).'

Dr. W. J. Miller, of the University of Georgia College of Agriculture gives†, for non-pregnant, non-lactating cows fed indoors, a figure of three to four pounds of water consumed for each pound of dry matter, when environmental temperature is between 10° and 40°F.

'It has been suggested that the water requirement for *grazing* cattle should be calculated as 50 per cent higher,' *i.e.* 4½ to 6 lb of water would be needed for each lb of dry matter eaten (at temperatures below 50°F). 'For each lb of *milk* produced, about 0·87 lb *more* water is considered to be needed.'

As the air temperature increases above 50°F, the water requirement rises rapidly.

Calves require much more water after they are weaned than before. A common mistake is to ignore this fact, with the result that the calves receive a check to their growth from which they may never fully recover.

Pigs are highly susceptible to water deprivation (*see* SALT POISONING). Approximate quantities required have been given by Professor King as 1 gallon per day for a litter of 3-week-old piglets, and up to 5 gallons per day for a nursing sow. The benefits of creep feeding may be lost if the piglets are denied water.

Quality of water. This is obviously of prime importance. Animals may suffer thirst and stress if the only drinking water available to them is disagreeable in taste. Where piped water is not available, and rain-water has to be stored in tanks, it is important to clean out gutters and the tanks themselves. Galvanised iron tanks should not be allowed to get rusty. Well-water may contain an excess of one or more minerals which may make it unpalatable or be harmful to the animal, so that sampling and analysis should be carried out.

Poisoning by water may result from the use of lead pipes or tanks. (*See* LEAD POISONING.) The use of lead paints in storage tanks is also a danger. (*See also* ZINC POISONING.) Stored rainwater containing decaying organic matter (leaves, bird droppings, etc.) has led to the death of pigs from nitrite poisoning.

Diseases spread by water. Apart from illness caused by some inorganic substance dissolved in the water, such as lead from lead pipes or tanks, arsenic from contamination with sheep-dip, water-borne infection may cause disease.

Among diseases that can be distributed in this manner are the following: Anthrax, from water used in tanneries or wool-washing premises, or when a carcase has been buried near a stream;

Johne's disease, salmonellosis, and coccidiosis in cattle, from contamination of streams, ditches, and ponds.

Washing water and water-tanks have been contaminated with, for example, *Bacillus subtilis*, leading to MASTITIS.

Water supply. A good stockman will ensure that the animals in his care are never short of water; that all automatic drinking bowls or nipple drinkers are in working order; that frost has not cut off the supply of piped water (lagging of exposed pipes is obviously necessary in winter), and that the water has not been allowed to freeze in troughs, tanks, etc. It is also necessary to ensure that the levers of automatic drinking bowls are not too stiff for young animals to operate, and that young stock are shown working nipple drinkers – not left to find them for themselves. (*See also* ALGAE.)

In one incident newly weaned pigs were put into a yard having automatic water-bowls fitted, but as the yard had been mucked out the bowls were out of reach of the young pigs.

Pigs deprived of water show nervous symptoms. They may walk in circles, or backwards, press their heads against a wall, champ their jaws, collapse and have convulsions. Of course, some pigs may be found dead without symptoms having been observed.

Sheep have shown symptoms suggestive of twin-lamb disease, and died, after being removed from a field where they had access to a stream and placed on pasture where the ball-valve of a drinking trough had been tied up. Sheep prefer to drink running water, and those of some breeds are so reluctant to drink anything else that, when housed, a running water supply must be arranged indoors.

A drop in milk yield may occur in dairy herds where the cows are moved periodically to a field too far from a water-trough; or where the water pressure is too low to ensure adequate supply.

Dogs, cats, and poultry should always be allowed an unlimited supply of water so

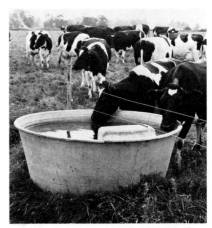

Designed for field use, this CemFil glass fibre-reinforced cement drinking trough is obtainable in sizes of up to 2000-litre capacity, and manufactured by Pilkington Brothers Ltd. The water supply is, of course, piped.

* *The UFAW Handbook on the care and management of Farm Animals.* (Churchill Livingstone, 1971.)
† *Dairy Cattle Feeding and Nutrition.* (Academic Press, Inc. 1979.)

arranged that they are unable to foul or upset the drinking vessels.

(*See also* DEHYDRATION.)

A point that should never be lost sight of in connection with watering of **horses** is that wherever possible *water should be given before the food*, or not for 1 to 2 hours after feeding. The horse's stomach is small, and cannot contain a full feed and several gallons of water simultaneously.

It would appear that it is neither necessary to heat water for tired horses nor to worry about its hardness as long as it is palatable. The best advice for the owners of horses is to offer the horse water in excess of requirements when at rest and to allow them to drink frequently when working. (Hinton, M. (1978). *Equine Veterinary Journal*, **10**, 27.)

Water intoxication. This may occur in farm livestock when, as a result of bad management, they have been deprived of adequate drinking water and then suddenly find themselves in circumstances which enable them to drink as much as they want.

One symptom may be a red discoloration of the urine. Convulsions, recumbency, hyperaesthesia, aimless wandering, and death have been seen in calves.

WATER BUFFALOES. In recent trials in such diverse countries as the United States, Papua New Guinea, Trinidad, and Australia, water buffalo herds have performed very well in growth rates, environmental adaptability, health, reproduction, and in the production of meat and milk.

But despite these apparent successes, widely held beliefs – that water buffaloes are mean and vicious, that their meat is tough and tasteless, and that the animals can only be raised near water – are helping to keep water buffaloes an under-utilized resource.

However, field experience reveals that these beliefs are not true. Unless wounded or severely stressed, most domesticated water buffaloes are quite gentle. In Egypt, water buffalo meat is the most common kind, and taste tests elsewhere indicate that it is considered similar to beef. And in Italy, water buffalo milk is the source of world-famous mozzarella cheese. It is also higher in butterfat and nonfat solids than is cow's milk.

Although water buffaloes must have shade nearby, they can reproduce and grow without being near a swamp or river.

Some of the steps needed to permit greater exploitation of this valuable resource are:

• trials to compare growth rate, feeding, nutrition, and other characteristics of water buffalo with those of cattle.

• selective breeding and protection of outstanding buffalo specimens, especially in Southeast Asia.

• replacement of the 1500-year-old inefficient wooden yoke (in rural Asia, where the water buffalo is the small farmer's 'tractor,' improved harnesses could increase pulling power by up to 25 per cent). (*See* ANIMAL TRANSPORT.)

The limitation of water buffaloes must be

taken into account. For instance, the animals suffer if forced to remain, even for a few hours, in direct sunlight. They cannot be worked for long periods during the heat of the day, and they are also susceptible to extreme cold. (*Source – The water buffalo: new prospects for an under-utilized animal*. Washington DC, US National Academy of Sciences, 1982.)

An important roundworm of the water buffalo (*Bubalus bubalis*) is *Paracooperia nodulosa*. This causes development of nodules in the intestine, and diarrhoea, anaemia, emaciation and sometimes death. (Sheikh-Omar, A. R. & others, *Veterinary Record* (1985) **116**, 134.) (*See* LIVESTOCK PRODUCTION IN THE TROPICS.)

WATER-DROPWORT. This is *Oenanthe fistulosa*, and while it and Parsley Water-Dropwort (*O. lachenalii* and also *O. aquatica*) are all poisonous, they are less so than **Hemlock Water-Dropwort** (*Oenanthe crocata*), a weed of marshy places, ditches, and other wet spots, is considered to be one of the most dangerous and poisonous of the commoner plants found in Great Britain, and many cases of poisoning, not only among animals but also among human beings, have been recorded. It is a member of the same botanical class as Cowbane, Hemlock, and Fool's Parsley, and like them the poisonous principle is found in all parts of the plant. In its leaves it has a great similarity to celery, and its rootsock has been mistaken for parsnip. The active toxic principle is called *Oenanthotoxin*, and is most abundant in the root.

SIGNS. The symptoms appear very quickly after the plant has been eaten, and death follows in from 1 to 4 hours when large amounts have been taken. Cattle become very depressed in general appearance, and their respiration is fast and laboured. The mucous membranes become con-

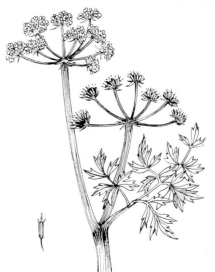

Water-dropwort (*Oenanthe crocata*). This should strictly be called Hemlock water-dropwort. The roots are the most poisonous part of the plant, and are often dislodged during severe floods or ditching or drainage work. Height: 4 ft or so.

gested, the eye rolls, the pulse is weak and fast, and there is a certain amount of foaming at the mouth. Convulsions follow.

In some cases that are not fatal one or more of the limbs may remain paralysed. In the horse the appearance of symptoms and the course of the illness are much more rapid and the nervous symptoms are exaggerated.

TREATMENT. Barbiturates may save life.

WATER-FLEAS. *Daphnia pulex*, a brown water-flea found in British ponds, is the intermediate host of the roundworms of ducks, *e.g. Acuaria uncinata*.

WATER HEMLOCK, a common plant of damp marshy places in all parts of the Northern hemisphere, has a short, stout hollow root-stock, and large much-divided leaves set on strong stems. Water Hemlock (*Cicuta virosa*), is also known as Cowbane.

The root in springtime contains the greatest amount of the poisonous principles, which are three in number: *viz.* an alkaloid, *cicutine*; an oil, *oil of cicuta*; and a bitter resinous substance, *cicutoxin*.

SIGNS. Salivation, dullness, vomiting in pigs; colic in horses; bloat in cattle; together with diarrhoea, a staggering gait. Sudden death or a few hours' illness.

FIRST-AID. Owing to the rapidity of the appearance of symptoms it is not often that treatment can be successfully carried out. Strong black

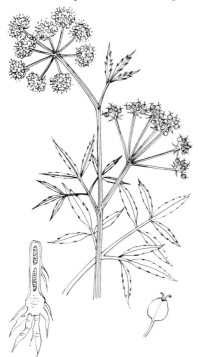

Water Hemlock or Cowbane (*Circuta virosa*), showing the dahlia-like roots attached to the enlarged base of the stem, seed capsule, leaves and greenish-white inflorescence. The flowering stem may be 5 to 10 ft tall.

coffee, tannic acid or gallic acid may be given. Veterinary help should be sought.

WATER, LOSS OF, from the tissues – a serious condition – is referred to under DEHYDRATION. It occurs especially during the course of diarrhoea.

WATERHAMMER PULSE. The peculiarly sudden pulse that is associated with incompetence of the aortic valves of the left side of the heart.

'WATERY MOUTH'. Probably caused by *E. coli*, affecting new-born lambs in Britain. The lambs appear strong and healthy but on taking milk from the ewe they soon show signs of abdominal pain, and a watery fluid drips from the mouth. There may be scouring. Death soon follows as a rule.

Clinical features of 102 cases of watery mouth in lambs are summarised. The majority of cases were observed in ram lambs (73 per cent) and within the first three days of life (80 per cent). The results suggest that the incidence of watery mouth may be reduced by delaying castration until lambs are at least three days old. (Collins, R. D., Eales, F. A. & Small, J., *British Veterinary Journal* (1985) **141**, 135.)

A similar condition occurs in calves due to *E. coli*.

WEALS are raised white areas of the skin which possess reddened margins. They may result from sharp blows or from continued pressure against some hard object. They are only visible upon the skins of pigs, as the hair of the other domestic animals hides the actual skin surface. (*See* URTICARIA.)

The term weal is also used in surgery in connection with the use of local anaesthetic solution. A primary weal is made, and when the local anaesthetic has taken effect, the needle of the syringe may be re-introduced into the now insensitive area and further injections made painlessly in order to anaesthetise a given area.

WEANING is a critical period in the life of the young animal unless carried out with care. Generally speaking, it is necessary to accustom the young growing animal to a diet in which its dam's milk takes a more and more secondary place for some weeks before actual separation occurs. In the case of dairy cattle there is an exception to this rule, in that newly-born calves are often taken away from their mothers as soon as they have had some colostrum, and are then reared from a pail. Sudden changes in the diet are to be avoided at all times, and the changes from a milk to a herbivorous or omnivorous diet should be gradual, for obvious reasons. In modern pig husbandry, creep-feeding is practised before weaning. (*See* CREEP-FEEDING, COLOSTRUM.)

Early weaning of calves. This is an alternative procedure to that of rearing dairy or beef calves on the bucket, using milk substitutes. The principle of early weaning is to provide an acceptable dry food which the calf will eat as early as 4 days of age. The rumen is thereby stimulated to growth and activity, and by the time the calf is 3 weeks old, the rumen is functioning – 2 or 3 weeks earlier than under normal conditions. By 5 weeks, bucket feeding can be dispensed with, and the calf reared on solid food only – together with a liberal supply of water. Kale or silage can be introduced at this period in small amounts.

The advantages of the system are that, from the farmer's point of view, 5 or 7 weeks' bucket-feeding is dispensed with – and that means less labour and adherence to special feeding times. Moreover, it is claimed that the risk of scouring is less, and that the earlier rumen development makes for sturdier calves, able to go on to an adult diet sooner.

On the other hand, early weaning has led in some instances to illness and death as a result of the imperfect functioning of the immature rumen and abomasum. Technically known as gastric dyspepsia, the main symptom is often persistent scouring. After several days' depression and lack of appetite, the calf dies. There may be staggering or fits, but hypomagnesaemia and not dyspepsia may be the cause of these.

Diagnosis is difficult. Lead poisoning and sal-monellosis have to be ruled out.

Early weaning of piglets 10 to 14 days old is now regularly practised on many farms. It obvi-ates the marked loss of condition which befalls sows which suckle their piglets to 8 weeks. Other advantages – from the farmer's point of view – are a quicker turn-round in the farrowing house, and consequently less accommodation needed; and the attainment of more than four litters in two years. Food costs per piglet are higher by this method, but weight at 8 weeks can be appreciably higher. The sow must be taken from the piglets, not *vice versa*, and housed out of earshot, as she will fret. Proprietary mixtures containing Vita-min B_{12} and an antibiotic are on the market.

Early weaning at 7–10 days, and transfer to cages for dry feeding at a temperature of 79–81°F, is a system introduced commercially into Britain in 1971. Except during twice-a-day feeding, the piglets are kept in darkness. On reaching about 15 lb weight when 3 weeks old, they are moved from the three-tier cages which hold 9 piglets, to single-tier ones holding 6, and remain for about 5 weeks (50 lb weight) when they are transferred to normal pens. (*See also under* SOW'S MILK.)

From a veterinary and animal welfare aspect, the darkness would seem highly questionable.

Early weaning of lambs (*see* SHEEP BREEDING).

WEATINGS. The particles finer than bran of the husk of wheat, containing not more than about 6 per cent crude fibre. They are also known as offals and middlings, and much confusion exists between these various terms.

WEAVING is a habit of horses – swinging the head and neck and the anterior parts of the body backwards and forwards, so that the weights rest alternately upon each fore-limb. Sometimes the feet remain upon the ground all the time, but in bad cases each foot is raised as the weight passes over on to the other.

CAUSES. Weaving appears to be most common in the lighter breeds of horses, and especially in those that are stabled for long periods in idleness. Unevenness of the stable floor has been blamed as a cause of weaving; the horse being unable to find a comfortable place for each of his feet, and con-sequently rests first upon one, and then upon the other.

The principal effect is fatigue, and a future ten-dency to stumble when at fast work. Like other bad habits it is likely to be imitated by other young horses in a stable and in some cases has been known to spread to all the horses under the same roof.

Young horses should not be left for long periods without exercise or work; it is better to turn them out to grass. Unevenness in the floor of the stable should be corrected.

Weaving starts as a habit, develops into a vice, and eventually becomes a nervous disease, so that it constitutes a radical unsoundness for which a warranted horse may be returned to the seller.

WEDDER (*see under* SHEEP).

WEDGE OSTEOTOMY. An operation for treating an angular deformity of the horse's fetlock of 8° or more.

WEEDKILLERS used in agriculture include: DNOC, DNP, PARAQUAT, DIQUAT. Hormone weedkillers: MCPA, Agroxone 4, and 2, 4-D. MCPA renders, it is claimed, pasture more pal-atable and has no ill effects upon cattle or their milk. Ragwort and buttercups also become more palatable, due to a temporary increase in their sugar content, and poisoning may consequently arise. (*See also* HERBICIDES.)

WEIGHTS OF CATTLE. At birth, calves of the larger breeds weigh 80 to 120 lb (170 lb has been recorded). The averages for heifer calves are about: British Friesian, 86 lb; Dairy Shorthorn, 80; Jersey, 56. Bull calves weigh about 5 lb more.

WEIGHTS OF HORSES. At birth, a Shire or Clydesdale foal averages 1¾ or 2 cwt.

WEIGHTS OF PIGS. Averages in Britain are as follows: at birth, 2 or 3 lb; at 3 weeks, 12 or 13 lb; at 8 weeks, 36 or 37 lb. (*See also* 'BACON WEIGHT'.)

WEIL'S DISEASE (*see* JAUNDICE, LEPTOSPIRAL OF DOGS).

WELFARE CODES FOR ANIMALS. Codes for cattle (including calves), pigs, domestic fowls, and turkeys were approved by Parliament in 1969, and published in 1970 (*see also under* BRAMBELL).

Regulations came into force on October 1, 1974. The regulations relating to cattle and poultry (1) prohibit tail docking of cattle, surgical castra-tion of poultry, operations on birds (other than feather clipping) to impede flight, and the fitting of blinkers to birds by a method involving mutilation of the nasal septum. Except in the case of blinkering, the performance by a veterinary surgeon of an operation he considers necessary for health reasons is unaffected.

The regulations relating to pigs (2) require that the docking of pigs shall be quick and complete severance of the part of the tail to be removed; and they prohibit the docking of pigs more than seven days old except when performed by a veterinary surgeon on health grounds or to prevent injury from tail-biting. These regulations are supplemented by the order (3), which prohibits the docking without anaesthetic of pigs more than seven days old.

(1) The Welfare of Livestock (Cattle and Poultry) Regulations 1974 (SI 1974 No 1062)
(2) The Welfare of Livestock (Docking of Pigs) Regulations 1974 (SI 1974 No 1061)
(3) The Docking of Pigs (Use of Anaesthetics) Order 1974 (SI 1974 No 798)

(*See also under* FARM ANIMAL WELFARE COUNCIL and LAW, PRODUCTIVITY.)

WELLS, WELL WATER (*see* WATER).

WESSELSBRON DISEASE.
CAUSE: a flavivirus. Transmitted by mosquitoes, and communicable to man, this infection was first reported in South Africa in 1955. It caused death of lambs, abortion, and some deaths of ewes; persistent muscular pain in man. It resembles Rift Valley fever.

WETHER (*see under* SHEEP).

WETTING AGENTS. Substances which lower the surface tension of water, so that the latter spreads out over the surface rather than remaining in the form of drops. Good wetting ability is necessary for detergents, which play such an essential part in the disinfection of vessels, pipes, glassware used for milk, fats, etc.

WHARTON'S DUCT is the name of the tube by which saliva secreted by the submaxillary gland reaches the cavity of the mouth. It opens in the floor of the mouth almost opposite to the canine tooth in the horse.

WHARTON'S JELLY, is the embryonic connective tissue that forms the basis of the umbilical cord in the fetus. In its substance are found the umbilical vessels and the other structures that constitute the umbilical cord.

WHEAT GLUTEN. For the adverse effect of this in some instances in calves, see under SOYABEAN.

WHEEZING (*see* BRONCHITIS *and also* BROKEN WIND).

WHELPING (*see under* PARTURITION, in the bitch).

WHEY can be a source of infection with tuberculosis in the pig. (*See* TUBERCULOSIS.) (*See also* HAEMORRHAGIC GASTRO-ENTERITIS, VOLVULUS.)

WHIPWORM is the popular name for the *Trichuris* found in caecum. (*See* ROUNDWORMS.)

WHISTLING is a defect affecting the respiratory system of the horse. In many respects it is similar to roaring, but the note emitted is higher pitched, It constitutes an unsoundness. (*See also* LARYNX, DISEASES OF, 'Roaring'.)

WHITE CELLS (*see under* BLOOD. For white cells in milk, *see under* MASTITIS).

WHITE DIARRHOEA, BACILLARY (*see under* PULLORUM DISEASE).

'WHITE HEIFER DISEASE'. A condition that is reputed to be most common in white heifers – usually Shorthorns – in which there is a rubberlike sheet of fibrous tissue and membrane stretching across the posterior part of the vagina – a 'persistent hymen'.

White heifer disease is not a very common condition, but when present it may be the cause of sterility by preventing service.
TREATMENT. The genital passage is made patent surgically. Where much débris has accumulated behind the membrane it may be necessary to irrigate the passage, using aseptic instruments and a boiled solution of 2 teaspoonfuls of common salt to the pint of water. For hypoplasia of the uterus nothing can be done. (*See diagram under* INFERTILITY.)

WHITE LINE is the margin of horn that runs round the outside of the sole, between it and the wall, in the horse's hoof. It acts as a slightly pliable cementing material between wall and sole. It is important as a guide to the shoeing smith, since it forms a line inside which it is unsafe to drive a nail without risk of pricking the sensitive parts of the foot.

'WHITE MUSCLE DISEASE' is another name for the result of Vitamin E deficiency. (*See* MUSCLES, DISEASES OF – NUTRITIONAL MUSCULAR DYSTROPHY.)

WHITE SCOUR IN CALVES is a disease affecting calves within the first 3 weeks of life. The disease is usually a rapid one. In the acute case the calf may be found dead or dying; in other cases death occurs in from 3 to 10 days after symptoms are first noticed.
CAUSE is usually *E. coli*, but other organisms may be involved, including *Proteus vulgaris* and *Pseudomonas pyocyanea, Salmonella* species.

Predisposing causes include exposure to cold and damp; deprivation of colostrum; sudden changes in diet; feeding with unsound milk or mouldy calf-meals from unclean utensils; overcrowding; and housing healthy calves in pens or boxes that have previously contained cases of the disease and have not been carefully disinfected afterwards.

White scour is very rare in beef cattle at pasture.

Calving-boxes should be disinfected and well littered before the pregnant cattle occupy them. A

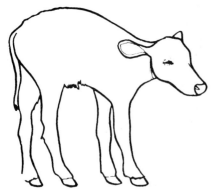

An arched back is characteristic of White Scour, also a dejected appearance.

protective serum has been used with encouraging results. Where bucket-feeding is adopted, colostrum must not be withheld.

TREATMENT. It is essential to overcome the dehydration resulting from the diarrhoea. (For details, *see* DEHYDRATION.)

Other treatment comprises the use of *E. coli* antiserum, sulphamezathine, or one of the other sulpha drugs, and in some cases the inclusion of yeast in the diet. Serum from the dam has been given by subcutaneous injection in default of colostrum. (*See also* DIARRHOEA.)

'WHITES' is another name for leukorrhoea, and is a term popularly used in connection with *C. pyogenes* infection in cows. (*See* LEUKORRHOEA; UTERUS, DISEASES OF; VAGINITIS.)

WHITESIDE TEST. This has been used for the detection of subclinical mastitis, by indicating an abnormally high white-cell count of the milk. A modified version consists in placing 1 drop of 4 per cent caustic soda and 5 drops of the milk on a glass plate, and stirring with a glass rod for 20 seconds or so. The presence of flakes indicates a positive result; a viscous mass at the end of the rod suggests a strong positive result. (For further details of this, the California Mastitis Test, and the Negretti Field Test, see *Veterinary Record* of September 22, 1962.)

WHORLS. These, as well as colour markings, assist in the identification of horses. A whorl is a pattern of hairs, often about an inch across.

WILD BIRDS. For unintended poisoning of these, *see under* GAME BIRDS. See also TEM.

WILD DOGS are an important source of human hydatid infection in New South Wales, where a sylvatic strain of *Echinococcue granulosus* circulates predominantly between them and wallabies. Between May and September 1986 only one of 76 domestic dogs was found to be infected. (Morrison, F. & others. *Australian Veterinary Journal* (1988) **65,** 97.)

WILTING of sugar beet tops is highly desirable before feeding in order to avoid poisoning, and

with a lush crop of grass on a new ley, cutting and allowing to wilt may obviate Bloat.

WINDBORNE INFECTION. Under favourable conditions the virus of foot-and-mouth disease may be carried from country to country, even where a long sea passage is involved. (*See* J. Gloster & others. *Vet. Record* (1982) **110,** 47.) (*See also* AUJESZKY'S DISEASE.)

WINDBREAKS (*see under* EXPOSURE).

WIND GALLS. Distensions of the joint capsules, or of tendon sheaths, in the region of the fetlock. (*See* SYNOVITIS.)

WIND-SUCKING (*see* CRIB-BITING).

WINTER DIET. It is often wise to incorporate 5 per cent of animal protein in the winter rations of dairy cattle, which otherwise may be getting too little protein and give milk low in SNF. Succulent food such as silage or kale forms a high proportion of the winter diet for cattle, which may be receiving too little carbohydrate. On self-fed silage the N I R D have recorded a 33 per cent reduction in dry matter intake compared with a diet of hay and concentrates.

'WINTER INFERTILITY' (*see* INFERTILITY).

WIRE (*see* FOREIGN BODIES IN RETICULUM, under STOMACH, DISEASES OF). Barbed wire is responsible for many small wounds of the cow's udder which predispose to mastitis, and for accidents in the hunting field.

WIRING (*see under* FRACTURES).

'WITCH'S MILK' is an old name for the abnormal secretion, in rare instances, of milk by the newborn of either sex.

'WOBBLER'. The name given to a horse which shows the following symptoms: a slight swaying action of the hindquarters, or stumbling, with worsening of the condition until, after 6 to 9 months, he cannot trot without rolling from side to side and falling. The cause is unknown, but possibly a spinal cord injury gives rise to these symptoms – seen in yearlings and two-year-olds; occasionally three-year-olds.

The **wobbler syndrome in the dog** is referred to under CERVICAL SPONDYLOPATHY, under SPINE, DISEASES OF.

WOMB (*see* UTERUS).

WOOD-ASH, EATING OF, by cattle is suggestive of a diet deficient in salt, calcium or magnesium.

WOOD PIGEONS (*see* TUBERCULOSIS in pigs; *also under* GAME-BIRDS, PIGEONS).

WOOD PRESERVATIVES. Some of these are a source of arsenical poisoning; others, containing chlorinated naphthalene compounds, of hyper-keratosis. Creosote and pentachlorophenol are very liable to cause poisoning in young pigs; and the latter has caused fatal poisoning in cats bedded on sawdust from treated timber. Cats have been killed also by DIELDRIN used for treating floorboards, etc., against woodworm.

WOOD'S LAMP is used in the diagnosis of ringworm; diseased hairs, etc., appearing fluor-escent in the case of *Microsporum canis* infection – but only to the extent of 50 per cent or so. A useful screening method nonetheless. The fluorescence is of an apple-green colour.

WOOL BALLS IN LAMBS. On opening a lamb's stomach after death from some unknown disease, if a mass of wool and greyish or greenish softer material is found in the first or fourth stomach and no other readily obvious symptoms are noticed, the shepherd or owner is very prone to reach the conclusion that the cause of death was this mass of wool. In some districts, so-called 'wool balls' have in the past been held to account for a high mortality among lambs, when the real cause was often lamb dysentery.

There is no doubt, however, that wool balls do occasionally kill in dry seasons or when ewes have for some other reason a reduced flow of milk. The hungry lamb withdraws all the milk available, but when it reaches the age of 2 to 4 weeks or so, this proves insufficient to satisfy its needs. It empties first one teat, then the other, and finally, searching for a further supply it finds a small tag of wool on the udder or near to it and sucks at it. The somewhat salty taste of the con-tained wool grease may possibly be pleasing, and in time the lock of wool comes away and is chewed and swallowed. Another lock is found, sucked, and also swallowed.

The mass of wool may occasionally result in blockage of the outlet from stomach to small intestine (pylorus).
PREVENTION. The removal of shed wool from the pastures, the 'udder-locking' (clipping all wool from the udder before or at lambing).

WOOL-EATING BY CATS may result from boredom (*e.g.* in Siamese) or from persistence of the sucking reflex, and cause an obstruction of pylorus or bowel.

'WOOL SLIP'. Alopecia occurring in housed ewes shorn during the winter, and reducing wool yield by up to 25 per cent.

In order to avoid this alopecia, it was suggested that sheep should be sheared at the same time as they are housed, to reduce the number of periods of stress; and that a better quality diet should be provided after shearing, and that the diet should be introduced before housing. 'Should these con-trol measures fail, and the association between "wool slip" and stress be proven, it may be necessary to cease winter shearing on welfare grounds.' (Morgan, K. L. and others. *Vet. Rec.* (1986) **119**, 621).

WOOL ROT (*see under* LUMPY WOOL).

WORKS CHIMNEYS (*see* FACTORY).

WORM EGG COUNTS. The use of faecal egg counts as a means of estimating the degree of in-festation can be misleading. With *Ostertagia* worms in calves, for example, the pattern of faecal egg counts tends to be the same whether the worm burden is large or small, increasing or de-creasing. Counts increase fairly rapidly to an early peak from which they decrease according to a logarithmic curve. This means that the egg count at any one point in time bears a constant relation to the egg count a given number of days before. The limit to total egg output evidently depends on the host's degree of immunity.

WORMS (*see* ROUNDWORMS, TAPEWORMS, LIVER FLUKES, RUMEN FLUKES, SCHISTOSOMIASIS for 'Blood flukes', HEARTWORMS; *and also* EARTH-WORMS.)

In cattle and sheep, parasitic gastro-enteritis and bronchitis (Husk) are important diseases caused by worms. (*See also* LIVERFLUKES, NEMATO-DIRUS, STEPHANOFILARIASIS, *and below.*)

In horses, strongyle worm larvae may cause a verminous arteritis with fatal results. (*See* HORSES, WORMS IN, EQUINE VERMINOUS ARTERITIS, DIARRHOEA; FOALS, DISEASES OF; HYDATID DISEASE.)

In dogs in Britain the worms usually en-countered comprise: ascarids, hookworms, whip-worms, and tapeworms. (*See also* ANTHELMINTICS, TOXOCARA, TRACHEAL WORMS, HEART-WORM, KID-NEY WORM, FLUKES.)

In pigs Ascaris worms in the intestine reduce growth rate, while their larvae, migrating through the lungs, may give rise to pneumonia and the symptom known as 'thumps'. Meta-strongylus lungworms cause bronchitis and sometimes pneumonia. (*See also* THIN-SOW SYN-DROME *and below.*)

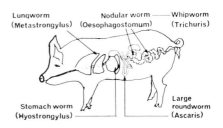

The principal parasitic worms of the pig and their habitat.

WORMS, FARM TREATMENT AGAINST. In recent years great progress has been made in the development of effective and safe drugs to con-trol infestation of farm livestock by parasitic worms. Today the choice is wide and farmers may sometimes have difficulty in deciding which drug to use.

There are anthelmintics which, given by mouth, kill or detach lungworms *in situ*, but also safer antifluke drugs and drugs effective against both flukes and the roundworms causing parasitic gastro-enteritis.

Does one use a dual-purpose drug or a single-purpose one? Does one resort to drenching or choose an anthelmintic which can be given in the feed – or by injection?

What follows is an attempt to offer a useful outline of the wide range of drugs currently available; to suggest certain criteria which might assist in any choice; and to comment on some aspects of worm control – it being understood that good pasture management, and the timing of anti-worm treatment, are as important as the anthelmintics themselves. In fact, they are complementary.

As to criteria, there are certain questions which have to be asked about an anthelmintic. Will the drug in question kill worm eggs? Is it effective against immature worms? Is it effective against adult worms of the economically important species?

Safety considerations are important, too. For example, can the operator use the anthelmintic 05without having to take special precautions against accidental contamination of skin, eyes, or mouth?

Smaller dosage rates. During the last three decades or so, the effective dose of anthelmintics has been steadily falling, owing to the development of more potent drugs.

MSD–AGVET (Merck Sharpe & Dohme) introduced the remarkable new avermectins, and their product Ivomec achieves control in cattle not only of PGE worms but also of lungworms, warble fly larvae, lice and sarcoptic mange mites! Moreover, the dose is exceedingly small, and can be given by an injection 'gun'.

Administration. The method of administering an anthelmintic is worth thinking about. No method is perfect – each having some disadvantage. Drenching can, if not done with care, lead to 'drenching pneumonia', and the necessary retraint may be undesirable with yarded cattle or in-lamb ewes. The smaller dosages now required make drenching less hazardous, but *see* DRENCHING.

Injection usually involves less restraint than drenching, but with any injection there is the slight risk of broken-off needles and an abscess at the site. Neither of these disadvantages applies to anthelmintics which can be given in the feed – a most convenient method which normally should not involve extra cost.

Pfizer's pioneered the anthelmintic use of a slow-release bolus, administered by means of a simple balling gun. The bolus lasts inside the reticulum/rumen 'for at least 90 days', it is claimed, so that with suitable grazing management a whole season's control of PGE worms in cattle can be achieved by a single dose, given at turnout to cattle weighing over 100 kg. The potential saving in labour costs through not having to dose more than once is a big advantage claimed by Pfizer.

Husk – drugs or vaccine? Parasitic bronchitis or verminous pneumonia (known coloquially as husk or hoose) is mainly thought of as a disease of ngyoungstockintheirfirstseasonatgrass.Recovery from an attack can be expected to result in a useful degree of immunity to the lungworm.

While the disease is a virtually permanent problem on many farms, and a risk on most others except where zero-grazing is practised, some farms do escape it altogether – at any rate for a time; but then one day it may suddenly appear out of the blue with devastating results. When this happens it may be cows in milk which suffer; losses to the farmer arising mainly as a result of a lowered milk yield but also of the extra feed needed for recuperation. There may be deaths, too, following symptoms common to those of an allergic condition. Indeed one shocked farmer, in his first encounter with husk, lost several dairy cows from oedema of the lungs – and his bull as well!

Especially on farms where the disease is a perennial problem, the farmer's own veterinary surgeon should be consulted concerning the use of Dictol vaccine as a preventative.

This vaccine consists of third-stage larvae of the lungworm, *Dictyocaulus viviparus*, exposed to a specified level of radiation by X-rays. This, the first anti-worm vaccine commercially available, was developed by veterinary research workers at the University of Glasgow.

The irradiated larvae are left with the ability to stimulate antibody production in the host animal, but are deprived of their power to cause disease. The vaccine is administered in two doses (each containing 1000 irradiated larvae) with a four week interval.

Certain precautions are necessary in using this vaccine. For example, calves should not be less than 2 months old when vaccinated and should be healthy. They should not be exposed to natural infestation with lungworms until 2 weeks after their second dose; and should be introduced gradually to heavily infested pasture. Vaccinated and non-vaccinated calves should not be mixed.

Where the vaccine is not used, reliance must be placed on anthelmintics. It will be readily appreciated, however, that once severe symptoms of husk have appeared, the most that any drug can do is to rid the animal of its lungworms. A drug cannot undo the lung damage, clear the blocked airways, or neutralise any subsequent infection; and the coughing will persist after the worms are gone. Vaccine can prevent such a situation arising. Drugs, however, are a valuable means of lung-worm control.

Liver-flukes. Years ago the problem with drugs intended to kill liver-flukes was their toxicity. The margin between an effective medicinal dose and a lethal dose was sometimes very small especially in an already seriously ill sheep.

The introduction of safer drugs still left the problem of resistance to them shown by immature flukes which, by their massive invasion of the liver, cause 'liver rot' and a high mortality in affected flocks. Later, however, came the introduction of diamphenethide, claimed to be effective against liver-flukes 3 days old and upwards; and the active ingredient of Coriban.

For routine dosing of sheep and cattle there is the less expensive drug rafoxanide, the active ingredient of Flukanide. This is active against liver-flukes younger than 4 weeks, and is claimed to remove over 99 per cent of adult flukes and up to 98 per cent of 6-week-old (immature) flukes.

Another drug with specific action on liver flukes is oxyclozanide, the active ingredient of Zanil, with which animals even in poor condition or those nearing calving or lambing or in milk, may be safely dosed according to the manufacturers' recommendations. It can be given as a drench or in the feed.

Dual-purpose and multi-purpose anthelmintics are available.

In 1983 ICI introduced 'Nilvax' for sheep. Given by injection as a single treatment it combined the properties of levamisole against intestinal and lungworms, with a multi-component vaccine against 8 clostridial diseases of sheep. Drugs in use during 1986 included the following:

against PGE worms in cattle and sheep	against liver flukes in cattle and sheep
levamisole	oxyclonazide
oxfendazole	rafoxanide
fenbendazole	nitroxynil
albendazole	
morantel tartrate*	

against lungworms in cattle and sheep	against worms in pigs†
fenbendazole	dichlorvos
oxfendazole	parbendazole
levamisole	thiophanate
febantel	levamisole
	thiabendazole

* a bolus, given by balling gun, for cattle only
  (see also ivermectin, for use against PGE worms
  and lungworms, in cattle and sheep; and against
  parasites of pigs)
† given in the feed

(PGE is used here as an abbreviation for parasitic gastro-enteritis.)

PARASITIC GASTRO-ENTERITIS. Advice from the Ministry's Central Veterinary Laboratory, Weybridge, is to the effect that calves should be dosed once with an efficient anthelmintic in mid-July and moved to pasture which has not been grazed that season by other cattle. Second-year cattle or sheep can then be grazed on the first pasture.

The second essential dose is in the autumn when cattle come in from grass. Limited ICI trails suggest that dosing 14 days after housing, rather than at housing, is preferable. (Intermediate dosing may be necessary on heavily infested pastures or where there is ill-health resulting from a particular species of worm.)

A 2-year study at Glasgow University, involving 39 calves, showed, stated Dr J. Parkin, that beef animals efficiently protected against gastrointestinal parasites gained almost 1 cwt extra liveweight – without the aid of growth promoters – compared with calves treated conventionally. Moreover better grading and leaner meat was achieved. The anthelmintic used was morantel tartrate in 'Paratect' CPfizer) slow-release boluses. (Control group 1 received no anthelmintic until symptoms appeared; control group 2 received fenbendazole every two weeks.) (Parkin, J., *Veterinary Times* (1985) November issue.)

Ostertagia worms, which are of considerable economic importance, are peculiar in that while most infective larvae living in the abomasum moult twice to become adults, some – especially perhaps those ingested by the calf during late summer and autumn – moult only once and remain as fourth-stage larvae in a dormant state. The larvae are resistant to many anthelmintics, but fenbendazole and albendazole are often effective. Later, they develop into adults causing a winter outbreak of gastro-enteritis, with scouring and other digestive disturbance. Accordingly, it is usually recommended that calves be dosed in September and moved to 'clean' land.

Ivomec is effective against immature and even inhibited Ostertagia larvae; and can be given to both beef and dairy cattle but not within 21 days of slaughter, or to dairy cows in milk or within 28 days prior to calving. Three doses a year – in spring, summer, and autumn – are recommended to make the best use of this multi-purpose anthelmintic.

Ivermectin ('Ivomec' being the brand name) has no action against flukes or tapeworms, but is highly effective against all the important roundworms, both adults and larval forms.

NEMATODIRUS IN LAMBS. Lambs 4–6 weeks old and upwards may become severely ill as a result of infestation with *Nematodirus* worms. A well recognised condition, it may show itself with dramatic suddenness in lowland flocks in spring, but – depending on locality and weather – the main period of incidence is probably the end of May until the second week in July.

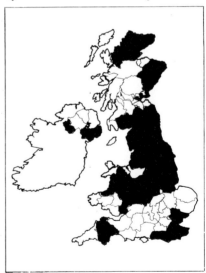

Areas where *Nematodirus* may be a problem. (With acknowledgements to ICI.)

The worms, each about 2/3 in long cause unthriftiness and poor liveweight gains; they may also cause a high mortality following 4 to 5 days' scouring which result in a lethal loss of body fluids, *i.e.* dehydration. Where recovery does take place, it is usually long drawn out and the animal may remain stunted.

These worms differ from others infesting the

stomach/intestine of sheep in Britain in that their life-cycle takes about 12 months to complete. This fortunate fact offers an obvious method of control – the well-known rule 'Never put lambs on the same pasture two years running.' On farms where it is impracticable to observe this rule, dosing three or four times with an appropriate anthelmintic is advisable. (*See also* 'CLEAN PASTURE'.)

WORMS IN PIGS. Anthelmintics, complemented by good hygiene, play an essential part in maintaining health in the intensively managed pig unit. Infestation by parasitic worms is best regarded as a herd problem, and the fact that anthelmintics are available in a palatable pellet form, or as a powder to mix in a meal, is a great help to the pig farmer. These are usually broad-spectrum drugs which will act against most of the species of worm normally found in the pig. Where a particular species has led to a severe health problem, an anthelmintic most effective against that species can be selected. For example, thiabendazole is particularly effective against Hyostrongylus, the stomach worm; diethyl-carbamazine against Metastrongylus, and dichlorvos against Ascaris; *and see* IVERMECTIN.

Steering a middle course. The farmer should, where necessary, seek veterinary advice on the spot, and aim to steer a middle course between inconveniently frequent dosing and high drug bills on the one hand, and tolerating poor live-weight gains, unthriftiness and even several deaths among his stock on the other hand. Internal parasites steal feed intended for their hosts, and often cause physical injury – sometimes very severe – as well.

WOUNDS. A wound may be defined as a breach of the continuity of the tissues of the body produced by violence. (*See also under* BRUISES.)

Varieties. Wounds may be classified according to the nature of the effect produced, viz. *incised, punctured, lacerated,* and *contused.*

Incised wounds are usually inflicted by some sharp instrument which leaves a clean cut; the tissues are simply divided without extensive damage to the surrounding parts. Bleeding from an incised wound is apt to be very profuse for a time, but it soon stops and is easily controlled.

Punctured wounds or stabs are inflicted with a pointed instrument or another animal's incisor or canine teeth. (A dose of tetanus antitoxin or toxoid is indicated in punctured wounds, especially in the horse, cow, and dog.)

Lacerated wounds are those in which great tearing takes place. They are usually very painful for a few days, and suppurate before they heal. They are usually followed by disfiguring scars when extensive.

Contused wounds are those accompanied by much bruising of the surrounding tissues, as in the case of blows from heavy sticks, kicks from shod horses, and from road accidents. There is usually little bleeding from the wound itself, but blood may be extravasated into the tissues (*see* HAEMATOMA).

Any one of these forms of wounds may become infected with pus-forming organisms, and develop into a suppurating, *septic wound.* (For other information *see under* ACCIDENTS, INJURIES; etc.)

First-aid treatment. With a serious wound involving much haemorrhage, the first consideration must obviously be to stop the bleeding. (*See* BLEEDING, ARREST OF.)

With all wounds it is advisable to clip away the hair – using preferably blunt-pointed surgical scissors; first inserting a piece of cotton-wool moistened in antiseptic into the cavity of the wound (if large enough), so that the cut hair does not fall into the wound.

If the hair is not cut away, it is apt to become matted by blood or oozing serum, and the wound may later be found to be suppurating instead of healing. (What may look to the animal-owner like a normal healthy scab may be, in fact, a crust of blood, matted hair and dirt.)

The surface of the wound may be cleaned by gentle application of a piece of cotton wool soaked in warm antiseptic such as diluted Dettol, Cetrimide, T C P, etc.

The wound may be covered in order to prevent contamination and infection by flies – in the case of farmyard animals – or to prevent excessive licking by dogs and cats. Before covering, a dry antiseptic dressing of sulphanilamide may be applied.

The covering of a wound cleaned and dressed as described, should be removed daily so that the progress of healing can be observed, and cleaning repeated if necessary. An open, granulating wound should have a clean, pink appearance.

Large, gaping wounds may require suturing, which should be done by a veterinary surgeon, who should also always be consulted concerning the treatment of punctured and lacerated wounds, and will prescribe an antibiotic.

The healing of wounds may be delayed by cortisone, and influenced by insulin. Vitamin A is used to promote or hasten healing of wounds.

Other points that should be noted are: (1) that stitches should be removed if they commence to suppurate, and in any case after being in position for a week, after which they serve no useful purpose; (2) that if pus burrows under the skin surrounding a wound it must be given drainage by incision below the level of the most dependent burrowing or by drainage tubes; (3) that if the granulation tissue (*i.e.* 'proud flesh') rises to a higher level than the skin around, it may need professional treatment; and (4) that in cases of injury to special parts, such as the eyes, nostrils, lips, genital organs, feet, etc., it is essential to seek skilled advice rather than to persist in rule-of-thumb methods which often lead the enthusiastic amateur astray, and cause the animal unnecessary distress. (*See also* BLEEDING, ARREST OF; FRACTURES; GRANULATION TISSUE; ULCER; *and* ANTISEPTICS; ANTIBIOTICS; SULPHONAMIDES; *and also under* ACCIDENTS, INJURIES, *and* CORTISONE.)

Professional treatment. Noxythiolin (oxymethylene methylthiourea) was recommended by Dr E. L. Gerring, Royal Veterinary College, for its effectiveness against antibiotic resistant strains of organisms including *Pseudomonas pyocyanea.*

Sometimes pieces of tissue need to be removed; e.g. for the treatment of a malignant growth, a wound, chronic infection, sinus formation, etc.

Marles mesh can be used. It is biologically inert, resistant to infection, and granulation tissue and capillaries will grow through it, and aid the building of a strong layer of connective tissue in 4 to 6 weeks. (Fox, S. M. & others. *Compendium of Continuing Education* (1988) **10,** 897).

Ultrasound. In human medicine, ultrasound has been shown to be beneficial for wound healing, both in the treatment of pressure sores and in the preparation of trophic ulcers for skin grafting. Studies have shown that it influences the activity of fibroblasts. (Callam, M. J. and others. *Lancet* (1987) **87, 204.)**

(*See also* SEROSAL.)

WOUNDS, HOW THEY HEAL. The blood clots. (*See* CLOTTING.) The clot consists of minute threads of fibrin, in which are enmeshed red blood cells and white blood cells. The threads of fibrin bridge the gap between the cut surfaces of the wound, at its base, forming a scaffolding, and harden into a scab under which tissue repair can take place.

From the neighbouring blood capillaries come white cells (especially neutrophils) which engulf dirt, bacteria, etc. (*See* PHAGOCYTOSIS.) Monocytes arrive later, especially if the wound has become infected. They become macrophages which remove any disintegrated neutrophils and also bacteria. Meanwhile, the cells of the epidermis begin to multiply in order to restore the skin covering. (*See* LYMPHOCYTES.)

Healing of wounds may be delayed if the animal is being treated with corticosteroids.

WRY-NECK (Torticollis), which occurs in foals particularly, is a lateral deviation of the head and neck to the right or left side of the body, usually so marked as to hinder or prevent foaling. The bones of the skull and neck are frequently distorted, and the ligaments, tendons, and muscles on the inside of the curve are shorter than those on the outside.

The condition may also be met with in cattle.

X

X-RAYS are capable of passing through considerable thicknesses of many substances which are opaque to ordinary light without undergoing material absorption, but other substances, even in very small thicknesses, are able to absorb the great majority of the rays: thus, flesh, is very transparent; healthy bone is fairly opaque.

Precautions. Guard screens of lead glass, rubber impregnated with lead, or sheet lead, are used to protect the operators of radiographic apparatus, and precautions are necessary to shield the testes and ovaries of young persons and animals from the sterilising effects of the rays.

Detailed precautions are as follows: 1. Persons under 16 years must not take part in radiological procedures. 2. Fluoroscopy or radiotherapy should not be carried out except under expert radiological guidance. Hand-held fluoroscopes must not be used in any circumstances. 3. Personnel radiation monitoring devices, such as film badges, must be worn by all persons who take part routinely in radiological procedures. 4. The animal should, if possible, be anaesthetised or tranquillised for radiography, and all persons should withdraw as far as practicable from the useful beam. 5. If it should be necessary to hold the animal for radiography, lead-protective gloves and aprons must be worn. Whenever possible, holding should be done by the owners, unless they are under 16 years or pregnant. 6. Persons should not expose any part of their bodies to the useful beam even when wearing protective clothing. 7. The useful beam should be restricted to the area being examined by means of a beam limiting device.

Notes on protection against radiation will also be found in the British Veterinary Association's guide to the Health & Safety at Work Act.

Regulations. In the UK the Ionising Regulations 1985 came into force at the beginning of 1986, and require veterinary surgeons using X-ray equipment to notify their local Health & Safety Executive. Many veterinary practices will have to employ a radiation protection adviser.

Uses. The chief use of X-rays is for diagnostic purposes. They are, as yet, mainly applicable to the smaller carnivora and to the limbs and heads of the larger animals, for, owing to the large mass of tissue in the trunks of these latter, an apparatus capable of producing rays powerful enough to penetrate is extremely costly.

EMI-Scanner. This British invention which has revolutionised radiography in human medicine, has also been found of great value in veterinary medicine. Godfrey Hounsfield F R S, the inventor, replaced X-ray film with crystal detectors, and arranged for these and the source of the X-ray beam to rotate through 180° at 10° intervals, providing 300,000 readings in 20 seconds. A mini-computer then selects from these readings and, in a further 20 seconds, puts a picture of a diseased bone, for example, or a tumour, on a television screen. The technique not only avoids pictures with one organ appearing superimposed on another, but can give an end-on view of a horse's trunk or limb. Foot and neck lesions can also be clearly viewed. Unfortunately the Scanner costs between a third and a half million pounds, so that it is financially out of reach even for veterinary faculties at universities.

Ordinary radiography. The production of a radiograph of the internal structure of a small animal is a comparatively simple matter once the difficulty of control is overcome. The animal is arranged upon the table in such a position as will allow the rays to pass down through the part and become registered upon a sensitive plate placed flat upon the table immediately below. The animal may lie upon its back, on one or the other side, or on its chest and abdomen with the legs pulled out from under it. To maintain this position it is always advisable to administer an anaesthetic, *e.g.* nembutal. The discharge tube is best arranged immediately above the animal in such a position as will allow the rays to fall perpendicularly down through the body on to the plate. (For screening, the tube must be below the table, and the screen held or supported above the animal.) The period of exposure to the passage of the rays varies according to the tissues, according to the softness or hardness of the tube, to the distance of the tube from the plate, and to whether or not an intensifying screen is used.

There are many conditions in which the actual extent of injury or disease can be accurately discovered *only* by the use of X-rays, but the most important are diseases and injuries of bones. Fractures of the limb bones are well shown, and their extent is better realised than is possible by palpation. Exostoses (overgrowths of bone) can also be clearly indicated, while tumour formation (usually sarcomatous) shows as a thinning and enlargement of the bone tissue. Where only one limb is affected it is advisable to arrange the animal so as to include a picture of the normal limb for comparison. Foreign bodies – especially needles, pins, nails, and other metallic substances – which have been swallowed are best shown by a profile view of the abdomen. Pieces of game bones (which are specially dense and show up well) can also be seen in the stomach or intestines, and are very often surrounded by gas, which, in the negative, appears as a dark shadow, the bone itself appearing light. Internal tumours can very often be diagnosed. They appear as more or less discrete pale areas in positions where a radiograph from a normal animal is denser under the same conditions of exposure, etc. A method has been devised whereby certain tumours can be made to show up well by giving the animal medicinal doses of a lead salt for a few days

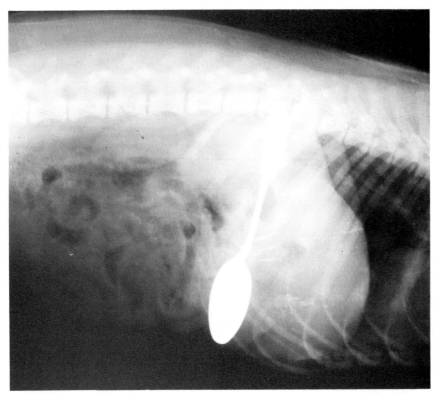

A teaspoon in the stomach of a Cocker Spaniel. The spoon was swallowed while the animal was being given cod-liver oil. (Reproduced by courtesy of Mr S. W. Douglas, University of Cambridge School of Veterinary Medicine.)

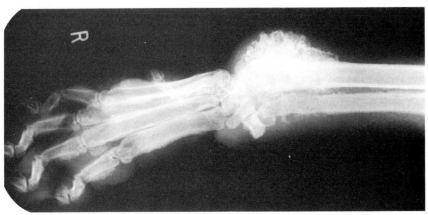

Radiography reveals that a painful swelling on the leg of a St Bernard is due to an osteosarcoma (see CANCER) involving the radius. (Reproduced by courtesy of Mr S. W. Douglas, University of Cambridge School of Veterinary Medicine.)

before taking the plate. Some of the lead becomes deposited in the tumour and intensifies the contrast. Where some displacement, stricture, or dilatation of the stomach or of part of the intestinal canal is suspected, the animal is given a feed or a draught containing an emulsion of bismuth or barium carbonate, or some other harmless metallic salt, or has some of the same material injected into the rectum. After waiting until the salt has become suitably distributed, a radiograph of the abdomen is taken, and the outlines of those organs to which the salt has been carried by peristalsis, can be made out as pale areas in the negatives.

Other conditions in which X-rays are useful are as follows: stones in the kidney, urinary or gallbladder; dilatation of the heart; solidification of a portion of a lung; pleurisy.

X-ray therapy has been applied to a limited extent in the treatment of certain tumours in the dog. The necessary apparatus is cumbersome and extremely costly.

XANTHOSIS is a yellowish brown pigmentation of meat, generally affecting the heart and the tongue. It gives the meat an objectionable colour, but is quite harmless.

XEROPHTHALMIA. A disease of the eye associated with a vitamin A deficiency. Blindness may be produced.

XYLAZINE. The active ingredient of 'Rompun'*, a sedative used to render farm livestock easier to handle. It is also a muscle relaxant and analgesic. For surgical operations, an anaesthetic is needed in addition.

Xylazine increases blood glucose levels and urine output. Side effects may include bradycardia, slower breathing, and lowered blood pressure. In cattle Tolazoline has been used as a xylazine antagonist.

*(Bayer.)

Y

YARDED CATTLE. Before yarding cattle in the autumn, it is wise to make a gradual change from sugar-poor autumn pasture to things like roots. Otherwise digestive upsets are very likely to occur.

Similarly, in spring it is a mistake to turn calves straight out on to grass. This means a sudden change from protein-poor food to the rich protein of the early bite, and the resulting effect upon the rumen will set them back. It is best to get them out before there is much grass for a few hours each day; let them have hay and shelter at night to protect them from sudden changes of weather. Hypomagnesaemia, too, is far less likely under these circumstances. (*See also* HOUSING OF ANIMALS.)

Boss cows can be a nuisance in yards, but the provision of yokes for feeding overcomes the main difficulty.

When self-feeding of silage is practised, precautions are necessary in order to prevent foot-troubles. (*See* SILAGE.)

Yarded animals fed on cereals, sugarbeet pulp, straw, and hay – but with little or no greenstuff – may go blind as a result of a vitamin A deficiency.

YAWNING is an important sign of KIMBERLEY HORSE DISEASE (which see); and may also be seen in cases of LABURNUM POISONING, and NARCOLEPSY.

YEAST is a valuable source of Vitamin B, but should not be fed in excessive amounts to pigs or it may give rise to rickets unless adequate Vitamin D is simultaneously available. Yeast has proved successful in the treatment of tropical ulcers in humans, and success has been reported in a limited number of cases in horses in the tropics. The human patients were mostly those whose diet was deficient in Vitamin B, a deficiency further increased by sweating. The yeast was applied directly to the ulcer, and a small quantity given internally also.

YEASTS sometimes cause enteritis, and are important in some cases of refractory otitis in the dog (*see* FUNGAL INFECTIONS.)

'YELLOW FAT DISEASE' OF CATS (*see* STEATITIS).

YELLOW FEVER. A virus disease affecting man and other vertebrates, principally monkeys, in large areas of tropical America and Africa. There are two known cycles of transmission, the urban and jungle cycles. In the urban cycle, man is the reservoir and *Aedes aegypti* probably the only vector. This cycle from man to *Aedes aegypti* to man is now virtually unknown in the Americas owing to efforts to eradicate the vector, but it is still common in Africa.

The jungle cycle, which was not discovered until the 1930s, has a primate reservoir maintained by various mosquitoes. Movement of virus from the monkey-mosquito-monkey cycle into man is accidental, and is the result of human penetration into jungle where the disease is endemic. (*World Health Organisation.*)

The causative organism is classified as a flavivirus.

YELT. A female pig intended for breeding, up to the time that she has her first litter.

YERSINIOSIS. Infection with *Yersinia pseudotuberculosis* or with *Y. enterocolitica.*

Up to 1960, states WHO, only the former organism was regularly isolated in man and animals in Europe; but since then most of the isolations have been of *Y. enterolitica.*

'Pseudotuberculosis' is still (1991) occasionally found in rodents and birds, especially in France and the UK, and is a zoonosis. People may become infected through pets such as guinea pigs, hamsters, and cats; all of which may have a subclinical infection only but excrete *Y. pseudotuberculosis.*

An investigation in Invermay, New Zealand, resulted in *Yersinia pseudotuberculosis* being isolated from 675 apparently healthy small mammals and birds. In descending order of prevalence were feral cats (27·8 per cent), Norway rats (8·6 per cent), mice, hares, rabbits, ducks, sparrows, seagulls and starlings. (Mackintosh, C. G. & Henderson, T. *New Zealand Veterinary Journal* (1984).)

In New Zealand yersiniosis has also emerged as a serious disease of farmed red deer. It appears to be triggered off by stress, and most cases occur during the winter.

Cats (which are liable to become infected by their prey) may also show clinical symptoms: loss of appetite, vomiting and diarrhoea. Loss of weight.

Pheasants. Yersiniosis is an important cause of death of these birds in the UK.

Yersinia enterocolitica infection in Europe was first found in hares, in outbreaks of disease on chinchilla farms, in monkeys in zoos, and in guinea pigs. There may be enteritis and other lesions, but symptomless carriers have been found among all the farmyard mammals and birds.

Occasionally *Y. enterocolitica* has been isolated from cases of mastitis in cows, endocarditis in bulls, and septicaemia in pigs.

Camels, foxes, and fleas may also carry the organism.

Public health. *Y. enterocolitica* infection is not regarded as a genuine zoonosis by WHO. Person-to-person infection occurs, and also infection from soil-contaminated vegetables. The human illness is characterised by enteritis, and as a cause of diarrhoea *Y. enterocolitica* is in Malmo,

Sweden, placed third after *Salmonella* and *Campylobacter*. Ileitis may be accompanied by acute pain, suggestive of appendicitis. A mesenteric adenitis is also seen, and sometimes polyarthritis, deep abscesses, eye lesions, and occasionally septicaemia.

In the UK in 1984 250 cases were reported. Outbreaks in North America have been linked to raw milk. (For *Y. pestis* see BUBONIC PLAGUE which can occur in cats and dogs in subclinical form.)

YEW POISONING. All varieties of the British yew trees are poisonous, but owing to its more frequent cultivation, the common yew (*Taxus baccata*) is most often responsible for outbreaks of poisoning among animals. The Irish yew (*Taxus baccata*, var. *fastigiata*) and the Yellow yew appear to contain less of the poisonous alkaloid, which is called *Taxine*. The bark, leaves, and seeds all contain it. The older dark leaves are more dangerous than the fresh green young shoots, which cattle have been known to eat in small amounts without harm. Cases of poisoning have been noted among horses, donkeys, mules, cattle, sheep, goats, pigs, deer, rabbits, and even pheasants, but the majority of cases occur in young store cattle and in dairy cows which have access to the shrubberies, graveyards, etc., where yew trees are most common.

SIGNS. In many cases cattle drop dead without showing any preliminary symptoms at all. They may fall while cudding almost as suddenly as if shot. In other cases where less has been eaten, excitement and paresis may be seen.

TREATMENT. Antidotes: as for alkaloids. If time allows, rumenotomy may be carried out.

YOLK SAC INFECTION (*see* OMPHALITIS).

YORKSHIRE BOARDING. Vertically arranged boards with a gap between each, used for partial cladding of a livestock building. It is a very useful means of improving ventilation and avoiding condensation; thereby reducing the risk or incidence of bronchitis and pneumonia.

Z

ZEARALENONE (F₂). A toxin from the fungus *Fusarium graminearum* of standing corn. The toxin has caused abortion in sows, and possibly a splayleg condition in piglets. (*Vet. Rec.* (1975) **97**, 279.)

ZEBU. *Bos indicus*, the cattle of India, E. and W. Africa, and S.E. Asia. The American name is Brahman; in South Africa, the Afrikaner.

ZERO GRAZING. Taking cut fodder to yarded cattle, or to cattle in exercise paddocks. Zero grazing has a place on heavy land, with high stocking rates, and large herds. It obviates poaching and the spoiling of grass, and a given acreage zero-grazed can provide more grass than if grazed. It means, however, cutting grass every day, and mechanical failures can upset the system. It is not yet considered economic for sheep.

ZINC is a trace element, and a deficiency has occurred in pigs. (*See* PARAKERATOSIS.) A zinc supplement to prevent or correct this condition must be used with care, as 1000 parts per million can cause poisoning. It seems that a high calcium intake by pigs aggravates a zinc deficiency.

A zinc deficiency may also occur in dogs, especially in those fed largely on flaked maize or 'loose cereal-based diets'. Signs include a predisposition to skin infections, a poor coat, localised alopecia, and hardening of the skin in places. Response to a zinc supplement is usually quick. (*See* SHEEPDOGS.)

A zinc supplement has been used to protect sheep against facial eczema due to ingestion of the mycotoxin sporidesmin. (Murray, R. & Manns, E. *New Zealand Veterinary Journal* (1989) **37**, 65.)

External uses. Zinc oxide is an ingredient of ointments; the carbonate an ingredient of Calamine Lotion used for moist eczema, etc. The sulphate in weak solution has been used in wound treatment and in eye lotions; the chloride – a caustic – to repress granulations.

ZINC BACITRACIN. Official clearance has been given for the use of zinc bacitracin without veterinary prescription as a 'feed' antibiotic, following the Government's acceptance of the Swann Committee report. Zinc bacitracin may now be included in feeds for growing pigs and poultry at approved levels of up to 125 g/ton.

In 1971 the permitted use of zinc bacitracin was extended to growth promotion in lambs and calves up to six months of age, up to 125 g/ton. (*See* ADDITIVES.)

ZINC POISONING. Chronic zinc poisoning has been reported in a dairy herd as a result of contaminated drinking water – caused by inter-action between copper pipes and newly galvanised tanks. The main symptom was chronic constipation throughout the herd, and a diminished yield from the cows in milk. (*See* above.)

Fatal zinc poisoning has occurred in dairy cattle fed on dairy nuts to which zinc oxide has been added instead of magnesium oxide. The first death occurred after 3 weeks.

Zinc-responsive skin disease. The most common cause of this is the feeding of soya or cereal-based diets; with little or no meat, which is rich in zinc. Some dogs may have an inherent defect which limits zinc absorption.
SIGNS: a dull, harsh coat; sometimes with whitish crusts on the skin. (Thoday, K. L. *J. of Small Animal Practice* (1989) **30**, 213.)

ZONDEK-ASCHEIM TEST (*see* PREGNANCY DIAGNOSIS TESTS).

ZOO LICENSING ACT 1981 is intended to promote animal welfare and public safety at zoos. It covers any collection of wild animals (including mammals, birds, reptiles, fish, and insects) in Great Britain to which the public has access for more than 7 days in any 12-month period; but exempts pet shops and circuses, as these are covered by the Pet Animals Act 1951 and the Performing Animals (Registration) Act 1952.

ZOONOSES. Diseases communicable between animals and man. Information about them will be found under the following headings; ARIZONA infection, BABESIOSIS (*e.g.* from cattle), ANTHRAX, B VIRUS (from monkeys), BRUCELLOSIS, CAT SCRATCH FEVER, CHAGAS' DISEASE, EQUINE ENCEPHALOMYELITIS, EQUINE INFECTIOUS ANAEMIA, FOOT-AND-MOUTH DISEASE (very rare in human beings), GLANDERS, HYDATID, LEPTOSPIROSIS, LISTERIOSIS, LIVER-FLUKES, LOUPING ILL, LYMPHOCYTIC CHORIOMENGITIS (from mice), NEWCASTLE DISEASE, ORNITHOSIS, ORF, PASTEURELLOSIS, Q FEVER, RABIES, RAT-BITE FEVER, RIFT VALLEY FEVER, RINGWORM, ROCKY MOUNTAIN FEVER, RUSSIAN SPRING-SUMMER VIRUS, SALMONELLOSIS, SCABIES, SCHISTOSOMIASIS, TAPEWORMS, TICK-BITE FEVER, TICK PARALYSIS, TOXOCARA, TOXOPLASMOSIS, TRICHINOSIS, TUBERCULOSIS, TULARAEMIA, VESICULAR STOMATITIS, MARBURG DISEASE, WESSELBRON DISEASE, YERSINIOSIS, YELLOW FEVER, SWINE VESICULAR DISEASE, PORCINE STREPTOCOCCAL MENINGITIS, ROTAVIRUS, LASSA FEVER, RIFT VALLEY FEVER, BOVINE ENCEPHALOMYELITIS, LEISHMANIASIS, BUBONIC PLAGUE, ENCEPHALOMYOCARDITIS.)

It should be added that typhus and plague may be transmitted, by flea-bite, from rats; and, in jungle areas, yellow fever, by mosquito-bite, from monkeys. (*See also under* RODENTS, MONKEYS, INFLUENZA.)

Among skin diseases, the parasite of follicular mange may occasionally infest the human eyelid. Among eye infections, INFECTIOUS BOVINE

KERATOCONJUNCTIVITIS should be mentioned. Human enteritis has followed contact with sheep affected with Campylobacter abortion.

(*See also* BIRD-FANCIER'S LUNG, MELIOIDOSIS, CAMPYLOBACTER IN DOGS, CHLAMYDIA (for PSIT-TACOSIS *and* ENZOOTIC ABORTION), BOUTONNEUSE FEVER, LEISHMANIASIS (for HANTAAN VIRUS, TICK-BORNE ENCEPHALITIS, LYME DISEASE, EHRLICHIA.)

ZOONOSES IN UK VETERINARIANS. A questionnaire was distributed to 1717 members of veterinary and support staff of the Ministry of Agriculture and the Institute for Research on Animal Diseases; 1625 (95 per cent) responded comprising 563 veterinary surgeons, 690 scientific staff and 372 technical support staff. A total of 1057 (61·5 per cent) had apparently not suffered any zoonotic infection. Animal ringworm was the commonest reported zoonosis. The incidences of ringworm, brucellosis and Newcastle disease were higher in the veterinary and support staff than in the laboratory workers. In contrast ornithosis, salmonellosis and Q fever occurred at least as often in the laboratory staff. Fourteen people developed tuberculosis during their employment although only one was caused by *Mycobacterium bovis*. The veterinarians reported 441 injuries that resulted from accidents at work; 397 (71 per cent) of these involved animal handling. The comparable figures for laboratory workers and technical staff were 329 and 103 (15 per cent) and 198 and 179 (42 per cent) respectively. Constable, P. J. & Harrington, J. M., *British Medical Journal* (1982) **284**, 246.

ZOONOSES ORDER 1975. A UK measure intended to help reduce the risk of salmonella infections in mammals and birds being transmitted to human beings. The Order also covers brucellosis.

The reserve powers conferred by this Order will probably seldom be used, but they do overcome the absurd situation previously prevailing where, if salmonellosis was rampant on a farm and nothing was being done to control it, neither veterinary nor medical authorities could go on to that farm if the owner/tenant refused consent. A serious outbreak of food-poisoning in people could then be unpreventable; now salmonellosis can be tackled at source, in time.

ZOOTECHNY. Animal management.

ZYGOMA is the bridge of bone which runs from near the base of the ear to the lower posterior part of the eye-socket. It protects the side of the bony orbit, forms part of the support of the outside of the joint of the lower jaw with the rest of the head, and serves as a base of attachment for part of the strong masseter muscle which closes the mouth and is important in the chewing of the food. The zygomatic arch (another name for the zygoma) is formed by projections from the temporal, zygomatic, and maxillary bones.

ZYGOTE. The body that results from the fertilisation of an egg cell by a sperm.

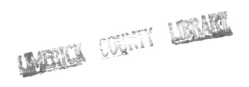

APPENDIX

ACTINOBACILLUS SEMINIS. This was discovered, in a sheep, in Australia. The infection, sometimes subclinical, has since been recognised in several countries including the UK, and causes polyarthritis. (Heath, P. J. & others. *Veterinary Record* (1991) **129**, 304.)

AEROSOL.
AEROSOLS AS A MODE OF INFECTION. Salmonella infection of veterinary surgeons through aerosols has occurred during uterine irrigation and embryotomies in cows.

'BLUE-EAR' DISEASE OF PIGS. The Central Veterinary Laboratory, Weybridge, UK, has developed a new serological test.

BOVINE SPONGIFORM ENCEPHALO-PATHY (BSE). Cases of this were being confirmed at a rate of about 550 per week in January 1992; but a reduction was expected later in the year.

CHIMERA. A sheep-goat chimera was found at the School of Veterinary Medicine, University of California, USA, to be capable of oestrus cycles, producing fertile ova, and carrying pregnancy to full term. (Anderson, G. D. & others. *Veterinary Record* (1991) **129** November 23rd issue.)

CRYPTOSPORIDIOSIS. This disease is now being increasingly recognised in both people and animals.

DOGS, WORKING (*see* SHEEPDOGS). Working dogs include also Guide Dogs for the Blind, Hearing Dogs for the Deaf, Avalanche Rescue Dogs, Dogs as Predictors of Human Epilepsy. (The way in which some dogs can detect the imminence of fits in people is as yet unknown. Further investigation is being undertaken in Canada and the USA. The service is a valuable one, because it allows the epileptic time to get to a safe place, and to take appropriate medication; or for the dog to warn the person's family.)

Huskies are used in the Arctic for transport purposes (and bred back to wild wolf stock every few generations). Refuse collection is yet another service performed by dogs, and was introduced in Milan, Italy. In 1992 demonstration dogs were shown picking up plastic and soft drink cans; and one bitch has learned to alert her handler by barking when she finds a hypodermic syringe on the ground.

ELISA. Additional tests have been developed for the diagnosis of 'Blue-ear' disease of pigs and Johne's disease.

EMERGENCY FOOD PROTECTION DIVISION. This forms part of the UK's Veterinary Investigation Service.

FELINE CORONAVIRUS. This is a common infection in cats. 'Five to 12 seropositive cats develop feline infectious peritonitis (FIP). In 1992 it was possible to differentiate these two infections only by their different clinical histories in infected catteries.' (Addie, D. D. & Jarrett, O. *Veterinary Record* (1992) **130**, 133.)

FEMUR, FRACTURES OF THE HEAD OF THE. In 38 dogs repair was achieved by means of divergent K wires or lag screws. (Gibson, E. L. & others. *JAVMA* (1991) **198**, 886.)

FOOD SAFETY DIRECTORATE. This came into being in 1991, through the amalgamation of the State Veterinary Service with its administrative counterpart within MAFF (Ministry of Agriculture, Fisheries and Food) to form the Animal Health and Veterinary Group. Both the Central Veterinary Laboratory and the Veterinary Medicines Directorate became executive agencies in 1991.

Over 45,000 samples of animal products are already being taken from slaughterhouses by staff of the State Veterinary Service to minimise the risk of harmful residues passing into the food chain.

HYPOCALCAEMIA. This occurs also in mares. The signs are a stiff gait, with the hindlegs placed forward when standing still, trismus, and dyspnoea. (Richardson, J. & others, University of Liverpool. *Veterinary Record* (1991) **129**, 98.)

LAW, THE.
Welfare of Livestock Regulations 1990. These were amended at the beginning of 1992. They require the training of stockmen and also the conditions under which animals in intensive units are kept.

The second amendment requires that alarm systems are installed for automatic ventilation systems; and that additional equipment is available to provide adequate ventilation in the event of a failure in the automatic system.

Anthrax Order 1938. It was updated at the beginning of 1992. Cleansing and disinfection of premises, and the disposal of slurry, are to be supervised by the divisional veterinary officer and carried out by the farmer and local authority; the cost being borne by the farmer. The DVO can compel the owner of an affected herd to treat and vaccinate his stock.

Other legislation.
Animal Health and Welfare Act 1984.
Animals and Fresh Meat (Examination for Residues) Regulations 1988.
Collection and Disposal of Waste Regulations 1989.
Dangerous Wild Animals Act 1978.
Dangerous Wild Animals Licensing Act 1981.
Diseases of Animals Act 1981.
Dogs (Protection of Livestock) Act 1953.

Endangered Species Act 1982. (An amendment in that same year relates to tortoises.)
Environmental Protection Act 1953.
Feeding Stuffs (Sampling and Analysis) Regulations 1982.
Importation of Birds, Poultry and Hatching Eggs Order.
Markets (Protection of Animals) Amendment Order 1965.
Meat (Sterilisation) Regulations 1969.
Milk and Dairy Regulations 1959.
Movement of Pigs Order 1973.
Performing Animals (Protection) Act 1952.
Pet Animals Act 1951.
Poultry and Hatching Eggs Order 1979.
Sale of Pigs Order 1975.
Slaughterhouses (Hygiene Amendment) Regulations 1987.
Tuberculosis (Deer) Order 1989.
Warble Fly Order 1989.
Welfare of Livestock (Cattle and Poultry) Order 1974.
Welfare of Livestock (Docking of Pigs) Regulations 1974.
Wildlife and Countryside Act 1981.

LENTIVIRUSES. Members of this group include EQUINE INFECTIOUS ANAEMIA, MAEDI/VISNA of sheep, and CAPRINE ARTHRITIS-ENCEPHALITIS, as well as the human AIDS virus.

LEUCOGEN. This is claimed to be the first vaccine to be produced by genetic engineering for use against a retrovirus. 'It has EC approval for the protection of cats against feline leukaemia, and has been used in France and the USA.' (Virbac Ltd., Tonbridge, Kent.)

LITHIUM POISONING occurred in two dogs whose sole source of drinking water for several months was a swimming pool chlorinated with lithium hypochlorite. One dog had fits. Both had diarrhoea, became weak, and dehydrated. They recovered after being provided with fresh, uncontaminated water. (Davies, N. L. *Journal of the South African Veterinary Association* (1991) **62,** 140.)

NATIONAL PET REGISTER. This provides a service for re-uniting lost pets with their owners,

third-party liability. Address: Heydon, Royston, Herts. SG8 8PN.

NORWEGIAN SCABIES. This is a form of sarcoptic mange. The skin becomes red, the hair falls out in patches, and there is intense pruritus.

NOTIFIABLE DISEASES. 'Blue-ear' disease of pigs has been added to the list.

OFFAL. Animal organs. Feeding of this to cattle was banned in the UK in 1988 because of the risk of transmitting Bovine Spongiform Encephalopathy (BSE).

PARVOVIRUS.
Human parvovirus infection. This is most common in children, and is associated with a rash and fever; and sometimes pain in the joints.
CAUSE. B19 virus, which is unrelated to canine or other parvoviruses. (Candlish, Irene and Thompson, Hal, Canine Infectious Disease Unit, University of Glasgow.)

PIGEONS. These must be vaccinated against paramyxoviruses within 24 hours of their arrival in the UK. Four weeks later they must receive a second dose of vaccine, and remain in quarantine for a further week.

PYRROLIZIDINE ALKALOIDS. These cause poisoning in animals which have eaten ragwort. (*See* RAGWORT POISONING.)

ULTRASONIC.
'Ultrasonic' flea collars. These are fitted with a small sound-generator, intended to produce an ultrasonic environment around a dog or cat. However, 'it seems unlikely that the collars are effective. The sounds emitted are well within the hearing range of many pets, and could be a source of stress to animals, especially while resting.' (Roe, D. J. & Sales, G. D. *Veterinary Record* (1992) **130,** 142.)

VOLCANIC GASES. Typically these comprise water vapour, carbon dioxide, sulphur dioxide, hydrogen sulphide, hydrochloric acid, hydrogen fluoride, and carbon monoxide. (*British Medical Journal* (1989) **298,** 1437.)

March 1992
LAW, THE.
The Veterinary Surgery (Epidural Anaesthesia) Order 1992 has amended the **Veterinary Surgeons Act 1966** to allow suitably trained lay persons to administer epidural anaesthetics.

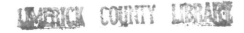